Foundations *of* Community Health Nursing
Community-Oriented Practice

Marcia Stanhope, RN, DSN, FAAN
Associate Dean
Good Samaritan Foundation Professor of Disease Prevention and Health Promotion
College of Nursing
University of Kentucky
Lexington, Kentucky

Jeanette Lancaster, RN, PhD, FAAN
Sadie Heath Cabaniss Professor and Dean
School of Nursing
University of Virginia
Charlottesville, Virginia

Illustrated

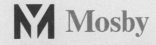 Mosby

A Harcourt Health Sciences Company

St. Louis   London   Philadelphia   Sydney   Toronto

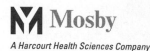

A Harcourt Health Sciences Company

Vice President, Publishing Director: Sally Schrefer
Executive Editor: Darlene Como
Managing Editor: Linda Caldwell
Project Manager: Deborah L. Vogel
Project Specialist: Ann E. Rogers
Book Design Manager: Bill Drone
Cover Design: Christine Fullgraf, Tempus Fugit

Mosby, Inc.
A Harcourt Health Sciences Company
11830 Westline Industrial Drive
St. Louis, Missouri 63146

Printed in the United States of America.

W 93
CH N

Library of Congress Cataloging in Publication Data

Stanhope, Marcia.
  Foundations of community health nursing: community-oriented practice/Marcia
Stanhope, Jeanette Lancaster.
    p.; cm.
  Includes bibliographical references and index.
  ISBN 0-323-00861-5
    1. Community health nursing. I. Lancaster, Jeanette. II. Title.
  [DNLM: 1. Community Health Nursing. 2. Community Health Services. WY 106
S786f 2002]
RT98 .S78197 2002
610.73'43—dc21

                                            2001031476

01 02 03 04 05 CL/RRDW 9 8 7 6 5 4 3 2 1

Foundations
of
Community
Health
Nursing
Community-Oriented
Practice

EXPAND YOUR KNOWLEDGE

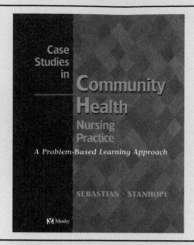

Sebastian & Stanhope
CASE STUDIES IN COMMUNITY HEALTH NURSING PRACTICE:
A Problem-Based Learning Approach

This unique text and workbook teaches nursing students to think critically and apply nursing knowledge to solving problems! A case-study approach helps them ask the right questions, gather supporting data, sort through options, and identify optimal solutions.

1999. 224 pp. Soft cover. **#0-323-00260-9**

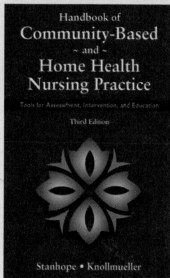

Stanhope & Knollmueller
HANDBOOK OF COMMUNITY-BASED AND HOME HEALTH NURSING
PRACTICE: Tools for Assessment, Intervention, and Education, 3rd Edition

This portable resource offers students quick access to all the information they need to provide care in a community-based setting.

Features...
• 295 tool and reference documents
• Many lists, tables, charts, and forms
• Clinical decision-making guides
• Teaching and assessment tools

1999. 686 pp. Soft cover. Illustrated. **#0-323-00875-5**

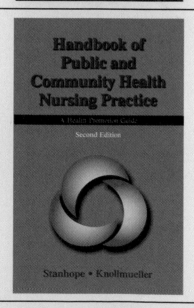

Stanhope & Knollmueller
HANDBOOK OF PUBLIC AND COMMUNITY HEALTH NURSING
PRACTICE: A Health Promotion Guide, 2nd Edition

This practical guide focuses on primary prevention. It offers comprehensive health promotion and disease prevention information that is easy to use in clinical settings.

Features...
• Assessment tools, risk indicators, and teaching tips
• Accessibility grid that cross-references like material
• A wealth of resource information

2001. 970 pp. Soft cover. Illustrated. **#0-323-01332-5**

About the Authors

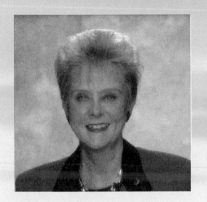

Marcia Stanhope, RN, DSN, FAAN

Marcia Stanhope is currently Associate Dean and Professor at the University of Kentucky College of Nursing in Lexington, Kentucky. Dr. Stanhope has been appointed to the Good Samaritan Foundation Professorship–Disease Prevention and Health Promotion. She has practiced community and home health nursing, as well as serving as an administrator and consultant in home health, and she has been involved in the development of two nurse-managed centers. She has taught community health, primary care nursing, and administration courses. Dr. Stanhope formerly directed the Division of Community Health Nursing and Administration at the University of Kentucky. She has been responsible for both undergraduate and graduate courses in community health nursing. She has also taught at the University of Virginia and the University of Alabama, Birmingham. Her presentations and publications have been in the areas of home health, community health and community-based nursing practice, and primary care nursing. Dr. Stanhope holds a diploma in nursing from the Good Samaritan Hospital in Lexington, Kentucky, and a bachelor of science in nursing from the University of Kentucky. She has a master's degree in public health nursing from Emory University in Atlanta and a doctorate of science in nursing from the University of Alabama, Birmingham. Dr. Stanhope is the co-author of four other Mosby publications: *Community and Public Health Nursing* (also with Dr. Lancaster), *Handbook of Community-Based and Home Health Nursing Practice, Public and Community Health Nurse's Consultant,* and *Case Studies in Community Health Nursing Practice: A Problem-Based Learning Approach.* Dr. Stanhope received the 2000 Public Health Nursing Creative Achievement Award from the Public Health Nursing Section of the American Public Health Association.

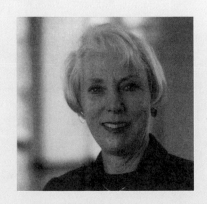

Jeanette Lancaster, RN, PhD, FAAN

Jeanette Lancaster is currently the Sadie Heath Cabaniss Professor of Nursing and Dean at the University of Virginia School of Nursing in Charlottesville, Virginia. She has practiced psychiatric nursing and taught both psychiatric and community health nursing. She formerly directed the master's program in community health nursing at the University of Alabama, Birmingham, and served as dean of the School of Nursing at Wright State University in Dayton, Ohio. Her publications and presentations have been largely in the areas of community and public health nursing, leadership and change, and the significance of nurses to effective primary health care. Dr. Lancaster is a graduate of the University of Tennessee, Memphis, College of Nursing. She holds a master's degree in psychiatric nursing from Case Western Reserve University and a doctorate in public health from the University of Oklahoma. Dr. Lancaster is the author of another Mosby publication, *Nursing Issues in Leading and Managing Change,* and co-author (with Dr. Stanhope) of *Community and Public Health Nursing.*

HEALTHY PEOPLE 2010
HEALTHY PEOPLE IN HEALTHY COMMUNITIES

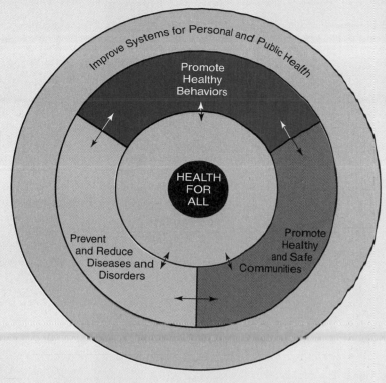

From *Healthy People 2010: Understanding and Improving Health,* March, 2001, available online: http://web.health.gov/healthypeople/

COMMUNITY NURSING DEFINITIONS

...munity-Oriented Nursing Practice is a philosophy of nursing service delivery that ...lves the generalist or specialist community health or public health nurse providing "health ...' through community diagnosis and investigation of major health and environmental prob-... health surveillance, and monitoring and evaluation of community and population health ...s for the purposes of preventing disease and disability and promoting, protecting, and main-...g "health" in order to create conditions in which people can be healthy.

...munity Health Nursing Practice is the synthesis of nursing theory and public health the-...applied to promoting, preserving, and maintaining the health of populations through the ...ery of personal health care services to individuals, families, and groups. The focus of prac-...s health of individuals, families, and groups and the effect of their health status on the health ...e community as a whole.

...munity-Based Nursing Practice is a setting-specific practice whereby care is provided for ...' individuals and families where they live, work, and go to school. The emphasis of prac-...s acute and chronic care and the provision of comprehensive, coordinated, and continuous ...ces. Nurses who deliver community-based care are generalists or specialists in maternal-...t, pediatric, adult, or psychiatric–mental health nursing.

Contributors

We gratefully acknowledge the following individuals who wrote chapters in the fifth edition of *Community and Public Health Nursing,* upon which the chapters in this book are based.

Dyan Aretakis, MSN, FNP
Project Director
Teen Health Center
University of Virginia Health Sciences Center
Charlottesville, Virginia

Ruth D. Berry, RN, MSN
Assistant Professor, Community Health Nursing
 Administration
University of Kentucky
Coordinator, Parish Nurse Services
Coordinator, Nurse-Managed Clinic for Homeless
Lexington, Kentucky

Christine Di Martile Bolla, RN, DNSc
Adjunct Professor
Department of Nursing
Western University of Health Sciences
Chico, California

Joyce Bonick, RN, JD
Nursing Regulation Consultant
Kentucky Board of Nursing
Louisville, Kentucky

Jacquelyn C. Campbell, PhD, RN, FAAN
Anna D. Wolf Endowed Professor
Associate Dean for Doctoral Education Programs and
 Research
School of Nursing
Johns Hopkins University
Baltimore, Maryland

Ann H. Cary, PhD, MPH, RN, A-CCC
Professor and Coordinator of Doctoral Nursing Program
George Mason University
College of Nursing
Fairfax, Virginia

Marcia K. Cowan, MSN, CPNP
Pediatric Nurse Practitioner
St. Thomas Pediatric Center
Tullahoma, Tennessee

Cynthia E. Degazon, PhD, RN
Associate Professor
Hunter Bellevue School of Nursing
Hunter College of the City University
New York, New York

Janna Dieckmann, PhD, RN
Visiting Assistant Professor
School of Nursing
University of North Carolina
Chapel Hill, North Carolina

Mary Eure Fisher, RN, MSN
Former Public Health Nurse Manager
Thomas Jefferson Health District
Clinical Instructor
University of Virginia School of Nursing
Charlottesville, Virginia

Kathleen Fletcher, RN, MSN, CS, GNP
Director, Geriatric Services
University of Virginia Health Systems
Charlottesville, Virginia

Beverly C. Flynn, PhD, RN, FAAN
Professor, Department of Environments for Health
Director, Institute of Action Research for Community
 Health
Head, World Health Organization Collaborating Center in
 Healthy Cities
Indiana University School of Nursing
Indianapolis, Indiana

Karen MacDonald Thompson, RN, MSN
Doctoral Candidate
University of Virginia
Consultant, The Epsilon Group
Charlottesville, Virginia

Sally P. Weinrich, PhD
Professor
College of Nursing
University of South Carolina
Columbia, South Carolina

Cynthia J. Westley, RN, MSN, ANP-C
Community Care Manager
University of Virginia Health System
Charlottesville, Virginia

Carolyn A. Williams, PhD, RN, FAAN
Dean and Professor
College of Nursing
University of Kentucky
Lexington, Kentucky

Judith Lupo Wold, PhD, RN
Associate Professor and Director
School of Nursing
Georgia State University
College of Health and Human Sciences
Atlanta, Georgia

Donna McGeogh Musselman, MS, RN, C
Professor of Nursing
Howard Community College
Columbia, Maryland

Debra Gartma
Instructor
Division of Ass
Hinds Commun
Jackson, Missis

Despite the fact that more money is spent per capita in the United States for illness care than in any other country, Americans are not the healthiest of all people. Life-style continues to play an enormous role in morbidity and mortality. For example, half of all deaths are still attributed to tobacco, alcohol, and illicit drug use; diet and activity patterns; microbial agents; toxic agents; firearms; sexual behavior; and motor vehicle accidents. Over the years the most significant improvements in the health of the population have come from advances in public health such as improved sanitation, food pasteurization, refrigeration, immunizations, and the emphasis on personal life-style and environmental factors that affect health. Changes in the public health system are essential if the health of the people in the United States is to improve.

The need to focus attention on health promotion, life-style factors, and disease prevention led to the development of a healthy public policy for the nation. This policy was designed by a large number of people representing a wide range of groups interested in health. The policy is reflected in the document *Healthy People 2000* and the updated document *Healthy People 2010,* which identify a comprehensive set of national health-promotion and disease-prevention objectives.

The most effective disease-prevention and health-promotion strategies designed to change personal life-styles are developed by the establishment of partnerships between government, business, voluntary organizations, consumers, communities, and health care providers. According to *Healthy People 2010,* these partnerships aim to eliminate health disparities among Americans by targeting care to children, minorities, elderly, and the uninsured; and to increase the span of healthy life among Americans. To develop healthy populations, individuals, families, and the communities must commit to those goals. In addition, society, through the development of health policy, must support better health care, the design of improved health education, and the financing of strategies to alter health status.

What does this mean for the community health nurse? Because people do not always know how to improve their health status, the challenge of nursing is to initiate change. Community health nursing is a practice that is focused on the health of individuals, families, and groups to change the health of the population as a whole. Community health nurses often focus on the delivery of personal health services directed toward all age-groups. Community health nursing takes place in a variety of public and private settings and includes disease prevention, health promotion, health protection, education, maintenance, restoration, coordination, management, and evaluation of care of individuals, families, and populations, including communities.

To meet the demands of a constantly changing health care system, nurses must be visionary in designing their roles and identifying their practice areas. To do so effectively, the nurse must understand concepts and theories of public health, the changing health care system, the actual and potential roles and responsibilities of nurses and other health care providers, the importance of a health-promotion and disease-prevention orientation, and the necessity to involve consumers in the planning, implementation, and evaluation of health care efforts.

This text was written to provide nursing students and practicing nurses with a comprehensive source book that provides a foundation for designing community health nursing strategies for individuals, families, and populations, including communities. The unifying theme for the book is the integration of health-promotion and disease-prevention concepts into the multifaceted role of community-oriented practice. The text emphasizes community health practice with increased attention to the effects of the internal and external environment on health. The focus on interventions for the individual and family emphasizes community health practice with attention to the effects of all of the determinants of health, including life-style, on personal health.

Organization

The text is divided into seven sections:
- *Part One,* **Perspectives in Health Care Delivery and Community Health Nursing,** describes the historical and current status of the health care delivery system and community health nursing practice.
- *Part Two,* **Influences on Health Care Delivery and Community Health Nursing,** addresses specific issues and societal concerns that affect community health nursing practice.
- *Part Three,* **Conceptual Frameworks Applied to Community Health Nursing Practice,** provides conceptual models

for community health nursing practice, and selected models from nursing and related sciences are also discussed.

- *Part Four,* **Issues and Approaches in Health Care Populations,** examines the management of health care and select community environments as well as issues related to managing cases, programs, disasters, and groups.
- *Part Five,* **Issues and Approaches in Family and Individual Health Care,** discusses risk factors and health problems for families and individuals throughout the life span.
- *Part Six,* **Vulnerability: Predisposing Factors,** covers specific health care needs and issues of populations at risk.
- *Part Seven,* **Community Health Nurse: Roles and Functions,** examines diversity in the role of community health nurses and describes the rapidly changing roles, functions, and practice settings.

Pedagogy

Each chapter is organized for easy use by students and faculty. Chapters begin with a list of **Objectives,** which guide student learning and assist faculty in knowing what students should gain from the content. The **Chapter Outline** alerts students to the structure and content of the chapter. **Key Terms** and their **definitions** are also provided at the beginning of the chapter to assist the student in understanding unfamiliar terminology. The Key Terms are in boldface within the text.

The following features are presented in most or all chapters:

Briefly Noted Boxes

Present notes to the student that may be a fact of interest, a special consideration for clinical practice, or a contemporary issue that stimulates debate and discussion.

HOW TO Boxes

Provide specific, application-oriented information.

 ### Evidence-Based Practice Boxes

Illustrate the use and application of the latest research findings in public health, community health, and nursing.

Clinical Applications

At the end of each chapter, these provide the reader with an understanding of how to apply chapter content in the clinical setting through the presentation of a case situation with questions students will want to think about as they analyze the case.

 ### *Remember This!*

Provides a summary in list form of the most important points made in the chapter.

 ### *What Would You Do?*

Stimulates student learning by suggesting a variety of activities that encourage both independent and collaborative effort.

In the back of the book you'll find additional important sources of information in the Appendixes and the Answers to Clinical Applications.

Numerous **Appendixes** provide additional resources and key information.

Answers to Clinical Applications. Answers are provided for each Clinical Application question.

Teaching and Learning Package

- A website, www.mosby.com/MERLIN/Stanhope/foundations, with instructor and student materials.
  For the instructor:
    1. Lecture Outlines and Chapter Summaries
    2. Critical Thinking activities and questions
    3. Test Bank, with 600 questions
    4. Electronic Image Collection, with 40 illustrations from the book
    5. Teaching Tips
  For the instructor and student:
    1. Frequently Asked Questions
    2. Chapter-specific WebLinks
- Mosby's Community Health Nursing Video Series (eight-part series)
- A CD-ROM workbook: *Real World Community Health Nursing: An Interactive CD-ROM*

Acknowledgments

We would like to thank our families, friends, and colleagues who supported us in the completion of this edition. Special thanks go to our co-workers at the University of Kentucky College of Nursing and the University of Virginia School of Nursing who provided generous support and assistance. We especially thank June Thompson and Linda Caldwell at Harcourt Health Sciences and the peer reviewers for their time and thoughtfulness in completing the revisions.

We would like to extend special thanks to the contributors of the 5th edition of *Community and Public Health Nursing* for their careful and thoughtful reviews and critique of the chapters of this book.

Marcia Stanhope   Jeanette Lancaster

Contents

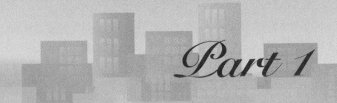

Part 1

Perspectives in Health Care Delivery and Community Health Nursing

Since the late 1800s, nurses have led many of the improvements in the quality of health care for individuals, families, and communities. Also, as nurses around the world meet and learn about one another, it is clear that, from one country to another, community health nursing has more similarities than differences.

Significant changes in health care occurred during the 1990s. Part 1 presents information about significant factors affecting health in the United States. Playing an instrumental role in changing the level and quality of services requires informed, courageous, and committed nurses. The chapters in Part 1 are designed to provide essential information so that community health nurses can make a difference in health care by understanding the roles of community health nurses and nurses in community-oriented practice as well as understanding how the public health system differs from the primary care system.

Part 1 offers explanations of exactly what makes community health nursing unique. Often people confuse community and public health nursing with community-based nursing practice. There is a core of knowledge known as "public health" that forms the foundation for community health nursing. Working with people in the community may not necessarily be community health or public health nursing. These nursing practice areas involve more than the care of a person or family whose care has been moved from the hospital to the community. It involves an emphasis on health promotion, disease prevention, health protection, and restoration using a variety of nursing strategies and interventions.

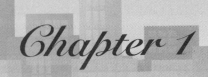

Community-Oriented Nursing and Community-Based Nursing

CAROLYN A. WILLIAMS

OBJECTIVES

After reading this chapter, the student should be able to:
- Describe the core functions of public health and the services generally provided by practitioners of public health.
- Discuss the role of the public health nursing specialist and how it influences nursing practice in the community.
- Explain community-based nursing practice.
- Describe community-oriented nursing practice.
- Examine how community-based nursing practice differs from community-oriented nursing.

CHAPTER OUTLINE

What is Public Health?
Population-Focused Nursing Practice
Practice Focusing on Individuals, Families, and Groups
Community-Oriented Community Health Nursing
Community-Based Nursing
Challenges for the Future

KEY TERMS

aggregate: a population group.

assessment: systematic data collection about a population. This includes monitoring of the population's health status and providing information about the health of the community.

assurance: the public health role of making sure that essential community-oriented health services are available.

community: People and the relationships that emerge among them as they develop and use in common some agencies and institutions and a physical environment.

community-based: occurs outside an institution; services are provided to individuals and families in a community.

community-based nursing: the provision of acute care and care for chronic health problems to individuals and families in the community.

community health nursing: nursing practice in the community, with the primary focus on the health care of individuals, families, and groups in a community. The goal is to preserve, protect, and promote or maintain health.

community-oriented nursing: nursing that has as its primary focus the health care of either the community or individuals, families, and groups.

community-oriented practice: Broader in scope than community-based practice. A form of care in which the nurse provides health care after doing a community diagnosis to determine what conditions need to be altered in order for individuals, families, and groups in the community to stay healthy.

policy development: providing leadership in developing policies that support the health of the population.

population: a collection of people who share one or more personal or environmental characteristics.

population-focused: emphasizes populations who live in a community.

population-focused practice: the core of public health, a practice that emphasizes health protection, health promotion, and disease prevention of a population.

Continued

TABLE 1-1	Select Examples of Similarities and Differences Between Community-Oriented and Community-Based Nursing—cont'd	
Community-Oriented Community Health Nursing		**Community-Based Nursing**
Roles—cont'd		
Group oriented:		**Group oriented:**
• Leader (personal health management)		• Leader (disease management)
• Change agent (screening)		• Change agent (managed-care services)
• Community advocate		
• Case finder		
• Community care agent		
• Assessment		
• Policy developer		
• Assurance		
• Enforcer of laws/compliance		
• Case finding		• Care management (direct care)
Priority of Nurse's Activities		
• Case finding		• Patient education
• Client education		• Individual and family advocacy
• Community education		• Interdisciplinary practice
• Interdisciplinary practice		• Continuity of care provider
• Case management (direct care)		
• Program planning, and implementation		
• Individual and family advocacy		

decreased stroke deaths by 50%, coronary heart disease deaths by 40%, and overall death rates for children by 25% (U.S. Public Health Service, 1993).

Another way of looking at the benefits of public health practice is to look at how early deaths can be prevented. The U.S. Public Health Service estimates that medical treatment can prevent only about 10% of all early deaths in the United States; whereas population-focused public health approaches could help prevent about 70% of early deaths in America through measures that influence the way people eat, drink, drive, engage in exercise, and treat the environment (U.S. Public Health Service, 1994/1995). Public health practice provides many benefits, especially considering the small portion of the health care budget in the United States that is used for this prevention and population-focused specialty. Some of this decline in the 1980s and 1990s occurred as public health agencies increasingly provided personal care services to people who were unable to obtain care elsewhere. Providing such care shifted resources and energy away from public health's traditional population-focused activities (U.S. Public Health Service, 1994/1995). As overall health needs improve in the United States, a stronger commitment to population-focused services is emerging (U.S. Department of Health and Human Services, 1999).

Briefly Noted

Despite many public health successes, funding for public health has decreased by about 25% over the last decade. Less than 1% of national health expenditures support population-focused initiatives.

Public health is described as what society collectively does to ensure that conditions exist in which people can be healthy (Institute of Medicine, 1988). Public health is a community-oriented, population-focused specialty area. The overall mission of public health is to organize community efforts that will use scientific and technical knowledge to prevent disease and promote health (Institute of Medicine, 1988). Figure 1-1 describes public health in America. The three **public health core functions** are assessment, policy development, and assurance.

• **Assessment** is systematic data collection on the population, monitoring the population's health status, and making information available about the health of the community.

• **Policy development** refers to efforts to develop policies that support the health of the population, including using a scientific knowledge base to make policy decisions.

• **Assurance** is making sure that essential community-oriented health services are available. These services might include providing essential personal health services for those who would otherwise not receive them. Assurance also includes making sure that a competent public health and personal health care workforce is available.

A working group within the U.S. Public Health Service developed the Health Services Pyramid (Figure 1-2). In this pyramid, population-focused public health programs with the goals of disease prevention, health protection, and health promotion should provide a foundation for **primary, secondary,** and **tertiary health care services.** Each service level in the pyramid is important to the health of

PUBLIC HEALTH IN AMERICA

Vision:

Healthy people in healthy communities

Mission:

Promote physical and mental health and prevent disease, injury, and disability

Public health

- Prevents epidemics and the spread of disease
- Protects against environmental hazards
- Prevents injuries
- Promotes and encourages healthy behaviors
- Responds to disasters and assists communities in recovery
- Ensures the quality and accessibility of health services

Essential public health services

- Monitors health status to identify community health problems
- Diagnoses and investigates health problems and health hazards in the community
- Informs, educates, and empowers people about health issues
- Mobilizes community partnerships to identify and solve health problems
- Develops policies and plans that support individual and community health efforts
- Enforces laws and regulations that protect health and ensure safety
- Links people to needed personal health services and ensures the provision of health care when otherwise unavailable
- Ensures a competent public health and personal health care workforce
- Evaluates effectiveness, accessibility, and quality of personal and population-based health services
- Researches for new insights and innovative solutions to health problems

Source: Essential Public Health Services Work Group of the Core Public Health Functions Steering Committee.
Membership: American Public Health Association
          Association of Schools of Public Health
          Association of State and Territorial Health Officials
          Institute of Medicine, National Academy of Sciences
          National Association of County and City Health Officials
          National Association of State Alcohol and Drug Abuse Directors
          National Association of State Mental Health Program Directors
          Public Health Foundation
          U.S. Public Health Service
            Agency for Healthcare Research and Quality
            Centers for Disease Control and Prevention
            Food and Drug Administration
            Health Resources and Services Administration
            Indian Health Service
            Office of the Assistant Secretary for Health
            Substance Abuse and Mental Health Services Administration

Figure 1-1   Public health in America.

the population. The base of the pyramid should provide effective services that will support the top tiers and contribute to better health. All tiers of the pyramid need to be adequately financed (U.S. Public Health Service, 1994/1995). In reality health care in the United States has been organized with the pyramid upside down. That is, more attention, support, and funding are given to tertiary and secondary care than to primary and preventive services including population-focused care. Box 1-1 lists the essential public health services.

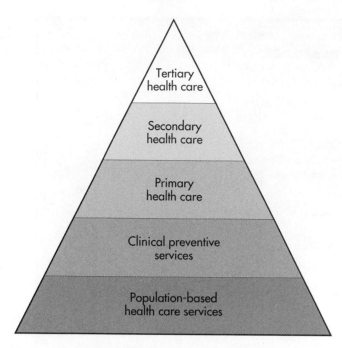

Figure 1-2   Health services pyramid.

POPULATION-FOCUSED NURSING PRACTICE

Public health nursing is a specialty with a distinct focus and scope of practice and it requires a special knowledge base. The role of the public health nurse has changed over the years in response to:

- Changes in health care
- Priorities for health care funding
- The needs of the population
- The educational preparation of nurses.

As readers will note in Chapter 2, public health nursing began more than 100 years ago; early public health nurses provided direct care to people, most often in their homes. The Henry Street Settlement established in New York City in the late 1900s by Lillian Wald was an early model for public health nursing. At Henry Street the nurses took care of the sick in their homes and also looked at the overall population of low-income people in the community from which their home care patients came. The primary focus that has differentiated public health nursing from other specialties has been the emphasis on the population rather than on single individuals or families. Following the examples of Lillian Wald, these nurses have:

- Looked at the community or population as a whole
- Raised questions about the overall health status and the factors associated with that status, including environmental factors such as physical, biological, social, economic, and cultural aspects
- Worked with the community to improve health status.

The primary goal of public health—the prevention of disease and disability—is achieved by ensuring that conditions exist in which people can remain healthy. The How To box on this page describes ways to distinguish what actually makes up the specialty of public health nursing.

Box 1-1	**Essential Public Health Services**

Public health providers engage in the following services:

- Monitoring the health status of the population to identify community health problems
- Diagnosing and investigating health problems and hazards in the community
- Informing and educating people about health issues
- Bringing together community partnerships to identify and solve health problems
- Developing policies and plans to support individual and community health
- Enforcing laws and regulations to protect health and ensure safety
- Linking people to needed services and ensuring that services are actually available
- Making sure there is an adequate and competent health care workforce
- Evaluating the effectiveness, accessibility, and quality of both personal and population-focused health services
- Conducting research to develop new solutions to health problems

From U.S. Public Health Service: *A time for partnership, prevention report,* Washington, D.C., Dec 1994/Jan 1995, Office of Disease Prevention and Health Promotion.

HOW TO Distinguish the Specialty of Public Health Nursing

- *Population-focused:* Primary emphasis is on *populations* that live in the *community,* as opposed to those that are institutionalized.
- *Community-oriented:*
  1. Concern for the connection between health status of the population and the environment in which the population lives (physical, biological, sociocultural)
  2. An imperative to work *with* members of the community to carry out core public health functions
- *Health and preventive focus:* Predominant emphasis on strategies for health promotion, health maintenance, and disease prevention, particularly primary and secondary prevention.
- *Interventions at the community and/or population level:* The use of political processes to affect public policy as a major intervention strategy for achieving goals.
- *Concern for the health of all members of the population or community, particularly vulnerable sub-populations.*

In 1981 the public health nursing section of the American Public Health Association defined public health nursing and described how this role contributes to health care delivery. This statement was reaffirmed in 1996 (APHA, 1996). **Public health nursing** is defined as a specialty that brings together knowledge from the public health sciences and nursing to improve the health of the **community.** Public health nursing is defined by the Quad Council of Public Health Nursing Organizations as "population-focused,

Box 1-2	The Process of Public Health Nursing

Public health nursing is a systematic process that:

- Assesses the health and health care needs of a population in collaboration with other disciplines to identify subpopulations (aggregates), families, and individuals at increased risk of illness, disability, or premature death.
- Plans interventions to meet these needs. The plan includes resources available and those activities that contribute to health and its recovery, the prevention of illness, disability, and premature death.
- Implements the plan effectively, efficiently, and equitably.
- Evaluates progress to determine the extent to which these activities have influenced the health status of the population.
- Utilizes the results to influence and direct the delivery of care, use of health resources, and the development of local, regional, state, and national health policy and research to promote health and prevent diseases.

Based on American Public Health Association: *The definition and role of public health nursing in the delivery of health care: a statement of the Public Health Nursing Section,* Washington, D.C., 1981, The Association; American Public Health Association: *The definition and role of public health nurses: A statement of the American Public Health Association's Public Health Nursing Section,* Washington D.C., 1996, The Association.

community-oriented nursing practice. The goal of public health nursing is the prevention of disease and disability for all people through the creation of conditions in which people can be healthy" (Quad Council of Public Health Nursing Organizations, 1999, p. 2). Box 1-2 presents the APHA definition of public health nursing.

Public health nurses, like others in public health, engage in assessment, policy development, and assurance activities. These functions are achieved when nurses work in partnerships with others including nations, states, communities, organizations, groups, and individuals. Public health nurses carry out this mission by participating in the essential public health services described earlier in the chapter.

Although population-focused practice is the central feature of public health nursing, many of the skills and activities are used when community health nurses and community-based nurses work in the community. For this reason, these practices are described in detail here. A **population** or **aggregate** is a collection of people who share one or more personal or environmental characteristics. Members of a community can be defined either in terms of geography (e.g., a county, group of counties, or a state) or a special interest (e.g., children attending a particular school). These members compose a population. Generally there are **sub-populations** within the larger population. Examples of a sub-population within a population of a county are high-risk infants under the age of 1 year, unmarried pregnant adolescents, or individuals exposed to a particular event such as a chemical spill.

In **population-focused practice,** problems are defined (assessments/diagnoses) and solutions (interventions), such as policy development or providing a given preventive service, are implemented for or with a defined population or sub-population as opposed to diagnoses, interventions, and treatment carried out at the individual level. This contrasts with basic professional education in nursing, medicine, and other clinical disciplines, which emphasizes developing competence in decision-making at the level of the individual client by assessing health status, making management decisions (ideally with the client), and evaluating the effects of care. The ways in which nurses provide care to people with high blood pressure can demonstrate how population-focused practice differs from the clinical direct care practice so often used in nursing. Specifically, in a clinical direct care situation a community health nurse might decide that a person is hypertensive based on certain clinical signs. The nurse would evaluate different interventions to find the best one for this person and implement an intervention like a change in diet. In contrast, a public health nurse engaged in population-focused practice would ask these questions:

- What is the prevalence rate of hypertension among various age, race, and gender groups?
- Which sub-populations have the highest rates of untreated hypertension?
- What programs could reduce the problem of untreated hypertension and decrease the risk of further cardiovascular morbidity and mortality?

Public health nurses are typically concerned with more than one sub-population, and they often deal with the health of the entire community. Assessment, one of the public health core functions, is a logical first step in examining a community setting to determine its suitability from a health perspective.

The core public health function of *assessment* includes the following:

- Activities involving the collection, analysis, and dissemination of information on both the health and health-relevant aspects of a community or a specific population
- Questions such as whether the health services of the community are available to the population and are adequate to address needs
- Monitoring of the health status of the community or population and the services provided over time
- Evaluation of the social, economic, environmental, and lifestyle characteristics and practices of a population as well as the health services and capacity available within the community to support good health for the population

Listed below is a general set of questions that can be used or modified to gather assessment data.

HOW TO Assess: Assessment Questions to Ask

- What are the major health problems in this community?
- Which population groups are at greatest risk?
- How are risks distributed geographically?
- What services are available?
- What services need to be provided but are unavailable?
- Of the available and needed services, what is their level of quality?
- What do citizens think are their most pressing health needs?
- Do providers view the most pressing health needs to be the same as the citizens do?
- What is the history of agency collaboration and cooperation in this community?

Healthy People 2010
Overview and Goals

In 1979, the Surgeon General issued a report that began a 20-year focus on promoting health and preventing disease for all Americans. The report, entitled *Healthy People,* used morbidity rates to track the health of individuals through the five major life cycles of infancy, childhood, adolescence, adulthood, and older age.

In 1989, *Healthy People 2000* became a national effort of representatives from government agencies, academia, and health organizations. Their goal was to present a strategy for improving the health of the American people. Their objectives are being used by public and community health organizations to assess current health trends, health programs, and disease-prevention programs.

Throughout the 1990s, all states used *Healthy People 2000* objectives to identify emerging public health issues. The success of the program on a national level was accomplished through state and local efforts. Early in the 1990s, surveys from public health departments indicated that 8% of the national objectives had been met, and progress on an additional 40% of the objectives was noted. In the mid-course review published in 1995, it was noted that significant progress had been made toward meeting 50% of the objectives.

Using the progress made in the past decade, the committee for *Healthy People 2010* proposed two goals:
- To increase years of healthy life
- To eliminate health disparities among different populations

They hope to reach these goals by such measures as promoting healthy behaviors, increasing access to quality health care, and strengthening community prevention.

The major premise of *Healthy People 2010* is that the health of the individual almost cannot be separated from the health of the larger community. Therefore the vision for *Healthy People 2010* is "Healthy People in Healthy Communities."

U.S. Department of Health and Human Services, 1999.

Evidence-Based Practice

This study describes an assessment by two public health nursing specialists that focused on a target population of 1-year-old Mexican-American and white non-Hispanic infants enrolled in a Medicaid-managed care demonstration project. It was found that despite the fact that the infants had access to care, there were differences between the immunization levels of the Mexican-Americans as compared to the white non-Hispanic infants. The Mexican-Americans completed fewer doses of both DPT and polio vaccine and were less likely to complete the recommended immunization series by 1 year of age than the white non-Hispanic infants. In fact, the Mexican-American infants received less than 60% of the three DPTs.

APPLICATION IN PRACTICE

This shows that continuous enrollment in a Medicaid-managed care system does not assure that there will be a high rate of immunization coverage. The strongest predictor of the number of immunizations received was the number of siblings. In both ethnic groups, infants with fewer siblings received more immunizations. After controlling for a set of potential explanations, the multi-regression analysis showed that the ethnic group was not a predictor of immunization levels. Significant predictors of a higher number of immunization levels included fewer siblings, for both the Hispanic and non-Hispanic groups, and higher maternal education for the white non-Hispanic, but not for the Hispanic group. This assessment clearly showed that factors other than enrollment in Medicaid influence immunization rates. This assessment process provided considerable information for the public health nursing specialists about which sub-group of infants in this target population were at risk for incomplete immunization coverage.

Moore P, et al: Indicators of differences in immunization rates of Mexican-American and white non-Hispanic infants in a Medicaid-managed care system, *Public Health Nurs* 13:21, 1996.

Excellent examples of assessment at the national level are the U.S. Department of Health and Human Services' efforts to organize the goal-setting, data collection and analysis, and monitoring necessary to develop the series of publications describing the health status and health-related aspects of the U.S. population. These efforts began with *Healthy People* in 1980, and continued with *Promoting Health, Preventing Disease: 1990 Health Objectives for the Nation* and *Healthy People 2000,* and most recently *Healthy People 2010* (U.S. Department of Health and Human Services, 1999).

In a local health department, public health nurses would participate in and provide leadership for assessing community needs, health status of populations within the community, and environmental and behavioral risks. They also look at trends in the health determinants, identify priority health needs, and determine the adequacy of existing community resources.

Policy development is a core function of public health and one of the core intervention strategies used by public health nursing specialists. Policy development relies heavily on

planning and begins with the identified needs and priorities set by the people involved. It also includes building constituencies who can bring about policy changes. It is important to know what the powerful people in the community think about a specific public health concern. Health and human service providers as well as the people who will be served or affected must be included. Public health nursing is a "with the people" not a "to the people" or "for the people" approach to planning. Historically, health care providers have been accused of providing care for or to people without actually involving the recipients in the decisions. The beneficiaries of services in public health need to be included from the very beginning in identifying the need, planning the intervention, and deciding on the format for the evaluation (Box 1-3).

The third core public health function, assurance, focuses on the responsibility of public health agencies to be sure that activities are appropriately carried out to meet public health goals and plans. Not only does public health nursing include assessment or investigative functions, but the role also requires skill in collaboration, consultation, and cooperation. The assurance function makes sure that the activities

The policy development function:

- Is essentially a planning process that uses the assessment data to define health needs, set priorities, identify alternatives, outline a plan including the determination of available and needed resources, and determine who needs to be involved to ensure some measure of success.
- Serves as a resource and/or catalyst to help elected officials or heads of community organizations develop population-based health plans.
- Assists people who make policies to do so in such a way that the needs of many people or groups are met. Also advises these individuals and/or groups about which needs are most important and should be handled first.
- Consistently advocates for better health conditions for the population as a whole.

| Box 1-4 | **Key Assurance Functions for Public Health Agencies** |

- Provide public nursing services
- Provide environmental health services
- Encourage, purchase, or provide additional population-based services (e.g., health promotion programs, educational programs, transportation services, bilingual services).
- Maintain emergency response capacity
- Administer quality assurance
- Help recruit and retain health care practitioners and
- Maintain administrative capacity (e.g., personnel, contracting, budgeting, accounting, legal)

From National Association of County Health Officials: *Core public health functions,* Olympia, Wash, 1993, The Association.

designed during the policy development or planning phase are carried out. This is done through collaboration with people in a variety of health and human service organizations to promote, monitor, and improve both the availability and quality of providers and services. Public health nursing is not a good field for people who like to work alone. While there is considerable opportunity for autonomy in thinking and planning, effective and consistent collaboration is vital to success. Assurance does not always mean to provide something. Rather, another agency may provide the needed service. Assurance means making certain that the services determined to be needed are provided by some agency within the community. Further, assurance includes assisting communities to implement and evaluate plans and projects. It includes maintaining the ability of both public health agencies and private providers to manage day-to-day operations as well as the capacity to respond to critical situations and emergencies (National Association of County Health Officials, 1993) (Box 1-4).

In public health nursing, the nurse often reaches out to those who might benefit from a service or intervention. In other forms of nursing, the client is more likely to seek out and request assistance. As will be discussed in later chapters, often the people or populations most in need of public

Evidence-Based Practice

An example of public health nursing leadership in assurance is seen in an account of a home visiting program (Resources, Education and Care in the Home [REACH]) designed to reduce preventable causes of morbidity among socially disadvantaged infants in selected high-risk, high-need Chicago communities. The target population was normal infants born into socially deprived homes and living in a high-risk environment. The intervention was designed to put in place a monitoring effort, as well as to provide clinical services and instruction. Information was provided to the mothers to help them reduce the development of preventable causes of morbidity and mortality. The results indicated that repeated home visits with ongoing infant monitoring and culturally sensitive teaching helped mothers maintain good health practices and early identification of infant problems.

APPLICATION IN PRACTICE

This project is an example of ensuring that a target group of infants in a high-risk environment received careful attention during an important and vulnerable period of their lives. It was designed and put in place by public health nursing specialists, but the actual clinical encounters were provided by teams consisting of community-based nurses working for a hospital and community lay workers. It is a clear example of a partnership between a public health agency and a hospital organization to meet the specific needs of a target population.

Barnes-Boyd C, Norr KF, Nacion KW: Evaluation of an interagency home visiting program to reduce postneonatal mortality in disadvantaged communities, *Public Health Nurs* 13:201, 1996.

health services are the least likely to ask for them. Examples include homeless, poor, and mentally ill people. The dominant needs of the population outweigh the expressed needs of one or a few people. Since resources often are limited, careful assessment to identify key needs is important.

However, the special contributions of public health nursing specialists include looking at the community or population as a whole, raising questions about its overall health status and factors associated with that status, including environmental factors (physical, biological and social-cultural) and working *with the community* to improve the population's health status.

PRACTICE FOCUSING ON INDIVIDUALS, FAMILIES, AND GROUPS

As has been mentioned, community-based nursing practice, with its focus on the provision or assurance of care to individuals and families in the community, is different from **community-oriented practice.** The latter is broader in scope and is a form of care in which the nurse provides health care after doing a community diagnosis to determine what conditions need to be altered for individuals, families, and groups in the community to stay healthy. While it is hoped that all direct care providers contribute to the community's health in the broadest sense, not all are primarily concerned with the population focus, or the "big picture." All nurses in a given community, including those working in hospitals, physicians' offices, and health clinics, contribute positively to the health of the community. Examples of community settings for treating individuals include ambulatory surgery, outpatient clinics, physician and advanced-practice nursing offices and clinics, employment and school sites, as well as preschool programs, housing projects, and migrant camps. These sites often provide individual-focused health care services. This contrasts to **population** (i.e., large group)-**focused** services. A specific example would be the federally-funded program for preschool children called Head Start. From a community-oriented nursing care perspective, nursing services could be provided to individual children such as by conducting developmental-level screening tests to evaluate each child's level of cognitive and psychomotor development in comparison to established standards for children of the same age while the community-based nurse may deliver illness care to the children in the school. In contrast, a public health or population-based approach would focus on looking at the entire group of children being served by the program as well as the characteristics of the facilities and its programs to see if they are effective in achieving the goals of making the school population healthier.

Community-Oriented Community Health Nursing

Most community health nurses and many staff public health nurses—both historically and at present—focus on providing direct care services, including health education, to persons or families outside of institutional settings, either in the home or in a clinic. Historically, the term *community health nurse* applied to all nurses who practiced in the community, regardless of whether they had preparation in public health nursing. Thus, nurses providing secondary or tertiary care in a home, school, or clinic, or any nurse who did not practice in an institutional setting, could be considered a "community health nurse." To a large extent the development of what is today called community health nursing was influenced by the development within medicine of the specialty of community medicine. At that time both community medicine and community health nursing reached out to the community and began doing community assessments to determine more effectively the needs of the people. Thus disease prevention and health promotion could be targeted to specific needs in a given community. Specifically, the community health nurse operates from a health care focus that is based on an understanding of broader community needs. The nurse is continually evaluating the community to see if changes are occurring that will influence the health of the people who live there. The American Nurses Association (1986) defines community health nursing as:

The practice of nursing which involves health promotion, health maintenance, health education, management, coordination and

continuity of care in the management of the health care of individuals, families and groups in a community. A holistic approach is used and the goal of this care is to promote and preserve the health of the community in which the clients live.

Evidence that community health nurses are practicing effectively in the community would include the provision of the following:

1. Provides quality services that can control costs
2. Focuses on disease prevention and health promotion
3. Organizes services where people live, work, play, and learn
4. Works in partnerships and with coalitions
5. Works across the life span and with culturally diverse populations
6. Works with at-risk populations to promote access to services
7. Develops the community's capacity for health
8. Works with policy makers for policy change
9. Works to make the environment healthier (Flynn, 1998, p. 168).

As can be seen, community health nursing emphasizes health protection and promotion and disease prevention, as well as self-reliance among clients. Regardless of whether the client is a person, a family, or a group, the goal is to promote health through education about prevailing health problems, proper nutrition, beneficial forms of exercise, and environmental factors such as safe food, water, air, and buildings. The community health nurse is likely to be involved in immunizing individuals as well as organizing the immunization programs for vaccinating the community for influenza, for example, and educating the community about the value of this service. Other individual and family services include maternal and child health care, treatment of common communicable and infectious diseases and injuries, and providing basic screening programs for such problems as lice, vision, hearing, and scoliosis (Zotti, Brown, and Stotts, 1996).

While community health nurses have always been involved in providing family-centered care to individuals, families and groups across the life span, they also work to identify high-risk groups in the community. Once such groups are identified, the community health nurse can work with others to develop appropriate policies and interventions to reduce risk and provide beneficial services. Both community health nurses and CBNs must be aware of cultural diversity and provide care that is appropriate to the needs of the recipient. Likewise, both groups of nurses provide care in homes.

Community-Based Nursing

As has been mentioned, the goal of community-based nursing is to manage acute or chronic conditions while promoting self-care among individuals and families (Zotti, Brown, and Stotts, 1996). In CBN the nursing care is family centered, which means that the nurse works to improve the competencies of families to enable them to take better care of

Community-Oriented Nursing Practice: a philosophy of nursing care delivery that involves generalist or specialist public health and community health nurses providing "health care" through community diagnosis and investigation of major health and environmental problems, health surveillance, monitoring, and evaluation of community and population health status, in order to prevent disease and disability, promote, protect, and maintain health to create conditions in which people can be healthy.

Public Health Nursing Practice: the synthesis of nursing and public health theory applied to promoting and preserving the health of populations. Practice focuses on the community as a whole, and the effect of the community's health status (resources) on the health of individuals, families, and groups. The goal is to prevent disease and disability and promote and protect the health of the community as a whole.

Community Health Nursing Practice: the synthesis of nursing and public health theory in order to promote, preserve, and maintain the health of the population through the delivery of personal health services to individuals, families, and groups. Focus is on the health of individuals, families, and groups, and how their health status affects the community as a whole.

Community-Based Nursing Practice: a setting-specific practice whereby care is provided for "sick" individuals and families where they live, work, and attend school. Emphasizes acute and chronic care and the provision of comprehensive, coordinated, and continuous care. These nurses may be generalists or specialists in maternal-infant, pediatric, adult, or psychiatric mental health nursing.

themselves. The nurse pays particular attention to the uniqueness of each family and works to plan the most useful interventions. A "cookbook" approach cannot be used since no one nursing approach will fit each family or individual. Cultural diversity is taken into account as are the situation and stressors facing the person or the family at a given time. The nurse promotes client autonomy and helps care recipients learn to do as much as possible for themselves.

The nurse practicing as a CBN is more likely to give direct care to people than are nurses who practice from a community-oriented framework. The nurse assesses client needs and also the services that are available in order to plan the most appropriate course of action. Throughout care delivery, the nurse teaches and counsels clients so they can more fully develop their own ways of taking care of themselves. Box 1-5 provides definitions of each of the four key modes of nursing practice seen in the community.

CHALLENGES FOR THE FUTURE

Over the past few years the places in which care is given have changed dramatically. In previous decades the majority of care was given in an inpatient setting. At present, the trend is to move as much care as possible into community settings. There are a variety of reasons for the change. First, community care is often much less expensive than hospital care. Since the cost of health care in the United States has risen considerably over the past decade, there is a significant need to find new ways to deliver care that is accessible to the recipients, less expensive, and with adequate quality to meet client needs. Also, care in the community is usually more appealing to people who prefer to remain at home rather than be treated in a hospital. Currently, care is given in homes, schools, and at the work-site, as well as in a variety of out-patient clinics. This trend is expected to grow, and it is expected that the role of the nurse in community settings will likewise grow and continue to change.

Clinical Application

Debate with classmates where and how public health nursing specialists practice and how their practice compares with what has been defined as community-based nursing.

Debate with classmates which of the nurses in the following categories are practicing population-focused nursing:

A. *School nursing*
B. *Staff nurses in home care*
C. *Director of nursing for a home care agency*
D. *Nurse practitioners in a health maintenance organization*
E. *Vice-president of nursing in a hospital*
F. *Staff nurses in a public health clinic or community health center*
G. *Director of nursing in a health department*

Choose three categories on the list above and interview at least one nurse in each category.

A. *Determine what their scope of practice is.*
B. *Are they carrying out population-focused practice?*
C. *Could they?*
D. *How?*
E. *Ask them if they would change their role if this were possible*
F. *Inquire whether they believe their role is either community-oriented nursing or community-based nursing practice.*

Answers are in the back of the book.

 ## *Remember This!*

- Public health is what members of a society do collectively to ensure that conditions exist in which people can be healthy.
- Assessment, policy development, and assurance are the core public health functions at all levels of government.
- Assessment refers to systematic data collection on the population, monitoring of the population's health status, and making information available on the health of the community.
- Policy development refers to the need to provide leadership in developing policies that support the health of the population, including use of the scientific knowledge base in decision-making about policy.
- Assurance refers to the way public health practice makes sure that essential community-wide health services are

available. This may include providing essential personal health services for those who would otherwise not receive them. Assurance also includes making sure that a competent public health and personal health care work force is available.

- Setting is frequently viewed as the feature that distinguishes public health nursing from other specialties. A more useful approach is to use characteristics such as the following: a focus on populations who live in the community, an emphasis on prevention, concern for the interface between health status of the population and the environment (physical, biological, socio-cultural), and the use of political processes to influence public policy in order to achieve one's goals.
- Specialization in public health nursing is seen as a subset of community health nursing.
- Population-focused practice is the focus of specialization in public health nursing. The focus on community-based populations and the emphasis on health protection, health promotion, and disease prevention are the fundamental factors that distinguish public health nursing from other nursing specialties.
- Population is defined as a collection of individuals who share one or more personal or environmental characteristics. The term *population* may be used interchangeably with the term *aggregate*.

? What Would You Do?

1. Define each of the following:
   a. The core functions of public health
   b. The specialist in public health nursing
   c. The nurse whose practice is community-based
   d. The community-oriented community health nurse
2. Discuss with classmates examples in your community where the community-based nursing role is the ideal role to meet client needs. Also identify examples in which the most useful nursing role would be that of the community-oriented community health nurse. How can you justify your opinion if classmates disagree?
3. With three or four of your classmates, develop a plan for identifying two or three nurses in your community who

are in an administrative role and discuss with them the following:
   a. How they define the populations they serve
   b. The strategies they use to monitor the population's health status
   c. The strategies they use to ensure that the populations are receiving basic needed services
   d. What initiatives they are taking to address problems.

REFERENCES

American Nurses Association: Standards of community health nursing practice, Kansas City, Mo, 1986, The Association.

American Public Health Association: *The definition and role of public health nurses: A statement of the American Public Health Association's Public Health Nursing Section,* Washington, D.C., 1996, The Association.

American Public Health Association: *The definition and role of public health nursing in the delivery of health care: a statement of the Public Health Nursing Section,* Washington, D.C., 1981, The Association.

Barnes-Boyd C, Norr KF, Nacion KW: Evaluation of an interagency home visiting program to reduce postneonatal mortality in disadvantaged communities, *Public Health Nurs* 13:201, 1996.

Flynn BC: Communicating with the public: community-based nursing research and practice, *Public Health Nurs* 15(3):165-170, 1998.

Institute of Medicine: *The future of public health,* Washington, D.C., 1988, National Academy Press.

Moore P, et al: Indicators of differences in immunization rates of Mexican-American and white non-Hispanic infants in a Medicaid-managed care system, *Public Health Nurs* 13:21, 1996.

National Association of County Health Officials: *Core public health functions,* Olympia, Wash, 1993, The Association.

Quad Council of Public Health Nursing Organizations: *Scope and standards of public health nursing practice,* Washington, D.C., 1999, American Nurses Association.

U.S. Department of Health and Human Services: *Healthy People 2010 Objectives,* Washington, D.C., 1999, U.S. Department of Health and Human Services.

U.S. Public Health Service: *A time for partnership, prevention report,* Washington, D.C., Dec 1994/Jan 1995, Office of Disease Prevention and Health Promotion.

U.S. Public Health Service: *The core functions project,* Washington, D.C., 1993, Office of Disease Prevention and Health Promotion.

Zotti ME, Brown P, Stotts RG: Community-based nursing versus community health nursing: what does it all mean? *Nurs Outlook* 44:21-217, 1996.

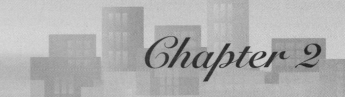

Chapter 2

The History of Community Health and Community Health Nursing

JANNA DIECKMANN

OBJECTIVES

After reading this chapter, the student should be able to:
- Discuss historical events that have influenced how health care is delivered in the community at the present time.
- Describe the contributions of Florence Nightingale, Lillian Wald, and Mary Breckinridge to establishing the foundation for current community health and community health nursing.

- Explain significant historical events in the development of contemporary community health nursing.
- Examine the ways in which community health nursing has been provided, including settlement houses, visiting nurse associations, official health organizations, and schools.
- Evaluate the status of community health nursing practice in the twenty-first century.

CHAPTER OUTLINE

Historical Roots of Public Health

America's Colonial Period and the Development of Systems for Health Care

Nursing in the Nineteenth Century

Public Health Nursing Comes of Age

The Importance of Public Health Nursing During the Early Twentieth Century

Economic Depression and the Effect on Public Health

From World War II Until the 1970s

Community and Public Health Nursing From the 1970s to the Present

KEY TERMS

American Nurses Association (ANA): a national association for registered nurses in the United States, founded in 1896 as the Nurses' Associated Alumnae of the United States and Canada.

American Public Health Association (APHA): national organization founded in 1872 to facilitate interdisciplinary efforts and promote public health.

American Red Cross: a national organization founded in 1881 through the efforts of Clara Barton that seeks to reduce human suffering through various health, safety, and disaster-relief programs in affiliation with the International Committee of the Red Cross.

Mary Breckinridge: pioneering nurse who established the Frontier Nursing Service to deliver much-needed community health services to families in rural Kentucky.

district nursing: in early public health nursing a nurse was assigned to each district in a town to provide home health care to needy people.

Frontier Nursing Service: provides community health services to rural families in Kentucky. Begun by Mary Breckinridge in 1925 with the development of outpost centers throughout the mountain area in Kentucky to provide midwifery and nursing, medical, and dental care. A hospital was established and operating in Hyden, Kentucky in 1935.

Continued

KEY TERMS—cont'd

instructive district nursing: an early term for visiting nursing; began in Boston, emphasizing that families were provided with health education and care.

Metropolitan Life Insurance Company: a life insurance company that provided home nursing services for its beneficiaries and their families.

National League for Nursing (NLN): a national nursing organization that began as the American Society of Superintendents of Training Schools of Nursing (later the National League for Nursing Education) to establish training standards and promote collegial relations among nurses.

Florence Nightingale: an English nurse who is credited with establishing nursing as a discipline.

official health agencies: those operated by state or local governments to provide a wide range of public health services, including community and public health nursing services.

William Rathbone: a British philanthropist who founded the first district nursing association in Liverpool. With Florence Nightingale, he advocated for district nursing throughout England.

settlement houses: neighborhood centers providing social and health services.

Social Security Act of 1935: Title VI, one part of this Act, was enacted to protect the health of people and included funds for education and employment of community health nurses.

visiting nurse associations: agencies staffed by nurses who provided care where the patient needed it and most often in the home.

visiting nurses: nurses who provide care wherever the client may be—home, work, or school.

Lillian Wald: the first public health nurse in the United States and an influential social reformer. One notable contribution was founding the Henry Street Settlement in New York.

One of the best ways to make plans for today and tomorrow is to look at the past. What worked? What did not work? What past lessons about health care, nursing, and communities can be used to plan for the future? Over the last few years, much of true public health has been lost. The current emphasis on the cost of health care and the heavy use of hospitals has reduced the funds available for community-oriented care. Since public health emphasizes prevention, measuring the outcomes of the work has always been a challenge. In the short run, it has been easier to document the effectiveness of a treatment or intervention than of prevention.

Most of the current health threats caused by communicable diseases, the environment, the pressures of a fast-paced life, chronic illness, and aging have been present over time. The specific ways in which these threats affect people have changed. Community health nurses have always needed to be flexible, creative, and able to work with people from many backgrounds and with varied skills. While a few historical figures are highlighted in this chapter since they clearly demonstrated these qualities, it is important to know that many nurses contributed to building organizations and providing services to improve the health of the public. Effective planning for the future is built upon learning from those who preceded us.

Community health nursing leaders have worked to improve the health status of individuals, families, and populations. They have spent time, energy, and effort working with high-risk or vulnerable groups. Part of the appeal of community health nursing has been its autonomy of practice and independence in problem solving and decision-making, as well as the interdisciplinary nature of the specialty. Many of the varied and challenging community health roles can be traced to the late 1800s when public health efforts focused on environmental conditions such as sanitation, control of communicable diseases,

education for health, prevention of disease and disability, and care of sick persons in their homes. This chapter describes the beginnings of public health, the role of nursing in community-oriented care, the contributions made by nurses to community and public health, and the influence of nurses on community-based and community-oriented practices.

HISTORICAL ROOTS OF PUBLIC HEALTH

All people and all cultures have been concerned with the events surrounding birth, death, and illness. People have tried to prevent, understand, and control disease. Their ability to preserve health and treat illness has depended on their knowledge of science, use and availability of technologies, and degree of social organization. For example, ancient Babylonians understood the need for hygiene and had some medical skills. They knew how to use medicine to treat sick people. The Egyptians of about 1000 BCE (before the common era) developed a variety of pharmaceutical preparations and constructed earth privies and public drainage systems. The Hebrew Mosaic law described in the Old Testament talked about many aspects of health including maternal health, communicable disease control, protection of food and water, and waste and sanitary disposal (Rosen, 1958).

The ancient Greeks were more concerned with personal rather than community health. They did practice many health behaviors that today are considered necessary for good health. The Greeks linked health to the environment; wealthy people valued personal cleanliness, exercise, diet, and sanitation. In contrast, less-privileged people had difficult lives and struggled to survive. The classical Roman civilization viewed medicine from a community health and

TABLE 2-1 Milestones in the History of Public Health, Public and Community Health Nursing: 1600-1865

Year	Milestone
1601	Elizabethan Poor Law written
1617	Sisterhood of the Dames de Charite organized in France by St. Vincent de Paul
1789	Baltimore Health Department established
1798	Marine Hospital Service established; later became Public Health Service
1812	Sisters of Mercy established in Dublin where nuns visited the poor
1813	Ladies Benevolent Society of Charleston, South Carolina, founded
1836	Lutheran deaconesses provide home visits in Kaiserwerth, Germany
1851	Florence Nightingale visits Kaiserwerth, Germany, for 3 months of nurse training
1855	Quarantine Board established in New Orleans; beginning of tuberculosis campaign in the United States
1859	District nursing established in Liverpool by William Rathbone
1860	Florence Nightingale Training School for Nurses established at St. Thomas Hospital in London
1864	Beginning of Red Cross

social medicine perspective. They emphasized regulation of medical practice and punishment for negligence; provision of pure water through a complex system of settling basins, aqueducts, and reservoirs; establishment of sewage systems and drainage of swamps; and supervision of street cleaning and public food preparation. During the period of the Roman Empire, women visited and cared for sick persons in their homes (Pellegrino, 1963).

The decline of the Greco-Roman civilization led to both a decay of urban culture and a disintegration of community health organization and practice (Rosen, 1958). As cities grew, people built large walls around the cities to protect themselves from invasions. These walls, while protecting from attacks, also led to crowding and poor sanitary conditions. Christianity brought with it the idea of personal responsibility for others, and care of the sick was one way of fulfilling this responsibility. During the Middle Ages between 500 and 1500 CE (common era), European cities had high population density, lack of clean water, and poor handling of refuse and body wastes. Poor sanitary conditions and residential crowding led to increases in communicable diseases such as cholera, smallpox, and bubonic plague. While most people were responsible for securing their own health care services, religious convents and monasteries established hospitals to care for the sick, poor, and neglected, including the aged, disabled, and orphaned (Rosen, 1958). During the latter part of the Middle Ages, there was interest in health education and personal hygiene knowledge, and healthful living and moderate eating was encouraged.

During the Renaissance (from the fourteenth through the sixteenth centuries CE), health practices were influenced by recognition of human dignity and worth (Kalisch and Kalisch, 1995). While the growth of science and technology during this period supported the advance of medicine and public health, public health measures remained modest. For example, while increased social organization led to better management of cities, many still depended upon private companies for their water supply and completely lacked systems of sewage disposal. In England, the Elizabethan Poor Law of 1601 guaranteed medical care for poor, blind, and "lame" individuals. This minimal care was generally provided in almshouses supported by local government. This care tried to regulate the poor as well as to provide care during illness. Table 2-1 presents milestones of public health efforts that occurred during the seventeenth, eighteenth, and nineteenth centuries.

The Industrial Revolution in nineteenth-century Europe led to social changes, while making great advances in transportation, communication, and other forms of technology. Previous care-giving structures, which relied on families, neighbors, and friends, became inadequate due to migration, urbanization, and increased demand. During this period, small numbers of Roman Catholic and Protestant religious women provided nursing care in institutions and sometimes in the home. For example, Mary Aikenhead, also known by her religious name, Sister Mary Augustine, started the Irish Sisters of Charity in 1812 in Dublin, where the nuns visited poor people (Kalisch and Kalisch, 1995).

Many lay women who performed nursing functions in almshouses and early hospitals in Great Britain were poorly educated and untrained. As the practice of medicine became more complex in the mid-1800s, hospital work required a more skilled caregiver. Physicians and hospital administrators began to be interested in the quality of nursing services. Early experiments led to some improvement in care, but it was due to the efforts of Florence Nightingale that health care was revolutionized and the discipline of nursing actually begun.

AMERICA'S COLONIAL PERIOD AND THE DEVELOPMENT OF SYSTEMS FOR HEALTH CARE

In the early years of America's settlement, as in Europe, the care of the sick was usually informal and provided by the women of the household. These women not only nursed members of their households during sickness and childbirth, but they also grew or gathered healing herbs in season for use throughout the year. This traditional system became insufficient as the number of urban residents grew in the early 1800s.

British settlers in the New World influenced the American ideas of social welfare and care of the sick. Just as the American legal system is based on English common law, colonial Americans established systems of care for the sick, poor, aged, mentally ill, and dependent based on the model of the Elizabethan Poor Law. Early county or township government was responsible for the care of all dependent residents, and they were strict about caring only for their own residents. Those who were residents elsewhere were returned to their home county for care. Few hospitals existed, and then only in the larger cities. Pennsylvania Hospital, the first hospital in the United States, was founded in Philadelphia in 1751.

Early colonial public health efforts included the collection of birth and death statistics, improved sanitation, and control of the many communicable diseases brought in at the seaports. The colonists did not have a system to ensure that public health efforts were supported and enforced. Epidemics often occurred and strained the limited local organization for health during the seventeenth, eighteenth, and nineteenth centuries (Rosen, 1958).

After the American Revolution, the threat of disease, especially yellow fever, led to public interest in establishing government-sponsored, or official, boards of health. By 1800, with a population of 75,000, New York City had established a public health committee for monitoring water quality, sewer construction, drainage of marshes, planting of trees and vegetables, construction of a masonry wall along the waterfront, and burial of the dead (Rosen, 1958).

With industrialization, the growth of cities, and inadequate housing and sanitation, disease increased, including epidemics of smallpox, yellow fever, cholera, typhoid, and typhus. Tuberculosis and malaria were always present, and infant mortality was about 200 per 1000 live births (Pickett and Hanlon, 1990). American hospitals in the early 1800s were generally unsanitary and staffed by poorly trained workers. Physicians had limited education, and medical care was scarce. Public dispensaries, similar to outpatient clinics, and private charitable efforts tried to provide some care for the poor.

The federal government focused its early public health work on providing health care for merchant seamen and protecting seacoast cities from epidemics. The Public Health Service, which remains a key federal public health agency in the twenty-first century, was established in 1798 as the Marine Hospital Service. The first Marine Hospital was opened in Norfolk, Virginia, in 1800.

Also during the early 1800s, nursing care began to be provided in homes. The Ladies' Benevolent Society of Charleston, South Carolina, provided charitable assistance to the poor and sick beginning in 1813. In Philadelphia, lay nurses were given a brief training program to teach them to care for postpartum women and their newborns in their homes and in Cincinnati, Ohio, the Sisters of Charity began

a visiting nurse service (Rodabaugh and Rodabaugh, 1951). Although these local programs provided useful services, they were not adopted elsewhere, and their influence on later community-based care is unclear.

By the mid-nineteenth century, national interest began to address public health problems in order to improve urban living conditions, and the few urban boards of health now focused on communicable disease as well as environmental health. In 1850 the Massachusetts Sanitary Commission published the famous Shattuck Report, which called for major changes in government action for public health. This landmark report recommended these changes:

1. The establishment of a state health department and local health boards in every town
2. Sanitary surveys and collection of vital statistics
3. Environmental sanitation
4. Food, drug, and communicable disease control
5. Well-child care and health education
6. Smoke and alcohol control
7. Town planning
8. Teaching preventive medicine in medical schools (Kalisch and Kalisch, 1995).

A few of the recommendations were implemented 19 years later. The Shattuck Report is important because it was the first effort that described a modern approach to public health organization.

NURSING IN THE NINETEENTH CENTURY

Florence Nightingale's vision of trained nurses and her model of nursing education influenced the development of professional nursing and, indirectly, community health nursing in the United States. In 1850 and 1851, Nightingale had carefully studied nursing "system and method" by visiting Pastor Theodor Fliedner at his Kaiserwerth, Germany, School for Deaconesses. Her work with Pastor Fliedner and the Kaiserwerth Lutheran deaconesses, with their systems of district nursing led her to include offering nursing care to the sick in their homes.

During the Crimean War (1854 to 1856), the British military established hospitals for sick and wounded soldiers in Scutari in Asia Minor. The care of soldiers was poor, with cramped quarters, poor sanitation, lice and rats, not enough food, and inadequate medical supplies (Palmer, 1983; Kalisch and Kalisch, 1995). When the British public demanded improved conditions, Florence Nightingale asked to work in Scutari. Because of her wealth, social and political connections, and knowledge of hospitals, the British government sent her to Asia Minor with 40 ladies, 117 hired nurses, and 15 paid servants. In Scutari, Nightingale progressively improved the soldiers' health using a population-based approach that improved both environmental conditions and nursing care. Using simple epidemiology measures, she documented a decreased mortality rate from 415 per 1000 at the beginning of the war to 11.5 per 1000 at the end (Cohen, 1984; Palmer, 1983). Like

Nightingale's efforts in Scutari, nurses who practice community oriented care identify health care needs that affect the entire population. They then mobilize resources and organize themselves and the community to meet these needs.

After the Crimean War and her return to England in 1856, with her fame established, Nightingale organized hospital nursing practice and nursing education in hospitals to replace untrained lay nurses with Nightingale nurses. She focused both on the role of hospital nursing and on community oriented nursing. She said that nursing should promote health and prevent illness, and she emphasized proper nutrition, rest, sanitation, and hygiene (Nightingale, 1894 and 1946).

In 1859, British philanthropist **William Rathbone** founded the first **district nursing** association in Liverpool, England. Based on the success of these "Friendly Visitors" who provided care to needy people (Kalisch and Kalisch, 1995), Nightingale and Rathbone recommended steps to provide nursing in the home, and district nursing was organized throughout England (Nutting and Dock, 1935).

With increased urbanization during the Industrial Revolution, the number of jobs for women rapidly increased. Educated women became teachers, secretaries, or saleswomen, while less-educated women worked in factories. As it became more acceptable to work outside the home, women were more willing to accept the rigors of nursing. The first nursing schools based on the Nightingale model opened in the United States in 1870. Early trained graduate nurses worked in private duty nursing or held the few positions of hospital administrators or instructors. The private duty nurses often lived with the families of patients receiving care. Since it was expensive to hire private duty nurses, only the well-to-do could afford their services. Community health nursing began in order to meet urban health care needs, especially for the disadvantaged by providing visiting nurses.

Visiting nurses took care of several families in one day, rather than attend only one as the private duty nurse did, which made their care more economical. The movement grew, and in the next few years, **visiting nurse associations** were established in Buffalo (1885), Philadelphia (1886), and Boston (1886). Wealthy people interested in charitable activities funded both settlement houses and visiting nurse associations. The first trained nurse to be hired as a visiting nurse was Frances Root. She was hired in 1887 by the Women's Board of the New York City Mission to care for sick people in their homes.

Briefly Noted

Wealthy upper-class women, freed from some of the social restrictions that had previously limited their social life and contributions, began to do charitable work and created, supported, and supervised early visiting nurses.

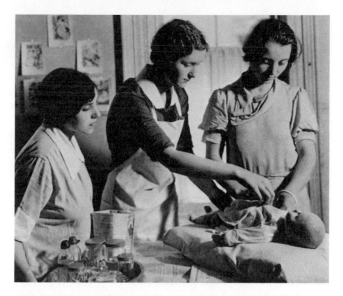

Figure 2-1   Public health nurse demonstrating well-child care during a home visit. (Courtesy the Visiting Nurse Service of New York.)

Visiting nurses spread the word about prevention through home visits and well-baby clinics. They worked with physicians, gave selected treatments, kept temperature and pulse records, and also taught family members how to care for the sick and also personal and environmental prevention measures, such as hygiene and good nutrition (Fig. 2-1). Many early visiting nurse agencies employed only one nurse, who was supervised by members of the agency board, whose members were wealthy or socially prominent women. These ladies were critically important to the success of visiting nursing through their efforts to open new agencies, financially support existing agencies, and make the services socially acceptable.

In 1886 in Boston, two women, in order to improve their chances of gaining financial support for their cause, coined the term **instructive district nursing** to emphasize the relationship of nursing to health education. Support was also secured from the Boston Dispensary, which provided free outpatient medical care. In February 1886 the first district nurse was hired in Boston, and in 1888 the Instructive District Nursing Association was incorporated as an independent voluntary agency. Sick poor persons, who paid no fees, were cared for under the direction of a trained physician (Brainard, 1922).

Nurses began to establish **settlement houses** and neighborhood centers, which became hubs for health care and social welfare programs. For example, in 1893 **Lillian Wald** and Mary Brewster, both trained nurses, began visiting the poor on New York's Lower East Side. The nurses' settlement they established became the Henry Street Settlement and later the Visiting Nurse Service of New York City. By 1905, public health nurses had provided almost 48,000 visits to more than 5,000 patients (Kalisch and Kalisch, 1995). Lillian Wald emerged as the established leader of public health nursing during its early decades (Box 2-1, Fig. 2-2).

| Box 2-1 | Lillian Wald: First Public Health Nurse in the United States |

Public health nursing evolved in the United States in the late nineteenth and early twentieth centuries largely because of the pioneering work of Lillian Wald. Born on March 10, 1867, Lillian Wald decided to become a nurse after Vassar College refused to admit her at 16 years of age. She graduated in 1891 from the New York Hospital Training School for Nurses and spent the next year working at the New York Juvenile Asylum. To supplement what she thought had been inadequate training in the sciences, she enrolled in the Woman's Medical College in New York (Frachel, 1988).

Having grown up in a warm, nurturing family in Rochester, New York, her work in New York City introduced her to an entirely different side of life. In 1883, while conducting a class in home nursing for immigrant families on the Lower East Side of New York, Wald was asked by a small child to visit her sick mother. Wald found the mother in bed, having hemorrhaged for 2 days. This home visit confirmed for Wald all of the injustices in society and the differences in health care for poor persons versus those persons able to pay (Frachel, 1988).

She simply could not tolerate seeing poor people with no access to health care. With her friend Mary Brewster and the financial support of two wealthy laypeople, Mrs. Solomon Loeb and Joseph H. Schiff, she moved to the East Side and occupied the top floor of a tenement house on Jefferson Street. This move eventually led to the establishment of Henry Street Settlement. In the beginning, Wald and Brewster helped individual families. Wald believed that the nurse's visit should be friendly, more like a friend than someone paid to visit (Dolan, 1978).

Wald used epidemiological methods to campaign for health-promoting social policies in order to improve environmental and social conditions that affected health. Not only did she write *The House on Henry Street* to describe her own public health nursing work, but also she led in the development of payment by insurance companies for nursing services (Frachel, 1988).

In 1909, along with Lee Frankel, Lillian Wald established the first community health nursing program for workers at the Metropolitan Life Insurance Company. Believing that keeping workers healthier would increase their productivity, she urged that nurses at agencies such as Henry Street Settlement provide skilled nursing care. Wald convinced the company that it would be more economical to use the services of community health nurses than to employ their own nurses. She also convinced them that services could be available to anyone desiring them, with fees graduated according to the ability to pay. This nursing service designed by Wald continued for 44 years and contributed several significant accomplishments to community health nursing, including the following (Frachel, 1988):

1. Providing home nursing care on a fee-for-service basis
2. Establishing an effective cost-accounting system for visiting nurses
3. Using advertisements in newspapers and on radio to recruit nurses
4. Reducing mortality from infectious diseases

Lillian Wald also believed that the nursing efforts at Henry Street Settlement should be aligned with an official health agency. Therefore she arranged for nurses to wear an insignia that indicated that they served under the auspices of the Board of Health. Also, she established rural health nursing services through the Red Cross. Her other accomplishments included helping to establish the Children's Bureau and fighting in New York City for better tenement living conditions, city recreation centers, parks, pure food laws, graded classes for mentally handicapped children, and assistance to immigrants (Backer, 1993; Dock, 1922; Frachel, 1988; Zerwekh, 1992).

Data from Backer BA: Lillian Wald: connecting caring with action, *Nurs Health Care* 14:122-128, 1993; Dock LL: The history of public health nursing [reprinted by the American Public Health Association] from *Pub Health Nurs* 1922; Frachel RR: A new profession: the evolution of public health nursing, *Pub Health Nurs* 5(2):86-90, 1988; Zerwekh JV: Public health nursing legacy: historical practical wisdom, *Nurs Health Care* 13:84-91, 1992.

Briefly Noted

Lillian Wald demonstrated an exceptional ability to develop approaches and programs to solve the health care and social problems of her times. How can we use today some of her creative tools for improving health care?

The public was interested in limiting disease among all classes of people, partly for religious reasons, partly as a form of charity, but also because the middle and upper classes were afraid of the diseases that seemed to be brought in by the large communities of European immigrants. During the 1890s in New York City, about 2,300,000 people were packed into 90,000 tenement houses. The environmental conditions of immigrants in tenement houses and sweatshops were familiar features of urban life across the northeastern United States and into the upper Midwest. From the beginning, community health nursing practice included teaching and prevention (Fig. 2-3). Community-oriented interventions led to improved sanitation, economic improvements, and bet-ter nutrition. These interventions were credited with reducing the incidence of acute communicable disease by 1910.

The **American Red Cross,** through its Rural Nursing Service (later the Town and Country Nursing Service) initiated home nursing care in areas outside larger cities. Lillian Wald obtained the initial donations to support this agency, which provided care to the sick, instruction in sanitation and hygiene in rural homes, and improved living conditions in villages and lonely farms. The Town and Country nurse addressed diseases such as tuberculosis, pneumonia, and typhoid fever with resourcefulness born of necessity. By 1920, Red Cross Town and Country Nursing Services numbered 1,800, and they eventually grew to almost 3,000 programs in small towns and rural areas.

Briefly Noted

The emphasis of community oriented nursing has been varied and has changed over time. Two early leaders whose legacy offers many ideas for the present and the future were Florence Nightingale and Lillian Wald.

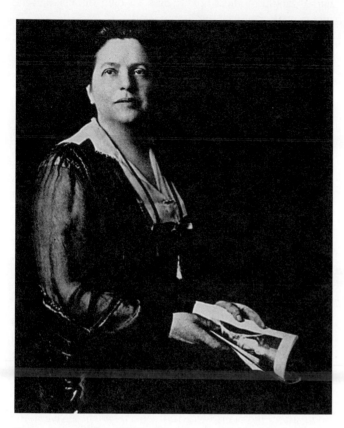

Figure 2-2 Lillian Wald. (Courtesy the Visiting Nurse Service of New York.)

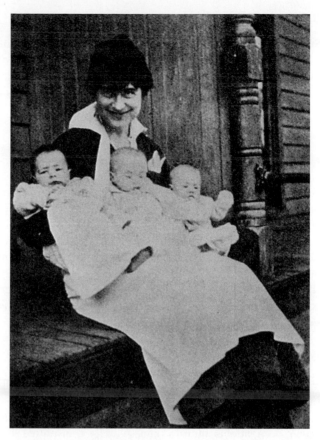

Figure 2-3 Teaching well-child care was a significant public health nursing role. (Courtesy Instructional Visiting Nurse Association of Richmond, Va.)

Occupational health nursing, beginning as industrial nursing, was an outgrowth of early home visiting efforts. In 1895, Ada Mayo Stewart began to work with employees and families of the Vermont Marble Company. As a free service for the employees, Stewart provided obstetric care, sickness care, and some post-surgical care. Interestingly, she provided few services for work-related injuries (Kalisch and Kalisch, 1995).

In New York City in 1902, more than 20% of children might be absent from school on a single day, due to conditions like pediculosis, head lice, ringworm, scabies, inflamed eyes, discharging ears, and infected wounds. School medical inspection began in 1897, but focused on excluding infectious children from school, rather than on providing or obtaining medical treatment so they could return to school. Lillian Wald tried to introduce English innovations by providing nurses for the schools. Lina Rogers, a Henry Street Settlement resident, became the first school nurse. She worked with the children in New York City schools and made home visits to teach parents and provide follow-up care to children absent from school. The new school nurses found that many children were absent because they had no shoes or adequate clothes; they were hungry, and many took care of younger or sick children (Hawkins, Hayes, and Corliss, 1994). School nursing was a big success, and in New York more nurses were added. Soon school nursing began in Los Angeles, Philadelphia, Baltimore, Boston, Chicago, and San Francisco.

PUBLIC HEALTH NURSING COMES OF AGE

Established by the Cleveland Visiting Nurse Association, the publication of the *Visiting Nurse Quarterly* in 1909 initiated a professional form of communication for clinical and organizational concerns. Also in 1909, the first nursing program associated with a university began at the University of Minnesota. In 1911 a joint committee of existing nurse organizations convened, under the leadership of Lillian Wald and Mary Gardner, to standardize nursing services outside the hospital. Recommending formation of a new organization to address public health nursing concerns, 800 agencies involved in community health nursing activities were invited to send delegates to an organizational meeting in Chicago in June 1912. Following a heated debate on its name and purpose, the delegates established the National Organization for Public Health Nursing (NOPHN) and chose Lillian Wald as its first president (Dock, 1922). Unlike other professional nursing organizations, the NOPHN membership included both nurses and their lay supporters. The NOPHN worked "to improve the educational and service standards of the public health nurse, and promote public understanding of and respect for her work" (Rosen, 1958, p. 381) and soon became a dominant force in public health nursing (Roberts, 1955).

Briefly Noted

Securing information about the organizational history of a practice agency, such as a visiting nurse association, may provide important perspectives on current agency values, decision-making structures, service areas, and clinical priorities.

It soon became obvious that graduate nurses were unprepared for home visiting. Nursing school courses were inadequate for teaching home care since diploma schools of nursing emphasized hospital care of patients. Community and public health nurses needed additional education. In 1914, Mary Adelaide Nutting working with the Henry Street Settlement, began the first postgraduate nursing course in public health nursing at Teachers College, New York City (Deloughery, 1977). The American Red Cross provided scholarships for graduates of nursing schools to attend the public health nursing course.

Public health nurses were also active in the **American Public Health Association (APHA),** which was established in 1872 to facilitate interdisciplinary efforts and promote the "practical application of public hygiene" (Scutchfield and Keck, 1997, p. 12). APHA focused on important public health issues, including sewage and garbage disposal, occupational injuries, and sexually transmitted diseases. In 1923, the Public Health Nursing Section was formed within APHA to provide a national forum for discussion of strategy for public health nurses within the context of the larger public health organization. Also in 1923, the Rockefeller Foundation endowed a School of Nursing at Yale University, and Frances Payne Bolton, a wealthy Cleveland woman established the School of Nursing at Western Reserve University.

Concurrently, public health organizations began in rural areas to target epidemics. For example, in 1911 efforts to control typhoid fever in Yakima County, Washington, and to improve health status in Guilford County, North Carolina, led to the establishment of local health units, or **official health agencies,** that were primarily staffed by public health nurses. These public health nurses assumed a leadership role on health care issues by collaborating with local officials, nurses, and other health care providers.

The experience of Orange County, California, during the 1920s and 1930s demonstrates the concerns of the public health nurse in the local health department. Following the efforts of a private physician, social welfare agencies, and a Red Cross nurse, the county board created the public health nurse position in 1922. Presented with a shining new Model T car, sporting the bright orange seal of the county, the nurse began her work by dealing with the serious communicable disease problems of diphtheria and scarlet fever. Typhoid became epidemic when a drainage pipe overflowed into a well, infecting those who drank the water, as well as those who drank raw milk from an infected dairy. Almost 3,000 residents were immunized. At weekly baby conferences, nurses taught mothers how to care for their infants, and the infants were weighed and immunized.

THE IMPORTANCE OF PUBLIC HEALTH NURSING DURING THE EARLY TWENTIETH CENTURY

In 1918 during World War I, the Vassar Camp School for Nurses started as a unique and patriotic aspect of nursing education. The American Red Cross and the Council of National Defense jointly supported this novel program, which proposed that nursing education be shortened from 3 years to 2 years for college graduates. The Vassar Camp School, modeled after the Plattsburg Military Camp in New York, intensively trained college graduates so that they could become Army Reserve officers and meet urgent wartime needs. A total of 435 graduates of this program represented many colleges across the United States. The program ended when peace was declared (Buhler-Wilkerson, 1989; Kalisch and Kalisch, 1995).

The personnel needs of World War I in Europe depleted the ranks of public health nurses, yet the NOPHN identified a need for a second and third line of defense at home. Jane Delano of the Red Cross, who was sending 100 nurses a day to the war, agreed that despite the sacrifice, the greatest patriotic duty of public health nurses was to stay at home. Soon after, the worldwide influenza epidemic swept the United States. The NOPHN and the Red Cross formed a coalition to aid those with influenza. Houses, churches, and halls were turned into hospitals, with loss of life also occurring among nurse volunteers. The NOPHN also loaned a nurse to the U.S. Public Health Service to establish a public health nursing program for military outposts, which led to the first federal government sponsorship (Shyrock, 1959; Wilner, Walkey, and O'Neill, 1978).

During the early twentieth century, the major obstacle to extending nursing services in the community was limited funding. Most early visiting nurse associations relied on contributions from wealthy and middle-class supporters. Even poor families were encouraged to pay a small fee for nursing services, reflecting social welfare concerns against promoting economic dependency by providing charity. In 1909, largely due to the advocacy of Lillian Wald, the **Metropolitan Life Insurance Company** began a program using visiting nurse organizations to provide care for sick policyholders. By 1912, 589 Metropolitan nursing programs provided care through existing agencies or through visiting nurses hired directly by Met Life. In 1918, Metropolitan Life calculated an average decline of 7% in the mortality rate of policyholders, and almost a 20% decline in the deaths of children under age 3. The insurance company attributed this improvement, as well as reduced costs for the insurance company, to the work of visiting nurses.

Community health nurses' efforts to influence public policy included advocacy for the Children's Bureau and the Sheppard-Towner Program. In 1912, Lillian Wald and other nursing leaders influenced the establishment of the

Evidence-Based Practice

The relationship between the nursing profession and Metropolitan Life Insurance Company is both interesting and reflective of a range of historical events in nursing. Metropolitan Life led the insurance industry in the provision of nursing care in the home for its policyholders. A friend of Lillian Wald's, Lee Frankel, headed the welfare department at Metropolitan. She proposed that nurses could assess illness, teach health practices, and effectively collect data from policyholders. On June 9, 1909, the first Henry Street nurse made a home visit to a policyholder. By 1914 Metropolitan provided home nursing care to policyholders in 1804 cities. The original idea was for the company to contract for services with existing nursing agencies. However, in 1910 the Metropolitan Visiting Nurse service was established in St. Paul, Minnesota, and these nurses became "Met nurses." They not only provided care to policy-holders that may have lengthened their lives, but also collected immense amounts of data that were invaluable to the insurance industry.

APPLICATION IN PRACTICE

The author describes the relationship among the insurance company, nurses, and policyholders in the study of tuberculosis that began in Framingham, Massachusetts, in 1916. The article is not about tuberculosis but rather is about nursing and how since the early 1900s other groups have tried to be in control.

Hamilton D: Research and reform: Community nursing and the Framingham tuberculosis project, 1914-1923, *Nurs Res* 41(1):8-13, 1992.

Children's Bureau, whose goal was to address national problems of maternal and child welfare. Children's Bureau experts investigated the effects of income, housing, employment, and other factors on infant and maternal mortality. Their work led to federal child labor laws and the 1919 White House Conference on Child Health.

Problems of maternal and child morbidity and mortality spurred the Maternity and Infancy Act (often called the Sheppard-Towner Act) in 1921, which provided federal matching funds to establish maternal and child health divisions in state health departments. Education during home visits by public health nurses included promoting the health of mother and child, as well as seeking prompt medical care during pregnancy. While credited with saving many lives, the Sheppard-Towner Program ended in 1929, in response to concerns by the American Medical Association and others that the legislation gave too much power to the federal government and too closely resembled socialized medicine (Pickett and Hanlon, 1990).

In contrast to significant changes in public support for community and public health nursing, some innovations resulted from individual commitment and private financial support. In 1925, **Mary Breckinridge** established the **Frontier Nursing Service** (FNS). This creative service was based on systems of care used in the Highlands and islands of Scotland (Box 2-2, Fig. 2-4). Breckinridge introduced the first nurse-midwives into the United States. The unique pio-

neering spirit of the FNS influenced the development of public health programs to improve the health care of the rural and often inaccessible population in the Appalachian sections of southeastern Kentucky (Browne, 1966; Tirpak, 1975) (Fig. 2-5). FNS nurses were trained in nursing, public health, and midwifery. Their work led to reduced pregnancy complications for their patients and one third fewer still-births and infant deaths in an area of 700 square miles (Kalisch and Kalisch, 1995). The Frontier Nursing Service continues to provide comprehensive health and nursing services to the people of that area and supports the Frontier School of Midwifery and Family Nursing.

ECONOMIC DEPRESSION AND THE EFFECT ON PUBLIC HEALTH

A continuing challenge to community oriented nursing was the tension between preventive care and care of the sick, and the related question of whether nursing interventions should be directed toward groups and communities or toward individuals and their families. While each nursing agency was unique and services varied from region to region, voluntary visiting nurse associations tended to emphasize care of the sick, while official public health agencies provided more preventive services. Not surprisingly, this splintering of services led to rivalry between "visiting," or community, and "public health" nurses. This splintering interfered with the development of comprehensive community nursing services (Roberts and Heinrich, 1985). In addition, one household could receive services from several community nurses representing different agencies. For example, in the same home there might be separate visits for a postpartum woman and new baby, for a child sick with scarlet fever, and for an elderly person sick in bed. This was confusing and duplicated services.

The "combination service" merged sick care services and preventive services into one comprehensive agency; often these were public agencies. However, compared to visiting nurse organizations, community health nurses in official agencies often had less control of the program, since physicians and politicians determined services and assignment of personnel. The "ideal program" of the combination agency was hard to administer, and many of the combination services implemented between 1930 and 1965 later reverted back to their former, divided structures of visiting nurse agencies and official health departments.

The economic crisis of the 1930s depression deeply influenced nursing. Not only were agencies and communities unable to meet the huge needs and numbers of the poor, but decreased funding for nursing services reduced the numbers of nurses in hospitals and in the community. The Federal Emergency Relief Administration (FERA) supported nurse employment through increased grants-in-aid for state programs of home medical care. FERA often purchased nursing care from existing visiting nurse agencies that supported the nurses and prevented agency closure. During this time more than 10,000 nurses were employed by the Civil

Box 2-2   Mary Breckinridge and the Frontier Nursing Service

Born in 1881 into the fifth generation of a well-to-do Kentucky family, Mary Breckinridge devoted her life to the establishment of the Frontier Nursing Service (FNS). Learning from her grandmother, who used a large part of her fortune to improve the education of southern children, Breckinridge later used money left to her by her grandmother to start the FNS (Browne, 1966).

Tutored in childhood and later attending private schools, Mary Breckinridge did not consider becoming a nurse until her husband died. She "yearned for adventure and struggled for the opportunity to 'do something useful'" (Hostutler, et al, 2000). In 1907, she enrolled at St. Luke's Hospital School of Nursing in New York. She later married for a second time and had two children. Her second marriage ended after her daughter died at birth and her son died at age 4. From the time of her son's death in 1918, she devoted her energy to promoting the health care of disadvantaged women and children (Browne, 1966).

After World War I and work in postwar France, she returned to the United States passionate about helping the neglected children of rural America. To prepare herself for what would become her life's work, she studied for a year at Teacher's College, Columbia University to learn more about public health nursing (Browne, 1966).

Early in 1925 she returned to Kentucky. She decided that the mountains of Kentucky were an excellent place to demonstrate the value of community health nursing to remote, disadvantaged families. She thought that if she could establish a nursing center in rural Kentucky, this effort could then be duplicated anywhere. The first health center was established in a five-room cabin in Hyden, Kentucky. Establishing the center took not only nursing skills but also the construction of the center and later the hospital and other buildings; it required extensive knowledge about securing a water supply, disposing of sewage, getting electric power, and securing a mountain area in which landslides occurred (Browne, 1966). Despite many obstacles inherent in building in the mountains, six outpost nursing centers were built between 1927 and 1930. The FNS hospital was built in Hyden, Kentucky, and physicians began entering service. Payment of fees ranged from labor and supplies to funds raised through annual family dues, philanthropy, and fundraising efforts of Mary Breckinridge (Holloway, 1975).

The FNS established medical, surgical, and dental clinics; provided nursing and midwifery services 24 hours a day; and served nearly 10,000 people spread out over 700 square miles. At the suggestion of a supportive physician, baseline data were obtained on infant and maternal mortality before beginning services. The reduced mortality following the inception of the FNS is especially remarkable considering the environmental conditions in which these rural Kentuckians lived. Many homes had no heat, electricity, or running water. Often physicians were located more than 40 miles from their patients (Tirpak, 1975).

During the 1930s, nurses lived in one of the six outposts, from which they traveled to see patients; often had to make their visits on horseback. Like her nurses, Mary Breckinridge traveled many miles through the mountains of Kentucky on her horse, Babette, providing food, supplies, and health care to mountain families (Browne, 1966).

Over the years several hundred nurses have worked for the FNS. Despite the fact that Mary Breckinridge died in 1965, the FNS has continued to grow and provide needed services to people in the mountains of Kentucky. This service continues today as a vital and creative way to deliver community health services to rural families.

Data from Browne H: A tribute to Mary Breckinridge, *Nurs Outlook* 14:54-55, May 1966; Holloway JB: Frontier Nursing Service 1925-1975, *J Ky Med Assoc* 13:491-492, Sept 1975; Hostutler J, Kennedy MS, Mason D, Schorr TM: Nurses: then and now and models of practice, *Am J Nurs* 100(2):82-83, 2000; Tirpak H: The Frontier Nursing Service—fifty years in the mountains, *Nurs Outlook* 33:308-310, 1975.

Works Administration Programs (CWA) and assigned to official health agencies. "While this facilitated rapid program expansion by recipient agencies and gave the nurses a taste of public health, the nurses' lack of field experience created major problems of training and supervision for the regular staff" (Roberts and Heinrich, 1985, p. 1162). Basic nursing education emphasized care of individuals, and students got little information on groups and the community as a unit of service. Thus new graduates were inadequately prepared to work in public health and required considerable agency orientation and teaching (National Organization for Public Health Nursing, 1944).

Changes at the federal level affected the structure of community health resources and led to a "new era in public health nursing" (Roberts and Heinrich, 1985, p. 1162). In 1933 Pearl McIver became the first nurse employed by the U.S. Public Health Service to provide consultation services to state health departments. McIver was convinced that the strengths and ability of each state's director of public health nursing would determine the scope and quality of local health services. Together with Naomi Deutsch, director of nursing for the federal Children's Bureau, and with the support of nursing organizations, McIver and her staff of nurse consultants influenced the direction of public health nursing. Between 1931 and 1938, more than 40% of the increase in public health nurse employment was in local health agencies. Even so, more than one third of all counties in the nation still lacked local public health nursing services.

The **Social Security Act of 1935** tried to remedy the national setbacks of the depression. Title VI of this act provided funding to expand opportunities for health protection and promotion through education and employment of public health nurses. More than 1,000 nurses completed educational programs in public health in 1936. Title VI also provided $8 million to assist states, counties, and medical districts to establish and maintain adequate health services, as well as $2 million for research and investigation of disease (Buhler-Wilkerson, 1985; Buhler-Wilkerson, 1989; Kalisch and Kalisch, 1995).

At this time Congress began to support categorical funding that provides federal money for priority diseases or groups rather than for a comprehensive community health program. Thus local health departments designed programs to fit the funding priorities. Included among these were maternal and child health services and crippled children (1935), venereal disease control (1938), tuberculosis (1944),

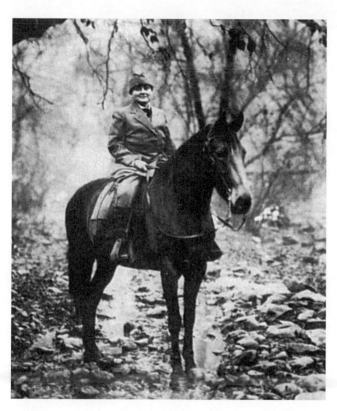

Figure 2-4 Mary Breckinridge, founder of the Frontier Nursing Service. (Courtesy the Frontier Nursing Service of Wendover, Ky.)

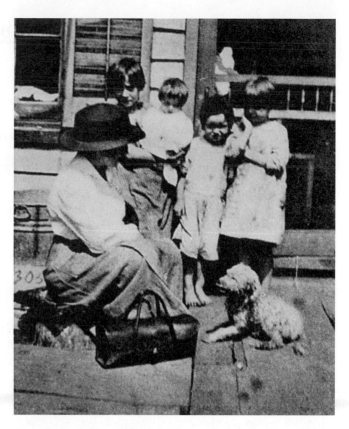

Figure 2-5 Early public health nurses provided a range of services for families. (Courtesy Instructional Visiting Nurse Association of Richmond, Va.)

mental health (1947), industrial hygiene (1947), and dental health (1947) (Scutchfield and Keck, 1997). This pattern of funding continues at the present time.

The war increased the need for nurses both for the war effort and at home. Many nurses joined the Army and Navy Nurse Corps. U.S. Representative Frances Payne Bolton of Ohio led Congress to pass the Bolton Act of 1943 that established the Cadet Nurses Corps. This legislation supported increased undergraduate and graduate enrollment in schools of nursing. Funding became more available to educate nurses by providing financial support for them to go to school, and many focused on public health.

Due to the number of nurses involved in the war, civilian hospitals and visiting nurse agencies shifted outpatient care to families and non-nursing personnel. "By the end of 1942, over 500,000 women had completed the American Red Cross home nursing course, and nearly 17,000 nurse's aides had been certified" (Roberts and Heinrich, 1985, p. 1165). By the end of 1946, more than 215,000 volunteer nurse's aides had received certificates. During this time community health nursing expanded its scope of practice. For example, more community health nurses practiced in rural areas, and many official agencies began to provide bedside nursing care (Buhler-Wilkerson, 1985; Kalisch and Kalisch, 1995).

The changes brought about by the war increased the need for services from local health departments, including sudden increases in demand for care of emotional problems, accidents, alcoholism, and other responsibilities new to official health agencies. Changes in medical technology improved the ability to screen and treat infectious and communicable diseases (e.g., using antibiotics to treat rheumatic fever and venereal diseases). Job opportunities for public health nurses grew since they made up a major portion of health department staff. At this time more than 20,000 nurses worked in health departments, visiting nurse associations, industry, and schools. Table 2-2 highlights significant milestones in community and public health nursing from the mid-1800s to the mid-1900s.

FROM WORLD WAR II UNTIL THE 1970s

By 1950 Americans were living longer, and the leading causes of death had changed from infectious diseases to heart disease, cancer, and cerebrovascular disease. Nurses were influential in the reduction of communicable diseases through their work with immunization campaigns, improved nutrition, and better hygiene and sanitation. Availability of more medications, better housing, and good emergency and critical care services also extended the lives of many people. The over-65 population grew from 4.1% in 1900 to 9.2% of the total in 1950. Chronic illnesses and longer lives brought new health

TABLE 2-2   Milestones in the History of Community Health and Public Health Nursing: 1866-1945

Year	Milestone
1866	New York Metropolitan Board of Health established
1872	American Public Health Association established
1873	New York Training School opens at Bellevue Hospital, New York City, as first Nightingale-model nursing school in United States
1877	Women's Board of the New York Mission hires Frances Root to visit the sick poor
1885	Visiting Nurse Association established in Buffalo
1886	Visiting nurse agencies established in Philadelphia and Boston
1893	Lillian Wald and Mary Brewster organized a visiting nursing service for the poor of New York, which later became the famous Henry Street Settlement; Society of Superintendents of Training Schools of Nurses in the United States and Canada was established (in 1912 became known as the National League for Nursing Education)
1896	Associated Alumnae of Training Schools for Nurses established (in 1911 became the American Nurses' Association)
1902	School nursing started in New York (Lina Rogers)
1903	First nurse practice acts
1909	Metropolitan Life Insurance Company provides first insurance reimbursement for nursing care
1910	Public health nursing program instituted at Teachers College, Columbia University, in New York
1912	National Organization for Public Health Nursing formed with Lillian Wald as first president
1914	First undergraduate nursing education course in public health offered by Adelaide Nutting at Teacher's College
1918	Vassar Camp School for Nurses organized; U.S. Public Health Service (USPHS) establishes division of public health nursing to work in the war effort; worldwide influenza epidemic begins
1919	Textbook, *Public Health Nursing,* written by Mary S. Gardner
1921	Maternity and Infancy Act (Sheppard-Towner Act)
1925	Frontier Nursing Service using nurse-midwives established
1934	Pearl McIver becomes first nurse employed by USPHS
1935	Passage of Social Security Act
1941	Beginning of World War II
1943	Passage of Bolton-Bailey Act for nursing education and Cadet Nurse Program established; Division of Nursing begun at USPHS; Lucille Petry appointed chief of Cadet Nurse Corps
1944	First basic program in nursing accredited as including sufficient public health content

challenges including the need to provide long-term care. Also, as mentioned earlier, categorical funding supported the development of programs to treat a narrow range of problems thus leading to duplication among agencies.

During the 1930s and 1940s, more people chose to get care in hospitals since this was where physicians worked and where technology was readily available to diagnose and treat illness. Health insurance was developed that allowed middle-class people to get care in hospitals that had previously been available only to those who could afford to pay their own bills. In 1952, Metropolitan Life Insurance and John Hancock Life Insurance Companies ended their support of visiting nurse services for their policyholders, and the American Red Cross ended its programs of direct nursing service.

Nursing organizations also continued to change. The functions of the NOPHN, the National League for Nursing Education, and the Association of Collegiate Schools of Nursing were distributed to the new **National League for Nursing.** The **American Nurses Association** continued as the second national nursing organization. In 1948 the National League for Nursing adopted the recommendations of Esther Lucile Brown's study of nursing education, *Nurs-*

ing for the Future, and this considerably influenced how nurses were prepared. She recommended that basic nursing education be done in colleges and universities.

In the 1950s, public health nursing became a required part of most baccalaureate nursing education programs, and in 1952, nursing education programs began in junior and community colleges. Louise McManus, a director of the Division of Nursing Education at Teachers College, Columbia University, wanted to see if bedside nurses could be prepared in a 2-year program. The intent was to prepare nurses more quickly than in the past in order to ease the prevailing nursing shortage (Kalisch and Kalisch 1995). This would also move more nursing education into American higher education. Mildred Montag, an assistant professor of nursing education at Teacher's College, became the project coordinator. In 1958, when the 5-year study was completed, this experiment was determined to be a success.

Currently, the largest number of nurses are prepared at the associate degree nursing (ADN) level. In recent years, just as health care has changed, so has ADN education. Both have moved away from a heavy focus on inpatient care to community-based care. Curricula in ADN programs have begun to add content and clinical experiences in management, community health, home health, and gerontology.

COMMUNITY AND PUBLIC HEALTH NURSING FROM THE 1970s TO THE PRESENT

During the 1970s, nurses made many contributions to improving the health care of communities including participation in the hospice movement, the development of birthing centers, daycare for elderly and disabled persons, drug-abuse treatment programs, and rehabilitation services in long-term care. Some significant changes occurred during the 1980s as health care costs grew. Health-promotion and disease-prevention programs were not as well supported since funding began to shift to meet the costs of acute hospital care, medical procedures, and institutional long-term care. The use of ambulatory services including health maintenance organizations was encouraged, and the utilization of nurse practitioners was increased. Although facing many reimbursement threats, home health care began to increase its role in care of the sick at home by the end of the 1980s. Individuals and families assumed more responsibility for their own health, and health education—always a part of community health nursing—became more popular. Consumer and professional advocacy groups urged the passage of laws to prohibit unhealthy practices in public such as smoking and driving under the influence of alcohol. Reduced federal and state funds led to decreases in the number of nurses in official public health agencies.

The National Center for Nursing Research (NCNR) was established in 1985 within the National Institutes of Health in Washington, D.C. This focused attention on the value of nursing research and has promoted the work of nurses. Nurses were later than some other professional groups in investigating how their work benefited the people for whom they cared. Actual nursing research began in the 1950s, which means that considerable growth and sophistication took place in the next 40 years leading up to the establishment of the NCNR. Another milestone took place in 1993 when the NCNR attained institute (rather than center) status and became the National Institute of Nursing Research (NINR).

By the late 1980s, public health had declined in its effectiveness in implementing its mission and affecting the health of the public. The reduced political support, financing, and effectiveness was clearly described by the Institute of Medicine (IOM) in *The Future of Public Health* (1988). The IOM study group who wrote the report found that public health in the United States was in disarray; while many agreed about what the mission of public health should be, there was much less agreement about how to turn the mission into action and effective programs.

The IOM report emphasized the core functions of public health as assessment, policy development, and assurance (see Chapter 1). Three additional U.S. Public Health Service documents, *Healthy People 2000: National Health Promotion and Disease Prevention Objectives* (1991), *Healthy*

Healthy People 2010
Overall Areas of Emphasis

Healthy People 2010 continues the trends set by the first report released in 1979 (see Chapter 1). More than *Healthy People 2000*, this document supports the work and the roles of all community health providers, including public health providers. The emphasis of *Healthy People 2010* is on:

- Active participation by individuals in decisions regarding their health and the health of their families.
- Encouraging leadership roles in promoting healthier behaviors in clients, neighborhoods, or communities.
- The goal to improve the nation's health.
- Nurses who can improve health by beginning with the self and one client.
- Those factors that encourage health.
- The factors determining health: the physical, social, environmental factors related to individuals and communities, as well as the policies and interventions used to promote health, prevent disease, and ensure access to quality health care.

Communities 2000: Model Standards (1991), and *Healthy People 2010: Understanding and Improving Health (2000)* emphasized the need for goal setting in public health. *Healthy People 2000* proposed a national strategy to improve the health of the public significantly by using strategies to prevent major chronic illness, injuries, and infectious diseases. Specific goals and objectives were established, and time frames for accomplishing them were determined. The degree to which these strategies were met have been described in the report, *Healthy People 2000 Review,* 1998-99 (2000), and new and/or revised objectives for health are set forth in *Healthy People 2010: Understanding and Improving Health (2000).*

During the 1990s concern focused on cost, quality, and access to services. Despite considerable interest in universal health insurance coverage, neither individuals nor employers are willing to pay for this level of service. The core debate of the economics of health care—who will pay for what—has emphasized the need for reform of medical care, rather than comprehensive reform of health care. In 1993, a blue-ribbon group assembled by President Clinton, with First Lady Hillary Rodham Clinton serving as chair, proposed the American Health Security Act. Although this act received insufficient support in Congress to be enacted, it did discuss many of the key issues and concerns in health care, especially the organization and delivery of medical care with an emphasis on managed care. Following the failure to pass the American Health Security Act, considerable change occurred in health care financing with control assumed by the private sector. Managed care grew, costs began to be contained, and constraints increased in terms of how to access care and how much and what kind of care would be paid for. Throughout this debate, the failure to pass the Act, and the assumption of considerable control of health

| TABLE 2-3 | Milestones in the History of Community Health and Public Health Nursing: 1946-2000 |

Year	Milestone
1946	Nurses classified as professionals by U.S. Civil Service Commission; Hill-Burton Act approved providing funds for hospital construction in underserved areas and requiring these hospitals to provide care to poor people; passage of National Mental Health Act
1950	25,091 nurses employed in public health
1951	National organizations recommend that college-based nursing education programs include public health content
1952	National Organization for Public Health Nursing merges into the new National League for Nursing; Metropolitan Life Insurance Nursing Program closes
1964	Passage of Economic Opportunity Act; public health nurse defined by the ANA as a graduate of a BSN program; Congress amended Social Security Act to include Medicare and Medicaid
1965	ANA position paper recommended that nursing education take place in institutions of higher learning
1977	Passage of Rural Health Clinic Services Act, which provided indirect reimbursement for nurse practitioners in rural health clinics
1978	Association of Graduate Faculty in Community Health Nursing/Public Health Nursing (later renamed as Association of Community Health Nursing Educators)
1980	Medicaid amendment to the Social Security Act to provide direct reimbursement for nurse practitioners in rural health clinics; both ANA and APHA developed statements on the role and conceptual foundations of community and public health nursing respectively
1983	Beginning of Medicare prospective payments
1985	National Center for Nursing Research established in National Institutes of Health (NIH)
1988	Institute of Medicine published *The Future of Public Health*
1990	Association of Community Health Nursing Educators published *Essentials of Baccalaureate Nursing Education*
1991	More than 60 nursing organizations joined forces to support health care reform and published a document entitled *Nursing's Agenda for Health Care Reform*
1993	American Health Security Act of 1993 published as a blueprint for national health care reform; the national effort, however, failed, leaving states and the private sector to design their own programs
1993	NCNR became the National Institute for Nursing Research, as part of the National Institutes of Health
1993	Public Health Nursing section of the American Public Health Association updates *The Definition and Role of Public Health Nursing*
1998	*The Public Health Workforce: An Agenda for the 21st Century* was published by the U.S. Public Health Service to look at the current workforce in public, health, educational needs, and use of distance learning strategies to prepare the future public health workers.
1999	The Public Health Nursing Quad Council through the American Nurses Association released a new scope and standards of public health nursing document that differentiates between community-oriented and community-based nursing practice.

care by the private sector, public health was once again mostly ignored. No one really looked at who would ensure that populations and the communities in which they lived were healthy. This omission meant there was a large gap in the design of a comprehensive program for health care.

In 1991 the American Nurses Association, the American Association of Colleges of Nursing, the National League for Nursing, and more than 60 other specialty nursing organizations joined to support health care reform. The document resulting from this historic joint effort of nursing organizations incorporated the key health care issues of access, quality, and cost, and set forth a range of efforts designed to build a healthy nation through improved primary care and public health efforts. Professional nursing support for revisions in health care delivery and extension of public health services to prevent illness, promote health, and protect the public continues (Table 2-3).

Public health nursing celebrated "A Century of Caring" in 1993, to mark the centennial of the establishment of the Henry Street Settlement. Two excellent photo essays, *A Cen-*

tury of Caring: a Celebration of Public Health Nursing in the United States, 1883-1993 (U.S. Public Health Service, Division of Nursing, 1993) and *Healing at Home: Visiting Nurse Service of New York, 1893-1993* (Denker, 1994) reflect on a century of caring and document 100 years of courage, caring, and commitment of public health nurses. The photos in both books depict how much work was done by community-oriented nurses who, often with minimal support and few resources, served people who often had enormous health problems. Public health nursing, historically and in the present, can be characterized by its reaching out to care for the health of people in need (U.S. Public Health Service, 1993). At present, many nurses work in the community. Some bring a public health population-based approach and have as their goal preventing illness and protecting health. Other nurses have a community-oriented approach and deal primarily with the health care of individuals, families, and groups in a community. Still other nurses bring a community-based approach that focuses on "illness care" of individuals and families in the community. Each type of nurse is needed in today's communities. The latter two groups are growing and will continue to do so since so much of health care is being provided in community rather than inpatient settings. Today, nurses who work in the community need to look to the past and learn how to avoid the mistakes of those who went before and also to gain inspiration and be able to explain and predict the current and future needs in nursing and health care.

Clinical Application

Mary Lipsky has worked for a visiting nurse association in a major, urban area for almost two years. Her nursing responsibilities include a wide variety of services, including caring for older and chronically ill clients recently discharged from hospitals, new mothers and babies, mental health clients, and clients with long-term health problems, such as chronic wounds.

When she leaves the field to return to her own home each evening, she finds she holds her clients in her thoughts. Why is it so difficult for mothers and new babies to qualify for and receive WIC (Women, Infant, and Children Nutrition) Services? Why must she limit the number of visits and length of service for clients with chronic wounds? Why are there so few services for clients with behavioral health problems? She especially has on her mind the burdens and challenges that families and friends face in caring for the sick at home.

A. *Why might it be difficult to solve these problems at the individual level, on a case-by-case basis?*
B. *What information would you need to build an understanding of the policy background for each of these various populations?*

Answers are in the back of the book.

 Remember This!

- A historical approach can be used to increase understanding of public and community health nursing in the past, as well as its contemporary dilemmas and future challenges.
- Public and community health nursing is a product of various social, economic, and political forces, and incorporates public health science, in addition to nursing science and practice.
- Federal responsibility for health care was limited until the 1930s, when the economic challenges of the Depression highlighted the need for local responsibility for care.
- Florence Nightingale designed and implemented the first program of trained nursing, while her contemporary, William Rathbone, founded the first district nursing association in England.
- Urbanization, industrialization, and immigration in the United States increased the need for trained nurses, especially in public and community health nursing.
- Increasing acceptance of public roles for women permitted public and community health nursing employment for nurses, as well as public leadership roles for their wealthy supporters.

- The first trained nurse in the United States who was salaried as a visiting nurse was Frances Root, who was hired in 1887 by the Women's Board of the New York City Mission to provide care to sick persons at home.
- The first visiting nurse associations were founded in 1885 and 1886 in Buffalo, Philadelphia, and Boston.
- Lillian Wald established the Henry Street Settlement, which became the Visiting Nurse Service of New York City, in 1893. She played a key role in innovations that shaped public and community health nursing in its first decades, including school nursing, insurance payment for nursing, national organization for public health nurses, and the United States Children's Bureau.
- Founded in 1902, with the vision and support of Lillian Wald, school nursing sought to keep children in school so that they could learn.
- Metropolitan Life Insurance Company established the first insurance-based program in 1909 to support community health nursing services.
- The National Organization for Public Health Nursing (founded in 1912) provided essential leadership and coordination of diverse public and community health nursing efforts, before the organization merged into the new National League for Nursing in 1952.
- Official health agencies slowly grew in numbers between 1900 and 1940, accompanied by a steady increase in public health nursing positions.
- The innovative Sheppard Towner Act of 1921 expanded community health nursing roles for maternal and child health during the 1920s.
- Mary Breckinridge established the Frontier Nursing Service in 1925 to provide rural health care.
- Tension between the community health nursing roles of caring for the sick and of providing preventive care, and the related tension between intervening for individuals or for groups, has characterized the specialty since at least the 1910s.
- The challenges of World War II sometimes resulted in extension of community health nursing care, and sometimes in retrenchment and decreased public health nursing services.
- By mid-twentieth century, the reduced incidence of communicable diseases and the increased prevalence of chronic illness, accompanied by large increases in the population over age 65, led to examination of the goals and organization of community health nursing services.
- Between the 1930s and 1965, organized nursing and community health nursing agencies sought to establish health insurance reimbursement for nursing care at home.
- Implementation of Medicare and Medicaid programs in 1966 established new possibilities for supporting community-based nursing care, but encouraged agencies to focus on post-acute care services rather than prevention.
- Efforts to reform health care organization, pushed by increased health care costs during the last 40 years, have focused on reforming acute medical care rather than on designing a comprehensive preventive approach.

- The 1988 Institute of Medicine report documented the reduced political support, financing, and impact that increasingly limited public health services at national, state, and local levels.
- In the late 1990s, federal policy changes dangerously reduced financial support for home health care services, threatening the long-term survival of visiting nurse agencies.
- *Healthy People 2000* and *Healthy People 2010* have brought renewed emphasis on prevention to public and community health nursing.

? *What Would You Do?*

1. Interview three nurses who work in a community setting. Ask them to describe the changes they have seen in the way in which care is delivered in the community. Ask if they think the changes have been positive or negative and to discuss specifically how they view the changes in regard to improving the health of the community residents.
2. Interview older friends or relatives to see if they have had any experiences with nursing care in the community. Next, meet with three or four classmates and discuss the following: If the older people had received nursing care in the community, what type of care was it? Was the care useful? What suggestions do they have for how care could be more useful to them if provided in a community setting?
3. What part of community-based practice interests you? If you were to work in a community setting, what would it be? What impact would your work likely have? If you prefer not to work in a community setting now or in the future, what are your primary reasons for this decision?
4. The chapter has described the work and enormous contributions of several leaders in community health nursing. Which one do you admire the most? Whose work would you like to continue in the present health care system? What do you see as strengths and limitations of previous community health nurses? Which one strikes you as most interesting? Why?

REFERENCES

Backer BA: Lillian Wald: connecting caring with action, *Nurs Health Care* 14:122-128, 1993.

Brainard A: *Evolution of public health nursing,* Philadelphia, 1922, WB Saunders.

Browne H: A tribute to Mary Breckinridge, *Nurs Outlook* 14:54-55, May 1966.

Buhler-Wilkerson K: Public health nursing: in sickness or in health? *Am J Pub Health* 75:1155-1161, 1985.

Buhler-Wilkerson K: *False dawn: the rise and decline of public health nursing, 1900-1930,* New York, 1989, Garland Publishing.

Cohen IB: Florence Nightingale, *Sci Am* 3:128-137, 1984.

Deloughery GL: *History and trends of professional nursing,* ed 8, St Louis, 1977, Mosby.

Denker EP (editor): *Healing at home: Visiting Nurse Service of New York, 1893-1993,* New York, 1994, The Carl and Lily Pforzheimer Foundation.

Dock LL: The history of public health nursing (reprinted by the American Public Health Association) from *Pub Health Nurs,* 1922.

Frachel RR: A new profession: the evolution of public health nursing, *Pub Health Nurs* 5(2):86-90, 1988.

Hawkins JW, Hayes ER, Corliss CP: School nursing in America— 1902-1994: a return to public health nursing, *Pub Health Nurs* 11(6):416-425, 1994.

Holloway JB: Frontier Nursing Service 1925-1975, *J Ky Med Assoc* 13:491-492, Sept 1975.

Hostutler J, Kennedy MS, Mason D, Schorr TM: Nurses: then and now and models of practice, *Am J Nurs* 100(2):82-83, 2000.

Institute of Medicine: *The future of public health,* Washington, D.C., 1988, National Academy of Science.

Kalisch PA, Kalisch BJ: *The advance of American nursing,* ed 3, Philadelphia, 1995, JB Lippincott.

National Organization for Public Health Nursing: approval of Skidmore College of Nursing as preparing students for public health nursing, *Pub Health Nurs* 36:371, 1944.

Nightingale F: Sick nursing and health nursing. In Billings JS, Hurd HM (editors): *Hospitals, dispensaries, and nursing,* Baltimore, 1894, Johns Hopkins Press, reprinted New York, 1984, Garland Publishing.

Nightingale F: *Notes on nursing: what it is, and what it is not,* Philadelphia, 1946, Lippincott.

Nutting MA, Dock LL: *A history of nursing,* 4 vols, New York, 1935, GP Putnam's Sons.

Palmer IS: *Florence Nightingale and the first organized delivery of nursing services,* Washington, D.C., 1983, American Association of Colleges of Nursing.

Pellegrino ED: Medicine, history, and the idea of man, *Ann Am Acad Pol Soc Sci* 346:9-20, 1963.

Pickett G, Hanlon JJ: *Public health: administration and practice,* St Louis, 1990, Mosby.

Roberts DE, Heinrich J: Public health nursing comes of age, *Am J Pub Health* 75:1162-1172, 1985.

Roberts M: *American nursing: history and interpretation,* New York, 1955, Macmillan.

Rodabaugh JH, Rodabaugh MJ: *Nursing in Ohio: a history,* Columbus, OH, 1951, Ohio State Nurses Association.

Rosen G: *A history of public health,* New York, 1958, MD Publications.

Scutchfield FD, Keck CW: *Principles of public health practice,* Albany, NY, 1997, Delmar Publishers.

Shyrock H: *The history of nursing,* Philadelphia, 1959, WB Saunders.

Tirpak H: The Frontier Nursing Service—fifty years in the mountains, *Nurs Outlook* 33:308-310, 1975.

U.S. Department of Health and Human Services: *Healthy people 2010 objectives,* Washington, D.C., 1999, U.S. Department of Health and Human Services.

U.S. Public Health Service, Division of Nursing: *A century of caring: a celebration of public health nursing in the United States, 1893-1993,* Washington, D.C., 1993, U.S. Government Printing Office.

U.S. Public Health Service: *Healthy communities 2000: model standards,* Washington, D.C., 1991, U.S. Government Printing Office.

U.S. Public Health Service: *Healthy people 2000: national health promotion and disease prevention objectives,* Washington, D.C., 1991, U.S. Government Printing Office.

Wilner, DM, Walkey RP, O'Neill EJ: *Introduction to public health,* ed 7, New York, 1978, Macmillan.

Zerwekh JV: Public health nursing legacy: historical practical wisdom, *Nurs Health Care* 13:84-91, 1992.

Chapter 3

The Public Health and Primary Health Care Systems

SUSAN B. HASSMILLER

OBJECTIVES

After reading this chapter, the student should be able to:

- Define public health, primary care, primary health care, and community-oriented primary care.
- Differentiate between primary care and primary health care.
- Describe the current public health system in the United States and compare and contrast the responsibilities of the federal, state, and local public health systems.

- Examine nursing roles in selected governmental agencies.
- Describe the steps of the community-oriented primary care (COPC) model.
- Define the nursing role in a COPC system of care.

CHAPTER OUTLINE

Society and Health Care: The Nature of the Relationship

Forces Stimulating Change in the Demand for Health Care
    Demographic Changes
    Health Workforce Trends
    Technological Trends

The Current Health Care System
    Cost
    Access
    Quality

Organization of the Health Care System
    The Primary Health Care System
    The Primary Care System
    The Public Health System

Forces Influencing the Health Care System of the Future

A Comprehensive Model: The Integration of Public Health and Primary Care
    Community-Oriented Primary Care

KEY TERMS

advanced-practice nurse: a nurse who holds graduate preparation in a nursing specialty area.

Community-Oriented Primary Care (COPC): a community-responsive model of health care delivery that integrates both primary care and public health by combining the care of individuals and family with a focus on the community.

community participation: involvement of members of the community in decision making and planning for meeting their needs.

cost shifting: making up lost revenue from patients who cannot pay (or fully pay) by charging more to those who can pay.

Declaration of Alma Alta: resolution supporting primary health care for all people by 2000.

Department of Health and Human Services (DHHS): federal agency most heavily involved in health and welfare.

health maintenance organization (HMO): a method for delivering health care whereby people pay a fixed fee for primary care, emergency, and hospital care that is provided by a designated group of providers.

Continued

KEY TERMS—cont'd

managed care: an integrated system for providing health care services so that consumers must abide by certain rules designed to achieve cost savings.

National Health Service Corps: a commissioned corps of health personnel who provide care in designated underserved areas.

preferred provider organization (PPO): an organization of health care providers who contract on a fee-for-service basis with third-party payers, such as an HMO, to provide comprehensive medical services to subscribers.

primary care: personal health care services that provide for first contact, continuous, comprehensive, and coordinated care for a person.

primary health care: essential care that is accessible to all people in a community and provided at an affordable cost.

public health: organized community efforts designed to prevent disease and promote health. It links disciplines, builds on the science of epidemiology, and focuses on the community.

The American health care system has done a good job in providing health care to the American people. Some would say, including former U.S. Surgeon General, Jocelyn Elders, that the U.S. is unsurpassed in providing health care to the sickest patients (Sullivan, 1998). However, what often seems to be lacking is a comprehensive health care system that begins with a public health approach with its emphasis on a healthy population. Clearly, during the last century many "wonder drugs" were developed. These drugs saved and prolonged lives, and a number of deadly and debilitating diseases were eliminated through effective immunizations and treatments. Sanitation, water supplies, and nutrition were vastly improved, and transplant surgery was begun. In addition, the latter part of the century saw the beginning of animal cloning. But the nation still has not embraced primary health care.

This chapter describes the current primary and public health systems in the United States. These two systems are compared and contrasted both to one another and also to the concept of primary health care. Before discussing the two systems, current social changes are described that influence the need for primary health care and the way care is planned, organized, delivered, and financed. The last part of the chapter looks toward the future and discusses the kind of health care system that might effectively meet the needs of the population.

SOCIETY AND HEALTH CARE: THE NATURE OF THE RELATIONSHIP

Even though the United States spends more than any other country in the world on health care, the goal of good health care for all is not being met. Despite talk about the importance of prevention and about personal responsibility for health care, the following facts address the inadequacies of the health care system:

1. One half of the population is considered to be either slightly overweight or obese
2. One fourth smokes in spite of widespread publicity about the dangers of smoking, and the rate of smokers is growing more rapidly among women and female teens than among males
3. The infant mortality rate remains high
4. Many children are not fully immunized against preventable diseases.

Also, despite the enormous gains made in the last century using antibiotics to treat disease, new strains of diseases have emerged that are resistant to many if not most of the current antibiotics. Old diseases once thought completely eliminated, like tuberculosis, have reemerged, and they are more virulent than in the past.

FORCES STIMULATING CHANGE IN THE DEMAND FOR HEALTH CARE

In the past 30 years, there have been enormous changes in society, both in the United States and most other countries of the world. The extent of interaction among countries is stronger than ever; when the economy in one country declines, many others feel the strain. The United States has felt the effects of rising labor costs as some companies have begun having their products made in other countries where labor costs are lower. It is often less expensive to assemble clothes, automobile parts, appliances, and so forth, in a less-industrialized country and pay the shipping charges than to have the items fully assembled in the United States. This has affected the employment rate in the United States as well as the number of people who have comprehensive insurance coverage. U.S. industry traditionally provided employees with good health insurance coverage.

Demographic Changes

Population demographics have also affected the demand for health care services. World population is expected to double by 2050, with 85% of the increase occurring in developing countries (Aschenbrener, 1998). The mean age of the global population is declining, with 50% being younger than 20 years of age. Yet Western industrialized nations are "graying," with an increasing percent of the population older than age 65 and a decreasing number of people in the wage-earner age-group.

The members of the "baby boom generation" who were born after World War II will greatly effect health care delivery. This group born between 1946 and 1964 represents 78 million people or the largest segment of the population. Between January 1, 1996, and January 2, 2014, a "boomer" will turn 50 every 18 seconds, and "his or her preferences will affect every aspect of American life" (Aschenbrener, 1998, p. 36). Boomers grew up in a period of unprecedented economic growth in the United States. They grew up thinking they were special; that they could question their teachers; that anything was possible if they were educated and worked hard. Gender roles blurred, and the American dream of a two-car, two-career family with two children became a reality for many. This group of assertive people followed parents who were considered part of the "silent generation." The parents of boomers grew up in a time of strong military and political leaders. They respected authority, and conformity was rewarded more than was aggressiveness or rebellion. The silent generation thinks that health care providers know all there is to know about taking care of them. If they "do what the doctor says," then they will be fine. In contrast, boomers read about health care and have many questions to ask their providers. They want to be partners in planning the course of their care, and they are not reluctant to blame health care providers when the outcome of treatment is not as expected.

The boomer generation has a special interest in lifestyle and self-responsibility for health. They spend money on nutrition, exercise, and complementary therapies, including herbal treatments, acupuncture, acupressure, massage, biofeedback, and chiropractic care. About 80% to 95% of all health problems are treated to some extent at home through self-care measures (Ory and DeFriese, 1998).

The aging of the population has implications for the health care system, not the least of which are increased costs. The U.S. Census Bureau projects that the number of people over 85 years of age will double from about 3.5 million to 7 million by 2020 (Waite, 1996). As people age, they have more illnesses including chronic illnesses. Thus older people simply consume more health care resources than do their younger counterparts.

Birth rates in the United States have been declining since the 1970s. Women are having children later in life, and families are smaller in size. Birth rates are expected to decline until 2000 when they should level off and remain stable through 2015 (U.S. Census Bureau, 1996b).

Immigration and the shift in majority versus minority populations also effect health care demand. Nearly half a million legal immigrants enter the United States annually (Haupt and Kane, 1997). The number of illegal immigrants is much harder to estimate, and the border states of California, Arizona, New Mexico, Texas and Florida are effected most. Blacks are currently the largest minority group in the US, but it is expected that by 2015, Hispanics will outnumber Blacks (U.S. Census Bureau, 1996a).

The U.S. household composition is also changing. Families constitute about 70% of all households, down from 81% in 1970 (Day, 1996). Single parents, usually a mother, head 3 out of 10 families. Single-parent families constitute 19% of all white families with children, while 31% of Hispanic families with children and 54% of black families with children reside with only one parent (U.S. Census Bureau, 1996b).

In the last decade, mortality rates for both sexes in all age-groups declined (U.S. Census Bureau, 1996b). As a result of medical progress, the leading causes of death have changed from infectious diseases to chronic and degenerative diseases. Substantial gains against infectious diseases have decreased mortality among children. The mortality rates for older Americans also declined, especially during the 1970s and 1980s. However, people 50 years of age and older have higher rates of chronic illness, and they consume a larger portion of health care services than other age-groups. While the distribution of income has dramatically changed over time, more than 12 million families—about 20% of households—receive only 5% of the total income. In addition, high costs and lower real wages, especially for black women, continue to add to the difficulty of rising out of poverty (Johnson, 1992). This means that a sizable proportion of low-income Americans will continue to rely on public support to maintain a minimum standard of living. Chapter 7 discusses the economics of health care and how finances influence decisions about public health services.

The number of people with health care insurance affects the demand for health care. Currently about 43 million Americans do not have coverage. Many of these people are employed. Either their employers do not provide health care coverage, or the amount that the family must pay is significant, and they cannot afford to pay the insurance premium.

Health Workforce Trends

In recent years there has been a mandated recommitment to the use of primary care providers including physicians and advanced-practice nurses, especially nurse practitioners. Many insurers insist that patients see a primary care provider before they can be approved to seek the services of a physician specialist. While the intent of this trend was financial in origin, it is also part of a comprehensive system of primary health care. Currently, there is an adequate supply of primary care providers and an oversupply of specialists in many parts of the country. The supply of primary care providers is not, however, uniform across the states. Rural and densely populated urban areas continue to need additional primary care providers.

Significant changes are expected in the nursing workforce in the first 5 to 10 years of the twenty-first century. The Bureau of Labor Statistics predicts that health care services will grow by 29% by 2008. This should lead to about 2.8 million new jobs (U.S. Bureau of Labor Statistics, 1999). Since nursing has the largest number of health professionals, a significant growth in nursing jobs is projected. These new jobs will not necessarily be in the same types of facilities as in the past. Hospitals may continue to close, and more people will be cared for in outpatient and other community settings. While the number of hospital beds will decrease, this will not be directly correlated with the number of registered nurses who are needed. It is expected that as more patients are cared for outside of the hospital, those who remain in the hospital will be sicker and need more intensive and highly skilled nursing care. Also, managed care emphasizes the quality of care. In hospitals, no good substitute for highly competent RNs has been found for most areas (Buerhaus, 1998). At present there are no precise ways to project the number of RNs that will be needed in public health, community health, and community-based practices. However, it seems logical that if more patients are cared for outside the hospital, then more RNs will be needed in home health, public health, and other non-hospital sectors.

A nursing shortage is projected based on the fact that the current employed nursing population is aging and will leave the profession at a faster rate than new RNs will enter nursing. In the future, it will be highly undesirable for a health care facility to have a shortage of nurses since market forces will increasingly demand quality care and positive outcomes for their patients.

Technological Trends

Advances in technology have influenced the demand for health care. The accelerating growth of new diagnostic equipment and the ability to use treatment and monitoring technology for things ranging from cosmetic surgery to telenursing has increased both demand and costs. Also, both community- and hospital-based facilities have made remarkable strides in the development of information technology systems. Although the costs of technology were expected to reach $18 billion in 2000, in the long run, technology is expected to provide better health care treatment and some reduced costs as machines replace people (Copeland, 1998).

Briefly Noted

The same sensors that are being developed for automobiles, video cameras, and all other electronics, will become cheap enough to be used in medical devices for the purpose of remote telemetry. Examples will include monitoring vital signs with wireless heart monitors, respiratory meters, blood pressure cuffs, blood glucose monitors, and alerts from pill dispensers that a needed pill hasn't been taken. Built into the sensors will be the software capabilities to analyze, report, and react to abnormal results, or the absence of them, which will ensure appropriate follow up by a nurse (Institute for the Future, 1997).

While advances in medical technology will continue, the emphasis is expected to shift from heavy use of expensive diagnostic and therapeutic technologies to simpler, cheaper, and more mobile tests and procedures that can be used in a range of settings.

THE CURRENT HEALTH CARE SYSTEM

Clearly the current health care system has extended the life for many people through advances in medical technology

and scientific discoveries, including new drugs. The system, though, continues to have many problems associated with cost, quality, and access to care. These problems, although heavily debated in the last several years, have yet to be resolved. "Media reports about people who lack access to medical care may push emotional buttons—the elderly man left unattended for hours in an emergency room, say, or the poor pregnant woman who receives no medical treatment until she goes into premature labor and delivers a one-and-a-half pound infant. . ." (Berk and Schur, 1997, p. 55).

Most industrialized nations want similar things from their health care system. They want effective services that improve the health and quality of life of their citizens. They want equitable access to health care for all citizens, and they want efficient use of resources. Industrialized nations have taken different routes to achieve these goals. The United States has relied heavily on market forces to shape how health care is provided. In contrast, Canada and the United Kingdom have given their governments a greater role in health care delivery. There are some trade-offs, depending on which choice was made. The American health care system is more flexible and innovative than the systems in Canada and the United Kingdom. However, the latter two countries have done a better job of controlling total health spending, ensuring access to basic health care for all people, and reducing preventable mortality and morbidity. As has been mentioned, the United States has relied in recent years more on market forces through the mechanism of managed care plans. These organizations have taken over many of the functions typically assigned to governments of rationing care, setting hospital and physician payment rates, and controlling costs (Davis, 1998).

Cost

In 1997, Americans spent $1.092 trillion dollars, nearly 14% of the gross domestic product (GDP) on health care (Health Care Financing Administration, 1998b). This amount is expected to grow to 17% of the GDP by 2007. The Health Care Financing Administration (HCFA) forecasts that health care expenditures will increase over 7% annually between 2001 and 2007. If health care expenditures in 2007 reach $2.133 trillion, this will nearly double what was spent in 1997. Per capita health expenditures are expected to increase yearly over the next decade and grow from $4,093 in 1998 to $7,100 per person by 2007. (Health Care Financing Administration, 1998). Although several cost containment measures have been initiated, this enormous problem of escalating health care costs has not been solved. The United States spends more than any other country in the world on health care. See Chapter 7 for additional information about the economics of health care.

Briefly Noted

With approximately 14% of the GDP spent on health care in the U.S., this is nearly double what is spent in the United

Kingdom (6.7%) and significantly greater than Canada with a spending of 9.3%, Australia who spends 8.3% and New Zealand with expenditures of 7.6% (Davis, 1998, p.6).

Access

Growing costs have been accompanied by another significant problem: uneven access to health care. According to the Center for Studying Health System Change (1997) nearly one quarter of all Americans report growing difficulty in getting good health care. The system is described as a two-class system: private and public. People with insurance or those who can personally pay for health care appear to get good care. In contrast, individuals who rely on public funds to pay for their care, or the working poor who do not have insurance nor qualify for public funds because they make too much money to qualify or are illegal immigrants, may receive less adequate health care. In 1996, 41.7 million Americans or 15.6% of the total population were uninsured (Haupt and Kane, 1997). The number of uninsured people is growing by 750,000 people per year and will reach an estimated 44 million by 2002. The rate will then begin to decrease due to shifting ages in the population (Institute for the Future, 1997). Young adults between 18 and 24 years (28.9% of all uninsured) are more likely than other age-groups to lack coverage, and the elderly (1.1% of all uninsured) are the least likely to lack coverage (U.S. Census Bureau, 1996b).

The gradual erosion of public health services has hampered access to adequate health care. For example, funding to clinics in rural and heavily populated urban areas has been reduced, leading many uninsured people to seek care at the emergency room. In order to care for the uninsured, hospitals automatically charge more for their services to those who have insurance. This process of making up for lost revenue by charging more to those who are able to pay is called **cost shifting.** Managed care allows much less cost shifting than was previously possible with fee-for-service funding.

Quality

Quality of care is the third major concern in the United States. Although managed care has begun to control health care costs, many would say that it has been at the expense of quality. Consumer advocates say that employers and managed care plans are more concerned with reducing costs than offering needed services (Copeland, 1998). At the other extreme, when medically unnecessary care is provided, quality is again affected. Both federal and state health insurance plans, (e.g., Medicare, Medicaid), and private managed care plans, have incorporated ways to improve the quality of care that they deliver. The best-known private group, the National Committee for Quality Assurance (NCQA), has developed a set of standard performance measurements that most managed care organizations are using. The Health Care Financing Administration (HCFA) that funds Medicare and Medicaid has also adopted quality mechanisms for the

populations they serve (Wilensky, 1997). Chapter 15 provides more detail about quality approaches in health care.

ORGANIZATION OF THE HEALTH CARE SYSTEM

A large number and variety of providers and facilities make up the health care system. These include physicians' and dentists' offices, hospitals, health maintenance organizations (HMOs), nursing homes and other related inpatient facilities, mental health centers, ambulatory care centers, rehabilitation centers, and local, state, and federal official and voluntary agencies. In general, however, the American health care system is divided into two somewhat distinct components: a private or personal care component and a public health component, with some overlap, as discussed below. The personal care component is composed of primary, secondary, and tertiary care. This chapter will discuss primary care and primary health care.

The Primary Health Care System

While there is disagreement about exactly what constitutes primary care and primary health care, they can be differentiated in several ways. **Primary health care (PHC)** is more broadly defined than primary care. PHC includes a comprehensive range of services including public health, prevention, diagnostic, therapeutic, and rehabilitative services. PHC is essential care made universally accessible to individuals and families in a community with full participation and at a cost that the community and country can afford. Full **community participation** means that individuals within the community participate in defining health problems and developing approaches to address the problems. Any community in any country can be a setting for primary health care (World Health Organization, 1978).

PHC encourages self-care and self-management of one's health and social welfare. People are taught to use their knowledge, attitudes, and skills to engage in activities that improve their health and the health of their families and neighbors. PHC promotes individual, family, and community self-reliance and competence.

The Primary Health Care Workforce

The primary health care workforce is made up of a multidisciplinary team of health care providers. Team members include professionals such as generalist and public health physicians, nurses, dentists, pharmacists, optometrists, nutritionists, community outreach workers, mental health counselors, and other allied health professionals. Community members are also considered to be team members. Chapter 16 provides an in-depth discussion of community groups, including teams made up partly of community residents.

The Primary Health Care Movement

The primary health care movement officially began in 1977 when the 30th World Health Organization (WHO) Health

Assembly adopted a resolution accepting the goal of attaining a level of health that permitted all citizens of the world to live socially and economically productive lives. At the 1978 International WHO conference in Alma Ata, USSR, the goal of health for all was to be met through PHC. This **Declaration of Alma Ata** resolution became known by the slogan "Health for All (HFA) by the Year 2000" and captured the official health target for all of the member nations of the WHO.

In 1981 the WHO established global indicators for monitoring and evaluating the achievement of HFA. The *World Health Statistics Annual* (1986b) grouped these indicators into four categories: health policies, social and economic development, provision of health care, and health status. An important part of the global indicators is the emphasis on health as an objective of socioeconomic development (Mahler, 1981). In this context, health improvements result from efforts in many areas including agriculture, industry, education, housing, communications, and health care. Because PHC is as much a political statement as a system of care, each UN member country interprets PHC in the context of its own culture, health needs, resources, and system of government. Clearly, the goal of PHC has yet to be met in most countries.

Promoting Health/Preventing Disease: Year 2010 Health Goals for the Nation

Although the United States, as a WHO member nation, endorsed primary health care as a strategy for achieving the goal of "Health For All by the Year 2000," this has not been seen as the primary strategy for improving the health of the American people. The national health plan for the United States focuses more on disease prevention and health promotion in the areas of most concern in the nation. This focus is seen in the nation's health goals, *Healthy People 2010* (U.S. Public Health Service, 2000). These objectives were published first by the Public Health Service of the Department of Health and Human Services in 1979 and again in 1990. Each time data were gathered from health professionals and organizations throughout the country.

The broad-reaching goals focus on two major themes:
- Increasing the quality and years of healthy life
- Eliminating health disparities (among racial and ethnic groups).

The *Healthy People 2010* goals are accompanied by leading health indicators that measure 10 areas of health status. In total, there are 467 health objectives grouped into 28 focus areas. Many of the objectives target interventions designed to reduce or eliminate illness, disability, and premature death among individuals and communities. Others deal with broader areas such as improving access to quality health care, strengthening public health services, and improving the availability and communication of health-related information. In general, the 10 leading health indicators refer to the following (U.S. Public Health Service, 2000):
- Physical activity
- Injury and violence
- Overweight and obesity
- Environmental quality
- Tobacco use
- Immunization
- Substance abuse
- Responsible sexual behavior
- Mental health
- Access to health care

The Primary Care System

Primary care refers to personal health care that provides for first contact and continuous, comprehensive, and coordinated care. It addresses the most common needs of patients within a community by providing preventive, curative, and rehabilitative services to maximize their health and well-being. Although primary care practitioners are encouraged to consider the patient's social and environmental attributes in diagnosing, interventions are directed primarily at an individual's pathophysiological process (Starfield, 1992). A comparison of primary health care and primary care is shown below.

HOW TO Differentiate Primary Care and Primary Health Care

Primary Care	Primary Health Care
Individual focused	Community focused
Preventive, rehabilitative, with emphasis on curative	Curative, rehabilitative, with emphasis on preventive
Care provided by generalist physicians, NPs, CNMs, and PAs with help of ancillary team members	Care provided by many members of the health care team
Professional dominance	Self-reliance

Primary care, an essential component of any primary health care system, is delivered in a variety of accessible community settings such as physician offices, managed care organizations, community health centers, and community nursing centers. In an effort to control health care costs, many areas of the country have moved into programs of managed care. **Managed care** uses primary care as its basis and the starting point for patients to access care. **Health maintenance organizations (HMOs)** and **preferred provider organizations (PPOs)** are two of the most common systems that manage care for a specified population. In 1997 more than 65 million Americans were enrolled in HMO plans and nearly 100 million Americans were enrolled in PPOs (Institute for the Future, 1997; Peterson, 1997).

HMOs in one form or another have operated for more than 30 years. Each HMO operates as an organized system of health care that, for a fixed fee, provides primary care services, emergency and preventive treatment, and hospital care to HMO enrollees for a specified period of time. HMOs can be a facility in which all health care workers are direct employees, or the organization or plan can consist of a more loosely organized system whereby providers contract with the HMO on a fee-for-service basis. In most HMOs specialty care is received (and paid for) only upon the recommendation of a primary care provider, sometimes referred to as the gatekeeper. HMOs keep costs under control by encouraging prevention, keeping referrals to a minimum, and reducing unnecessary hospitalization.

Briefly Noted

A primary care provider in an HMO should refer patients to specialists only as outlined in the referral guidelines set forth by their employing organization, whether they agree with the guidelines or not.

A PPO is an organization of providers that contracts on a fee-for-service basis with third-party payers, such as an HMO, to provide comprehensive medical services to subscribers. The agreement between the PPO and the third-party payer allows subscribers to receive medical services at lower-than usual rates (Roble, Knowlton, and Rosenberg, 1984). Physicians and other primary care providers can belong to several preferred provider plans. Other health care delivery organizations include community nursing centers and community health centers.

The Primary Care Workforce

Primary care began to grow as a specialty area in the 1960s. The medical specialty of family practice and the arrival of nurse practitioners and physician assistants emerged in response to the need to provide primary care. Currently, primary care providers include generalists who possess skills in health promotion and disease prevention, assessment/evaluation of undiagnosed symptoms and physical signs, management of common acute and chronic medical conditions, and identification and appropriate referral for other needed health care services (U.S. Department of Health and Human Services, 1992). The health care personnel trained as primary care generalists include family physicians, general internists, general pediatricians, nurse practitioners, physician assistants, and nurse midwives. Some physicians with special training in preventive medicine/public health and obstetrics/gynecology also deliver primary care. It is interesting to note that, per capita, the United States has more specialists and fewer primary care physicians than any other industrialized country (Davis, 1998).

In addition to community health and public health clinical nurse specialists (see Chapters 25 through 29), nurse practitioners (NPs) and certified nurse midwives (CNMs), all considered **advanced-practice nurses,** are key members of the primary care and primary health care team. Nurse practitioners receive advanced training—usually at the master's level—with most taking a certification examination in a specialty area such as pediatrics, adult, gerontology, obstetrics/gynecology, or family. Training emphasizes clini-

Evidence-Based Practice

A study of the utilization of emergency room services of a population of public housing residents determined that a significant number of emergency room visits were for needs that could be more appropriately met in primary care settings. The study found that 68% of the emergency room visits made by this population were between 7:00 AM and 7:00 PM, when primary care services were readily available. These daytime emergency room visits tended to be less acute, suggesting that those who utilized the emergency room as a source of non-urgent care were more likely to do so during the day. The study also found wide variation in the amount of services consumed during an emergency room visit; however, of all visits by this population, 41% consumed no services. In consuming no services, the visit likely consisted of either health assessments, counseling, or patient education suggesting a need for primary care services to address these individuals' ability to cope with the problems of daily living. Age was a strong predictor of emergency room use, with the very young and very elderly consuming the most services.

APPLICATION IN PRACTICE

The author points out that to better serve children, primary care services should focus on prompt treatment of infectious diseases, and to better serve the elderly, primary care should focus on health promotion and chronic disease management. This study found that a large percentage of emergency room visits among low-income groups were not urgent and required no immediate assistance. Previous studies have revealed that the most significant barrier to seeking primary care services was the lack of an accessible primary care provider. To address this barrier, this study endorses the use of community-based primary care clinics. If primary care clinics are more accessible and available, it can be hypothesized that inappropriate use of the emergency room will decline, which will allow for lower costs and more efficient and effective use of health care services.

From Glick DF, Thompson KM: Analysis of emergency room use of primary care needs, *Nurs Economics* 15[1]:42-49, 1997.

cal medical skills (history, physical examination, and diagnosis), pharmacology, and pathophysiology in addition to the psychosocial and disease-prevention skills that are part of nursing. Studies have shown that 60% to 80% of primary care traditionally done by physicians can be delivered by a NP for less money and with equal or better quality (Office of Technology Assessment, 1986).

Nurse midwifery is defined as "the independent management and care of essentially normal newborns and women antepartally, intrapartally, postpartally, and gynecologically, occurring within a health care system that provides for medical consultation, collaborative management, and referral . . ." (Rooks and Haas, 1986, p. 9). The mother is the primary focus of care for nurse midwives, who spend the majority of their time on prenatal care, labor, delivery, and postpartum care, as well as family planning services. Nurse midwives receive advanced training either at the master's level or by attending a

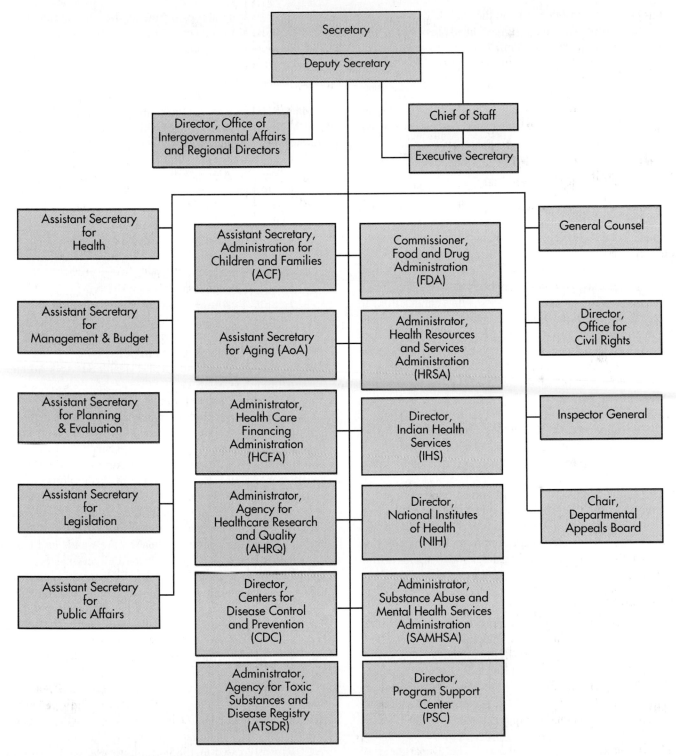

Figure 3-1 Organizational chart of the U.S. Department of Health and Human Services. (From U.S. Department of Health and Human Services; available online at www.hhs.gov/about/orgchart.html.)

school of nurse midwifery. All CNMs are certified based on a national examination.

Physician assistants (PAs) operate under the license of a physician. This is different from NPs and CNMs, who operate as independent practitioners. Most PAs receive their training at the baccalaureate level and are able to sit for their certification boards once they have graduated. PAs assist or substitute for physicians in the performance of specific medical tasks. Like NPs, PAs are proficient in taking the history, performing physical examinations, and diagnosing and treating uncomplicated medical conditions. Both are trained to prescribe a limited numbers of drugs. The scope of their prescriptive authority depends on the state laws where they live. In the past, CNMs and NPs have been pressured to limit their practice in order to avoid infringing on what physicians perceive as their role. Many state practice laws for NPs and PAs have changed and now allow both of these groups and also CNMs more independence in implementing their roles. In general, the federal government has supported this expansion of practice for what are considered competent yet economical providers.

The Public Health System

Although the goal of the public health system is to ensure that the health of the community is protected, promoted, and assured, there is overlap between this system and the personal care system. The overlap comes not only from the personal care system providing health promotion and disease prevention, but also through the public health system providing personal care services for those who cannot afford to receive their care elsewhere. For example, the Department of Health and Human Services supports a commissioned corps of uniformed health personnel, the **National Health Service Corps,** to serve residents of medically underserved areas.

Local, state, and national laws mandate the services that will be provided by the **public health** system. Two examples of public health laws instituted to protect the health of the community include mandatory immunizations for all children entering kindergarten and constant monitoring of the local water supply to ensure that the water supply meets certain standards.

The public health system is organized into multiple levels comprising the federal, state, and local systems. Most, but not all, local governmental units are involved in health care. There is also wide variation in both the financial support for public health and the organizational structure from state to state and from one local area to another.

The Federal System

U.S. DEPARTMENT OF HEALTH AND HUMAN SERVICES. The **Department of Health and Human Services (DHHS)** is the agency most heavily involved with the health and welfare of U.S. citizens. As mentioned earlier, the organizational chart of DHHS (Figure 3-1) shows the office of the Secretary, eleven agencies, and a program-support center. Although not shown on the organizational chart, in 1998 the U.S. Surgeon General's position was combined with that of the Assistant Secretary for Health. The Department of Health and Human Services is charged with regulating health care and overseeing the health status of Americans. This department is the largest health program in the world. Its mission is to protect and advance the health of the American people through the following means (U.S. Public Health Service, 1994):

- Medical research
- Disease tracking and identification
- Health care to American Indians and Alaska Natives and medically underserved populations

- Alcohol, drug abuse, and mental health programs
- Identification and correction of health hazards
- Promotion of exercise and healthy habits
- Protection of the nation's food and drug supply
- Medical assistance after disasters.

The major components of the Department of Health and Human Services are shown in Figure 3-1. The DHHS is directed by the Secretary for Health and is organized into the following twelve functional units:

1. Administration for Children and Families (ACF)
2. Agency on Aging (AoA)
3. Health Care Financing Administration (HCFA)
4. Agency for Health Care Policy and Research (AHCPR)
5. Centers for Disease Control and Prevention (CDC)
6. Agency for Toxic Substances and Disease Registry (ATSDR)
7. Food and Drug Administration (FDA)
8. Health Resources and Services Administration (HRSA)
9. Indian Health Service (IHS)
10. National Institutes of Health (NIH)
11. Substance Abuse and Mental Health Services Administration (SAMHSA)
12. A Program Support Center (PSC) that supports the Secretary and all of the previous agencies named.

Ten regional offices are maintained to provide more direct assistance to the states. Table 3-1 presents their locations. The Health Resources and Services Administration of the DHHS contains the Bureau of Health Professions, which includes separate divisions for Nursing, Medicine, Dentistry, and Allied Health Professions. Within this bureau, the Division of Nursing administers nurse education legislation; interprets nursing and health care trends and nursing needs of the nation's health care delivery system; and maintains liaison with the nursing community and with local, state, and international health groups and interests. The Division of Nursing identifies current and future nursing education and practice issues and needs. The Division works collaboratively with other federal agencies and with national nursing organizations (Division of Nursing, 1993).

Two other agencies within the DHHS—the National Institute for Nursing Research (NINR) and the Agency for Healthcare Research and Quality (AHRQ)—involve nurses. Specifically, the National Center for Nursing Research (NCNR) was created in 1985 within the National Institutes of Health. The research and research-related training activities previously supported by the Division of Nursing were transferred to this new Center. In 1993 the NCNR was renamed the National Institute for Nursing Research (NINR). This Institute is the focal point of the nation's nursing research activities. It promotes the growth and quality of research in nursing and patient care, provides important leadership, expands the pool of experienced nurse researchers, and serves as a point of interaction with other bases of health care research.

TABLE 3-1	Regional Offices of the U.S. Department of Health and Human Services	
Region	**Location**	**Territory**
1	Boston	Connecticut, Maine, Massachusetts, New Hampshire, Rhode Island, Vermont
2	New York	New Jersey, New York, Puerto Rico, Virgin Islands
3	Philadelphia	Delaware, District of Columbia, Maryland, Pennsylvania, Virginia, West Virginia
4	Atlanta	Alabama, Florida, Georgia, Kentucky, Mississippi, North Carolina, South Carolina, Tennessee
5	Chicago	Illinois, Indiana, Michigan, Minnesota, Ohio, Wisconsin
6	Dallas	Arkansas, Louisiana, New Mexico, Oklahoma, Texas
7	Kansas City	Iowa, Kansas, Missouri, Nebraska
8	Denver	Colorado, Montana, North Dakota, South Dakota, Utah, Wyoming
9	San Francisco	American Samoa, Arizona, California, Guam, Hawaii, Nevada, N. Mariana Islands, Trust Territories
10	Seattle	Alaska, Idaho, Oregon, Washington

The Agency for Health Care Policy and Research (AHCPR) was created in 1990. Its name is now the Agency for Healthcare Research and Quality (AHRQ). The mission of this agency is to conduct research on the effectiveness of medical services, interventions, and technologies, including research related to nursing interventions and outcomes that contribute to the improved health status of the nation.

Briefly Noted

Nurses can apply for support for research, projects, or training from a variety of agencies within the federal government in addition to the National Institute for Nursing Research and the Division of Nursing of the U.S. Health Resources and Services Administration.

OTHER FEDERAL GOVERNMENT AGENCIES. DHHS has primary responsibility for federal health functions. The cabinet departments of the federal government carry out certain other functions related to the health of the nation. Those departments include Commerce, Defense, Labor, Agriculture, and Justice.

Department of Commerce. The U.S. Census Bureau, within the Department of Commerce, provides health care information. Established in 1902, this bureau conducts a census of the population every 10 years. The National Oceanic and Atmospheric Administration, also in this department, provides special services to support the control of urban air quality, a major factor in community health today.

Department of Defense. The Department of Defense delivers health care to members of the military and their dependents. The Assistant Secretary of Defense for Health Affairs administers the Civilian Health and Medical Program of the Uniformed Services (CHAMPUS). The departments within Defense (Army, Navy, Air Force, and Marines) each have a surgeon general. Health services, including community health services for members of the military, are delivered by a Health Services Command in each department. In each command, high-ranking military nurses are part of the health services administration.

Department of Labor. The Department of Labor has two agencies with health functions: the Occupational Safety and Heath Administration and the Mine Safety and Health Administration. Both are charged with writing safety and health standards and ensuring compliance in the workplace. This includes conducting inspections, investigating complaints, and issuing citations if necessary. Each agency coordinates its activities with state departments of labor and health.

Department of Agriculture. The Department of Agriculture is involved in health care primarily through administering the Food and Nutrition Service. Although plant, product, and animal inspection by the Department of Agriculture is also related to health, the Food and Nutrition Service oversees a variety of food assistance activities. This service collaborates with state and local government welfare agencies to provide food stamps to needy persons to increase their food purchasing power. Other programs include school breakfast and lunch programs; the Supplemental Food Program for Women, Infants, and Children (WIC); and grants to states for nutrition education training.

Department of Justice. Health services to federal prisoners are administered within the Department of Justice. The Health Services Division of the Bureau of Prisons includes medical, psychiatric, dental, and health support services. It also administers environmental health and safety, farm operations, and food service, along with commissary, laundry, and other personal services for inmates.

The State System

Although varying considerably in their roles, state health departments play a substantial role in health care financing (such as Medicaid), providing mental health and professional education, establishing health codes, licensing facilities and personnel, and regulating the insurance industry. They also are involved in direct assistance to local health departments, including ongoing assessment of health needs. Box 3-1 provides examples of typical state health department programs.

As in international and federal agencies, nurses serve in many capacities in state health departments such as in: consultation, direct services, research, teaching, supervision, planning,

Box 3-1	Typical Programs Found Within a State Health Department

Legal services
Service to the chronically ill and aging
Juvenile services
Medical assistance: policy, compliance operations
Mental health and addictions
Mental retardation and developmental disabilities
Environmental programs
Departmental licensing boards
Division of vital records
Media: public relations and educational information
Health services cost review
Case management
Sexually transmitted diseases: screening and treatment
AIDS services
Referrals to resources
Quality assurance
Health planning and development
Preventive medicine and medical affairs

Box 3-2	Examples of Programs Provided by Local Health Departments

Addictions and alcoholism clinics
Adult health
Birth and death records
Child daycare and development
Child health clinics
Crippled children's services
Dental health clinic
Environmental health
Epidemiology and disease control
Family planning
Geriatric evaluation
Health education
Home health agency
Hospital discharge planning
Hypertension clinics
Immunization clinics
Information services
Maternal health
Medical social work
Mental health
Mental retardation and developmental disabilities
Nursing
Nursing home licensure
Nutrition
Occupational therapy
School health
Speech and audiology

and evaluation of health programs. Many health departments have a division or department of community health nursing.

Every state has a board of examiners of nurses. The board may be found either in the department of licensing boards of the health department or in an administrative agency of the governor's office. Created by legislation known as a State Nurse Practice Act, the examiners' board is made up of nurses and consumers. A few states have other providers or administrators as members. The functions of this board are described in the practice act of each state and generally include licensing and examination of registered nurses and licensed practical nurses; approval of schools of nursing in the state; revocation, suspension, or denial of licenses; and writing of regulations about nursing practice and education.

The Local System

The local health department has direct responsibility to the citizens in their community or jurisdiction. Services and programs offered by local health departments vary depending on the state and local health codes that must be followed, the needs of the community, and available funding and other resources. For example, one health department might be more involved with public health education programs and environmental issues, while another health department might emphasize direct patient care. Local health departments vary in their level of involvement with sick care or even primary care. A list of health department programs, taken from an urban-suburban county health department in a mid-Atlantic state, is shown in Box 3-2. At the local level, just as at the state level, coordination of health efforts between health departments and other county or city departments is essential. For example, local boards of education and departments of social services are an integral part of

activities of local governments. More often than at other levels of government, community health nurses at the local level provide direct services. Some deliver special or selected services, such as follow-up of contacts in cases of tuberculosis or venereal disease, or providing child immunization clinics. Others have a more generalized practice, delivering services to families in certain geographical areas. This method of delivery of nursing services involves broader needs and a wider variety of nursing interventions.

FORCES INFLUENCING THE HEALTH CARE SYSTEM OF THE FUTURE

At present few people are satisfied with the health care system. Costs are high, and quality and access are uneven across the country and within communities depending on whether people have adequate insurance. What then, are some of the factors that can potentially influence health care? First, as a country, citizens must decide both what is important to provide for all people, who will be in charge of the system, and what method of payment will be used. In recent years federal and state services have been reduced, and there has been a growth in the private sector. Health care delivery has become big business. Stocks in health care management companies are now traded on major stock exchanges; corporate directors receive benefits when profits are high, and the locus of control has shifted from providers to those who pay for the care.

Four major competing forces will influence the future shape of health care: consumers, employers/purchasers, managed care organizations, and state and federal legislation. First, consumers want lower costs, quality health care without so many restrictions and limitations, and greater choice in selecting providers. Consumers are becoming more informed and better organized and can be a powerful force for change.

Second, employers, or purchasers of health care, want accessible basic health care plans at reasonable costs. They put continual pressure on HMOs to decrease costs and are always threatening to change plans if their costs are not low enough or their benefits do not fit the needs of their employees. Employers expect employees to pay a greater share of the cost of health insurance; some employers have dropped health care coverage for family members and cover only the worker.

Briefly Noted

Mandating small business owners to purchase health insurance for their employees is one way to help ensure that the health needs of more people are met.

Third, managed care plans and other major health care systems want a better balance between consumer and purchaser demands. They also are insisting on a positive financial bottom line. In order to stay financially sound while providing quality care, HMOs and other health care systems are downsizing as well as creating alliances, mergers, and other joint ventures.

Finally, legislation, especially concerning access and quality issues, continues to be enacted, thus creating yet another force helping to shape a health care system based on incremental changes. Legislators feel the pressure not only from their own constituents who might be seeking changes due to an unsatisfactory experience with a health care system or provider, but from consumer groups representing the uninsured to find ways of creating equitable health care systems. Legislators also receive pressure from employers who continually fight against mandated coverage for their employees, as well as from the managed care industry that is trying to remain profitable.

A COMPREHENSIVE MODEL: THE INTEGRATION OF PUBLIC HEALTH AND PRIMARY CARE

What is needed to improve health care? First, delivery systems, as they attempt to deliver the most cost-effective care possible, must also find ways to improve access and quality in the communities they serve, especially to the underserved. Second, students must be prepared to work together with other health professionals to understand the needs of

the community and how to promote prevention. Third, *Healthy People 2010* (U.S. Public Health Service, 2000) and the World Health Organization's Health For All by the Year 2000 documents call for increased attention to population-based preventive activities as a means of increasing the health status of Americans. The systems must also become integrated as a means of controlling the cost of personal health care. In addition, there has been a call for all health professions' education to be more responsive in preparing students for a greater understanding of the needs of the community and prevention-oriented care (O'Neil, 1993). One model for integrating the public health and primary care systems is called community-oriented primary care.

Community-Oriented Primary Care

Community-Oriented Primary Care (COPC) is a community-responsive model of health care delivery that integrates aspects of both primary care and public health. It combines the care of individuals and families in the community with a focus on the community and its subgroups when services are planned, provided, and evaluated (Abramson, 1984). This model recommends allocating more resources into community care in order to save money, increase access, and create better health outcomes in personal care (Hattis, 1993). As former DHHS Assistant Secretary for Health, Philip Lee, M.D., said, "When the public health system is not maintained and falls into disrepair, the health of the community suffers and, inevitably, the health risks, volume of care, and cost of care to the individual increases as well" (in Ketter, 1994, p. 17).

Wright (1993), in speaking of health care transformation and the evolving competitive marketplace, states that COPC is the most effective model for emphasizing prevention, utilizing a planning process that targets resources to high priority needs, and for empowering communities to encourage individual responsibility. Wright (1993) describes the tools required to use the COPC model as follows:

1. A *community-based* primary care practice
2. An identifiable population or community for which the practice assumes responsibility for effecting change in health status
3. A planning, monitoring, and evaluation process for identifying and resolving health problems.

Although COPC systems in this country may attempt to invite and maintain community participation, this aspect of the plan cannot be overemphasized. The COPC process of inviting participation by members of the community, although effective, differs from what has generally been called the "community-based" health care approach, which is a process initiated by community members. The most effective and sustainable individual and system changes come when there is active participation from the people who live in the community regardless of who initiates the process. This is an important element in primary health care as well.

The W.K. Kellogg Foundation (1993), a foundation that financially supports efforts to improve the health of communities, states that a community-based practice must involve community members by allowing them to set their own priorities and solutions. Kellogg has found that when the right tools—such as power, information, and financial support—are shared with community members, they become more actively involved in the process. Building a consensus among the many diverse community leaders who have a vested interest in the process helps to ensure a more accurate and comprehensive representation of the community's health needs as well as a wider array of solutions to these needs. In this context, it must be remembered that health care cannot be separated from the broader scope of community development, such as housing and economic development. Consider the example of a young mother who has been scolded by a health professional for allowing several insect bites on her child to become infected without ever determining if the windows in the family's apartment had screens.

The strategies for using COPC are similar to the nursing process, using the community as the client. The steps are shown below.

HOW TO Use the COPC Model

1. Define and characterize the community. Use personal knowledge (including observations) of the community in conjunction with data obtained from community leaders. Data should include morbidity and mortality rates, existing health care services, and accessibility, transportation services, cultural diversity, environmental issues, and more.
2. Identify a list of community health problems and needs, and from that list formulate a community diagnosis. The process of formulating a diagnosis should develop as a consensus from key members of the delivery team and community leaders who truly represent the diverse needs and resources of the community.
3. Assist community leaders in the development of interventions corresponding to the community diagnosis. This would include personal care services, as well as health promotion and disease prevention activities. Encourage interdisciplinary teamwork to gain maximum benefits from human resources. Maintain community input to determine feasibility and resources.
4. Coordinate and manage services. Work in partnership with social service agencies, health professionals, and community leaders to provide comprehensive care and encourage networking.
5. Evaluate the interventions with the input of community leaders. The system should allow for continuous feedback to allow for intermittent modification and redirection of resources.

Role of the Community Health Nurse in COPC

Nurses move in and are trusted in the community like few other professionals. They can be found in schools, homes, churches,

and on street corners developing relationships, collecting data, assessing needs, and providing care. In addition, with the knowledge that community health nurses have regarding community resources, they make excellent case managers (Bower, 1992). Nurses are ideally suited to practice using a COPC model. Although community health nurses will continue to be used for some hands-on services, a generalist, prevention-oriented, public health background will allow them to bridge the gap between personal care and the health of the community.

Clinical Application

During a well-child clinic visit, Jenna Wells, R.N., met Sandra Farr and her 24-month-old daughter, Jessica. The Farrs had recently moved to the community. Mrs. Farr stated that she knew Jessica needed the last in a series of immunizations and because they did not have health insurance, she brought her daughter to the public health clinic. Upon initial assessment, Mrs. Farr told the nurse that her husband would soon be employed, but the family would not have any health care coverage for the next 30 days. The Farrs also need to decide which health care package they want. Mr. Farr's company offers a preferred provider option (PPO), a health maintenance organization (HMO), and a community nursing clinic plan to all employees. Neither Mr. or Mrs. Farr have ever used an HMO or a community nursing clinic and they are not sure what services are provided.

Mrs. Farr asks Nurse Wells what she should do.

Along with directing Mrs. Farr to other sources of health care should the family need to see a provider while they are uninsured, Nurse Wells should:
A. *Encourage Mrs. Farr to choose the HMO, as it will pay more attention to the family's preventive needs.*
B. *Encourage Mrs. Farr to choose the PPO as it will have a greater number of qualified providers to choose from.*
C. *Encourage Mrs. Farr to choose the local community nursing center since it is staffed with well-qualified nurse practitioners who can provide comprehensive health care with an emphasis on health education.*
D. *Explain the differences between a PPO, HMO, and community nursing clinic and encourage Mrs. Farr to discuss the options with her husband.*

Answer is in the back of the book.

 ### *Remember This!*

- Health care in the U.S. is made up of a personal care system and a public health system, with overlap between the two systems.
- Primary care is a personal health care system that provides for first contact and continuous, comprehensive, and coordinated care.
- Primary health care is essential care made universally accessible to individuals and families in a community. Health care is made available to them through their full

participation, and it is provided at a cost that the community and country can afford.

- Primary care is part of primary health care.
- Although primary care practitioners are encouraged to consider the client's bio-psycho-social needs, interventions are directed primarily at the pathophysiological process.
- Public health refers to organized community efforts designed to prevent disease and promote health.
- Several important trends affecting the health care system are demographic, social, economic, political, and technological trends.
- There are approximately 43 million uninsured people in this country and many more who simply lack access to adequate health care.

 ## What Would You Do?

1. Compare the local and state services where you live with those presented in this chapter. What are the similarities? What are the main differences? What changes would you recommend to your local officials to improve public health and primary health care in your area?
2. Debate the following with a classmate: The major problem with the health care system is (choose one of the following topics):
   a. Escalating costs (including those from increased use of technology)
   b. Fragmentation of services
   c. Access to care
   d. Quality of care
3. Interview both a nurse practitioner and a physician assistant to determine any philosophical differences in their scopes of practice. What does each consider the most stressful part of the job? What are the key job challenges for each? What are the biggest areas of job satisfaction for each?
4. If there is an HMO in your community, interview three providers and three consumers to determine what each sees as the advantages and disadvantages of this type of care delivery system. Meet with a classmate to compare and contrast what you learned in your interviews.

REFERENCES

Abramson JH: Application of epidemiology in community oriented primary care, *Public Health Rep* 99(5):437-442, 1984.

Aschenbrener CA: Leadership, culture and change: critical elements for transformation. In Rubin ER: *Mission management,* vol 2, Washington, D.C., 1998, Association of Academic Health Centers, pp. 33-65.

Bennefield RL: *Health insurance coverage: 1996: current population reports of the Census Bureau,* Washington D.C., Sept 1997, U.S. Department of Commerce, Economics and Statistics Administration.

Berk ML, Schur CL: A review of the national access-to-care surveys. In Isaacs SL, Knickman JR (editors): *To improve health and health care 1997,* San Francisco, 1997, Jossey-Bass.

Bower KA: *Case management by nurses,* Kansas City, Missouri, 1992, American Nurses Publishing.

Buerhaus PI: Is another RN shortage looming? *Nurs Outlook* 46(3):103-108 May/June 1998.

Center for Studying Health System Change: *Data bulletin from the Community Tracking Study,* Washington, D.C., 1997, The Center.

Copeland C: Issues of quality and consumer rights in the health care market, *Employee Benefit Research Institute Issue Brief,* April, 1998, The Institute.

Davis K: *President's message: Common concerns: international issues in health care system reform,* Annual Report, New York, 1998, Commonwealth Fund.

Day JC: *Projections of the number of households and families in the United States: 1995-2010,* U.S. Census Bureau, Current Population Reports, 25-1129, Washington, D.C., 1996, U.S. Government Printing Office.

Division of Nursing of the Health Resources and Services Administration: *Information booklet on the Division of Nursing,* November, 1993, U.S. Department of Health and Human Services.

Glick DF, Thompson KM: Analysis of emergency room use of primary care needs, *Nurs Economics* 15(1):42-49, 1997.

Hattis PA: Retooling for community benefit, *Health Progress* 74(7):38-41, 1993.

Haupt A, Kane TT: *The Population Reference Bureau's population handbook,* ed 4, Washington, D.C., 1997, Population Reference Bureau, Inc.

Health Care Financing Administration. "Table 1: National Health Expenditures Aggregate and per Capita Amounts, Percent Distribution, and Average Annual Percent Growth, by Source of Funds: Selected Calendar Years 1960-97" 13 November, 1998b, website: http://www.hcfa.gov/stats/NHE-Proj/tables/t01.htm.

Health Care Financing Administration. "Table 1: National Health Expenditure Amounts, Percent Distribution, and Average Annual Percent Growth, by Source of Funds: Selected Calendar Years 1970-2007" 06 November 1998a, website: http://www.hcfa.gov/stats/NHE-Proj/tables/t01.htm.

Institute for the Future: *Piecing together the puzzle: the future of health and health care in America,* a commissioned report to the Robert Wood Johnson Foundation, 1997, The Institute.

Institute of Medicine: *The future of public health,* Washington, D.C., 1998, National Academy Press.

Johnson T: Changing demographics in minority populations of the United States. In *Caring for the emerging majority: creating a new diversity in nurse leadership,* 1992, Division of Nursing and the Office of Minority Health.

Ketter J: Is there a cure for our ailing public health system? *Am Nurse* vol 26, June 17, 1994.

Mahler H: The meaning of "Health for all for the year 2000," *World Health Forum* 2(1):5-22, 1981.

Office of Technology Assessment: *Nurse practitioners, physicians' assistants, and certified nurse-midwives: a policy analysis,* health technology case study no 37, Washington, D.C., 1986, U.S. Government Printing Office.

O'Neil EH: *Health professions education for the future: schools in service to the nation,* 1993, San Francisco, Pew Health Professions Commission.

Ory MG, DeFriese GH: *Self care in later life: research, program and policy perspectives,* 1998, New York, Spring Publishing.

Peterson MA: Health care into the next century, *J Health Politics Policy Law* 22(2):291-313, 1997.

Roble DT, Knowlton WA, Rosenberg GA: Hospital-sponsored preferred provider organizations. *Law, Medicine and Health Care* 12(5):204-209, 1984.

Rooks J, Haas JE (editors): *Nurse midwifery in America,* 1986, Washington, D.C., Report of the American College of Nurse Midwives Foundation.

Starfield B: *Primary care: concept, evaluation and policy,* New York, 1992, Oxford University Press.

Sullivan E: *The future: imagine the possibilities,* part II, Health Care, *J Prof Nurs* 1(5):261-262, 1998.

U.S. Bureau of Labor Statistics: Industry employment, *Occupational Outlook Q* 43(4):25-30, 1999.

U.S. Census Bureau: *Household and family characteristics,* Washington, D.C., pp. 20-488, 1996a, U.S. Government Printing Office.

U.S. Census Bureau: *Population projections of the United States by age, sex, race and Hispanic origin (1995-2050),* Washington, D.C., 1996b, U.S. Government Printing Office.

U.S. Department of Health and Human Services: *Health personnel in the United States:* eighth report to Congress 1991 (DHHS pub. no. HRS-P-OD-92-1), Washington, D.C., 1992, U.S. Government Printing Office.

U.S. Department of Health and Human Services: *The registered nurse population,* Rockville, Md, 1996, Health Resources and Services Administration.

U.S. Public Health Service: *Healthy people 2010: understanding and improving health,* Washington, D.C., 2000, U.S. Government Printing Office, website: www.health.gov/healthypeople.

U.S. Public Health Service: *Keeping America healthy* (brochure), Washington, D.C., 1994, U.S. Government Printing Office.

Waite LJ: The demographic face of America's elderly, *Inquiry* 33:220-224, 1996.

Wilensky GR: Promoting quality: a public policy view, *Health Affairs* 16(3):77-81, May/June 1997.

WK Kellogg Foundation: *Lessons learned in community-based health programming,* Battle Creek, Mich, 1993, The Foundation.

World Health Organization: *Primary health care,* Geneva, Switzerland, 1978, The Organization.

World Health Organization: *Basic documents,* ed 36, Geneva, Switzerland, 1986a, The Organization.

World Health Organization: *World health statistics annual,* Geneva, Switzerland, 1986b, The Organization.

Wright RA: Community-oriented primary care: the cornerstone of health care reform, *JAMA* 269(19):2544-2547, 1993.

Part 2

Influences on Health Care Delivery and Community Health Nursing

In recent years the U.S. health care system has been criticized for its rapidly rising health care costs, inconsistency in the level and quality of services provided from one area of the country to another, and a general inconsistency in accessibility of health services. With 44 million Americans uninsured and 12% of the remaining population underinsured, it has been recognized that equal access to health care services is not a right, as most Americans think it should be. The inconsistency in health care is more significant when cost is considered. Specifically, health care costs in the United States increased from $24 million in 1960 to more than $1 trillion in 2000.

These factors have led to major health care reform debates at the national and state levels. The health care delivery system has moved into a managed care system that seeks to control costs. As a result of the debates, legal, economic, ethical, social, cultural, political, and health-policy issues have become extremely important. Now more than ever in the history of community health nursing, nurses must understand how these issues affect their practice and the outcomes of care.

The chapters in Part 2 provide the community health nurse with an understanding of the economic, ethical, cultural, environmental, and policy issues that affect nursing in general and community health nursing specifically.

Concern currently exists that the environment's effects on health and social conditions are causing an increase in the rate of infectious diseases. Community health nurses must be concerned with prevention, control, case-finding, reporting, and maintenance strategies as they relate to both communicable and infectious disease processes and to environment-related problems. Technological advances increasingly influence the environment and make it a potential threat to many aspects of health maintenance. Nurses must help others recognize how their actions as individuals—as well as in a composite group (aggregate) or community—are destroying vital parts of the environment.

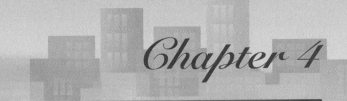

Chapter 4

Ethical and Cultural Influences

SARA T. FRY

CYNTHIA E. DEGAZON

OBJECTIVES

After reading this chapter, the student should be able to:

- Describe professional responsibilities in community health care.
- Identify the relationship of ethical rules, principles, and theories in community health nursing decisions.
- Discuss the application of ethical principles, including their potential conflicts.
- Discuss clients' rights in today's health care system.
- Identify the effect of culture on nursing practice.
- Evaluate methods for developing cultural competence.
- Examine the effects of cultural organization factors on health and illness.
- Conduct a cultural assessment of a person from a cultural group other than one's own.

CHAPTER OUTLINE

KEY TERMS

accountability: being answerable legally, morally, ethically or socially, to someone for something one has done.

advance directive: written or oral statements by which a competent person makes known treatment preferences and/or designates a surrogate decision maker.

Continued

KEY TERMS—cont'd

advocacy: activities for the purpose of protecting the rights of others while supporting the client's responsibility for self-determination; involves informing, supporting, and affirming a client's self-determination in health care decisions.

aggregate: a population or defined group.

beliefs: statements of convictions or tenets of truth of a society or culture.

caring: behavior that is directed toward the protection and maintenance of the health and welfare of clients. Indication of a commitment toward the protection of human dignity and the preservation of human health.

clients' rights: services, programs, goods, and health provider behaviors that consumers are entitled to in order to maintain or achieve health or to exist.

Code for Nurses: the American Nurses Association's professional statement prescribing moral behavior and actions of nurses based on moral principles.

codes of ethics: set of statements encompassing rules that apply to people in professional roles.

confidentiality: information kept private, such as between health care provider and client.

culture: learned ways of behaving that are communicated by one group to others in order to provide solutions to problems.

cultural accommodation: adapting or adjusting to a culture that is different than one's own.

cultural awareness: an appreciation of and sensitivity to a client's values, beliefs, practices, lifestyle, and problem-solving strategies.

cultural blindness: differences between cultures are ignored and persons act as though these differences do not exist.

cultural brokering: advocating, mediating, negotiating, and intervening on behalf of the client between the health care culture and the client's culture.

cultural competence: an interplay of factors that motivate persons to develop knowledge, skill, and ability to care for others.

cultural conflict: a perceived threat that may arise from a misunderstanding of expectations between clients and nurses when neither is aware of their cultural differences.

cultural encounter: interactions with clients related to all aspects of their lives.

cultural imposition: the process of imposing one's values on others.

cultural knowledge: the information necessary to provide nurses with an understanding of the organizational elements of cultures and to provide effective nursing care.

cultural preservation: use by clients of those aspects of their culture that promote healthy behaviors.

cultural repatterning: working with clients to make changes in health practices when the client's cultural behaviors are harmful or decrease their well-being.

cultural skill: the effective integration of cultural knowledge and awareness to meet client needs.

culture shock: feelings of helplessness, discomfort, and disorientation experienced by a person attempting to understand or effectively adapt to a different cultural group because of dissimilarities in practices, values, and beliefs.

ethics: the science or study of moral values; a code of principles and ideals that guide action.

ethical decision making: making decisions in an orderly process that considers ethical principles, client values, and professional obligations.

ethnicity: shared feeling of belonging among a group of individuals.

ethnocentrism: belief that one's own group or culture is superior to others.

moral: refers to standards of what is good and right about character, conduct, intentions, social relationships.

multiculturism: the process of becoming adapted to or involving more than one culture.

Patient's Bill of Rights: a document prepared by the American Hospital Association that defines the provider-client relationship within an organization.

prejudice: the emotional manifestation of deeply held beliefs about other groups; involves negative attitudes.

principles: fundamental truths that serve as the foundation for rules.

public health ethic: a principle of providing health care services that will offer the greatest benefit for the greatest number of people.

race: a biological designation whereby group members share distinctive features.

racism: a form of prejudice. Refers to beliefs that persons who are born into particular groups are inferior in intelligence, morals, beauty, and self-worth.

right to health: right to not have one's health affected by others (a negative right).

right to health care: right to goods, resources, and services to maintain and improve one's state of health (a positive right).

rule of utility: rule derived from the principle of beneficence. Includes the moral duty to weigh and balance benefits and reduce the occurrence of harms.

rules: guidelines or regulations that govern actions or behaviors.

stereotyping: the basis for ascribing certain beliefs and behaviors about a group to an individual without giving adequate attention to individual differences.

surrogate: a person who has been appointed to speak for another.

theories: a collection of principles and rules.

values: ideas of life, customs, and ways of behaving that members of a society or a culture regard as desirable.

veracity: a duty to tell the truth and not lie or deceive others.

ETHICAL INFLUENCES

Community health nurses observe many ethical conflicts in today's health care delivery system. The nursing profession has traditionally upheld the rights and needs of the individual client. Today, however, this focus on the individual includes the additional goal of improving the health of populations, or **aggregates.** Populations identified as being at risk, however, are not well served by community health nursing efforts because of a lack of funds to work with aggregates. Nurses often feel this conflict between the individual focus of the professional ethic and the aggregate focus in community health settings. The first part of this chapter will look at traditional **ethics** of professional nursing and apply these principles to the practice of community health nursing. Since the client is the focus of all nursing actions, clients' rights are discussed first as well as general ethical principles, moral rules, and the various theories of social justice. These principles, their definitions, and applications in community health nursing are presented, and their priority in nursing is discussed.

Accountability—being answerable to someone for what has been done in the nursing role—is a strong value in nursing and directs the nurse's practice. The developing of methods to measure accountability is a high priority in nursing. It is a priority because nursing must show that services in promoting health and preventing illness and meeting normal requirements for professional practice will increase the community's health and the nurse's accountability to individual clients.

ETHICAL DECISION MAKING

Ethical decision making in the clinical area follows an orderly process using ethical principles, client values, and professional obligations. The need for this orderly process is demonstrated by the increasing use of ethical decision-making frameworks in nursing practice. Although such frameworks should not be used as foolproof formulas for ethical decision making, they help individual nurses to seek out **moral** issues and relevant **values** to come to a specific decision (Fry, 1994a).

Jameton's Method for Resolving Nursing Ethics Problems is an example of a framework that can be used in community health nursing practice (1984). His framework has six steps (see box below). The use of ethical decision-making frameworks can help the community health nurse in situations of conflict in values. They are not used to "solve" moral conflict, but they do provide an orderly means for assessing the issues.

HOW TO Make an Ethical Decision

1. Identify the problem. The nurse should clarify what is at issue: values, conflicts, and matters of conscience.
2. Gather additional information. The nurse should decide who the main decision maker is and what the clients or their surrogate decision makers want.
3. Identify all the options open to the decision maker. All possible courses of action and their outcomes should be considered. The likelihood of whether future decisions might have to be made should also be evaluated.
4. Think the situation through. Consider the basic values and the professional obligations involved. Explore the ethical principles and relevant rules.
5. Make the decision. The decision maker should choose the course of action that reflects his or her best judgment.
6. Act and assess the decision and its outcomes. The nurse should compare the actual outcomes of the situation with the projected outcomes. Can the process of decision making be improved for further situations having similar characteristics? Can this decision be generalized to other client care situations?

Modified from Jameton A: *Nursing practice: the ethical issues,* Englewood Cliffs, NJ, 1984, Prentice-Hall.

HOW TO Manage an Ethical Conflict

Discuss the client care situation with the following:
• Another nurse
• Nurse administrator or supervisor
• A representative from the Ethics Committee of the agency or the health department
• The client or the client's family
• The client's physician
• A religious counselor

CLIENTS' RIGHTS AND PROFESSIONAL RESPONSIBILITIES IN COMMUNITY HEALTH CARE
Clients' Rights

A right to health and a right to health care are often thought to be basic human rights, but it is not clear that they are. Other **clients' rights,** such as rights to informed consent, to refuse treatment, or to privacy, have been aided and made clear by consumer groups and health care providers such as the American Hospital Association (AHA) (Annas, 1996).

Briefly Noted

One of the earliest recognitions of a right to health was made by the National Convention of the French Revolution in 1793. The leaders of the revolution declared that there should be only one patient to a bed in hospitals and that hospital beds should be placed at least 3 feet apart. When introducing the Public Health Act of 1875 to the British Parliament, Prime Minister Disraeli noted that "the health of the people is really the foundation upon which all their happiness and all their powers of state depend" (Brockington, 1956, p. 47). In modern times, the right to health has been considered comparable to the rights of life and liberty. The right to health obligates "the State to prevent individuals from depriving each other of their health" (Szasz, 1976, p. 478).

Right to Health

A **right to health** has been historically recognized as one of the basic human rights. In the United States, early nineteenth-century public health measures, such as sanitation and water supply regulations to control the spread of disease, are examples of early protective laws of human health and hygiene. However, most of these measures protected a negative right to health: the right to not have one's health endangered by the actions of others. The negative right to be free to enjoy good health may lead to the positive right to obtain certain services or have community health safeguards. The negative right to not have one's health endangered by others led to:

- Public health measures developed for sewage disposal, safe water supply, and the regulation of prostitution (Brockington, 1956)
- Housing safety and measures protecting children's health
- Federally supported programs and services to protect citizens against preventable diseases and disability (in particular, alcoholism and smoking-related illness), such as driving under the influence laws and smoke-free restaurant regulations.

Thus advocacy, in the guise of protecting a negative right to health, has helped open the door to consideration of the right to health as a positive right. It has been aided by documents such as the Universal Declaration of Human Rights of the United Nations Assembly. This document acknowledges the right of all persons to a standard of living adequate to provide for health and well-being and the right "to food, clothing, housing, and medical care" (United Nations Educational, Scientific, and Cultural Organization, 1949).

Right to Health Care

Even though one may think that the *right to health* means *right to health care,* the two terms explain different kinds of rights. The right to health is a negative right to a natural human state, which can be of various degrees, for example, fair, good, or excellent health. It is a right not to have one's health interfered with by others. However, the **right to health care** is a positive right to goods and services to maintain and improve whatever state of health the client has. Examples are:

- Immunization programs
- Kidney dialysis services
- Home health services for Medicare and Medicaid recipients
- Federally-funded prenatal and family-planning services

The distinction between the two terms is often blurred for two reasons. First, the World Health Organization (WHO) defines *health* as "a state of complete physical, mental, and social well-being and not merely the absence of disease or infirmity" (World Health Organization, 1958, p. 459). The emphasis on complete physical, mental, and social well-being in this definition suggests that one is unhealthy without complete well-being. However, persons have varying degrees of health but are not necessarily "unhealthy." The WHO definition of health should be thought of as an ideal state of health, one that very few persons actually have over a long term. As a definition of an ideal state of health, it does not dictate that health care services are a right of all persons.

A second reason why the distinction between the terms *right to health* and *right to health care* has become blurred

stems from the recent advances of modern medicine and the willingness of government to support medical treatment for specific disorders such as renal disease (Public Law 92-603, 1972) and genetic disorders, like sickle-cell anemia (Public Law 92-278, 1976). This tendency has created an increase of expectations for services to achieve optimal health. Therefore by supporting treatment of some diseases and genetic disorders, government has created the idea that the right to health means a right to good health, a state that can be achieved only through the providing of health care services that meet the needs of all clients. This idea is clearly wrong. Recognizing the right to health does not mean simply that the government is obligated to offer health services to maintain health or improve it. Although there may be other reasons why the differences between the right to health and the right to health care are not clear, these two reasons are certainly important.

Other Rights

Other basic human rights of clients recognized by the health care delivery system include the basic human right of all clients to refuse treatment. In the Omnibus Budget Reconciliation Act (OBRA) of 1990, The Patient Self-Determination Act (PSDA) was passed. This act requires all health care agencies who receive Medicare or Medicaid funds to inform clients that they have the right to refuse medical and surgical care. Clients also have the right to a written **advance directive.** This is a written or oral statement by which competent persons make known their treatment preferences. They can also name a **surrogate** decision maker if they should become unable to make medical decisions on their own behalf. Box 4-1 lists the specific requirements of the PSDA.

Briefly Noted

In 1972 the American Hospital Association issued its study entitled the ***Patient's Bill of Rights.*** Soon, health care facilities began to use this document for health care providers to communicate rights to their clients. The bill affirmed the basic human rights of all clients who seek health care services (American Hospital Association, 1973). It included the rights to:

1. Receive considerate and respectful care
2. Obtain complete medical information
3. Receive information necessary for giving informed consent
4. Refuse treatment
5. Request services
6. Refuse participation in research projects
7. Expect reasonable continuity of care
8. Be informed of institutional regulations
9. Have privacy
10. Have personal information and medical records treated confidentially
11. Be provided with information about other institutions and individuals related to care and treatment
12. Examine and obtain explanations of financial charges.

- Provide written information to adult clients about their rights to make medical decisions, including the right to accept or refuse treatment and the right to formulate advance directives.
- Document in each client's record whether the client has previously executed an advance directive.
- Implement written policies regarding the various types of advance directives.
- Ensure compliance with state laws regarding medical treatment decisions and advance directives.
- Refrain from discriminating against individuals regarding their treatment decision specified in an advance directive.
- Provide education for staff and the community on issues and the law concerning advance directives.

From Omnibus Budget Reconciliation Act of 1990, sections 4206 and 4751, PL 101-508, Nov 5, 1990.

Societal Obligations

The issue of client rights is a problem in health care delivery because society does not make clear its obligations to citizens regarding health. As a result, health care providers fail to recognize and protect clients' basic rights. To correct this problem, health professionals need to consider what society's obligations are to citizens regarding health and what kind of responsibilities health care providers have in response to client rights.

Differences in available health services by income or place of residence were reported by the President's Commission for the Study of Ethical Problems in Medicine and Biomedical and Behavioral Research in a lengthy document entitled *Securing Access to Health Care* (President's Commission, 1983). The commission reached several conclusions concerning current patterns of access to health care and made significant recommendations for changes noting that "society has an ethical obligation to ensure equal access to health care for all" (President's Commission, 1983, p. 4) and that this obligation "rests on the special importance of health care and is derived from its role in relieving suffering, preventing premature death, [and] restoring functioning" (p. 29) (Box 4-2).

Case 1

What Are Society's Obligations to the Client?

Mr. Hall is a 48-year-old man referred to the visiting nurse association for evaluation and treatment of stasis ulcers on his legs and for maintenance of a weight-reduction program for both Mr. Hall and his wife. Mr. Hall is 6 feet tall and weighs more than 380 pounds. Mr. and Mrs. Hall have a 27-year-old mentally retarded son.

When she visited the home, Karla Lowe, the visiting nurse, found large, oozing, sticky areas of raw tissue on Mr. Hall's legs. Ms. Lowe cleaned and dressed the ulcers and continued visiting every other day for the next 3 months. As the ulcers

| Box 4-2 | Ethical Framework of the President's Commission |

The Commission concluded the following:
- Society has an ethical obligation to ensure equal access to health care for all.
- Society's obligation is balanced by individual obligations.
- Equal access to health care requires that all citizens be able to secure an adequate level of care without excessive burdens.
- When equity occurs through the operation of private forces, there is no need for government involvement, but the ultimate responsibility for ensuring that society's obligation is met, through a combination of public- and private-sector arrangements, rests with the federal government.
- The cost of achieving equal access to health care should be shared fairly.
- Efforts to contain rising health care costs are important but should not focus on limiting equal access for the least-served portion of the public.

From President's Commission for the Study of Ethical Problems in Medicine and Biomedical and Behavioral Research: *Securing access to health care*, vol 1: Report on the ethical implications of differences in the availability in health services, Washington, D.C., 1983, U.S. Government Printing Office.

began to heal, Ms. Lowe attempted to talk to the Halls in discussion about nutrition and hygiene and to encourage them to start a weight-reduction program. Mr. and Mrs. Hall were not interested and chose not to participate in any type of weight-reduction program.

Several months went by and Mr. Hall's ulcers stopped healing. When they began to deteriorate, he was hospitalized. Within a few weeks, they had healed enough that he could return home. Ms. Lowe visited his home to change dressings as before, but despite her efforts the ulcers deteriorated once again. It was too soon for him to return to the local hospital under his Social Security Supplemental Income benefits, so it was arranged to have him admitted to the state hospital. Two days later he signed himself out of this hospital. "It was too far away, and I didn't know anybody. Besides, they were too rough on me," he stated.

Angered by Mr. Hall's decision, his physician refused to continue treating him, and Ms. Lowe was left without any current physician orders. This meant that she could no longer give Mr. Hall physical care or receive reimbursement for her visits. Mr. Hall's unwillingness to cooperate in the development of "healthy behaviors" made him ineligible for the agency's health maintenance program. When Ms. Lowe explained the situation to her client, Mr. Hall said that Mrs. Hall could wash his legs and apply the medicine that Ms. Lowe had been applying. Besides, he did not think that his physicians had really helped him, and he had no intention of ever going to one again. He would miss Ms. Lowe's visits but thought he could manage. Ms. Lowe left a number to call if they ran into any unforeseen problems.

Nearly a year passed. One summer day Mrs. Hall called Ms. Lowe. She said that Mr. Hall was "awful sick" and had been in bed for nearly a month. The Visiting Nurse Association (VNA) policy allowed a one-time evaluation visit, so Ms. Lowe visited the home. She found Mr. Hall's legs alive with the larvae of the summer flies attracted to the steamy bedroom. She urged Mr. Hall to seek hospitalization. He would not be turned away, even if he no longer had a physician. Mr. Hall agreed, an ambulance was called, and Mr. Hall was transported to the local hospital. Because of the condition of his legs, a bilateral leg amputation was performed.

When news of Mr. Hall's general condition got out (he had created quite a sensation in the emergency department of the local hospital), the people of the small town were aghast. How could a man be allowed to rot away? Where were all the services? Who was responsible? The mayor appointed a special task force to investigate the matter. Months (and endless newspaper columns) later, "no fault" was found, and it was announced that the town's health services "had sufficient mechanisms to prevent such a thing from ever happening again." Mr. Hall recovered, obtained prostheses, and moved to another state where he had family to help him.

Yet Ms. Lowe was not satisfied. Did the system fail clients such as Mr. Hall? Did clients have an obligation to accept the services offered to them and the recommendations of health workers who took care of them? If they refused to follow recommendations, did it mean that health care services should be totally withdrawn? Could the amputations have been prevented if Ms. Lowe had at least continued her visits and prevented the extreme condition of Mr. Hall's legs before his last hospitalization?

1. *What are society's health care obligations to Mr. Hall?*
2. *What are the VNA's obligations to Mr. Hall according to the Patient Self-Determination Act?*
3. *Can the conclusions in the report of the President's Commission, Securing Access to Health Care (1983), help Ms. Lowe?*
4. *Is it reasonable for clients such as Mr. Hall to refuse treatments in advance by executing a written advance directive? Why or why not?*

Professional Responsibilities

In response to clients' rights, health care professionals have particular duties or responsibilities. Some of these duties are supported by professional codes of ethics and correlate with the client's basic rights.

Code Duties

Professional **codes of ethics** are statements of rules that apply to persons in professional roles. The rules contained in professional codes of ethics for nurses are specific applications of more universal moral principles. The professional code of ethics for nurses prescribes moral behavior and actions based on moral principles (Fry, 1994b). Thus the professional nurse has a moral obligation to follow the rules in a code of ethics such as the ***Code for Nurses* With Interpretive Statements** of the American Nurses Association (2000) (Box 4-3).*

Some of the rules in the Code for Nurses have legal ties to licensure requirements concerning professional acts. For example, the rules of respecting client confidentiality and accountability are mentioned in the Code for Nurses as both morally obligatory and legally required.

---

*Hereafter referred to as Code for Nurses.

Box 4-3   Code for Nurses With Interpretive Statements

- The nurse provides services with respect for human dignity and the uniqueness of the client, unrestricted by considerations of social or economic status, personal attributes, or the nature of health problems.
- The nurse safeguards the client's rights to privacy by judiciously protecting information of a confidential nature.
- The nurse acts to safeguard the client and the public when health care and safety are affected by the incompetent, unethical, or illegal practice of any person.
- The nurse assumes responsibility and accountability for individual nursing judgments and actions.
- The nurse maintains competence in nursing.
- The nurse exercises informed judgment and uses individual competence and qualifications as criteria in seeking consultation, accepting responsibilities, and delegating nursing activities to others.
- The nurse participates in activities that contribute to the ongoing development of the profession's body of knowledge.
- The nurse participates in the profession's efforts to implement and improve standards of nursing.
- The nurse participates in the profession's efforts to establish and maintain conditions of employment conducive to high-quality nursing care.
- The nurse participates in the profession's effort to protect the public from misinformation and misrepresentation and to maintain the integrity of nursing.
- The nurse collaborates with members of the health professions and other citizens in promoting community and national efforts to meet the health needs of the public.

From American Nurses Association: *Code for nurses with interpretive statements,* Kansas City, Mo, 2000, American Nurses Publishing.

Codes of ethics also prescribe duties that are required of the professional in response to clients' rights (Fry, 1994b). The duties of veracity, advocacy, confidentiality, caring, and accountability are specifically mentioned in the Code for Nurses as correlating with clients' rights.

Veracity

Truthfulness has long been known to be the fundamental basis for trust among human beings. **Veracity** is a duty to tell the truth and not lie or deceive others. In health care relationships, several arguments are usually given in support of veracity (Beauchamp and Childress, 1994).

- Veracity is part of the respect that is owed other persons, including the right to be told the truth and not be lied to or deceived. An example is being truthful to clients regarding the nature of the care they are receiving.
- The duty of veracity is derived from, or is a way of expressing, the duty of keeping promises.
- Relationships of trust are necessary for cooperation between clients and health care professionals.

Nurses often have difficulty observing a duty of veracity. The truth is sometimes withheld or filtered because a nurse may think certain information will cause a client anxiety.

Nurses also withhold information because they think that clients, particularly if very sick or dying, do not really want to know the truth about their conditions.

Case 2
When the Family Asks the Nurse Not to Tell the Truth

Ralph Bradley, a recently widowed man in his mid-60s, was discharged from the hospital after exploratory surgery that disclosed colon cancer with metastasis to the lymph nodes. His physician referred him to a home health agency for nursing care follow-up. In reading the referral, the nurse learned that Mr. Bradley had been living with a married daughter and her family since his wife's death. An unmarried daughter apparently lived nearby, visiting him regularly and helping with his daily care. The referral did not explain what, if anything, the client had been told by his physician concerning his condition.

During the first home visit, it became apparent that Mr. Bradley did not know that the tumor removed from his body had been diagnosed as cancerous or that it had metastasized to the lymph nodes. He did not realize the seriousness of his condition, but he did express concern about his health. He complained of vague pain in the abdomen, asked for information about the results of the tests performed before discharge from the hospital, and wanted to know how soon he would be able to return to his work as a cabinetmaker. When the nurse avoided a direct answer to these questions, Mr. Bradley asked directly, "Is everything all right?" The married daughter, who was present when her father was asking these questions, assured him that everything was all right and that he would soon be up and around.

Walking the nurse to her car when the visit was over, the married daughter confided that it was the family's wish that their father not be told how serious his condition was. She said that her mother's recent death had been very difficult for him to accept. They did not want him to be further burdened with the knowledge of his condition. The nurse listened, acknowledging the difficulties posed by the wife's recent death and the father's serious condition. She told the daughter, however, that it would be very difficult, if not impossible, for anyone from her agency to continue to provide nursing care to Mr. Bradley without his knowledge of his condition.

When she returned to her office, the nurse discussed Mr. Bradley's situation with her supervisor. The nurse did not want to continue visiting the client knowing he was being deceived by the physician and family. The supervisor suggested that she consult with the attending physician as soon as possible and explain that Mr. Bradley was asking questions about his condition. Luckily, the nurse was able to reach the physician before it was time to make the next home visit. She asked the physician what the client had been told about his condition. The physician said that at the family's request, Mr. Bradley had not been told that he had cancer. He said he agreed with the family that Mr. Bradley could probably not withstand the anxiety of knowing he had a terminal illness so soon after his wife's death. The physician also expressed concern about Mr. Bradley's daughters who, as he put it, "need a little time to accept the mother's death, as well as accept the impending death of the old man." The physician said that he would con-

sider any act of disclosure on the nurse's part at this time to be inappropriate to her role as a visiting nurse and inconsistent with the well-being of the client and his family.

1. *What is the professional duty of veracity?*
2. *What reasons might the nurse give for telling Mr. Bradley the truth?*
3. *What reasons might the nurse give for not telling Mr. Bradley the truth?*
4. *How does not telling the truth constrain nursing care in the community?*

Modified from Veatch RM, Fry ST: Case studies in nursing ethics, Philadelphia, 1987, JB Lippincott.

Confidentiality

In general social interaction, certain information is regarded as confidential. Regarding information as confidential enables control of the disclosure of personal information and limits the access of others to sensitive information (Fry, 1994a).

In community health care relationships, **confidentiality** of information is maintained for several reasons.

- If health care professionals did not follow a rule of confidentiality, clients might not seek help when they need it, or reveal necessary information that aids treatment (e.g., family-planning clients might not reveal information about their reproductive history).
- It helps protect the nurse-client relationships.
- Privacy is recognized as a basic human right. Because of respect for persons, nurses respect clients' rights to privacy by maintaining the moral rule of confidentiality.

Advocacy

The nursing profession recognizes a strong duty of **advocacy** where the care or safety of clients is concerned. In the role of *advocate*, the nurse speaks for or in support of the best interests of the individual client or vulnerable client populations.

Caring

The value of **caring** is widely recognized as important to the nurse-client relationship (Fry, 1994a). Since nurses have special relationships with their clients, they are called upon and expected to provide caring behaviors to those who have health needs. Caring is a form of involving self with others that is directly related to concern about how other individuals experience their world.

Accountability

Nursing has long recognized the need for moral accountability in responding to basic human rights in practice.

- Accountability includes providing an explanation to oneself, the client, the employing agency, and the nursing profession for what one has done in the role of nurse.
- It is an obligation that has both moral and legal components and implies that a contract exists between two parties.

- When a nurse enters into an agreement to perform a service for a client, the nurse will be answerable for performing this service according to agreed-upon terms, within a determined time period, and with use of certain resources and performance standards. The nurse as contractor is responsible for the quality of the services and is accountable to the individual client, the health service agency, the nursing profession, and even his or her own conscience for what has been done (Fry, 1994a).

ETHICAL PRINCIPLES IN COMMUNITY HEALTH
Relationship of Ethical Rules, Principles, and Theories

In making moral decisions, various rules, principles, or theories apply. **Moral** judgments are evaluations of what is good or bad, right or wrong, and have certain characteristics that separate them from nonmoral evaluations such as personal preferences, beliefs, or matters of taste. Moral judgments are generally made about human actions, character traits, or institutions. Nurses frequently make moral judgments:

- When the nurse decides to arrange a home visiting schedule on the basis of need or seriousness of illness
- When the nurse decides to refer a client to a physician for further evaluation based on the expressed wishes of the client and his or her condition
- When in response to a request for an abortion a nurse decides, regardless of personal beliefs, to inform the client of all the options available
- When a nurse, resisting pressure from other individuals, decides not to participate in political activities that might reduce health care coverage for vulnerable populations

Rules state that certain actions should (or should not) be performed because they are right (or wrong). An example would be that "Nurses ought to always tell the truth to clients." **Principles** are more abstract than rules and serve as the foundation of rules. For example, the ethical principle of autonomy is the foundation for such rules as "Always support the right to informed consent," "Tell the truth," and "Protect the privacy of the client." Likewise, the principle of justice serves as the foundation of rules such as "Treat equals equally" and "Divide your time on the basis of needs." **Theories,** however, are collections of principles and rules and will not be discussed in this text.

Principles

Three principles—beneficence, autonomy, and justice—will be discussed here, with examples of the rules that relate to them.

BENEFICENCE. The principle of **beneficence** is that one ought to do good and prevent or avoid doing harm. Beneficence is a duty to help others gain what is of benefit to them but does not carry the obligation to risk one's own welfare or interests in helping others. Care should not be expected if clients' needs infringe either upon nurses' personal lives or upon their responsibilities to other clients or their own families.

Balancing Harms and Benefits. Service that brings about the greatest balance of good over evil, or benefit over harm, is in accordance with a **rule of utility** (Beauchamp and Childress, 1994). In community health, a rule of utility may be the basis for deciding whether to conduct screening programs for communicable diseases, for example. The decision is made by balancing the possible harm and benefit of the course of action. The nurse should accurately assess the known benefits and harms to clients from the point of view of nursing care and should present them with other relevant facts that might enter into the decision-making process, for example, the benefit of reduced possibility of a communicable disease like "flu" while the harm may be a mild case of flu-like symptoms or an allergic reaction to the vaccine.

AUTONOMY. *Autonomy* refers to freedom of action that an individual chooses. Persons who are autonomous are capable of choosing and acting on plans they themselves have selected. To respect persons as autonomous individuals is to acknowledge their personal rights to make choices and act accordingly (Fry, 1994a).

The principle of autonomy is applied in rules related to the following issues:

1. Respect for persons
2. Protection of privacy
3. Provision of informed consent
4. Freedom of choice, including treatment refusal
5. Protection of diminished autonomy.

Briefly Noted

Some ethical conflicts experienced by nurses have been the same over time. For example, in an early research study about nurses' ethical conflicts conducted by Vaughan in 1935, 2265 moral problems, 67 problems of etiquette, and 110 questions about ethical behavior were found in the diaries of 95 nurses working in various localities in the United States. This was an average of 23.4 moral problems experienced by each nurse over a period of 3 months. The most frequently mentioned problem was cooperation—between nurses and physicians, among nurses in general, with and among supervisors, between nurses and clients' relatives, in giving medications and treatments, and in maintaining asepsis. In a 1994 study of ethical conflicts experienced by 462 practicing nurses in the state of Maryland, Fry and Damrosch (1994b) found that 40% of the nurse participants had direct involvement with ethical issues either one to four times weekly or daily to almost daily. One of the most frequently experienced ethical issues was conflict in the nurse-physician relationship.

Respect for Persons. Clients are respected because they are persons and have the right to determine their own plan of life. Community health nurses acknowledge respect by seriously considering the opinions and choices of clients and not obstructing their actions unless they are harmful to themselves or others. Denying clients freedom to act on their own

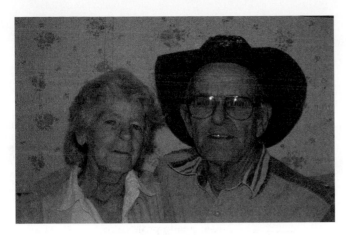

Figure 4-1 Age does not render clients less worthy of respect.

judgments or withholding information necessary to make judgments demonstrates a lack of respect for clients.

Elderly clients provide an example. Community health nurses often find it easier and quicker to communicate with family members than with the clients themselves. They may simply tell the client what treatment has to be performed, not giving them choices or even involving them in deciding on the treatment plan. Age, however, does not render a client less worthy of respect (Fig. 4-1). Elderly persons have the right to determine their life and health plans as long as they have the capacity to do so.

Protection of Privacy. Community health nursing care involves close observation of clients, physical touching, and access to personal health and economic information about clients and their families. All of these aspects of nursing care may invade the privacy of clients or threaten their right to control personal information.

Since the relationship between nurse and client is built on trust, the nurse has a responsibility to protect the privacy of clients and their families insofar as their health is concerned. Personal information gathered in the home assessment of clients must be recorded in a manner that acknowledges respect for clients' privacy and is communicated only to those directly concerned with client care.

When personal economic information must be shared with third parties for payment of nursing care, clients have the right to authorize or withhold information. Even though the information may be essential for continuity of nursing care services, the client retains control of all information.

Using health records in determining funding levels for community health nursing services does not justify using nurse-generated information about the client without the client's knowledge and permission. Health record information can only be used for quality-assurance purposes or research studies. This information can be shared with others only under clearly defined policies and written guidelines protecting client privacy.

Provision of Informed Consent. Clients are provided the opportunity to choose what will or will not happen when adequate disclosure standards for informed consent are included in the contract for nursing services. Three elements are essential for adequate informed consent:

- *Information.* The nurse must disclose information about treatment procedures, their purposes, any discomforts and anticipated benefits, alternative procedures for therapy, and options for questioning procedures or ending the contract at any time. Clients should also be adequately informed about health records confidentiality.
- *Comprehension.* The manner and context in which information is conveyed to clients is also important for informed consent requirements. Clients must be allowed time to consider information provided by the nurse and time to ask questions. If the client is unable to comprehend because of a language barrier, the nurse must provide an interpreter. The client must be competent to understand and make decisions rationally.
- *Voluntariness.* Any contract or agreement with the client constitutes valid consent only if it is given voluntarily and is free of coercion or undue influences. Voluntariness includes the freedom to choose one's own health goals without the controlling influence of another person or certain conditions, such as debilitating disease, psychiatric disorders, and drug addictions (Beauchamp and Childress, 1994).

These three elements—information, comprehension, and voluntariness—constitute informed consent in nursing practice. Informed consent is not valid without all elements, and no contract between client and nurse is ethically acceptable without valid informed consent.

Individual Freedom of Choice. Respecting the client's right to self-determination includes respecting a decision to refuse treatment. Factors the nurse must weigh include the client's personal freedom, the potential harm to the client or other citizens, the cost of treatment refusal, and the values of society. The right of the client to refuse treatment and the right to initiate written advance directives are protected by the Patient Self-Determination Act (OBRA, 1990).

In situations of questionable competency, decisions have generally been made opting for the preserving of life (Beauchamp and Childress, 1994). Nurses should recognize that respect for persons may involve allowing clients and their legal guardians to make decisions concerning their lives and health that may be very difficult for the nurse to accept.

Protection of Diminished Autonomy. The principle of autonomy is generally applied only to persons capable of making choices. Factors such as immaturity or physical or psychological incapacities may diminish one's autonomy. The nurse may have difficulty recognizing when diminished capacities render clients incapable of self-determination. The capacity for self-determination is related to:

- Maturity
- Chronological age
- Presence or absence of illness
- Mental disability
- Social factors

However, respect for the principle of autonomy requires that nurses recognize when persons lack the capacity to act

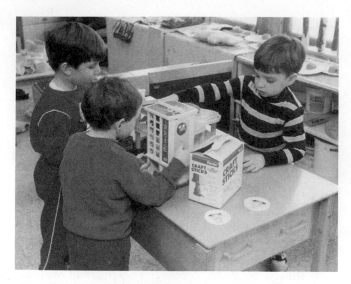

Figure 4-2 Children have diminished autonomy and are entitled to protection in health care delivery. (From Wong DL: *Nursing care of infants and children,* ed 6, St Louis, 1999, Mosby.)

autonomously and therefore are entitled to protection in health care delivery (Fig. 4-2).

Invasion of Privacy. In protecting the health of vulnerable populations, the nurse may infringe on the rights to privacy rule by actively gathering private information. For example, a sharp rise in the incidence of venereal disease among a high-school population may require interviewing teenagers diagnosed with the disease and accurately following up with all named contacts. This action may lead to invasion of individual privacy through discussion of sexual habits and preferences and potential disclosures to adults, including parents. Privacy may also be invaded by the assessment and recording of personal client information. For example, the community health nurse may record information about the social habits and lifestyles of pregnant women. Subsequently, that information may be used in research studies correlating neonatal mortality and morbidity with social habits during pregnancy. This type of personal information is often freely communicated because of the trust relationship between nurse and client. It may also be recorded in the client's record without full understanding of the potential effect of this information if, in fact, a child is born with anomalies related to social habits or lifestyles during pregnancy. The presence of this information in prenatal records means that it might eventually be shared with other health professionals and members of the client's family, constituting further invasion of the client's right to privacy of personal information. All of these actions infringe on self-determining behavior but are considered justifiable because of potential harm to others.

Briefly Noted

REQUESTS FOR EUTHANASIA OR ASSISTANCE TO COMMIT SUICIDE

Clients frequently ask nurses for information about euthanasia and/or assistance in bringing about their own death. Such a request may create conflict for a nurse, especially when the nurse feels that the client has a right to decide when and how he or she dies, or the nurse does not think that the client's quality of life is very good. Nurses must remember that *euthanasia* (i.e., any action that intentionally brings about the client's death for reasons of mercy) and *professionally assisted suicide* (i.e., providing assistance to a client in ending his or her own life) are very controversial acts for the nurse. The ANA *Code for Nurses* states that it is unethical and illegal to participate in acts of euthanasia. It is also considered unethical for a nurse to assist a client to end his or her life (although some states have enacted legislation permitting clients, under certain circumstances, to legally make such requests from health professionals).

JUSTICE. The formal principle of *justice* holds that persons should be treated fairly (Beauchamp and Childress, 1994). In considering a community's health, material principles of justice are considered (e.g., need, merit, contributions to society) to determine which social burdens and benefits, including health goods (such as access to care, doctors, hospitals, nurses, EMS), should be distributed among all individuals in the community.

The application of a principle of justice creates conflicts in two areas. First, it creates challenges about priorities for distributing basic goods and health services in the community. Second, it creates conflicts in determining which population or individuals should obtain available health goods and nursing services.

Distributing Basic Goods and Services. In deciding how to apply the rule to distribute basic health care goods or resources within a community, there are several decisions to be made:

1. *How should priorities be set?* Should the protection and promotion of health be the main consideration, or should a major portion of resources be set aside for other social goods, such as housing or education?

2. *What are the most effective and efficient methods of meeting this basic right while preventing catastrophic events that need immediate and more concentrated attention?* Such events may lead to death or disability. Should the emphasis be placed on direct health care services (e.g., clinics, programs) to care for illness, or should indirect services (e.g., health education, transportation services) to prevent illness or promote health receive equal emphasis?

3. *What is the appropriate relationship between rescue services and preventive services?* Is it more effective to concentrate on kidney dialysis and terminal cancer services, or should concentrated effort and economic resources be devoted to preventing disease and disability through, for example, hypertension and diabetes screening?

4. *Should certain diseases or categories of illness receive more emphasis than others?* For example, should the preventing and treating of coronary heart

disease be a priority over the prevention and treatment of venereal disease?

5. *In establishing certain priorities, will these priorities compromise important values or principles?* For example, preventive strategies aimed at discouraging alcohol use or smoking may involve emphasis on behavioral change or the altering of lifestyles. The nurse might question whether these preventive strategies would have a substantial effect on the autonomy of community members, particularly regarding their choice to engage in behaviors that are health risks.

Distributing Nursing Resources. Once the priorities for health are known, nurses need to decide how to deliver health care equally according to client needs. Several strategies can be implemented:

1. *Focus services on those who have the most reasonable chance of benefiting from services.* Examples are children and childbearing families. This is aimed at providing the greatest overall benefit.

2. *Provide basic services in all categories in limited amounts, and accommodate requests for nursing care services on a first-come, first-served basis.* This approach may certainly cost more in terms of services provided. It may even overlap with similar services provided in the community. It does meet the basic requirement of providing the opportunity for everyone to have equal access to services, even though they may have to wait a long time to be served.

3. *Focus nursing services on those who are most able to pay for services.* This approach is all too frequently used in today's health care delivery system. This approach has been fostered by legislation and funding by government and its agencies. Unfortunately, this approach may have limits when looking at the needs of a particular community.

4. *Categorize those in the community according to health needs, and decide who should receive first priority.* Individuals who cannot survive without nursing resources (those receiving kidney dialysis or respiratory therapy at home) have first priority. Those who can be assisted to prevent long-term disability (e.g., populations at high risk, preeclamptic clients, children with minor cardiac anomalies) would come next. Last priority would be given to those who do not have an acute disabling illness or are not at risk of long-term disability (e.g., school-age children, the elderly, or some persons with chronic diseases). Other groups who may be given a high priority include those whose health needs can be easily met and who can benefit the health of others (e.g., women with uncomplicated pregnancy, mothers with children under 2 years of age). This approach limits the access of some groups to nursing services according to their priority (Fig. 4-3).

As can be demonstrated by all of these various approaches to distributing nursing care resources, the moral requirements of justice create numerous conflicts of interest for health providers when they face specific choices.

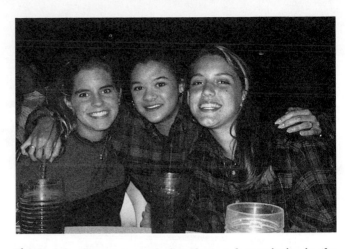

Figure 4-3   Teenage populations have a low priority in the allocation of health and nursing services. (From Wong DL: *Nursing care of infants and children,* ed 6, St Louis, 1999, Mosby.)

APPLICATION OF ETHICS TO COMMUNITY HEALTH NURSING PRACTICE
Priority of Ethical Principles

In community health nursing, ethical principles direct and guide nursing actions with individuals and aggregates. The professional ethic in most nursing actions places a greater emphasis on observing the principles of autonomy, freedom of choice, and beneficence (do good and do no harm), than on the principle of justice (treat everyone fairly).

In the community, nursing actions are guided not only by the professional ethic and its priority of ethical principles, but also by the **public health ethic,** which has a different priority of principles. This ethic is strongly modeled on the priority of the principle of beneficence—do good and do no harm—follows the rule of utility (the greatest good for the greatest number), in disease detection and prevention, as well as health maintenance. Following a rule of utility in matters of health might influence the practice of community health nursing. For example, it might encourage the nurse to identify the needs of aggregates in order to provide population groups with net benefit over possible health harms, such as in the case of spending money for a flu vaccine program rather than facing the prospect of increased deaths among the elderly from respiratory infections and pneumonia (Fry, 1994a). Emphasizing the moral requirements of the principle of beneficence, with a community focus, does not easily align with the individual client focus of the Code for Nurses, with its emphasis on respect for client autonomy.

Briefly Noted

Meeting accountability requirements in community health nursing will be different than meeting accountability requirements in other spheres of nursing practice. For example, the professional ethic clearly indicates that all nurses are morally accountable for how they respect the client's right to self-determination and provide health services with respect for "the uniqueness of the client." However, in community health, nurses are also morally accountable for how they provide health services to maximize total net health in population groups. Rather than being primarily accountable for how the moral requirements of the principle of autonomy are met in individual client care, the nurse is accountable for maximizing the total net health benefits of the community.

Healthy People 2010 addresses ethical and cultural issues. The *Healthy People 2010* box gives examples of how these issues are addressed.

Healthy People 2010
Related to Cultural and Ethical Issues

GOAL:

To eliminate health disparities among different segments of the population as defined by gender, race or ethnicity, education, income, disability, living in rural areas, and sexual orientation.

OBJECTIVES:

* Increase proportion of persons with health insurance.
* Increase the proportion of insured persons with clinical preventive services coverage.
* Increase the proportion of persons who have a specific source of ongoing care.
* Increase the proportion of persons with a usual primary care provider.
* Reduce the proportion of families that experience difficulties or delays in obtaining health care for one or more family members.
* Increase the proportion of all degrees awarded in the health professions to members of underrepresented racial and ethnic groups.

CULTURAL INFLUENCES

Caring for culturally diverse groups has been a focus of nursing from its beginning. As early as 1893, nurses in New York City provided home care to immigrants, particularly recent arrivals (Denker, 1994). These nurses were not from the same cultural background as the immigrants and had to deal with the cultural differences between themselves and the persons in their care.

The United States has always been a multicultural society. Recent changes in immigration laws have increased migration and the volume of cultural groups entering the United States (Battle, 1998) (Table 4-1).

If the current immigration trend continues, the United States will soon consist of a greater variety of cultural groups. About 51.1% of the total population, or more than 135 million people, will be of a culture other than Caucasian and will make up the nation's majority (U.S. Department of Commerce, 1997). About 25% of them will speak languages other than English at home.

There is great diversity among cultural groups in values and **beliefs.** In turn, their beliefs about health and illness also differ. Enormous challenges face nurses who want to understand clients' health and illness beliefs, as they provide interventions that promote and maintain wellness. However, an obstacle to helping clients promote and maintain their wellness is an insufficient number of nurses who understand the experiences and needs of diverse cultural groups (Bernal, 1993).

The purpose of the second part of this chapter is to look at cultural competence among community health nurses. Emphasis is on four cultural groups: African-Americans, Asian-Americans, Hispanic-Americans, and Native Americans. These groups have been consistently identified in the literature as having more economic difficulties, poorer health, and less-accessible health care than other groups (Giger and Davidhizar, 1999; Spector, 1996).

TABLE 4-1	Immigrants by Country of Birth: 1981 to 1995*			
Continent/Country	**1981-1990**	**1991-1993**	**1994**	**1995**
All countries	7338.1	3705.4	804.4	720.5
Europe[†]	705.6	438.9	160.9	128.2
Asia[†]	2817.4	1073.5	292.6	267.9
North America				
Canada	119.2	45.9	16.1	12.9
Mexico	1653.3	1286.5	111.4	89.9
Caribbean[†]	892.7	337.0	104.8	96.8
Central America[†]	458.7	226.8	39.9	31.8
South America[†]	455.9	189.2	47.4	45.7
Africa[†]	192.3	91.0	26.7	42.5
Other countries[‡]	41.9	16.4	4.6	4.7

Data from U.S. Census Bureau: *Statistical abstract of the United States: 1997,* ed 117, Washington, D.C., 1997, U.S. Government Printing Office.
*In thousands; for fiscal years ending in year shown.
[†]Includes countries not shown separately.
[‡]Includes Australia, New Zealand, and unknown countries.

Briefly Noted

As human beings, we have more similarities than differences with one another.

CULTURE, RACE, AND ETHNICITY

The concepts of culture, race, and ethnicity play a strong role in understanding human behavior. In everyday living, these three terms are often used incorrectly. Nurses are expected to understand the meaning of each when providing culturally relevant health care to clients of diverse cultures.

Culture

Culture is a learned set of ideals, values, and assumptions about life that are widely shared among a group of people (Leininger, 1995). It is a dynamic process that develops over time and changes with difficulty. In response to the needs of its members and their environment, culture provides guidance to help them solve life's problems.

Individuals learn about their culture during the process of learning language and being socialized, usually as children (Battle, 1998). Parents and family, the most important sources for the transfer of traditions, teach both obvious and implied behaviors of the culture. The *obvious behaviors,* such as language, interpersonal distance, and kissing in public, can be observed and allow the individual to identify the self with other persons of the culture. This way people share traditions, customs, and lifestyles with others. The *implied behaviors* are less visible and include the way individuals perceive health and illness, their body language, difference in language expressions, and the use of titles. These behaviors are subtle and may be difficult for persons to explain, yet they are very much a part of the culture. For example, deferring to the elderly, standing when they enter the room, or offering them a seat in which to sit suggests a cultural value related to the elderly. Another example of an implied aspect of culture is the use of language to communicate. For example, in one culture a sign might read "No smoking is permitted." In another culture the sign might read "Thank you for not smoking." The former statement represents a culture that values directness, whereas the latter values indirectness.

Each culture has a structure that distinguishes it from another and provides the elements for what members of the cultural group determine as appropriate or inappropriate behavior. Such elements include child-rearing practices, religious practices, family structure and values, and attitudes (Locke and Hardaway, 1992). In the case of language, there are expressions that are unique to each language (Phillips, Luna de Hernandez, and Torres de Ardon, 1994). It is important that nurses know these organizing elements to provide appropriate care to persons of diverse cultures. This does not mean, however, that one should overlook or fail to recognize the individuality of any person within any culture when developing a plan of care. Just as all cultures are not alike,

Box 4-4	**Factors Influencing Individual Differences Within Cultural Groups**

- Age
- Religion
- Dialect and language spoken
- Gender identity roles
- Socioeconomic background
- Geographic location in the country of origin
- Geographic location in the current country
- History of the subcultural group with which clients identify in their current country of residence
- History of the subcultural group with which clients identify in their country of origin
- Amount of interaction time among older and younger generations
- The degree of assimilation in the current country of residence
- Immigration status*
- Conditions under which migration occurred*

Except where noted with an asterisk (*), from Orque M: Orque's ethnic/cultural system: a framework for ethnic nursing care. In Orque MS, Bloch B, Monrroy LSA, editors: *Ethnic nursing care: a multi-cultural approach,* St Louis, 1983, Mosby.

all individuals within a culture are not alike. Box 4-4 summarizes factors that may contribute to individual differences within cultures.

Race

Race is primarily a social classification that relies on physical markers such as skin color to identify group membership (Bhopal and Donaldson, 1998). Individuals may be of the same race but differ in culture. For example, African-Americans are usually born in Africa, the Caribbean, or North America. Although they are different groups, they are often viewed as culturally and racially similar. This often blurs understanding of these culturally diverse groups.

A factor that highlights race's diminishing importance and makes *ethnic* identity more important is the interracial family. Physical changes in biracial and multiracial generations lead to changes in physical appearances of individuals and make race less important than ethnic identity.

Ethnicity

Ethnicity is the shared feeling of peoplehood among a group of individuals. Ethnicity reflects cultural membership and is based on individuals sharing similar cultural patterns (such as values, beliefs, customs, behaviors, and traditions) that over time create a common history that is very resistant to change. Ethnicity represents the identifying characteristics of culture such as race, religion, or national origin. It is influenced by education, income level, location, and association with ethnic groups other than one's own. Members of an ethnic group give up aspects of their own identity and society when they adopt characteristics of the group's identity. When there is a strong ethnic identity, the group maintains the values, beliefs, behaviors, practices, and ways of thinking of the group.

CULTURAL COMPETENCE

Many people are taught by and have knowledge of a dominant culture (Brislin, 1993). As long as the person is operating within that culture, one responds without thinking to a variety of situations. In today's climate of **multiculturism,** nurses are caring for a greater number of culturally diverse clients than ever before, which requires an understanding of cultural competence to provide nursing care that meets the needs of these persons.

Cultural competence is a set of knowledge-based and interpersonal skills that nurses use to effectively care for the client, individual, family, or community (Campinha-Bacote, Yahle, and Langenkamp, 1996; Frei, et al, 1994). Culturally competent nursing care is guided by four principles (American Academy of Nursing Expert Panel, 1992):

1. Care is designed for the specific client.
2. Care is based on the uniqueness of the person's culture and includes cultural norms and values.
3. Care includes self-empowerment strategies to facilitate client decision making in health behavior.
4. Care is provided with sensitivity based on the cultural uniqueness of clients.

Nurses must be culturally competent for the following reasons:

- *The nurse's culture often differs from that of the client.* Nurses come from a variety of cultural backgrounds and have their own cultural traditions. With such differences of beliefs and values, when the client and the nurse interact they may have a different understanding as to the meaning of the problem and different expectations about what to do to promote and protect health.
- *Care that is not culturally competent may further increase the cost of health care and decrease opportunities for positive client outcomes.* In the current health care climate of cost constraints, the health care industry is very focused on cost effectiveness. *Cost effectiveness* means that there is a balance between cost and quality (Irvine, Sidani, and Hall, 1998). *Quality of care* means that positive health outcomes are achieved. Care that is not focused on the clients' values and ideas is likely to increase cost and diminish quality. For example, when clients are using both folk medicine and traditional medicine and nurses fail to assess and use this information in teaching, the clients may not get the full benefits of the treatment protocol.

- *Specific objectives for persons of different cultures need to be met as outlined in Healthy People 2010.* Achievement of *Healthy People 2010* objectives requires that clients' lifestyles and personal choices be considered. For example, the American health care system views excessive drinking as a sign of disease. However, many Native Americans view alcohol consumption as an acceptable way to participate in family celebrations and tribal ceremonies (Orlandi, 1992). Refusal to drink with family may be viewed as a sign of rejection. Table 4-2 gives examples of *Healthy People 2010* health promotion objectives for selected minority groups who are at risk.

Developing Cultural Competence

Developing cultural competence is an ongoing life process. It is challenging and at times painful as the nurse struggles to break with the old and adopt new ways of thinking and performing (Frei, et al, 1994). Nurses develop cultural competence in different ways, but development occurs mainly by working with clients of other cultures and through the nurses' awareness of these experiences.

Campinha-Bacote, Yahle, and Langenkamp (1996) offer a model to explain the development of cultural competence. The components of the model are as follows:

- Cultural awareness
- Cultural knowledge
- Cultural skill
- Cultural encounter

Cultural Awareness

Cultural awareness is an appreciation of and sensitivity to the client's values, beliefs, practices, lifestyles, and problem-solving strategies (Campinha-Bacote, Yahle, and Langenkamp, 1996). To be aware suggests that nurses want to

---

TABLE 4-2 Selected Risk-Reduction 2010 Objectives for Target Groups	
Objectives	**1995 Baseline**
1. Reduce homicides to less than 3.2 per 100,000 people	6.2 (age adjusted)
Target group: African-American	25.2
2. Decrease coronary heart disease deaths to no more than 166 per 100,000	208.0
Target group: African-American	257.0
3. Decrease hepatitis B rates to 2.4 per 100,000 in persons less than 25 years of age (except perinatal infections)	124.0
Target group: Asian/Pacific Islander	42.4
4. Reduce to 12% the proportion of adults (18 and older) who use tobacco products	24.0
Target group: Native American	34.2

From U.S. Department of Health and Human Services, Office of Public Health and Science: *Healthy people 2010 objectives: draft for public comment,* Washington, D.C., 1998, U.S. Government Printing Office.

Evidence-Based Practice

Eliason reported in the 1998 study referenced in the footnote that there is a significant positive relationship between students' comfort level and the amount of experience they have had in caring for culturally diverse clients.

APPLICATION IN PRACTICE

This supports the need for nurses' education to include exposure to a variety of cultures.

Eliason J: Correlates of prejudice in nursing students, *J Nurs Educ* 37(1):27, 1998.

learn more about the cultural dimensions of the client. Cultural awareness means the nurse is willing to examine the nurse's personal values and biases (Misener, et al, 1997). Nurses who are culturally aware understand the basis for their own behavior and how it helps or hinders the delivery of competent care to persons from cultures other than their own. The nurse recognizes that health is expressed differently across cultures and that care can be delivered using a variety of modes consistent with the client's health values. For example, at a community outreach program, the nurse was teaching a racially mixed group the screening protocol for breast and cervical cancer detection. An African-American woman in the group refused to give the return demonstration for breast self-examination. When encouraged to do so, she said "my breasts are much larger than those on the model. Besides, the models are not like me. They are all white." After hearing the client's comments, the nurse realized that she had not considered the influence of culture or race on screening for breast and cervical cancer.

The nurse talked with the client, asked for her recommendations, and encouraged her to return the demonstration. The nurse coached the client through the self-examination process while pointing out that regardless of breast size, shape, and color, the technique is the same for feeling the tissue and squeezing the nipple to make certain that there is no discharge. Because this nurse was culturally aware, she did not become angry with herself or with the client and she did not impose her own values on the client. Rather, she encouraged the client to talk about her culture so that she could learn the appropriate intervention strategies to help the client meet her cultural needs. Box 4-5 identifies a number of questions nurses may ask as they try to know their own culture and the implications of their own cultural values.

Cultural Knowledge

Cultural knowledge is necessary to care for a multicultural society. **Cultural knowledge** provides nurses with an understanding of the elements of cultures and the information necessary to provide effective nursing care. Emphasis is on learning about the client's world view from an native perspective. Knowledge of the client's culture decreases misinterpretations by the nurse and supports the client's cooperation with the health care regimen. Nurses who lack cultural knowledge may develop feelings of inadequacy and helplessness because they are often unable to effectively help their clients. It is unrealistic to expect that nurses will have knowledge of all cultures. Instead they should be aware of and know how to obtain the knowledge of cultural influences that affect groups with whom they work. There are many ways one can obtain such knowledge: observe a culturally diverse or specific community group; watch how persons of a specific culture relate to each other, interview key leaders of the cultural group of interest, or read about the culture at the local library (Leininger, 1995).

Cultural Skill

Cultural skill reflects the effective use of cultural awareness and cultural knowledge to meet clients' needs. When communicating, culturally skillful nurses use appropriate touch during conversation, modify the physical distance between themselves and others, and use strategies to avoid cultural misunderstandings while meeting mutual goals.

Cultural Encounter

A **cultural encounter** is the final step in becoming culturally competent. In this step, nurses integrate the importance of culture at all levels of care as they make changes to meet the culturally unique needs of the client. Cultural encounters involve all interactions, not only those that are health related (Jezewski, 1993). The most important encounters are those in which nurses learn directly from clients about their life experiences and the significance of these experiences for health (Leininger, 1995) (Fig. 4-4).

Developing cultural competence comes from reading, taking courses, and discussing within multicultural settings the different cultures and their ideas about health, illness,

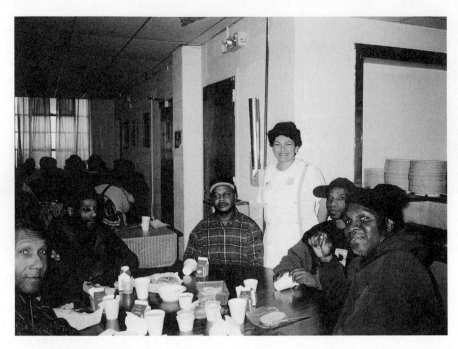

Figure 4-4   **A Hispanic nursing student interacting with African-American men at a nutrition center. To interact in a culturally competent manner, the student needs to have an awareness of and knowledge about the differences between her culture and the men's culture and the skill to portray this in her behavior toward them.**

and health care. Having cultural competence and being a cultural expert are two different things. Successfully working with clients from different cultures (cultural competence) is judged on four aspects (Brislin, 1993):

1. Nurses feel successful with established relationships with the client.
2. Clients feel that the interactions are warm, cordial, respectful, and cooperative.
3. The tasks are done efficiently.
4. The nurse and client experience little or no stress.

Briefly Noted

Nurses can help clients who come from different cultures as they attempt to recover from similar illnesses. Through educational groups, the clients from these different cultures can learn from each other new survival strategies and a variety of ways to relate to families, community, and workplace.

Dimensions of Cultural Competence

Four strategies are used by the culturally competent nurse to provide quality holistic nursing care:

- Cultural preservation
- Cultural accommodation
- Cultural repatterning
- Cultural brokering

Cultural Preservation

The goal of **cultural preservation** is to support the use by clients those aspects of the clients' culture that promote

healthy behaviors. For example, Mrs. Lin, a 73-year-old Chinese woman, is discharged to home care after surgery for cancer of the large intestine. The nurse found her at home alone with her 76-year-old husband. After the physical assessment, the nurse discussed making a referral for Mrs. Lin to have a home health aide to assist her with physical care and light housekeeping chores. The family was gracious but seemed hesitant to accept the referral. The nurse knew that in China, the extended family network and family decision making are valued.

She asked the couple if they would like to discuss the situation with their daughters. Both the client and her husband seemed pleased with the idea, and the nurse promised to get back to them the next day. When the nurse returned for her visit, one of Mrs. Lin's daughters was present and told the nurse that the family could manage without additional help. The three daughters had made a schedule to take turns in caring for their parents. The nurse demonstrated acceptance and support for the family's decision and told them that if they decide at a later time to have the home health aide, they should call the agency. She then gave them the telephone number and scheduled the next follow-up visit with them.

Cultural Accommodation

Cultural accommodation means that the nurse negotiates with clients to include aspects of their folk practices with the traditional health care system to implement essential treatment plans. The emphasis should be to make sure that the practice is not harmful, is safe, and has health benefits for the client. For example, Ms. Etienne is a 36-year-old Haitian woman who is pregnant and diagnosed with hypertension. For each of her last three visits at the neighborhood health clinic, the client was hypertensive. When questioned, Ms. Etienne confided in the nurse that she was drinking special teas that were prescribed by her voodoo priest to support her having a "strong baby." The nurse asked for the names of the herbs that she was using. The nurse than scheduled a conference with the pharmacist to discuss the specific ingredients in the herbs and ways that they might help the client to meet her cultural needs. The nurse found out that one of the herbs led to the client's high blood pressure and negotiated with the client not to drink that specific tea.

Cultural Repatterning

Cultural repatterning means that the nurse works with clients to make changes in health practices when these behaviors are harmful or decrease the clients' well-being. For example, a culturally competent nurse knows of the high incidence of obesity among Mexican-American women 20 years of age and over (U.S. Department of Health and Human Services, 1998). While respecting the client's tradition, the nurse must teach the client about weight loss and about ways of including cultural foods that would support a healthier lifestyle.

Culture Brokering

Culture brokering is another strategy used by culturally competent nurses to make certain that clients receive culturally appropriate care (Jezewski, 1993). Culture brokering is advocating, mediating, negotiating, and intervening between the health care culture and the client's culture on behalf of the client. Culturally competent nurses are in a position to understand both cultures and may use knowledge to resolve or lessen problems that may have resulted from individuals in either culture not understanding the other person's values. To illustrate, migrant workers tend to have high occupational mobility; many are poor and may have limited formal education. They may seek health care only when they are ill and cannot work. Whenever nurses interact with them, they should use every opportunity to teach them about prevention and health maintenance, environmental sanitation, and nutrition, because it may be the only opportunity that the nurse will ever have to treat a particular migrant worker. Nurses should also advocate for the rights of the migrant worker to receive quality health care. For example, the nurse may contact the Migrant Health Services for follow-up or referral care for the migrant worker.

INHIBITORS TO DEVELOPING CULTURAL COMPETENCE

When nurses fail to provide culturally competent nursing care, it may be because they have had minimal opportunity for learning about transcultural nursing, their supervisors are pressuring them to increase productivity by increasing their case loads, or they are pressured by colleagues who are not knowledgeable about other cultures and who are offended. Any of these factors may result in nurse behaviors

 Evidence-Based Practice

A study was conducted in South Carolina to determine differences in functional status, health status, and use of community services between elderly African-Americans and Caucasians diagnosed with diabetes. Data were collected over an 8-year period from the agency records for a four-county non-retirement and non-resort region. Results showed that there were no significant differences between the groups in functional status or health status. However, the elderly Caucasians had significantly more difficulty in specific activities of daily living, such as house cleaning, food preparation, and transportation. Although both groups under-used the community services, the use of services was significantly lower for the African-Americans elders. Community services included case management, outreach, group meals, home-delivered meals, food distribution, recreation, and transportation.

Under-use of community services is a significant finding, particularly as it relates to the elderly who live alone. The elderly who do not use community services are likely to be at increased risk for developing diabetic complications and a poorer quality of life, and as a consequence, increased mortality.

APPLICATION IN PRACTICE

The findings suggest that nurses should explore reasons for the failure to use and develop interventions that would increase use of services, especially to vulnerable groups such as elderly African-Americans with diabetes.

Witucki J, Wallace DC: Differences in functional status, health status, and community-based service use between black and white diabetic elders, *J Cult Divers* 6(3):94, 1998.

such as stereotyping, prejudice, racism, ethnocentrism, cultural blindness, cultural imposition, cultural conflict, and cultural shock.

- **Stereotyping** means one attributes certain beliefs and behaviors about a group to an individual without giving adequate attention to individual differences (Brislin, 1993).
- **Prejudice** is the emotional reaction to deeply held beliefs (stereotypes) about other groups (Brislin, 1993). It usually refers to negative feelings.
- **Racism** is a form of prejudice and refers to the belief that persons who are born into a particular group are inferior, for example, in intelligence, morals, beauty, or self-worth (Brislin, 1993).
- **Ethnocentrism,** a type of cultural prejudice at the cultural population level, is the belief that one's own group determines the standards for behavior by which all other groups are to be judged. Ethnocentric nurses are unfamiliar and uncomfortable with anything that is different from their culture.
- **Cultural blindness** is the tendency to ignore all differences between cultures and to act as though the differences do not exist.
- **Cultural imposition** is the process of imposing one's values on others. Nurses impose their values on clients when they forcefully promote Western medical

traditions while ignoring the clients' value of non-Western treatments such as acupuncture.

- **Cultural conflict** is a perceived threat that may arise from a misunderstanding of expectations between clients and nurses when either group is not aware of cultural differences (Andrews and Boyle, 1998).
- **Culture shock** is the feeling of helplessness, discomfort, and disorientation experienced by an individual attempting to understand or effectively adapt to another cultural group that differs in practices, values, and beliefs.

Being aware of the clients' own cultural beliefs and having knowledge of other cultures may help nurses to be less judgmental, more accepting of cultural differences, and less likely to engage in the negative behaviors listed previously.

CULTURAL NURSING ASSESSMENT

A *cultural nursing assessment* is "a systematic way to identify the cultural beliefs, meanings, symbols, and practices of individuals or groups using a holistic perspective including a world view, life experiences, environment, ethnohistory, and social structure factors" (Leininger, 1995, p. 118). Skills such as listening, explaining, acknowledging, recommending, and negotiating help the nurse to be non-judgmental. It is vital that nurses listen to clients' perceptions of their problems and, in turn, that nurses explain to clients the nurse's perceptions of the problems. Nurses and clients should acknowledge and discuss similarities and differences between the two perceptions to develop suggestions and recommendations for managing problems. Nurses also negotiate with clients on nursing care actions to meet clients' needs.

Many tools are available to assist nurses in conducting cultural assessments (Andrews and Boyle, 1998; Leininger, 1995; Ludwig-Beymer, et al, 1998; Tripp-Reimer, Brink, and Saunders, 1997). The focus of such tools varies, and selection is determined by the dimensions of culture to be assessed.

During initial contacts with clients, nurses should perform a cultural assessment that may be brief or may be just the beginning of an in-depth assessment (Tripp-Reimer, Brink, and Saunders, 1997). In a brief cultural assessment, nurses ask clients about the following issues:

- Ethnic background
- Religious preference
- Family patterns
- Food patterns
- Health practices

Such basic data help nurses understand the client from the client's point of view and recognize what is unique about the client, thus avoiding stereotyping. Data from a brief assessment help determine the need for an in-depth cultural assessment.

An in-depth cultural assessment should be conducted over a period of time and should not be restricted to the first encounter with the client. This gives both clients and nurses time to get to know each other and gives clients a chance to see nurses in helping relationships. Tripp-Reimer, Brink, and

Saunders (1997) suggest that an in-depth cultural assessment should be conducted in two phases: a data-collecting phase and an organizing phase (see Appendix B.2 for cultural assessment tool).

The key to a successful cultural assessment lies in nurses being aware of their own culture. Randall-David (1989) developed a variety of principles that may be helpful as nurses conduct cultural assessments. Nurses should do the following:

1. *Always be aware of the environment.* They should look around and listen to what is being said and understand nonverbal communications before taking action.
2. *Know about community social organizations* such as schools, churches, hospitals, tribal councils, restaurants, taverns, and bars.
3. *Know the specific areas that the nurse wants to focus on* before beginning the cultural assessment.
4. *Select a strategy to help gather cultural data.* Strategies may include in-depth interviews, informal conversations, observations of everyday activities or specific events in the life of the client, survey research, and a case method approach to study certain aspects of a client.
5. *Identify a confidante* who will help "bridge the gap" between cultures.
6. *Know the appropriate questions* to ask without offending the client.
7. *Interview other nurses or health care professionals* who have worked with the specific client to get their input.
8. *Talk with formal and informal cultural leaders* to gain a comprehensive understanding about significant aspects of community life.
9. *Be aware that all information has both subjective and objective data,* and verify and cross-check the information that is collected before acting on it.
10. *Avoid pitfalls* in making premature generalizations.
11. *Be sincere, open, and honest* with self and the clients.

Using an Interpreter

Communication with the client or family is required for a cultural assessment. When nurses do not speak or understand the client's language, they should make every effort to obtain an interpreter. Nurses should be aware of the powerful role that interpreters play in determining information shared between clients and nurses. Interpreters may emphasize their personal preferences by influencing both nurses' and clients' decisions to select and participate in treatment modalities. Nurses may minimize this by learning basic words and sentences of the most commonly spoken languages in the community. Strategies that nurses may use to select and effectively use an interpreter are listed in the box below.

HOW TO Select and Use an Interpreter

1. When feasible, select an interpreter who has knowledge of health-related terminology.
2. Use family members with caution because it may be inappropriate to discuss intimate health matters in the presence of certain family members.

3. The gender of the interpreter may be of concern, particularly when asking questions about sexuality or childbirth. In some cultures women may prefer a female interpreter and men may prefer a male.
4. The age of the interpreter may also be of concern. For example, older clients may want a more mature interpreter. Children tend to have limited language skills, and when used as interpreters, they may have difficulty interpreting the information.
5. Differences in socioeconomic status, religious affiliation, and educational level between the client and the interpreter may lead to problems in translation of information.
6. Identify the client's birth origin and language or dialect before selecting the interpreter. For example, Chinese clients speak different dialects depending on the region in which they were born.
7. Avoid using an interpreter from the same community as the client to avoid a breach of confidentiality.
8. Avoid using professional jargon, colloquialisms, abstractions, idiomatic expressions, slang, similes, and metaphors. Speak slowly and use words that are common in the client's culture.
9. Clarify roles with the interpreter.
10. Introduce the interpreter to the client, and explain to the client what the interpreter will be doing.
11. Review the situation and information to be translated before and at the end of each health care encounter.
12. Observe the client for non-verbal messages, such as facial expressions, gestures, and other forms of body language. If the client's responses do not fit with the question, the nurse should check to be sure that the interpreter understands the question.
13. Increase accuracy in transmission of information by asking the interpreter to translate the client's own words, and ask the client to repeat the information that was communicated.
14. At the end of the interview, review the material with the client to ensure that nothing has been missed or misunderstood.

Briefly Noted

Health care agencies have a responsibility to effectively communicate with their clients. When an interpreter is not available to translate, the client may view this behavior as unacceptable and bring legal action against the agency.

CULTURAL GROUPS' DIFFERENCES

Although all cultures are not the same, all cultures have the same basic organizing factors (Giger and Davidhizar, 1999). These factors should be explored in a cultural assessment because of the potential for differences among groups. Some of these differences among cultural groups are presented in Table 4-3.

Communication

Understanding variations in patterns of verbal and nonverbal communication is the basis for achieving therapeutic goals. Variations among cultures are reflected in verbal styles—such as pronunciation, word meaning, voice quality, and humor—and in nonverbal styles such as eye contact, gestures, touch, interjecting during conversation, body posture, facial expression, and silence.

Briefly Noted

Respect all information that a client shares with you even though the information may be in conflict with your own value system.

Space

Personal space is the physical area that persons need between themselves and others to feel comfortable. When this space is violated, the client may experience discomfort. Nurses should take cues from clients to place themselves in the appropriate spatial zone and avoid misinterpretation of clients' behavior as they handle their spatial needs.

Social Organization

Social organization, especially that of the family, is defined differently across cultural groups. The significance of family also varies across cultures. Nurses should advocate for the individual, so that when families make decisions, the individual's needs are also being considered.

Time Perception

Cultures are considered to be either future oriented, present oriented, or past oriented. The American middle-class culture tends to be future oriented, and individuals are willing to delay immediate gratification until future goals are accomplished. When nurses discuss health promotion and disease prevention strategies with persons from a present orientation, they should focus on the immediate benefits these clients would gain rather than emphasize future outcomes. Nurses socialized in the Western culture may view time as money and equate punctuality with goodness and being responsible. Working with clients who have a different time perception than the nurse can be problematic. Nurses should clarify the clients' perception to avoid misunderstanding. It is not feasible to expect that clients will change their behavior and adopt the nurse's schedule.

Environmental Control

Environmental control refers to the relationships between humans and nature. Cultural groups might perceive humans as having mastery over nature, being dominated by nature, or having a harmonious relationship with nature.

TABLE 4-3	Variations Among Selected Cultural Groups			
	African-Americans	**Asians**	**Hispanics**	**Native Americans**
Verbal communication	Asking personal questions of someone that you have met for the first time is seen as improper and intrusive	High level of respect for others, especially those in positions of authority	Expression of negative feelings is considered impolite	Speaks in a low tone of voice and expects the listener to be attentive
Nonverbal communication	Direct eye contact in conversation is often considered rude	Direct eye contact among superiors may be considered disrespectful	Avoidance of eye contact is usually a sign of attentiveness and respect	Direct eye contact is often considered disrespectful
Touch	Touching another person's hair is often considered offensive	It is not customary to shake hands with persons of the opposite sex	Touching is often observed between two persons in conversation	A light touch of the person's hand instead of a firm handshake is often used when greeting a person
Family organization	Usually have close extended family networks; women play key roles in health care decisions	Usually have close extended family ties; emphasis may be on family needs rather than individual needs	Usually have close extended family ties; all members of the family may be involved in health care decisions	Usually have close extended family; emphasis tends to be on family rather than on individual needs
Time	Often present oriented	Often present oriented	Often present oriented	Often past oriented
Perception	Harmony of mind, health, body, and spirit with nature	Balance between the "yin" and "yang" energy forces	Balance and harmony among mind, body, spirit, and nature	Harmony of mind, body, spirit, and emotions with nature
Alternative healers	"Granny," "root doctor," voodoo priest, spiritualist	Acupuncturist, acupressurist, herbalist	*Curandero, espiritualista, yerbero*	Medicine man, shaman
Self-care practices	Poultices, herbs, oils, roots	Hot and cold foods, herbs, teas, soups, cupping, burning, rubbing, pinching	Hot and cold foods, herbs	Herbs, corn meal, medicine bundle
Biological variations	Sickle cell anemia, mongolian spots, keloid formation, inverted T waves, lactose intolerance, skin color	Thalassemia, drug interactions, mongolian spots, lactose intolerance, skin color	Mongolian spots, lactose intolerance, skin color	Cleft uvula, lactose intolerance, skin color
Food preferences	Fried foods, greens, bread, lard, pork, rice, foods with high sodium and starch content	Soy sauce, rice, pickled dishes, raw fish, tea, balance between yin (cold) and yang (hot) concepts	Fried foods, beans and rice, chili, carbonated beverages, high-fat and high-sodium foods	Blue corn meal, fruits, game and fish
Nutritional excess	Cholesterol, fat, sodium, carbohydrates, calories	Cholesterol, fat, sodium, carbohydrates, calories	Cholesterol, fat, carbohydrates, calories	Carbohydrates, calories
Risk factors	Coronary heart disease, obesity	Coronary heart disease, liver disease, cancer of the stomach	Coronary heart disease, obesity	Diabetes, malnutrition, tuberculosis, infant and maternal mortality

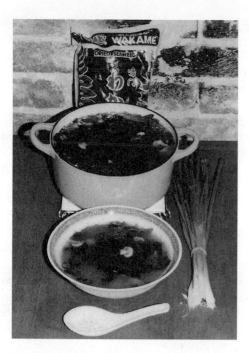

Figure 4-5   Mi-Yuk Gook (seaweed soup) is a Korean dish eaten by postpartum women to stop bleeding and to clean up body fluids. It is also eaten every birthday.

Briefly Noted

Some clients may view their illness as punishment for misdeeds and may have difficulty accepting care from nurses who do not share their belief.

Biological Variations

Biological variations distinguish one racial group from another. They occur in areas of growth and development, skin color, enzymatic differences, and susceptibility to disease (Andrews and Boyle, 1998; Giger and Davidhizar, 1999). Other common and obvious variations include eye shape, hair texture, adipose tissue deposits, shape of ear lobes, thickness of lips, and body configuration.

Nutrition

Nutritional practices are an integral part of the assessment process for all families, especially since they play a prominent role in health problems of some groups (Greenberg, et al, 1998). Efforts to understand dietary patterns of clients should go beyond relying on membership in a defined group. Knowing clients' nutrition practices makes it possible to develop treatment regimens that would not conflict with their cultural food practices (Fig. 4-5). Box 4-6 identifies several questions that nurses should ask when conducting a nutritional assessment.

Socioeconomic Factors

Socioeconomic factors contribute greatly to understanding perceptions of health and illness among minority groups.

Box 4-6	Assessment of Dietary Practices and Food-Consumption Patterns

- What is the social significance of food in the family?
- What foods are most frequently bought for family consumption? Who makes the decision to buy the food?
- What foods, if any, are taboo or prohibited for the family?
- Does religion play a significant role in food selection?
- Who prepares the food? How is it prepared?
- How much food is eaten? When is it eaten and with whom?
- Where does the client live and what types of restaurants does he or she frequent?
- Has the family adopted foods of other cultural groups?
- What are the family's favorite recipes?

These groups may not have similar opportunities for education, occupation, income earning, and property ownership as the dominant group. Socioeconomic status is a critical factor in determining access to health care and the development of some chronic health problems (Kington and Smith, 1997). Nurses should be able to distinguish between culture and socioeconomic class issues and not misinterpret behavior as having a cultural origin, when in fact it should be attributed to socioeconomic class. Nurses must conduct a cultural assessment for all individuals when they first come in contact with them. Nurses should have guidance in integrating cultural concepts with other aspects of client care to meet their clients' total health care needs.

Clinical Application

Mr. Nguyen, a 64 year old from rural Vietnam, entered the United States with his family 3 years ago through the displaced persons program. Mr. Nguyen was a farmer in his homeland, and since his arrival he has been unable to obtain a stable job that allows him to adequately care for his family. His financial resources are limited and he has no insurance. He speaks enough English to interact directly with people outside his family and community. His oldest daughter, Shu Ping, is enrolled in a 2-year program to become a registered nurse.

The Nguyen family attends the neighborhood church where there are other Vietnamese families. Mr. Nguyen has also been attending the clinic at the hospital but refuses to discuss with his family, even with Shu Ping, the reason for these visits. Shu Ping became increasingly concerned as she observed her father having insomnia, retarded motor activity, an inability to concentrate, and weight loss. However, Mr. Nguyen denied that he was not well. Shu Ping decided to discuss her concerns with a nurse she had befriended at the church. She invited the nurse to her home for lunch on a Saturday so the nurse could meet her father and validate her impressions.

After several visits with the family, the nurse was able to establish a close enough relationship with Mr. Nguyen so that she could engage him in a discussion of his health. Because of her extensive work with other Vietnamese immigrants, the nurse was familiar with themes of loss and decided to focus her conversation with Mr. Nguyen on his adjustment to the new community, gains and losses as a result of immigration, and coping strategies. After several discussions, Mr. Nguyen, confided in the nurse that he feared that he was dying because he had been diagnosed with cancer of the small intestine. He further revealed that he did not share the diagnosis with the family as he did not want them to know of his "bad news." Mr. Nguyen had refused treatment because he knew that people never got better after they had cancer; they always died.

Which of the following actions best characterizes the nurse's willingness to provide culturally competent care to Mr. Nguyen and his family?
A. *Discuss with the client his understanding of his diagnosis.*
B. *Discuss with the client the prognosis for a person diagnosed with cancer of the small intestine in Vietnam.*
C. *Discuss with the client the prognosis for a person diagnosed with cancer of the small intestine in the United States.*
D. *Discuss the medical treatment and surgical intervention for cancer of the small intestine.*

Consider the following ethical questions.

A. *What is the role of the nurse in assisting individuals to reach a decision with which they can live?*
B. *What does it mean to respect Mr. Nguyen as an autonomous individual?*
C. *Do clients really have the right to refuse services or treatment? Does such refusal limit future treatment? Why or why not?*
D. *Is there any happy medium for aging parents when they can no longer live independently?*

Answer is in the back of the book.

⚠ Remember This!

- Because clients have rights, health care professionals have responsibilities to tell the truth, respect confidentiality, function as client advocates, and accept accountability for providing proper health care.
- The development of methods to measure accountability is a high priority in nursing.
- A right to health has been historically recognized as a basic human right.
- The negative right to be free to enjoy good health may lead to the positive right to obtain certain services or community health safeguards.
- "Right to health" and "right to health care" are different kinds of rights and should be kept separate.
- Health care providers do not often communicate rights to their clients.
- Clients have the right to accept or refuse treatment and the right to formulate advance directives.
- According to a recent presidential commission, "society has an ethical obligation to ensure equitable access to health care for all."
- The professional code of ethics for nurses prescribes moral behavior and actions based on moral principles.
- The ethical principles operable in community health nursing are beneficence, autonomy, and justice.

- The four major theories of justice used to decide how to allocate health care resources are the entitlement theory, the utilitarian theory, the maximin theory, and the egalitarian theory.
- The moral requirements of justice create numerous conflicts of interest for health providers when specific choices must be made.
- The professional ethic generally places a greater emphasis on observing the principles of autonomy and beneficence than on the principle of justice in most nursing actions.
- In community health nursing, moral accountability means being answerable for how the health of aggregate groups has been promoted, protected, and met.
- Clients' rights to equal access to health care and the aggregate's needs and interests in health matters will often compete for the attention and services of the nurse.
- The United States is an increasingly diverse population, and it is key that nurses, particularly community-oriented nurses, learn about the culture of the individuals for whom they give care.
- Culture is a learned set of behaviors that are widely shared among a group of people that helps guide individuals in problem solving and decision making.
- Nurses should include the clients' cultural beliefs and practices to improve the clients' health status and reduce health care costs.
- Culturally competent nursing care is designed for a specific client, reflects the individual's needs and experiences, and is provided with sensitivity.
- *Culturally competent* means that the nurse is culturally aware and culturally knowledgeable, and is able to use cultural skills with culturally diverse clients.
- There are four strategies that nurses may use to negotiate with clients and promote culturally competent care: cultural preservation, cultural accommodation, cultural repatterning, and culture brokering.
- Barriers to providing culturally competent care are stereotyping, prejudice, racism, ethnocentrism, cultural imposition, cultural blindness, cultural conflict, and culture shock.
- Nurses should complete a cultural assessment on every client with whom they interact. They use cultural assessments to help them understand clients' perspectives of health and illness and to guide them in discussing culturally appropriate interventions with the client. The needs of clients are based on age, education, religion, and socioeconomic status.
- When nurses do not speak or understand the client's language, they should make every effort to obtain an interpreter. In selecting an interpreter, nurses should consider the clients' cultural needs and respect their right to privacy.
- Members of minority groups are greatly represented on the lower tier of the socioeconomic ladder. Nurses should be able to distinguish between culture and socioeconomic class issues and not interpret behavior as having a cultural origin when in fact it is attributed to socioeconomic class.

What Would You Do?

1. Hold a conference among two or three nursing students and two or three practicing community health nurses. Discuss how these nurses assume responsibility and accountability for individual nursing judgments and actions in their areas of practice. Be sure to distinguish moral accountability from legal accountability.

2. Suggest three ways by which nursing might extend the scope of accountability for nurses in delivering nursing care services to aggregate groups in the community.

3. Determine how clients' rights to privacy are respected and protected in a community health care agency. To what extent do nurses contribute to the protection of client privacy? Are client records used in research studies? If so, how is personal information about the client protected?

4. Suggest two methods by which client privacy could be more adequately protected. What would be the relative costs and benefits of your proposed methods?

5. Summarize the role of nurses in discussing and implementing advance directives in community health settings.

6. A 90-year-old South American woman refuses to have her nursing care provided by an African-American nurse. Should the community agency assign a nurse from another racial group to care for the client, or should the client be transferred to another community health agency?

7. What strategies would you use when caring for clients who do not speak your language and for whom no translator is readily available?

8. In public-opinion surveys about professional aid in dying, 50% to 75% of adults favor allowing health care professionals to euthanize or to assist the suicide of those who are terminally ill. Nurses, however, are ethically and legally prohibited from assisting the suicide of anyone and participating in acts of euthanasia. What should the nurse do when a terminally ill and suffering client asks the nurse to help him die?

9. Mr. Jeff Williams, team leader in Home Health Care Services at the county health department, was preparing to visit Mr. Chisholm, a 59-year-old client recently diagnosed as having emphysema. Mr. Chisholm, who was unemployed because of a farming accident several years earlier, was well known to the health department. Hypertensive and overweight, he was also a heavy, long-term cigarette smoker despite his decreased lung function. Mr. Williams visited Mr. Chisholm to find out why the client had missed his latest chest clinic appointment. He also wanted to find out if the client was continuing his medications as ordered.

As Mr. Williams parked his car in front of his client's house, he could see Mr. Chisholm sitting on the front porch smoking a cigarette. A flash of anger made him wonder why he continued trying to teach Mr. Chisholm reasons for not smoking and why he took the time from his busy home care schedule to follow up on Mr. Chisholm's missed clinical appointments. This client certainly did not seem to care enough about his own health to give up smoking.

During the home visit, Mr. Williams determined that Mr. Chisholm had discontinued the use of his prophylactic antibiotic and was not taking his expectorant and bronchodilator medication on a regular basis. Mr. Chisholm's blood pressure was 210/114 mm Hg, and he coughed almost continuously. Although he listened politely to Mr. Williams's concerns about his respiratory function and the continued use of his medications, Mr. Chisholm simply made no effort to take responsibility for his health care. Even so, another clinic appointment was made, and Mr. Williams encouraged the client to attend.

As he drove to his next home visit, Mr. Williams wondered to what extent he was obligated as a nurse to spend time on clients who took no personal responsibility for their health. He also wondered if there was a limit to the amount of nursing care a noncooperative client could expect from a community health service.

1. *What are Mr. Williams's professional responsibilities for Mr. Chisholm's rights to health care?*
2. *Is there a limit to the amount of care nurses should be expected to give to clients?*
3. *What authority defines the moral requirements and moral limits of nursing care to clients?*

(Modified from Veatch RM, Fry ST: Case studies in nursing ethics, Philadelphia, 1995, JB Lippincott.)

REFERENCES

American Academy of Nursing Expert Panel on Culturally Competent Health Care: Culturally competent health care, *Nurs Outlook* 40:277, 1992.

American Hospital Association: Statement on a patient's bill of rights, *Hospitals* 47:41, 1973.

American Nurses' Association: *Code for nurses with interpretive statements,* Kansas City, Mo, 2000, The Association.

Andrews MM, Boyle JS: *Transcultural concepts in nursing care,* ed 3, Philadelphia, 1998, JB Lippincott.

Annas JG: Patients rights movement. In Reich WT (editor): - Encyclopedia of bioethics, ed 2, New York, 1996, Simon & Schuster.

Battle DE: *Community disorders in multicultural populations,* ed 2, Boston, 1998, Butterworth-Heinemann.

Beauchamp TL, Childress JF: *Principles of biomedical ethics,* ed 4, New York, 1994, Oxford Press.

Bernal H: A model for delivering culture-relevant care in the community, *Public Health Nurs* 10(4):228, 1993.

Bhopal R, Donaldson L: White, European, Western, Caucasian, or what? Inappropriate labeling in research on race, ethnicity, and health, *Am J Public Health* 88(9):1303, 1998.

Brislin R: *Understanding culture's influence on behavior,* Fort Worth, Tx, 1993, Harcourt Brace.

Brockington C: *A short history of public health,* London, 1956, Churchill.

Campinha-Bacote J, Yahle T, Langenkamp M: The challenge of cultural diversity for nurse educators, *J Contin Educ Nurs* 27:59, 1996.

Denker EP (editor): *Healing at home: Visiting Nurse Service of New York,* 1893-1993, Dalton, Mass, 1994, Studley Press.

Frei F, et al: *Work design for the competent organization,* Westport, Conn, 1994, Quorum Books.

Fry ST: *Ethics in nursing practice: a guide to ethical decision making,* Geneva, 1994a, International Council of Nurses.

Fry ST, Damrosch S: Ethics and human rights issues in nursing practice: a survey of Maryland nurses, *Maryland Nurse* 13(7):11, 1994b.

Giger JN, Davidhizar R: *Transcultural nursing: assessment and intervention,* ed 3, St Louis, 1999, Mosby.

Greenberg MR, et al: Region of birth and Black diets; the Harlem household survey, *Am J Public Health* 88:1199, 1998.

Irvine D, Sidani S, Hall LM: Finding value in nursing care: a framework for quality improvement and cultural evalutation, *Nurs Econ* 16(3):110, 1998.

Jameton A: *Nursing practice: the ethical issues,* Englewood Cliffs, NJ, 1984, Prentice-Hall.

Jezewski MA: Culture brokering as a model for advocacy, *Nurs Health Care* 14(2):78, 1993.

Kington RS, Smith JP: Socioeconomic status and racial ethnic differences in functional status associated with chronic diseases, *Am J Public Health* 8(5):805, 1997.

Leininger MM: *Transcultural nursing: concepts, theories, research, and practices,* New York, 1995, McGraw Hill.

Locke DC, Hardaway YV: Moral perspectives in interracial settings. In Cochrane D, Manley-Casimir M (editors): *Moral education: practical approaches,* New York, 1992, Praeger.

Ludwig-Beymer P, et al: Community assessment in a suburban Hispanic community: a description of method, *J Transcultural Nurs* 8(10):19, 1998.

Misener TR, et al: Sexual orientation: a cultural diversity issue for nursing, *Nurs Outlook* 45:178, 1997.

Omnibus Budget Reconciliation Act of 1990, sections 4206 and 4751, PL 101-508, Nov 5, 1990.

Orlandi MA (editor): *Cultural competence for evaluations,* Washington, D.C., 1992, U.S. Department of Health and Human Services.

Phillips LA, Luna de Hernandez I, Torres de Ardon E: Focus on psychometrics: strategies for achieving cultural equivalence, *Res Nurs Health* 17:149, 1994.

President's Commission for the Study of Ethical Problems in Medicine and Biomedical and Behavioral Research: *Securing access to health care,* vol 1: report on the ethical implications of differences in the availability in health services, Washington, D.C., 1983, U.S. Government Printing Office.

Public Law 92-603, Social Security amendments of 1972, 92nd Congress, Oct 30, 1972.

Public Law 92-278, The national sickle cell anemia, Cooley's anemia, Tay-Sachs and Genetic Disease Act, Title IV, 90 stat, Section 410, 1976.

Randall-David E: *Strategies for working with culturally diverse communities and clients,* Bethesda, Md, 1989, Association for the Care of Children's Health.

Spector RE: *Cultural diversity in health and illness,* ed 4, Norwalk, Conn, 1996, Appleton & Lange.

Szasz T: The right to health. In Gorovitz S, et al (editors): *Moral problems in medicine,* Englewood Cliffs, NJ, 1976, Prentice-Hall.

Tripp-Reimer T, Brink PJ, Saunders JM: Cultural assessment: content and process. In Spradley BW, Allender JA (editors): *Readings in community health,* ed 5, Philadelphia, 1997, JB Lippincott.

United Nations Educational, Scientific, and Cultural Organization: Human rights, a symposium, New York, 1949, Allan Wingate.

U.S. Department of Commerce: *Statistical abstract of the United States,* ed 117, Washington, D.C., 1997, U.S. Government Printing Office.

U.S. Department of Health and Human Services, Office of Public Health and Science: *Healthy people 2010 objectives: draft for public comment,* Washington, D.C., 1998, U.S. Government Printing Office.

Vaughan RH: *The actual incidence of moral problems in nursing: a preliminary study in empirical ethics* (thesis), Washington, D.C., 1935, Catholic University of America.

World Health Organization: *The first ten years of the World Health Organization,* New York, 1958, World Health Organization.

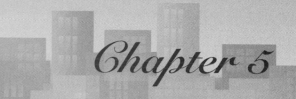

Chapter 5

Environmental Health

ANN H. CARY

LILLIAN H. MOOD

OBJECTIVES

After reading this chapter, the student should be able to:
- Identify the relationship between the environment and human health and disease.
- Apply the nursing process to the practice of environmental health.
- Describe legislative and regulatory policies that have influenced the effect of the environment on health and disease patterns in communities.
- Include environmental principles in practice.

CHAPTER OUTLINE

Human Dependence on the Environment

Healthy People 2000/2010 Objectives and Environmental Health

Protecting the Environment
    Prevention
    Control
    Environmental Standards
    Monitoring

Citizen Roles

Nursing's Environmental Heritage

Environmental Health Competencies for Nurses
    Basic Knowledge
    Assessment and Referral
    Advocacy, Ethics, and Risk Communication
    Legislation and Regulation

Roles for Nurses in Environmental Health

KEY TERMS

bio-unavailable: in a physical or chemical state that is not accessible or cannot be taken up by air, water, plants, or animals.

biodegradation: the process of breaking down or decomposing under natural conditions.

compliance: process for ensuring that requirements for environmental protection, as stated in environmental permits, are met.

deforestation: destruction of forests.

determinant: factor that influences risk or outcomes.

dose: amount of chemical or radiation exposure received at one time or over a stated interval.

ecological: the relationship between living things to one another and their environment.

enforcement: federal, state, or local legal actions to obtain compliance with environmental laws, rules, regulations, or

agreements and/or to obtain penalties or criminal sanctions for violations.

estuaries: areas where fresh water meets salt water. Examples include bays, mouths of rivers, salt marshes, and lagoons. Estuaries are delicate ecosystems. They serve as nurseries and spawning and feeding grounds for large groups of marine life, and they provide shelter and food for birds and wildlife.

incineration: a treatment technology involving destruction of waste by controlled burning at high temperatures.

landfilling: burial of waste in the soil.

land use planning: authority for planning and zoning of land use to promote livable and sustainable communities and minimize waste.

Continued

leachate: a liquid that results from water collecting contaminants as it trickles through waste, pesticides, or fertilizers: leaching may occur in farming areas, feedlots, and landfills and may result in hazardous substances entering ground water, surface water, or soil.

non-point sources (NPSs): a pollution source that does not have a single point of origin, for example, water pollution from parking-lot run off or air pollution from motor vehicles (mobile sources).

outrage factors: characteristics of risk that contribute to the public's response to environmental hazards.

ozone: a chemical oxidant and major component of photochemical smog; produced through complex chemical reactions of nitrogen oxides and hydrocarbons (products of combustion of petroleum projects) and sunlight.

permitting: process of issuing an authorization, license, or equivalent control document to implement the requirements of an environmental regulation.

remediation: implementation of environmental cleanup procedures at a contaminated site.

risk assessment: the qualitative and quantitative evaluation performed in an effort to define the risk posed to human health and the environment by the presence or potential presence and/or use of specific pollutants.

risk communication: sending and receiving information on the magnitude and probability of harm from an environmental hazard, an exposure, or a health threat.

waste minimization: processes that increase efficiency and reduce waste.

water discharge: disposal of waste into surface water by treating the waste so that the dosage of pollutants is not great enough to cause harm or by altering the waste product to a less toxic form.

Why should a textbook for nurses have a chapter on environmental health? It would not be too dramatic to say that the reason is because lives depend on it. From the smallest one-cell organisms in the food chain to the global issues of warming, **ozone** depletion, the loss of living species, and **deforestation,** the environment affects and alters lives.

HUMAN DEPENDENCE ON THE ENVIRONMENT

The science of public health has long recognized environment as a primary determinant of health (Pope, Snyder, and Mood, 1995). Dependence of the human species can be seen through the lens of each of the environmental media: air, water, soil, and food.

Life depends upon pure *air.* Polluting the air affects breathing and life and health. Life depends on the oxygen exchange with green leafy trees and on the temperature of the air. Scientists know that even a one-degree change in the average temperature on the planet makes a difference in the melting of glaciers, water temperatures, sea levels, and plant life. The recent experiences with El Niño and La Niña, the weather phenomena created by changes in temperatures of the Pacific waters, is one example of the planet-wide effect of changes in temperatures of water and air.

Not every scientist agrees about global warming, but in the book *Earth in the Balance,* then Senator and now former Vice President Al Gore could have been writing for nurses. He said, "Global warming is the fever that accompanies a victim's desperate effort to fight off an invading virus whose waste products have begun to contaminate the metabolic processes of the host" (Gore, 1993, p. 216).

Water is necessary for all life forms. Human bodies are made up of 75% water. Only 2.5% of the water on this planet is freshwater, not salt water. Much of the freshwater is in the ice of the polar ice caps; groundwater makes up most of what remains, leaving only 0.01% in lakes, creeks,

streams, rivers, and rainfalls (Gore, 1993). Life depends on freshwater and water's drinkable quality to survive.

Discharges into water bodies from industries and from wastewater treatment systems contribute to decline in water quality. Water quality is also affected by **non-point sources (NPSs)** of pollution, such as storm water run-off from paved roads and parking lots, erosion from clear-cut tracts of land for timbering and mining, run-off from chemicals added to soils as fertilizers and pesticides (whether as large-scale farming operations or from individual lawns and gardens). Animal waste from wildlife or confined animal industries for food production (swine and poultry) can get into nearby water bodies and result in contamination. The result can be illness from ingesting contaminated water and the creating of conditions that allow toxic algae growth (South Carolina Task Group on Toxic Algae, 1998).

Water is necessary for the production of *food* and is also necessary for life. Rudy Mancke, a noted naturalist, has said that any life form that is not a chlorophyll-producing organism is a consumer on this planet, and that includes humans (Mancke, 1998). The quality of the *soil* in which plants grow is essential to the safety of the food chain. The quality of the soil is affected by its water supply and by the potential for disposing of contamination from the air. Soil that is free from harmful contamination and pathogens is basic to life and health.

Human actions affect basic **ecological** shifts and cause insult to the environment. One example is the destruction of forests, which disrupts the basic oxygen exchange and the stability of soil and pollutes bodies of water with sediment. Industry waste discharged into the air affects its quality, as do individually controlled discharges, such as automobile exhaust, which is the largest contributor to ground-level ozone pollution (South Carolina Department of Health and Environmental Control, 1998), and which can cause problems with the human respiratory system.

The chain of potential damage to life continues in the additives to farm produce and to animal diets, such as pesticides, growth hormones, and antibiotics, which become secondary additives to humans who eat the end products. Food preparation, washing food and hands, cooking temperatures, and time all contribute to either prevention or catching of food-borne illnesses. Public health scares have been raised about *alar* in apples and *salmonella* and *Escherichia coli* in chicken, eggs, and hamburger (American Public Health Association, 1995). The sanitary preparation of food is important to health whether it takes place in home kitchens, in public eating places, or in the handling of food and milk in canning, freezing, and packaging for eating.

The bottom line is that life depends on the environment, and what humans do collectively affects that vital resource for present and future generations. A central theme in Native American cultures is that humans are stewards, not owners, of the environment. Native Americans make the "Rule of Seven"—What will be the effect on the seventh generation?—central to all environmental decisions. This long-term view is essential to environmental health.

Briefly Noted

The number of waterborne disease outbreaks from infectious agents and chemical poisoning increased in the 1990s. These have become major community health issues.

HEALTHY PEOPLE 2000 AND 2010 OBJECTIVES AND ENVIRONMENTAL HEALTH

Environmental health was one of the 22 priority areas of the *Healthy People 2000* objectives. The federal government is recognizing the importance of environmental risks and the underlying factors causing diseases; therefore 17 environmental health objectives were found in this report. These objectives are listed in the *Healthy People 2010* box. As of the mid-1990s, three of the objectives were progressing in the correct direction:

1. Increase the number of people with clean air in their communities
2. Increase the number of people with radon-tested houses
3. Elimination of the incidence of children with blood lead levels of 25 mcq/dl (U.S. Public Health Service, 1995).

Box 5-1 presents *Healthy People 2010* environmental health target improvements.

Briefly Noted

Factors contributing to the reduction of lead levels in the United States include eliminating lead in gasoline; reducing the number of manufactured foods, cans, and household plumbing components containing lead solder; passing lead screening laws; and conducting lead paint abatement programs in communities.

PROTECTING THE ENVIRONMENT

Sanitarians or civil engineers were the first workers to be hired by government to protect the environment, usually addressing

Healthy People 2010 Objectives Related to Environmental Health

- Reduce the proportion of persons exposed to air that does not meet the U.S. EPA health based standards for harmful air pollutants.
- Increase use of alternative modes of transportation to reduce motor vehicle emissions and improve the nation's air quality.
- Improve the nation's air quality by increasing the use of cleaner alternative fuels.
- Reduce air toxic emissions to decrease the risk of adverse health effects caused by airborne toxic substances.
- Increase the proportion of persons served by community water systems who receive a supply of drinking water that meets the regulations of the Safe Drinking Water Act.
- Reduce the waterborne disease outbreaks arising from water intended for drinking among persons served by community water systems.
- Reduce the per capital domestic water withdrawals.
- Increase the proportion of assessed rivers, lakes, and estuaries that are safe for fishing and recreational purposes.
- Reduce the number of beach closings that result from the presence of harmful bacteria.
- Reduce the potential human exposure to persistent chemicals by decreasing fish contaminant levels.
- Eliminate elevated blood lead levels in children.
- Minimize the risks to human health and the environment posed by hazardous sites.
- Reduce pesticide exposures that result in visits to a health care facility.
- Reduce the amount of toxic pollutants released, disposed of, treated, or used for energy recovery.
- Increase recycling.

From U.S. Public Health Service: *Healthy people 2010: understanding and improving health,* Washington, D.C., 2000, available online at www.health.gov/healthypeople.

Box 5-1   Targets of Environmental Health Improvements in *Healthy People 2010*

- Asthma hospitalizations
- Prevalence of serious mental retardation
- Waterborne diseases
- Blood lead levels exceeding 15 and 25 mg/dl
- Counties exceeding standards for air pollution
- Radon testing
- Toxic agent releases
- Solid waste production and disposal
- Safe drinking water
- Impaired surface waters: rivers, lakes, estuaries
- Home testing for lead-based paint
- Construction standards to minimize radon levels
- State disclosure laws for radon levels and lead-based paint
- Health risks from hazardous waste sites
- Household hazardous waste collection
- State laws and funds to track sentinel environmental diseases
- Children's exposure to tobacco smoke at home

From U.S. Public Health Service: *Healthy people 2010: understanding and improving health,* Washington, D.C., 2000, available online at www.health.gov/healthypeople.

safety of wastewater. Others were added, for example, hydrogeologists (water geologists), chemists, biologists, and climatologists (weather experts) to the environmental health team to improve progress in solving environmental problems. Nurses and others who are medical and community experts add to the interdisciplinary work of environmental health. There are some differences among states in the organization and approach to environmental protection, but the common essential strategies of prevention and control are found in every state.

Prevention

As in every community intervention, prevention is a basic value. Preventing problems is less costly than correcting them, whether the cost is measured in resources, like money spent, or human effects, like morbidity. Education is a primary preventive strategy. State and local environmental protection agencies educate individuals, groups, and communities about environmental issues and ways to prevent environmental problems.

Examples of education interventions are numerous. Environmental staff meet with and speak to individuals, neighborhood and civic organizations, and schools. Educational materials that cover a wide range of topics and are tailored to the needs of different groups in the population are developed and distributed. In some states (e.g., South Carolina) curricula for teaching environmental protection have been developed with classroom teachers from the kindergarten level through high school, and training in their use is provided to school districts.

Many initiatives to reduce the production of wastes that require disposal target the general population, but some states also have organized units to assist industry, in a nonregulatory capacity, to identify ways to reduce wastes in their operations. This is called **waste minimization.** Industries participate as partners with health and environmental advocates and regulators because they recognize that less waste means more efficient operations, less cost for waste disposal, and improved health in their community.

Land use planning is another effective prevention strategy. Authority for planning and zoning of land use is usually given to local (city and county) governments. Thoughtful attention to separating industry and residential areas; preserving green space with parks, greenways, and land trusts; and limiting the types of industries recruited and welcomed can result in more livable and healthy communities. Good planning can also expand the opportunity for the location of industries that can partner with others to dispose of waste or provide raw materials.

Federal and state governments can support local planning processes. State initiatives, like Maryland's "Smart Growth," promote planning through incentives to reduce urban sprawl (Glendening, 1998). Both state and federal support for mass-transit systems and walking/biking paths can prevent pollution from too many automobiles with harmful emissions and an over-dependence on automobile use.

Control

Potentially harmful pollution that cannot be prevented must be controlled. Control involves *permitting, setting standards,*

monitoring, compliance, enforcing, and *remediating.* The first step in the process of controlling pollution is **permitting.** Industries and businesses whose processes will result in releases (discharges or emissions) that have the potential for harm are required to obtain environmental permits to build and operate a plant with standards that are protective of the environment and the public's health. Many permits may be required (e.g., stormwater control, construction, procedures for air and wastewater discharges, and waste management). It is in the government's permitting process that some of the previously mentioned prevention strategies can be exercised. For example, waste minimization can be included as a permit condition, with the agreement of the industry, even if it is not required by law or regulation. Once a condition exists in the permit, it has the force of law.

There is usually some form of public participation required or included voluntarily in the permit process and can include public notice, public comment, public meetings, and hearings initiated by the government regulatory agency. Limits on what an industry or business can lawfully release into the air or water are based on environmental standards.

Environmental Standards

A standard is often reflective of a level of pollution that will limit the number of excess deaths at a given level of exposure over a specified period of time. The primary goal of environmental standards is protecting human health, as well as considering the cost and feasibility to the industry. It is obvious that standards protective of human health cannot be developed through broad population research experiments, using standard scientific methods, with one population group exposed to various doses and another matched group used as controls. The options for setting standards that are protective of human health and safety include the following:

- *Using laboratory animal experiments.* This option has the advantage of a relatively short timeline, which is also one of the drawbacks. In laboratory experiments, small animals are exposed to large doses of chemicals over a short time period and results are observed and measured. General assumptions are made about how humans would react to the chemicals in smaller doses over longer periods of time.
- *Using data from worker studies.* Conclusions are drawn from data on relatively healthy adults who work with chemicals at close range in enclosed controlled environments for a limited time during a day. It is difficult to know if reactions would be the same in a population, varying in age and health status, living 24 hours a day at some distance in an open environment, subject to differing weather conditions.
- *Learning from the effects on persons exposed through disasters.* Examples would be tracking the health effects of persons exposed to bombing of Hiroshima in World War II and the more recent nuclear plant accident at Chernobyl in the former Soviet Union.

The uncertainty in conclusions from any of these imperfect methods requires that a significant safety factor be built into the standard. For example, the standard level of acceptable contamination of drinking water may be the level of exposure that would produce one excess (over the expected rate) cancer death if a person drank 1 liter of the water each day for 70 years. Cancer deaths have been the most frequently used outcome measure in environmental standards, but the outcome measures are now expanding to include birth defects, reproductive disorders, immune function disorders, and morbidity (kidney, liver, respiratory, neurotoxic conditions) (Pope, Snyder, and Mood, 1995) (Box 5-2 and Table 5-1). There is no situation in which the need for research is more evident than in setting environmental standards. The costs for good-quality studies are very high.

Monitoring

Once environmental standards are set, the next step in control is monitoring. Any monitoring process must use methods approved by the federal Environmental Protection Agency (EPA) or by consensus of the environmental scientific community. Monitoring procedures must follow accepted protocols, for example, maintaining a documented chain of custody of samples (may be water, air, soil) to ensure accuracy and protection from post-sampling contamination at a laboratory. Environmental monitoring takes two main forms. One is actual inspections of permitted industries to observe first-hand whether the plans submitted in the permit application are being conducted as approved. In addition to unannounced inspections, continuous monitoring of data and operating procedures required in permits are studied for any differences from what is allowed. Finally, periodic measures of the industries' air and water emissions are measured directly for compliance with laws and regulations.

An alternative monitoring method is self-reported data from the regulated industry. Factors such as costs, reliability, public trust, and acceptance must be considered in deciding how much of the monitoring requirement can be met through self-reporting.

Beyond the monitoring of individual permitted facilities, official regulatory agencies design sampling networks for measuring the quality of water and air throughout the geographic area for which they have responsibility. Routine samples are taken at specific monitoring sites and analyzed for contamination; levels are measured nationwide for air and water (Boxes 5-3 and 5-4).

Compliance and enforcement are the next building blocks in controlling environmental damage. **Compliance** refers to the processes for seeing that permitting requirements are met. When violations of permits or other legally defined restrictions are found, the first effort is to get quick, voluntary compliance from the violator (the industry). Incentives in the form of reducing or eliminating fines and

Box 5-2 Cancer Deaths Attributable to Selected Factors

LIFESTYLE
Alcohol
Tobacco
Diet
Infection
Reproduction and sexual behavior

SOCIETAL
Occupation
Industrial products
Food additives
Medicines and medicinal procedures

ENVIRONMENTAL
Pollution
Geophysical factors
Cumulative attributable

Based on data from U.S. Public Health Service: *Healthy people 2010*, Washington, D.C., 2000, Department of Health and Human Services.

Box 5-3 Criteria Air Pollutants (National Ambient Air Quality Standards)

- Ozone (ground level)
- Sulfur dioxide
- Nitrogen dioxide
- Particulate matter
- Carbon monoxide
- Lead

TABLE 5-1 Environmental Agents Implicated in Adverse Reproductive Outcomes

Exposure	Known or Suspected Effect
Anesthetic compounds	Infertility, spontaneous abortion, fetal malformations, low birth weight
Antineoplastics	Infertility, spontaneous abortion
Dibromochloropropane	Sperm abnormalities, infertility
Ionizing radiation	Infertility, microcephaly, chromosomal abnormalities, childhood malignancies
Lead	Infertility, spontaneous abortion, developmental disabilities
Manganese	Infertility
Organic mercury	Developmental disabilities, neurologic abnormalities
Organic solvents	Congenital malformations, childhood malignancies
PCBs, PBBs	Fetal mortality, low birth weight, congenital abnormalities, developmental disabilities

From Aldrich T, Griffith J: *Environmental epidemiology and risk assessment*, New York, 1993, Von Nostrand Reinhold.

Box 5-4	Routine Water Analysis (Private Well)

BACTERIOLOGICAL	CHEMICAL
Total coliform	Lead
Fecal coliform	Hardness
Chlorine residual	Nitrates
	Chloride
	Alkalinity
	Iron
	pH
	Copper
	Calcium
	Manganese
	Magnesium
	Zinc

penalties may be negotiated in return for rapid and effective action to correct the problem. Formal **enforcement** actions are taken when voluntary compliance is not achieved, including fines or penalties, suspended operations, or closing the facility. If the violation is found to be willful, with full knowledge that it was unlawful, criminal law may provide for prison terms for the owners and/or operators in addition to other consequences.

Clean-up or **remediation** of environmental damage is the final control step. The authority to direct and see that actions are taken to restore adequate environmental quality may lie directly with state or federal government agencies, or it may be contracted out to private companies who are given official government oversight. For example, a contaminated site like the Love Canal in New York, where waste was illegally dumped and houses had to be removed, may meet the requirements for the federal "Superfund" National Priority List (Comprehensive Environmental Response Compensation and Liability Act [CERCLA]). In this case the EPA would assume the lead responsibility for clean-up. In contrast, at a site where an operating industry is violating air and water standards, the state may take the lead, either under state law or by delegated responsibility from the EPA.

Public information and involvement, such as citizen advisory panels or community forums, are necessary to select remedial action that fits plans for future land use. These remedies must be acceptable to the affected community as part of the decision process.

CITIZEN ROLES

Where do nurses enter this picture? It is best to begin with the basic roles of nurses as informed citizens and to consider the actions each person takes to protect and conserve water and trees, to reduce waste, to recycle, and to prevent and clean up litter in the environment.

In the citizen role, nurses are respected and trusted messengers. There are several examples of community groups depending on nurses as providers of accurate information

and as spokespersons on environmental issues. In one example, a citizen group led by a nurse was organized to protect the quality of the air. This group not only had an effect on a local industry but also influenced the passing of a state air toxicity law. In another community, a nurse organizer and spokesperson influenced a county land use decision that prevented the location of an asphalt plant in a neighborhood. As informed citizens, nurses can foster community action to address environmental dangers that can be threats to health.

NURSING'S ENVIRONMENTAL HERITAGE

Within the profession, there is widespread recognition that nurses, like physicians, are taught very little about the environment and environmental threats to health. This recognition and the concern it generates led to two separate studies by the Institute of Medicine (IOM) in the National Academy of Science. The IOM conducted a study of environmental medicine (Warren and Goldstein, 1988) and a study of nursing, which produced the report *Nursing, Health, and Environment* (Pope, Snyder, and Mood, 1995).

Briefly Noted

"Freedom from illness or injury is related to lack of exposure to toxic agents and other environmental conditions that are potentially detrimental to human health" (Pope, Snyder, and Mood, 1995, p. 3).

The IOM nursing study recognized that concern for the environment as a **determinant** of health is deeply rooted in nursing's heritage. Pictures of and quotes from Florence Nightingale are used throughout the report, not only because she is a recognized symbol of nursing (as the lady with the lamp), but also because she taught that environmental conditions can lead to illness.

Briefly Noted

"In watching diseases, both in private homes and in public hospitals, the thing which strikes the experienced observer most forcibly is this, that the symptoms or the sufferings generally considered to be inevitable and incident to the disease are very often not symptoms of the disease at all, but of something quite different—of the want of fresh air, or of light, or of warmth, or of quiet, or of cleanliness, or of punctuality and care in the administration of diet, of each or of all of these. . ." (Nightingale, 1859, p. 8).

Lillian Wald spent her life improving the environment of the Henry Street neighborhood and working her broad network of influential contacts to make changes in the physical environment and social conditions that had direct health effects on her clients. A twentieth-century nurse leader, Virginia Henderson offered a definition of nursing that many nurses were taught in their first "fundamentals" course. That definition provided a broad and reliable direction for practice that fostered prevention and moving toward self-sufficiency, two key elements in environmental health.

Briefly Noted

"The unique function of the nurse is to assist the individual, sick or well, in the performance of those activities contributing to health or its recovery (or to a peaceful death) that the client would perform unaided if he/she had the necessary strength, will, or knowledge. It is likewise the function of nurses to help people gain independence as rapidly as possible" (Henderson, 1966, p. 15).

ENVIRONMENTAL HEALTH COMPETENCIES FOR NURSES

If nurses believe that they belong in the picture of environmental health, what do nurses need to know to be effective partners in the enterprise? The 1995 IOM study *Nursing, Health, and Environment* (Pope, Snyder, and Mood, 1995) identifies four general environmental health competencies for nurses, which are presented in Box 5-5 and discussed in the following sections.

Basic Knowledge

No single chapter in a book can provide all the environmental science needed for competent nursing practice. The science base is too large and is constantly undergoing change. Interdisciplinary practice makes it unnecessary for the nurse to be an in-depth expert in environmental science. It is essential to have a basic understanding of four principles and how they explain environmental threats to health and environmental protection needs. Nurses will want to have a working knowledge of how to access other information as the situation demands.

Environmental Principle 1: *Everything is connected to everything else.*

This principle is introduced in elementary school science, in which students are taught about the water cycle of evaporation and condensation. The consequences of the connectedness of all things in the environment can be seen in Figure 5-1. Lead in paint is a good example, banned in 1978 but still present in older homes in poorer neighborhoods, and in restored homes in more affluent communities. More than 80% of U.S. homes built before 1978—some 64 million—contain lead paint (Environmental Protection Agency, 1996). The lead-containing paint chips are scraped, become airborne in breathing space for a brief time, and then end up in nearby soil. Children play in the soil, where their hand-to-mouth activity results in exposure to lead that has develop-

Box 5-5	General Environmental Health Competencies for Nurses

BASIC KNOWLEDGE AND CONCEPTS

All nurses should understand the scientific principles and underpinnings of the relationship between individuals or populations and the environment (including the work environment). This understanding includes the basic mechanism and pathways of exposure to environmental health hazards, basic prevention and control strategies, the interdisciplinary nature of effective interventions, and the role of research.

ASSESSMENT AND REFERRAL

All nurses should be able to successfully complete an environmental health history, recognize potential environmental hazards and sentinel illnesses, specific illnesses related to the environmental hazard (e.g., "black lung" in coal miners), and make appropriate referrals for conditions with probable environmental causes. An essential component is the ability to access and provide information to clients and communities and to locate referral sources.

ADVOCACY, ETHICS, AND RISK COMMUNICATION

All nurses should be able to demonstrate knowledge of the role of advocacy (case and class), ethics, and risk communication in client care and community intervention with respect to the potential adverse effects of the environment on health.

LEGISLATION AND REGULATION

All nurses should understand the policy framework and major pieces of legislation and regulations related to environmental health.

From Pope AM, Snyder MA, Mood LH (editors): *Nursing, health, and environment,* Washington, D.C., 1995, Institute of Medicine, National Academy Press.

mental and behavioral effects, both known and being discovered through research (Box 5-6).

Lead poisoning is a top environmental health hazard in young children, affecting as many as 1.7 million children 5 years of age and under (Environmental Protection Agency, 1996). The remedies for lead contamination have a required chain of their own: education for prevention, screening (both the victim and the source), treatment (in the individual and the environment), and authority for regulatory and remedial action in public policy. The principle of connectedness is the essence of tracking exposures and risks (Box 5-7).

Environmental Principle 2: *Everything has to go somewhere.*

Again this principle can be traced to science taught in elementary education: matter cannot be created or destroyed. Once waste products are generated, they must be disposed of in one of three ways:

- **Incineration.** Burning can change the chemical composition through heat, but the products of burning such as ash and air emissions must be controlled and disposed of in one of the other options below.
- **Water discharge.** To interrupt the exposure pathway, the products to be disposed of in water must be treated

<table>
</table>

Box 5-6   Example of Principle 1

A citizen calls the local health department to report that his drinking water, from a private well, "smells like gasoline." A water sample is collected, and analysis reveals the presence of petroleum products. A nearby rural store and service station has removed its old underground gasoline storage tanks and replaced them, as required by law. Contaminated soil from the old leaking tank has been removed, and a well to monitor groundwater contamination is scheduled for installation. Sandy soil has allowed more rapid movement of the contamination through the groundwater, and the plume has reached the neighbor's drinking-water well in levels that exceed the drinking-water standard. Possible responses to the problem are short-term alternate drinking water (bottled), long-term extension of water lines from a nearby municipality, monitoring and clean-up of the contaminated groundwater (including testing other wells), testing children for lead poisoning, and informing the community of the risks and remedies.

Box 5-7   Environmental Harm

For persons to be harmed by something in the environment, several factors must be in place and connected (see Fig. 5-1):
- A source of harm that has chemical and/or physical properties
- An environmental medium for transport—air, water (surface and/or groundwater), or soil
- A receptor population within the exposure pathway for harm to human health
- A route of exposure. Humans can be exposed to environmental contaminants through only three routes: inhalation, ingestion, and skin absorption
- An adequate amount (**dose**) of the chemical to result in human harm

to ensure that the dose in the water is not great enough to do harm.
- **Landfilling** or burial in the soil. Protections must be put in place, such as liners and **leachate** pumps and monitors, to avoid seepage of harmful doses into groundwater or air.

Each of the options for waste disposal is intended to either provide a way to alter the waste product to a less toxic form through chemical intervention (**biodegradation**), or store the product in a **bio-unavailable** form or place. Since either of the options for disposal can be a problem, prevention becomes more appealing.

The principles of connectedness and matter occupying space become more important when the issues of population growth and density are considered, as shown in Fig-

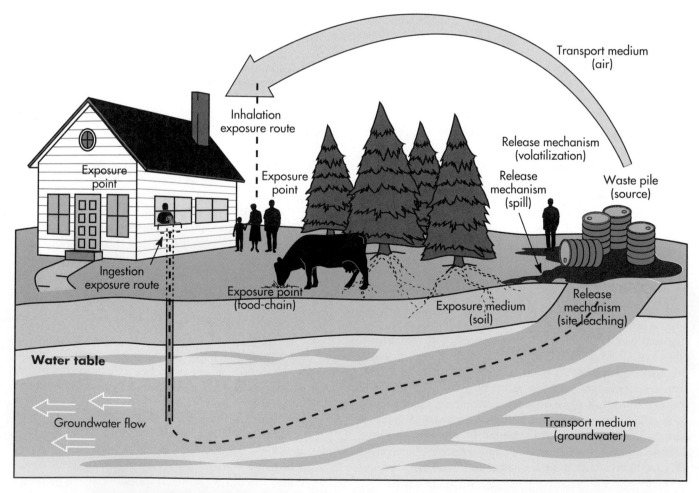

Figure 5-1   Exposure pathways. (From Agency for Toxic Substances and Disease Registry: *Public health assessment guidance manual,* Washington, D.C., 1992, Department of Health and Human Services.)

Evidence-Based Practice

The article referenced in the footnote is a case study of childhood lead exposure in a family living at the poverty level. It is known that child lead exposure is common among those living in poverty and substandard housing. Children and families living along the U.S.-Mexico border experience multiple exposures to environmental hazards, especially lead. The impact of lead exposure on fetuses, infants, and children is dramatically compounded by poor nutrition, extreme poverty, inadequate access to health care, hazardous occupational exposures of other family members, social isolation, language and legal barriers, high-risk home environments, lead-laden herbal home remedies, and medicinal and cultural practices.

In this case of Hispanic children and their families, the authors found evidence to support exposure to lead for many of the reasons listed above, as well as likely exposure pathways, such as inhaling and ingesting lead-laden dust from auto repair, wire recycling, and paint chips.

APPLICATION IN PRACTICE

This research supports the role that nurses can play in doing routine assessments of individuals and groups known to be at risk and providing community health services to reduce the long-term effects of lead exposure.

Amaya MA, et al: Childhood lead poisoning on the US-Mexico border: a case study in environmental health nursing lead poisoning, *Public Health Nurs* 14(6):353, 1997.

ure 5-2. One surprising conclusion may be that family planning could be an important nursing intervention in environmental health. Family planning helps to control the population growth and therefore affects the environmental consequences.

One additional point of emphasis is that human effects are intensified in the most sensitive, vulnerable environments, such as **estuaries,** the nurseries for much of sea and coastal plant and animal life. Some of the most valued food sources are also the most sensitive to pollution. Shellfish are very efficient filters of contaminants in the water in which they live. For example, oysters filter and retain almost all contaminants from the water in which they grow. It is impossible to rid them of contaminants after harvesting. The only protection for humans is to grow oysters in environments free from harmful contamination. Safe seafood depends on clean water. This example leads to the third principle.

Environmental Principle 3: *The solution to pollution is dilution.*

Reflecting on the element of dose in human exposure reveals the truth in this principle. The use of this principle can be seen in historic environmental and sanitation measures. Garbage was moved from streets to the nearest body of water. Early industries went from dumping wastes outside their buildings to piping them to the nearest stream or river. Human wastes followed the same paths and pipelines. The problem with this principle is that it was tied to a world view that saw the environment as an unlimited resource, a limitless repository for

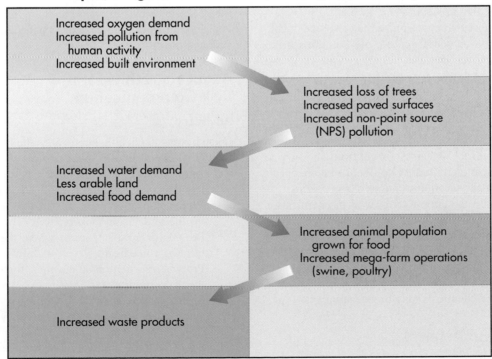

Figure 5-2   Connectedness of population growth and environmental consequences.

whatever was useless. The dilution capacity of large rivers and certainly the ocean seemed boundless. The belief in the capacity of air to dilute resulted in such "solutions" as taller smoke stacks to release pollutants higher into the atmosphere. The reality, which becomes more evident every day, is that this planet's capacity to assimilate by-products of human civilization is far from limitless. It is, in fact, fragile and delicately balanced, and the knowledge and practice about how to live peacefully within that balance without doing harm is far from adequate. The fourth principle reflects this insight.

Environmental Principle 4: *Today's solution may be tomorrow's problem.*

As in almost every aspect of life, environmental scientists and regulators are dealing with incomplete information and insufficient science. The brief history of organized environmental protection is filled with examples. Garbage that went from the streets into unlined landfills is now a source of groundwater contamination. Gasoline tanks that were buried underground to avoid an ugly landscape were found to leak over time. New solutions of lined landfills and double-walled storage tanks, with sensors for leaks and monitoring wells, have emerged, as has the increasing work of cleaning up the earlier "mistakes."

What can now be called mistakes were not necessarily the result of malicious carelessness or insensitivity. Decisions were based on the best information available at the time. The "best information" is often likely to be incomplete and imperfect. That is why research continues to be so necessary. An encouraging trend in industry's new product development is engineering analysis of the full life-cycle of the product, from raw material to waste disposal. Up-front consideration of the costs and effects throughout the cycle can lead to choices that prevent future problems.

One of the greatest challenges and a major source of concern in today's environmental picture are solutions themselves. The growing number and complexity of chemicals that are part of everyday life exemplify this. Citizens have enthusiastically embraced "better living through chemistry," with more than 65,000 new chemical compounds introduced into the environment between 1950 and 1984 (Pope, Snyder, and Mood, 1995). An estimated 1000 or more have been added each year since. The uses range from industry to household to medical, and there is no doubt that chemicals have been a part of the solution to numerous problems.

The problem with the enormous growth in chemicals is that the effects of new chemicals on the environment are unknown. Neighborhoods that are in close proximity to industrial parks express concern that, even when only allowable levels of each chemical are released, no one is able to say what the health effects of exposure to the combination of small amounts of chemicals may be over time.

Assessment and Referral

The second general environmental health competency cited in the IOM study is assessment and referral. Both of these activities are familiar parts of nursing practice, but they have specific meaning in environmental health.

Assessment activities of nurses can range from individual health assessments to being full participants in community assessment or partners in a specific environmental site assessment. The skills and tools may range from developing and using computer-assisted geographic information systems (GIS) to small area analysis or individual exposure history. This section focuses on assessing environmental factors for the effects on an individual's health and using these factors in all health histories and physical examinations.

There are many forms and formats for taking environmental exposure histories. One form is shown in Appendix G.5. The key questions in any assessment should cover past conditions in work, home, and community environments (Pope, Snyder, and Mood, 1995):

1. What are your longest held jobs, current and past?
2. Have you been exposed to any radiation or chemical liquids, dusts, mists, or fumes?
3. Is there any relationship between current symptoms and activities at work or at home?

Referral resources may vary in communities. One starting point may be the environmental epidemiology or toxicology unit of the state health department or environmental agency. Another local or state resource may be environmental medicine experts in medical schools. The Association of Occupational and Environmental Clinics is a network of specialty clinics that are housed in medical schools and are available for consulting about or assessing individual cases and for providing of educational programs for health professionals.

Box 5-8 lists many general referral sources. Table 5-2 lists several major toxic agents and symptoms that may be associated with past exposure to them. Further investigation is needed to determine the exact connection between exposure and the problem.

Advocacy, Ethics, and Risk Communication

Advocacy

In environmental health, nurses are called on to advocate for individual clients and to speak and act on behalf of groups and communities concerning their environment. The nurse advocate may:

- Work from an agency to make community concerns visible to decision makers
- Provide or arrange forums where the community can have its voice heard
- Provide information on technical matters as well as on the decision process
- Speak on behalf of the community in policy discussions when community members may not be present.

Citizen involvement in regulatory decisions that affect the public is often a requirement of environmental law and regulation. Communities and the public can be passionate advocates for the protection of their health, their homes, and

TABLE 5-2	Toxic Agents and Symptoms That May Be Associated With Past Exposure

Agent	Primary Manifestations
Arsenic	Peripheral neuropathy, sensorimotor changes; nausea and vomiting, diarrhea, constipation; dermatitis, fingernail and toenail striations, skin cancer; nasal septum perforation; lung cancer
Lead	Anemia; nephropathy; abdominal pain ("colic"); palsy ("wrist drop"); encephalopathy, behavioral abnormalities; spontaneous abortions
Mercury (organic)	Dermatitis; sensorimotor changes, visual field constriction, tremor
Benzene	Acute CNS depression; leukemia, aplastic anemia; dermatitis
Formaldehyde	Irritant and contact dermatitis; eye irritation; respiratory tract irritation, asthma
Trichloro-ethylene (TCE)	Acute CNS depression; peripheral and cranial neuropathy; irritation; dermatitis; arrhythmias
Ozone	Delayed pulmonary edema (generally 6 to 8 hours after exposure)

Modified from Pope AM, Snyder MA, Mood LH (editors): *Nursing, health, and environment,* Washington, D.C., 1995, Institute of Medicine, National Academy Press.

Box 5-8	Information and Guidance Sources for Referrals

FEDERAL AGENCIES

Agency for Toxic Substances and Disease Registry (ATSDR)
Centers for Disease Control and Prevention (CDC)
Consumer Product Safety Commission
Environmental Protection Agency (EPA)
    Office of Children's Environmental Health
Food and Drug Administration (FDA)
National Institute for Occupational Safety and Health
National Institute of Environmental Health Sciences
National Institutes of Health (NIH)
    National Cancer Institute
    National Institute of Nursing Research
Occupational Safety and Health Administration (OSHA)

STATE AGENCIES

State Health Departments
State Environmental Protection Agencies

ASSOCIATIONS AND ORGANIZATIONS

National Environmental Education and Training Foundation, Inc.
Association of Occupational and Environmental Clinics
Society for Occupational and Environmental Health (SOEH)
American Association of Poison Control Centers
Pesticide Education Center
Teratogen Exposure Registry and Surveillance
American Cancer Society
American Lung Association
American College of Occupational and Environmental Medicine

their neighborhoods. They may see threats to their safety and quality of life in proposed new or expanded industry and many times do not see the benefits. They may be openly vocal about their distrust of the government charged with protecting them.

Because forums for public participation cause adversity and conflict and can become verbally abusive, regulatory agencies have sometimes looked for ways to avoid or min-

imize the opportunities to hear directly from the public. The nurse can be a welcomed partner in the public input process, which may be the activity that is most uncomfortable for environmental scientists. The public generally has known and had experience with nurses as empathic listeners and professionals with the community's interests at heart. Having a nurse as a facilitator of the dialogue allows people to relax a little, knowing they will be heard. Calm and respectful attention can lead to better outcomes in public dialogue. The most positive outcome may be opening the lines of communication between the community and the industry as neighbors, all interested in the well-being of their surroundings.

Ethics

A grounding in ethics is essential for nurses making their own choices, in describing issues and options within groups, and in advocating for ethical choices. When the sticking points are around competing "goods" such as jobs versus environmental protection, or production versus conservation, the skillful nurse can change the discussion from "either/or" to "both" by opening new possibilities for both ethical and mutually satisfactory outcomes. Ethical issues likely to arise in environmental health decisions are as follows:
- Who has access to information and when?
- How complete and accurate is the available information?
- Who is included in decision making and when?
- What and whose values and priorities are given weight in decisions?
- How are short- and long-term consequences considered?

Risk Communication

Sandman, Chess, and Hane (1991) noted that, in their experience, the reaction to things that scare people and the things that kill people are often not related to the actual hazard. They have gone further to probe what is behind those differences and identified a list of 20 **outrage factors** to explain people's responses to risk (Table 5-3). They maintain that the outrage is just as predictable and open to intervention as the science of addressing the hazard (Box 5-9).

TABLE 5-3   Outrage Factors: Characteristics of Risk That Contribute to the Public's Feeling of More or Less Outrage

Safer = Less Outrage	Less Safe = More Outrage
12 Primary Outrage Factors	
Voluntary	Involuntary (coerced)
Natural	Industrial (artificial)
Familiar	Exotic
Not memorable	Memorable
Not dreaded	Dreaded
Chronic	Catastrophic
Knowable (detectable)	Unknowable (undetectable)
Individually controlled	Controlled by others
Fair	Unfair
Morally irrelevant	Morally relevant
Trustworthy sources	Untrustworthy sources
Responsive process	Unresponsive process
8 Secondary Outrage Factors	
Affects average populations	Affects vulnerable populations
Immediate effects	Delayed effects
No risk to future generations	Substantial risk to future generations
Victims statistical	Victims identifiable
Preventable	Not preventable (only reducible)
Substantial benefits	Few benefits (foolish risk)
Little media attention	Substantial media attention
Little opportunity for collective action	Much opportunity for collective action

Communication of risk involves understanding the outrage factors of risk so they can be included in the message—the information—to either reduce unnecessary fear or produce action to ensure safety or prevent harm. An example of raising outrage to produce action can be seen in the shift from emphasis on smokers (voluntary risk) to victims of passive smoking (involuntary risk) to stimulate policies that limit or ban smoking in public places. When the emphasis on risk went from a voluntary choice of smokers to an involuntary exposure of nonsmokers, the outrage level of the non-smoking public became high enough to lead to legislation guaranteeing smoke-free public spaces such as public buildings, airplanes, and restaurants.

Outrage diminishes when people get information on the situation from a trusted source, and nurses can be trusted sources of information on environmental risks. The public trust is a compelling incentive to match professional knowledge and skills to a community's expectations. Reducing the outrage factor can also be a driving force in building credibility and trustworthiness in every person whose work involves interacting with the public.

Box 5-9   **Example of Reducing Outrage**

Consider the situation that occurred in a neighborhood of apartment residents with a stream nearby where children played. During a routine sample testing of the stream water, a local environmental staff discovered a chemical known to be used by a neighboring industry. The industry was notified and immediately began a search for the source. A sign was posted that warned persons to avoid contact with the stream—"No swimming or wading." The apartment management was contacted, and a meeting with residents was arranged.

The early meeting meant that a lot of information was not yet known—how the chemical got into the stream, how much had been released or spilled, and how long it would take to restore the stream to a safe level. However, the rapid response, the obvious concern of the industry, the availability of a qualified toxicologist skilled in public interactions, and the rationale for early contact ("We thought it would be irresponsible not to alert you early, to protect your children's safety, even though we do not have full information on the problem to give to you") resulted in a reassured rather than an outraged community. Plans were made for what would be done, and arrangements were made for updating the residents as new information became available. The citizens left the meeting knowing that their government was acting quickly in their best interests and that their industrial neighbors were taking their responsibility for correcting the problem seriously. Using the language of the risk formula (i.e., risk = hazard + outrage), the outrage was addressed before the hazard itself could be resolved.

Risk communication includes all the principles of good communication in general. It is a combination of the following:
- *The right information*—accurate, relevant, in a language that audiences can understand
- *To the right people*—those affected and those who are worried but may not be affected
- *At the right time* for timely action or to allay fear.

Five themes recur in communicating with the public as presented below.

HOW TO Interact With the Public

1. *Listen.* Really listen; do not just wait your turn to speak.
2. *Take the public seriously.* Even when the hazard is minimal, their concern is real and deserves a serious response.
3. *Treat people with respect.* Even, perhaps especially, when outrage is high. Underlying the loud voices and the anger will almost always be feelings of fear and power-lessness. Do not give away your power as a knowledgeable, caring, and responsible professional by reacting to anger or blaming with anger or defensiveness.
4. *Give the public "straight" information.* Tell them what is known, when it was known, what is not known, and what is being done to learn more. Always provide information in language that is understandable.
5. *Do what you say you will do.* This includes everything from returning phone calls to taking major action steps.

From Mood LH: Environmental health policy: environmental justice. In Mason SW, Leavitt JK (editors): *Policy and politics in nursing and health care*, ed 3, Philadelphia, 1998, WB Saunders.

Evidence-Based Practice

The purpose of the study listed in the footnote was to look at differences in environmental tobacco smoke exposure between smokers and nonsmokers. The study method used a diary of 1 full day's activities. The presence of smoke in their environment was reported on in this way by 1579 Californians. Active smoke and passive smoke from tobacco are chemically similar.

This study concluded that clients who smoke incur greater exposure to the harmful effects of smoking since they report up to four times more passive smoke exposure than nonsmokers. Smokers tend to associate with other smokers and/or spend more exposure time in the company of others who smoke. Therefore smokers are exposed to the chemical effects of their own active smoking as well as the passive smoking of others. There smokers have two risk factors from the ill effects of tobacco: the number of tobacco products they actively use and the passive smoke inhalation from other smokers.

APPLICATION IN PRACTICE

A suggestion may be that the workplace construct separately ventilated smoking lounges to meet the needs of the smoking workforce and to protect the health of nonsmoking workers.

Robinson JP, Switzer P, Ott W: Daily exposure to environmental tobacco smoke: smokers vs nonsmokers in California, *Am J Public Health* 86(9):1303, 1996.

Box 5-10 Major Federal Environmental Laws

- Clean Air Act (CAA)
- Clean Water Act (CWA)
- Safe Drinking Water Act (SDWA)
- Comprehensive Environmental Response, Compensation, and Liability Act (CERCLA)
- Resource Conservation and Recovery Act (RCRA)
- Federal Insecticide, Fungicide, and Rodenticide Act (FIFRA)
- Toxic Substances Control Act (TSCA)
- Marine Protection, Research, and Sanctuaries Act (MPRSA)
- Uranium Mill Tailings Radiation Control Act (UMTRCA)
- Pollution Prevention Act (PPA)

ify that no environmental permit application will be considered that is inconsistent with local zoning ordinances.

Environmental laws are generally written separately for each medium (air, water, and soil) and have been enacted and amended at different times. The patchwork result means that there may be differences among laws and regulations, particularly in public participation requirements, and there may be gaps where no specific law or rule exists. A working knowledge of environmental laws and regulations is essential if the nurse is to provide access to accurate information for communities, guide communities through public participation and decision-making processes, inform communities of their rights, and recognize advocacy needs and opportunities.

ROLES FOR NURSES IN ENVIRONMENTAL HEALTH

Nurses can be involved in a number of roles in environmental health, in full-time work, as a part of existing responsibilities, and as informed citizens. These roles include:
- Community involvement and public participation
- Individual and population **risk assessment**
- Risk communication
- Teaching others.

HOW TO Apply the Nursing Process to Environmental Health

If you suspect that a client's health problem is being influenced by environmental factors, follow the nursing process and note the environmental aspects of the problem in every step of the process:
1. *Assessment.* Include inventories and history questions that have environmental items as a part of the general assessment.
2. *Diagnosis.* Relate the disease and the environmental factors in the diagnosis.
3. *Goal setting.* Include outcome measures that change or eliminate the environmental factors.
4. *Planning.* Look at community policy and laws as methods to facilitate the care needs for the client; include environmental health personnel in planning.

These are good-quality indicators in risk communication and a means of becoming a trustworthy source of information in the public's eyes. These actions are always within the health professional's control, and they always make a difference.

Legislation and Regulation

The fourth general competency in environmental health practice is to be familiar with the laws and regulations of environmental health. Some environmental laws relating to sanitary practices have been a part of public health for a long time. The EPA was not established until 1970, followed by major federal environmental laws, such as the Clean Air Act and the Safe Drinking Water Act, and the "Superfund" legislation that provides funding for environmental clean-up of the most seriously contaminated sites where no responsible party can be found (Environmental Protection Agency, 1993) (Box 5-10).

Sources of laws and ordinances bring variety to regulation among states and local areas. State laws supplement federal laws in addressing water quality, air quality, and waste management and may impose stricter requirements than federal statutes, with some exceptions, but may not be more lenient. Local ordinances can impose additional requirements to protect communities from environmental hazards of pollution and growth. Some state statutes require that local requirements be met before considering an industry's permit application. For example, a state law may spec-

5. *Intervention.* Coordinate medical, nursing, and community health actions to meet the client's needs.
6. *Evaluation.* Examine criteria that include the immediate and long-term responses of the client as well as a recurrence of the problem for the client.

Clinical Application

At the county health department, a 3-year-old boy named Billy is brought in because of gastric upset and behavior changes. These symptoms have persisted for several weeks. Billy's parents report that they have been renovating their home to remove lead paint. They had been discouraged from routinely testing their child because their insurance does not cover testing and they could not find information on where to have the test done. Their concern has heightened with the persistent symptoms in their child.

The nurse tests Billy's blood-lead level and finds that it is high. She researches lead poisoning and discovers that children are at great risk because of their inclination to absorb lead into their central nervous systems. The nurse also finds that chronic lead poisoning may have long-term effects, such as developmental delays and impaired learning ability. She refers Billy to his primary care physician. On further investigation, the nurse finds that Billy's home was built before 1950 and is still under renovation. The sanitarian tests the interior paint and finds a high lead content. Ample amounts of sawdust from sanding are noted in various rooms of the home. The nurse determines that a completed exposure pathway exists.

A. *What would the nurse include in an assessment of this situation?*
B. *What prevention strategies would you use to resolve this issue?*
* *At the individual level?*
* *At the population level?*

Answers are in the back of the book.

 Remember This!

* Nurses have responsibilities to be informed consumers and to be advocates for citizens in their community regarding environmental health issues.
* Proving a connection allows for the identification of risk and exposure in environmental health.
* Incineration, discharge, and landfills allow waste products to be altered to a less toxic or bio-unavailable form.
* There is a lack of scientific evidence of the health effects of many new and existing chemical compounds.
* Prevention activities include education, minimizing waste, and land use planning.
* Control activities include environmental permitting, environmental standards, monitoring, compliance and enforcement, and clean up and remediation.

* Every nursing assessment should include questions and observations concerning intended and unintended environmental exposures.
* Advocacy skills are important for nurses in environmental health practice.
* Risk communication is an important skill and must acknowledge the outrage factor experienced by individuals and groups facing environmental hazards.
* Federal, state, and local laws and regulations exist to protect the health of citizens from environmental hazards.
* Environmental health practice engages multiple disciplines, and nurses are important members of the environmental health team.
* Environmental health practice includes principles of health promotion, disease prevention, and health protection.
* *Healthy People 2000* and *Healthy People 2010* objectives both address targets for the reduction of risk factors and diseases related to environmental causes.

 What Would You Do?

1. Do you believe that waste materials from outside the United States should be accepted into the landfills in the United States as one method of increasing revenue sources for state budgets? Explain your answer.
2. Should access to information on toxic substances leaching into the water table of a community be withheld from the public until the government completes negotiations with the party responsible for the toxic substance? Why?
3. Discover if your jurisdiction has a law or regulation for the disclosure of radon levels for personal property as part of the act of sale for real estate. If your community does not, what would you do?

REFERENCES

American Public Health Association: *Control of communicable diseases manual,* ed 16, Washington, D.C., 1995, The Association.

Environmental Protection Agency: *Access EPA,* EPA pub no 220-B-93-008, Washington, D.C., 1993, Environmental Protection Agency.

Environmental Protection Agency: *Environmental health threats to children,* Washington, D.C., 1996, Environmental Protection Agency.

Glendening PN: *Smart growth and neighborhood conservation,* Annapolis, Md, 1998, Maryland Office of Planning (www.op.state.md.us/smart growth).

Gore A: *Earth in the balance,* New York, 1993, Penguin Books.

Mancke R: Nature walk lecture, Congaree Swamp National Monument, SC, April, 1998.

Pope AM, Snyder MA, Mood LH (editors): *Nursing, health, and environment,* Washington, D.C., 1995, Institute of Medicine, National Academy Press.

Sandman PM, Chess C, Hane BJ: *Improving dialogue with communities,* New Brunswick, NJ, 1991, Rutgers University.

South Carolina Department of Health and Environmental Control: *quality of the environment in South Carolina,* Columbia, SC, 1998, South Carolina Department of Health and Environmental Control.

South Carolina Task Group on Toxic Algae: State task group studies *P. fiesteria,* 1:1, 1998.

U.S. Public Health Service: *Healthy people 2000: midcourse review and revisions,* Washington, D.C., 1995, U.S. Department of Health and Human Services.

Warren JV, Goldstein BD: *Role of the primary care physician in occupational and environmental medicine,* Washington, D.C., 1988, Institute of Medicine, National Academy Press.

Chapter 6

Political and Legal Influences

JOYCE BONICK

OBJECTIVES

After reading this chapter, the student should be able to:

- Describe the trends and roles of several levels of government.
- Identify the effect of changing governmental roles and structures on health care.
- Describe the major governmental functions in health care.

- Discuss nursing roles in selected governmental agencies.
- Influence health policy by participating in the regulation-making process and the political arena.
- Describe selected laws that affect community health nursing practice, both generally and in specialty areas of practice.

CHAPTER OUTLINE

Political and Legal Influences

Important Terms in Policy and Politics

Governmental Role in Health Care
    Trends and Shifts in Governmental Roles
    Governmental Health Care Functions

Organization of Government Agencies
    International Organizations
    Federal Agencies
    State and Local Government Departments
    Social Welfare Programs

The Nurse's Role in the Political Process

Private-Sector Influence on Regulation and Health Policy

Laws Affecting Community-Oriented Nursing Practice
    Types of Laws
    General Community Health Nursing Practice and the Law
    Specialty Community-Oriented Nursing Practice and the Law

KEY TERMS

Code of Regulations: federal and state legal documents in which finalized regulations are published.

Division of Nursing: a component of the Public Health Service, part of the Health Resources and Services Administration, that oversees nursing education and special nursing demonstration projects in the United States.

Federal Register: a legal document in which all U.S.-government–proposed new regulations are published.

government: the ultimate authority in society, designated to enforce the policy whether it is related to health, education, economics, social welfare, or any other societal issue.

health policy: a set course of action to get a desired health outcome for an individual, family, group, community, or society.

law: the sum total of man-made rules and regulations by which society is governed in a formal and legally binding manner.

legislative process: the process used within governments to make laws.

National Institute of Nursing Research: one of the National Institutes of Health charged with promoting the growth and quality of research in nursing.

nurse practice acts: state laws that govern the practice of nurses and set boundaries that limit the practice of nursing by others.

Occupational Safety and Health Administration (OSHA): federal agency charged with improving worker health and safety by establishing standards and regulations and by educating workers.

police power: states' power to act to protect the health, safety, and welfare of their citizens.

policy: settled course of action to be followed by a government or institution to obtain a desired end.

KEY TERMS—cont'd

politics: the art of influencing others to accept a specific course of action.

Public Health Service (PHS): an arm of the Department of Health and Human Services that fulfills the function of overseeing health care services within the United States.

regulations: specific statements of rules or orders having the force of laws that relate to and clarify individual pieces of legislation

respondeat superior: when nurses or other health care workers are employed and functioning within the scope of that job, the employer is responsible for the employee's negligent actions. By directing an employee to carry out a particular function, the employer becomes responsible for negligence, along with the individual employee, including nurses.

scope of practice: the usual and customary practice of a profession taking into account how legislation defines the practice of that profession within a particular jurisdiction (local, state, community, or nationally).

sovereign immunity: doctrine by which an agency may be exempt from a lawsuit for particular kinds of actions. As an example, in some instances government health care agencies cannot be sued for negligence.

U.S. Department of Health and Human Services (USDHHS): a regulatory agency of the executive branch of government charged with overseeing health and welfare needs of U.S. citizens.

World Health Organization (WHO): an arm of the United Nations that provides worldwide services to promote health.

POLITICAL AND LEGAL INFLUENCES

Nurses and their practice are affected by the political system and the government of the United States, state and local governments, and other institutions responsible for implementing health policy. To promote and protect the practice of nursing and to be certain that nursing's clients receive high-quality care, nurses must be involved in politics and in seeing that appropriate health policies are developed. Politics are a part of the nurse's personal and professional life, including family, the professional organization, the health care agency, and government. For example, recently at the U.S. government level a new Patient's Bill of Rights was developed by a task force appointed by the President. A nurse served on that task force. In one state, a nurse organized a group of health workers and consumers to get a new policy developed to ensure that prenatal care would be available for all women in poverty. Recently a group of nurses joined together in a hospital and challenged the administrators about the numbers of nurses per shift needed to provide safe care to clients in the hospital. Advanced-practice nurses have organized throughout the United States to influence legislators to change laws about prescriptive privilege and reimbursement for nurses. Regardless of the educational preparation or years of experience, all nurses are needed to create changes that are important to both nurses and their clients.

IMPORTANT TERMS IN POLICY AND POLITICS

To understand the relationship between health policy, politics, and laws, one must first understand these terms. **Policy** is a settled course of action to be followed by a government or institution to obtain a desired end. **Health policy** is a set course of action to obtain a desired health outcome, either for an individual, family, group, community, or society. Policies are made not only by governments but also in families and in such institutions as a health department or other health care agency, or a professional organization.

Politics plays a role in the development of such policies. Politics is found in families, professional and employing agencies, and governments. **Politics** is the art of influencing others to accept a specific course of action. Therefore political activities are used to arrive at a course of action (the policy). **Law** is a system of privileges and processes by which people solve problems based on a set of established rules; it is intended to minimize the use of force. Laws govern the relationships of individuals and organizations to other individuals and to government. Through *political action* a policy becomes a law. After a law is established, **regulations** further define the course of action (policy) to be taken by organizations or individuals in reaching an outcome. **Government** is the ultimate authority in society and is designated to enforce the policy whether it is related to health, education, economics, social welfare, or any other society issue. The following discussion explains the role of government in health care.

GOVERNMENT ROLE IN HEALTH CARE

In the United States, the federal and most state governments are composed of three branches: the executive branch is composed of the President (or governor), cabinet, and regulatory units, such as the U.S. Department of Health and Human Services (USDHHS) at the federal level. The executive branch administers and regulates policy. For example, the Division of Nursing of the USDHHS writes criteria to fund nursing education. The legislative branch is made up of two houses of Congress: the Senate and the House of Representatives. The legislative branch passes laws that become policy (e.g., the Medicare amendments of the 1966 Social Security Act). The judicial branch is composed of a Supreme Court. The judicial branch interprets laws and the meaning of policy, as in its interpretation of states' rights to grant abortions.

Briefly Noted

Government has a great deal of influence on the way health care services are delivered and on who receives care. For example, when a government agency makes a change in services that will be covered by Medicare, private insurance companies soon adopt the same policy.

Most legal bases for congress to act in health care are found in Article I, Section 8 of the U.S. Constitution. These include:

1. Providing for the general welfare, for example, in education and safety.
2. Regulating commerce among the states, for example, through the interstate commerce commission, which provides controls on transporting food and other supplies across state lines.
3. Raising funds to support the military.
4. Providing through taxes spending power that gives the government the right to collect taxes and establish a federal budget.

These statements have been interpreted by the Court to include a wide variety of federal powers and activities. State power concerning health care is mostly **police power.** This means that states may act to protect the health, safety, and welfare of their citizens. Such police power must be used fairly, and the state must show that it has a compelling interest in taking actions, especially actions that might infringe on individual rights. Examples of a state using its police powers include requiring immunizations of children before school admission and requiring casefinding, reporting, follow-up care, and treatment of tuberculosis. These activities protect the health, safety, and welfare of state citizens.

Trends and Shifts in Governmental Roles

Government involvement in health care at both the state and federal levels began gradually. Many historical events link closely with the role that has developed. Wars, economic instability, depressions, different viewpoints, and political parties all have shaped the government's role.

- Before the 1930s the only major government action relating to health was the creation in 1798 of the Public Health Service (PHS).
- In 1930 federal laws were passed to promote the public health of merchant seamen and Native Americans.
- The Social Security Act of 1935 was a substantial piece of legislation that, through the years, included amendments on child welfare, health department grants, maternal and child health projects, Medicare, and Medicaid.
- In 1934 Senator Wagner of New York initiated the first national health insurance bill.
- In 1946 Congress enacted a mental health bill and the Hospital Survey and Construction Act.
- The National Institutes of Health (NIH) were created 1948. These institutes provide funds for research and client service in a number of health care areas, for example, the National Heart, Blood, and Lung Institute (NHLBI) provides funds for research in these areas. This particular institute has established guidelines for defining and monitoring hypertension.

These legislative acts created arms of the executive branch, now within the USDHHS. The USDHHS—a regulatory agency known until 1980 as the Department of Health, Education, and Welfare (HEW)—was not created until 1953.

In a democracy the role of government in health care depends on the beliefs of its citizens. Strong beliefs of self-determination and self-sufficiency mixed with beliefs about social responsibilities are hallmarks of a multiple approach to solving society's problems. Political party platforms demonstrate how different beliefs yield different approaches to problems. A good example of this was the debate in the 1990s between the Democratic and Republican parties over health care reform. The Democratic platform called for a health care system that was universally accessible and affordable. The Republican platform supported continuing the current system and reducing government's role in health care delivery through cuts in Medicare and Medicaid benefits. However, in an effort to begin health care reform, both parties passed the Health Portability and Accountability Act in 1997. This act was designed to ensure that workers will have health insurance coverage when they change or lose employment. This also applies to persons who may have preexisting medical conditions.

Nurses are becoming more aware of the influence of political parties on health care delivery. Nurses are citizens and professionals and can influence the changing role of government. For example, in 1991 the American Nurses Association, the National League for Nursing, the American Association of Colleges of Nursing, and more than 60 nursing specialty organizations published nursing's agenda for health care reform. This "white paper" was the profession's response to the political parties' attempts to reform health care, indicating the direction in which organized nursing wanted to see the new policy developed (see Box 7-5 on p. 124.)

Freedom of individuals must be balanced with government powers. Citizens express their views on the amount of governmental interference that will be tolerated. For example, the issue of sex education in public schools shows at least two viewpoints on the government-individual relationship:

- Ever since the legislative branch of government established a system of education, some citizens believe that education should include content on sex.
- Some citizens believe that sex education belongs in the family and should not be interfered with by public schools, which are governmentally established.

There are strong feelings about this issue, and the example presented in the Evidence-Based Practice box shows how opinions about government versus individual responsibilities can be divided.

Governmental Health Care Functions

Federal, state, and local governments all carry out four general categories of health care functions: *direct services, financing, information,* and *policy setting.*

Evidence-Based Practice

The purpose of the study referenced in the footnote was to determine whether a shift has occurred in popular attitudes toward federal policies that correspond with an increasing political interest in health care reform. Survey data collected between 1975 and 1989 were used to answer the following questions:

1. Who supports and who opposes an active federal role in health care reform?
2. How do those who support such policies differ from those who oppose them?
3. How do patterns of public support for health care compare with patterns of support for social policy?
4. How are these differences changing over time?

This study concluded that there is a higher level of popular support for government action in health care and that it is distributed among population groups differently than for other federal policies.

Support for federal health policy has grown over time. The gaps in support between rich and poor, educated and uneducated, and old and young are reduced for health policy. Characteristics that make a difference in how one responds to federal policies are age, gender, race, education, marital status, income level, employment status, and rural vs. urban residence. Gaps in support for antipoverty programs and general domestic policies still exist.

There is some evidence that growing support for health policy may be a result of the political ideology of the Reagan and first Bush administrations. Support for such policy does not translate into a willingness to pay for new health programs.

APPLICATION IN PRACTICE

Nurses can use this study to form strategies for promoting health care reform. Nurses will want to show others (clients, communities, legislators) how health care reform is an investment in society by improving the health of the nation, that health care reform promotes equal opportunity for all citizens to have health care, and that supporting investments in health care for all will eventually reduce the cost of health care for every citizen.

Schlesinger M, Lee TK: Is health care different? Popular support of federal health and social policies, *J Health Polit Policy Law* 18 (3 part 2):551, 1993.

Direct Services

Federal, state, and local governments provide *direct health services* to certain individuals and groups. For example, the federal government provides health care to Native Americans, members and dependents of the military, veterans, and federal prisoners (Box 6-1). State and local governments employ nurses to deliver services to individuals and families, usually based on financial need. State and local governments also may provide direct, specific services to all individuals, such as hypertension or tuberculosis screening, immunizations for children, and primary care for inmates in local jails or state prisons.

Financing

Governments pay for some health care services, training of personnel, and research. *Financial support* in these areas has sig-

Box 6-1 Public Health Care Programs

- *Military Medical Care System.* Provides health care coverage to military personnel and their dependents at no direct cost to the recipient. The system is composed of hospitals and clinics, typically located at military bases.
- *Civilian Health and Medical Program of the Uniformed Services (CHAMPUS).* Provides coverage for military families and dependents to obtain private-sector care if service is unavailable in the military system. The program is provided, financed, and supervised by the military system.
- *Veterans Administration (VA).* Health care system provided as a benefit for retired, disabled, and other specified categories of military service veterans. The system is composed of 172 hospitals and more than 200 outpatient departments.
- *Indian Health Service (IHS).* An agency within the Public Health Service that provides direct care to improve the health status of native Americans living on reservations. This agency operates approximately 50 hospitals and 340 clinics to serve more than 1 million Native Americans.

Modified from U.S. Department of Health and Human Services: *Health: United States, 1998,* DHHS pub no (PHS) 98-1232, Washington, D.C., 1998, U.S. Government Printing Office.

nificantly affected consumers and health care providers. State and federal governments finance the direct care of clients through the Medicare, Medicaid, and Social Security programs. Many nurses have been educated with government funds; schools of nursing have been built and equipped through federal capitation funds. Governments have also financially supported other health care providers. Monies in the form of grants have been given by governments for specific research and demonstration projects. One of the best-known centers of medical research is the federally funded National Institutes of Health. In 1993 the **National Institute of Nursing Research** was established by Congress to promote nursing research. This provides a substantial sum of money to the discipline of nursing for the purpose of defining the knowledge base of nursing.

Information

All branches and levels of government have collected, analyzed, and made available data about health care and health status in the United States. Collection of vital statistics, including mortality and morbidity data, gathering of census data, and sponsoring of health care status surveys are all government activities. An example is the annual report, *Health: United States,* compiled by the USDHHS (1998). Table 6-1 lists examples of available international and federal government data sources on the health status of the total U.S. population. These sources are available in the government documents sections of most large libraries. This information is especially important because it can help nurses understand the major health problems in the United States and those in their own state.

Policy Setting

Policy setting relates to all government functions. Decisions about health care are made by governments at all levels and within all branches. Governments often show preference

TABLE 6-1	International and National Sources of Data on the Health Status of the U.S. Population
Organization	**Data Source**
International	
United Nations	Demographic Yearbook
World Health Organization	World Health Statistics Annual
Federal	
Public Health Service	National Vital Statistics System
	National Survey of Family Growth
	National Health Interview Survey
	National Health Examination Survey
	National Health and Nutrition Examination Survey
	National Master Facility Inventory
	National Hospital Discharge Survey
	National Nursing Home Survey
	National Ambulatory Medical Care Survey
	National Morbidity Reporting System
	U.S. Immunization Survey
	Surveys of Mental Health Facilities
	Estimates of National Health Expenditures
	AIDS Surveillance
	Abortion Surveillance
	Nurse Supply Estimates
Department of Commerce	U.S. Census of Population
	Current Population Survey
	Population Estimates and Projections
Department of Labor	Consumer Price Index
	Employment and Earnings

Healthy People 2010
An Example of Current National Health Policy

Healthy People 2010 is an example of a health policy that has been influenced by a diverse group of individuals and organizations concerned with the nation's health, including nursing. A consortium was formed that included:

- 350 national organizations
- 250 state public health, mental health, substance abuse, and environmental agencies
- 11,000 individuals who provided comment by mail, internet, or in person
- Teams of experts from a number of federal agencies.

The work done by many on the *Healthy People 2000* objectives showed that, through business, private, government, professional, voluntary, charitable, and individual partnerships, progress could be made in improving the nation's health. This work resulted in:

- Increased childhood immunizations
- Decreased teen pregnancy
- Substance abuse stabilized
- Decreased deaths from heart disease and stroke
- Reduced unintentional injuries

Healthy People 2010 will continue to emphasize community partnerships to achieve the new objectives.

---

between groups when giving financial support. Such decisions affect the health care resources of each group and show the influence of government policy setting. Health policy decisions, or courses of action, usually have broad implications for financial growth, resource use, and development in the health care field. The law that has had the most significant impact on the development of public health policy, community health nursing, and social welfare policy in the United States is the Sheppard-Towner Act of 1921.

In 1912 the Child Health Bureau was established as part of the USPHS. In 1917 the Bureau published a report, *Public Protection of Maternity and Infancy,* to highlight findings of studies on infant and maternal mortality and consequently on the plight of women and children in the United States. In 1918 the first congresswoman, Jeanette Rankin, introduced a bill that later became the *Sheppard-Towner Act.* This act made nurses available to provide health services for women and children, offered well-child and child-development services, provided adequate hospital services and facilities for women and children, and provided grants-in-aid for the establishment of maternal and child welfare programs.

The Sheppard-Towner Act helped to establish:

- Precedent and set patterns for the growth of modern-day public health policy
- The federal government's involvement in health
- The role of the federal government in creating standards to be followed by states in programs such as today's Women, Infants, and Children (WIC) program and Early and Periodic Screening, Diagnosis, and Treatment (EPSDT) program
- The consumer as an important person in influencing, formulating, and conducting public policy
- The government's role in research
- A system for collecting national health statistics
- The integrating of health and social services (Pickett and Hanlon, 1990)
- The importance of prenatal care, anticipatory guidance, client education, and nurse-client conferences

ORGANIZATION OF GOVERNMENT AGENCIES

Nurses are actively involved with many levels of international and national government. This section discusses international organizations and the roles of nurses in different national government agencies.

International Organizations

In June 1945 many national governments joined together to create the *United Nations* (UN). Aims and goals described in its charter include several dealing with human rights, world peace, security, and promotion of economic and social advancement of all people. The UN is headquartered in New York City and is made up of subgroups, many specialized agencies and autonomous organizations. One of the autonomous organizations is the **World Health Organization (WHO),** located in Geneva, Switzerland.

Its goal is the highest possible level of health for all citizens throughout the world. Although its headquarters are in Geneva, Switzerland, the Office for the Americas is located in Washington, D.C., and is known as the Pan American Health Organization (PAHO).

The WHO services, which benefit all countries, include:
- A day-to-day information service on the occurrence of internationally important diseases
- Publication of the international list of causes of disease, injury, and death
- Monitoring of adverse reactions to drugs
- Establishing world standards for antibiotics and vaccines.

Assistance that is available to individual countries includes:
- Supporting national programs to fight disease
- Training workers
- Strengthening health services

The number of nursing roles in international health is increasing to include:
- Direct health services
- Consultants
- Educators
- Program planners
- Evaluators

Nurses focus their work on a variety of public health concepts:
- Environment
- Sanitation
- Communicable disease
- Wellness
- Primary care

In 1978 the *International Conference on Primary Health Care* sponsored by the WHO and held in Alma Ata, USSR, declared that the world community's goal should be the attainment of a level of health by the year 2000 that would permit all people to live socially and economically productive lives (World Health Organization, 1978). The conference resolved that primary health care was the key to attaining this goal (see Appendix A.3). At about the same time, the WHO Expert Committee on Community Health Nursing convened and outlined the broad role of community health nurses in primary health care. The WHO is encouraging strengthened regulation of nursing education and practice related to primary health care, and it is in support of nurses in their efforts to become forces in attaining the goal of "health for all" (World Health Organization, 1986).

Federal Agencies

Many federal agencies are involved in governmental health care functions. Legislation passed by Congress may be delegated to any regulatory agency within the executive branch for implementation, surveillance, regulation, and enforcement. Congress decides which agency will monitor specific laws. For example, most health care legislation is delegated to the USDHHS; however, legislation concerning the environment or occupational health would probably be monitored by the Environmental Protection Agency (EPA) or the Labor Department. Examples of those departments most involved with health care are included in the following discussion.

The **U.S. Department of Health and Human Services** is the agency most heavily involved with the health and welfare concerns of U.S. citizens. It touches more lives than any other federal agency. As mentioned previously, the organizational chart of the USDHHS (see Figure 3-1 on p. 93) depicts the office of the Secretary and four principal operating components: the Social Security Administration, the Health Care Financing Administration, the Administration for Children and Families, and the Public Health Service (PHS). The PHS is charged with regulating health care and overseeing the health status of Americans.

The **Public Health Service** has been a longstanding, significant contributor to the improved health status of Americans. The Health Resources and Services Administration (HRSA) of the PHS contains the Bureau of Health Professions (BHPr), which includes a Division of Nursing, as well as Divisions of Medicine, Dentistry, and Allied Health Professions.

The **Division of Nursing** has these specific goals (U.S. Department of Health and Human Services, Division of Nursing, 1995):
- Enhancing nursing's contribution to primary care and public health.
- Developing and promoting innovative practice models for improved and expanded nursing services.
- Enhancing racial and ethnic diversity and cultural competency in the nursing workforce.
- Promoting improved and expanded linkages between education and practice.
- Improving and expanding nursing services to high-risk and underserved populations.
- Enhancing nursing's contributions to achieving the *Healthy People 2010* objectives and health care reform.
- Capacity building for meeting the nursing service needs of the nation.

A significant addition to the PHS in 1990 was the creation of the *Agency for Health Care Policy and Research (AHCPR),* now called the *Agency for Healthcare Research and Quality (AHRQ).* This agency is charged with conducting research on effectiveness of medical services, interventions, and technologies, including research related to nursing interventions and outcomes that contribute to the improved health status of the nation.

The AHRQ has published protocols for care of clients with a variety of health problems. These protocols will become the future standards of health care delivery. In addition, the AHRQ has a project called "Put Prevention Into Practice" to promote the use of standardized protocols for primary care delivery for clients across the age span (see Appendix A.2). These protocols can be used by nurses in planning disease-prevention and health-promotion activities for their clients.

Other Federal Government Agencies

The USDHHS has primary responsibility for federal health functions. Several other cabinet departments of the federal government carry out certain other health-related functions. These departments include Commerce, Defense, Labor, Agriculture, and Justice.

- *Department of Commerce.* Within the Department of Commerce is the Census Bureau, which carries out an information function in health care. Also a part of the DOC is the National Oceanic and Atmospheric Administration, which provides special services in support of controlling urban air quality, a major factor in community health today.
- *Department of Defense.* The Department of Defense delivers health care to members of the military and their dependents. In each command, nurses of high military rank, including brigadier general, are part of the administration of health services.
- *Department of Labor.* The Department of Labor has two agencies with health functions: the Occupational Safety and Health Agency (OSHA) and the Mine Safety and Health Administration. Both are charged with writing safety and health standards and ensuring compliance in the workplace.
- *Department of Agriculture.* The Department of Agriculture is involved in health care primarily through administering the Food and Nutrition Service. This service collaborates with state and local government welfare agencies to provide food stamps to needy persons to increase their food purchasing power. Other programs include school breakfast and lunch programs, the WIC program, and grants to states for nutrition education and training.
- *Department of Justice.* Health services to federal prisoners are administered within the Department of Justice. The Medical and Services Division of the Bureau of Prisons includes medical, psychiatric, dental, and health support services.

State and Local Government Departments

Most state and local (county and city) areas perform governmental activities that affect the health care field. At the state level, three executive branch departments are described: health, education, and corrections. The organization of a local health department is outlined, and community health roles are discussed below.

State Health Departments

In most state health departments, nurses serve in capacities similar to those in international and federal agencies:

Box 6-2	Selected Programs Within a Typical State Health Department

Legal services
Services to the chronically ill and aging
Juvenile services
Medical assistance: policy, compliance, operations
Mental health and addictions
Mental retardation and developmental disabilities
Environmental programs
Departmental licensing boards
Division of vital records
Health services cost review
Health planning and development
Preventive medicine and medical affairs

- Consultation
- Direct services
- Research
- Teaching
- Supervision
- Planning
- Evaluation of health programs

Most health departments have a division or department of public health nursing. Box 6-2 lists typical programs in a state health department, which includes community and public health nursing.

Every state has a board of examiners of nurses. The board may be found either in the department of licensing boards of the health department or in an administrative agency of the governor's office. Created by legislation known as a *state nurse practice act,* the examiner's board is made up of nurses and consumers. A few states have other providers or administrators as members. The functions of this board are described in the practice act of each state and generally include licensing and examination of registered nurses and licensed practical nurses; approval of schools of nursing in the state; revocation, suspension, or denial of licenses; and writing of regulations about nursing practice and education. **Nurse practice acts** will be discussed later in a section on the scope of nursing practice.

State Education Departments

Some state departments of education coordinate health curricula and services provided within local school systems. Other state legislatures mandate that services be coordinated solely within the health department or jointly between the health and education departments.

State Departments of Corrections

Nurses work in state departments of corrections as planners and coordinators and sometimes as supervisors of health and nursing services for inmates in state prisons.

Local Health Departments

Depending on funding and other resources, programs offered by local health departments vary greatly. A fairly

Box 6-3	Examples of Programs Provided by Local Health Departments

Addiction and alcoholism clinics
Adult health
Birth and death records
Child daycare and development
Child health clinics
Crippled children's services
Dental health clinic
Environmental health
Epidemiology and disease control
Family planning
Geriatric evaluation
Health education
Home health agency
Hospital discharge planning
Hypertension clinics
Immunization clinics
Information services
Maternal health
Medical social work
Mental health
Mental retardation and developmental disabilities
Nursing
Nursing home licensure
Nutrition division
Occupational therapy
Physical therapy
School health
Speech and audiology
Vision and hearing screening

comprehensive list of such programs, taken from an urban-suburban county health department in a mid-Atlantic state, is shown in Box 6-3.

More often than at other levels of government, nurses at the local level provide direct services. Some nurses deliver special or selected services, such as follow-up of contacts in cases of tuberculosis or venereal disease or providing care through child immunization clinics. Other nurses have a more general practice, delivering services to families in certain geographic areas.

Social Welfare Programs

In addition to health programs, federal, state, and local governments also provide social welfare programs. Generally these programs provide money to the poor, elderly, disabled, and unemployed.

The federal Social Security Act established a number of programs, including the social insurance programs, Social Security, unemployment insurance, and welfare. The Social Security Administration, which is within the USDHHS, administers the following programs:

- Old Age Survivors and Disability Insurance (OASDI)
- Aid to Families with Dependent Children (AFDC)
- Supplemental Security Income (SSI)

OASDI provides monthly benefits to retired and disabled workers, their spouses and children, and survivors of insured workers. AFDC, which is a federal and state program, helps needy families with children. AFDC subsidizes children deprived of the financial support of one of their parents as a result of death, disability, absence from the home, or in some states, unemployment. SSI is a federal program for the aged, blind, and disabled that may be supplemented by state support.

In addition, there are human development services coordinated by the *Division of Administration for Children and Families* within USDHHS. Programs are focused on the following groups:

- Aging
- Children, youth, and families
- Native Americans
- Developmentally disabled

Specifically, one law passed to support this division was the *Older Americans Act.* The program is designed to promote the welfare and needs of older people. Social programs focused on children and families include programs on:

- Adoption opportunities
- Head Start services
- Runaway-youth facilities
- Child-abuse prevention and treatment
- Juvenile justice
- Delinquency prevention

THE NURSE'S ROLE IN THE POLITICAL PROCESS

The number and types of laws influencing health care are increasing; this makes the political process very important to nursing.

Briefly Noted

The nurse's basic understanding of the political process should include knowing who the lawmakers are, how bills become laws, the regulation-writing process, and methods of influencing the process used for shaping health policy. With this knowledge nurses can shape nursing practice. Figure 6-1 depicts how a bill becomes a law.

The federal and state legislatures are composed of two houses that together are called an assembly, which usually comprises a house and a senate. Representatives and senators are elected by the people within geographic jurisdictions. Each state has two federal senators and one or more representatives, depending on the state's population. Each state has its own rules for deciding on the number of senators and representatives within the state for the state legislature.

Although Congress meets throughout the year, state legislatures have sessions of different lengths. Each legislature has its own leadership, usually dominated by either the Democratic or

The Federal Level

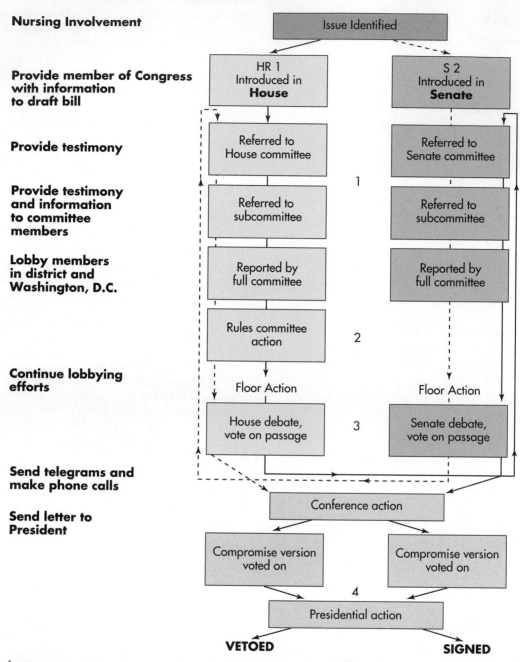

Nursing Involvement

Provide member of Congress with information to draft bill

Provide testimony

Provide testimony and information to committee members

Lobby members in district and Washington, D.C.

Continue lobbying efforts

Send telegrams and make phone calls

Send letter to President

[1] A bill goes to full committee first, then to special subcommittees for hearings, debate, revisions, and approval. The same process occurs when it goes to full committee. It either dies in committee or proceeds to the next step.

[2] Only the House has a Rules Committee to set the "rule" for floor action and conditions for debate and amendments. In the Senate, the leadership schedules action.

[3] The bill is debated, amended, and passed or defeated. If passed, it goes to the other chamber and follows the same path. If each chamber passes a similar bill, both versions go to conference.

[4] The President may sign the bill into law, allow it to become law without his signature, or veto it and return it to Congress. To override the veto, both houses must approve the bill by a 2/3 majority vote.

Figure 6-1   **How a bill becomes a law.** (From Mason DJ, Talbott SW, Leavitt JK: *Policy and politics for nurses: action and change in the workplace, government, organizations, and community,* ed 2, Philadelphia, 1993, WB Saunders.)

the Republican party. Roles include the presiding officer, party floor leaders, and committee chairpersons.

The legislative process follows these steps:

- The process begins with ideas that are developed into bills.
- After a bill is drafted, it is introduced to the legislature, given a number, read, and assigned to a committee.
- Hearings, testimony, lobbying, education, research, and informal discussion follow.
- If the bill is passed from the committee, the entire house hears the bill, amends it as necessary, and votes on it.
- A majority vote in one house moves the bill to the other house, where it is read, amended, and voted on.
- Nurses can be involved in this process at any point.

An important part of this **legislative process** is the work of the staff members of the legislatures. These individuals do the legwork, research, paperwork, and other activities that develop policy ideas into bills and then into law. In addition to the individual legislators' staff, committee staff are also important. Both of these can provide valuable information for citizens and their legislators. Nurses often serve as staff to legislators or are constituents (citizens) of a legislator and will want to give information to (or get information from) that legislator about health policy.

Many professional nursing associations have professional lobbyists, legislative committees, and political action committees (PACs) to shape health policy.

Common methods of lobbying include:

- Face-to-face encounters
- Personal letters (via mail or Internet)
- Mailgrams, telegrams
- Telephone calls
- Testimony
- Petitions
- Reports
- Position papers (white papers)
- Fact sheets
- Letters to the editor
- News releases
- Speeches
- Coalition-building
- Demonstrations
- Law suits

Depending on the issue, each of these methods can be equally effective. Tips on communication are provided in the following How To boxes. Tips on writing to and visiting legislators and general tips on political action are presented in Boxes 6-4, 6-5, and 6-6.

HOW TO Build a Professional Image

Several points should be considered in building a professional image. What images do you have of yourself: strong, assertive, confident, competent, powerful? To be politically influential requires being an effective image shaper. What images do you convey in the workplace, the community, the government, and professional organiza-

---

Box 6-4 Tips for Writing to Legislators

1. Use your own stationery, not hospital or agency stationery. A letter is better than a postcard or telegram. Use your own words; form letters are not as effective as original ones.
2. Identify your subject clearly. State the name (and bill number if possible) of the legislation you are writing about.
3. Be brief, giving the reasons that you are for or against the legislation.
4. Explain how the issue would affect you, the nursing profession, clients, and/or your community.
5. Know what committees your legislators serve on and indicate in the letter if the bill will be brought before any of those committees. Know the current status of the bill (where it is in the legislative process).
6. Sign your name with "R.N." after it. Be sure your correct address is on the letter and the envelope. (Envelopes sometimes get thrown away before the letter is answered.)
7. Be courteous. A rude letter neither makes friends nor influences the legislator. Be sure to express your appreciation for work well done, a good speech, a favorable vote, or fine leadership in committee or on the floor.
8. Timing is important. Try to write your positions on a bill while it is in committee. Your legislators will usually be more responsive to your appeal at that time rather than later, when the bill has already been dealt with by a committee.
9. Limit your letter to one issue.
10. Keep a copy of all correspondence for your files. Send a copy of your letter and any response from the legislator to the government relations' staff at your professional nursing organization.
11. Address written correspondence as follows (the same general format applies to state and local officials):

U.S. Senator	U.S. Representative
Honorable Jane Doe	Honorable Jane Doe
United States Senate	House of Representatives
Washington, DC 20510	Washington, DC 20515
Dear Senator Doe:	Dear Representative Doe:

12. You may be able to send a facsimile transmission (fax) or e-mail to your legislator if you both have the necessary technology. This technique offers speed and conveys a sense of urgency. If you choose this method, follow up by sending the original letter through the mail.

Modified from Mason DJ, Talbott SW, Leavitt JK: *Policy and politics for nurses: action and change in the workplace, government, organizations, and community,* ed 2, Philadelphia, 1993, WB Saunders.

---

tions? The following checklist will help you identify some of your messages.

- In your daily encounters with clients and their families, do your verbal and nonverbal behaviors convey your professional pride and confidence?
- Do you carry business cards to facilitate contacts with persons you meet?
- Do you share your expertise through the local and national media?
- Do you thoroughly document your nursing care?
- Do you spend time every day teaching and listening to the concerns of your clients and their families?

Box 6-5   Tips for Visiting Legislators

1. Call ahead to make an appointment to meet with the legislator. If the legislator is unavailable, ask to meet with the staff person who handles health issues.
2. Prepare. Know the background of the legislator and the history of the bill or issue you are discussing. Contact the government relations staff at your professional nursing organization to let them know about the visit. They may be able to provide important information about the issue, the political climate, your legislator's previous record on this issue, and the overall lobbying strategy on this issue.
3. At the beginning of the visit, introduce yourself and state what you want to discuss. Specify the issues and bills.
4. Ask the legislator what his or her position is on the issue or bill.
5. Many legislators and staff may not be familiar with nursing practice or legislative concerns. Be prepared to discuss them in basic terms. If possible, be prepared with facts about nursing practice in your state or district.
6. Ask if he or she has heard from others who support this issue or bill. Ask what the supporters are saying.
7. Ask if he or she has heard from opponents. Ask who the opponents are and what their arguments are.
8. Offer to provide additional information if you do not have data at hand, but do not make promises you cannot keep. It is better to admit that you do not know than to promise and not deliver or to convey erroneous information.
9. Follow up with a thank-you note, and share your reflections on the visit.
10. Keep a written record of your visit. Notify the government relations staff of your professional nursing organization so that they can follow up with the legislator.
11. Spend more time with your legislators even if their position is not in agreement with yours. You might lessen the intensity of their positions and maintain contact for subsequent issues.
12. Invite legislators to meet you and your colleagues at your work site to help expand their understanding of nursing and health care issues.

From Mason DJ, Talbott SW, Leavitt JK: *Policy and politics for nurses: action and change in the workplace, government, organizations, and community,* ed 2, Philadelphia, 1993, WB Saunders.

- At staff meetings, do you set the tone for serious collaboration by asking questions and giving your opinions?
- Do you regularly communicate your ideas, concerns, and suggestions to your supervisors, public officials, and organizational leaders?
- Do you vote in every national and local election?
- What does your body language communicate?
- Do you call or write to supervisors, community members, public officials, and organizational leaders to thank them when they have helped you with a problem or issue?
- Does your attire communicate that you are a serious, businesslike professional?

From Mason DJ, Talbott SW, Leavitt JK: *Policy and politics for nurses: action and change in the workplace, government, organizations, and community,* ed 2, Philadelphia, 1993, WB Saunders.

Box 6-6   Tips for Action

- Get to know your legislators and the chair of your state board of nursing. Make sure you meet the governor and know the governor's chief executive aide.
- Apply the problem-solving and negotiation skills you have developed in nursing to the process of making and implementing laws. They are the same skills you use to convince a diabetic client to let you help him or her develop a care plan.
- Cultivate relationships with people who make the rules or pass the laws.
- Run for office.
- Develop a bipartisan nurse advisory council to assist your local legislator. (One state organized a statewide advisory group for a U.S. Senator. This group previewed U.S. health legislation for the Senator, and several nurses testified before the U.S. Senate Appropriations Subcommittee on Health and Human Services.)
- Spend an hour or two a week to upgrade your knowledge of political developments, health policy initiatives, legislators, and state government executives.

From Mason DJ, Talbott SW, Leavitt JK: *Policy and politics for nurses: action and change in the workplace, government, organizations, and community,* ed 2, Philadelphia, 1993, WB Saunders.

HOW TO Refine Your Communication Skills

Since communication is a key aspect of political activity and policy development, it is imperative to possess finely honed skills:

- Get assistance in developing your writing and speaking; they are indispensable in sending messages that will be taken seriously.
- Attend continuing education sessions on public speaking, writing, and media training.
- Volunteer to speak at programs in your workplace, at nursing association meetings, and in the community.
- Testify at public hearings.
- Write short articles in your areas of expertise for your local newspapers and workplace newsletters.
- Team up with colleagues when you visit legislators, write an article, testify, or speak on a radio show or at a workshop. You will learn from the shared experience and bolster each other's confidence.
- Learn invaluable influence skills through committee work and involvement in nursing organizations, work-related committees, political action committees, multidisciplinary and consumer groups, and political clubs.
- Vote and encourage others to vote.

From Mason DJ, Talbott SW, Leavitt JK: *Policy and politics for nurses: action and change in the workplace, government, organizations, and community,* ed 2, Philadelphia, 1993, WB Saunders.

Behind the scenes is the political party activity in which nurses can be involved. A wide variety of activities are available:

- Voting
- Participating in the party organization
- Registering voters

- Encouraging citizens to vote
- Fundraising
- Building networks or communication links
- Participating in political action committees

The passage of the *National Health Research Extension Act* of 1985 is one example of how nurses can use their influence. This act included establishing the *National Center for Nursing Research.* The Center began as the idea of a small group of nurses who worked to gain the support of colleagues and major national nursing organizations. Individual nurses provided testimony to Congress on the importance of nursing research. Some visited their congressional representatives to lobby for the bill. Many wrote letters and provided position papers and fact sheets to help legislators understand the need for the Center. Although the process took several years, the idea became a reality. Both the nursing profession and the client will benefit from the research and the knowledge base developed through the Center. In 1993, the Center became one of the National Institutes of Health, now called the **National Institute of Nursing Research.**

More recently, the American Nurses Association, through its national organization and state nursing associations, was a strong lobbyist for the *Patient Safety Act of 1997.* This law requires health care facilities to make public some information on nurse staff levels, staff mix, and outcomes, and requires the USDHHS to review and approve all health care organization acquisitions and mergers. All of these requirements are to determine any long-term effect on the health and safety of clients, communities, and staff.

PRIVATE-SECTOR INFLUENCE ON REGULATION AND HEALTH POLICY

In each level of government the executive branch can, and in most cases must, prepare regulations. These regulations are detailed, and they establish, fix, and control standards and criteria for carrying out certain laws. Figure 6-2 shows the steps in the typical regulation-writing process.

When the legislature passes a law and delegates its administration to an agency like the USDHHS, it gives that agency the power to make regulations. Because regulations flow from legislation, they have the force of law. Nurses, including students, can influence these regulations by writing letters to the regulatory agency in charge or by speaking at public hearings.

The proposed regulations are put into final draft form and printed in the legally required publication, which at the federal level is the *Federal Register.* Similar registers exist in most states where regulations from state departments, including state health departments, are published.

Regular surveillance of the *Federal Register* or state registers is essential. Once proposed resolutions are published, members of the private sector may influence regulations by attending hearings, providing comments, testifying, and engaging in lobbying aimed at individuals involved in the writing. Final regulations, published in a **Code of Regula-**

Evidence-Based Practice

The purpose of the observational research study referenced in the footnote was to do a case analysis to look at the policies and the potential implications for seven states that, by 1995, had made legislative changes to reform their health care systems: Florida, Hawaii, Massachusetts, Minnesota, Oregon, Vermont, and Washington. Common problems across states were identified, as were common factors that helped states survive. Three major factors appeared to lead to success in reforming health policy:

1. Taking advantage of a window of opportunity (i.e., people must be ready for change)
2. A need for policy entrepreneurship (i.e., an individual citizen, nurse, or legislature must be willing to emerge as a leader in the legislative process and must have a passion for change, understanding of the issue, a positive and objective outlook, and be willing to take a risk)
3. Involving key persons and groups affected by the change

APPLICATION IN PRACTICE

Nurses can use these three factors in promoting legislation, regulatory change, or in introducing new public health policy.

Paul-Shaheen P: The states and health care reform: the road traveled and lessons learned from seven that took the lead, *J Health Polit Policy Law* 23:2, 1998.

tions (both federal and state), usually lead to changes in practice. For example, Medicare regulations setting standards for nursing homes and home health are incorporated into these agencies' manuals and influence how nurses practice.

LAWS AFFECTING COMMUNITY-ORIENTED NURSING PRACTICE

The community health nurse is subject to the laws relating to nursing practice and public health practice. This section discusses the various types of laws, how they affect nurses, and the legal resources available.

Types of Laws

Several definitions of law are available. However, many of these tend to describe *what law is not* rather than what it is. Definitions of law include the following:

- A rule established by authority, society, or custom
- The body of rules governing the affairs of people within a community or among states
- Social order (the common law)
- A set of rules or customs governing a discrete field or activity (e.g., criminal law, contract law)
- Laws of a society are supported by the system of courts, judicial process, and legal officers or lawyers.

These definitions reflect the close relationship of law to community and to society's customs and beliefs. Since community-oriented nursing reflects society's beliefs and

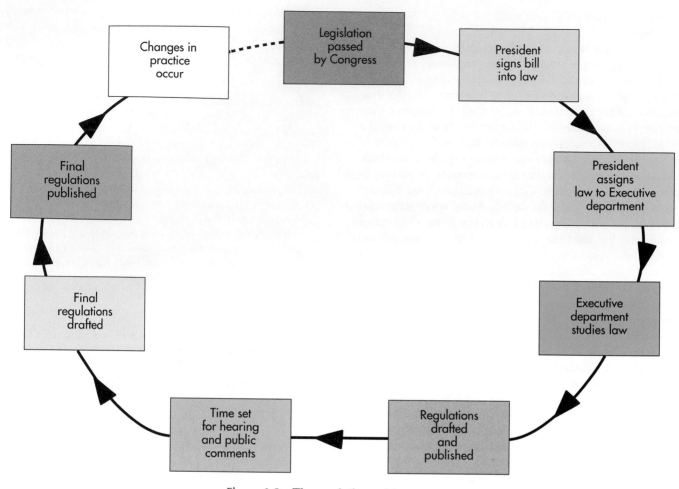

Figure 6-2   **The regulation writing process.**

customs, law has had a major effect on this practice. Although community health nursing practice emerged from individual voluntary activities, society soon recognized the need for it. Through laws, positions and functions for nurses in community settings were created, which, in many instances, carry with them the "force of law." For example, if the nurse discovers a person with tuberculosis, the law directs the nurse and others legally designated in the community to take specific action. This is just one example of how the law has shaped nursing practice.

Briefly Noted

As a former Speaker of the House of Representatives noted, "all politics is local." Therefore should nurses focus their political activities only in the local community?

There are three types of law in the United States: *constitutional law, legislation and regulation,* and *judicial and common law.*

Constitutional law emerges from federal and state constitutions. From this type of law nurses can get answers to questions in selected practice situations. For example, on what basis can the state require quarantine or isolation of individ-

uals with tuberculosis? The answer to this question can be found in constitutional law. The major power of the states relating to nursing practice is the right to intervene in a reasonable manner to protect the health, safety, and welfare of the citizenry, as through the state's "police power." For example, isolating an individual from a community because he or she has a communicable disease has been deemed an appropriate exercise of state powers. The state can isolate an individual even though it infringes on individual rights (freedom, autonomy) under the following conditions:

1. The isolation is done in a reasonable manner.
2. There is a compelling state interest in the prevention of an epidemic.
3. The isolation is necessary to protect the health, safety, and welfare of individuals in the community or the public as a whole.

Briefly Noted

The community's rights are more important than the individual's rights when there is a threat to public health.

Legislation is the type of law that comes from the legislative branches of federal, state, or local government. Much legislation has an effect on nursing. Regulations are very specific statements of rules or orders that relate to individual pieces of legislation. For example, state legislators have enacted laws (statutes) establishing boards of nursing and defining terms such as *licensed registered nurse* and *nursing practice.* The boards of nursing, through regulation, enforce the law by writing rules on how to become a licensed registered nurse and such practice issues as delegation and continuing-education requirements.

Judicial and common law is the last group of laws having an effect on nursing. Judicial law is based on court or jury decisions. The opinions of the courts are judicial opinions and are referred to as *case law.* The court uses other types of laws to make its decisions, including previous court decisions or cases. *Precedent* is one principle of common law. Judges are bound by previous decisions unless they are convinced that the "old law" is no longer relevant or valid. These play an important role in decisions made by courts.

General Community Health Nursing Practice and the Law

Despite the broad nature and varied roles of nursing practice, two legal aspects apply to most practice situations. The first aspect is *professional negligence,* or *malpractice;* the second is the *scope of practice* defined by custom and state practice acts.

Professional negligence, or malpractice, is defined as an act or failure to act on behalf of a client that leads to injury of that client. To prove that a nurse was negligent, the client must prove all of the following:

1. The nurse owed a duty to the client or was responsible for the client's care.
2. The duty to act as a reasonable, prudent nurse or as another nurse would act under the circumstances was breached or not fulfilled.
3. The failure to be reasonable under the circumstances led to the alleged injuries.
4. The injuries provided the basis for a monetary claim through the legal system.

Reported cases involving negligence and community health nurses are almost nonexistent. As one example, a case involving an occupational health nurse is discussed. Although occurring some years ago, this example clearly represents the four criteria that must be present to prove negligence. Since nurses still use standing orders, a similar problem could happen to a nurse today.

Briefly Noted

In the eyes of the law, the "prudent nurse" used as an example, or standard, to judge the competency of a nurse's practice can be practicing anywhere in the United States and not just in the community in which the nurse actually works.

The California case of Cooper *versus* Motor Bearing Co., 288P 2d 581, involved an occupational health nurse who negligently implemented standing orders on an injury involving a puncture wound. The nurse, by her own testimony, did not examine or probe the wound, nor did she refer the worker to a physician; she simply swabbed and bandaged it. Only after 10 months, in which time there were many documented visits to the dispensary and complaints by the worker that the wound was not healing, did the nurse refer him to the company doctor. On referral, basal cell carcinoma was found and surgery followed.

The fact that the nurse was employed by the industry to render first aid established the first element of negligence: a duty was owed to the worker. The nurse acknowledged that it was her duty to refer any unfamiliar or questionable condition or injury to the doctor for diagnosis. The standard of good nursing care in the community was to examine the wound for the presence of foreign bodies. The nurse knew that the normal healing time was 1 to 2 weeks. If a wound persisted and did not heal, proper nursing care would indicate referral to a physician. Testimony was given that the practice of an occupational health nurse in this particular type of industry is to probe wounds for foreign bodies. According to the nurse's education and experience, she should have been aware of the possibility of foreign objects being present in such a wound.

In this case the nurse's failure to detect the foreign body was the proximate cause of the basal cell carcinoma. The pain, suffering, lost time and wages, and bodily disfigurement were all injuries that could be calculated and totaled as a monetary amount. The nurse and the company were found negligent by the California Court.

An integral part of negligence suits is the question of who should be sued. Obviously, those who made the mistakes should be sued, but part of the consideration has to do with who can best pay for the injuries. When a nurse is employed and functioning within the scope of that job, the employer is responsible for the nurse's negligent actions. This is referred to as the doctrine of *respondeat superior.* By directing a nurse to carry out a particular function, the employer becomes responsible for negligence, along with the individual nurse. Nurses employed by government agencies need to know whether that agency has **sovereign immunity.** Under this doctrine the agency may be exempt from suit for particular kinds of actions, such as negligence. However, sovereign immunity will not protect nurses who are acting under the agency's immunity when the negligence occurs. In some states the legislature has granted personal immunity to nurses employed by public agencies to cover all aspects of their practice.

Nursing students need to be aware that they are governed by the same laws and rules governing the professional nurse.

The issue of **scope of practice** involves differentiating among the practices of physicians, nurses, and other health care providers. Scope of practice is assessed by examining the usual and customary practice of a profession and taking into account how legislation defines the practice of a particular profession in a state. The issue is especially important to community health nurses who have traditionally practiced with much autonomy.

The usual and customary practice of nursing can be determined through a variety of sources, including the following:

1. Content of nursing educational programs, general and specific
2. Experience of other practicing nurses (peers)
3. Activities and statements, including standards, of nursing professional organizations
4. Policies and procedures of agencies employing nurses
5. Needs and interests of the community
6. Literature, including books, texts, and journals

Every nurse should know and follow closely the proposed changes in practice acts in nursing, medicine, pharmacy, and other related professions. These pieces of state legislation define the scope of practice for professionals in these areas. The nurse should always examine all definitions related to nursing practice. For example, a review of the Pharmacy Act will let the nurse know whether to question the right to dispense medications in a family planning clinic in a local health department.

Specialty Community-Oriented Nursing Practice and the Law

Legal aspects of community health nursing vary depending on the setting where care is delivered, the clinical specialty, and the functional role. Four special areas of practice and their respective legal aspects are discussed to illustrate how the law affects specific practice areas.

School and Family Health

School and family health nursing may be delivered by nurses employed by health departments or boards of education. School health legislation establishes a minimum of services that must be provided to children in public and private schools, for example:

- Children must have had immunizations against certain communicable diseases before entering school
- Children must have had a physical examination before entering school
- Some types of health screening are conducted in schools (e.g., vision and hearing testing)
- Most states require nurses to notify police or a social service agency of any situation in which they suspect a child is being abused or neglected

Child abuse and neglect is one instance in which society permits a professional to breach confidentiality to protect someone who may be in a helpless and vulnerable position. There is civil immunity for such reports, and the nurse may be called as a witness in any court hearing. The majority of legal cases involving community health nurses concern child abuse.

Other examples of federal legislation affecting nursing practice in schools and families are:

- Head Start
- Early diagnostic screening programs
- Nutritional programs
- Services for the handicapped
- Special education

Occupational Health

Occupational health is another special area of practice that is affected greatly by state and federal laws. The **Occupational Safety and Health Administration (OSHA)** imposes many requirements on industries. These requirements shape the functions of nurses and the types of services given to workers:

- A required reporting system for workers exposed to toxic agents in the workplace
- A required record-keeping system for health records in the workplace
- State monitoring and inspecting of industries, as well as the health services rendered to them by nurses
- A "worker's right to know" law requiring employers to provide employees with information concerning the nature of toxic substances in the workplace (most states)
- Compensation statutes that provide a legal opportunity for claims of workers injured on the job

Access to records, confidentiality, and the use of standing orders are legal issues of great significance to nurses employed in industries.

Home Care and Hospice

Home care and hospice services rendered by nurses are affected greatly by state laws that require licensing and certification. Compliance with these laws is directly linked to the method of payment for the services. For example, a provider must be licensed and certified to obtain payment for services through Medicare. Federal regulations implementing Medicare have an effect on much of nursing practice, including how nurses record details of their visits.

Legislation affecting home care and hospice services has related to such issues as:

- The right to death with dignity
- Rights of residents of long-term facilities and home-health clients
- Definitions of death
- Required use of living wills, specifically advance directives
- Requirement that nurses report elder abuse to the proper authorities

Correctional Health

Nursing practice in correctional health systems is controlled by federal and state laws and regulations and by recent Supreme Court decisions. The laws and decisions relate to the type and amount of services that must be provided for incarcerated individuals. For example, physical examinations are required of all prisoners after they are sentenced. Regulations specify basic levels of care that must be provided for prisoners, and care during illness is particularly addressed. Court decisions requiring adequate health services are based on constitutional law.

Legal Resources

There are many resources in public libraries and law libraries, including the following:

- State bar association publications
- State code
- State annotated code
- Indexes to codes
- Supplements to codes and indexes
- *Federal Register* and state registers
- *Code of Regulations* (federal and state)
- Administrative agency rules and decisions
- Case law
- Opinions of attorney generals
- Legal dictionaries
- Legislative histories
- Legal periodicals
- *Lexis* (a computerized search tool)
- *Scorpio* (Library of Congress computerized search tool)

Each nurse working within a service based on legislation should be oriented to the legislation. It is advisable that the legislation and its regulations be included in the nursing agency's manual of policies and procedures so that the nurse may refer to it. Box 6-7 lists some general resources for legal information.

Briefly Noted

Persons with communicable diseases such as tuberculosis may be confined to a prison hospital if they are considered a threat to their community by failing to follow their treatment regimen.

Clinical Application

Larry was in his final rotation in the Nursing program at State University. He was anxious to complete his community health nursing course because upon graduation he would begin a position as a staff nurse specializing in school health at the local health department. His wife was expecting their first child, and she had been receiving prenatal care at the health department.

Larry was aware that a few years ago the federal government had, by law, provided grants to states for primary care, maternal child health programs, and other health care needs of states. He had read the *Federal Register* and knew that the regulations for these grants had been written through U.S. DHHS departments. He was aware that these regulations did not require states to fund specific programs.

Larry read in the local paper that the health department was closing its prenatal clinic at the end of the month. When this state had received its block grant, they decided to spend the money for programs other than prenatal care. Larry found that a 3-year study in his own state showed improved pregnancy outcomes as a result of prenatal care. The results were further

improved when the care was delivered by community health nurses.

Larry was concerned that, as a student, he would have little influence. However, he decided to call his classmates together to plan a course of action.

What would such an action plan include?

Answer is in the back of the book.

 Remember This!

- Many historical events have been significant in developing the role of government in health care.
- The legal basis for most congressional action in health care can be found in Article I, Section 8 of the U.S. Constitution.
- The four major health care functions of the federal government are direct service, financing, information, and policy setting.
- The goal of the World Health Organization is the attainment by all people of the highest possible level of health.
- Many federal agencies are involved in government health care functions. The agency most directly involved with the health and welfare of Americans is the U.S. Department of Health and Human Services (USDHHS).
- Most state and local jurisdictions have government activities that affect the health care field.
- The variety and range of functions of government agencies have had a major effect on nursing. Funding in particular has shaped the role and tasks of nurses.
- The private sector can influence legislation in many ways, especially through influencing the process of writing regulations. Nurses are a part of the private sector.
- The number and types of laws influencing health care are increasing. Because of this, being involved in the political process is important to nurses.
- Professional negligence and the scope of practice are two legal aspects particularly relevant to nursing practice.
- Nurses must consider the legal implications of their own practice in each clinical encounter.
- The federal and most state governments are composed of three branches: the executive, the legislative, and the judicial.
- Each branch of government plays a significant role in health policy.
- The U.S. Public Health Service was created in 1798.
- The first national health insurance bill was introduced in Congress in 1934.
- The political party platforms are good sources of information to find out how a government will respond to a health policy issue.
- *Health: United States* is an important source of data about the nation's health care problems.
- In 1912 the Child Health Bureau was established.
- In 1921 the Sheppard-Towner Act was passed and had an important influence over child health programs and community health nursing practice.

- The Division of Nursing, the National Institute of Nursing Research, and the Agency for Healthcare Research Quality are governmental entities important to nursing.
- Nurses through state and local health departments function as consultants, direct care providers, researchers, teachers, supervisors, and program managers.
- The state governments are responsible for regulating nursing practice within the state.
- Federal and state social welfare programs have been developed to provide monetary benefits to the poor, elderly, disabled, and unemployed.
- Social welfare programs affect nursing practice. These programs improve the quality of life for special populations, thus making the nurse's job easier in assisting the client with health needs.
- The nurse's scope of practice is defined by legislation and by standards of practice within a specialty.

 What Would You Do?

1. Select a community nursing role you would like to examine more closely. Interview a person in that role, asking questions about job function, organizational structure, agency goals, salary, mobility within the agency, and potential contributions of this role to the health of the community.
2. Locate your state register or other documents, such as newspapers, that publish proposed regulations. Select one set of proposed regulations and critique them. Submit your opinion in writing as public comment, or attend the hearing and testify on the regulations. Be sure to submit something in writing. Evaluate your participation by stating what you learned and whether the proposed regulations were changed in your favor.
3. Find and review your state nurse practice act and define your scope of practice.
4. Contact your local public health agency to discuss the state's official powers in regulating epidemics, such as AIDS. Explore the state's right to protect the health, safety, and welfare of the citizens. Ask about the conflict between the state's rights and individual rights and how such issues are resolved. Ask about the standards of care that apply to this issue and how it is decided which services offered to clients should be mandatory and which should be voluntary. Explore how the role of public health differs in these epidemics compared with the past epidemics of smallpox and tuberculosis.

REFERENCES

Mason DJ, Talbott SW, Leavitt JK: *Policy and politics for nurses: action and change in the workplace, government, organizations, and community,* ed 2, Philadelphia, 1998, WB Saunders.

Paul-Shaheen P: The states and health care reform: the road traveled and lessons learned from seven that took the lead, *J Health Polit Policy Law* 23:2, 1998.

Pickett G, Hanlon J: *Public health administration and practice,* St Louis, 1990, Mosby.

Schlesinger M, Lee TK: Is health care different? popular support of federal health and social policies, *J Health Polit Policy Law* 18(3 part 2):551, 1993.

Smith S, et al: The Health Expenditures Projection Team: the next ten years of health spending: what does the future hold? *Health Affairs* 17(5):128, 1998.

U.S. Department of Health and Human Services, Division of Nursing: Washington, D.C., 1995, U.S. Department of Health and Human Services.

U.S. Department of Health and Human Services: *Health: United States, 1998,* DHHS pub no (PHS) 98-1232, Washington, D.C., 1998, U.S. Government Printing Office.

U.S. Department of Health and Human Services: *Healthy people 2010,* Washington, D.C., 2000, U.S. Department of Health and Human Services.

World Health Organization, United Nations Children's Fund: *Primary health care: a joint report,* Geneva, Switzerland, 1978, World Health Organization.

World Health Organization: Technical report series, 738, Geneva, Switzerland, 1986, World Health Organization.

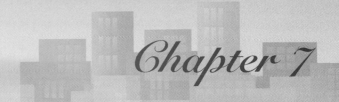

Chapter 7

Economic Influences

CHERYL BLAND JONES
KAREN MACDONALD THOMPSON

OBJECTIVES

After reading this chapter, the student should be able to:

- Relate economics to nursing and health care.
- Describe the economic theories of microeconomics and macroeconomics.
- Trace the evolution of health care service delivery.
- Identify major factors influencing national health care spending.
- Identify the role of government and other third-party payers in health care financing.
- Identify mechanisms for financing health care services delivery.
- Discuss the implications of health care rationing from an economic perspective.
- Evaluate the effect of health care financing on poverty.
- Relate primary prevention to health economics.

CHAPTER OUTLINE

Definitions

Economic Issues

Health System Evolution: The Context of Care Delivery

Trends in Health Care Spending

Factors Influencing Health Care Costs
    Price Inflation
    Changes in Demographics
    Technology and Intensity

Financing of Health Care
    Public Support
    Private Support

Health Care Payment Systems

Other Factors Affecting Resource Use in Health Care
    The Uninsured
    The Poor
    Access to Care
    Health Care Rationing

Primary Prevention

Implications for Nursing Practice

KEY TERMS

capitation: a payment system whereby one fee is charged the client to pay for all services received or needed.

diagnosis-related groups (DRGs): a patient classification scheme that defines 468 illness categories and the corresponding health care services that are reimbursable under Medicare.

economics: social science concerned with the problems of using or administering scarce resources in the most efficient way to attain maximum fulfillment of society's unlimited wants.

fee-for-service: list of health care services with monetary or unit values attached that specifies the amounts third parties must pay for specific services.

Continued

KEY TERMS—cont'd

health economics: branch of economics concerned with the problems of producing and distributing the health care resources of the nation in a way that provides maximum benefit to the most people.

human capital: the combined human potential of the people living in a community.

inflation: a sustained upward trend in the prices of goods and services.

macroeconomic theory: branch of economics that deals with the total or aggregate consumption and spending of all individuals and organizations.

managed care: a method of organizing a number of different health care services together along a continuum of care from physician's office, to hospital, home health, and nursing home, for example. The client pays for services through an insurance plan.

Medicaid: a jointly sponsored state and federal program that pays for medical services for the aged, poor, blind, disabled, and families with dependent children.

Medicare: a federally funded health insurance program for the elderly, disabled, and persons with end-stage renal disease.

microeconomic theory: the branch of economics that deals with the consumption and spending behaviors of individuals and organizations and the effects of those behaviors on prices, costs, and the allocation and distribution of resources.

prospective reimbursement: method of payment to an agency for services to be delivered based on predictions of what an agency's costs will be for the coming year.

retrospective reimbursement: method of payment to an agency based on units of service delivered.

third-party payment: reimbursement made to health care providers by an agency other than the client for the care of the client (e.g., insurance companies, governments, or employers).

The history of the nation's health care delivery system shows a changing health care market. While the U.S. health care system once supported and encouraged expanding, unlimited spending and a booming job market, the system is now very different. Today's health care system is:

- Constantly changing
- Very competitive
- Limited in resources
- Restricting resource use, available services, and access to new technologies
- Encouraging providers to deliver care outside of traditional settings and discipline boundaries

The changing nature of health care has polarized various groups that come into contact with the system—clinicians, administrators, providers, payers, consumers, and policy makers—causing reactions and anticipations of further system problems.

McCloskey (1995) notes that the health care system cycles periodically between a focus on either cost or quality. For example, during the 1960s when Medicare and Medicaid were implemented, the social and health care emphasis was on providing quality health care for the elderly and poor; during the late 1980s and early 1990s the focus was on containing the increasing costs of health care. In between these periods, the system has cycled, to differing degrees, between cost and quality.

With health care shifting between cost and quality, nurses are challenged to implement changes in practice to provide the best care for health care dollars spent. These activities require a basic understanding of economics and the health care system and awareness of the effects of nursing practice on the delivery of cost-effective care (Pew Health Professions Commission, 1993).

DEFINITIONS

Economics is the area of social science concerned with allocating scarce resources and providing the means to evaluate how society gets its wants and needs met when resources are scarce. Thus **health economics** is concerned with the allocating of scarce resources within health care and focuses on producing and distributing health care (services). The allocating of public money or a decision of an individual to spend money for health care is a sensitive issue and often meets resistance from individuals and groups within society because that means there is less money available for other needs, such as education, transportation, recreation, housing, and defense.

This chapter provides an overview of important economic issues in health care. These issues are particularly relevant to community health nurses whether they work with individuals, families, or groups.

Economic issues frequently deal with the influences of health care costs, quality, access, levels of income, and policies on the overall U.S. economy and the behaviors of individuals related to prices, costs, and purchases of health care services. The amount of money the individual person or organization is willing to pay, to a degree, reflects consumer choice and decision making.

Specifically, *willingness to pay* for a good or service reflects the consumer's choice to make a "trade-off," or to purchase a particular good or service, and not other things like buying a new car rather than a new house (Folland, Goodman, and Stano, 1993). Thus willingness to pay reflects individual desires, choices, and the level of satisfaction that is expected for a good or service (Gold, et al, 1996).

The nation's aggregate and industry factors are examined in considering health care financing, national health insurance, rationing, and managed care and in comparing the U.S. health care system with that of other countries. **Human capital** is a way of measuring the value society places on the worth of individuals. Human capital values health in terms of the productive years people have in the job market (Gold, et al, 1996). The value is expressed in dollars and it places a real limit on how much money either people or society will pay for health care. Using human capital methods as a way of making decisions about spending money for health care may mean possible losses of people to death or poor health that result from not investing in a health program or service. For example, as more people died from AIDS, more money has been spent on health programs.

Briefly Noted

When the media refers to "the economy," the phrase typically is used to describe the wealth and financial performance of the nation as a whole. Health care contributes to the economy through goods and services produced and employment of providers.

ECONOMIC ISSUES

Nurses face economic issues every day. For example, when working with an individual, they are influenced by **microeconomics** when:
- Referring clients for available services
- Informing clients and others of the cost of services
- Evaluating client access to services.

Nurses who work with aggregates of individuals and groups are faced with **macroeconomic** issues such as:
- Health policies that make the development of new programs possible
- Local, state, and federal budgets that support certain programs
- The effect that services have on improving the health of the individual or group.

An understanding of economics helps nurses to understand and argue a position for meeting the needs of their clients. It is often argued that unique aspects of the health care sector make the application of economic principles impossible or inappropriate. These arguments, often made by passionate health care professionals, include the following (Folland, Goodman, and Stano, 1993):
- The health care consumer is "captive" because the health care market is not competitive.
- There is not enough public information such that consumers cannot adequately make health care decisions.
- The financing of health care in the United States does not allow consumers to make trade-offs in costs and quality of care.
- Health services are subject to the influence of special-interest groups.
- Illness and vulnerability require health care services and therefore costs do not go down when more service is available.

HEALTH SYSTEM EVOLUTION: THE CONTEXT OF CARE DELIVERY

From the 1800s through the late 1900s, the U.S. health care delivery system experienced four developmental stages, each with a differing emphasis on health care economics. A developmental framework for health services is useful to describe the evolving organization of health care delivery and to provide the framework for a discussion of health economics. Figure 7-1 shows the four basic categories included in the framework for health services delivery: *service needs and intensity, facilities, technology,* and *labor.*

Intensity is the use of technologies, supplies, and health care services by or for the client (Banta, 1995a). *Medical technology* refers to the techniques, drugs, equipment, processes, and procedures used by health care professionals in delivering medical care to individuals (Banta, 1995a).

Developmentally, the health services delivery framework acknowledges that the four framework categories have changed over time, reflecting total society changes in morbidity and mortality rates, national health policy, and economics. The developmental framework captures four time periods, or stages, as shown in Figure 7-2. Each element of the framework is used to show changes within stages to illustrate the growth and development of the U.S. health care system.

The *first developmental stage* (1800 to 1900) was characterized by:
- Epidemics of infectious diseases, such as cholera, typhoid, smallpox, influenza, malaria, and yellow fever
- Health concerns related to social and public health issues including contaminated food and water supplies, inadequate sewage disposal, and poor housing conditions (Banta, 1995b; Pickett and Hanlon, 1990)
- Most health care being provided in the home by family and friends
- Hospitals few in number and characterized by overcrowding, disease, and unsanitary conditions
- Sick persons cared for in hospitals often died from poor hospital conditions
- Most people avoiding care in a hospital unless there was no alternative
- Health care paid for by individuals who could afford health care, through bartering with physicians, or through charitable contributions from individuals and organizations
- Very basic and practical technology to aid in disease control but in keeping with knowledge development of the time
- The physician's "black bag" with few medicines and tools available for treatment
- A labor force composed mostly of physicians and nurses who attained their skills through apprenticeships or on-the-job training
- Predominantly female nurses in the United States whose education was linked to religious orders, with expectations of service, dedication, and charity (Kovner, 1999)
- The focus of nursing primarily on the support of physicians and assisting clients with activities of daily living

The *second developmental stage* (1900 to 1945) of U.S. health care delivery focused on:
- The control of acute infectious diseases
- Improving environmental conditions that influenced major advances in water purification, sanitary sewage disposal, milk and water quality, and urban housing quality
- Health problems changing from mass epidemics to

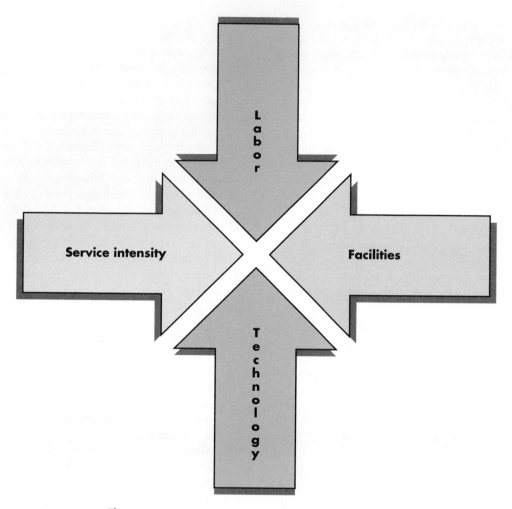

Figure 7-1   Components of health services development.

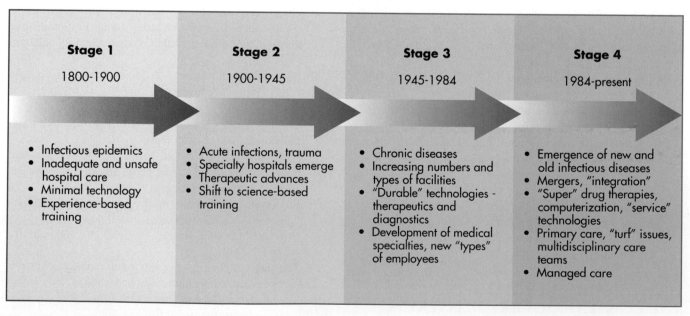

Figure 7-2   Developmental framework for health services delivery: service needs and intensity, facilities, technology, and labor.

individual acute infections or traumatic episodes (Pickett and Hanlon, 1990)

- Hospitals and health departments experiencing rapid growth during the late 1800s and early 1900s as technological advances in society were made (Kovner, 1999)
- City, county, and state governments beginning to contribute to health care by providing services for poor persons, state mental institutions, and other specialized hospitals, such as tuberculosis hospitals in addition to private and charitable financing of health care
- Public health departments emphasizing case finding and quarantine
- Health care paid for primarily by individuals
- The federal government's increasing interest in addressing social welfare problems, signified by The Social Security Act of 1935
- Clinical medicine entering its "golden age"
- Major technology advances in surgery and childbirth
- The identification of disease processes—such as the cause of pernicious anemia—that enhanced the ability to diagnose and treat diseases
- The discovery and development of pharmacologic advances—such as insulin in 1922 for control of diabetes, sulfa drugs in 1932 for treatment of infectious diseases, and antibiotics such as penicillin in the 1940s that eradicated certain infectious disease—increased treatment options, and decreased morbidity and mortality rates (Rice, 1994)
- Technology and new knowledge as physician education shifted away from apprenticeships to scientifically based college education, which occurred after the publication of the Flexner Report in 1910
- Nurses training primarily in hospital schools of nursing, with an emphasis on following and executing physicians' orders
- Nurses in training, unmarried and under the age of 30, providing the bulk of care in hospitals (Kovner, 1999)
- Public health nurses tracking infectious diseases and implementing quarantine procedures and working more collegially with physicians (Kovner, 1999)
- University-based nursing programs emerging to establish and to accommodate the expanding practice base of nursing
- Client education being assumed as a nursing function
- Roughly 40 types of other health care providers before 1940, such as pharmacists

The *third developmental stage* (1945 to 1984) included:

- A shift away from acute infectious health problems to chronic health problems such as heart disease, cancer, and stroke, resulting from increasing affluence and lifestyle changes in the United States
- The number and types of facilities expanding to include, for example, hospital clinics and long-term care facilities, to meet society's needs
- The Joint Commission on Accreditation of Hospitals, established in 1951 and later renamed the Joint Commission on Accreditation of Healthcare Organizations (JCAHO), focused on the safety and protection of the public and the delivery of quality care (Weitzman, 1990)
- Major technological advances such as the development of chemotherapeutic agents, immunizations, anesthesia, and electrolyte and cardiopulmonary physiology
- Expansion of diagnostic laboratories and complex equipment such as the computerized tomography (CT) scanner
- Organ and tissue transplants
- Radiation therapy
- Laser surgery
- Specialty units for critical care, coronary care, and intensive care
- The first "test tube baby" born via in vitro fertilization, and other fertility advances
- Health care providers constituting more than 5% of the total U.S. workforce
- The three largest health care employers: hospitals, convalescent institutions, and physicians' offices
- Between 1970 and 1984 alone, a growth in the number of persons employed in the health care industry by 90%
- Increasing the number of personnel employed in the community
- Physician assistants being trained under the supervision of physicians and employed to assist physicians in delivering routine medical care
- Care organized around specialties because of increasing technology and knowledge
- Nursing shortages in the 1970s and early 1980s
- Nursing education expanding from hospital-based diploma and university-based baccalaureate training to include associate degree preparation at the entry level
- The closure of nursing diploma schools beginning in the early-to-mid 1980s
- The number of baccalaureate and associate degree programs increasing
- Graduate nursing education expanding to include nurse practitioner (NP) and clinical nurse specialty (CNS) training to meet increasing societal demands, specialization, and technological advances
- The first doctoral programs in nursing to build the scientific base for nursing and to increase the number of nursing faculty
- The increasing role of the commercial health insurance industry, and a strong link between employment and the provision of health care benefits emerged
- The federal government's role expanding through landmark policy making that would affect health care delivery well into the twenty-first century, specifically, the passage of Titles XVIII and XIX of the Social Security Act in 1965 creating the Medicare and Medicaid programs, respectively
- The health care system appearance of unlimited resources for growth and expansion.

The *fourth developmental stage* (1984 to present) is a period of:

- Limited resources, with emphasis on cost containment, restricted growth in the health care industry, and reorganization of care delivery

- Escalating health care costs
- Limited public and private resources taking priority in policy discussions
- Increasing interest in the financing of health care
- Amendments to the Social Security Act in 1983 creating diagnostic-related groups and a prospective system of paying for health care provided to Medicare recipients
- The 1997 and 1999 Balanced Budget Act legislating additional federal mandates for Medicare and Medicaid
- Private-sector employer concerns about the rising costs of health care for employees
- Fear of profit losses spurring a major change in the delivery and financing of health care known as managed care
- Drastic changes in the settings and organization of health care delivery
- Commonplace transformation in health care organizations, and buzzwords of the period of reorganization, reengineering, restructuring, and downsizing
- Organizational mergers at an accelerated rate in an effort to consolidate care, find ways to reduce costs, the management of care, and coordinate care across the continuum (i.e., from "cradle to grave")
- Merger discussions about the union of similar agencies (e.g., acute care hospital mergers)
- Mergers between different types of acute care hospitals, long-term care facilities, and home health facilities
- Hospital closings and a shift of care from hospitals to other settings, such as ambulatory and community-based clinics and specialty diagnostic centers that offer traditional technologies like magnetic resonance imaging (MRI) and sonography
- Rehabilitative, restorative, and palliative care shifting from hospitals to other settings, such as sub-acute care hospitals, specialty rehabilitation hospitals, long-term care, and even to individual homes
- Patients admitted to the traditional acute care hospital who were more acutely ill
- Length of stay for patients declining and care delivery becoming more intense
- Technological advances, such as the widespread use of computers and the Internet, which have enabled society to become increasingly sophisticated about health
- The public's increasing knowledge about health care and awareness of health care advances influencing their demand for health care, such as diagnostic and therapeutic services for treatment
- Pharmaceutical companies and other technological suppliers actively marketing their products through television, printed advertisements, the Internet, and other sources so that clients rapidly become aware of the availability of new technologies
- Health professionals dependent upon technology to care for clients
- Distance as a barrier to the diagnosis and treatment of disease being overcome through the use of telehealth
- Health care professionals, along with payers, becoming the principal purchasing agents of technology for the client, often making decisions about when and if a certain technology will be used in a given situation
- Nurses becoming dependent upon technologies to monitor client progress, making decisions about client care, and delivering care in new and innovative ways

Health professionals of this stage were forced to consider alternative models of care delivery that run counter to traditional approaches. The consideration of these alternatives was prompted by economic and policy pressures to correct for the excesses of the health care system created during the previous developmental periods. The shift away from traditional hospital-based care to the community and the need to consider new models of care brought about:

- Increased emphasis on primary care
- The development of care delivery teams
- Collaboration in practice and education
- The substituting of one type of health personnel for another to control care delivery costs at two major levels: the substitution of NPs for primary care providers and the substitution of unlicensed personnel for staff nurses in hospitals and long-term care facilities
- "Turf" battles fueled by these substitutions
- The increase in specialization of health professionals leading to changes in certification, qualifications, education, and standards of care in health professions
- Increased number and kinds of providers to meet the demands of the health care system
- Between 1990 and 1996 alone, health service employment increasing by 19%, more than twice the increase of the total U.S. workforce
- The number of types of health care personnel rising to more than 200

The Bureau of Labor Statistics (BLS) predicts that two sectors of health care employment will be among the top ten industries with fast employment growth between 1996 and 2006: the health services sector in general is ranked second (behind computer and data processing services) with a projected job growth of 68%, and offices of health practitioners are ranked ninth, with a projected growth of 47% (Bureau of Labor Statistics, 1998). Box 7-1 presents the numbers of certain active health care professionals in 1997.

| Box 7-1 | Number of Health Care Professionals in the United States |

In 1997, the numbers of active health professionals included the following:
- 756,710 physicians
- 29,500 optometrists
- 185,000 pharmacists
- 11,121 podiatrists
- 2,161,700 registered nurses
- 154,900 dentists

From U.S. Department of Health and Human Services, Health Resources and Services Administration Bureau of Health Professions, National Center for Health and Workforce Information and Analysis, 2000, online: www.hrsa.gov.

The registered nurse labor market is the largest sector of health care professionals, representing 2.3 million practicing registered nurses (Health Resources and Services Administration, 2000). Of those practicing nurses, approximately 18% were employed in community and public health. The nursing profession is identified as one of five occupations projected to have the largest number of new jobs going into the twenty-first century, with above average anticipated earnings (Bureau of Labor Statistics, 1998). The continuing shift in emphasis to preventive health care and health promotion is clearly in line with community health nursing and an increasing role for nursing within community settings and care delivery programs such as managed care.

Finally, during this period:
- The United States experienced an increase in the number and types of communicable, infectious, and environmental illnesses
- Infant mortality is at a record low in the United States
- Life expectancy is at a record high
- Chronic illnesses resulting from environmental and lifestyle influences are increasing

With the resurgence of communicable and infectious diseases, such as tuberculosis, acquired immunodeficiency syndrome (AIDS), and new strains of streptococcus, major challenges in health care delivery are anticipated in the twenty-first century.

TRENDS IN HEALTH CARE SPENDING

Much has been written in the popular and scientific literature about the costs of U.S. health care and how society makes decisions about allocating available and scarce resources. Given that economics in general and health care economics in particular are concerned with resources, any discussion of the economics of health care must consider past and current health care spending. The trends documented here reflect past public and private decisions about health care and health care delivery.

Figure 7-3 shows U.S. health care expenses between 1970 and 2001. Spending for health care increased from approximately $24 million in 1980 to over $1 trillion in 2000.

Figure 7-4 provides a breakdown of the distribution in health care expenses for 1999 (U.S. Department of Health and Human Services, 2000). The largest proportions of health care expenses were for hospital care and physician services. Only a small fraction of health care dollars was spent on home health, public health, and research and construction. Health care spending was almost $14 of every $100 spent in the United States in 1999 (Health U.S., 1999).

While the costs of health care have decelerated in recent years, predictions suggest that health care spending may increase in the future (Smith, et al, 1998). In 2000, health care costs are on the rise (Health Care Financing Administration, 2000). The basis of this prediction was that cost savings from managed care would be achieved. This appears to have become true. Smith and colleagues suggested that health care spending may reach $2.1 trillion by the year 2007, almost doubling current spending within less than 10 years. If these projections are true, health care will represent approximately 17 cents of every dollar. Box 7-2 presents a more in-depth overview of predicted changes in health care spending.

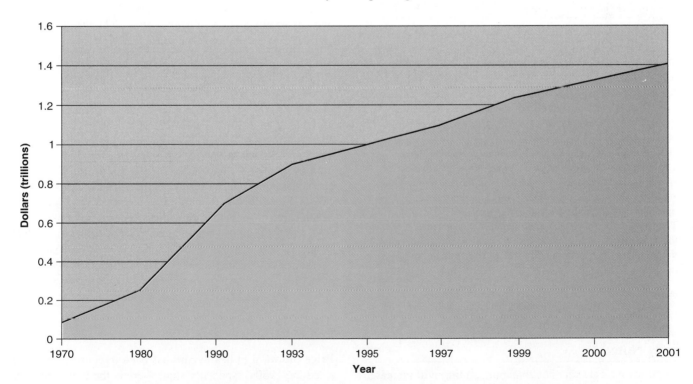

Figure 7-3 **U.S Health Care Expenses from 1970 to 2001 (data projected for 2000 and 2001).** (Data from Health Care Financing Administration: National health expenditures tables, 2000, available online at www.hcfa.gov/stats/nhe-oact/tables/.)

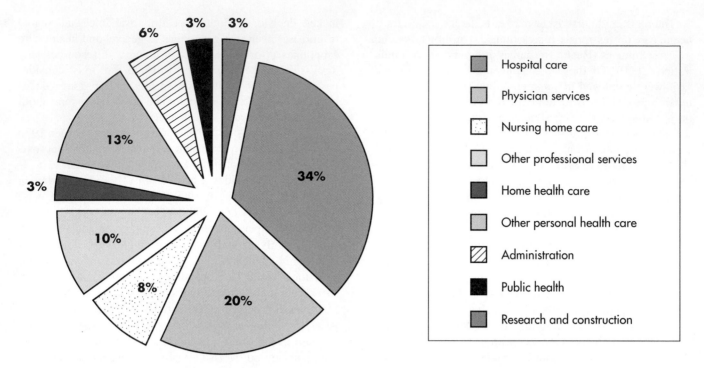

Notes: 1) Percentages have been rounded upward to add to 100. 2) "Other professional services" includes dental and other non-physician health care services. 3) "Other personal services" includes drugs and other non-durable health care goods, vision products and other durable health care goods, and any other personal health care.

Figure 7-4   **Distribution of U.S. health care expenditures for 1999.** (Data from U.S. Department of Health and Human Services: *Health: United States, 2000,* DHHS pub no [PHS] 00-1232, Washington, D.C., 2000, U.S. Government Printing Office.)

Box 7-2   Predicted Changes in Health Care Spending

Researchers predict that between 1996 and 2007, health care spending will change in the following ways:

- Hospital spending growth will be lower than all other health care spending.
- Spending for physician services will be substantially increased.
- Spending on pharmaceuticals is expected to accelerate.
- Spending for nursing home care will initially accelerate, then decelerate.
- Home health care spending will be greater than all other spending growth; however, in 2000 the home health care spending declined because of changes in federal regulations.
- Annual spending for specialists such as podiatrists, optometrists, and chiropractors will increase.
- The overall costs of health care benefits will increase faster than the growth in total salary compensation, suggesting that the numbers of uninsured will grow as individual employees increasingly become more responsible for benefit payments.

Data from Smith, et al: The Health Expenditures Projection Team: the next ten years of health spending: what does the future hold? *Health Affairs* 17(5):128, 1998.

Briefly Noted

Projections indicate that health care spending will increase, perhaps even double, in less than 10 years and that health care will represent approximately 17% of all monies spent in the U.S. for goods and services. If this happens, what impact will this increase have on the U.S. society and economy? Is spending 17% of every dollar on health care a concern? Provide a rationale for your position.

FACTORS INFLUENCING HEALTH CARE COSTS

Health economists, providers, payers, and politicians have explored different explanations for the rapid rate of increase in health expenses in contrast to population growth. The explanation that individuals, over time, have consumed more health care is not sufficient. A more plausible possibility is that the health care consumed by individuals became more expensive for a combination of complex reasons. The following factors frequently are considered the causes of spending increases over the past 40 years (Levit, et al, 1997): *inflation, changes in population demography,* and *technology and intensity of services.* Discussion of each factor is presented here.

Price Inflation

Price inflation in health care has been a recurring concern since the 1950s, especially since there is the belief, usually backed up by documented proof, that increasing amounts and portions of public resources have been allocated to

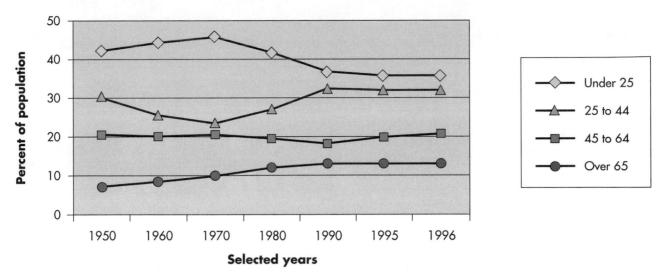

Figure 7-5   U.S. population by age-group for selected years from 1950-1996. (Data from U.S. Department of Health and Human Services: *Health: United States, 1998,* DHHS pub no [PHS] 98-1232, Washington, D.C., 1998, U.S. Government Printing Office.)

health care rather than to other society investments. Inflation occurs when there is a sustained upward trend in the prices of goods and services (Boyes, 1992). General inflation in the U.S. economy affects the prices of all goods and services in the United States, including health care. However, there is a certain amount and/or proportion of inflation that is specific to the health care industry.

Changes in Demographics

Another factor often associated with rising health care costs is the *change in demographics.* The changing demographics, in turn, affects the ways in which health care resources are used and what technologies are developed. The first notable demographic change is that the U.S. population, in general, has increased in size. This means that, across all age-groups and segments of society, the sheer number of people requiring health services has increased.

Second, while all age-groups are increasing in number, an important demographic shift is the aging of the society. In 1996, approximately 13% of the U.S. population was over the age of 65; the same age-group made up approximately 9% of the total U.S. population in 1960 (U.S. Department of Health and Human Services, 1998). By the year 2030, the over-65 age-group will compose roughly 20% of the U.S. population (Health Care Financing Administration, 1998). This shift in the age of the population, shown in Figure 7-5, places increasing pressure on society to allocate and spend more money on age-related health issues, including long-term care, research, and preventing and treating chronic diseases.

This trend will continue and become more profound as the baby boom generation ages. The baby boom generation refers to individuals born between 1946 and 1964. The first of the baby boomers is now over 55 years old. This well-educated generation is more oriented to preventive health

care and is just beginning to move into the time of life when long-term care will be needed. Just as this group increased the need for pediatric health care in the 1950s, they now will increase the need for long-term care for chronic conditions (Pew Health Professions Commission, 1993). In 1996 the cost of 1 year in a nursing home averaged more than $37,500 (U.S. Department of Health and Human Services, 1998). To receive Medicaid long-term care benefits, elderly persons must "spend down" their life savings to poverty levels, including selling their homes. The decreasing size of the younger and college-aged population, usually the healthiest group requiring less health care service, will mean fewer persons to help pay for the cost of elder care through insurance premiums (Pew Health Professions Commission, 1993).

Other demographic factors potentially will add to increasing health care costs. There has been an increase in racial diversity within the United States. Table 7-1 documents this trend of increasing diversity in the population: the proportion of Caucasians has decreased, and the proportion of all other racial groups has increased. Recent reports suggest that the ethnic mix in the United States will continue to shift as, for example, the proportion of Hispanics surpasses the proportion of African-Americans in the year 2010 (U.S. Census Bureau, 1996).

Given that racial diversity varies by state and geographic region, the emphasis and relative importance of these issues also varies across the United States. For example, in 1994 California voters passed the controversial Proposition 187, an initiative that restricts the use of public-supported services by illegal immigrants.

Increased racial diversity presents certain health care challenges. Individuals of other nationalities often immigrate to the United States to escape social hardships within their country of origin, many of which, such as poor sanitation and over-crowding, are known detriments to health.

TABLE 7-1   U.S. Population (in thousands) by Ethnicity (%)

Year	All Persons	Caucasian	African-American	American Indian or Alaska Native	Asian Pacific Islander	Hispanic White
1950	149,984	134,942 (90%)	15,042 (10%)	—	—	—
1960	177,704	158,832 (89%)	18,872 (11%)	—	—	—
1970	200,679	178,098 (89%)	22,581 (11%)	—	—	—
1980	226,545	194,713 (86%)	26,683 (12%)	1,420 (0.6%)	3,729 (2%)	14,609 (6%)
1990	248,765	208,727 (84%)	30,511 (12%)	2,065 (0.8%)	7,462 (3%)	22,372 (9%)
1995	270,299	223,001 (83%)	34,431 (13%)	2,360 (0.9%)	10,507 (4%)	30,250 (10%)
1997	267,744	221,317 (83%)	33,973 (13%)	2,324 (0.9%)	10,130 (4%)	29,160 (11%)
1998	270,300	223,001 (83%)	34,431 (13%)	2,361 (0.9%)	10,507 (4%)	30,250 (11%)

From U.S. Census Bureau: *Statistical abstract of the United States: 1999,* Washington, D.C., 1999, U.S. Government Printing Office.

TABLE 7-2   Examples of Federal Regulatory Mechanisms Contributing to Technology Costs and Control

Year	Federal Regulation
1906	Prescription drug regulation passes (Food, Drug, and Cosmetic Act [now FDA])
1938	Manufacturers are required to prove drug safety (Food, Drug, and Cosmetic Act)
1952	Hill-Burton Act provides construction monies for new hospitals
1965	Amendments made to Social Security Act providing Medicare and Medicaid to support health care services provided to certain groups
1972	Social Security Act amendments: (1) extend coverage for end-stage renal disease to provide payment for use of treatment technologies; and (2) provide for professional standards review organizations to review appropriateness of hospital care for Medicare/Medicaid recipients
1974	Health Planning and Resources Development Act introduces certificate-of-need to limit major health care expansion at local and state levels
1976	Medical devices amendments regulate safety and effectiveness of medical equipment, such as pacemakers
1978	Medicare End-Stage Renal Disease Amendment provides home dialysis and kidney transplantation; Health Services Research, Health Statistics, and Health Care Technology Act establishes national council on health care technology to develop standards for use
1982	Tax Equity and Fiscal Responsibilities Act establishes prospective payment system for hospitalized Medicare patients by DRG category
	Omnibus Reconciliation Act created: (1) physician resource-based fee schedule to be implemented by 1992, with emphasis on high-tech specialties of surgery; and (2) the Agency for Health Care Policy and Research to perform research on effectiveness of medical services, interventions, and technologies, including nursing
1996	Health Insurance Portability and Accountability Act enacted to protect health insurance coverage for laid-off or displaced workers
1998	Third-party reimbursement for Medicare Part B services under Public Law 105-33 established for advanced-practice nurses

Individuals who could be considered members of the following groups have entered the United States:

- In poor health
- Lived in poverty
- Lived under poor circumstances after arriving
- Have not had access to needed health care services

Beyond those just entering the United States, there are U.S.-born individuals of all racial and ethnic groups who:

- Live in poverty
- Receive little or no education
- Have a low-paying job or no job at all
- Are homeless
- Lack access to needed health care services

When these demographic issues coexist, many health care problems often exist. As a result, individuals across all racial groups will continue to need services to meet even the most basic of health care necessities. Providing access to such services adds to the overall health care costs (Pew Health Professions Commission, 1993) and creates an important, yet fundamental, question for society: How can and should the United States allocate its money to get the best return on investment? The investment is the health of the population. The return would be a healthier nation. Many complexities and strong opposing viewpoints surround this question, making it historically difficult for the nation to take a definite stand on this sensitive issue.

Technology and Intensity

The introduction of new *technology* improves the delivery of care, but it also has the potential to increase the costs of care. As new and more complex technology is introduced into the

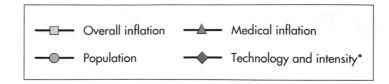

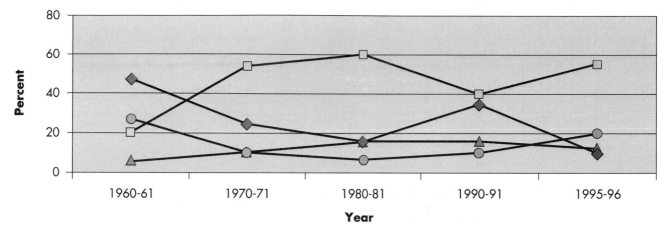

* Residual of growth that cannot be attributed to price increases or population growth; represents changes in use or kinds of services and supplies

Figure 7-6   **Factors affecting growth of health care expenditures.**   (Data from U.S. Department of Health and Human Services: *Health: United States, 1998,* DHHS pub no [PHS] 98-1232, Washington, D.C., 1998, U.S. Government Printing Office.)

system, the cost is typically high. However, clients often demand access to the technology, and providers want to use the technology. In an effort to keep health care costs down, however, payers have attempted to restrict use and availability of certain technologies. For example, the drug Viagra, developed for the treatment of impotence by Pfizer Pharmaceuticals, is an example of a controversial technology that, upon immediate availability to the public, was in high demand and prescribed by providers, yet restricted in use by payers.

The adoption of new technology increases the need for personnel, equipment, and facilities. Furthermore, new technology adds to administrative costs, especially if the federal government provides financial coverage for the service or is involved in regulating the technology. Table 7-2 outlines federal regulations that have, over time, contributed to the use of technology.

A health care problem that has contributed to the overall cost of health care through medical care, research, development of new technology, and cash assistance to clients is AIDS. AIDS is a problem that has affected a large number of people requiring a wide array of services (intensity), expensive treatments (technologies), and care. Money spent by the federal government alone for AIDS increased from approximately $6 million in 1982 to approximately $6 billion in 1999 (Centers for Disease Control and Prevention, 2000).

Chernew and colleagues (1998) identify technology as the "predominant factor" behind health care cost increases. They note that managed care plans, while restricting use of certain technologies, have failed to contain the health care cost increases.

Figure 7-6 summarizes the influence of demographic changes, service intensity and technology, along with infla-

tion on health care costs (U.S. Department of Health and Human Services, 1998). In 1996 overall national inflation, and changes in the population, contributed most to cost, while medical cost inflation and technology and intensity tied for third place in contributing to health care costs.

FINANCING OF HEALTH CARE

Health care financing has evolved during the twentieth century from a system in which the client was the primary payer to a system financed by third-party payers: publicly by state and federal governments, and privately through insurers and managed care. Figure 7-7 shows changes in the percentages of financing by source. From 1950 to 1999, out-of-pocket spending decreased, charitable (other private) payments increased slightly, and third-party federal public and private health insurance payments increased dramatically.

Public Support

The federal government became involved in health care financing for population groups early in U.S. history. In 1798 the federal government created the Marine Hospital Service to provide medical service for sick and disabled sailors and to protect the nation's borders against the importing of disease through seaports. The Marine Hospital Service is considered the first national health insurance plan in the United States. The original plan cost each sailor 20 cents per month in a payroll deduction for illness care.

Medicare and Medicaid, two federal programs administered by the Health Care Financing Administration (HCFA), account for the majority of public health care spending

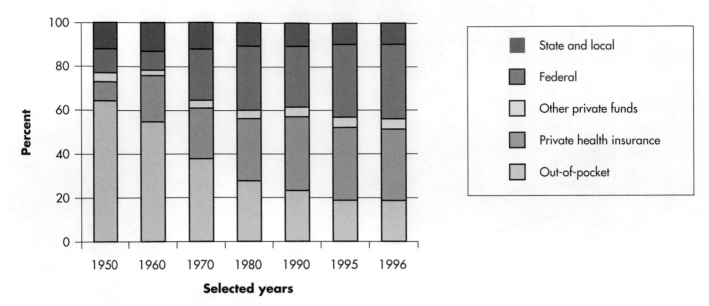

Figure 7-7   **Personal health care expenditures by source of funds.** (Data from U.S. Department of Health and Human Services: *Health: United States, 1998*, DHHS pub no [PHS] 98-1232, Washington, D.C., 1998, U.S. Government Printing Office.)

TABLE 7-3	Comparison of Medicare and Medicaid Programs	
Feature	**Medicare**	**Medicaid**
Obtain information	Local Social Security Administration office	State welfare office
Recipients	People who are 65 years old, are disabled, or have permanent kidney failure	Certain low-income and needy people, including children; the aged, blind, and/or disabled and those eligible to receive federally assisted income
Type of program	Insurance	Insurance
Government	Federal affiliation	Joint federal/state partnership
Availability	All states	All states
Financing of hospital insurance	Medicare Trust Fund, mandatory payroll deductions (1.45% employed persons; 2.9% self-employed); recipient deductibles; trust fund interest	Federal and state governments
Financing of medical insurance	Recipient premium payments ($45.50 per month in 2000); general revenue of the U.S. Treasury	Federal and state governments
Types of coverage	Inpatient and outpatient hospital services, skilled nursing facilities, partial home health services coverage; hospice care, physician services, medical and health services equipment and supplies	Inpatient and outpatient hospital services; prenatal care; vaccines for children; physician, dental, NP and nurse midwifery services; skilled nursing facility services for persons 21 years of age or older; family services; rural health clinic services; diagnosis; and treatment of children under 21 years of age

today. The HCFA is the federal regulatory agency within the USDHHS that is responsible for overseeing and monitoring Medicare and Medicaid spending. This agency routinely collects and reports actual health care use and spending and projects future spending trends.

Table 7-3 provides an overview and comparison of these programs. Through these programs, the federal government purchases health care services for population groups provided through independent health care systems,

such as managed care organizations, private physicians, and hospitals.

Medicare

The **Medicare** program, established in Title XVIII of the Social Security Act of 1965, provides hospital insurance and medical insurance to elderly persons, permanently and totally disabled persons, and people with end-stage renal disease. Currently 38.4 million people are enrolled in

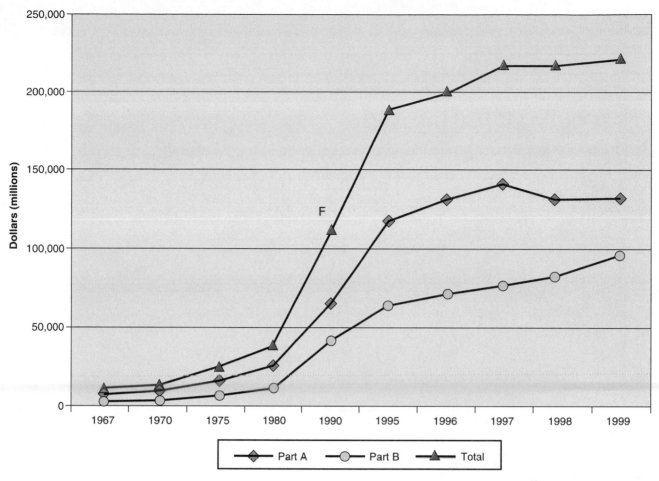

Figure 7-8 Medicare Expenditures for 1967-1999. (Data from Health Care Financing Administration: National health expenditures tables, 2000, available online at www.hcfa.gov/stats/nhe-oact/tables/)

Medicare, or more than 10% of the total U.S. population (Health Care Financing Administration, 2000).

The hospital insurance package, Part A, is available to all elderly individuals who have paid Social Security taxes. Estimates indicate that 98% of the elderly population are covered by Part A, which provides payment for:

- Hospital services
- Home health services
- Extended-care facilities

Part A requires a deductible from recipients of $776 for the first 60 days of services and a coinsurance payment of $194 for 61 to 90 days of service based on a rate equal to a 1-day stay in the hospital. That deductible has increased over the years as daily hospital costs have increased (Health Care Financing Administration, May 2000).

The medical insurance package, Part B, is available to all eligible people who wish to pay a monthly premium for the coverage. Approximately 96% of the elderly population is covered. The premium cost was $45.50 per month in 2000 (Health Care Financing Administration, May 2000).

Part B provides coverage for services other than hospitalization, such as:

- Physician care
- Outpatient hospital care
- Outpatient physical therapy

- Home health care not covered by Part A
- Laboratory services
- Ambulance transportation
- Prostheses
- Equipment
- Some supplies

After a deductible, up to 80% of reasonable charges are paid for these services. Part B resembles the major medical insurance coverage of private insurance carriers.

Figure 7-8 shows total expenses of the Medicare program from 1967 to 1996. With the passing of the Medicare amendments to the Social Security Act in 1965, the cost of Medicare has increased dramatically.

Hospital care continues to be the major factor contributing to Medicare costs; however, with shorter hospital stays, home health and nursing home costs have increased dramatically.

As a result of increasing costs, Congress passed a law in 1983, the Social Security amendments of 1983 (Public Law 98-21) to end cost-plus reimbursement by Medicare and instituted a prospective payment system (PPS) for inpatient hospital services. The purpose of the new hospital payment scheme was to shift the financial incentives away from the provision of more care, the use of more technology, and the use of more hospital care. Reimbursement is based on a

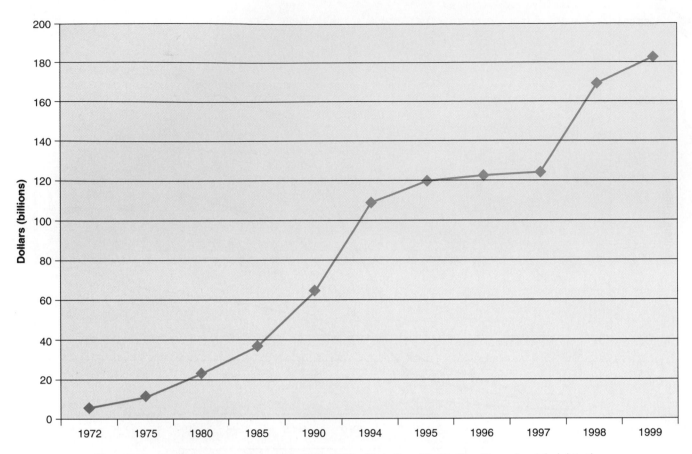

Figure 7-9   Medicaid Expenditures for 1972-1999. (Data from Health Care Financing Administration: National health expenditures tables, 2000, available online at www.hcfa.gov/stats/nhe-oact/tables/)

fixed price per case for clients in 468 **diagnosis-related groups (DRGs).** The objective of this system was to reduce hospital costs while maintaining quality health care and access. Although this type of reimbursement originally was mandated for hospitals only, the Balanced Budget Act (BBA) of 1997 determined that payments to Medicare skilled nursing facilities (SNFs) would be made based on the PPS, and began July 1, 1998. The PPS payment rates cover SNF services, including routine, ancillary, and capital-related costs (Health Care Financing Administration, 1998). Payments to physicians, home health, and ambulatory care are being considered.

Medicaid

The **Medicaid** program, Title XIX of the Social Security Act of 1965, provides financial assistance to states and counties to pay for medical services for the aged poor, the blind, the disabled, and families with dependent children. The Medicaid program is jointly sponsored and financed with matching funds from the federal and state governments. Currently, 37.5 million people are enrolled in Medicaid (Health Care Financing Administration, 2000). Medicaid expenditures from 1972 to 1996 are shown in Figure 7-9.

Full payment for five types of service was provided at the beginning of Medicaid (U.S. Department of Health and Human Services, 1994, 1998):

1. Inpatient and outpatient hospital care
2. Laboratory and radiology services
3. Physician services
4. Skilled nursing care at home or in a nursing home for people over 21 years of age
5. Early and Periodic Screening, Diagnosis, and Treatment (EPSDT) services for those under 21 years of age (U.S. Department of Health and Human Services, 1994, 1998).

The 1972 Social Security amendments added family planning as a program requirement and as program options:

- Prescriptions
- Dental services
- Eyeglasses
- Intermediate care facilities
- Coverage for the medically indigent

By law, the medically indigent are required to pay a monthly premium. Any state participating in the Medicaid program is required to provide the six basic services to participants who are below state poverty income levels. The optional programs are provided at the discretion of each state. In 1989, changes in Medicaid required states to provide care for children under 6 years of age and to pregnant women under 133% of the poverty level. For example, if the poverty level were $12,000, a pregnant woman could have a household income as high as $16,000 representing 100% of poverty, and still be eligible to receive care under Medicaid, with $4,000 additional representing 33% of poverty. These changes also provided for pediatric and family nurse practitioner reimbursement.

In the 1990s, states were allowed to petition the federal government for a waiver. If the waiver was approved, the states could use their Medicaid monies for programs other than the six basic services. The first waiver to be approved was given to Oregon for their health care reform plan. Other states have received waivers to develop Medicaid managed care programs for special populations.

The major expense categories for the Medicaid program historically have been skilled and intermediate nursing home care and inpatient hospital care. When combined, today these two categories account for 49% of all costs to the program (U.S. Department of Health and Human Services, 1998).

Public Health

Most public government agencies operate on an annual budget and plan for costs by estimating salaries, expenses, and costs of services for a year. Public health agencies, such as health departments and WIC programs, receive primary funding from tax revenues, with additional money for select goods and services through private third-party payers. Selected public health programs receive reimbursement for services as follows:

- Through grants given by the federal government to states for prenatal and child health
- Through Medicare and Medicaid for home health, nursing homes, WIC, and EPSDT programs
- Through collection of fees on a sliding scale for select client services, such as immunizations

Private Support

There are several private health care payer sources: insurance, employers, managed care, and individuals. Although insurance and consumers have been prominent health care payment sources for some time, the role of employers and managed care has become increasingly prominent and powerful during the last two decades of the twentieth century.

Insurance

Insurance for health care was first offered by the private sector in 1847 by a commercial insurance company. The purpose of the insurance was to provide security and indemnity for health care services to individuals. The idea behind insurance was that it provided security, guaranteeing (within certain limits) monies to pay for health care services to defray potential financial losses from unexpected illness or injury related to accidents, catastrophic communicable diseases, such as smallpox and scarlet fever, and recurring (but unexpected) chronic illnesses.

The Depression of the 1930s, rising medical costs, and the need to spread financial risk across communities spurred the development of the **third-party payment** system.

The system began as a major industry in the 1930s with the Blue Cross system, which initially provided prepayment for hospital care. It was modeled on the Baylor University prepayment plan established in 1929 to provide teachers with hospital coverage. In 1939 Blue Shield created plans to provide physician payment. The Blue Cross plans, which began as tax-free, nonprofit insurance organizations, were established under special legislation in various states.

In the 1940s and 1950s hospital and medical-surgical coverage increased substantially. Employee group coverage appeared, and profit-making commercial insurance underwriters began offering health insurance packages with competitive premiums.

Premium competition, the offering of health insurance as a fringe benefit, and the use of health insurance as a negotiable collective bargaining item led to an increase in covered benefits, payment of higher portions of medical care expenses, and increased employer-paid premiums. In turn, these factors pushed up premium costs and health care costs and enabled insurance plans to financially cover high-risk segments of the population, such as aged, poor, or disabled persons.

Employers

Since the beginning of Blue Cross and Blue Shield, health insurance became tied to employment and the business sector. This tie was strengthened during World War II to compensate, attract, and retain employees (Folland, Goodman, and Stano, 1993). Since that time, employers have become increasingly prominent in determining health insurance benefits, and they receive a tax break for providing these benefits.

Receiving health insurance through an employer is unlike the way an individual gets other types of insurance (Folland, Goodman, and Stano, 1993). For example, automobile insurance is a product that individuals purchase out of pocket; they choose a plan by making comparisons among insurers, specific plans offered, levels of coverage, premiums required, and individual needs. The link between health insurance and employers causes difficulties, for example, when one loses a job, changes jobs, or is between jobs.

Any additional insurance that individuals choose to purchase, above and beyond what the employer provides, usually comes out of "pre-tax" dollars, such that employees taxable wages are reduced. Employers, on the other hand, can deduct employee health insurance premiums as a cost of doing business, which reduces taxable income. Both employees and employers, to a certain degree, are better off if the employer purchases health insurance, as long as the costs of providing benefits does not become too costly for the employers, outweighing the tax benefits of doing so.

Employers, in essence, add another "layer" to the health care payment scheme:

- Individuals gain access to insurance to pay for health care services through their employers
- Employers make decisions about the level of care and plan of coverage that will be offered to employees
- Insurers make decisions about services that will be covered through various plan options offered to employers
- Providers deliver care to individuals within these limits.

One can argue that with the addition of each "layer" comes added costs and less choice by the client. Employers have incentives to keep costs down. Disadvantages of high health care costs include:

- Additional costs of doing business, which decrease profits
- A decrease in their ability to make other investments
- A decrease in money paid to stockholders

In an effort to bypass the costs added by insurers, some employers have found it less costly to "self-insure," an arrangement whereby an employer contracts directly with providers to provide health care services to employees rather than going through health insurance companies to purchase employee insurance. Some large businesses directly employ on-site providers for care delivery or offer on-site wellness programs. These programs within the private sector offer opportunities for nurses to provide wellness programs, perform health assessments, and screen and monitor employees and their families. This move to self-insure has resulted in savings to companies and has reduced overall sick care costs (Knickman and Thorpe, 1999).

These and other efforts by employers have strengthened their health care buying power. In fact, employers' quest to keep health care costs and employee benefit costs down brought about the increase in managed care in the United States.

Managed Care

Managed care is a philosophy of health care that integrates the financing, delivery, and use of care. This philosophy often gets misinterpreted as a source of financing exclusively because the managed care movement has overemphasized costs and underemphasized quality, and subsequently, reports in the popular press have focused on denials of care to individuals, clients' dissatisfaction with care, and a general lack of trust in the system of care. Negative press has also focused on the costs of providing administrative support to oversee managed care plans, providers, and others involved in the delivery of managed care.

Managed care offers a set of services to purchasers, such as employers or Medicare, for a set fee. This fee, in turn, is used to pay providers through predetermined arrangements for services delivered to covered individuals (U.S. Department of Health and Human Services, 1998). Managed care is based on the notion that the use of costly care could be reduced through consumer education on illness prevention and health maintenance. Therefore managed care is also based on the underlying values of disease prevention, health promotion, wellness, and consumer education, all of which are important principals that often get overlooked.

Types of arrangements commonly used in managed care are health maintenance organizations (HMOs) and preferred provider organizations (PPOs). Box 7-3 provides an overview of HMOs and PPOs. Although HMOs and PPOs seem like relatively new arrangements in health care, HMOs have actually been around since the 1940s.

The Health Maintenance Organization Act was passed in 1972, and since that time, the number of individuals receiving care through HMOs and other types of managed care organizations has increased considerably: between 1976 and

---

Box 7-3 Types of Managed Care

A health maintenance organization (HMO) is a provider arrangement whereby comprehensive care is provided to plan members for a fixed, "per member per month" fee. Common features include the following:
A. Capitation
B. Use of designated providers
C. Point-of-service care or receiving care from nondesignated plan providers
D. One of the following models:
 1. Staff model, whereby physicians are HMO employees
 2. Group model, whereby a physician group practice contracts with the HMO to provide care
 3. Individual practice association (IPA), whereby the HMO contracts with physicians in solo, small group practices, or physician networks to provide care
 4. Mixed model, whereby the HMO uses a combination group/IPA arrangement

A Preferred Provider Organization (PPO) is a provider arrangement whereby predetermined rates are established for services to be delivered to members. Common features include the following:
A. Hospital and physician providers
B. Discounted rate setting
C. Financial incentives to encourage plan members to select PPO providers
D. Expedited claims payment to providers

From Folland S, Goodman AC, Stano M: *The economics of health and health care,* New York, 1993, Macmillan; U.S. Department of Health and Human Services: *Health: United States, 1998,* DHHS pub no (PHS) 98-1232, Washington, D.C., 1998, U.S. Government Printing Office.

1997, the number of individuals enrolled in an HMO increased from 6 million to almost 67 million (U.S. Department of Health and Human Services, 1998).

Individuals

Before 1930 and the beginning of Blue Cross, the client, or consumer of health care, had more control and influence over health care costs because nearly all health care costs were paid using out-of-pocket money. In this scenario, consumers had to make decisions about how they would spend their money, making certain "trade-offs," for example, about the type and price of health care they were willing to buy. Furthermore, entering the system was restricted in large part to those who could afford to pay for care or to those few who could find care financed through charitable and philanthropic organizations. However, with the beginning of the U.S. health care third-party payer system and up until the late 1980s, health care was for the most part a seller's market. The services offered and price was controlled by the provider, who decided the type and level of care or service that would be offered.

In the purest sense, "consumer" implies that money is exchanged for goods and services purchased and used. Under the third-party system, however, this meaning becomes blurred because the one making purchasing and payment decisions for health care services is typically not the person receiving care. Specifically, the third party makes decisions about the level and type of care that will be purchased for clients and determines how payment will be made, and the client has limited influence on how services will be reimbursed. However, the consumer does affect the provider and payment through political channels.

In 1996, individuals paid out-of-pocket for approximately 17% of total health expenditures (Levit, et al, 1997). However, these figures do not reflect the amount of money the consumer pays in taxes to finance government-supported programs such as Medicare and Medicaid, insurance premiums coming out of paid wages that decrease the size of paychecks, or the direct insurance premiums paid for supplemental insurance to plug the gaps in the primary health insurance policy and Medicare (U.S. Department of Health and Human Services, 1994, 1998).

The average monthly cost for private health insurance is increasing. These premium increases reflect a shift of the health care cost burden from employers to employees, with the percentage of employer contributions to health care declining. The decrease in employer contribution to health insurance premiums parallels the move away from traditional insurance plans by small and large employers to managed care plans (Levit, et al 1998).

Given that access to health insurance is tied to employment, there was growing concern in the late 1980s and early 1990s about employment layoffs and downsizing occurring in private business. Those who lost their jobs also lost their ability to pay for health insurance and to qualify to purchase insurance privately. The Health Insurance Portability and Accountability Act of 1996 (HIPAA) was enacted to protect health insurance coverage for workers and families after a job change or loss (Health Care Financing Administration, Feb 1999). The most important point in this act was the ability of employees to continue their employer's insurance coverage for eighteen months until coverage could be obtained through a new program.

Another insurance reform discussion at the political level concerns medical savings accounts (MSAs). MSAs are touted as a way of turning health care decision-making control over to individuals receiving care. MSAs are tax-exempt accounts available to individuals who work for small companies, established usually through a bank or insurance company, that enable individuals to save money for future medical needs and expenses (Internal Revenue Service, 1998).

Money contributed to an MSA comes out of "pre-tax" dollars and employer contributions, so initial set-aside money does not come out of taxable income. Furthermore, interest earned in MSAs are tax-free, and any unused money in an MSA can be held in the account from year to year until the money is used. MSAs, in theory, would allow individuals to make cost/quality "trade-offs" but would mean that individuals would need to become knowledgeable about health care, become involved in health care decision making, and take responsibility for the decisions made. Providers, in turn, must be willing to provide and disclose information to individuals and relinquish control of health care decision making. The HIPAA and MSAs are examples of current health insurance reform efforts, and these efforts will likely remain in the forefront of political discussions for some time to come.

| Box 7-4 | **Elements of the Patient Protection Act** |

- Guaranteeing a Patient Right-to-Know will allow free and open communications between patients and doctors in order to make fully-informed decisions about the best course of treatment. This is commonly referred to as lifting "gag rules" placed on medical providers.
- Ensuring Access to Emergency Care by Applying Prudent Layperson Standards will guarantee that patients will be treated in emergency departments when they need care most by prohibiting health plans from arbitrarily refusing to pay for covered emergency benefits.
- Providing Direct Access for OB/GYNs will allow women the opportunity to bypass the insurance company's gatekeeper and go directly to their provider.
- Disclosing Plan Information will make it easier for patients to learn what their health plan covers specifically, including benefits, doctors, and facilities. It also enables patients to better compare coverage information between health plans.
- Expediting Internal Review will hold insurance companies accountable by giving patients access to immediate decisions from doctors about what is covered for emergency, urgent, and routine services without preventing legal options already provided under current law.
- Providing Independent Medical Expertise in External Appeals will guarantee unprecedented patient protection by requiring that an independent doctor decides if a requested service is medically necessary, if originally turned down by internal review.
- Creating Association Health Plans will provide avenues so small businesses can pool together for their employees to enjoy the kinds of coverage afforded in big businesses.
- Guaranteeing Patient Choice of Doctors will allow new avenues to health care coverage where quality and choice are unavailable by requiring health plans to offer point-of-service options.
- Improving Medical Savings Accounts will make it easier for patients to increase access to health care services and have greater control over their health care dollars.
- Creating HealthMarts will increase consumer choice by serving as a cooperative group marketplace where working families may choose from a menu of benefit options.
- Creating Community Health Organizations will promote expansion of health coverage to all patients within their communities.
- Reforming Health Care Lawsuits will hold down costs by ensuring that doctors are free to practice medicine responsibly without the fear of unnecessary litigation, excessive legal damages, or greedy trial lawyers.
- Safeguarding Medical Record Confidentiality will protect personal and sensitive health care data from abuse.

From HR 4250 Patient Protection Act of 1998, 105th US Congress, July 16, 1998.

Accounts of mistreatments in health care frequently are reported in the press. In response, numerous bills were introduced at the state and federal levels in 1996 and 1997 to regulate managed care and/or consumer protection. Notable enactments include the Patient Protection Act (Box 7-4) and the HIPAA. The President's Advisory Commission on Consumer

Protection and Quality in the Health Care Industry in 1998 also developed a Consumer Bill of Rights and Responsibilities, and current congressional efforts are under way to protect the public against unsafe service delivery practices and to ensure quality.

Briefly Noted

Americans report concern about the U.S. health care system, particularly managed care reform, yet they are generally satisfied with the care they receive personally (HMO reform, 1998). What are possible explanations for this conflicting information?

HEALTH CARE PAYMENT SYSTEMS

Several methods have been used by public and private sources to pay health care providers for health care services. These include retrospective and prospective reimbursement for paying health care organizations and fee-for-service and capitation for paying health care practitioners (Knickman and Thorpe, 1999).

Retrospective reimbursement is the traditional reimbursement method whereby fees for the delivery of health care services in an organization are set after services are delivered (Knickman and Thorpe, 1999). For example, the unit of service in home health is the visit, and the agreed-on price is a set amount of money that the home health agency will be paid for a home visit in the region of the United States in which the agency is located.

Prospective reimbursement is a more recent method of paying an organization whereby the third-party payer establishes the amount of money that will be paid for the delivery of a particular service before offering the services to the client (Knickman and Thorpe, 1999). Since the establishment of prospective payment in Medicare (DRGs) in 1983, private insurance has followed suit by requiring pre-approvals before clients can receive certain services, such as hospital admission or mammograms more than once per year (Knickman and Thorpe, 1999).

Contracting for health care services, designed to create incentives for providers to compete on price, has occurred as managed care has increased in health care markets. Managed care organizations also use this approach to negotiate with health care organizations, such as hospitals, for coverage of services to be provided to covered enrollees, often called *covered lives.*

Fee-for-service, the traditional method of paying health care practitioners (Knickman and Thorpe, 1999), is known as and is analogous to the retrospective method described above. The practitioner determines the costs of providing a service, delivers the service to a client, and submits a bill for services delivered to a third-party payer, and the payer pays the bill. This method is based on *usual, customary, and reasonable (UCR) charges* for specific services in a given geographic region, determined by periodic regional evaluations of physician charges across specialties (Knickman and Thorpe, 1999). Historically, Medicare, Medicaid, and private insurance companies have used this method of reimbursing physicians.

Capitation is similar to prospective reimbursement for health care organizations. Specifically, third-party payers determine the amount that practitioners will be paid for a unit of care, such as a client visit, before the delivery of the service, thereby placing a limit on the amount of reimbursement received per client (Knickman and Thorpe, 1999).

In capitated arrangements, physicians and other practitioners are paid a set amount to provide care to a given client or group of clients for a set period of time and amount of money. This arrangement, typically used by managed care organizations, is one whereby the practitioner contracts with the managed care organization to provide health care services to plan members for a predetermined and negotiated fee, like $100 per month per client.

Reimbursement for nursing services. Historically, practitioners eligible to receive reimbursement for health care services included physicians only. However, nurses who function in certain capacities, such as nurse practitioners, clinical specialists, and midwives, also provide primary care to clients and receive reimbursement for their services. However, being recognized as primary care providers and eligible to receive reimbursement has not been an easy achievement. Hospital nursing care costs traditionally have been included as part of the overall patient room charge and reimbursed as such. Other agencies, such as home health care agencies, include nursing care costs with administrative costs, supplies, and equipment costs. Nursing organizations, such as the American Nurses Association, have long advocated that nursing care should become a separate budget item in all organizations.

OTHER FACTORS AFFECTING RESOURCE USE IN HEALTH CARE
The Uninsured

In 1999 the number of uninsured Americans was 46.8 million. The typical uninsured person is a member of the workforce or their dependent. Uninsured workers are likely to be in low-paying, part-time, or temporary jobs, or jobs at small businesses (Kaiser Commission on Medicaid and the Uninsured, 1998).

These uninsured workers cannot afford to purchase health insurance, and/or their employers may not offer health insurance as a benefit. Others who are typically uninsured are young adults, especially males, minorities, persons under 65 years of age in good or fair health, and the poor or near-poor. These individuals may be unable to afford insurance, lack access to job-based coverage, or because of their age and/or good health status, may not perceive the need for insurance. Because of the eligibility requirements for Medicaid, the near-poor are actually more likely to be uninsured than the poor.

The Poor

"Health disparities between poor people and those with higher incomes are almost universal for all dimensions of health"

(U.S. Department of Health and Human Services, 1991, p. 29). In fact, socioeconomic status (SES) is inversely related to mortality and morbidity for almost every disease. Poor Americans with an income below $10,000 a year have a mortality rate nearly three times that of Americans with incomes of $30,000 or more even after accounting for age, gender, race, education, and risky health behaviors (smoking, drinking, overeating, and lack of exercise) (Lantz, et al, 1998). Historically, the link between poor health and SES resulted from:

- Poor housing
- Malnutrition
- Inadequate sanitation
- Hazardous occupations

Today, explanations for this phenomenon include the cumulative effects of a constellation of characteristics that explain the concept of "poverty." These characteristics include low educational levels, unemployment or low occupational status ("blue collar" or unskilled laborer), and low wages.

Access to Care

Medicaid is intended to improve access to health care for the poor. Although Medicaid recipients have improved access (approximately twofold) when compared with the uninsured, Medicaid recipients are only about half as likely to obtain needed health services (medical/surgical care, dental care, prescription drugs, and eyeglasses) as the privately insured (Berk and Schur, 1998). Specifically, "the poorest Americans have Medicaid insurance, yet they also have the worst health" (Income and health, 1998).

Insurance coverage is often used as a ticket to access to health care (i.e., insurance coverage provides the opportunity to get health services). In reality, access to care extends beyond insurance coverage. The poor and near-poor are:

- More likely to lack a usual source of care
- More likely to postpone needed medical care
- Less likely to use preventive services
- More likely to be hospitalized for avoidable conditions than those who are not poor (USDHHS, 1998).

The primary reasons for delay, difficulty, and/or failure to access care include:

- Inability to afford health care
- Insurance-related reasons, including insurer not approving, covering, or paying for care
- Having preexisting conditions
- Doctors' refusing to accept the insurance plan.

Other barriers include:

- Lack of transportation
- Physical barriers
- Communication problems
- Childcare needs
- Lack of time or information
- Refusal of services by providers (Weinick, Zuvekas, and Drilea, 1997)
- Lack of after-hours care
- Long office waits
- Long travel distance (Forrest and Starfield, 1998).

Community characteristics also contribute to individuals' ability to access care. For example, the prevalence of managed care and the number of safety net providers, as well as the wealth and size of the community, affect accessibility (Cunningham and Kemper, 1998).

Because reimbursement for services provided to Medicaid recipients is low, physicians are discouraged from providing services to this population. Thus people on Medicaid frequently have no primary care provider and often rely on the emergency department for primary care services (McNamara, Witte, and Koning, 1993; Nadel, 1993). Consequently, the uninsured and people on Medicaid and Medicare use disproportionately more emergency department services than those who have private third-party coverage (Nadel, 1993). Additional members of racial and ethnic minority groups and those of low SES are often dependent upon emergency departments as a regular source of care. Such inappropriate use of services is inefficient and costly.

Health Care Rationing

Escalating health care spending has spurred renewed interest in health care rationing, as health care costs continue to grow. Rationing is not new to health care. For decades the uninsured and those who do not qualify for federal programs have been denied care or have been eligible only for limited services. The absence of universal health care and federal program eligibility criteria are other examples of health care rationing.

By 1990, Oregon had passed the Basic Health Services Act to ensure basic health care to all state citizens. This plan, recognized as a model health plan, used a priority ranking system of health services according to their effectiveness and benefit. The key point in the Oregon plan is that a minimum set of covered services was established. Through limiting coverage to basic services, cost increase is managed.

Since demands for health care are insatiable while resources are limited, decisions regarding distribution of care must be made. Although there is still social support for national universal coverage for basic services, no agreement in terms of implementing such a plan has emerged. As a result, decisions regarding resource use are predominately based on how the care of individuals is financed.

Rand Corporation studies have shown that clients and providers will make choices based on who pays. The ability and willingness of individuals to pay through a fee-for-service system, or any cost sharing such as insurance deductibles, decrease contact with the health care system (client self-rationing). "Free care" results in quicker decisions by clients to seek health care. Conversely, when the client is paying, quicker decisions are made by the provider to offer more complex care. Such provider practices are often affected, however, in a managed care system with set capitation payments. Insurers also determine allocation of care through preexisting condition clauses and through selective coverage of individuals and services. The ability of an individual to receive a certain medical technology, such as laser angioplasty, may depend upon the health plan in which the individual is enrolled since health insurance plans vary dramatically in their coverage of new technologies (Steiner, et al, 1997). In addition, insurance companies may either deny coverage or increase premiums based on lifestyle risks such as lack of seat belt use, drinking, and smoking habits.

PRIMARY PREVENTION

Society's investment in the health care system has been based on the premise that more health services equal better health. There are, however, other non–health care factors that affect health. There are four major factors that affect health levels:

1. Personal behavior and lifestyle
2. Environmental factors (including physical, social, and economic environments)
3. Human biology
4. The health care system

Of these four major factors, medical services are said to have the least effect on good health. Attempts to quantify the effect of these four factors on health reveals that behavior and lifestyle have the greatest effect on health, followed by environment and biology, accounting for 70% of all illnesses (U.S. Department of Health and Human Services, 1991). Despite the significant role of behavior and environment on health, estimates indicate that 97% of health care dollars are spent on secondary and tertiary prevention. Such a reactionary, secondary-prevention system results in high cost, high technology, and disease-specific care and is consistent with the U.S. system's historical emphasis on "sickness care." A more proactive investment in disease prevention and health promotion targeted at improving health behaviors, lifestyle, and the environment has the potential to improve health status, thereby improving quality of life while reducing health care costs. The USDHHS has argued that a higher value should be placed on primary prevention. The goal of this approach is to preserve and maximize human capital through providing health promotion and social practices that result in less disease. An emphasis on primary prevention may reduce dollars spent and increase quality of life.

The reality is that health care resources are limited, and this has resulted in health care rationing. The return on investment in primary prevention through gains in human capital has, unfortunately, not been acknowledged. As a consequence, significant investments in primary prevention and public health care have not been made. Reasons given for lack of emphasis on prevention in clinical practice and lack of financial investment in prevention include the following (Young, Griffith, and Kamerow, 1994):

- Provider uncertainty concerning which clients should receive services and at what interval
- Lack of education about preventive services
- Negative attitudes about the importance of preventive care
- Lack of time for delivery of preventive services
- Delayed or absent feedback regarding success of preventive measures
- Lack of reimbursement for these services
- Lack of organization to deliver preventive services

In addition, C. Everett Koop (Fries, et al, 1998), former U.S. Surgeon General, notes that greed in the health care industry is a significant factor in the lack of investment in primary prevention. Ways that several organizations are promoting health can be found in Box 7-5.

| **Box 7-5** | **HOW TO** Promote the Health and Well-Being of the American People: Efforts by Several Organizations |

PEW CHARITABLE TRUSTS

Pew's Health and Human Services program's (Public Voices, Public Choices) foci:
- Public health
- Bioethics
- Health care delivery systems
- Welfare reform

Pew Health Professions Commission
- Access to care for all
- Cost-effective use of resources
- Market efficiency coupled with public compassion
- Orientation to health rather than medical care
- Participation by the public, both individually and collectively
- Evidence-based decision making

FEDERAL RECOMMENDATIONS

Public Health Service: *Healthy People* (U.S. Department of Health, Education, and Welfare, 1979)
- Elimination of cigarette smoking
- Reduction of alcohol use
- Moderate dietary changes to reduce intake of excess calories, fat, salt, and sugar
- Moderate exercise
- Periodic screening for major causes of morbidity and mortality, such as cancer
- Adherence to speed laws and use of seat belts

Public Health Service: *Healthy People 2000* (U.S. Department of Health and Human Services, 1991)
- Health promotion
- Family planning
- Mental health
- Health protection

NURSING'S AGENDA FOR HEALTH CARE REFORM (AMERICAN NURSES ASSOCIATION, 1991)

- Restructured health care system emphasizing access, primary care, and community care
- Use of cost-effective providers
- Personal health and self-care
- A standard package of essential health care services for all citizens, phased in
- Planned health care services representing national demographics
- Steps to reduce health care costs based on managed care
- Case management
- Long-term care
- Insurance reforms
- No payment at point of care
- Establishing a public or private review to monitor the system

Today, the third-party payers are beginning to cover preventive services, recognizing that the growth of the health care system can no longer be supported. Under capitated health plans, health care providers stand to make money by keeping clients healthy and reducing health care use. Only through aligning client interests with financial interests of the health care industry will primary prevention and public health be raised to the status and priority of acute care and chronic care.

IMPLICATIONS FOR NURSING PRACTICE

Nurses must plan for future changes in health care financing by becoming aware of the costs of nursing services, identifying aspects of care where cost savings can be safely achieved, and developing knowledge about how community nursing practice affects and is affected by the principles of economics. In this century, nursing must continue to focus on improving the overall health of the nation, defining its contribution to the health of the nation, deriving the value of nursing care, and ensuring its economic viability within the health care marketplace. Nurses must effect health care system change by providing leadership in developing new models of care delivery that provide effective, high-quality care and assuming a greater role in evaluating client care and nurse performance. It is through their leadership that nurses will contribute to improved decision making about the allocation of scarce health care resources.

Clinical Application

Connie, a community health nursing student, has identified a caseload of five families in a home health nursing program offered by the local public health department. She is interested in assessing the costs of care to her clients and to the agency. Connie approaches the public health nurse administrator and asks the following questions:

A. *How is the agency reimbursed for home health visits?*
B. *How is the payment for the visit determined?*
C. *Are nursing care costs known?*
D. *Are client visits rationed?*

Answers are in the back of the book.

 Remember This!

- From 1800 to 2000 the U.S. health care delivery system experienced four developmental stages, with different emphasis on health care economics.
- Four basic categories provide the framework for the development of health care services delivery: service needs and intensity, facilities, technology, and labor (workforce).
- Three major factors have been associated with the growth of the health care delivery system: price inflation, changes in population demographics, and technology and service intensity.

- Health care financing has evolved through the twentieth century from a system financed primarily by the consumer to a system financed primarily by third-party payers.
- To solve the problems of rising health care costs, a number of plans for future payments of health care are being considered; all include some form of rationing.
- Excessive and inefficient use of goods and services in health care delivery has been viewed as the major cause of rising health care costs.
- The concept of human capital has evolved in economics as a way to measure the value society places on the worth of an individual.
- Nurses need to understand basic economic principles to avoid contributing to rising health care costs.
- Social, economic, and communicable disease epidemics mark the problems of the twenty-first century.
- Medicare and Medicaid are two government-funded programs that help meet the needs of high-risk populations in the United States.
- Health care reform that focuses primarily on health insurance reform will change the way health care is delivered and financed in the twenty-first century.
- The uninsured represent millions of people, mostly the working poor, elderly persons, and children.
- Poverty has a detrimental effect on health.
- Health care rationing has always been a part of the U.S. health care system.
- *Healthy People 2010* is a document that has established U.S. health objectives.
- Human life is valued in health economics, like money. An emphasis on changing lifestyles and preventive care will reduce the unnecessary years of life lost to early and preventable death.

 What Would You Do?

1. Review Chapter 4. Debate in the class the ethical implications of the goal of rationing. Focus your debate on the implications for nursing practice.
2. Invite a community or public health nurse administrator to meet with your class or clinical conference group. Ask how inflation, changes in population, and technology have changed the public health care delivery system and nursing practice.

REFERENCES

Agency for Health Care Policy and Research: Medical Expenditure Panel Survey highlights: health insurance coverage in America 1996 (AHCPR pub no 98-0031), Rockville, Md, 1998, Agency for Health Care Policy and Research.

American Nurses Association: *Nursing's agenda for health care reform,* Washington, D.C., 1991. American Nurses Publishing.

Banta HD: Technology assessment in health care. In Kovner A (editor): *Health care delivery in the United States,* New York, 1995a, Springer.

Banta HD: What is health care? In Kovner A (editor): *Health care delivery in the United States,* New York, 1995b, Springer.

Berk ML, Schur CL: Access to care: how much difference does Medicaid make? *Health Affairs* 17(3):169, 1998.

Boyes WJ: *Macroeconomics: intermediate theory and policy,* ed 3, Cincinnati, 1992, South-Western Publishing.

Bureau of Labor Statistics, U.S. Department of Labor: *Occupational outlook handbook,* 1998-99 edition, Washington, D.C., 1998, U.S. Government Printing Office (Bulletin 2500).

Centers for Disease Control and Prevention: *HIV/AIDS surveillance report,* Washington, D.C., 2000, U.S. Government Printing Office.

Centers for Disease Control National Prevention Information Network, online: www.cdcnpin.org.

Chernew ME, et al: Managed care, medical technology, and health care cost growth: a review of the evidence, *Med Care Res Rev* 55(3):259, 1998.

Cunningham PJ, Kemper P: Ability to obtain medical care for the uninsured: how much does it vary across communities? *JAMA* 280(10):921, 1998.

Folland S, Goodman AC, Stano M: *The economics of health and health care,* New York, 1993, Macmillan.

Forrest CB, Starfield B: Entry into primary care and continuity: the effects of access, *Am J Public Health* 88(9):1330, 1998.

Fries JF, et al: Beyond health promotion: reducing need and demand for medical care, *Health Affairs* 17(2):70, 1998.

Gold MR, et al: *Cost-effectiveness in health and medicine,* New York, 1996, Oxford University Press.

Health Care Financing Administration: 1998 Medicare chartbook: a profile of Medicare, online: www.hcfa.gov/pubforms/chartbk.htm.

Health Care Financing Administration: HIPAA: the Health Insurance Portability and Accountability Act of 1996, Feb 22, 1999, online: www.hcfa.gov/HIPAA/HIPAAHm.htm.

Health Care Financing Administration, 2000, online: www.hcfa.gov/stats/enr/trnd.html.

HMO reform: still high on voters' list of concerns, *American HealthLine* Sept 17, 1998.

Income and health: poor are left behind in health gains, *American HealthLine* July 30, 1998.

Internal Revenue Service: Understanding MSAs, Nov 19, 1998, online: www.irs.gov/forms_pubs/pubs/p96901.htm.

Kaiser Commission on Medicaid and the Uninsured: *Uninsured facts: the uninsured and their access to health care,* Washington, D.C., 1998, The Commission.

Knickman J, Thorpe K: Financing for health care. In Kovner A (editor): *Health care delivery in the United States,* New York, 1999, Springer.

Kovner C: The health care workforce in the United States. In Kovner A (editor): *Health care delivery in the United States,* New York, 1999, Springer.

Lantz PM, et al: Socioeconomic factors, health behaviors, and mortality: results from a nationally representative prospective study of US adults, *JAMA* 279(21):1745, 1998.

Levit KR, et al: National health care expenditures, 1996, *Health Care Fin Rev* 19(1):161, 1997.

Levit KR, Lazenby HC, Braden BR: National health spending trends in 1996, *Health Affairs* 17(1):35, 1998.

McCloskey J: Breaking the cycle, *J Prof Nurs* 11(2):67, 1995.

McNamara P, Witte R, Koning A: Patchwork access: primary care in EDs on the rise, *Hospitals* 67(10):44, 1993.

Moses EG: *The registered nurse population, findings from the national sample survey of registered nurses, March 1996,* Washington, D.C., 1997, Division of Nursing, U.S. Department of Health and Human Services.

Nadel MV: *Emergency departments: unevenly affected by growth and change in patient use* (GAO/HRD-93-4), Washington, D.C., 1993, U.S. General Accounting Office, Human Resources Division.

Pew Health Professions Commission: *Contemporary issues in health professions, education and workforce reform,* San Francisco, 1993, UCSF Center for the Health Professions.

Pickett G, Hanlon J: *Public health administration and practice,* St Louis, 1990, Mosby.

Rice D: The health status and national health priorities. In Lee P, Estes C (editors): *The nation's health,* ed 4, Boston, 1994, Jones & Bartlett.

Smith S, et al: The Health Expenditures Projection Team: the next ten years of health spending: what does the future hold? *Health Affairs* 17(5):128, 1998.

Steiner CA, et al: Technology coverage decisions by health care plans and considerations by medical directors, *Medical Care* 35(5): 472, 1997.

U.S. Census Bureau: *Resident population of the United States: middle series projections 2006-2010 by sex, race, and Hispanic origin with median age, March 1996,* online: www.census.gov/population/projections/nationa/nsrh/nprh0610.txt.

U.S. Census Bureau: *Statistical abstract of the United States: 1999,* Washington, D.C., 1999, U.S. Government Printing Office.

U.S. Department of Health, Education, and Welfare: *Healthy people: the Surgeon General's report on health promotion and disease prevention,* DHEW pub no (PHS) 79-55071, Washington, D.C., 1979, U.S. Department of Health, Education, and Welfare.

U.S. Department of Health and Human Services: *Healthy people 2000: national health promotion and disease prevention objectives,* Washington, D.C., 1991, U.S. Department of Health and Human Services.

U.S. Department of Health and Human Services: *Health: United States, 1993,* DHHS pub no (PHS) 94-1232, Washington, D.C., 1994, U.S. Government Printing Office.

U.S. Department of Health and Human Services: *Health: United States, 1998,* DHHS pub no (PHS) 98-1232, Washington, D.C., 1998, U.S. Government Printing Office.

U.S. Department of Health and Human Services: *Health: United States, 1999,* DHHS pub no (PHS) 98-1232, Washington, D.C., 1999, U.S. Government Printing Office.

U.S. Department of Health and Human Services, Health Resources and Services Administration, Bureau of Health Professions, National Center for Health and Workforce Information and Analysis, 2000, online: www.hrsa.gov.

Weinick RM, Zuvekas SH, Drilea SK: *Access to health care: sources and barriers, 1996,* Rockville, Md, 1997, Agency for Health Care Policy and Research. MEPS Research Findings No 3, AHCPR pub no 98-0001.

Weitzman BC: The quality of care: assessment and assurance. In Kovner A (editor): *Health care delivery in the United States,* New York, 1990, Springer.

Young S, Griffith H, Kamerow D: Put prevention into practice: a program for community health centers, 1994, online: www.hhs.gov.

Part 3

Conceptual Frameworks Applied to Community Health Nursing Practice

In 1988 the National Center for Nursing Research (NCNR) was established under the National Institutes of Health to facilitate nursing research. In 1993 the United States Congress expanded the scope and functions of the NCNR and made it one of the National Institutes of Health and renamed it the National Institute of Nursing Research (NINR). The NINR is crucial to the profession's movement to build a stronger base for practice. Although no conceptual or theoretical model will meet the needs of all community health nurses, several nursing and public health models serve as frameworks for organizing educational programs and for making practice decisions.

The scientific base provided by public health as a specialty remains the foundation for community health nursing. In Part 3, three chapters provide information about how to use conceptual models, epidemiology, research, and principles of education to organize community health practice to meet the needs of clients in the community. Each chapter provides both theory and practical application of the specific topic to the clinical area. This section provides readers with tools that can be used to influence community health nursing practice.

It has been estimated that the effect of the medical care system on usual indices for measuring health of all clients is about 10%. The remaining 90% is determined by factors over which health care providers have little or no direct control, such as lifestyle and social and physical environmental conditions. This text focuses on the processes and practices for promoting health, principally by the nurse, who is considered to be an ideal person to demonstrate and teach others how to promote health. To be effective, health promotion requires that people cease focusing on how to "fix" themselves and others only when they detect physical and emotional problems and that they instead assume personal responsibility for health promotion. Such a change in emphasis requires that health care providers incorporate health-promotion techniques into their practice.

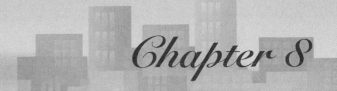
Chapter 8

Epidemiological Applications in Community Health Nursing

ROBERT E. McKEOWN

SALLY P. WEINRICH

OBJECTIVES

After reading this chapter, the student should be able to:
- Define epidemiology and describe how it has developed over time.
- Explain how nurses use epidemiology in clinical practice.
- Describe the steps of the epidemiological process.
- Discuss the basic epidemiological concepts of populations at risk, natural history of disease, levels of prevention,

host-agent-environment relationships, and web of causation model.
- Differentiate between descriptive and analytic epidemiology.
- Explain how to set up and evaluate a screening program.

CHAPTER OUTLINE

KEY TERMS

agent: causative factor invading a susceptible host through an environment favorable to produce disease, such as a biologic or chemical agent.

analytic epidemiology: a form of epidemiology that investigates causes and associations between factors or events and health.

Continued

KEY TERMS—cont'd

attack rate: a type of incidence rate defined as the proportion of persons exposed to an agent who develop the disease, usually for a limited time in a specific population.

bias: in determining causality, a systematic error due to the way the study is designed, how it was carried out, or some factors related to the variable(s) being studied.

case-control study: an epidemiologic study design in which subjects with a specified disease or condition (cases) and a comparable group without the condition (controls) are enrolled and assessed for the presence or history of an exposure or characteristic.

causality: the determination based on evidence or reasoning process that an event or state resulted from (or was caused by) some other events, exposure, characteristics, or a combination of them.

cohort study: an epidemiologic study design in which subjects without an outcome of interest are classified according to past or present (or future) exposures or characteristics and followed over time to observe and compare the rates of a particular health outcome in the various exposure groups.

confounding: a bias that results from the relation of both the outcome and study factor (exposure or characteristic) with some third factor not considered in analysis.

cross-sectional study: an epidemiologic study in which health outcomes and exposures or characteristics of interest are simultaneously ascertained and examined for association in a population or sample, providing a picture of existing levels of all factors.

cyclical time patterns of disease: one example is seasonal fluctuation of diseases.

descriptive epidemiology: a form of epidemiology that describes a disease according to its person, place, or time.

determinants: factors that influence the risk for or distribution of health outcomes.

distribution: pattern of a health outcome in a population; the frequencies of the outcome according to various personal characteristics, geographic regions, and time.

environment: all factors internal and external to a client that constitute the context in which the client lives and that influence and are influenced by the host and agent-host interactions.

epidemic: a rate of disease clearly in excess of the usual or expected frequency in that population.

epidemiology: study of the distribution and factors that determine health-related states or events in a population, and the use of this information to control health problems.

event-related cluster: disease patterns measured from a point of exposure, event, or experience.

host: human or animal that provides adequate living conditions for any given infectious agent.

incidence rate: the frequency or rate of new cases of an outcome in a population; provides an estimate of the risk of disease in that population over the period of observation.

levels of prevention: a three-level model of interventions based on the stages of disease, designed to halt or reverse the process of pathological change as early as possible, thereby preventing damage.

natural history of disease: course or progression of a disease process from onset to resolution.

negative predictive value: proportion of persons with a negative test who are disease free.

point epidemic: a concentration in space and time of a disease event, such that a graph of frequency of cases over time shows a sharp point, usually suggestive of a common exposure.

positive predictive value: proportion of persons with a positive screening or diagnostic test who do have the disease (the proportion of positives among those who test positive).

prevalence rate: the proportion of existing cases of a health outcome in a population at a given time.

primary prevention: a type of intervention that seeks to promote health and prevent disease from developing.

rate: a measure of the frequency of a health event in a defined population during a specified period of time.

reliability: refers to the precision of a measuring instrument, specifically its consistency from one time of use to another and its accuracy.

risk: the probability of some event or outcome within a specified period of time.

screening: application of a test to people who are as yet asymptomatic for the purpose of classifying them with respect to their likelihood of having a particular disease.

secondary prevention: intervention that seeks to detect disease early in its progression (early pathogenesis) before clinical signs and symptoms become apparent in order to make an early diagnosis and begin treatment.

secular trends: long-term patterns of morbidity or mortality (i.e., over years or decades).

sensitivity: the extent to which a test identifies those individuals who have the condition being examined.

specificity: the extent to which a test identifies those individuals who do not have the disease or condition being examined.

surveillance: systematic and ongoing observation and collection of data concerning disease occurrence in order to describe phenomena and detect changes in frequency or distribution.

tertiary prevention: intervention that begins once the disease is obvious; the aim is to interrupt the course of the disease, reduce the amount of disability that might occur, and begin rehabilitation.

validity: the accuracy of a test or measurement; how closely it measures what it claims to measure. In a screening test, validity is assessed in terms of the probability of correctly classifying an individual with regard to the disease or outcome of interest, usually in terms of sensitivity and specificity.

web of causality: complex interrelations of factors interacting with each other to influence the risk for or distribution of health outcomes.

Epidemiology is the study of the distribution of various states of health in the population and the conditions including environment, lifestyle, and other circumstances that influence health. The term originally referred to infectious epidemics such as cholera or tuberculosis. It now includes infectious diseases as well as chronic diseases, such as cancer and cardiovascular disease, and also mental health and other health-related events, such as accidents, injuries and violence, occupational and environmental exposures and their effects, and positive health states.

DEFINITIONS

Epidemiology investigates the **distribution** or the patterns of health events in populations and the determinants or the factors that influence those patterns. **Descriptive epidemiology** looks at health outcomes in terms of what, who, where, and when. That is: What is the disease? Who is affected? Where are they? When do events occur? Descriptive epidemiology discusses a disease in terms of person, place, and time. **Analytic epidemiology** looks at the etiology (origins or causes) of the disease and deals with determinants of health and disease (i.e., how and why). The **determinants** of health events are the factors, exposures, characteristics, and behaviors that determine (or influence) the patterns: How does it occur? Why are some people affected more than others? Determinants may be individual, relational or social, communal, or environmental.

Epidemiology, like both the research process and nursing process, has a set of steps. The first step is to define a health outcome. The health outcome can be a disease, injury, accident, or even wellness. Using epidemiologic methods a nurse describes the distribution (or the who, where, and when) of a disease, event, or injury, and searches for factors that explain the pattern or risk of occurrence. The nurse asks what influences the occurrence of this disease or injury or why and how events occurred as they did.

Like nursing, epidemiology builds on and draws from other disciplines and methods, including clinical medicine and laboratory sciences, social sciences, quantitative methods (especially biostatistics), and public health policy and goals. Epidemiology focuses on populations, while clinical medicine focuses on the diagnosis and treatment of disease in *individuals*. Epidemiology studies *populations* in order to understand the causes of health and disease in communities and to investigate and evaluate interventions that will prevent disease and maintain health.

HISTORY

In the fourth century BCE (before common era), Hippocrates was one of the first people to use the ideas that are now part of epidemiology (Timmreck, 1994). He examined health and disease in a community by looking at geography, climate, the seasons of the year, the food and water consumed,

and the habits and behaviors of the people. His approach, like descriptive epidemiology, looked at how health is influenced by personal characteristics, place, and time.

During the nineteenth century Louis Pasteur developed both the germ theory and pasteurization. Pasteur also recognized the role of personal characteristics, such as immunity and host resistance, in explaining why some people were susceptible to disease and others were not (Vandenbroucke, 1990). Other major discoveries during this century were made by Joseph Lister, the British surgeon who developed antiseptic surgery, and Robert Koch, a German scientist who developed pure culture and identified the organisms that cause tuberculosis, anthrax, and cholera. In the eighteenth and nineteenth centuries comparison groups began to be used to measure change or the effects of some action or treatment on an experimental group. Also at that time, quantitative methods (numeric measurements or counts) began to be used. One of the most famous studies using a comparison group is the mid-nineteenth century investigation of cholera by John Snow, whom some call the "father of epidemiology" (Lilienfeld and Stolley, 1994). Snow drew a map of the cases of cholera that developed and were clustered around a single public water pump to show how the water supply was related to the development of cholera. He later observed that cholera rates were higher among households supplied by water companies whose water came from downstream than among households whose water came from further upstream, where it was subject to less contamination. Because in some areas households near each other had different sources of water, differences observed in rates of cholera could not be attributed to location or economic status. Snow showed that households receiving water from the Lambeth Company, whose intake had been moved away from sewage contamination, had cholera rates considerably lower than those supplied by Southwark and Vauxhall, a company whose water intake was still in a contaminated section of the river. Snow conducted a "natural experiment," and as seen in Table 8-1 documented that foul water was the vehicle for transmission of the agent that caused cholera.

In nursing, Florence Nightingale contributed to the development of epidemiology in her work with British soldiers during the Crimean War (1854 to 1856). At this time, sick soldiers were cared for in cramped quarters that had poor sanitation, were overrun with lice and rats, and provided insufficient food and medical supplies. She looked at the relationship between the conditions of the environment and the recovery of the soldiers. Using simple epidemiology measures of rates of illness per 1000 soldiers, when she

TABLE 8-1	Household Cholera Death Rates by Source of Water Supply in John Snow's 1853 Investigation		
Company	**Number of Houses**	**Deaths From Cholera**	**Deaths per 10,000 Households**
Southwark and Vauxhall Company	40,046	1,263	315
Lambeth	26,107	98	37
Rest of London	256,423	1,422	59

From Snow J: On the mode of communication of cholera. In *Snow on cholera*, New York, 1855, The Commonwealth Fund, p. 86.

TABLE 8-2   Significant Milestones in the History of Epidemiology

Date	Investigator	Contribution
1662	John Graunt	Used Bills of Mortality (forerunner of modern vital records) to study patterns of death in various populations in England. Published early form of life table analysis
1747	James Lind	Studied scurvy using observation and comparison of response to various dietary treatments; early precursor of clinical trial
1760	Daniel Bernoulli	Used life table technique to demonstrate that smallpox inoculation conferred life-long immunity
1775	Percival Pott	First "cancer epidemiologist." Noted that a high proportion of patients presenting with cancer of scrotum were chimney sweeps. Inferred the exposure to soot was the cause. (Lack of a comparison group would reduce validity of inference by today's standards)
1798	Edward Jenner	Demonstrated effectiveness of smallpox vaccination
		Marine Hospital Service was opened; forerunner of U.S. Public Health Service (1912)
1836	Pierre Charles-Alexandre Louis	Used comparative observational studies to demonstrate ineffectiveness of bloodletting. Emphasized the importance of statistical methods ("*la méthode numerique*"). Influenced many of the pioneers in epidemiology in England and the United States
1836		Establishment of Registrar-General's Office in England as registry for births, deaths, marriages
1840s	William Farr	Developed forerunner of modern vital records system in Registrar-General's Office. Study of mortality in Liverpool led to significant public health reform. Pioneered mortality surveillance and anticipated many of the basic concepts in epidemiology. His data provided much of the basis for Snow's work on cholera
1850	Lemuel Shattuck	Reported on sanitation and public health in Massachusetts
		London Epidemiological Society founded. Known for influential reports on smallpox vaccination and studies of cholera
1850s	John Snow	Conducted epidemiologic research on transmission of cholera. Used mapping and natural experiment, comparing rates in groups exposed to different water supplies
1870-1880s	Robert Koch	Discovered causal agents for anthrax, tuberculosis, and cholera; development of causal criteria
1887	Joseph Kinyuon	Founded "Laboratory of Hygiene," forerunner of the National Institutes of Health (1930)
		The United States Public Health Service (USPHS) assumed the work previously done by the Marine Hospital Service
1921	Wade Hampton Frost	Founded first U.S. academic program in epidemiology at Johns Hopkins
		National Institutes of Health (NIH) created
1942		Office of Malarial Control in War Areas established; became Communicable Disease Center (CDC) in 1946; then Centers for Disease Control (1973); now Centers for Disease Control and Prevention
1948		Framingham Heart Study began

improved the environmental conditions and added nursing care, she was able to decrease the mortality rates of the soldiers (Cohen, 1984; Palmer, 1983).

Table 8-2 lists several key events or discoveries that led to major advances in epidemiology. Several changes in society influenced the further development of epidemiology during the twentieth century. Some of these were the Great Depression of the 1920s in the United States, World War II, a rising standard of living for many but abject poverty for others, improved nutrition, new vaccines, better sanitation, the development of antibiotics and cancer chemotherapies,

decreased birth rates in some countries, and decreases in infant and child mortality in many nations. People began to live longer, and the rates of several chronic diseases such as coronary heart disease, stroke, cancer, and senile dementia increased (Susser, 1985). Figure 8-1 shows the 10 leading causes of death in the United States in 1900 and in 1996, with the percentage of all deaths attributed to each.

During the twentieth century a shift occurred from looking for single agents, such as the infectious agent that causes cholera, to seeking multifactorial etiology or the many factors or combinations of factors that contribute to disease. An

TABLE 8-2   Significant Milestones in the History of Epidemiology—Cont'd

Date	Investigator	Contribution
1950s	A. Bradford Hill and Richard Doll	Pioneering studies on smoking and lung cancer conducted
	Jerome Cornfield	A Method of Estimating Comparative Rates from Clinical Data (use of odds ratio from case-control study as estimate of relative risk)
1964		Surgeon General's report on smoking and health released
1975		CDC Biomedical Scientists/Epidemiologists identified *Legionella* bacteria as case of outbreak of a "flu-like" syndrome, later named Legionnaire's disease, after the American Legion commanders who fell ill at a meeting in Philadelphia from this then-unknown disease
1981		The CDC's *Morbidity and Mortality Weekly Report (MMWR)* ran an article on *Pneumocystis* pneumonia that announced the new disease of AIDS
1983		The Public Health Service (PHS) published its first guidelines on AIDS prevention, recommending that people refrain from donating blood and modify their sexual practices
1988		The Institute of Medicine published *The Future of Public Health*. This report says that the core public health functions are assessment, policy development, and assurance. Epidemiology and statistics are established as the basis for the assessment function
1991		Publication of Healthy People 2000: National Health Promotion and Disease Prevention Objectives by the U.S. Department of Health and Human Services Public Health Service
1993		*Cryptosporidium* was found in the water supply coming to Milwaukee, Wisconsin, from Lake Michigan. In a country proud of its clean water, the estimated 403,000 sick people and 54 deaths was a terrible threat to health and safety
1995		Hantavirus respiratory disease, an acute disease usually fatal and caused by human exposure to mouse droppings, was declared a notifiable disease by the CDC
1999		The CDC published the "top ten" list of great public health accomplishments of the twentieth century. Many relied on epidemiological methods to assess and gather information
2000		Establishment of a task force to prepare the Guide to Community Prevention Services to spell out ways to implement the objectives of *Healthy People 2010*
		Publication of *Healthy People 2010: Understanding and Improving Health* by the U.S. Department of Health and Human Services

Based on data from Benedict I, Truman C, Smith-Akin K, Hinman AR, et al: Developing the guide to community preventive services: overview and rationale, *Am J Preventive Med* 18(1S):18-26, 2000; Institute of Medicine: *The future of public health,* Washington, D.C., 1988, National Academy Press; Lilienfeld DE, Stolley PD: *Foundations of epidemiology,* ed 3, New York, 1994, Oxford University Press; Mullan F: *Plagues and politics: the story of the United States Public Health Service,* New York, 1989, Basic Books; Schneider MJ: *Introduction to public health,* Gaithersburg, Md, 2000, Aspen; Susser M: Epidemiology in the United States after World War II: the evolution of technique, *Epidemiol Rev* 7:147, 1985; Timmreck TC: *An introduction to epidemiology,* Boston, 1994, Jones & Bartlett; U.S. Department of Health and Human Services: *Public Health Service Fact Sheet,* Washington, D.C., 1984, U.S. Department of Health and Human Services, Public Health Service.

example of multifactorial etiology would be looking at the complex number and type of factors that cause cardiovascular disease. People observed that not all the diseases of older people were due to the degenerative process of aging. Rather, it became clear that there were many behavioral and environmental factors that supported or encouraged the development of diseases. If this were true, then some diseases could be prevented and others could at least be delayed (Susser, 1985).

Also, the development of genetic and molecular techniques increased the epidemiologist's ability to classify persons in terms of exposures or inherent susceptibility to dis-

ease. Examples included the identification of genetic traits that indicated an increased risk for breast cancer and markers that identified exposures to environmental toxins, such as lead or pesticides. These developments are of particular interest to nurses who work with people in their living and work environments and understand the interaction of environment(s) on health and well-being. Further, nurses in the community can assess a broad range of health outcomes as well as factors that contribute to wellness and illness.

Unfortunately, in recent years new infectious diseases such as Lyme disease, Legionnaire's disease, and HIV/AIDS,

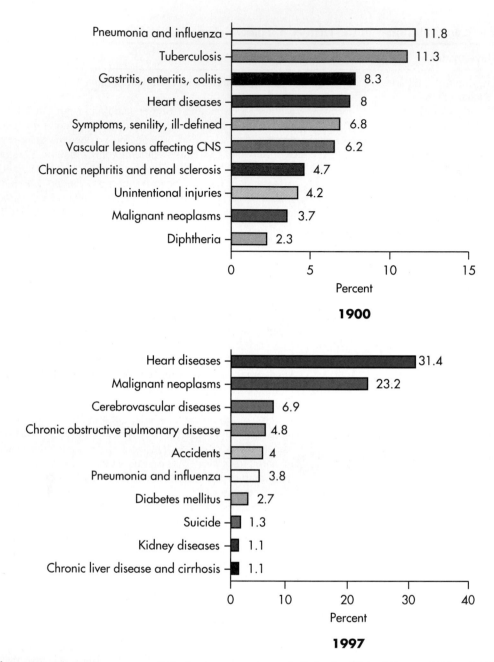

Figure 8-1 Ten leading causes of death as a percentage of all deaths, United States, 1900 and 1997. (Data from Brownson, et al: *Chronic disease epidemiology and control,* Washington, D.C., 1993, American Public Health Association; Ventura SJ, et al: Births and deaths: preliminary data for 1997, *National Vital Statistics Reports* 47:4, 1998.)

as well as new forms of old diseases such as resistant strains of tuberculosis have once again placed infectious-disease epidemiology in the spotlight. The tools provided by epidemiology can improve the control and management of health care, and they can be used to examine accidents, injuries and violence, occupational and environmental exposures, psychiatric and sociological phenomena, health-related behaviors, and in health services research.

HOW NURSES USE EPIDEMIOLOGY

Nurses are part of the interdisciplinary team in community-based settings who look at health, disease causation, and

how to both prevent and treat illness. In the community, nurses often use epidemiology since the factors that affect the individual, family, and population cannot be as easily controlled as in acute care settings. That is, it is difficult to control environmental elements such as water and food supplies, air conditions including pollutants, disposal of garbage and trash, and quality of paint used to ensure that it contains no lead. Therefore, clients in the community have more factors affecting their health than individuals in a more specific setting.

Nurses are involved in the surveillance and monitoring of disease trends. Working in homes, clinics, schools, occupational health, and health maintenance organizations, nurses can identify patterns of disease in a group. For example, if several children in a school develop abdominal problems within a short period of time (e.g., a 24-hour period), the nurse can trace what these children had in common. That is, did they eat the same food, drink from the same source of water, swim in the same pool, and so forth. Likewise, if workers in a plant displayed a similar pattern of symptoms, the nurse would look for factors in the workplace to locate the cause. The workplace would be examined first because that is the setting the individuals have in common.

Care of patients, families, and population groups in the community uses the following steps of the nursing process:

1. Assessment
2. Planning
3. Implementation
4. Evaluation

When using the nursing process, epidemiology provides baseline information for assessing needs, identifying problems, designing appropriate strategies to evaluate the problems, setting priorities in order to develop and implement a plan of care, and evaluating how effective the care was. The remainder of the chapter discusses the "tools of epidemiology" that are needed by nurses who work in community settings.

BASIC CONCEPTS IN EPIDEMIOLOGY
Epidemiologic Triangle: Agent, Host, and Environment

Epidemiologists understand that disease results from complex interactions among causal agents, susceptible persons, and environmental factors. These three elements—agent, host, and environment—are called the epidemiologic triangle (Figure 8-2). The natural life history of a disease focuses on an examination of the relationships among these three elements. Specifically, these elements or variables are defined as:

> **Agent:** an animate or inanimate factor that must be present or lacking for a disease or condition to develop.
>
> **Host:** a living species (human or animal) capable of being infected or affected by an agent.
>
> **Environment:** all that is internal or external to a given host or agent and that is influenced and influences the host and/or agent.

Changes in one element of the triangle can influence the occurrence of disease by increasing or decreasing a person's risk for disease. Risk is the probability or likelihood that a person will become ill (Last, 1995). As shown in Figure 8-2, the agent, the host, and their interaction are influenced by the environment in which they exist. Likewise, the agent and host influence the environment. Some examples of these three components are listed in Box 8-1.

Causal relationships (one thing or event causes another) are often more complex than the epidemiologic triangle conveys. The term **web of causality** recognizes the complex interrelationships of many factors interacting, sometimes in subtle ways, to increase (or decrease) risk of disease. Fur-

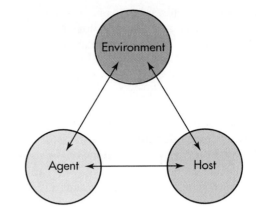

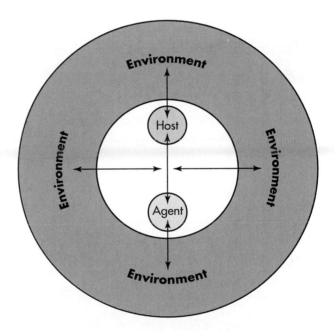

Figure 8-2 Two models of the agent-host-environment interaction (the "epidemiologic triangle").

ther, associations are sometimes mutual, with lines of causality going in both directions.

Stages of Health and Intervention

The goal of epidemiology is to understand causal factors well enough to devise interventions to prevent adverse events before they start (prevent initiation of the disease process or prevent injury). Public health professionals describe three levels of prevention related to specific stages in the **natural history of disease.** The natural history of disease is the course of the disease process from onset to resolution or from beginning to end (Last, 1995). Table 8-3 illustrates the relationship among the stages of disease and **levels of prevention.** Nurses who work in the community use the three levels of primary, secondary, and tertiary prevention.

Primary prevention refers to interventions that promote health and prevent disease processes from developing. These activities are directed toward individuals who are susceptible to disease but have no apparent pathology (prepathogenesis). Diet and exercise are examples of primary prevention for cardiovascular disease. Nurses implement primary prevention programs such as immunizations, provision of and training in use of barrier contraceptives, and health education about diet, physical activity, parenting, and avoiding high-risk behavior such as unsafe sexual practices or using drugs or alcohol.

Secondary prevention aims to detect disease in the early stages (early pathogenesis) before clinical signs and symptoms become apparent, in order to intervene with early diagnosis and treatment. The goal is to reverse or reduce the severity of the disease or provide a cure. Early stages of cardiovascular disease may be detected by treadmill stress tests or screening for hypertension. Screening programs, such as blood pressure

checks or Pap smears to detect cervical dysplasia, can be used to detect early disease in symptom-free persons. Similarly, family counseling is a form of secondary prevention designed to intervene before problems become serious. Since nurses play key roles in secondary prevention, a more detailed discussion of one form of secondary prevention—screening programs—is presented later in the chapter.

Tertiary prevention is directed toward persons with clinically apparent disease. The aim is to intervene in the course of disease, reduce disability, or rehabilitate the person. For example, persons with diagnosed heart disease may have coronary artery bypass surgery or enter cardiac rehabilitation programs. Other examples of tertiary prevention include treatment of patients with tuberculosis, the use of physical therapy to prevent contractures in patients with stroke or head or spinal cord injuries, or rehabilitating an injured worker through physical therapy and other techniques so the person can return to work. Rehabilitative job training through counseling for juvenile offenders is an additional form of tertiary prevention. Nurses who work in community settings are involved in teaching clients, monitoring compliance and progress, and providing services that will aid in recovery and improve quality of life.

| Box 8-1 | Examples of Agent, Host, and Environment Factors in the Epidemiologic Triangle |

AGENT

- Infectious agents: bacteria, viruses, fungi, parasites
- Chemical agents: heavy metals, toxic chemicals, pesticides
- Physical agents: radiation, heat, cold, machinery

HOST

- Genetic susceptibility
- Immutable characteristics: age, gender
- Acquired characteristics: immunologic status
- Lifestyle factors: diet, exercise, smoking

ENVIRONMENT

- Climate: temperature, rainfall
- Plant and animal life: may be agents or reservoirs or habitats for agents
- Human population distribution: crowding, social support
- Socioeconomic factors: education, resources, access to health care
- Working conditions: levels of stress, noise, job satisfaction, pollutants

BASIC METHODS IN EPIDEMIOLOGY
Sources of Data

An epidemiologic researcher must decide early in the process how to obtain study data (Kelsey et al, 1996). Three major categories of data sources are commonly used in epidemiologic investigations:

1. Routinely collected data, such as census data, vital records (birth and death certificates), and surveillance data (systematic collection of data about disease occurrence) that are often gathered by the Centers for Disease Control and Prevention (CDC)
2. Data collected for other purposes (such as medical, health department, and insurance records)

TABLE 8-3   Relation of the Stages of Disease to Levels of Prevention

Stage of Disease Process			
Pre-pathogenesis ↓	Pathogenesis ↓	↓	Resolution ↓
Susceptibility	Preclinical	Clinical	Death, disability, recovery
Levels of Prevention			
Primary prevention	Secondary prevention		Tertiary prevention
Examples of Intervention Related to Cardiovascular Disease			
Diet and exercise	Blood pressure and cholesterol screening, treadmill stress test		Cardiac rehabilitation, medication, surgery
Other Examples of Interventions			
Immunization, water treatment	Pap smear, screening for HIV		Physical therapy, surgery, medical treatment

3. Original data collected for specific epidemiologic studies.

Routinely Collected Data

The census, conducted every 10 years in the United States, provides population data, including distribution by demographic features (age, race, sex), as well as geographic distribution and additional information concerning economic status, housing, and education. These data provide denominators for various rates (discussed later).

Vital records are the primary source of birth and mortality (death) statistics. Although registration of births and deaths is mandated in most countries, providing one of the most complete sources of health-related data, the quality of the information varies from one country to another. For example, on birth certificates, sex and date of birth are usually reliable, whereas gestational age, level of prenatal care, or smoking habits of the mother during pregnancy are less reliable. On death certificates, the quality of the cause of death information varies over time and from place to place and depends on diagnostic capabilities and custom. Vital records are readily available in most areas; they are inexpensive and convenient, and they allow people to study the long-term trends. Mortality data, however, are informative only for fatal diseases.

Data Collected for Other Purposes

Hospital, physician, health department, and insurance records provide information on morbidity, as do **surveillance** systems, such as cancer registries and health department reporting systems, which collect reports of all cases of a particular disease within a geographic region. Other information, such as occupational exposures, may be available from employer records.

Epidemiologic Data

The National Center for Health Statistics sponsors periodic health surveys and examinations in carefully drawn samples of the U.S. population. These surveys provide information on the health status and behaviors of the population. For many studies, however, the only way to get the needed information is to collect the required data in a study specifically designed to investigate a particular question. The design of such studies is discussed below.

Measures of Morbidity and Mortality

Rates in Epidemiology

Epidemiologic studies usually rely on **rates.** Rates are a measure of the frequency (number of times something occurs) of a health event in a defined population during a specified period of time (Last, 1995). Epidemiology looks at the distribution of health events. Because people differ in their probability or risk of disease, it is important to know how they differ. Mapping cases of a disease in an area, as John Snow mapped cases of cholera in one area of London, and as many epidemiologists now map various health-related events, is useful. However, mapping cases is

limited in what it can reveal. A higher number of cases may be due to a larger population with more people who can potentially have the disease or be a case. Any description of disease patterns needs to take into account the size of the population at risk for the disease (i.e., look not only at the numerator, the number of cases, but also at the denominator, the number of people in the population at risk). For example, 50 cases of influenza may be a serious epidemic in a population of 250, but would indicate a rather low rate in a population of 250,000. Using rates instead of simple counts of cases takes the size of the population at risk into account.

An **epidemic** occurs when the rate of disease, injury, or other condition clearly exceeds the usual (endemic) level of that condition. There is no specific threshold of incidence that indicates an epidemic exists. Because smallpox has been eliminated, any occurrence of smallpox is considered to be an epidemic. In contrast, because there is a high rate of ischemic heart disease in the United States, it would take an increase of many cases before an epidemic was present.

The Concept of Risk

Risk refers to the probability an event will occur within a specified time period. A population at risk includes those individuals for whom there is some finite probability (even if small) that the event will occur. For example, although the risk of breast cancer in men is small, a few men do develop breast cancer and therefore could be considered part of the population at risk. There are some outcomes for which certain people would never be at risk (e.g., men cannot be at risk of ovarian cancer, nor can women be at risk of testicular cancer). A high-risk population, on the other hand, would include those persons who, because of exposure, lifestyle, family history, or other factors, are at greater risk of disease than the population at large. For example, since it appears that all people are susceptible to HIV infection, everyone is in the population at risk for HIV/AIDS. However, persons who have multiple sexual partners without adequate protection or who use IV drugs are in the high-risk population for HIV infection.

Briefly Noted

Genetic testing is becoming more common; however, most tests indicate only a susceptibility to a disease, not certainty that the disease will develop. Similarly, screening tests are not perfect, so there is always a possibility that a person will be classified improperly and misadvised.

Mortality Rates

Several key mortality rates are shown in Table 8-4. Many commonly used mortality rates are not true rates but rather are proportions. Although measures of mortality reflect serious health problems and changing patterns of disease, they have limited usefulness. They only provide information about fatal diseases and do not provide direct information about either the level of existing disease in the population or the risk of getting

TABLE 8-4   Common Mortality Rates

Rate	Definition	Example
Crude mortality rate	Usually an annual rate, represents the proportion of a population who die from any cause during the period	In 1991 there were 2,169,518 deaths in a total population of 252,177,000. 2,169,518 ÷ 252,177,000 = 8.6 deaths per 1000 people.
Age-specific rate	Number of deaths among persons of given age-group *divided by* Midyear population of that age-group	In 1991 the age-specific rate for 15- to 24-year-olds was 36,452. 36,452 ÷ 36,399,000 = 100.1 deaths per 100,000 15- to 24-year-olds.
Cause-specific rate	Number of deaths from a specific cause *divided by* Midyear population	In 1991 the cause-specific rate for HIV was 29,555 HIV deaths. 29,555 ÷ 252,177,000 = 11.7 per 100,000 people.
Case-fatality rate	Number of deaths from a specific disease in a given period *divided by* Number of persons diagnosed with that disease	If 87 of every 100 persons diagnosed with lung cancer die within 5 years, the 5-year case fatality rate is 87%. The 5-year survival rate would then be 13%.
Proportionate mortality ratio	Number of deaths from a specific disease *divided by* Total number of deaths in the same period	In 1991 720,862 deaths were from diseases of the heart out of 2,169,518 deaths from all causes. 720,862 ÷ 2,169,518 = 0.332 or 33.2% of all deaths were due to heart disease.
Infant mortality rate	Number of infant deaths under 1 year of age in a year divided by Number of live births in the same year	In 1991 there were 36,766 deaths under 1 year of age and 4,110,907 live births. 36,766 ÷ 4,110,907 = 0.0089 or 8.9 deaths per 1000 live births.
Neonatal mortality rate	Number of infant deaths under 28 days of age in a year divided by Number of live births in the same year	In 1991 there were 22,978 neonatal deaths and 4,110,907 live births. 22,978 ÷ 4,110,907 = 5.59 per 1000.
Postneonatal mortality rate	Number of infant deaths from 28 days to 1 year in a year *divided by* Number of live births in the same year	In 1991 there were 13,788 postneonatal deaths and 4,110,907 live births. 13,788 ÷ 4,110,907 = 3.35 per 1000.

From National Center for Health Statistics: *Health, United States, 1998,* Hyattsville, Md, 1998, U.S. Public Health Service.

a particular disease. Also, a person may have one disease (e.g., prostate cancer) yet die *from* a different cause (e.g., stroke).

Because the population changes during the course of a year, the population is estimated at midyear to get the denominator for annual rates. The crude annual mortality rate is an estimate of the risk of death for a person in a given population for that year. These rates are multiplied by a scaling factor, usually 100,000, to avoid small fractions. The result is then expressed as the number of deaths per 100,000 persons. A crude mortality rate, while easy to calculate and representative of the actual death rate for the total population, does have limitations. It does not reveal specific causes of death, which change in relative importance over time. Also, the mortality rate is affected by the population's age distribution, since older people are at much greater risk of death than younger people are. Mortality rates can be calculated for specific groups (e.g., age, gender, race).

The cause-specific mortality rate is an estimate of the risk of death from some specific disease in a population. It is the number of deaths from a specific cause divided by the total population at risk, usually multiplied by 100,000. Two related measures should be distinguished from the cause-specific

mortality rate. The case fatality rate (CFR) is the proportion of persons diagnosed with a particular disorder (i.e., cases) who die within a specified period of time. The CFR is an estimate of the risk of death within that period for a person newly diagnosed with the disease (e.g., the proportion of persons with breast cancer who die within 5 years). Since the CFR is the proportion of diagnosed persons who die within the period, 1 minus the CFR yields the survival rate. For example, if the 5-year CFR for lung cancer is 86%, then the 5-year survival rate is only 14% (Brownson et al, 1998). Persons diagnosed with a particular disease often want to know the probability of surviving. These rates provide that information.

The second measure to be distinguished from the cause-specific mortality rate is the proportionate mortality ratio (PMR), the proportion of all deaths that are due to a specific cause. The denominator is not the population at risk of death but the total number of deaths in the population; therefore, the PMR is not a rate, nor does it estimate the risk of death. The magnitude of the PMR is a function of both the number of deaths from the cause of interest and the number of deaths from other causes. If deaths from certain causes decline over time, deaths from other causes that remain fairly constant may have increasing PMRs. For example, motor vehicle accidents accounted for 5.2 deaths per 100,000 persons ages 5 to 14 in the United States in 1996. This was 24% of all deaths in this age-group (the PMR). By comparison, motor vehicle accidents caused 23.0 deaths per 100,000 persons 65 years of age and older in 1996, which was less than 0.5% of all deaths in the older age-group (Peters et al, 1998). This demonstrates that, although the *risk* of death from a motor vehicle accident was more than four times as great in the older group (based on the rates), such accidents accounted for a far greater proportion of all deaths in the younger group (based on the PMR). This is because of the much greater risk of death from other causes in the older group.

Infant mortality is used around the world as an indicator of overall health and availability of health care services. The most common measure, the infant mortality rate, is the number of deaths of infants in the first year of life divided by the total number of live births. Because the risk of death declines considerably during the first year of life, neonatal (newborn) and postneonatal mortality rates are also of interest.

Rate Adjustment

Rates are important in epidemiologic studies. However, rates can be misleading when they are compared across different populations. For example, since the risk of death increases dramatically after age 40 years, a higher crude death rate is expected in a population of older people compared with a population of younger people (Gordis, 1996). It is misleading to compare the overall mortality rate in an area with a large elderly population with the rate in a younger population. There are methods that adjust for differences in populations in order to compare death rates. Age adjustment is based on the assumption that a population's overall mortality rate is a function of the *age distribution* of the population and the *age-specific mortality rates*.

Age adjustment can be performed by *direct* or *indirect* methods. Both methods require a "standard population," which can be an external population, such as the U.S. population for a given year, a combined population of the groups under study, or some other standard chosen for relevance or convenience. A *direct* adjusted rate applies the age-specific death rates from the study population to the age distribution of the standard population. The result is the (hypothetical) death rate of the study population if it had the same age distribution as the standard population.

The *indirect* method is more complicated. The age-specific death rates of the standard population applied to the study population's age distribution produce an index rate that is used with the crude rates of both the study and standard populations to produce the final indirect adjusted rate, which is also hypothetical. The indirect method may be the best approach when the age-specific death rates for the study population are unknown or unstable (i.e., based on relatively small numbers). Often, instead of an indirect adjusted rate, a standardized mortality ratio (or SMR) is calculated. The SMR is the number of observed deaths in the study population divided by the expected number of deaths, based on the age-

specific rates in the standard population and the age distribution of the study population (Gordis, 1996).

Measures of Morbidity

PREVALENCE RATE. Epidemiologists and other health professionals pay close attention to measures of morbidity, especially prevalence and incidence rates, since these rates provide information about the levels of disease in a population, the rate of disease development, and the risk of disease. The **prevalence rate** is a measure of existing disease in a population at a particular time (i.e., the number of *existing* cases divided by the current population). The prevalence of a specific risk factor or exposure also can be calculated. For example, a health department and community hospital might jointly begin a screening program in an area with overcrowded housing, limited access to services, and under-utilization of preventive health practices. The program could include physical examinations; tuberculin skin tests followed up by chest x-rays when indicated; cardiovascular, glaucoma, and diabetes screening; as well as mammography for women and prostate screening for men over age 45. Of the 8,000 women screened, 35 had previously been diagnosed with breast cancer, and 20 who had no history of breast cancer were later determined to have confirmed cancer of the breast. The prevalence of breast cancer in this population of women would be:

$$\frac{55}{8000} = 0.006875 \text{ or } 687.5 \text{ per } 100,000$$

A prevalence rate is not an estimate of the risk of *developing* disease because it is a function of both the rate at which new cases of the disease develop and how long those cases remain in the population. In this example, the prevalence of breast cancer in this population of women is a function of how many new cases develop and how long women live with the cancer. A disease with a short duration (e.g., an intestinal virus) may not have a high prevalence rate even if the rate of new cases is high, because cases do not accumulate (see later Point Epidemic section). A disease with a long course will have a higher prevalence than a rapidly fatal disease that has the same rate of new cases. The box below discusses how to determine the prevalence of very-low–birth-weight infants in a community.

HOW TO Determine if a Problem Exists in a Community

Planning for resource and personnel needs requires that you know the extent of a given problem(s) in the community. For example, if you wanted to know how different counties in a state compared in terms of very-low–birth-weight infants, you would calculate the prevalence of these births in each county by:

- Determining the number of live births in each county by looking at birth certificate data in the Vital Records department of the health department.
- Listing the number of infants born weighing less than 1500 grams in each district based on the birth weight information.

- Calculating the prevalence of these very-low–birth-weight infants by county as the number of infants under 1500 grams at birth divided by the total number of live births.
- Using several recent years' data to get a more stable estimate if the number of very-low–birth-weight births in each county is small.

INCIDENCE RATE. The **incidence rate** is the number of *new* cases developing in a population at risk during a specified time. A cumulative incidence rate or incidence proportion estimates the risk of developing the disease in a population during a specific time. The population at risk is individuals who do not presently have the disease of interest but are at risk of acquiring it. Existing (or prevalent) cases are excluded from the population at risk for this calculation, since they already have the condition and are no longer at risk of developing it. Incidence counts new cases in a disease-free group (or *cohort*) of persons who are followed for some period. The risk of disease is a function of both the rate of new disease development and the length of time the population is at risk. In the example above, one could follow the 7945 women in whom no breast cancer was detected and chart the number of new cases of breast cancer detected over the next 5 years. Assuming no losses to follow-up, if 44 women were diagnosed over the 5-year period, then the 5-year cumulative incidence of breast cancer in this population would be:

$$\frac{44}{7945} = 0.005538 \text{ or } 553.8 \text{ per } 100,000$$

INCIDENCE AND PREVALENCE COMPARED. The prevalence rate measures existing cases of disease. This rate is roughly proportional to the incidence times the duration of disease, and it is affected by factors that influence risk and by factors that influence survival or recovery. In mathematical notation:

$$P \approx I \times D, \text{ where } P = \text{prevalence}, I = \text{incidence},$$
$$\text{and } D = \text{duration.}$$

For that reason, prevalence measures are less useful when looking for factors related to disease etiology. Because prevalence rates reflect duration in addition to the risk of getting the disease, it is difficult to sort out what factors are related to risk. Risk factors may be masked by differences in survival or cure. For example, the 5-year survival rate for breast cancer is about 85%, but the 5-year survival rate for lung cancer in women is only about 15%. Even if the incidence rates of breast and lung cancer were the same in women (and they are not), the prevalence rates would differ because on average women live longer with breast cancer (that is, it has a longer duration) than they do with lung cancer. Incidence rates, on the other hand, are the measure of choice to study etiology because incidence is affected only by factors related to the risk of developing disease and not to survival or cure. Prevalence is useful in planning health care services, since it is an indication of the level of disease existing in the population and therefore of the size of the population in need of services.

In the screening example, the health department needs to know both the existing level of tuberculosis in the area (the prevalence) in order to plan services and establish prevention and control measures, and the rate at which new cases are developing (the incidence) in order to study risk factors and evaluate the effectiveness of prevention and control programs.

ATTACK RATE. One final measure of morbidity, often used in infectious disease investigations, is the **attack rate.** This rate is a form of incidence rate defined as the proportion of persons exposed to an agent who develop the disease. Attack rates are often specific to one exposure. A food-specific attack rate would be the proportion of persons becoming ill after eating a specific food.

Comparison Groups

Comparison groups are often used in epidemiology. To decide if the rate of disease is due to a suspected risk factor, you should compare the exposed group with a group of comparable unexposed persons. To illustrate, one might investigate the effect of smoking during pregnancy on the rate of low birth weight by calculating the rate of low-birth-weight infants born to women who smoked during their pregnancy. However, the hypothesis that smoking during pregnancy is a risk factor for low birth weight is supported only when the low-birth-weight rate among smoking women is compared to the (lower) rate of low-birth-weight infants born to non-smoking women. The box below describes ways to assess community health problems.

Briefly Noted

Lung cancer has surpassed breast cancer as the leading cause of cancer mortality among women. This seems to coincide with the increased number of women who smoke.

HOW TO Assess Community Health Problems

- Identify major causes of disease through incidence, morbidity, and mortality rates.
- Evaluate major causes of hospitalizations and emergency room visits.
- Ask key community leaders to discuss critical community health problems.
- Hold focus groups with community groups involved in health.
- Analyze community environmental health hazards and pollutants such as water, sewage.
- Examine how much community residents know about and practice good health habits such as use of seat belts, helmets when riding bikes, lighted streets for safety.
- Identify cultural beliefs and values about health.
- Assess how the community understands and trusts federal, state, and local assistance programs.
- Conduct community surveys to assess for specific problems.

HOW TO Assess Individual Health Problems

- Take a history of physical and mental health problems.
- Ask people to identify their major health problems. Begin intervening with what the person considers most important.
- Take a family history of disease to identify potential genetic links or family patterns of disease.
- Perform a clinical examination, including lab work.
- Evaluate health risks based on lifestyle.
- Identify immediate and long-range safety concerns.
- Assess cultural beliefs about health.
- Assess availability of social support.
- Inquire about the knowledge and practices of good health habits.
- Do age-appropriate screening for diseases such as hypertension and cancer for adults.

DESCRIPTIVE EPIDEMIOLOGY

Descriptive epidemiology refers to the *distribution* of disease, death, and other health outcomes in the population according to person, place, and time. This type of epidemiology provides a picture of how things are or have been—the who, where, and when of disease patterns. *Analytic epidemiology,* on the other hand, searches for the *determinants* of the patterns observed—the how and why. That is, epidemiologic concepts and methods are used to discover what factors, characteristics, exposures, or behaviors may account for differences in the observed patterns of disease occurrence. Descriptive and analytical studies are observational. The investigator observes events as they are or have been and does not intervene to change anything or to introduce a new factor. Experimental or intervention studies, on the other hand, include interventions to test preventive or treatment measures, techniques, materials, policies, or drugs.

Person

Personal characteristics of interest in epidemiology include race, sex, age, education, occupation, income (and related socioeconomic status), and marital status. The most important predictor of overall mortality is age. The mortality curve by age drops sharply during and following the first year of life to a low point in childhood. The curve then begins to increase through adolescence and young adulthood (Gordis, 1996).

Mortality and morbidity differ by sex. Female infants have lower mortality than comparable male infants, and the survival advantage continues throughout life (National Center for Health Statistics, 1998; Peters et al, 1998). However, patterns for specific diseases vary. For example, women have lower rates of coronary heart disease until menopause, after which the gap narrows. For rheumatoid arthritis, the prevalence among women is greater than among men (Brownson et al, 1998).

Though the concept of race as a variable for public health research has been questioned (Centers for Disease Control and Prevention, 1993; Fullilove, 1998), there are clear differences in morbidity and mortality by race in the United States (National Center for Health Statistics, 1998; Peters et al, 1998). The 1996 U.S. age-adjusted death rate for African-Americans was 1.6 times higher than for white Americans. Death rates were also higher among blacks for 12 of the 15 leading causes of death in 1996 (Peters et al, 1998). The infant mortality rate for African-American infants, though declining, is still more than twice as high as the rate among whites. The NCHS report *Health, United States, 1998* provides further information about health disparities across socioeconomic levels.

Place

When considering the distribution of a disease, consider geographic patterns: does the rate of disease differ from place to place (e.g., with local environment)? If geography has no effects on disease occurrence, we might expect to see random geographic patterns. That is often not the case. For example, at high altitude there is a lower oxygen tension, which may result in smaller babies. Other diseases reflect distinctive patterns by place, for example Lyme disease is often found in areas where there are reservoirs of the disease (a large tick population as the vector for transmission to humans) and contact occurs between the human population and the tick vectors (Benenson, 1995).

Often variations by geographic location (place) are due to differences in the chemical, physical, or biological environment. However, variations by place also may result from differences in population densities or customary patterns of behavior and lifestyle or other personal characteristics. For example, one might find variations by place because of high concentrations of a religious, cultural, or ethnic group that practices certain health-related behaviors. The high rates of stroke found in the southeastern United States may be due to several social and personal factors that have little to do with geographic features per se. Neighborhood level variables, such as unemployment and crimes rates, social cohesion, and access to important services also affect rate variations (O'Campo et al, 1995; Sampson et al, 1997). These factors are of particular interest to nurses who work in community settings.

Time

Time is the third component of descriptive epidemiology. That is, is there an increase or decrease in the frequency of the disease over time or are other temporal patterns evident? Long-term patterns of morbidity or mortality are called **secular trends.** Secular trends may reflect changes in social behavior or practices. For example, the recent increase in lung cancer mortality that has been observed in recent years is a delayed effect of smoking in prior years, and the decline in cervical cancer deaths is primarily due to widespread screening using a Pap test (Brownson, et al, 1998).

Some secular trends may result from better diagnostic capability or changes in survival (or case fatality) rather than in incidence. Mortality data alone do not accurately depict the true situation. Changes in case definition or revisions in the coding of a disease according to International Classification of Diseases (ICD) also affect secular trends. Such changes can produce an artificial change in the rate (Peters et al, 1998).

Point epidemic is a time- and space-related pattern that is important in infectious disease investigations and as an indicator for toxic exposures in environmental epidemiology. A point epidemic is shown when the frequency of cases is graphed against time. The sharp peak characteristic of such graphs indicates a concentration of cases over a short interval of time. The peak often indicates the population's response to a common source of infection or contamination to which they were all simultaneously exposed. Knowledge of the incubation or latency period (the time between exposure and development of signs and symptoms) for the specific disease entity can help determine the probable time of exposure. An outbreak of gastrointestinal illness from a food-borne pathogen is an example of a point epidemic. Nurses who are alert to a sudden increase in the number of cases of a disease can chart the outbreak, determine the probable time of exposure, and, by careful investigation, isolate the probable source of the agent.

In addition to secular trends and point epidemics, there are also **cyclical time patterns of disease.** Seasonal fluctuation is a common type of cyclical variation in some infectious illnesses. Seasonal changes may be influenced by changes in the agent itself, changes in population densities or behaviors of animal reservoirs or vectors, or changes in human behaviors resulting in changing exposures (being outdoors in warmer weather and indoors in colder months). There also may be artificial seasons created by calendar events, such as holidays and tax-filing deadlines that are associated with patterns of stress-related illness. Patterns of accidents and injuries also may be seasonal, reflecting differing employment and recreational patterns. Some disease cycles, such as influenza, have patterns of smaller epidemics every few years, depending on strain, with major pandemics occurring at longer intervals (Benenson, 1995). Attention to cyclical patterns is especially important for people who work in public health to enable them to prepare adequately to meet possible increased demands for service.

A third type of temporal pattern is an **event-related cluster.** These are patterns in which time is not measured from fixed dates on the calendar but from the point of some exposure, event, or experience that affects some people, though not at the same time. An example of this pattern would be vaccine reactions during an immunization program. If vaccinations are given on a regular basis, one might see nonspecific symptoms, such as fever, headaches, or rashes, fairly consistently over time, making identification of a cluster related to the vaccinations difficult. If, however, the occurrence of symptoms is plotted against the amount of time since vaccination, the number of vaccine reactions is likely to peak at some period after the immunization.

ANALYTIC EPIDEMIOLOGY

While *descriptive* epidemiology deals with the *distribution* of health outcomes, *analytic* epidemiology tries to discover the *determinants* of outcomes—the how and the why. Analytic epidemiology deals with the factors that influence the observed patterns of health and disease, and increase or decrease the risk of adverse outcomes. This section will discuss analytic study designs and the related measures of association derived from them. Table 8-5 summarizes the advantages and disadvantages of each design.

Ecological Studies

An ecological study bridges descriptive and analytic epidemiology. The descriptive component looks at variations in disease rates by person, place, or time. The analytic component tries to determine if there is a relation of disease rates to variations in rates for possible risk (or protective) factors or characteristics. Ecological studies use only aggregate data, such as population rates, rather than data on individuals' exposures, characteristics, and outcomes. Examples include the following:

1. Information on per capita cigarette consumption can be examined in relation to lung cancer mortality rates in several countries, or several groups of people, or in the same population at different times
2. Comparisons of the rates of breast feeding and of breast cancer
3. Average dietary fat content and rates of coronary heart disease
4. Unemployment rates and level of psychiatric disorder.

Ecological studies are attractive because they often make use of existing, readily available rates, and are therefore quick and inexpensive to conduct. They are often a good first study. They are subject, however, to ecological fallacy (i.e., associations observed at the group level may not hold true for the individuals that compose the groups, or associations that actually exist may be masked in the grouped data). This can occur when other factors operate in these populations for which the ecological correlations do not account. For that reason, ecological studies may suggest possible answers, but they require confirmation with additional studies that use individual data (Gordis, 1996; Lilienfeld and Stolley, 1994).

Cross-Sectional Studies

The **cross-sectional study** provides a snap shot, or cross section, of a population or group (Gordis, 1996; Lilienfeld and Stolley, 1994). Information is collected on current health status, personal characteristics, and potential risk factors or exposures all at once. In the cross-sectional study there is simultaneous collection of information necessary for

TABLE 8-5	Comparison of Major Epidemiologic Study Designs	
Study Design	**Advantages**	**Disadvantages**
Ecological	• Quick, easy, and inexpensive first study • Uses readily available existing data • May prompt further investigation, suggest other/new hypotheses • May provide information about contextual factors not accounted for by individual characteristics	• Ecological fallacy; the associations observed may not hold true for individuals • Problems in interpreting temporal sequence (cause and effect) • More difficult to control for confounding, and "mixed" models (ecologic and individual data) more complex statistically
Cross-sectional (correlational)	• Gives general description of scope of problem, provides prevalence estimates • Often based on population (or community) sample, not just those who sought care • Useful in health service evaluation and planning • Data obtained at once; less expense and quicker than cohort because no follow-up • Baseline for prospective study or identify cases and controls for case-control study	• No calculation of risk; prevalence, not incidence • Temporal sequence unclear • Not good for rare disease or rare exposure unless large sample size or stratified sampling • Selective survival can be major source of selection bias. Surviving subjects may differ from those who are not included (death, institutionalization, etc.) • Selective recall or lack of past exposure information can bias
Case-control (retrospective, case comparison)	• Less expensive than cohort, smaller sample required • Quicker than cohort, no follow-up • Can investigate more than one exposure • Best design for rare diseases • If well designed can be important tool for etiologic investigation • Best suited to diseases with relatively clear onset (timing of onset can be established so that incident cases can be included)	• Greater susceptibility than cohort studies to various types of bias (selective survival, recall bias, selection bias in choice of both cases and controls) • Information on other risk factors may not be available, resulting in confounding • Antecedent-consequence (temporal sequence) not as certain as in cohort • Not well suited to rare exposures • Gives only an indirect estimate of risk • Limited to a single outcome because of sampling on disease status
Prospective cohort (concurrent cohort, longitudinal, follow-up)	• Best estimate of disease incidence • Best estimate of risk • Fewer problems with selective survival and selective recall • Temporal sequence more clearly established • Broader range of options for exposure assessment	• Expensive in time and money • More difficult to organize • Not practical for rare diseases • Attrition of participants can bias estimate • Latency period may be very long; may miss cases • May be difficult to examine several exposures
Retrospective cohort (nonconcurrent cohort)	• Combines advantages of both prospective cohort and case-control • Shorter time (even if follow-up into future) than prospective cohort • Less expensive than prospective cohort because relies on existing data • Temporal sequence may be clearer than case-control	• Shares some disadvantages with both prospective cohort and case-control • Subject to attrition (loss to follow-up) • Relies on existing records, which may result in misclassification of both exposure and outcome • May have to rely on surrogate measures of exposure (such as job title) and vital records information on cause of death

the classification of exposure and outcome. Historical information can also be collected (e.g., past diet, or history of radiation exposures).

Cross-sectional studies are sometimes called prevalence studies because they provide the frequency (number) of existing cases of a disease in a population (Kelsey et al,

1996). Cross-sectional studies can evaluate the association of a factor with a health problem by comparing the prevalence of the disease in those with the factor (or exposure) to the prevalence in the unexposed. The ratio of the two prevalence rates shows the association between the factor and the outcome. If the prevalence of coronary heart disease (CHD)

Evidence-Based Practice

The research article referenced below described an educational program on prostate cancer, which is a major cause of morbidity and mortality in men. Free prostate cancer screening was given to 179 men at their work sites. Only 16% of the African-Americans had obtained a digital rectal examination (DRE) in the last 12 months; 44% of the men participated in the free screening, and this was an increase of nearly four times. Similarly, only 6% of the African-American men had received a prostate-specific antigen (PSA) screen in the past 12 months, yet 42% got PSA screening after the educational program; this represented a seven-fold increase.

APPLICATION IN PRACTICE

The nurses who participated in this research helped to identify risk factors and encouraged screening and preventive health practices. Occupational health nurses could easily use this type of screening. Work sites are good places to carry out health promotion and diagnostic screening. There are many helpful forms of information that are easily understood by lay people available from voluntary organizations such as the American Heart Association, American Lung Association, or the American Cancer Society, as well as from the federal government.

Weinrich S, Greiner E, Reis-Starr C, Weinrich M, Yoon S: Work sites: effective sites for recruitment of African American men into prostate cancer screening, *J Community Health Nurs* 15(2):113-129, 1998.

in smokers were twice as high as the prevalence among non-smokers, the prevalence ratio would be 2. If a factor is unrelated to the prevalence of a disease, the prevalence ratio will be close to 1. A value less than 1 may suggest a protective association. For example, the prevalence of coronary heart disease (CHD) is lower among physically active people than among sedentary persons. Thus the prevalence ratio for the association between physical activity and CHD should be less than 1.

Cross-sectional studies are subject to bias resulting from selective survival, that is, existing cases who have survived to be in the study may be different from cases diagnosed about the same time who have died and are not available for inclusion. Suppose physical activity not only reduced the risk of heart disease, but also markedly improved survival among those with heart disease. Sedentary persons with heart disease would then have higher fatality rates than physically active persons who developed heart disease. One might observe higher rates of physical activity in a group of heart disease survivors than in a general population without heart disease. This might occur both because of the survival advantage and also participation of survivors in cardiac rehabilitation programs. It might, however, erroneously appear that physical activity was a risk factor for heart disease.

Case-Control Studies

In the **case-control study** design, subjects are enrolled *because* they are known to have the outcome of interest

(these are the cases) or they are known *not* to have the outcome of interest (these are the controls). Case-control status is verified using a clear case definition and some previously determined method or protocol (e.g., by an examination, laboratory test, or medical chart review). Information is then collected on the exposures or characteristics of interest, frequently from existing sources, subject interview, or questionnaire (Kelsey et al, 1996). The question in a case-control study is "Do persons with the outcome of interest (cases) have the exposure characteristic (or a history of the exposure) more frequently than those without the outcome (controls)?"

Given the way subjects are selected for a case-control study, neither incidence nor prevalence can be calculated directly. In a case-control study, an odds ratio tells us how much more (or less) likely the exposure is to be found among cases than among controls. The odds of exposure among cases (*a* to *c* in the table below) are compared to the odds of exposure among controls (*b* to *d*). The ratio of these two odds provides us with an estimate of the relative risk (discussed below).

Suppose a research group wanted to study risk factors for suicide attempts among adolescents. They enrolled 100 adolescents who had attempted suicide and selected 200 adolescents from the same community with no history of suicide attempts. The research group wanted to determine if the adolescents had a history of substance abuse (SA). Through a questionnaire and use of medical records they learned that 68 of the 100 adolescents who had attempted suicide had a history of substance abuse. They also found that 36 of the 200 adolescents with no suicide attempt had a substance abuse history. The information could be presented as follows:

	Suicide Attempt	No Attempt
History of substance abuse	68 a	36 b
No history of substance abuse	32 c	164 d
	100	200

The odds of a history of substance abuse among suicide attempters are *a/c* or 68/32, while the odds of substance abuse among controls are *b/d* or 36/164. The odds ratio (equivalent to *ad/bc*) is:

$$\frac{68 \times 164}{36 \times 32} = 9.68$$

This would be interpreted to mean that adolescents who attempted suicide are almost 10 times more likely to have a history of substance abuse than adolescents who have not attempted suicide. Note that, as with the prevalence ratio, an odds ratio of 1 is indicative of no association (i.e., the odds of exposure are similar for cases and controls). An odds ratio less than 1 suggests a protective association, that cases are less likely to have been exposed than controls.

Because the number of cases is known or actively sought out, case-control studies do not require large samples or the long follow-up time often required for prospective cohort studies. For these reasons, many important cancer studies have used the case-control design.

Cohort Studies

In epidemiology, cohort refers to a group of persons who are born at about the same time. In analytic studies, cohort refers to a group of persons, generally sharing some characteristic of interest, who are enrolled in a study and followed over time to observe some health outcome. Because of this ability to observe the development of new cases of disease, **cohort study** designs allow for calculation of incidence rates and therefore estimates of risk of disease. Cohort studies may be prospective or retrospective (Kelsey et al, 1996; Rothman and Greenland, 1998).

Prospective Cohort Studies

In a prospective cohort study (also called a longitudinal or follow-up study), subjects determined to be free of the outcome under investigation are classified on the basis of the exposure of interest at the beginning of the follow-up period. The subjects are then followed for some period of time to determine the occurrence of disease in each group. The question is "Do persons with the factor (or exposure) of interest develop (or avoid) the outcome more frequently than those without the factor (or exposure)?"

For example, one might recruit a cohort of subjects who would be classified as physically active ("exposed") or sedentary ("not exposed"). These subjects would be followed over time to see if they developed coronary heart disease. The cohort study avoids the problem of selective survival and also has the advantage of allowing estimation of the risk of acquiring disease for those who are exposed compared to those who are unexposed (or less exposed). This ratio of cumulative incidence rates is called the relative risk.

For example, suppose 1000 physically active and 1000 sedentary middle-aged men and women were enrolled in a prospective cohort study. All were free of coronary heart disease (CHD) at enrollment. Over the next 5 years, regular examinations detect CHD in 120 of the sedentary men and women and in 48 of the active men and women. Assuming no other deaths or losses to follow-up, the data could be presented as follows:

	CHD	No CHD	
Physically active	48 a	952 b	1000
Sedentary	120 c	880 d	1000

The incidence of CHD in the active group is $[a/(a + b)] = 48/1000$, and the incidence of CHD in the sedentary group is $[c/(c + d)] = 120/1000$. The relative risk is:

$$\frac{48/1000}{120/1000} = 0.4$$

As in the example of prevalence ratio, because physical activity is protective for CHD, the relative risk is less than 1. The interpretation for this hypothetical example is that, over a 5-year period, persons who are physically active had about 0.4 the risk of CHD compared to sedentary persons. If the risk were greater for those exposed, the relative risk would be greater than 1. For example, if the relative risk of CHD for smokers compared to nonsmokers were 3.5, it would be interpreted to mean that the risk of CHD among smokers is 3.5 times the risk among nonsmokers. The null value indicating no association is 1, since the incidence rates and thus the risk would be equal in the two groups if there were no association.

In the cohort study design, subjects are enrolled prior to disease onset. This pattern of subject recruitment allows the researcher to study more than one outcome, calculate incidence rates and estimate risk, and establish the temporal sequence of exposure and outcome with greater clarity and certainty. As a result, the researcher may avoid many of the problems of the earlier study designs with selective survival or exposure misclassification. On the other hand, large samples are often necessary to ensure that enough cases are observed to provide statistical power to detect meaningful differences between groups. This is complicated by the long period required for some diseases to develop (the latency period). Also, the number of subjects required to observe sufficient cases make longitudinal studies unsuitable for very rare diseases unless they are part of a larger study of a number of outcomes.

Retrospective Cohort Studies

Retrospective cohort studies combine some of the advantages and disadvantages of case-control studies and prospective cohort studies. They use existing records, such as employment, insurance, or hospital records, to define a cohort that is classified as having been exposed or unexposed at some time in the past. The cohort is followed over time, using the records to determine if the outcome occurred. Retrospective cohort studies (also called historical cohort) may be conducted entirely using past records, or they may include current assessment or additional follow-up time after study initiation. This approach saves time since researchers do not have to wait for new cases of disease to develop. The disadvantages are largely related to the reliance on existing historical records. Retrospective cohort studies frequently are used in occupational epidemiology where industrial records are available to investigate work-related exposures and health outcomes.

EXPERIMENTAL STUDIES

The study designs discussed so far are called observational studies because the investigator observes the association between exposures and outcomes as they exist, but does not intervene to alter the presence or level of any exposure or behavior. In contrast, in experimental or intervention studies, the investigator initiates a treatment or intervention to influence the risk or course of disease. These studies test whether interventions are effective in preventing disease or improving health. Both observational and experimental studies generally use comparison (or control) groups. In experimental studies persons can be randomly assigned to a particular group; an intervention (a treatment or exposure) is applied, and the effects of the intervention are measured. Intervention studies are of two general types: clinical trials and community trials (Gordis, 1996; Lilienfeld and Stolley, 1994).

Briefly Noted

Epidemiology uses a process much like the nursing process. It is essentially a systematic investigative process.

Clinical Trials

Clinical trials typically try to evaluate the effectiveness of an intervention such as a treatment for disease, a new or existing drug used in a new or different way, surgical technique, or other treatment. Randomization avoids the bias that may result if subjects self-select into one group or the other or if the investigator or clinician chooses subjects for each group.

A second aspect of treatment allocation is the use of masking or "blinding" treatment assignments. Generally, it is best to use the double-blinded study in which neither subject nor investigator knows who is receiving which treatment. Clinical trials generally are the best way to show causality because of the objective way in which subjects are assigned and the greater control over other factors that could influence outcome. Like cohort studies, they are prospective and provide the clearest evidence of time sequence. They tend to be conducted in a contrived (versus natural) situation, under controlled conditions, and with patient populations. The contrived situation may not be exactly like more realistic clinical or community conditions with a diverse patient population. Ethical issues need to be considered in experimental studies. For example, is it fair to withhold a treatment if the treatment may have great potential to intervene in a disease in order to systematically evaluate this treatment using both an experimental and a control group? Finally, clinical trials tend to be costly in time, personnel, facilities, and in some cases, supplies.

Community Trials

Community trials are similar to clinical trials in that an investigator determines what the exposure or intervention will be. However, community trials often deal with health promotion and disease prevention rather than treatment of existing disease. The intervention is usually undertaken on a large scale, and the unit of treatment allocation is a community, region, or group, rather than individuals. Although a pharmaceutical product may be involved in a community trial, such as fluoridation of water or mass immunizations, community trials often involve educational, programmatic, or policy interventions. Examples of community interventions would be measuring the rates of diabetes or cardiovascular disease in a community in which the availability of exercise programs

and facilities was increased or where a much larger supply of healthful, fresh foods was made available.

Although community trials provide the best means of testing whether changes in knowledge or behavior, policy, programs, or other mass interventions are effective, they do present some problems. For many interventions, it may take years for their effectiveness to be evident, such as the effect of changing the availability of exercise and healthful food on the rate of either diabetes or heart disease. Comparable community populations without similar interventions for comparative analysis are often difficult to find. Even when comparable comparison communities are available—especially when the intervention is improved knowledge or changed behavior—it is difficult and unethical to prevent the control communities from making use of generally available information, effectively making them less different from the intervention communities. Finally, because community trials are often undertaken on a large scale and over long periods of time, they can be expensive, require large staff, have complicated logistics, and need extensive communication about the study.

SCREENING

Screening is the assessment or evaluation of people who have no symptoms of disease in order to classify them as to their likelihood of having a particular disease. Screening may be a component of secondary prevention efforts. From a clinical perspective, the aim of screening is early detection and treatment in order to detect any problem early when there is a greater chance of successful intervention and a more favorable prognosis. From a public health perspective, the objective is to sort out efficiently and effectively those who *probably* have the disease from those who *probably* do not have the disease. The public health purpose is to detect cases early for treatment or initiate public health prevention and control programs. A screening test is not a diagnostic test. Screening programs require referral and diagnostic evaluation for those who are found to be positive in order to determine whether they actually have the disease and need treatment.

As seen in Box 8-2, successful screening programs have several characteristics that depend on both the tests and population screened. It is desirable to use reliable and valid screening tests (Gordis, 1996).

Reliability and Validity

Reliability

Any researcher needs to be concerned about the precision or **reliability** of a measure (its consistency or repeatability) and the accuracy of a measure. Accuracy refers to whether the study measures the intended variable and how closely it does so. Suppose you want to do a blood pressure screening in a community. You will take blood pressure readings on a large number of people, perhaps following up with repeated measures for individuals with higher pressures. If the sphygmo-

Evidence-Based Practice

Race- and age-specific values for prostate-specific antigen (PSA) levels have been suggested by the findings in the article referenced below. The race- and age-specific distribution of serum PSA levels in men in South Carolina was compared with distributions obtained in data from the Olmsted County Study and from the Walter Reed Army Medical Center/Center for Prostate Disease Research study. The sample had 1,127 healthy blacks and whites ages 40 to 69 years from a cross section of the general population in 11 counties of central South Carolina who participated in prostate cancer educational programs and subsequently obtained a physical examination including a PSA determination.

Higher PSA levels were found in older men and among the black men. Within each of the three studies, there were considerable age- and race-related differences in serum PSA levels, and for that reason, each study supports the use of age- and race-normed reference ranges for normal PSA that are specific to the population from which the norms were derived.

APPLICATION IN PRACTICE

Nurses need to know that reference ranges for normal serum PSA levels can vary from one setting to another. Men with questionable PSA levels need to be referred to a physician, especially if they have the increased risks that come from family history or race.

Weinrich M, Jacobsen S, Weinrich S, Osterling J, Jacobsen D, Wise R: Reference ranges for serum prostate specific antigen in black and white men without cancer, *Urology* 52(6):967-973, December 1998.

manometer used for the screening varies in its readings so that the readings vary when taken twice in a row on the same person, then it lacks precision. The instrument would be unreliable even if the overall mean of repeated measurements were close to the true overall mean for the persons measured. The problem would be that the readings would not be reliable for any individual, which is what a screening program requires.

On the other hand, suppose the readings are reproducible, that is, you get the same reading on the same person when you repeatedly take the blood pressure. However, unknown to you, the readings are about 10 mm Hg too high. This instrument is producing precise and reliable readings. However, the uncorrected (or uncalibrated) instrument lacks accuracy (does not give a valid reading). In short, a measure can be consistent without producing valid results.

There are three major sources of error affecting the reliability of tests:

1. Variation inherent in the trait itself (e.g., blood pressure that changes with time of day, activity, level of stress, and other factors)
2. Observer variation, which can be divided into intraobserver reliability (consistency by the same observer) and interobserver reliability (consistency from one observer to another)
3. Inconsistency in the instrument, which includes the internal consistency of the instrument (e.g., whether all items in a questionnaire measure the same thing) and the stability (or test-retest reliability) of the instrument over time.

Validity: Sensitivity and Specificity

Validity in a screening test is measured by sensitivity and specificity. **Sensitivity** quantifies how accurately the test identifies those individuals *with* the condition or trait. In other words, sensitivity represents the proportion of persons with the disease whom the test correctly identifies as positive (true positives; these people do have the disease). High sensitivity is needed both when early treatment is important and when identification of every case is important such as

when the disease is highly contagious or is crippling or fatal if not treated early.

Specificity indicates how accurately the test identifies those people *without* the disease (i.e., the proportion of persons without the disease whom the test correctly identifies as negative [true negatives]). High specificity is needed when rescreening is impractical and when reducing false positives is important.

The sensitivity and specificity of a test are determined by comparing the results from the test with results from a definitive or proven diagnostic procedure (sometimes called the "gold standard"). For example, the Pap smear is a common screening procedure for detection of cervical dysplasia and carcinoma. The definitive diagnosis of cervical cancer requires a biopsy with histological confirmation of malignant cells. The ideal for a screening test is 100% sensitivity and 100% specificity. This level of sensitivity and specificity would mean that the test results are positive for 100% of those who actually have the disease and the test results are negative for all those who do not have the disease. In practice, sensitivity and specificity are often inversely related. That is, if the test results are such that one can choose some point beyond which a person is considered positive (a "cutpoint"), as in a blood pressure reading to screen for hypertension or a serum glucose reading to screen for diabetes, then moving that critical point to improve the sensitivity of the test will result in a decrease in specificity, or an improvement in specificity can be made only at the expense of sensitivity.

A third measure associated with sensitivity and specificity is the predictive value of the test. The **positive predictive value** is the proportion of persons with a positive test who actually have the disease, interpreted as the probability that an individual with a positive test has the disease. The **negative predictive value** is the proportion of persons with a negative test who are actually disease-free. Although sensitivity and specificity are relatively independent of the prevalence of disease, predictive values are affected by the level of disease in the screened population, as well as by the sensitivity and specificity of the test. When the prevalence is low, the positive predictive value will be low, even with tests that are sensitive and specific. In addition, lower specificity produces lower positive predictive values because of the increase in the proportion of false-positive results.

Two or more tests can be combined to enhance sensitivity or specificity. They may be combined in *series* or in *parallel.* In series testing, the person is considered positive only if results are positive on *all* tests in the series, and one is considered negative if results are negative on *any* test. For example, if a blood sample were screened for HIV, a positive enzyme-linked immunosorbent assay (ELISA) might be followed up with a Western Blot, and the sample would be considered positive only if *both* tests were positive. Series testing improves specificity, producing fewer false positives, but sensitivity may be low. In series testing, sequence is important: researchers often use a very sensitive test first to pick up all cases plus false positives, then a second test that is very specific to eliminate false positives.

In parallel testing one is considered positive if positive results are found on *any* test and is considered negative only if results are negative on *all* tests. To return to the example of a blood sample being tested for HIV, a blood bank might consider a sample positive if it were positive on *either* the ELISA *or* the Western Blot. Parallel testing enhances sensitivity, leaving fewer false negatives, but specificity may be low.

CAUSALITY
Statistical Associations

One of the first steps in assessing the relation of some factor with a health outcome is determining whether a statistical association exists. That is, to assess if eating habits affect the onset of hypertension, you would need to establish a statistical association between the factor (diet) and the health outcome (hypertension). If the probability of disease seems unaffected by the presence or level of the factor, no association is apparent. If, on the other hand, the probability of disease does vary according to whether the factor is present, then there is a statistical association. When an observed measure of association (such as a relative risk) does not differ from the null value, there is no evidence for an association between the factor and outcome under investigation.

To say a result is statistically significant means that the observed result is unlikely to be due to chance. Note that statistical significance is also determined by sample size. In other words, the difference between 34.3% and 35.9% in a study group of 1000 is not statistically significant at $\alpha = 0.05$. However, in a much larger sample, a difference of this amount would be significant.

Bias

One also may observe a statistically significant result because of **bias,** a systematic error due to the study design, execution, or confounding. For example, if there were a gum ball machine with colors randomly mixed, and you got three red ones in a row, that would be due to chance. If, however, the person loading the gum ball machine had poured in a bag of red ones first, then green ones, then yellow, it would not be surprising to get three red ones in a row because of the way the machine was loaded. In epidemiologic studies, results often occur because of the way the study was "loaded" (i.e., the way the study was designed or subjects were selected or information collected and subjects classified). Although the types of bias are numerous, there are three general categories of bias.

Bias attributable to the way subjects enter a study is called *selection bias.* It has to do with selection procedures and the population from which subjects are drawn. It may involve self-selection factors as well. For example, are teenagers who agree to complete a questionnaire on alcohol, tobacco, and other drug use representative of the total teenage population?

Bias attributable to misclassification of subjects once they are in the study is information or *classification* (or misclassification) bias. It is related to how information is collected, including the information that subjects themselves supply or how subjects are classified.

Bias resulting from the relation of the outcome and study factor with some third factor not accounted for is called **confounding.** For example, there is a well-known association between maternal smoking during pregnancy and low-birth-weight babies. There is also an association between alcohol consumption and smoking that is not due to chance, nor is it causal. (That is, drinking alcohol does not cause a person to smoke, nor does smoking cause a person to drink alcohol.) If one were to investigate the association of alcohol consumption and low birth weight, smoking would be a confounder because it is related to both alcohol consumption and low birth weight. Failure to account for smoking in the analysis of the study's data would bias the observed association between alcohol use and low birth weight. In practice we can often identify potentially confounding variables in order to adjust for them in analysis.

Criteria for Causality

The existence of a statistical association does not necessarily mean there is a causal relation. As the previous sections have shown, the observed association may be a random

Healthy People 2010 Objectives Related to Epidemiology

1. Access to Quality Health Services
2. Arthritis, Osteoporosis, and Chronic Back Conditions
3. Cancer
4. Chronic Kidney Disease
5. Diabetes
6. Disability and Secondary Conditions
7. Educational and Community-Based Programs
8. Environmental Health
9. Family Planning
10. Food Safety
11. Health Communication
12. Heart Disease and Stroke
13. HIV
14. Immunization and Infectious Diseases
15. Injury and Violence Prevention
16. Maternal, Infant, and Child Health
17. Medical Product Safety
18. Mental Health and Mental Disorders
19. Nutrition and Overweight
20. Occupational Safety and Health
21. Oral Health
22. Physical Activity and Fitness
23. Public Health Infrastructure
24. Respiratory Diseases
25. Sexually Transmitted Diseases
26. Substance Abuse
27. Tobacco Use
28. Vision and Hearing

From U.S. Department of Health and Human Services: *Healthy People 2010: Understanding and improving health,* Washington, D.C., 2000, U.S. Government Printing Office; available online at www.health.gov/healthypeople.

event (due to chance) or may be due to bias from confounding or in the study design or execution. Statistical associations, although necessary to an argument for **causality,** are not sufficient proof. The criteria for causality, originally established to evaluate the link between an infectious agent and a disease, have been revised and elaborated to apply also to other outcomes.

HEALTHY PEOPLE 2010 AND EPIDEMIOLOGY

In *Healthy People 2010,* Objective 23-14, the need for epidemiology services and use of data is addressed. It is important to be able to "quickly detect, investigate, and respond to disease in order to prevent unnecessary transmission" (p. 23-18). The 28 focus areas on which data will be collected are listed in the box above.

Clinical Application

You are working in a local health department when Mr. Jones, a 46-year-old African-American man, comes in for a routine

blood pressure check. He comments that his father has recently died from prostate cancer, and this worries him. As you ask more questions, you learn that his father was diagnosed with prostate cancer when he was 52, and Mr. Jones' 56-year-old brother was just diagnosed with this disease. Mr. Jones has previously said that he still smokes a pack of cigarettes a day, eats considerable amounts of fried food, and likes to add extra salt to his vegetables.

What would the best action be?
A. *Give Mr. Jones a digital rectal examination and draw blood for a prostate-specific antigen (PSA) test immediately to screen for prostate cancer.*
B. *Do not mention prostate screening since Mr. Jones is still under 50 years of age and likely not at high risk.*
C. *Advise Mr. Jones to be tested immediately for prostate cancer since he has a strong family history for this disease.*
D. *Inform Mr. Jones of the risk and benefits of prostate screening and also talk with him about the health risks that he may experience from smoking and a high-fat, high-salt diet.*

Answer is in the back of the book.

Remember This!

- Epidemiology is the study of the distribution and determinants of health-related events in people, and the application of this information to improving health.
- Epidemiology is a multidisciplinary science that acknowledges the complex interrelations of factors that influence health and disease.
- Epidemiology uses a systematic process that is similar to that used in both the nursing process and the research process.
- Some of the basic epidemiological concepts include the interrelationships of agent, host, and environment (the epidemiological triangle); the interactions of factors, exposures, and characteristics in a causal web that affect the risk of disease; and levels of prevention that correspond to the natural history of disease.
- Primary prevention refers to interventions to reduce the incidence of disease by promoting health and preventing disease.
- Secondary prevention is designed to detect disease in its early stages and begin treatment immediately.
- Tertiary prevention provides treatments to people who have an apparent disease in order to interrupt, if possible, the course of the disease, reduce disability or rehabilitate.
- Basic epidemiologic methods include using existing data to study health outcomes and related factors and also using comparison groups to examine the association of exposures or characteristics to health outcomes.
- Epidemiologists use rates to determine levels of morbidity (illness) and mortality (deaths).
- Prevalence rates demonstrate the level of existing cases in a population at a certain time.

- Incidence rates measure the rate of new cases in a population and estimate the risk of disease.
- Descriptive epidemiology provides information about the distribution of disease and health states according to personal characteristics, geographic area, and time.
- Analytic epidemiology investigates associations between exposures or characteristics and health or disease outcomes. The goal is to understand what caused the disease.
- Epidemiological methods are used to design screening programs.

 What Would You Do?

1. Read your local newspaper for a week and see if you can find any reports that use epidemiologic methods. If yes, what was the health risk? What was the intervention? What might have prevented the disease or accident? Discuss this with two classmates to see if they agree or disagree.
2. During the winter months, keep a journal to evaluate the pattern of illness such as from colds or the flu. What seems to be the common carrier of the virus? How might transmission be interrupted? What do you do on a regular basis to prevent getting a cold or the flu?
3. Recall a time when you rode in a form of public transportation (bus, train, airplane). What were likely sources of disease transmission? How could you protect yourself from getting a disease if you rode on a bus, train, or airplane with one or more individuals who had a cough? Discuss this with a classmate to see when either/both of you got a disease and if you can trace the transmission.

REFERENCES

Benenson AS: *Control of communicable diseases in man,* ed 16, Washington, D.C., 1995, American Public Health Association.

Brownson RC, Remington PL, Davis JR: *Chronic disease epidemiology and control,* ed 2, Washington, D.C., 1998, American Public Health Association.

Centers for Disease Control and Prevention: Use of race and ethnicity in public health surveillance: summary of the CDC/ATSDR workshop, *MMWR* 42(RR-10), 1993.

Cohen IB: Florence Nightingale, *Sci Am* 3:128-137, 1984.

Fullilove MT: Comment: abandoning "race" as a variable in public health research: an idea whose time has come, *Am J Public Health* 88(9):1297, 1998.

Gordis L: *Epidemiology,* Philadelphia, 1996, WB Saunders.

Institute of Medicine: *The future of public health,* Washington, D.C., 1988, National Academy Press.

Kelsey JL, et al: *Methods in observational epidemiology,* ed 2, New York, 1996, Oxford University Press.

Krieger N: Epidemiology and the web of causation: has anyone seen the spider? *Soc Sci Med* 39(7):887, 1994.

Last JM: *A dictionary of epidemiology,* ed 3, New York, 1995, Oxford University Press.

Lilienfeld AM: Epidemiology and health policy: some historical highlights, *Public Health Rep* 99(3):237, 1984.

Lilienfeld DE, Stolley PD: *Foundations of epidemiology,* ed 3, New York, 1994, Oxford University Press.

Mullan F: *Plagues and politics: the story of the United States Public Health Service,* New York, 1989, Basic Books.

National Center for Health Statistics: *Health, United States,* 1998, Hyattsville, Md, 1998, Public Health Service.

O'Campo P, et al: Violence by male partners against women during the childbearing year: a contextual analysis, *Am J Public Health* 85(8):1092, 1995.

Palmer IS: *Florence Nightingale and the first organized delivery of nursing services,* Washington, D.C., 1983, American Association of Colleges of Nursing.

Peters KD, Kochanek KD, Murphy SL: *Deaths: Final data for 1996: national vital statistics reports,* 47:9, Hyattsville, Md, 1998, National Center for Health Statistics.

Rothman KJ, Greenland S: *Modern epidemiology,* ed 2, Philadelphia, 1998, Lippincott-Raven.

Sampson RJ, Raudenbush SW, Earls F: Neighborhoods and violent crime: a multilevel study of collective efficacy, *Science* 277(15 August):918, 1997.

Schneider MJ: *Introduction to public health,* Gaithersburg, Md, 2000, Aspen.

Snow J: *On the mode of communication of cholera.* In *Snow on cholera,* New York, 1855, The Commonwealth Fund.

Susser M: Epidemiology in the United States after World War II: the evolution of technique, *Epidemiol Rev* 7:147, 1985.

Timmreck TC: *An introduction to epidemiology,* Boston, 1994, Jones & Bartlett.

U.S. Department of Health and Human Services: *Healthy people 2010: understanding and improving health,* Washington, D.C., 2000, U.S. Government Printing Office.

U.S. Department of Health and Human Services: *Public Health Service Fact Sheet,* Washington, D.C., 1984, Public Health Service.

Vandenbroucke JP: Epidemiology in transition: a historical hypothesis, *Epidemiol* 1(2):164, 1990.

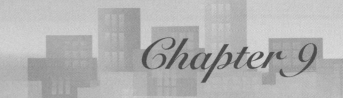

Chapter 9

Using Research in Community Health Nursing

BEVERLY C. FLYNN

JOYCE SPLANN KROTHE

OBJECTIVES

After reading this chapter, the student should be able to:
- Describe the stages of the research process.
- Describe the role of the community health nurse in research.
- Evaluate several nursing research studies using both quantitative and qualitative methods.

- Explain ways that nurses who work in the community can participate in research.
- Discuss relationships, communications, and ethics in nursing research.

CHAPTER OUTLINE

The Research Process
Assessment or Conceptual Stage
Planning or Design Stage
Implementation or Empirical Stage
Evaluation or Analytical Stage
Action or Dissemination Stage

Practice-Generated Questions for Research
Accessible Health Care
Community Involvement
Disease Prevention and Health Promotion

Appropriate Technology
Multisectoral Approach

Roles and Issues in Research
Relationships
Communication
Ethics and the Researcher Role
Funding of Research

Suggestions for Participation in Research
Healthy People 2010: Prevention Research

KEY TERMS

assumptions: statements that are believed to be true without proof or scientific testing of them.

deductive reasoning: a reasoning approach that develops specific predictions or ideas from general principles.

health promotion: "the process of enabling people to increase their control over and to improve their health" (World Health Organization, 1986, p. 1).

human subjects review committees: individuals who represent various disciplines or departments who come together

to review research proposals that involve using people as research subjects. Their major concerns are to protect subjects from physical or mental harm and to protect researchers from undue complaints.

inductive reasoning: a reasoning approach that develops general rules or ideas from specific observations.

limitations: in quantitative research, the uncontrollable elements of the research that limit the certainty of the findings or their applicability to the population in general.

Continued

national health objectives: major health concerns for different age-groups and specific standards that researchers can use to evaluate program success.

practice-generated research: questions and key concepts of health care and health promotion that can guide research.

qualitative methods: a tool of science that is characterized by inductive reasoning, subjectivity, discovery, description, and the meaning that an experience or phenomenon has for an individual or group.

quantitative methods: scientific inquiry characterized by deductive reasoning, objectivity, quasi-experiments, statistical methods, and control.

research process: a problem-solving method of scientific inquiry that involves assessment, planning, implementation, evaluation, and new action.

In a health care environment that focuses on outcomes or the results of nursing interventions, it is important for nurses to know how to use research in their practice. Nurses need to regularly read research studies to learn new approaches to practice, to learn basic research skills, and to be able to apply research findings to practice. Research may be done by one person or a group of nurses, or it may be conducted by an interdisciplinary group. To participate effectively in research, it is necessary to know what research is and how to follow a research process.

THE RESEARCH PROCESS

The term *research* means literally "to search again." The goal of research is to engage in a systematic and objective process of generating information to aid in making decisions. The **research process** is similar to both the nursing process and the epidemiological process discussed in Chapter 8. The nursing process, epidemiological process, and research process are all problem-solving methods of scientific inquiry. Each involves assessment, planning, implementation, evaluation, and action. Each also is like a cycle in that the last phase leads back to the initial phase. That is, the action phase leads to ongoing reassessment, followed by additional planning and implementation. The epidemiological and research processes develop knowledge. The nursing process uses knowledge to provide health and health-related services to individuals, families, groups, and communities.

The goals of the research process are:
1. Specify what information is needed
2. Design a method to collect that information
3. Collect the information (data)
4. Analyze the results
5. Communicate the findings of the research and explain the implications of these findings.

The stages of the research process are summarized in Box 9-1. Although the stages are listed in a sequence, the researcher actually goes back and forth among the various stages of the research process. Decisions made in any one stage must be consistent with decisions made in other stages. All stages are viewed as part of the total study and are arrived at logically and systematically. In quantitative research, the researcher needs to remain detached and impersonal about the study, with precon-

ceived ideas, prejudices or biases put aside in order to be objective in carrying out the research. In contrast, in qualitative research, the researcher acknowledges subjective ideas and opinions.

Research relies on sound decision-making. At each step in the process, important decisions must be made. Decision-making is a process for solving a problem or choosing from the alternatives and opportunities available. Three decision-making terms influence the research process: *certainty, uncertainty,* and *ambiguity.* Certainty means that decision-makers have all the information that they need to make the decision. The decision-maker knows the exact nature of the problem or need that the research will address. Unfortunately, in most situations, a person does not have absolute certainty or all possible information. Most situations have some degree of uncertainty. In an uncertain situation, the researcher understands the general nature of the desired goal, yet the information about all possible alternatives is incomplete. Ambiguity means that the nature of the problem to be solved is unclear. If ambiguity is present, the objectives of the research may be vague, and the decision alternatives are difficult to define. Obviously it is important to reduce the uncertainty and ambiguity and gain as much certainty as possible before the research is fully designed and implemented. Box 9-2 defines some key research terms.

Assessment or Conceptual Stage

The assessment or conceptual stage involves translating a hunch or curiosity about a clinical problem into a research question. For example, a nurse may wonder why some elderly people can live independently in the community while others enter a nursing home. The nurse begins the research by reading several research articles in professional journals to better understand the situation for older people and the current stage of research in this area. This initial literature review helps the nurse select a purpose and scope for the study. In this example, the nurse might decide that the purpose of the study is to determine how community health nursing services assist elderly persons to live successfully in the community. The next step identifies the characteristics of the study population. For example, the study population may include elderly people within a specific age range who live

---

Box 9-1   Stages of the Research Process

ASSESSMENT OR CONCEPTUAL STAGE

Identify a problem for study
Conduct an initial review of related literature
Identify the purpose of the research
Select the population to be studied

PLANNING OR DESIGN STAGE

Formulate the research problem
Continue review of related literature
Select a conceptual framework
Select a research design and appropriate methodology
Design the data-collection plan
Finalize and review the research plan
Follow human subjects review process
Conduct pilot studies and revise design if needed

IMPLEMENTATION OR EMPIRICAL STAGE

Invite community members to participate
Implement the data-collection plan
Prepare the data for analysis

EVALUATION OR ANALYTICAL STAGE

Analyze the data
Interpret the results
Draw conclusions

ACTION OR DISSEMINATION STAGE

Communicate the research findings
Use the findings in practice
Inform health policy makers
Take action for social change
Plan additional research

Selected stages of the research process are modified from Polit DF, Hungler BP: *Essentials of nursing research: methods, appraisal, and utilization,* ed 4, Philadelphia, 1997, JB Lippincott.

---

in a specified geographical area served by a particular community health agency.

Planning or Design Stage

Once a relevant purpose, scope, and study population are selected, the researcher begins the planning or design stage. This is a logical, organized process that proceeds in a step-by-step sequence. Planning involves critical thinking and communicating ideas in a clear and logical way, consistent with the format required by potential funding sources. Following the research process is a little like reading a map. On maps, some paths are better charted than others. Some routes arc difficult to travel while others are more interesting and easier to follow. In quantitative research, to successfully find your destination when reading a map, you must know exactly where you want to go. Usually when using a map to take a trip or research a destination, there is no one right way to go. There may be a best route, but usually more than one route will get you to your destination. The route

---

Box 9-2   Research Terms in Review

Research: means literally to "search again" or the systematic and objective process of generating information to assist in making decisions.

Decision making: process of solving a problem or choosing one alternative from several options.

Certainty: in decision making refers to having available all the information that the person making the decision needs in order to know the exact nature of the problem (need).

Uncertainty: in decision making refers to having some but not all of the needed information about all possible alternatives.

Ambiguity: in decision making means that the nature of the problem to be solved is unclear. The objectives are vague and the decision alternatives are hard to define.

---

you take depends on such things as: how many alternatives you have considered, how much time you have, and how much money you have for such things as gasoline, food, and lodging along the way. Similarly, in the research process, there are several paths to follow. Throughout the remainder of the chapter, there will be discussions of criteria to consider in choosing the route to take to design the research process.

Designing a research project, like accurately reading a map, is a problem-solving process. After identifying a problem for study and formulating a question about the problem, the researcher continues to review related literature, decides on a method to use that is consistent with the research question, and then writes a clear proposal. Tornquist and Funk (1990) provide some useful information about how to write a research proposal. Not all questions can or need to be answered by research. Brink and Wood define a researchable question as "an explicit query about a problem or issue that can be challenged, examined, and analyzed and that will yield useful new information" (1994, p. 2). Potential topics for research come from the thoughts, observations, and practice experiences of the nurse. These topics can be investigated using quantitative or qualitative methods.

Briefly Noted

Although the dominant methodology used in nursing research has been quantitative, there is a growing acceptance of nursing science as a composite of different perspectives and thereby of quantitative and qualitative research methodologies (Munhall and Boyd, 1993).

The specific focus of the research is stated during the planning stage. In the previous example, the nurse decides that the problem to be investigated is a lack of information about the relationship between community health nursing services and the ability of elderly people to live independently in the community.

Next, key terms are defined. In the example, the nurse decides that for the purpose of the study, elderly people will be defined as individuals 75 years of age or older who live in the geographical area served by a specific home health agency. The literature review helps to define terms and select the conceptual framework to provide structure for the study. Also, the literature review provides examples of how research and data analyses were carried out in previous research studies. It is important to know about the results of similar research and where possible, how they have actually been used in nursing practice.

The conceptual framework that the nurse selects needs to fit the problem being investigated. A conceptual framework is a group of concepts and a set of propositions that spell out the relationships between them. Some conceptual frameworks are abstract, while others draw on more precise phenomena. For example, the concept of caring can have many different meanings. The researcher needs to be clear which conceptual definition of caring is being used in a study. In the example, the nurse selects an ecological conceptual framework. This framework would look at the community as a system. It would take into account how all parts of the environment, including the people, affect the population being studied. That is, an ecological framework would look at how each part affects every other part of the system. Next, the nurse identifies specific research questions or hypotheses for the research. These statements include the key variables of the study. Variables are anything that can be changed. The national health objectives may be helpful in specifying and defining key variables (U.S. Department of Health and Human Services, 1997). The **national health objectives** indicate major health concerns for different age groups and provide specific standards that researchers can use to evaluate program progress.

In the example, the nurse wants to know if the range of services available for elderly people will enable them to live independently in the community. One goal of the current national health objectives states that independence among older people is preserved when no more than 90 per 1000 people age 65 years and older have difficulty performing two or more personal care activities (U.S. Department of Health and Human Services, 1997). Perhaps the greater the range of nursing services available, the greater the number of elderly people able to live independently in the community. The key variables are (1) the range of nursing services and (2) elderly people's performance of personal care activities.

Next the nurse selects a research approach that fits the phenomenon (i.e., any observable fact or event) being investigated. The research approach may be historical, survey, or experimental. Each approach has different requirements for a research design. Considerations include whether the data will be collected at one point in time or longitudinally over time and whether the data will be collected from a single group or from several groups in the population. Historical research data are considered secondary data since the information was originally gathered for some other purpose. This form of data may be more accessible and quicker to obtain. Survey data collection involves asking people questions either by a pencil-and-paper format or through a telephone or personal interview. In quantitative research, it is often possible to examine cause-and-effect relationships. This type of research allows researchers to isolate and manipulate one variable while holding the others constant. In contrast, qualitative research does not look at cause and effect but rather tries to understand the phenomenon more clearly.

In the example, the nurse decides that a historical approach, or a review of past information, will not adequately address the problem. An experimental approach is not feasible because the study cannot be conducted under controlled conditions. Instead, the nurse decides that a survey is the most appropriate approach for comparing elderly people living independently in the community and their use of services. Using a survey allows the nurse to collect the information from all participants within the same time period. The nurse might hold focus groups as a first step in designing the survey. A focus group includes 6 to 10 people in a loosely structured format. The leader plans carefully for the group meeting and asks a few general questions. Members can say whatever they think. There is opportunity for give and take among the members, and new ideas will often emerge as people discuss their thoughts and points of view.

The planning stage is the time to select the methodology or way of handling the research information. The research question determines the choice of methodology. Traditional scientific inquiry is usually referred to as quantitative research. Quantitative research can measure the effects of the research using numbers. Researchers objectively gather information that can be verified by another researcher and generalized to other populations. **Quantitative methods** of research usually are characterized by **deductive reasoning** (i.e., reasoning from the general to the specific), objectivity, reducing prejudice or bias as much as possible, and the use of control groups who do not participate in the research events. They are also quasi-experiments and use statistics to measure their effectiveness. Quantitative methods are used often in nursing research.

Although many nursing research questions can be measured using quantitative methods, others require a different approach. Some research questions are more effectively answered using **qualitative methods.** This method is characterized by **inductive reasoning** (reasoning from specific facts to the general), subjectivity (influenced by one's feelings), discovery, description, and the meaning that the experience has for an individual or group (Brockopp and Hastings-Tolsma, 1994).

Quantitative methods use standardized procedures to gather data, while qualitative methodology allows for more variability (Popay, Rogers, and Williams, 1998). This does not mean that qualitative research is loose and haphazard. There are explicit methods used when conducting a qualitative study. The qualitative approach does provide greater opportunity to understand the client's perspective than does a quantitative approach. Box 9-3 presents definitions of key research terms that explain this stage of the research process.

<table>
<tr><td>

Box 9-3   **Terms to Remember**

</td></tr>
</table>

Conceptual framework: the theoretical background that provides the foundation for the research.

Variable: anything that can be changed; may assume different numerical values.

Phenomenon: an observable fact or event that can be described.

Focus group: an unstructured, free-flowing interview with a small group of people who meet at a central location.

Inductive reasoning: thinking that progresses from the specific to the more general.

Deductive reasoning: thinking that progresses from the general to the specific.

Once a research method is chosen, the next stage is to select a data-gathering method, such as observing, measuring, or interviewing. Observing means that the researcher records what is seen without relying on reports from the subjects. This is a more complex method than simply counting the replies on a questionnaire. Interviewing is time consuming but has the advantage of providing clarification by using aids such a pictures or objects as well as observing nonverbal communication. The techniques or instruments selected should be consistent with the research design. For example, if a questionnaire is used for data collection, a specific instrument can be selected that respondents will understand. That is, the questionnaire should be about the same reading level as that of the people who will fill it out. Or if the participants cannot read, then picture questionnaires, can be used instead of print.

The researcher may use more than one instrument to gather data about each of the major study variables. In the example of the elderly people in the community, the nurse may use both observing and interviewing methods. That is, the nurse researcher could observe nurses who provide services to elderly people in order to determine the scope and range of services they currently provide. To avoid making nurses and clients feel uncomfortable about being observed, the nurse researcher can use the qualitative methodology of participant observation. In this method, the nurse researcher makes the purpose of the study clear to clients and also participates while collecting data. In addition to observation, the nurse could also use the quantitative method of an interview questionnaire to determine the level of physical functioning of the elderly clients.

The research questions and the method for collecting data will help to identify the appropriate plan for data analysis. At this time the researcher should identify the computer software available to assist with data analysis and also decide how findings will be presented. For example, the researcher may want to design sample tables to be used when the data are collected. These tables will help ensure that all the data necessary to answer the research questions have been collected.

The research questions and plan for data analysis guide sample selection. The research method to be used determines the sample size. There are many methods of sample selection, but two are considered here: random and deliberate sampling. Random sampling means that each participant has an equal opportunity to be included in the study. Deliberate sampling means that specific persons are invited to participate in the study. Choice of research methodologies will determine the characteristics of the sample population.

In the example, the nurse decides to study elderly persons within the geographical boundaries served by a community health agency. After consultation with a statistician, the nurse decides that the sample should consist of 100 persons over 75 years of age living in the community. This number of people is based on an estimated sample size required for the statistics selected. The researcher may use power analysis software that can help to determine sample size. Of course, it is impossible to know the exact number of elderly people living in the community, so the nurse estimates the total elderly population based on census data. A deliberate sample of persons 75 years of age and older is selected until 100 are included in the sample.

Research approval by an institutional **human subjects review committee** should be obtained at this time. These committees are made up of representatives of various disciplines or departments who meet to review research proposals. Their major concerns are protecting human research participants from physical or mental harm, as well as protecting the researcher from undue complaints. Funding agencies and federal, state, and institutional regulations often require that researchers document institutional human subject's review committee approval.

In the example, the home health agency has a committee that reviews research proposals involving agency services. The nurse researcher must obtain approval from the committee before the research begins. The first step is to communicate clearly in writing to the review committee what is planned, how participants will be involved in the research, and whether their participation will put them at risk for physical or mental harm. The researcher is ethically responsible for carrying out these plans as directed or approved by the committee. Changes that occur in the plans as the research progresses need to be reported to the committee for further review and approval. Many committees have specific, detailed forms that need to be completed and that list the questions that must be answered.

Pilot studies can be used to test on a small scale the data-gathering methods and the data-analysis plan. A pilot study is simply a small-scale exploratory research technique that does not necessarily apply the rigorous standards that will be expected in the actual data-collection stage. The pilot study typically uses a small number of subjects who are similar to those who will be used in the full study. A pilot study is especially important when the data-gathering technique is unfamiliar to the researcher because the instrument is new or it has not been used with the population under study, or because the study is going to be conducted in an unfamiliar environment. The nurse researcher in the example decides to pilot test the study with five elderly clients from a neighboring county after obtaining permission from both the nurse and the clients.

Next, the assumptions and limitations of the research are identified. **Assumptions** are statements that are believed to be true without proof or scientific testing of them. Usually, this is because they have been documented in previous research. An assumption of the study example is that some community services enable elderly people to live independently in the community.

The **limitations** are uncontrollable elements of the research. These elements limit the certainty of the findings or their applicability to the population in general. In this study, a limitation is that deliberate sampling does not ensure that all elderly people are equally represented. As a result, the study findings may not be applicable beyond the study sample.

Implementation or Empirical Stage

The implementation or empirical stage of the research plan refers to carrying out the research procedures. This stage includes inviting the members of the sample population to participate, obtaining their informed consent, collecting and verifying the data, and analyzing the data. The nurse researcher may send a letter to potential participants inviting them to participate. Or the nurse may go door-to-door and personally ask the elderly people to participate if they live near one another and if such a labor-intensive approach to subject selection is feasible. After a follow-up phone call, an appointment is arranged with the client and the nurse. At this meeting the participants, both the client and nurse, are asked to give their signed informed consent to participate in the study.

The nurse researcher then collects data through observation and interviews. Information collected in qualitative studies is validated with the participants. Depending on the methods chosen, data analysis occurs at the same time as the data collection (qualitative methodology) or at the end of the data collection phase (quantitative methodology).

In both quantitative and qualitative research methods, data collection and analysis follow specified guidelines. They both follow certain steps, in a certain order and according to specific rules. Merely interviewing people does not mean that a study is necessarily qualitative (Munhall and Boyd, 1993). In qualitative research there is prolonged contact between the subjects and the researcher that allows the researcher to become more of an insider.

Evaluation or Analytical Stage

The evaluation or analytical stage includes analyzing the findings and comparing them with previous research results. Conclusions are then drawn, building on a body of previous knowledge. Research reports should provide clear documentation of what was done and when. The results of the research for the specific problem, research questions, or hypotheses under study are presented. If the research design is quantitative, hypotheses that were not supported also need to be reported. Recommendations for future research should be clear and con-

sistent with the study results. The need for replication studies should be specified. Replication studies with other populations are useful because recommendations for practice should be based on more than one set of study results. The research findings are presented to professional colleagues; to persons in decision-making positions, such as administrators, policy makers, and legislators; and to the general public, which might be affected by any decisions made.

In the hypothetical research example, the study findings indicated that the greater the range of nursing services, the greater the ability of elderly people to live independently. Future research could examine information regarding severity of health problems among the elderly group and how they affect the ability of these individuals to remain in the community, or a qualitative study might yield information that does not suggest adding services but rather shows that ways need to be found to inform elderly citizens and their families about the services that are already available. Next, it is important for the nurse researcher to communicate the results of the study to all those who need the information. This would include the administrators and staff at the home health agency; the county senior citizen organization; professional colleagues; reporters for the local newspaper, radio, or television stations; and the state legislative committee responsible for policies for community-based care.

Action or Dissemination Stage

The results of nursing research should be used in practice to improve the health of people in the community and to stimulate social change. This means that nurses should make specific recommendations based on what they find in their research. Policy makers, other professionals, and community members will soon learn that nursing research findings are relevant and guide practice. In the example of the study of elderly people in the community, the nurse can explain to policy makers what services are needed to enable elderly people to stay in their homes.

For example, the results of a well-designed study of older people in a given community could support the expansion of community health nursing services (Krothe, 1997). The economic difference between keeping elderly clients in their homes versus placing them in an institution might provide a compelling argument in support of expanded home health care services. Research documenting the cost effectiveness of community-based nursing care, the quality of care, client and family satisfaction, and the ability for these older people to remain independent is needed. Research results can assist agencies to develop new programs within their organizations and also identify the need for additional research in the organization.

PRACTICE-GENERATED QUESTIONS FOR RESEARCH

Significant questions for research can be generated from community health nursing practice in response to everyday observations in the field. Practicing nurses may not consider research a part of their practice; they may have difficulty identifying potential questions for research that arise from their practice. What individuals observe stops being a normal part of the routine observations people make and becomes research when it is systematically planned and recorded (Brink and Wood, 1994).

Briefly Noted

Research is a problem-solving process that provides quantitative evidence. You can identify researchable questions by asking "what is the scientific basis for how I do things"?

The following discussion provides examples of **practice-generated research** questions. These questions are grouped according to several key primary care concepts that are important in community health nursing: accessibility, community involvement, disease prevention and health promotion, appropriate technology, and multisectoral approach.

Accessible Health Care

Accessibility of health services refers to the extent to which nursing services are available to the people who need them the most and also how equitably these services are distributed throughout the population. A research question might be:

- Are nursing services accessible to people with the greatest need? For example, are the services available at times and in locations where the people who need them the most can use them?
- Are the personnel adequate to meet the needs?
- Are these services available in both urban and rural areas?
- Who uses the services and who does not use them?
- What are the health care needs of the people who use the services compared with those who do not?
- What are the barriers to the use of services?
- Are the costs too high?
- Are the services relevant to consumers' perceived needs?
- Are the nurses sensitive to the concerns of consumers?
- Do consumers have transportation to reach the services?
- Are services offered at times when those most in need of them are able to use them?

HOW TO Identify Nursing Research Questions

Community health nursing practice presents us with daily problems and successes. The following questions can help identify researchable problems:
- What examples from your clinical practice seem to lead to successful outcomes?
- Are there examples from your clinical practice that continue to cause problems?
- What differences are there in access to health services or health status in the population you are serving? Why do you think these differences exist?
- What can you do to address these discrepancies?

- What *Healthy People 2010* national health objectives standards pertain to populations you work with?
- What does the research literature say about identifying problems for research? What has worked or not worked in practice?
- What questions for research come to mind?
- How would you compare two or more different approaches for dealing with the same problem?
- How would you design a study with a control group?
- What are the ethics of such a comparison?
- Can you offer different services to different populations without jeopardizing the quality of care?

Community Involvement

Community involvement is concerned with the level of participation of community residents in health care decision making. To promote community development and self-reliance, residents need to participate in decisions about the community's health. Residents and health providers need to work together to identify problems and to seek solutions.

Practice-related research questions applicable to the level and mechanism of community involvement in health decision making might include the following:
- To what extent are community residents involved in the various stages of assessing health care needs, planning, management, and monitoring community health nursing services?

 Evidence-Based Practice

The study referenced below explores the mental and physical health status and utilization of services among the informal caregivers of the chronically ill, elderly, disabled, and mentally ill in Ontario, Canada. Research participants were identified by stratification and multistage probability sampling of respondents in the Ontario Health Survey, a community-based epidemiological survey. The main objectives of the study were to compare characteristics of caregivers with non-caregivers in the community and determine whether being a caregiver is associated with various physical or mental health problems and utilization of services. The following statistical tests were used: chi-square statistic; t tests; and proportions (95% confidence intervals around the proportions).

APPLICATION IN PRACTICE

This study shows that caregivers had higher rates of mental health disorders than non-caregivers and utilized mental health services at twice the rate of non-caregivers. It provided important information about potential unmet needs of caregivers, as well as implications for community health nursing practice and policy considerations for governments that increasingly advocate community-based care.

Cochrane JJ, Goering PN, Rogers JM: The mental health of informal caregivers in Ontario: an epidemiological survey, *Am J Public Health* 87(12):2002-2007, 1997.

- What mechanisms and processes can people use to be actively involved and to take joint responsibility, along with nurses, for decisions?
- In particular, what decisions involving the community have been implemented and evaluated?
- Is utilization of services improved as a result?

Briefly Noted

Nurses conduct research that addresses significant issues. For example, in the Institute of Medicine's study, *Nursing, Health and Environment,* Pope, Snyder, and Mood (1995) reported that nursing research focused on populations at risk for health problems including agricultural workers, industrial workers, health service providers, pregnant women, new mothers, and disabled people. Health hazards studied by nurses included pesticides, accidents, lead exposure, and natural disasters.

Disease Prevention and Health Promotion

Community health focuses on **health promotion** and prevention of disease rather than on curative services. Examples include physical exercise, seat belt use, smoking cessation, and other healthful lifestyle changes. Key research questions might include the following:

- What are the major preventable health problems in the community? For example, are there high rates of automobile accidents or heart disease in a particular community?
- Are problems being addressed by preventive and health-promoting measures?
- What measures are being taken to reduce or control these problems?
- Are these measures appropriate for the culture(s) of the community residents?
- Do the community health nursing services include recommendations and educational programs about infant car seat use, ways to reduce alcohol intake among drivers, smoking cessation programs, and how to promote health in schools?

Appropriate Technology

Appropriate technology refers to health care that is both relevant and acceptable to people's health needs and concerns. It includes issues of cost and affordability of services given the current resources, such as the number and type of health professionals and other providers, equipment, and supplies, and their pattern of distribution throughout the community. The National Science Foundation's definition of appropriate technology summarizes these considerations: "Appropriate technologies are defined as those which are decentralized, require low capital investment, conserve natural resources, are managed by their users, and are in harmony with the environment" (1979, p. 1). What this means is that just

Evidence-Based Practice

In the study referenced below, the authors trace commonalities in philosophies of the nursing profession and faith communities through history to empower people and enhance their self-care capacity to the present day model of parish nursing. They note an absence in the literature of evidence-based research on parish nursing and outcome-based practice. The purpose of this exploratory study was to document implementation by parish nurses of the *Healthy People 2000* objectives to build partnerships to enhance the health of the community. The method used was a descriptive retrospective study utilizing monthly parish nurse reports and interviews with parish nurses.

APPLICATION IN PRACTICE

This study shows how *Healthy People 2000* objectives had been identified across the lifespan from retrospective review of reports and validation during interviews. Community partnerships developed, for example, when parish nurses addressed the objective related to home and fire safety and formed a partnership with firefighters to secure smoke detectors for individuals who needed them. Results of this study support parish nursing as a model to address challenges set forth in *Healthy People 2000* for effective delivery of health services in the community and building community coalitions to address health needs.

Weis D, Matheus R, Schank MJ: Health care delivery in faith communities: the parish nurse model, *Public Health Nurs* 14(6):368-372, 1997.

because a technology is available, does not mean that it is the best or most appropriate one for a given group of people or a community. Some technology might be useful in an urban area but irrelevant in a rural area. It also might be useful as long as it works well, but if the machine breaks down and there is no way to get repairs in a particular area, its use is lost to the community.

The overriding questions to be answered include the following:

- Do the services use the simplest and least costly technology available?
- Are the services acceptable to the community?
- Are they affordable initially and over time?
- What is the cost effectiveness of alternative approaches or strategies for community health services?
- Are family home visits as effective as working with families in groups?
- Are nonprofessionals, such as home health aides and community health workers, effective in providing some aspects of the nursing services?
- What are the most effective management and supervisory techniques for nonprofessionals and professionals within a community health agency?

There are technology changes that affect community health nursing practice and research. For example, more people have access to computers. Community health nurses may have computerized record systems that offer new opportunities for data collection and analysis (Figure 9-1).

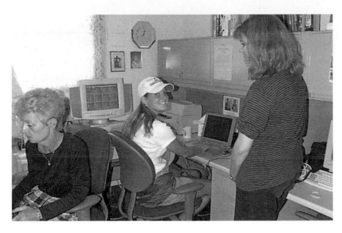

Figure 9-1   Computerized nursing record systems are an example of technological changes that affect nursing practice and research.

Multisectoral Approach

The health of a community cannot be improved by intervention only within the health sector. Other sectors are equally important in promoting the community's health and self-reliance. For example, education, business, environment, the faith community, industry, housing, and nutrition are interrelated with health. Therefore, these sectors need to work together to coordinate their goals, plans, and activities to ensure that they contribute to the health of the community and to avoid conflicting or duplicating efforts.

Relevant research questions include the following:

- What mechanisms are available that can promote or hinder multisectoral collaboration?
- Do the committees or task forces that address community-wide concerns represent various fields, such as education, industry, housing, transportation, and health?
- What are two examples of multisectoral efforts to solve a community problem?
- How were successful solutions derived in the past?
- What factors contributed to their success?
- What conflicts exist across sectors?
- How are conflicting activities across the various sectors resolved?
- What are the gaps in efforts across the various sectors in solving community health problems?

ROLES AND ISSUES IN RESEARCH

Although some of the roles of the nurse researcher and the issues related to research are presented in other sections of this chapter, additional areas need to be considered. These include relationships, communication, ethics, and sources of funds to conduct research.

Relationships

The practicing nurse may conduct research or work with a researcher or an administrator within an organization to carry out a study. Partners each have their own areas of expertise,

Evidence-Based Practice

The author examines the health-promotion beliefs and practices of immigrant women and how their cultural values influence their health-promotion behaviors. The methodology for the research study was a descriptive ethnographic study, permitting an emic view yielding data within a cultural context that could not be gained from a standardized survey instrument.

APPLICATION IN PRACTICE

In this study, health-promotion activities were found to be closely tied to activities of daily living and contextually related to the health and well-being of the entire family, rather than for individual well-being per se. The effects of migration were found to interfere with women's ability to continue some health-promoting behaviors; for example, climatic changes between India and Canada significantly decreased walking activities. Community health nurses should be aware of the effects of migration and culture on health behaviors and integrate these into health-promotion activities.

Choudry UK: Health promotion among immigrant women from India living in Canada, *Image* 30(3):269-274, 1998.

and they benefit from the expertise of the others. For example, community nurses, who are experts in practice, can identify research problems and examine the feasibility of various research designs. Administrators can help identify policy issues related to the research and can provide organizational and financial support. The researcher can help develop practice problems into researchable questions, suggest appropriate research methods, and collect and analyze data.

The nurse may also work with the community group concerned with the research problem. Citizens, professionals, and other persons interested in community health may identify a priority problem for research. In this case, persons in the group have expertise about the community, and the researcher and the nurse work as resources to the group in conducting the research.

Involving others in the research process can present problems and be inconvenient. Sometimes it is hard for participants to agree on the specific question(s) to be asked. Because community health nursing research often takes place in a dynamic setting in which the chief responsibility is health care (e.g., a neighborhood clinic), priority may be given to clinical commitments rather than to research. Access to records and files may be controlled by people other than the researcher, and the agency may withhold client information that is needed for the research. As a result, a variety of dynamics and political processes may take place. Researchers need to recognize these dynamics and work to ensure that the study is conducted with proper attention to sound research principles. Skills in communication and collaboration are essential to the process.

Communication

Communication with participants, co-researchers, nursing practitioners, administrators, community residents, and policy makers is important throughout the research process. Communication can take many forms. The researcher needs to consider the appropriateness of verbal, written, and visual aids in clarifying any information being presented. Often the researcher has an academic background and appointment and has been socialized differently from practitioners and community citizens. The researcher may use different terms to describe things in the setting than do the practitioners and citizens. It is important for the researcher to carefully consider how information is presented, including taking into account the level of understanding of the reader or listener. The researcher also needs to be attentive to issues that concern the audience. The presentation format varies depending on whether the audience is a group of academic researchers, practicing nurses, policy makers, or community citizens.

Information must be provided about the research early in the study and throughout the project. Negative findings, such as the discovery that nursing intervention did not reduce costs, must be presented along with positive results. A focus on concepts rather than on the specific program being studied may facilitate the acceptance of negative findings.

Ethics and the Researcher Role

Ethical issues need careful attention in any research. Ethical issues arise from conflicting social pressures between the profession and the larger society. For example, should the researcher publish the results when the findings reflect negatively on a particular group? This information may be taken out of context and used to limit government funding of services to a particular group. In addition, it may promote victim blaming.

Ethical issues also must be considered in the design stage of the study. For example, community health nurses may want to evaluate the effectiveness of a home health agency's policies for the care of clients with acquired immunodeficiency syndrome (AIDS). It would be unethical to assign a group of clients with AIDS to a control group and then withhold information about the diagnosis from the nurses providing care to these clients.

Dilemmas may arise over ensuring the confidentiality of responses, disclosing the actual purpose of the research to the respondents, or even disseminating research results to the respondents. As mentioned, institutional human subjects review committees evaluate whether a study can be conducted. The researcher is ethically responsible for carrying out the research consistent with the plans that the committee approved. Changes that occur in research plans must be reported to the committee for further review.

There are also ethical considerations in data reporting. This issue is important in nursing research because few replication studies exist. Fraudulent research data and results of health-related research have been published. The effects of this can be widespread, affecting not only the profession but also, and more important, persons in the community and those involved in policy formulation.

Briefly Noted

The nurse researcher has an ethical responsibility to report both positive and negative results of research despite possible consequences to the programs being studied. The researcher needs to carefully note the strengths and limitations of the study.

Funding of Research

A final issue is obtaining funds for research. Some federal funding is available for nursing research through agencies such as the National Institute of Nursing Research and the Agency for Healthcare Research and Quality. However, obtaining money for research, especially federal funding, is increasingly competitive. For this reason, the pursuit of funding from voluntary foundations and organizations should not be overlooked. Private foundations, such as the Robert Wood Johnson Foundation or the W.K. Kellogg Foundation, offer program funding that can include evaluation research.

State and local funding sources include community foundations, local chapters of Sigma Theta Tau, regional nursing research societies, the March of Dimes, the American Heart Association, the American Cancer Society, hospitals, and corporations. Universities may offer small grants for faculty to initiate research. Local and state health departments offer program grants through maternal child health or various preventive block grants that have evaluation research components. Finally, employers can sometimes grant release time from work so that educators, administrators, consultants, and practitioners can conduct research. Table 9-1 provides a summary of selected examples of funding sources. Researchers need to explore alternative funding sources, be aware of new funding initiatives, and design creative financing options.

SUGGESTIONS FOR PARTICIPATION IN RESEARCH

Practicing nurses can participate in each stage of the research process. They are in key positions to identify clinical problems to be researched. Nurses can take anecdotal notes about clinical situations that will help in identifying key variables for study. They also can read research on the topic of concern and discuss observations with other nursing colleagues, including researchers. Frequently, nurse researchers work in universities and are more than willing to collaborate in joint research efforts. Practicing nurses can assist researchers in securing institutional approval to conduct research and in facilitating access to research participants. They also may be involved in data collection, whether for pilot studies, replication studies, or original research. The nurse may be a participant in research by answering questionnaires and participating in interviews or by being observed in practice.

TABLE 9-1	Examples of Funding Sources for Research
National	
Federal government	National Institutes of Health
	National Institute for Nursing Research
	National Cancer Institute
	Agency for Healthcare Research and Quality
Private/voluntary	W.K. Kellogg Foundation
	Robert Wood Johnson Foundation
	Pew Charitable Trusts
	Rockefeller Foundation
	American Cancer Society
	American Heart Association
	American Diabetes Foundation
State	
Public	State department of health
	Department of family and social services
	State universities
Private/voluntary	March of Dimes
	State hospital association
	State cancer society
	State heart association
	State nurses association
	Corporations
Local	
Public	Health department
Private/voluntary	Sigma Theta Tau chapters
	Regional nursing research societies
	March of Dimes
	Business and industry

- Describe the research findings and your application to practice to nursing administrators and policy makers
- Post brief summaries of research findings in prominent locations in the work place
- Distribute research findings that have application to practice to colleagues via electronic mail

Community health nurses can provide valuable insights into study findings, often explaining relationships, or a lack thereof, to researchers. They can apply relevant research findings in practice. They also can explain or report on research findings to community members, administrators, policy makers, and others, thus initiating action for social change.

Community health nurses work with community members to improve their health. They can help seek and identify scientifically oriented solutions to health and nursing problems; thus, they are in a key position to develop knowledge that can be used in practice and that has implications for health policy.

Healthy People 2010: Prevention Research

Healthy People 2010 objective 23-17 emphasizes the need for population-based prevention research. The document points out that research is the nation's investment in the future. While most past research has focused on biomedical research for individual diseases or risk factors, it is now recognized that to improve the nation's health, the value of including diverse populations and communities in studies is a high priority (HP 2010, 2000). Prevention research will direct evidence-based guidelines for practice, as can be seen in examples throughout the text.

HOW TO Apply Research in Practice

Ways of applying research findings in practice:
- Read journals that report research relevant to your practice, for example, *Public Health Nursing, Nursing Research,* or the *American Journal of Public Health*
- Begin a research discussion group with your colleagues and identify who is responsible for reviewing research in these journals
- Form a journal club
- Discuss the quality of research studies
- Obtain research assistance, such as with statistical analysis and research methods, if needed
- Identify research findings that can be applied to practice
- Discuss clinical practice situations in which you can apply the findings
- Apply the findings and evaluate results
- Discuss what you have found

Clinical Application

Laura and Jennifer had their clinical experience during their community health course at an outreach site of a rural nurse-managed clinic. They were involved with the owner of a local sock factory in planning for disease-prevention and health-promotion activities for the employees. After consulting with the faculty members responsible for the course and the nurse-managed clinic, they designed a survey to distribute to employees to assess their needs for health-education programming. The students submitted the survey to the university's Institutional Review Board for approval before distributing it to the employees.

One of the employee priorities identified from the survey data was to establish a smoking-cessation program for factory employees. The students met with the factory owner, their faculty members, and a representative of the local chapter of the American Lung Association to plan how to implement this initiative. They set a timeline to notify employees of an opportunity to participate in the smoking-cessation program. This included notices distributed in employee paychecks and signs posted in prominent locations throughout the factory. The students discussed plans for conducting a research study related to implementation and evaluation of the smoking-cessation program with the faculty members.

Which action would be a logical first step in planning for the research study?
A. Distribute written materials to all employees summarizing the harmful health effects of smoking.
B. Design a data-collection plan to gather a smoking history from participants before they enroll in the program.
C. Discuss with the factory owner incentives for employees who complete the program.
D. Implement a phase-in plan for a smoke-free work environment, including a smoke-free lounge.

Answer is in the back of the book.

 Remember This!

- Although community health nursing practice research has developed over the years, community health nurses need to increase their scientific research base.
- Community health nursing, primary health care, and health promotion are complementary. Research conducted by community health nurses can make a significant contribution to nursing practice and also to primary health care.
- The research process is a problem-solving process involving assessment, planning, implementation, evaluation, and action.
- Significant questions for research can be generated from community health nursing practice and linked with the key concepts of primary health care.
- Community residents can be involved in various stages of the research process.
- Potential research questions can address the basic concepts of primary health care and health promotion.
- The ethical issues in research need thoughtful attention by the nurse researcher.
- Federal money for research is competitive. Researchers need to locate alternative funding sources and use creative financing options.

 What Would You Do?

1. Identify one priority problem that has relevance to community health nursing practice and that could be researched in the community. Who would you involve in selecting the problem? What information would you gather? What problems might you encounter? Who might support your investigation? Who might oppose your investigation? Would you need funds to carry out your investigation?

2. Looking at current nursing journals, find two research articles that can be applied in community-based care. Choose one that uses a qualitative approach and one that uses a quantitative approach to research.
3. Find a nursing research study that supports community-based care. Design a plan to explain the findings of this study to a policy maker at the local, state, or national level. Who could help you? What obstacles might you expect? List your steps in the most logical sequence for success.

REFERENCES

Brink PJ, Wood MJ: *Basic steps in planning nursing research: from question to proposal,* Boston, 1994, Jones & Bartlett.

Brockopp DY, Hastings-Tolsma MT: *Fundamentals of nursing research,* Boston, 1994, Jones & Bartlett.

Choudry UK: Health promotion among immigrant women from India living in Canada, *Image* 30(3):269-274, 1998.

Cochrane JJ, Goering PN, Rogers JM: The mental health of informal caregivers in Ontario: an epidemiological survey, *Am J Public Health* 87(12):2002-2007, 1997.

Krothe JL: Giving voice to elderly people: community-based long-term care, *Public Health Nurs* 14(4):217-226, 1997.

Munhall PL, Boyd CO: *Nursing research: a qualitative perspective,* New York, 1993, National League for Nursing.

National Science Foundation: NSF announcements for December, *NSF Bulletin,* Washington, D.C., 1979, The Foundation.

Polit DF, Hungler BP: *Essentials of nursing research: methods, appraisal, and utilization,* ed 4, Philadelphia, 1997, JB Lippincott.

Popay J, Rogers A, Williams G: Rationale and standards for the systematic review of qualitative literature in health services research, *Qualitative Health Res* 8(3):341-351, 1998.

Pope AM, Snyder MA, Mood L (editors): *Nursing health and environment: strengthening the relationship to improve the public's health,* Washington, D.C., 1995, Committee on Enhancing Environmental Health Content in Nursing Practice, Division of Health Promotion and Disease Prevention, Institute of Medicine, National Academy Press.

Tornquist EM, Funk SG: How to write a research grant proposal, *Image* 22:44-51, 1990.

U.S. Department of Health and Human Services, Office of Disease Prevention and Health Promotion: *Developing Objectives for Healthy People 2010,* Washington, D.C., 1997, U.S. Department of Health and Human Services.

U.S. Department of Health and Human Services: *Healthy people 2010 objectives,* Washington, D.C., 2000, U.S. Department of Health and Human Services.

Weis D, Matheus R, Schank MJ: Health care delivery in faith communities: the parish nurse model, *Public Health Nurs* 14(6):368-372, 1997.

World Health Organization: Ottawa charter for health promotion, Copenhagen, 1986, World Health Organization.

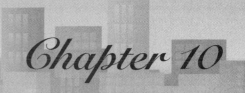

Chapter 10

Using Health Education in the Community

LISA L. ONEGA

OBJECTIVES

After reading this chapter, the student should be able to:
- Describe six educational theories that explain health education in the community.
- Explain three health education models.

- Discuss educational principles that support the use of health education.
- Explain the five steps of the educational process.
- Describe the importance of evaluating the educational product.

KEY TERMS

affective domain: the learning domain that deals with feelings, attitudes, values, and interests.
behavioral theory: has the goal of changing behavior and uses target behavior, reinforcers, withdrawal of a reinforcer, and punishment.

cognitive domain: the learning domain that deals with the recall or recognition of knowledge and the development of intellectual skills.
cognitive theory: states that by changing thought patterns and providing information, learners can change their behavior.

Continued

critical theory: considers learning to be an "ongoing dialogue" in which the educator tries to change the learner's beliefs by questioning the learner.

developmental theory: states that changes occur in human development according to certain stages, phases, levels, direction, and forces.

health belief model: a model that describes health based on perceptions about susceptibility, seriousness, and the advantages or disadvantages of certain actions.

health promotion model: a model that is organized like the health belief model and has the goal of improving the level of well-being of the person.

humanist theory: views individuals as unique, self-determined, worthy of respect, and guided by basic human needs.

long-term evaluation: a form of evaluation designed to follow and assess the behavior of an individual, family, or community over time.

PRECEDE-PROCEED model: a health education model that is oriented toward outcomes and asks "why" before it asks "how"; can be used with individuals, families, groups, or communities.

psychomotor domain: the learning domain that includes performance of skills that require some degree of neuromuscular coordination.

short-term evaluation: a form of evaluation that identifies behavioral effects of health education programs and determines if changes are caused by the educational program.

social learning theory: an explanation of motivation theory that emphasizes the extent to which individuals are motivated by learning from others with whom they identify.

Health education, a vital part of nursing, can help individuals, families, groups, and communities improve and maintain their health. This form of education assists people to make knowledgeable decisions, cope more effectively with health and life-style alterations, and assume greater personal responsibility for their health (Graham, 1992).

As health costs grow and collaboration between health service providers and consumers increases, clients are assuming more responsibility for their own health maintenance. As people live longer, they experience the chronic illnesses related to aging that require changes in diet, exercise, and life-style along with increased medical treatments. Nurses have both the skills and opportunities to educate consumers about ways to manage their health more effectively (Clarke, Beddome, and Whyte, 1993). Also, attainment and maintenance of the objectives of *Healthy People 2000* and *Healthy People 2010* depend heavily on community-based programs to promote healthy habits and life-styles (U.S. Department of Health and Human Services, 2000).

Initially, Healthy *People 2000* set forth a strategy for improving national health by describing objectives that, if attained and maintained, could prevent major chronic illness, injuries, and infectious diseases. Education, a primary strategy in assisting people to change their habits, is provided in a wide variety of community health settings including schools, homes, the workplace, and ambulatory and inpatient health care facilities (U.S. Department of Health and Human Services, 1991).

The accomplishment and maintenance of many of the national health objectives relies on educational strategies (U.S. Department of Health and Human Services, 2000). Two key goals are to (1) increase quality of years and healthy life and (2) eliminate health disparities. Objectives are organized into four categories, with each requiring health education:

1. Promote healthy behaviors
2. Promote healthy and safe communities

3. Improve systems for personal and public health
4. Prevent and reduce diseases and disorders

While health education can take place in almost any setting, four settings are often used. They are the community, workplace, schools, and various health care sites. Primary health care sites are especially useful locations to teach clients about healthy behaviors, risk factors, and the advantages of a healthy life-style (Visser, Thurmond, and Stinson, 1998). Nurses practicing in the community use learning theories in a variety of settings to teach health concepts and self-care skills in understandable ways.

Learning is defined in a variety of ways. Most definitions of the learning process include a measurable change in behavior that persists over time. Newly learned knowledge and behaviors are practiced and thus are repeatedly reinforced (Padilla and Bulcavage, 1991). Although many learning theories and principles related to learning are applicable to nursing, only samples of the most useful and readily adaptable ones are included here. A good understanding of health education enables nurses to educate clients successfully. See Figure 10-1 for the sequence of actions that a nurse follows when developing an educational program.

GENERAL EDUCATIONAL THEORIES

Knowing about educational theories helps nurses understand how people learn and aids in the design and implementation of client education. Table 10-1 provides an overview of six major educational theories. It is important to understand each of these educational theories and be able to choose and then apply the most appropriate theory to a wide variety of health education situations. Often it is necessary to combine several of these theories in the education process.

Behavioral Theory

Behavioral theory focuses on learning by concentrating on behaviors that can be observed, measured, and changed. The educator identifies a *target behavior* to either increase or

The author wishes to thank Douglas C. Forness for his assistance with designing and developing the boxes, figure, and tables for this chapter.

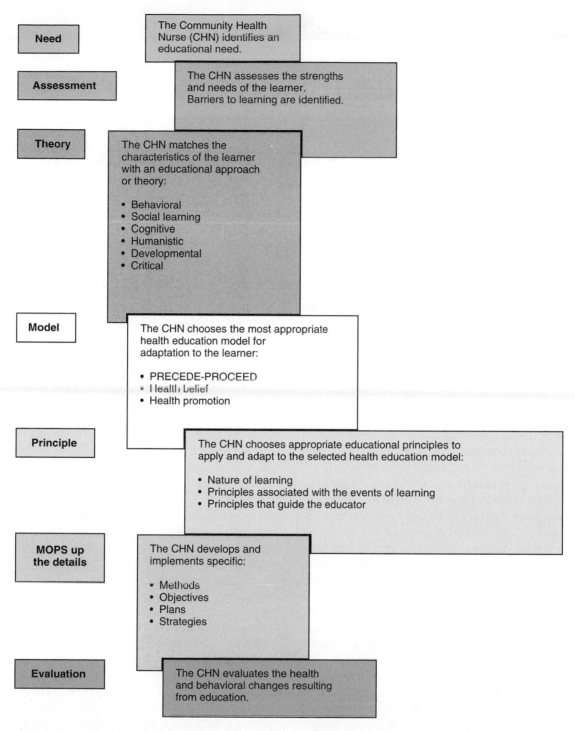

Figure 10-1   The sequence of actions that a community health nurse follows when developing an educational program.

decrease. The way to increase a behavior is to identify and consistently use a *reinforcer* to modify the target behavior. Decreasing a behavior is accomplished by identifying and consistently using *withdrawal of a reinforcer (punishment)* to modify the target behavior (Dembo, 1994; Dignam, 1992; Driscoll, 1994).

The behavioral approach is useful when the educator can control the reward and consequences, that is, the feedback system. This approach is also useful when the learner has cognitive limitations since the behavioral approach requires only the most elementary use of cognition. For example, a nurse working in a school system might want to decrease the number of adolescent deaths associated with alcohol use. The nurse identifies the target behavior as use of a designated driver. The nurse works to increase the use of designated drivers for transporting students from school-related functions. Therefore, after every school-related sporting or social event, four trained adults sit at the exit

TABLE 10-1   Overview of Six General Educational Theories

Theory	Focus	Method
Behavioral	Change behavior	Reinforcement/punishment
Social learning	Change expectations and beliefs	Link information, beliefs, and values
Cognitive	Change thought patterns	Variety of sensory input and repetition
Humanist	Utilize feelings and relationships	Learners will do what is best for themselves (self-determination)
Developmental	Consider human developmental stage	Educational opportunities match readiness to learn
Critical	Increase depth of knowledge	Ongoing dialogue and open inquiry

Based on data from Driscoll MP: *Psychology of learning for instruction,* Boston, 1994, Allyn and Bacon; Edwards L: Health education. In Edelman CL, Mandle CL (editors): *Health promotion throughout the lifespan,* ed 5, St Louis, 1998, Mosby.

doors, evaluate the sobriety of designated drivers, and assign designated drivers to cars. Designated drivers each receive $10 for gasoline, have their names printed in the weekly school newspaper, and are eligible for a weekly prize drawing of $20.

Social Learning Theory

Social learning theory builds on the principles of behavioral theory by stating that behavior is a function of a person's expectations about the value of an outcome (Do I want the outcome?) or self-efficacy (Can I achieve the outcome?). If clients think an outcome is desired and attainable, they are more likely to change their behavior to achieve that goal. Thus, educators may use this theory to change behaviors by enabling clients to either change their expectations about the value of a certain outcome or their ability to achieve the desired outcome or both (Blair, 1993; Dembo, 1994). For example, if a nurse wants to help a group of obese women lose weight, the nurse instructs the women to eat less, select healthful foods, and exercise more. Through the presentation of scientific data describing balanced eating and the positive effects of exercise, the nurse helps the women develop the expectation that decreased food intake and increased exercise will lead to weight loss. Thus, through case study presentations and before-and-after photos, the nurse helps the women change their expectations about their power to achieve the goal of weight loss. Without a belief in their power to change, the women may be unable to remain motivated to change their target behaviors.

Cognitive Theory

Cognitive theory says that by changing thought patterns and providing information, learners will change their behavior. This theory states that people's thought patterns undergo constant change as they interact with their environment. Thus, the educator should provide information in a variety of ways that will change clients' thought patterns and ultimately lead to behavior changes (Dembo, 1994; Dignam, 1992; Driscoll, 1994).

For example, if a woman does not do monthly breast self-examinations (BSEs), the nurse instructs the client to begin doing so. The nurse tries to change the woman's thought patterns by providing information about BSE in a variety of ways. The nurse teaches the client about the procedure and explains the reasons for doing BSE, shows the woman a video about BSE, and observes as the client practices BSE on a breast model. Finally, the nurse gives the woman a handout with the procedure written and drawn on it and instructs her to hang the handout next to the bathroom mirror as a reminder to do monthly BSEs. Thus, by using a variety of environmental cues and sensory input, the client's thought patterns can be changed, thereby influencing her behavior related to BSE.

Humanist Theory

Humanist theory describes the influence that *feelings, emotions,* and *personal relationships* have on behavior. Humanistic theorists believe that learners should be encouraged to examine their feelings and engage in various forms of self-expression. In addition, humanists think that people need to be aware of and able to clarify their values. If people are given *free choice,* they will choose the best approach. Humanists encourage health educators not to be overly controlling and restrictive with learners, but rather to help them grow and develop according to their natural inclinations (Dembo, 1994; Dignam, 1992).

For example, if members of a retirement community want to develop a health promotion program, they may invite the nurse to schedule meetings to assist them. At the meetings, the nurse helps the group discuss the goals and strategies of the program and provides a variety of handouts related to health promotion. Finally, the nurse answers questions and offers encouragement to group members as they develop their own health promotion program.

Developmental Theory

According to **developmental theory,** learning occurs in concert with developmental stages. Each stage is a major transformation from the previous stage; therefore, learning occurs quite differently in each developmental period. *Readiness to learn* depends on the individual's developmental stage (Hancock and Mandle, 1998).

For example, to help the parents of a 2-year-old prevent accidents in the home, the nurse teaches safety practices. The nurse also teaches the parents how to educate the toddler simply and clearly about safety according to the toddler's developmental stage and readiness to understand concepts and behavioral patterns. The nurse recognizes that the parents' and the toddler's levels of readiness to learn are quite different. Since the toddler cannot reach the top of the stove, teaching about the dangers of a hot stove at this stage of physical development is unnecessary. However, the toddler is at risk for accidental poisoning. Although the parents may teach the toddler not to open bottles and jars without their help, all poisons must be removed from the toddler's possible reach as a necessary precaution. The risk of poison ingestion is incomprehensible to the toddler because of the stage of the child's language and cognitive development as well as the child's inability to understand cause-and-effect relationships.

Critical Theory

Critical theory approaches learning as an ongoing dialogue. An individual holds a belief about a health matter. The educator attempts to change this belief by *questioning* the learner. As the learner answers the questions, the learner's beliefs begin to change, new questions arise, and the learner then asks the educator more questions. The educator replies, and this process of discourse ultimately changes thinking and behavior (Welton, 1993).

For example, the nurse wants a newly diagnosed group of diabetic clients to assume responsibility for managing their diabetes. The nurse asks them what they know about diabetes. The clients demonstrate that they can check their own blood sugar and prepare their own insulin injections. However, on further questioning, the nurse sees that they do not know the long-term complications of diabetes. The nurse then educates them about these complications. As a result, the clients begin to see an ophthalmologist annually and check their feet daily for changes in skin color or integrity.

HEALTH EDUCATION MODELS

Conceptual models organize global ideas and simplify systems of thought into more concise formats. Thus, conceptual models provide meaningful descriptions to guide the thinking, observations, and practice of educators (Edwards, 1998). Three health education models that can be used in the community are:

1. PRECEDE-PROCEED
2. Health belief
3. Health promotion

Box 10-1	PRECEDE and PROCEED Acronyms
PRECEDE IS AN ACRONYM FOR:	**PROCEED IS AN ACRONYM FOR:**
P redisposing,	P olicy,
R einforcing, and	R egulatory, and
E nabling	O rganizational
C auses in	C onstructs in
E ducational	E ducational and
D iagnosis and	E nvironmental
E valuation	D evelopment

Based on data from Green LW, Kreuter MW: CDC's planned approach to community health as an application of PRECEDE and an inspiration for PROCEED, *J Health Educ* 23(3):140-147, 1992.

PRECEDE-PROCEED Model

The **PRECEDE-PROCEED model** focuses primarily on planning and evaluating community health education programs. The PRECEDE-PROCEED acronym is shown in Box 10-1. One strength of the PRECEDE-PROCEED model is that it consistently includes the client in problem-solving to provide health education for an identified area of need. This model focuses on helping groups change their behaviors. It begins by assessing the environment in which the group lives and considering the social factors that influence health behaviors. Next, the model examines both the internal and external environmental factors of the group that predispose it (PRECEDE) to certain behaviors or health problems. The model then identifies factors that will help the group adopt healthy actions. Priorities are set. The program is developed, implemented, and finally evaluated (PROCEED). The PRECEDE-PROCEED model is easy to use; its steps serve as a checklist for ensuring that all stages of the problem-solving process are followed (Edwards, 1998; Green and Kreuter, 1992).

Health Belief Model

The **health belief model** can provide a framework for understanding why some people take specific actions to avoid illness, whereas others fail to protect themselves. When the model was developed, both the public and the private health sectors were concerned that people were reluctant to be screened for tuberculosis, to have Pap smears to detect cervical cancer, to be immunized, or to take other preventive measures that were either free or available at nominal cost. The model was designed to predict which people would and would not use preventive measures and to suggest interventions that might reduce client reluctance to use health care (Padilla and Bulcavage, 1991). Box 10-2 outlines the three major components of the health belief model: (1) individual perceptions, (2) modifying factors, and (3) variables affecting the likelihood of action. In addition, cues to action such as mass media campaigns, advice from others, reminder postcards from health care providers, illnesses of family members or friends, and newspaper or magazine articles help motivate clients to take action (Salazar, 1991).

The health belief model can be used to:

1. Assess health protection or disease-prevention behaviors
2. Organize information about clients' views of their state of health and what factors may influence them to change their behavior.
3. Provide organized assessment data about clients' abilities and motivation to change their health status. Health education programs can then be developed to better fit client needs (Salazar, 1991).

Health Promotion Model

The **health promotion model** was developed as a complement to other health-protecting models such as the health belief model. The health promotion model explains the likelihood that healthy life-style patterns or health-promoting behaviors will occur (Palank, 1991; Simmons, 1990). Box 10-3 outlines the three major categories of determinants of health-promoting behavior:

1. Cognitive-perceptual factors
2. Modifying factors
3. Variables affecting the likelihood of action.

Although these three categories are similar to the three factors of the health belief model, the health promotion model expands and modifies them.

Nurses can use this model, as with the health belief model, as a framework for client assessment. However, the health promotion model expands the principles of the health belief model and says that individuals are likely to change their behavior to feel better physically, psychologically, socially, and spiritually.

Briefly Noted

One in four adolescents in the United States suffers as a result of pregnancy, drug use, dropping out of school, depression, suicidal thoughts, or violence. Of U.S. high school students, 54% have had sexual intercourse, 72% do not always wear seat belts, 51% are not enrolled in physical education, 42% were in a physical fight during the last year, 31% had five or more alcoholic drinks on one occasion in the past month, and 28% smoked cigarettes in the past month. Clearly health education reform is needed to improve the health of the nation's teens. Comprehensive health education programs need to begin in children's early school years (Andrews, 1994).

EDUCATIONAL PRINCIPLES

A variety of educational principles guide the selection of health information for individuals, families, and communities. Three of the most useful categories of educational principles include those associated with (1) the nature of learning, (2) the events of instruction, and (3) guidelines for the effective educator.

The Nature of Learning

The nature of learning refers to the cognitive, affective, and psychomotor domains of learning (Rankin and Stallings, 1996). Each domain has specific behavioral components that form a hierarchy of steps or levels. Each level builds on the previous one. An understanding of these three learning domains forms the background for providing effective health education.

The **cognitive domain** includes memory, recognition, understanding, and application, and is divided into a hierarchical classification of behaviors. Learners master each level of cognition in order of difficulty and move from the simple to the complex (Dembo, 1994). The effective health educator begins by assessing the cognitive abilities of the learner so that the instructor's expectations and plans tar-

---

Box 10-2	The Three Major Components of the Health Belief Model

INDIVIDUAL PERCEPTIONS	MODIFYING FACTORS	VARIABLES AFFECTING THE LIKELIHOOD OF INITIATING ACTION
Person's *beliefs* about his/her own *susceptibility* to disease	*Demographic variables* • Age • Gender • Race • Ethnicity	Person's *perceived benefits* of action
PLUS		MINUS
The *seriousness* with which he/she views the disease	*Sociopsychological variables* • Personality • Social class • Peer pressure	His/her *perceived barriers* to accomplishing action
EQUALS		EQUALS
The *perceived threat* of an illness for each person	*Structural variables* • Knowledge about the disease • Prior contact with the disease	The *likelihood* that a person will take action to change his/her behaviors

Based on data from Salazar MK: Comparison of four behavioral theories, *AAOHN J* 39(3):128-135, 1991.

Box 10-3 — Three Categories of Determinants of Health Promoting Behavior

COGNITIVE-PERCEPTUAL FACTORS

Definition of health
- Importance of health
- Perceived health status
- Perceived control of health
- Perceived self-efficacy
- Perceived benefits of health-promoting behavior
- Perceived barriers to health-promoting behavior

MODIFYING FACTORS

Demographic factors
- Age
- Gender
- Race
- Ethnicity
- Education
- Income

Biological characteristics
- Body weight
- Body fat
- Height

Interpersonal influences
- Expectations of significant others
- Family patterns of health care
- Interactions with health professionals

Situational (environmental) factor
- Access to care

Behavioral factors
- Cognitive and psychomotor skills necessary to carry out healthy behaviors

VARIABLES AFFECTING THE LIKELIHOOD OF INITIATING ACTION

Depend on internal and external cues
- The desire to feel well
- Individualized health teaching
- Mass media health-promotion campaigns

Based on data from Palank CL: Determinants of health-promotive behavior: a review of current research, *Nurs Clin North Am* 26(4):815-832, 1991; Simmons SJ: The Health-Promoting Self-Care System Model: directions for nursing research and practice, *J Adv Nurs* 15(10):1162-1166, 1990.

get the correct level. Teaching above or below a person's level of understanding leads to frustration, irritation, and discouragement.

The **affective domain** includes changes in attitudes and the development of values. In affective learning, the teacher considers and tries to influence what individuals, families, and communities think, value, and feel. Since the nurse's values and attitudes may differ from those of the clients, nurses need to listen carefully to detect clues to feelings that may influence learning. As with cognitive learning, affective learning consists of a series of steps (Dembo, 1994). Table 10-2 compares steps in the affective domain with those in the cognitive domain. It is difficult to change deep-seated characteristics such as values, attitudes, beliefs, and interests. To make such changes, people need support and encouragement from those around them to reinforce new behaviors.

The **psychomotor domain** includes the performance of skills that require some degree of neuromuscular coordination. Community health clients are taught a variety of psychomotor skills including giving injections, taking blood pressures, measuring blood sugars, bathing infants, changing dressings, and walking with crutches. Psychomotor learning occurs when three conditions are met (Dembo, 1994):

1. *The learner has the necessary ability.* For example, a person with Alzheimer's disease may be capable of following instructions of only one or two steps. Therefore, the nurse must adapt the education plan to fit the client's abilities. In assessing a client's ability to learn a skill, the nurse must evaluate physical, intellectual, and emotional ability. For example, a tremulous person with poor eyesight may be unable to learn insulin self-injection. Similarly, some people do not have the intellectual ability to learn the steps that make up a complex procedure. Therefore, it is important to teach at the level of the learner's ability.

2. *The learner has a sensory image of how to carry out the skill.* For instance, when educating a group of pregnant women about techniques to manage labor,

TABLE 10-2 — Steps in the Cognitive Domain as Compared with the Affective Domain

	Cognitive Domain	Affective Domain
Knowledge	Requires *recall* of information	Learner *receives* the information
Comprehension	*Combines* recall with understanding	Learner *responds* to what is being taught
Application	Takes new information and *uses it in a different way*	Learner *values* the information
Analysis	Breaks down communication into constituent parts in order to understand the parts and their *relationships*	Learner *makes sense* of the information
Synthesis	Builds on the previous four levels by putting the parts back together into a *unified whole*	Learner *organizes* the information
Evaluation	*Judges the value* of what has been learned	Learner *adopts behaviors* consistent with the new value system

Based on data from Dembo MH: *Applying educational psychology,* ed 5, New York, 1994, Longman Publishing Group.

the nurse asks the clients to visualize themselves in calm control of their delivery.

3. *The learner has opportunities to practice the new skills being learned.* Practice sessions should be provided during the program because many clients do not have the facilities, motivation, or time to practice at home what they have learned. To facilitate skill learning, nurses show the learners the skill either in person, on a video, or with pictures. Then they allow learners to practice and immediately correct any errors in performing the skill.

The Events of Instruction

To educate effectively, the nurse needs to understand the basic sequence of instruction. When nurses consider the following nine steps of instructing others, they can systematically plan health education so that learners gain as much as possible from the instruction (Driscoll, 1994).

1. *Gain the learner's attention.* Before learning can take place, the educator must gain the learner's attention. One way to do this is by convincing the learner that the information about to be presented is important and beneficial.

2. *Explain the goals and objectives of the instruction.* Before beginning to teach, outline the major goals and objectives of instruction so learners develop expectations about what they are supposed to learn.

3. *Ask learners to recall prior learning.* Have learners recall previous knowledge related to the topic of interest so they can link the new knowledge with prior knowledge.

4. *Present the stimulus.* Present the essential elements of a topic in as clear, organized, and simple a manner as possible. Present the material in a way that is congruent with the learner's strengths, needs, and limitations.

5. *Provide learning guidance.* Long-lasting behavioral changes depend on learners' storing information in long-term memory. The educator's job is to help the learner transform new general information into meaningful information that can be recalled.

6. *Demonstrate what is learned.* Practice or repeat performance helps to see what the learner really knows; it also allows the learner to correct errors and improve skills.

7. *Provide feedback.* Provide feedback to learners to assist them to improve their knowledge and skills by changing their thinking patterns and behaviors based on this feedback.

8. *Assess performance.* Evaluate the learning. Knowledge and skills should be formally assessed to see if the new information was understood.

9. *Aid with retention and transfer of knowledge.* Once a baseline level of knowledge and skills has been attained, educators can help learners apply this information to new situations.

Box 10-4	Six Principles That Guide the Educator

1. *Message:* Sending a clear message to the learner.
2. *Format:* Selecting the most appropriate learning format.
3. *Environment:* Creating the best possible learning environment.
4. *Experience:* Organizing positive and meaningful learning experiences.
5. *Participation:* Engaging the learner in participatory learning.
6. *Evaluation:* Evaluating and giving objective feedback to the learner.

Modified from Knowles M: *The adult learner: a neglected species,* ed 5, Houston, 1998, Gulf Publishing.

By using these instructional principles, nurses may help clients to get the most from learning experiences. If steps of this process are omitted, superficial and fragmented learning may occur.

The Effective Educator

Nurses who work in the community must be effective teachers. Six basic principles that guide the effective educator are listed in Box 10-4 and are discussed next.

Sending a Clear Message

Even when the content is important and the learner is interested, the material must be presented in a clear and organized manner for effective learning to occur. Educators must continually reassess learner readiness and watch for possible barriers to effective communication (Hamachek, 1995). Both emotional stress and physical illness can limit the amount of information a learner can absorb. Educators need to be aware of possible factors affecting the learner and recognize that the needs and barriers influencing the learner's receptivity may vary from session to session. Educational strategies and activities can be developed and adjusted to fit the changing needs of the learner.

Educators need to provide information that is understandable. Medical jargon and technical terms may interfere with the clarity of the intended message. For example, in helping clients understand diet control for hypertension, the nurse might use the phrase "high blood pressure" rather than the term "hypertension" to tailor the message to the learner's ability to understand. See Box 10-5 for communication guidelines in educational interactions.

Selecting the Learning Format

The educator must decide how to teach, and this includes selecting an appropriate learning format, or strategy, for implementing the learning program. The format needs to match the goals and objectives of the program and correspond to the learning needs of the client. In addition, teaching tools such as printed materials or audiovisual aids that will enhance learning can be used (MacDonald, 1999). Three examples of learning formats are outlined in Box 10-6.

Box 10-5	Communication Guidelines for Educational Interactions

Begin strongly. People remember the first point.

Use a clear, direct, and succinct style. This helps the learner to remain focused.

Use the active voice. For example, the educator may say, "We will discuss relaxation techniques" instead of "Relaxation techniques will be discussed."

Accentuate the positive. For example, the educator may say, "The majority of individuals are able to lose weight with a well-balanced diet and exercise" instead of "A few people have not been able to lose weight with a well-balanced diet and exercise."

Use vivid communication, not statistics or jargon. Specific case histories are often more meaningful than general, nonspecific terms or dry statistics.

Refer to trustworthy sources. For example, "the surgeon general" is a more credible source than "some people."

Base strategies on a knowledge of the audience. Be aware of the perceptions and perspectives of the audience.

Make points explicitly. Be direct and give clear instructions.

End strongly. The last point made is likely to be remembered.

Modified from Damrosch S: General strategies for motivating people to change their behavior, *Nurs Clin North Am* 26(4):833-843, 1991.

Creating the Best Learning Environment

The environment influences the effectiveness of learning. Establishing the appropriate learning climate for an educational event begins when announcements of the program are made. The tone and appearance of letters, flyers, and media messages announcing the program provide a mental picture for participants of what the activity will be like. By carefully considering program objectives and information about the culture, beliefs, and educational level of learners, the nurse can develop preparatory materials that appeal to the target population (Knowles, 1998). During the program, the educator must create a positive, supportive, and pleasant atmosphere for clients.

Briefly Noted

Regardless of the methods of evaluation the nurse uses to determine teaching and program effectiveness, a helpful concept to keep in mind is the curve of normal distribution. In any group of learners, about 2% will be extremely negative, and 2% will be extremely positive in their evaluation of the program. Another 14% will be fairly negative, and 14% will be quite enthusiastic. The majority of participants (68%) will be somewhat neutral in their responses. Therefore, even though the nurse should consider the extremely negative responses, alarm or discouragement should not develop until the proportion of extremely negative responses rises above 16% (Knowles, 1988).

Box 10-6	Examples of Learning Formats

1. The client is a large class of university students studying communicable diseases. The selected format is a lecture to be followed by a question-and-answer period.
2. The client is a group from a shelter for victims of domestic violence. The chosen format is an informal, open, small-group discussion following a short poster presentation.
3. The client is a family with a newly diagnosed insulin-dependent, diabetic 6-year-old child. The objectives are different for each family member. Therefore, the format must be adapted to each member as well. The child requires materials appropriate to his/her developmental stage. The objectives for the child are to overcome fear of injections and to begin to deal with possible life-style changes. The material will be presented in the form of a picture book and storytelling that provides a realistic yet nonthreatening look at both the illness and the treatment. The objectives for the parents are to understand both the short- and long-term ramifications of their child's disease and to learn the specific skills needed in order to manage the illness at home.
   a. Informational handouts will be gathered and several medical journal articles will be copied and given to the parents to read.
   b. Insulin injection demonstrations and practice sessions will be provided.
   c. The nurse will provide the phone number to the clinic for follow-up questions as well as phone numbers for several diabetes associations.
   d. The family will be introduced to a local chapter of a support group appropriate to their specific needs. This will help them process their fears and concerns.

Organizing Learning Experiences

Regardless of the educator's level of knowledge or the quality of the interpersonal relationship that the educator has developed with the learner, sound organization of the material is essential if learning is to occur. Materials should be presented in a logical and integrated manner, from simple foundational concepts to more complex ideas. These should represent building blocks in a well-designed structure with a clear and unambiguous blueprint. The educator should reduce difficult or confusing concepts to their component parts and show the learner how to reassemble them one at a time. The pace of the presentation should match the ability of the learner and leave adequate time for the learner to absorb the material.

The principles of continuity, sequence, and integration are important aids in the organization of educational programs. A lack of *continuity* causes a break in the flow of logical thought and may confuse the learner. One valuable technique that helps maintain continuity for the learner is repeated emphasis of essential points.

Sequencing means that each learning experience builds on the previous one and requires a higher level of functioning. Learning activities should be sequenced so that participants start with simple, easy-to-master exercises or materials and progress to more complex ones requiring greater skill, coordination, or understanding.

Integration of various aspects of the material demonstrates how each component fits into the whole. Without integration, the learner is left with a puzzle of disjointed facts or concepts that is difficult to assimilate in a productive way (Knowles, 1998).

Encouraging Participatory Learning

People learn better when they are actively involved in the learning process. Participation increases motivation, flexibility, and learning rate. Participatory learning includes more than the psychomotor domain. The cognitive and affective domains also call for a teaching strategy in which the instructor enlists the active involvement of the learner. Verbal response or feedback, as long as it engages the learner, is participatory. Merely sitting and listening is not as effective as is discussion, even when the presentation is stimulating, interesting, and dynamic. Role-playing, acting out an experience, storytelling, "hands-on" training, and similar activities are good examples of participatory learning. Immediate feedback, an important advantage of participatory learning, ensures that errors are corrected before problematic habits or misconceptions develop. Computer-assisted learning provides immediate feedback to learners (Knowles, 1998).

Educators can structure learning activities and the environment to facilitate participatory learning. Proper teaching materials can provide learners with adequate prompting and modeling to ensure their ability to practice and to demonstrate mastery of the material. Participatory learning often makes the material more accessible and meaningful to learners and is more likely to be retained and used in the future (Knowles, 1988).

Providing Evaluation and Feedback

It is essential to evaluate learning and provide constructive and helpful feedback to learners throughout the educational process to avoid discouraging or offending the learner. Through clear and behaviorally focused feedback, clients can monitor their progress, level of knowledge, and learning needs. The educator may use tools such as quizzes, tests, completed study sheets, observation of skills, small-group tasks, and competency rating scales to evaluate learning outcomes. Not only should learners receive feedback, but the educator should also elicit feedback from learners throughout the educational process. Modifications in the implementation and presentation of the educational program are made based on the feedback that the educator receives from learners (Knowles, 1998).

THE EDUCATIONAL PROCESS

In addition to understanding the nature of learning, the events of instruction, and strategies for effective education, nurses need to understand the educational process. Interestingly, the educational and nursing processes are similar, and both are used at the individual, family, and community levels (Bigbee and Jansa, 1991). A comparison of the two processes is outlined in Table 10-3. The steps of the educational process are also discussed below.

Identifying Educational Needs

Nurses working in the community determine client health education needs by performing a systematic and thorough client needs assessment. The steps of a needs assessment are in the box below. Once needs are identified, they are prioritized so that the most critical educational needs are met first (Strodtman, 1984).

 Evidence-Based Practice

Most psychiatric nurses know that learner readiness is an important part of patient education; however, many psychiatric patients deny their illness, refuse treatment, cannot concentrate, and appear disinterested. Freed evaluated the stories that 12 psychiatric nurses told about educating psychiatric patients who did not exhibit typical signs of learner readiness. The primary pattern that emerged from these psychiatric nurses' stories was *perseverance*. She determined that perseverance is composed of elements of trust, patience, acceptance, caring, and hope.

APPLICATION IN PRACTICE

Nurses must to recognize that psychiatric patients will not accept new information as quickly as members of the general population. It is important to watch for verbal and nonverbal signs of things such as skepticism, fear, doubt, or a tendency to begin believing and thinking in new ways and accepting information.

Freed PE: Perseverance: the meaning of patient education in psychiatric nursing, *Arch Psychiatric Nurs* 2:107-113, 1998.

TABLE 10-3	A Comparison of the Nursing and Educational Processes

Nursing Process	Educational Process
Assessment	Identify educational needs
Diagnosis	Establish educational goals and objectives
Planning	Select appropriate educational methods
Implementation	Implement the educational plan
Evaluation	Evaluate the educational process and product

Based on data from Edwards L: Health education. In Edelman CL, Mandle CL (editors): *Health promotion throughout the lifespan,* ed 5, St Louis, 1998, Mosby; Hawe P, Degeling D, Hall J: *Evaluating health promotion: a health worker's guide,* Philadelphia, 1990, MacLennan & Petty; Strodtman LK: A decision-making process for planning patient education, *Patient Educ Counseling* 5(4):189-200, 1984.

HOW TO Do a Needs Assessment

1. Identify what the client wants to know.
2. Determine how the client wants to learn.
3. Discern what will enhance the client's ability and motivation to learn.
4. Collect data systematically from the individual, family, community, and other sources to assess learning needs, readiness to learn, and situational and psychosocial factors influencing learning.
5. Analyze assessment data to identify cognitive, affective, and psychomotor learning needs.
6. Encourage client participation in the process.
7. Assist the client in prioritizing learning needs.

Based on data from Volker DL: Patient education: needs assessment and resource identification, *Oncol Nurs Forum* 18(1):119-123, 1991.

Several factors influence clients' learning needs and ability to learn. Demographic, physical, geographical, economic, psychological, social, and spiritual characteristics of learners influence learning needs. The educator must also understand how the learner's existing knowledge, skills, and motivation influence learning. Identify resources for and barriers to learning. Resources include printed materials, equipment, agencies, and other individuals. Barriers include lack of time, money, space, energy, confidence, and organizational support (Edwards, 1998; Rankin and Stallings, 1996). Communication barriers may result from cultural and language differences between the nurse and the client or from printed materials that are inappropriate to the client's reading level. Educators need to understand the population for whom a program is being planned so that the planning can take into account any cultural or language needs and the medium for providing information fits the abilities of the learners (Gallivan, et al, 1998).

Briefly Noted

Nurse educators need to consider the setting in which community education will take place. Currently, school, work, and health care settings are common sites of health education. The educational setting has an impact on the teaching plan; cost-effectiveness; individual, family, and community behavioral changes; participation; and health care education policies.

Establishing Educational Goals and Objectives

Once learner needs are determined, educators identify the goals and objectives to guide the educational program. Goals are broad, long-term expected outcomes such as, "Mr. Williams will be able to independently take care of his ostomy bag within 3 months." Program goals need to directly address the client's overall learning needs (Rankin and Stallings, 1996).

Objectives are specific, short-term criteria that need to be met as steps toward achieving the long-term goal such as,

"Mr. Williams will properly reattach his own ostomy bag after the nurse has cleaned the site five consecutive times within 2 weeks." Objectives are written statements of an intended outcome or expected change in behavior and should define the minimum degree of knowledge or ability needed by a client (Green and Ottoson, 1994; Rankin and Stallings, 1996). Objectives must be stated clearly. Expected outcomes must be defined in measurable terms. The four parts of an objective are outlined in Table 10-4.

Selecting Appropriate Educational Methods

Educational methods should be chosen to assist in an efficient and successful accomplishment of program goals and objectives. Methods need to appropriately match the client's strengths and needs. Nurses should try to avoid educational designs; instead it is best to choose the simplest, clearest,

TABLE 10-4 **The Four Parts of an Objective**

Question	Phrase
Instructions:	String all "a" phrases together as one sentence for one example. String all "b" and "c" phrases together in like manner.
Who is to exhibit the behavior?	a. Each member of the Jones family b. Ms. Smith c. Eighty percent of the target population
What behavior is expected?	a. Will give an insulin injection to Billy b. Will perform a blood sugar test on herself c. Will take their children to receive immunizations
Conditions and qualifiers of behavior:	a. With accuracy regarding dosage b. With accuracy regarding the blood sugar reading c. Within 1 month of the immunization due date
Standards of behavior or performance:	a. 100% of the time for ten consecutive trials. b. Within 10 points of the educator's reading for ten consecutive trials. c. For 100% of standard childhood disease immunizations.

Based on data from Green LW, Ottoson JM: *Community health*, ed 7, St Louis, 1994, Mosby; Hawe P, Degeling D, Hall J: *Evaluating health promotion: a health worker's guide*, Philadelphia, 1990, MacLennan & Petty.

and most succinct manner of presentation. They must also know how to use a variety of tools. Examples of strategies to enhance learning are listed below. When selecting educational methods, developmental disabilities, age, educational level, knowledge of the subject, and size of the group must be considered in order to match media and other tools to the needs of the learner.

HOW TO Enhance Learning

1. Printed materials
2. Audiovisual materials
3. Computer-assisted learning
4. Demonstrations
5. Guest speakers
6. Role play
7. Field trips
8. Peer presentations
9. Peer counseling and tutoring

Modified from Knowles M: *The adult learner: a neglected species,* ed 5, Houston, 1998, Gulf Publishing.

For example, visually impaired clients may need more verbal description. Clients with hearing impairments may need more visual material or presenters able to use sign language. Also, if learners have limited ability to concentrate and pay attention, creative methods and tools for keeping the learner focused may be required. Such methods and tools include frequent breaks; plain, non-distracting surroundings; small-group interactions that keep the learner involved and interested; and "hands-on" equipment such as mannequins, models, and other materials the learner can physically manip-

Evidence-Based Practice

Printed educational materials are convenient and economical methods of health education. The authors evaluated reading materials developed at both the fifth- and the ninth-grade levels with general medical and surgical patients. They used the Wide Range Achievement Test-Revised (WRAT-R) to assess the reading levels of patients and the Cloze test to determine the reader's level of comprehension. They found that more subjects were able to understand the materials written at the fifth-grade reading level than those written at the ninth-grade level.

APPLICATION IN PRACTICE

Nurses need to be aware that many clients read at a lower comprehension level than one would assume. Often we assume that people who appear competent in life have mastery of basic skills like reading when they do not. One way to evaluate skill in reading in a nonthreatening manner is to ask the client to read a set of simple directions, a chart, or headlines in a newspaper or magazine.

Estey A, Musseau A, Keehn L: Comprehension levels of patients reading health information, *Patient Educ Counsel* 18:165-169, 1991.

ulate. Comprehension and retention are related to the depth or intensity of the learner's involvement. The educator tries to involve the learner appropriately and creatively in a variety of ways and to keep the involvement as active as possible.

Briefly Noted

Patient-centered education is a term used to define education based on what the individual, family, or community identify that they need to learn. Traditionally, health care professionals have designed educational programs based on their agenda, not on that of their patients (Dunbar, 1998; Gallagher and Zeind, 1998).

Implementing the Educational Plan

Once educational methods are selected, they can be implemented through management of the educational process. Implementation includes:

1. Control over starting, sustaining, and stopping each method and strategy in the most effective and appropriate time and manner
2. Coordinating and controlling environmental factors, the flow of the presentation, and other contributory parts of the program
3. Keeping the materials logically related to the core theme and overall program goals.

Educators must be flexible. They will need to modify educational methods and strategies to meet unexpected challenges that arise. External influences such as time limitations, expense, administrative and political factors, and learner needs require an ongoing evaluation of their impact on the educational program (Knowles, 1998). See below for ways to effectively teach clients.

HOW TO Effectively TEACH Patients

Tune in. *Listen before you start teaching. Patient's needs should direct the content.*

Edit information. *Teach necessary information first. Be specific.*

Act on each teaching moment. *Teach whenever possible. Develop a good relationship.*

Clarify often. *Make sure your assumptions are correct. Seek feedback.*

Honor the patient as a partner. *Build on the patient's experience. Share responsibility with the patient.*

Modified from Hansen M, Fisher J: Patient-centered teaching from theory to practice, *Am J Nurs* 98(1):56,58,60, 1998.

Evaluating the Educational Process

Evaluation is as important in the educational process as it is in the nursing process. Evaluation provides a systematic *and* logical method for making decisions to improve the educational program. There will be evaluation of the educator, process, and product (Hawe, Degeling, and Hall, 1990). *Educator evaluation* allows for modifications in the teaching process to better meet the learner's needs. The learner's evaluation of the educator occurs continuously throughout the educational program. The educator may receive feedback from the learner in written form, such as an evaluation sheet, as well as verbally or nonverbally, as in return demonstrations and by facial expressions (Knowles, 1998). Inadequate learner responses generally reflect an inadequate program, not an inadequate learner. When evaluation reveals that the learning objectives are not being met, the nurse determines why the instruction is not effective and reconsiders ways to present the material creatively and meaningfully (Knowles, 1998). Ultimately, the educator must assume responsibility for the success or failure of the educational process and the development of learner knowledge, skills, and abilities.

Process evaluation looks at the components of the educational program. It follows and assesses the movements and management of information transfer and attempts to keep the objectives on track. Process evaluation is necessary *throughout* the educational program to determine if goals and objectives are being met and how much time is needed for their accomplishment. Ongoing evaluation also allows the teacher to correct misinformation, misinterpretation, or confusion. Goals and objectives should be periodically reconsidered. It is also important to periodically ask if the desired health behavior change is really necessary. Such a question inevitably leads back to the original learning objectives and motivates the educator to rethink the practicality and merit of each objective. Finally, if teaching seems ineffective, factors that influence learner readiness and motivation should be reassessed. Process evaluation uses information gathered from the educator as well as from learner evaluations and assesses the dynamics of their interactions (Hawe, Degeling, and Hall, 1990).

The educational program will follow these steps:

1. Identify the goals clearly
2. Analyze the environment including client needs, services, and programs provided by other agencies or people
3. Identify the target group to receive the health education
4. Define the roles of team members
5. Choose the program topic and make sure that it fits the needs of the learners
6. Select the way to present the material
7. Create the program materials and do not forget the "voice of the learner" (i.e., continue to seek input from participants)
8. Implement the program and remember to be simple, direct, and concise in the information presented
9. Evaluate the program (Gallivan, et al, 1998; Visser, Thurmond, and Stinson, 1998)

THE EDUCATIONAL PRODUCT

The educational product or outcome of the educational process is measured both qualitatively and quantitatively. For instance, a qualitative assessment should answer the question, "How well does the learner appear to understand the content?" A quantitative assessment should answer the question, "How much of the content does the learner retain?" Thus, the quality of the product is measured by an improvement and increase in the learner's knowledge, skills, and abilities related to the content of the educational program. In nursing the educational product is assessed as a measurable change in the health or behavior of the client. Evaluation of the educational product can be divided into three components:

1. Evaluation of health and behavioral changes
2. Short-term evaluation
3. Long-term evaluation

Evaluation of Health and Behavioral Changes

A variety of approaches, methods, and tools can be used to evaluate health and behavioral changes. These include questionnaires, surveys, skill demonstrations, testing, subjective client feedback, and direct observation of improvements in client mastery of materials. Qualitative or quantitative strategies may be used, depending on the nature of the expected educational outcome. Evaluation of outcomes measured includes changes in knowledge, skills, abilities, attitudes, behavior, health status, and quality of life (Hawe, Degeling, and Hall, 1990).

Approaches to evaluating health education effects will vary, depending on the situation. For example, when considering a client's ability to perform a psychomotor skill, such as changing a dressing, watching the person perform the skill is the most appropriate means of evaluation. Another more complex example is the nurse's completion of the implementation phase of a family education program. The nurse might use a specific tool, such as the Family Assessment Device—a self-report instrument designed specifically to evaluate the effects of clinical interventions for families—to measure learning. The family functioning components that the Family Assessment Device measures are problem solving, communication, roles, affective responsiveness, affective involvement, behavior control, and general functioning (Reeber, 1992). This type of evaluation tool is necessary to measure a wide array of variables; when working with families, educational outcomes may sometimes be manifested in unexpected ways.

If evaluation of the educational product shows positive changes in health status and health-related behaviors, the educator can expect good results in similar health educational programs. If evaluation of the educational product shows that either no changes or negative changes in health status and health-related behaviors resulted, then various components of the educational process can be examined and modified to produce better results in the future (Redman, 1993).

Short-Term Evaluation

It is important to evaluate short-term health and behavioral effects of health education programs and to determine if they

Box 10-7   Why Long-Term Evaluation Is Challenging

COOPERATION

Clients may not follow up with return appointments or calls.
Clients may show a lack of interest in their own health care.
Clients may think it is too time-consuming or expensive to follow-up.

TIME

Follow-up requires making phone calls, evaluating clients, and reviewing and analyzing the results of the evaluation.

ENERGY

Follow-up requires the educator to keep track of clients and to relocate those who have moved.
The nurse must obtain the cooperation of clients.
The nurse must balance long-term evaluation responsibilities with other demands.

EXPENSE

Travel, phone calls, mail, and staff time can be costly.

Based on data from Redman BK: Patient education at 25 years; where we have been and where we are going, *J Adv Nurs* 18(5):725-730, 1993.

are really caused by the educational program. Short-term objectives are often easy to evaluate (Edwards, 1998; Green and Ottoson, 1994). For example, a **short-term evaluation** of whether or not a client can perform a return demonstration of breast self-examination requires minimal energy, expense, or time; skill mastery can be determined in minutes. If the short-term objective is not met, the nurse determines why and identifies possible solutions so that successful learning can occur. If the short-term objective is met, the nurse can then focus on long-term evaluation designed to assess the lasting effects of the education program. In this case, long-term evaluation would include ongoing monthly breast self-examinations performed by the learner independently at home.

Long-Term Evaluation

The ultimate goal of health education is to help clients make lasting behavioral changes that will improve their overall health status. Long-term follow-up with clients is a challenging task. Even though clients make positive behavioral changes and their health status improves, they often no longer use the health care services of the nurse (Redman, 1993). Box 10-7 lists some of the other reasons long-term evaluation can be challenging. **Long-term evaluation** means following and assessing the status of an individual, family, or community over time. The evaluation tools must identify whether specific goals and objectives were met, as well as the extent and direction of changes in client health status and health behaviors (Redman, 1993).

For nurse educators, the goal of long-term evaluation is to analyze the effectiveness of the education program, not the specific health status of the individual client. Nurses track the client's (who may be an entire community) performance of objectives over time. Thus, in a changing popula-

Healthy People 2010
Educational Community-Based Programs

Goal
- Increase the quality, availability, and effectiveness of educational and community-based programs designed to prevent disease and improve health and quality of life.

School Setting
- Increase high school completion.
- Increase the proportion of middle, junior high, and senior high schools that provide comprehensive school health education to prevent health problems in the following areas: unintentional injury; violence, suicide; tobacco use and addiction; alcohol or other drug use; unintended pregnancy, HIV/AIDS, and STD infection; unhealthy dietary patterns; inadequate physical activity; and environmental health.
- Increase the proportion of college and university students who receive information from their institution on each of the six priority health-risk behavior areas.
- Increase the proportion of the nation's elementary, middle, junior high, and senior high schools that have a nurse-to-student ratio of at least 1:750.

Worksite Setting
- Increase the proportion of worksites that offer a comprehensive employee health-promotion program to their employees.
- Increase the proportion of employees who participate in employer-sponsored health-promotion activities.

Health Care Setting
- Increase the proportion of health care organizations that provide patient and family education.
- Increase the proportion of patients who report that they are satisfied with the patient education they receive from their health organization.
- Increase the proportion of hospitals and managed care organizations that provide community disease-prevention and health-promotion activities that address the priority health needs identified by their community.

Community Setting and Select Populations
- Increase the proportion of Tribal and local health service areas of jurisdictions that have established a community health-promotion program that addresses multiple *Healthy People 2010* focus areas.
- Increase the proportion of local health departments that have established culturally appropriate and linguistically competent community health promotion and disease prevention programs for racial and ethnic minority populations.
- Increase the proportion of older adults who have participated during the preceding year in at least one organized health-promotion activity.

From U.S. Department of Health and Human Services: *Healthy people 2010*, Washington, D.C., 2000, U.S. Department of Health and Human Services.

tion, long-term evaluation of the results of an education program is still possible. The percentage of objectives and goals met by sampling the target population gives valid statistics for program assessment, even though the individual population may have experienced a complete turnover.

For example, a nurse working in the community notes that according to annual health department data, 60% of all pregnant women in the area where the nurse works received some prenatal care. Wanting to increase this percentage to 100%, the nurse tries an educational intervention in which radio and television stations make public service announcements about the importance and availability of prenatal services. After 1 year, the nurse notes that 80% of all pregnant women now receive prenatal care. The nurse continues to use public service announcements the following year because good results are evident. However, the long-term goal of the education program to influence the behavior of 100% of the pregnant women in the community has still not been met. Therefore, the nurse asks volunteers to put informational posters in shopping malls, grocery stores, public transportation stops, laundries, and on public transportation vehicles. The second year after implementing the revised educational program, again using the statistics from the health department, the nurse finds that 95% of all pregnant women in the target area now receive prenatal care. The nurse can thus evaluate and modify a community educational program over time to increase the rate, range, and consistency of progress made toward meeting the long-term goals of the project.

HEALTHY PEOPLE 2010 AND EDUCATIONAL AND COMMUNITY-BASED PROGRAMS

Healthy People 2010 has 12 objectives related to health education in schools, worksites, health care settings, and community settings with select populations. These are listed in the *Healthy People 2010* box. Meeting these objectives is fundamental to health promotion and improving quality of life. The health of communities depends on the health of individuals as well as the quality of the physical and social aspects of communities. The models described in this chapter can be used in health education within the four settings that the objectives address.

Clinical Application

In this section the educational concepts that have been highlighted in this chapter are applied to a clinical situation. Refer to Figure 10-1, which shows the sequence of actions that a community health nurse follows when developing an educational program.

IDENTIFYING AN EDUCATIONAL NEED

During an initial survey of a school, the nurse finds in the records that an unusually large percentage of elementary school children are not receiving standard immunizations for communicable childhood diseases. The nurse identifies education about immunizations as a need in the community.

ASSESSING STRENGTHS, NEEDS, AND BARRIERS

The nurse's assessment shows that the majority of the parents are of a certain ethnic group, are single, work full time, and are of a lower socioeconomic status. The nurse designs a simple verbal questionnaire that includes questions about attitudes and beliefs related to immunizations and assigns several pollsters to speak with a sampling of the parents. The following barriers to learning are identified:
1. Lack of awareness about the need for and the benefits of immunization
2. Belief that immunizations can be harmful to children
3. Belief that immunizations are expensive
4. Inability to get time off from work to have children immunized

The nurse next develops a strengths-and-needs list from the information gathered in the survey. Strengths that the nurse finds in the community members are their desire to be good parents and their involvement in the parent-teacher organization. The survey also demonstrates that the average education of the parents is at a tenth-grade level. The nurse identifies the following as client needs: knowledge about the existence and benefits of immunization, valid information about the risks of immunization, knowledge that immunizations are free, and information about the availability and accessibility of immunizations through the school system. Parents also need to know that the community has a mobile immunization unit that operates in the evenings for families with infants and preschoolers or who do not have transportation.

CHOOSING AN EDUCATIONAL THEORY

The nurse next matches the characteristics of the learner to an educational theory. In this case, the nurse educator chooses to combine and apply three theories to the educational situation. Social learning theory is chosen because of the desire to influence the parents' beliefs and expectations. Cognitive theory is chosen because the nurse thinks that the parents will respond to a variety of information. Humanistic theory is selected because the client is a close-knit, supportive community and is strongly devoted to its children.

CHOOSING A HEALTH EDUCATIONAL MODEL

Next the nurse educator selects a health education model for adaptation to the learner. The health belief model is chosen because of the need to change many of the parents' beliefs about immunizations. Based on the principles of this model, the nurse expects that the behaviors of the parents will change once their beliefs change.

CHOOSING EDUCATIONAL PRINCIPLES

The nurse considers educational principles and determines that the educational format should be that of a "town meeting." The best place to support the concentration and comfort of the group is the local high-school auditorium. Next the nurse plans an informal lecture about immunizations. A local family physician, who grew up in the neighborhood and has family still living in the community, will give the lecture. After the talk, parents will be invited to ask questions and discuss issues. The program will conclude by asking parents to enjoy snacks and socialize with each other. Small discussion groups will be encouraged to develop into community action groups of those who think that immunizations are important.

MOP UP THE DETAILS

The community health nurse also organizes other educational methods, objectives, plans, and strategies (MOPS). For example, the nurse may ask interested parents to volunteer to help arrange further meetings. Once the previously listed plans and strategies have been developed, the nurse then implements them. First, the nurse arranges a meeting with as many of the target group as possible through the local parent-teacher organization. The meeting is widely advertised through direct mailing to the target group and through notices that the children take home with their report cards. Public service announcements on the local television news and radio broadcasts are made. Carpools and shuttle vans are arranged for those who call for assistance with transportation. The date and time of the program are made as convenient as possible.

EVALUATING THE EDUCATIONAL PROGRAM

Soon after the strategies for these objectives have been implemented, the nurse educator develops an evaluation program for 3 months, 6 months, 9 months, and 1 year after the initiation of the educational program to evaluate the success of the program. The central criterion for the determination of success is the number of children receiving immunizations. Thus, even as the specific individuals change over time, the program evaluation process can be applied far into the future without the need for fundamental revision.

A. *What aspect(s) of this clinical application indicate that the nurse educator needs to have a solid foundation in community health nursing?*

B. *How would the program have differed if the nurse had used behavioral theory to understand how individuals learn instead of social learning theory, cognitive theory, and humanistic theory?*

C. *What strategy might the nurse use to determine whether the program attendees enjoyed and benefited from the program?*

D. *Would the evaluation process be adequate if long-term evaluation were omitted?*

Answers are in the back of the book.

 Remember This!

- Health education is a vital component of nursing care provided in the community since the promotion, maintenance, and restoration of health rely on clients' understanding of health care requirements.
- Six important general educational theories used to guide the nursing practice of health educators are behavioral, social learning, cognitive, humanist, developmental, and critical theories.
- Three current and useful models for organizing health education are the PRECEDE-PROCEED, health belief, and health promotion models.
- Three domains of learning are cognitive, affective, and psychomotor. Depending on the needs of the learner, one

or more of these domains may be important for nurse educators to consider as learning programs are developed.

- Nine instructional principles are gaining attention, informing the learner of the objectives of instruction, stimulating recall of prior learning, presenting the stimulus, providing learning guidance, eliciting performance, providing feedback, assessing performance, and enhancing retention and transfer of knowledge.
- Principles that guide the effective educator include message, format, environment, experience, participation, and evaluation.
- The five phases of the educational process are identifying educational needs, establishing educational goals and objectives, selecting appropriate educational methods, implementing the educational plan, and evaluating the educational process and product.
- Evaluation of the product includes the measurement of short-term and long-term goals and objectives related to improving health and promoting behavioral changes.

 What Would You Do?

1. Review the general theories of learning summarized in the chapter. Discuss with a classmate which one would most effectively fit the learning needs of a person who has been recently diagnosed with lung cancer, a family caring for an individual with Alzheimer's disease, and a community in which adolescent cigarette smoking is on the rise.
2. Recall an educational interaction with a client that did not seem to go well. Using educational principles, identify what might have been the problem. Working with a classmate, develop a plan to improve interaction.
3. Recall a learning experience in which either the message, format, environment, experience, participation, or evaluation was problematic. Then, develop a plan for how the problem could have been overcome and turned from a negative or neutral learning situation into a positive one.
4. Working alone or in a small group, review the phases of the educational process. Apply this process to an individual with hypertension, a family with a child who has attention deficit disorder, and a community in which tuberculosis is on the rise.

REFERENCES

Andrews DJ: Comprehensive health education: primary prevention's best hope, *J Med Assoc Georgia* 83:397-399, 1994.

Bigbee JL, Jansa N: Strategies for promoting health protection, *Nurs Clin North Am* 26(4):895-912, 1991.

Blair JE: Social learning theory: strategies for health promotion, *AAOHNJ* 41(5):245-249, 1993.

Clarke HF, Beddome G, Whyte NB: Public health nurses' vision of their future reflects changing paradigms, *Image* 25(4):305-310, 1993.

Damrosch S: General strategies for motivating people to change their behavior, *Nurs Clin North Am* 26(4):833-843, 1991.

Dembo MH: *Applying educational psychology,* ed 5, New York, 1994, Longman Publishing Group.

Dignam D: Cinderella and the four learning theories, *Nurs Praxis NZ* 7(3):17-20, 1992.

Driscoll MP: *Psychology of learning for instruction,* Boston, 1994, Allyn & Bacon.

Dunbar CN: Developing a teaching program, *Am J Nurs* 98(8):16B-16D, 1998.

Edwards L: Health education. In Edelman CL, Mandle CL (editors): *Health promotion throughout the lifespan,* ed 5, St Louis, 1998, Mosby.

Estey A, Musseau A, Keehn L: Comprehension levels of patients reading health information, *Patient Educ Counsel* 18:165-169, 1991.

Freed PE: Perseverance: the meaning of patient education in psychiatric nursing, *Arch Psychiatric Nurs* 2:107-113, 1998.

Gallagher S, Zeind SM: Bridging patient education and care, *Am J Nurs* 98(8):16AAA-16DDD, 1998.

Gallivan LP, Lundberg ME, Fiedelholtz JB, Andringa K, Stableford S, Visser L: Promoting opportunities for community based health education in managed care, *J Health Educ* 29(5):S-28-33, 1998.

Graham KY: Health care reform and public health nursing, *Public Health Nurs* 9(2):73, 1992.

Green LW, Kreuter MW: CDC's planned approach to community health as an application of PRECEDE and an inspiration for PROCEED, *J Health Educ* 23(3):140-147, 1992.

Green LW, Ottoson JM: *Community health,* ed 7, St Louis, 1994, Mosby.

Hamachek D: *Psychology in teaching, learning, and growth,* ed 5, Boston, 1995, Allyn & Bacon.

Hancock LA, Mandle CL: Overview of growth and developmental framework. In Edelman CL, Mandle CL (editors): *Health promotion throughout the lifespan,* ed 5, St Louis, 1998, Mosby.

Hansen M, Fisher J: Patient-centered teaching from theory to practice, *Am J Nurs* 98(1):56,58,60, 1998.

Hawe P, Degeling D, Hall J: *Evaluating health promotion: a health worker's guide,* Philadelphia, 1990, MacLennan & Petty.

Knowles M: *The adult learner: a neglected species,* ed 5, Houston, 1998, Gulf Publishing Company.

Knowles MS: *The modern practice of adult education: from pedagogy to andragogy,* ed 5, Chicago, 1988, Follett.

MacDonald RE: *A handbook of basic skills and strategies for beginner teachers: facing the challenge in today's schools,* Reading, Mass, 1999, Addison Wesley Longman.

Padilla GV, Bulcavage LM: Theories used in patient/health education, *Semin Oncol Nurs* 7(2):87-96, 1991.

Palank CL: Determinants of health-promotive behavior: a review of current research, *Nurs Clin North Am* 26(4):815-832, 1991.

Rankin SH, Stallings KD: *Patient education: issues, principles, practices,* ed 3, New York, 1996, JB Lippincott.

Redman BK: Patient education at 25 years: where we have been and where we are going, *J Adv Nurs* 18(5):725-730, 1993.

Reeber BJ: Evaluating the effects of a family education intervention, *Rehabil Nurs* 17(6):332-336, 1992.

Salazar MK: Comparison of four behavioral theories, *AAOHN J* 39(3):128-135, 1991.

Simmons SJ: The health-promoting self-care system model: directions for nursing research and practice, *J Adv Nurs* 15(10):1162-1166, 1990.

Strodtman LK: A decision-making process for planning patient education, *Patient Educ Counseling* 5(4):189-200, 1984.

U.S. Department of Health and Human Services: *Healthy people 2000: national health promotion and disease prevention objectives,* Washington, D.C., 1991, U.S. Department of Health and Human Services.

U.S. Department of Health and Human Services: *Healthy people 2010,* Washington, D.C., 2000, U.S. Department of Health and Human Services; available online at http://web.health.gov/healthypeople/.

Visser L, Thurmond L, Stinson N: Health education: a "primary" component to the delivery of comprehensive primary care, *J Health Educ* 29(5):S-10-14, 1998.

Volker DL: Patient education: needs assessment and resource identification, *Oncol Nurs Forum* 18(1):119-123, 1991.

Welton MR: The contribution of critical theory to our understanding of adult learning. In Merriam SB (editor): *An update on adult learning theory,* San Francisco, 1993, Jossey-Bass.

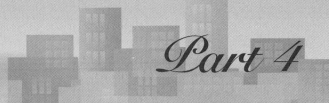

Part 4

Issues and Approaches in Health Care Populations

The primary orientation of health care delivery has been toward care and cure of the individual. There is increasing evidence that life-style and personal health habits influence the health of individuals, families, groups, and communities.

Community health nurses must identify health risk factors among individuals and groups in the community so that health problems of the total community can be identified. Healthy communities provide greater resources for growth and nurturing of individuals and families than do their unhealthy counterparts.

Certainly, community-oriented nurses use a public health approach to work with individuals and families in promoting health, intervening in disease onset or progression, and assisting with rehabilitation. Likewise, nurses often find that strategies used to introduce health behaviors directed at illness prevention and life-style changes are applicable to groups in the community and the community at large. Promoting health behaviors through groups, identifying community groups and their contributions to community life, and helping groups work toward community health goals are essential to community-oriented nursing practice.

A community assessment provides the basis for helping communities establish their goals. Case management and program management are approaches that have been used since the inception of community health nursing to match the most appropriate services and health care delivery interventions to client needs. Although all communities strive to protect their populations and provide a safe living environment, natural and human-made disasters may occur; community health nurses can play a significant role in helping a community through such a crisis. The chapters in this section help the nurse learn how to work with clients to develop quality services that will promote healthy communities.

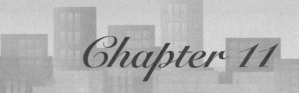

Chapter 11

The Community as Client and Partner

GEORGE F. SHUSTER

JEAN GOEPPINGER

OBJECTIVES

After reading this chapter, the student should be able to:
- Decide whether nursing practice is community oriented.
- Understand selected concepts basic to community-oriented nursing practice: community, community client, community health, and partnership for health.

- Compare the nursing process to community-oriented nursing practice.
- Decide which methods of assessment, intervention, and evaluation are most appropriate in selected situations.
- Develop a community-oriented nursing care plan.

CHAPTER OUTLINE

KEY TERMS

aggregate: population or defined group.

change agent: nursing role that facilitates change in client or agency behavior to more readily achieve goals. This role stresses gathering and analyzing facts and implementing programs.

change partner: nursing role that facilitates change in client or agency behavior to more readily achieve goals. This role includes the activities of serving as an enabler-catalyst, teaching problem-solving skills, and activist advocate.

community: people and the relationships that emerge among them as they develop and use in common some agencies and institutions and a physical environment.

community assessment: process of critically thinking about the community and getting to know and understand the community as a client. Assessments help identify community needs, clarify problems, and identify strengths and resources.

community health: meeting collective needs by identifying problems and managing interactions within the community and larger society. The goal of community-oriented practice.

community health problem: actual or potential difficulties within a target population with identifiable causes and consequences in the environment.

community health strength: resources available to meet a community health need.

Continued

community-oriented practice: a clinical approach in which the nurse and community join in partnership and work together for healthful change.

community partnership: collaborative decision making process participated in by community members and professionals.

confidentiality: information kept private, such as between health care provider and client.

database: collection of gathered and generated data.

data collection: the process of acquiring existing information or developing new information.

data gathering: the process of obtaining existing, readily available data.

data generation: the development of data, frequently qualitative rather than numerical, by the data collector.

evaluation: provision of information through formal means, such as criteria, measurement, and statistics, for making rational judgments necessary about outcomes of care.

goals: the end or terminal point toward which intervention efforts are directed.

implementation: carrying out a plan that is based on careful assessment of need.

informant interviews: directed conversation with selected members of a community about community members or groups and events; a direct method of assessment.

interdependent: the involvement among different groups or organizations within the community that are mutually reliant upon each other.

intervention activities: means or strategies by which objectives are achieved and change is effected.

objectives: a precise behavioral statement of the achievement that will accomplish partial or total realization of a goal; includes the date by which the achievement is expected to be completed.

participant observation: conscious and systematic sharing in the life activities and occasionally in the interests and activities of a group of persons; observational methods of assessment; a direct method of data collection.

partnership: a relationship between individuals, groups, or organizations in which the parties are working together to achieve a joint goal. Often used synonymously with *coalitions* and *alliances,* although partnerships usually have focused goals, such as jointly providing a specific program.

problem analysis: process of identifying problem correlates and interrelationships and substantiating them with relevant data.

problem prioritizing: evaluation of problems and establishment of priorities according to predetermined criteria.

secondary analysis: analysis using previously gathered data.

setting for practice: the community.

surveys: method of assessment in which data from a sample of persons are reported to the data collector.

target of practice: population group for whom healthful change is sought.

value: ideas of life, customs, and ways of behaving that members of a society regard as desirable.

windshield surveys: a community assessment, the motorized equivalent of a physical assessment for an individual; *windshield* refers to looking through the car windshield as the community health nurse drives through the community collecting data.

In the past nurses have viewed the community as a client and as a partner in improving health status of its citizens. Since the days of Florence Nightingale and Lillian Wald, nurses have looked at what is going on in the communities in which they found their clients. Florence Nightingale defined her community as Wartown America and discovered that the lack of fresh air, sanitation, and hygiene were contributing to the illnesses of the soldiers. Lillian Wald found that the neighborhoods around the Henry Street Settlement were impoverished with poor housing conditions, sanitation, improper nutrition, and crowding contributing to the problems of new mothers and children. Both women became political activists, worked with the leaders in their communities, and even solicited help from their respective governments to help change the conditions for the individuals and families in their communities. Many public health nurses consider the community their most important client and, more recently, their partner (Anderson and McFarlane, 1999). Guidelines for nursing practice with the community as client and as partner emphasize the use of the nursing process from assessment through evaluation to promote the community's health. This process begins with **community assessment,** which involves getting to know the community. It is a logical, systematic approach to identifying community needs, clarifying problems, and identifying community strengths and resources. Community health nurses are interested in these concepts because they want to know how the community's health affects their individual, family, and group clients.

WHAT IS A COMMUNITY?

The concept of *community* varies widely. The Expert Committee Report on community health nursing of the World Health Organization (WHO, 1974, p. 7) includes this definition: "A community is a social group determined by geographic boundaries and/or common values and interests. Its members know and interact with one another. It functions within a particular social structure and exhibits and creates norms, values and social institutions."

While the most often used single definition of community is "community of place" or geographic boundaries with agency interactions (such as between schools, social services, and governmental agencies), and the ability to solve problems, nurses working in communities quickly learn that society consists of many different kinds of communities. Neighborhood and face-to-face communities are two examples. Some other types of communities are listed in Box 11-1.

Other communities, such as communities of special interest or resource communities, are spread out across widely scattered geographic areas. They are brought together by common concerns and interests that can be long term or

TABLE 11-1	The Concept of Community Specified

Dimensions	Indicators
Space and time	Geopolitical boundaries Local or folk name for area Size in square miles, acres, blocks, or census tracts Transportation avenues such as rivers, highways, railroads, and sidewalks Physical environment such as land use patterns and condition of housing History
People or person	Number and density of population Demographic structure of population such as age, sex, socioeconomic, and racial distributions; rural and urban character; and dependency ratio Informal groups such as block clubs, service clubs, and friendship networks Formal groups such as schools, churches, businesses, industries, government bodies, unions, and health and welfare agencies Linking structures (intercommunity and intracommunity contacts among organizations)
Function	Production, distribution, and consumption of goods and services Socialization of new members Maintenance of social control Adaptation to ongoing and expected change Provision of mutual aid

Box 11-1   Types of Communities

Face-to-face community
Neighborhood community
Community of identifiable need
Community of problem ecology
Community of concern
Community of special interest
Community of viability
Community of action capability
Community of political jurisdiction
Resource community
Community of solution

From Blum HL: *Planning for health,* New York, 1974, Human Sciences Press.

short term in nature. An example of another type of community is a community of problem ecology, which is created when environmental problems affect a widespread area. For instance, a problem such as water pollution can bring people together from areas that would not normally share a common interest. Nurses also may work in partnership with political communities, such as school districts, townships, or counties. Because the nature of each type of community varies, nurses planning interventions with communities must take into account the characteristics of that specific community. Each community is unique, and its defining characteristics will affect the nature of the partnership.

In most definitions, the concept of *community* includes three dimensions: *people, place,* and *function.*

- The *people* are the community residents.
- *Place* refers both to geographic and time dimensions.
- *Function* refers to the aims and activities of the community.

Community health nurses regularly need to examine how the personal, geographic, and functional dimensions of community shape their nursing practice with individuals, families, and groups. They can use both a conceptual definition and a set of indicators for the concept of *community* in their practice.

In this chapter, the following conceptual definition is used: **Community** is a locality-based entity, composed of systems of formal organizations reflecting society's institutions, informal groups, and aggregates. As defined in Chapter 1, an **aggregate** is a collection of individuals who have in common one or more personal or environmental characteristics. The components of community are **interdependent,** and their function is to meet a wide variety of collective needs. This definition of community includes personal, geographic, and functional dimensions and recognizes interaction among the systems within a community. Indicators of the dimensions of this definition are listed in Table 11-1.

The next section describes the community as client and partner of the nurse. The community is first the **setting for practice** for the community health nurse practicing health-promotion and disease-prevention interventions with individuals, families, and groups. Second, the community is the target of practice for the nurse whose practice is focused on the broader community rather than on individuals, like the public health nurse.

COMMUNITY AS CLIENT

Community-oriented nursing has often been considered unique because of its **target of practice.** The idea of health-related care being provided within the community is not new. At the turn of the century most persons stayed at home during illnesses. As a result, the practice environment for all nurses was the home rather than the hospital.

As the range of community nursing services expanded, many different kinds of agencies were started, and their services often overlapped. For instance, both privately established voluntary agencies and official local health agencies worked to control tuberculosis. The nurses employed by these agencies were called *community health nurses, public health nurses,* or *visiting nurses.* Nurses practiced in clients' homes and not in the hospital. Early public health nursing textbooks included lengthy descriptions of the home environment and tools for assessing the extent to which that environment promoted the health of family members. Health education about the domestic environment was often a major part of home nursing care.

By the 1950s, schools, prisons, industries, and neighborhood health centers, as well as homes, had all become areas of practice for community health nurses. Many of the new community health nurses did not consider the environments in which they practiced. Although their practices took place within the community, they focused on the individual client or family seeking care.

When the *location of practice* is the community and the *target of practice* is the individual or family living in the community, then the client is the individual or family, not the whole community. Although the clients may be individuals, families or other interacting groups, aggregates, institutions, and communities, the resulting changes are intended to affect the whole community. For example, an occupational health nurse's target might be preventing illness and injury for the individual worker. This would result in maintaining or promoting the health of an entire company workforce. This means that because the nurse works with individuals through health education to teach them safety, the numbers of industry accidents decline from one year to the next. Because of this focus, the nurse not only would help the individual worker seeking service to overcome an injury but also would become involved with promoting vocational rehabilitation and would seek reasonable employment policies for all workers to promote safety.

Briefly Noted

Many nurses believe that home health nursing is focused on the individual and therefore should not be considered a part of community health nursing. Other nurses argue that home health nursing focuses on the family, takes place in the community, and should be considered a part of community health nursing.

The Community as Client and Partner in Nursing Practice

The concept of community as client and partner makes direct clinical care an aspect of community health practice (Abraham and Fallon, 1997). For instance, sometimes direct nursing care is provided to individuals and family members because their health needs represent common community-related problems rather than problems that are unique to their situations. Changes in their health will affect the health of their communities (Courtney, 1995). In such cases, decisions are made at the individual level because the individual's health is related to the health of the population as a whole and because the individual has an effect on community health. Improved health of the community remains the overall goal of nursing intervention. Interventions to stop spouse abuse and elder abuse are two examples of nursing interventions done primarily because of the effects of abuse on society and therefore on the population as a whole.

The concept of community as client and partner also highlights the complexity of the change process. Change for the benefit of the community client often must occur at several levels, ranging from the individual to society as a whole. In his classic work, Ryan (1976) points out that the "victim" cannot always be blamed and expected to correct the problem without changes also being made at the same time in the helping professions and in public policy. For instance, lifestyle–induced health problems, such as smoking, overeating, and speeding, cannot be solved simply by asking individuals to choose health-promoting habits. Society also must provide healthy choices. Most individuals cannot change their habits alone; they require the support of family members, friends, community health care systems, and relevant social policies.

A commitment to the health of individuals, families, and groups who make up the community client requires a process of change at each of these levels. Both collaborative practice models involving the community and nurses in joint decision making and specific nursing roles are required for each of the types of clients (Courtney, 1995). Community health nursing roles emphasize individual and direct personal care skills and focus on the family as the unit of service. The public health nursing role focuses on the community as a unit of service, especially constituent community groups.

Viewing the community client as partner and thus as the target of service means embracing two key concepts: community health and partnership for community health. Together these form not only the goal but also the means of community-oriented practice.

GOALS AND MEANS OF COMMUNITY-ORIENTED PRACTICE

In **community-oriented practice** the nurse and community seek healthful change together (Shiell and Hawe, 1996). Their common goal of community health involves an ongoing series of health-promoting changes rather than a fixed state. The most effective means of completing healthy changes in the community is through this same partnership.

Community Health

Like the concept of community, *community health* has three common characteristics or dimensions: status, structure, and process. Each dimension has a unique effect on a community's health as the goal of community-oriented practice.

Status

Community health in terms of status or outcome is the most well-known and accepted approach; it involves biological, emotional, and social components. The *physical component* of community health often is measured by traditional morbidity and mortality rates, life-expectancy indices, and risk-factor profiles. *Morbidity and Mortality Weekly Report* published the work of a consensus committee involving representatives from a number of community-health–related organizations. This committee identified by consensus 18 community health status indicators, which are presented in Box 11-2.

The *emotional component* of health status can be measured by consumer satisfaction and mental health indices.

Box 11-2	Consensus Set of Indicators* for Assessing Community Health Status

INDICATORS OF HEALTH STATUS OUTCOME

1. Race-specific and ethnicity-specific infant mortality, as measured by the rate (per 1000 live births) of deaths among infants less than 1 year of age

Death rates (per 100,000 population)[†] for:

2. Motor vehicle crashes
3. Work-related injury
4. Suicide
5. Lung cancer
6. Breast cancer
7. Cardiovascular disease
8. Homicide
9. All causes

Reported incidence (per 100,000 population) of:

10. Acquired immunodeficiency syndrome (AIDS)
11. Measles
12. Tuberculosis
13. Primary and secondary syphilis

INDICATORS OF RISK FACTORS

14. Incidence of low birth weight, as measured by percentage of total number of live-born infants weighing less than 2500 g at birth
15. Births to adolescents (females 10 to 17 years of age) as a percentage of total live births
16. Prenatal care, as measured by percentage of mothers delivering live infants who did not receive prenatal care during the first trimester
17. Childhood poverty, as measured by the proportion of children less than 15 years of age living in families at or below the poverty level
18. Proportion of persons living in counties exceeding U.S. Environmental Protection Agency standards for air quality during the previous year

---

From Consensus set of health status indicators for the general assessment of community health status–United States, *MMWR* 40(27):449, 1991.
*Position or number of the indicator does not imply priority.
†Age-adjusted to the 1940 standard population.

Crime rates and functional levels reflect the *social component* of community health. Other status measures, such as worker absenteeism and infant mortality rates, reflect the effects of all three components.

Structure

Community health, when viewed from the structure of the community, is usually defined in terms of *services* and *resources*. A structural perspective also defines the characteristics of the community structure itself. Indicators used to measure community health services and resources include service use patterns, treatment data from various health agencies, and provider/client ratios. These data provide information, such as the number of available hospital beds or the number of emergency room visits to a particular hospital.

Attributes of the community structure are commonly identified as social indicators, or correlates, of health. Measures of community structure include demographic characteristics, such as age, gender, socioeconomic and racial distributions, and educational levels. Their relationships to health status have been thoroughly documented. For instance, studies have repeatedly shown that health status decreases with age and improves with higher socioeconomic levels.

Process

The view of community health as the process of effective community functioning or problem solving is well established. However, it is especially appropriate to community-oriented nursing because it directs the study of community health to promote effective community action for health promotion, which is an important aim of community-oriented nurses.

The term **community health** as used in this chapter is the meeting of collective needs by identifying problems and managing interactions within the community itself and between the community and the larger society (Hemstrom, 1995). This definition emphasizes the process dimension but also includes the dimensions of status and structure. Indicators for all three dimensions are listed in Table 11-2.

The use of status, structure, and process dimensions to define community health is an effort to develop a broad definition of community health, involving indicators that are often not included when discussions focus only on individual and family risk factors as the basis for community health.

There are several different community-oriented health-promotion approaches, but regardless of what approach is taken, specific strategies to improve community health often depend on whether the status, structure, or process dimension of community health is being emphasized (Courtney, 1995; Freudenberg, et al, 1995). If the emphasis is on the *status dimension,* the best strategy is usually at the levels of primary or secondary prevention at the community level because the objective is either to prevent a disease or treat it in its early stages. Immunization programs are an example of a nursing intervention at the primary prevention level.

TABLE 11-2   The Concept of Community Health Specified

Dimension	Indicators
Status	Vital statistics (live births, neonatal deaths, infant deaths, maternal deaths)
	Incidence and prevalence of leading causes of mortality and morbidity
	Health risk profiles of selected aggregates
	Functional ability levels
Structure	Health facilities such as hospitals, nursing homes, industrial and school health services, health departments, voluntary health associations, categorical grant programs, and prepaid health plans
	Health-related planning groups
	Health providers available, such as physicians, dentists, nurses, environmental sanitarians, social workers, and others
	Health resource use patterns, such as bed occupancy days and client/provider visits
Process	Commitment
	Awareness of self and others and clarity of situational definitions
	Articulateness
	Effective communication
	Conflict containment and accommodation
	Participation
	Management of relationships with society
	Machinery for facilitating participant interaction and decision-making

Nursing intervention strategies focused on the *structural dimension* are directed to either health services or population demographic characteristics. Intervention aimed at altering health services might include program planning like developing a new program in occupational health nursing because of all the illnesses and injuries identified through an assessment at a certain industry. Interventions aimed at affecting demographic characteristics might include community development. A group of community leaders may come together in a country because they have recognized that children ages 6 to 17 do not have adequate health care in the schools. The leaders in partnership with the health departments may be able to plan for school health clinics.

When the emphasis is on the *process dimension*—usually the level of intervention of the community health nurse—the best strategy is usually health promotion, also a primary prevention strategy. For example, if family-life education is lacking in a community because of ineffective communication among families, children, school board members, religious leaders, and health professionals, then the most effective strategy may be to open discussion among these groups and help community members develop education programs.

Healthy People 2010

One important guideline that is available for nurses working to improve the health of the community is *Healthy People 2010,* a publication from the U.S. Department of Health and Human Services (2000) that offers a vision of the future for healthy communities and specific objectives to help attain that vision. The *Healthy People 2010* vision recognizes the need to work collectively, in community partnerships, to bring about the changes that will be necessary to fulfill this vision. "The final message of this report is one of shared responsibility among the many partners in prevention. It is

Healthy People 2010 and Community as Partner

Healthy People 2010 promotes partnerships with communities, states, and national organizations and suggests:
- Taking a multidisciplinary approach to achieving health equity
- Using approaches to improving not only health but education, housing, labor, justice, transportation, agriculture, and the environment
- Empowering individuals to make informed health care decisions
- Promoting community-wide safety, education, and access to health care
- Tailoring approaches to prevention for the type of community and ensuring community participation in the process

what we do collectively and personally that will move us as individuals and as a Nation towards a healthier future" (U.S. Department of Health and Human Services, 1991, p. 88).

Briefly Noted

There is a valuable *Healthy People 2010* website that can be accessed on the Internet through the WebLinks of this book's website (www.harcourthealth.com/MERLIN).

Community Partnerships

Community partnership is crucial because community members and professionals who are active participants in a collaborative decision-making process have a vested interest in the success of efforts to improve the health of their community (Courtney, 1995). Consequently, successful

1. *Informed.* Lay and professional partners must be aware of their own and other's perceptions, rights, and responsibilities (Jackson and Parks, 1997).
2. *Flexible.* Lay and professional partners must recognize the unique and similar contributions that each can make to a given situation. For example, professionals often contribute important knowledge and skills that laypersons lack. On the other hand, laypersons' definitions of community health problems are often more accurate than those of professionals.
3. *Negotiated.* Because contributions vary and each situation is different, the distribution of power must be negotiated at every stage of the change process.

strategies for improving community health must include community partnership as the basic means, or key, for improvement (McClowry, et al, 1996).

Partnership means the active participation and involvement of the community or its representatives in healthful change (Eng, Parker, and Harlan, 1997). Partnership is defined here as the informed, flexible, and negotiated distribution (and redistribution) of power among all participants in the processes of change for improved community health. The three main characteristics of partnership are captured in Box 11-3.

Partnership, as defined here, is a concept that is as essential for nurses to know and use as are the concepts of community, community as client partner, and community health. Experienced nurses know that partnership is important because health is not always a reality, but rather it is generated through new and increasingly effective means of lay-professional collaboration at the individual, family, group, or community level. For example, safety is an issue for many urban neighborhoods. Active efforts by neighborhood residents can make neighborhoods cleaner and safer places to live (Hemstrom, 1995).

However, such changes also require active professional service providers, such as school teachers, public safety officers, and horticulturists. Partnership in identifying problems and setting goals is especially important because it brings commitment from all persons involved, which is essential to successful change.

The significance and effectiveness of partnership in improving community health is supported by a growing body of literature. Studies document the use of partnership models involving urban areas (Parker, et al, 1998) and lay advisors (Baker, et al, 1997; Schulz, et al, 1997). The roles of these partners-in-health have included listening sympathetically, offering advice, making referrals, and starting programs (Aguirre-Molina and Parra, 1995; Bechtel, Garrett, and Grover, 1995; Courtney, 1995; Goeppinger, et al, 1995). Recent work by Hildebrandt (1998) and Kroeger and colleagues (1997) shows the continuing use of partnership models for improving health in other countries. In international health, partnership models generally are viewed as empowering people, through their lay leaders, to control their own health destinies and lives. In the United States, partnership models have often involved churches and informal community leaders.

COMMUNITY-FOCUSED NURSING PROCESS: AN OVERVIEW OF THE PROCESS FROM ASSESSMENT TO EVALUATION

Most nurses are familiar with the nursing process as it applies to individually focused nursing care. Using it to promote community health makes this same nursing process community focused (Flick, Reese, and Harris, 1996). The phases of the nursing process that directly involve the community client as partner begin at the start of the contract or partnership and include assessment, diagnosis, planning, implementation, and evaluation.

Assessing Community Health

Community assessment is the process of critically thinking about the community and involves getting to know and understand the community client as partner. This helps the community health nurse to understand the individual, family, and group problems, and to know what community strengths and resources are available to help the nurse solve the client's problems. The community assessment phase involves a logical, systematic approach to the initial phase of the nursing process. Community assessment helps:
- Identify community needs
- Clarify problems
- Identify strengths and resources.

There are different types of community assessment. Community assessments can be short and simple or long and complex. One example of a short and simple community assessment is the windshield survey, which is discussed in this section. Comprehensive community assessment is the necessary initial phase of the community nursing process with the community client as partner.

Assessing community health requires three steps:
1. Gathering relevant existing data and generating missing data
2. Developing a composite database
3. Interpreting the composite database to identify community problems and strengths

Data Collection and Interpretation

The primary goal of **data collection** is to get usable information about the community and its health. The systematic collection of data about community health requires:
- Gathering or compiling existing data
- Generating missing data
- Interpreting data
- Identifying community health problems and community abilities.

DATA GATHERING. **Data gathering** is the process of obtaining existing, readily available data. These data usually describe the demography of a community:

- Age of residents
- Gender distribution of residents
- Socioeconomic characteristics
- Racial distributions
- Vital statistics, including selected mortality and morbidity data
- Community institutions, including health care organizations and the services they provide
- Health personnel characteristics.

Often these data have been collected by others via structured interviews, questionnaires, or surveys and are available in published reports at the library or local public health department. These data give the nurse a snapshot of how the clients receiving services fit into the community.

DATA GENERATION. Data generation is the process of developing data that do not already exist through interaction with community members, individuals, families, or groups. This type of information is harder to get and is generally not statistical in nature. Data that often must be generated include information about a community's knowledge and beliefs, values and sentiments, goals and perceived needs, norms, problem-solving processes, power, leadership, and influence structures. These data are more likely to be collected by interviews and observation (Ludwig-Beymer, et al, 1996).

COMPOSITE DATABASE ANALYSIS. Combining the gathered and generated data creates a composite **database.** Data analysis seeks to make sense of the data. First, data are analyzed and synthesized and themes are noted. **Community health problems,** or needs for action, and **community health strengths,** or abilities, are determined. Next, the resources available to meet the needs are identified. Problems are indicated by differences between the nurse's and community's goals for community health. Strengths, on the other hand, are suggested by similarities between the nurse's and community's concepts of community health and available data. Next, the resources available to meet the needs are identified.

Data-Collection Methods

Several methods to collect data are needed. Methods that encourage the nurse to consider the community's perception of its health problems and abilities are as important as those methods structured to identify knowledge that the nurse considers essential.

Five useful methods of collecting data are:

1. Informant interviews
2. Participant observation
3. Windshield surveys
4. Secondary analysis of existing data
5. Surveys.

These methods can be grouped into two distinct but complementary categories:

- Methods that rely on what is directly observed by the data collector
- Methods that rely on what is reported to the data collector.

COLLECTION OF DIRECT DATA. *Informant interviews, participant observation,* and *windshield surveys* are three methods of directly collecting data. All three methods require:

- Sensitivity
- Openness
- Curiosity
- Ability to:
  - Listen
  - Taste
  - Touch
  - Smell
  - See life as it is lived in a community.

Informant interviews, which consist of directed talks with selected members of a community about community members or groups and events, are basic to effective data collection. Talking to key informants is a critical part of the community assessment. Key informants are not always people who have a formal title or position. Key informants often have an informal role within the community.

Also basic is **participant observation,** the deliberate sharing, if conditions permit, in the life of a community. For example, if the nurse lives in the community, activities such as participating in clinical organizations, church life, and reading the newspaper give the nurse "observations" of the community's life. Informant interviews and participant observation are good ways to generate information about community beliefs, norms, values, power and influence structures, and problem-solving processes. Such data can seldom be reported in numbers, so often they are not collected. Even worse, conclusions that are based on intuition and unchecked are sometimes used to replace this type of data. Conclusions from direct data collection methods should be confirmed by those people providing the information.

HOW TO Identify a Key Informant for Interviews

Key informants may be:
- County health department nurses or church leaders
- Nurses also know many community members and can identify other key informants
- The president of the parent-teacher organization
- The mayor or other local politicians
- The mother who organized the local chapter of Mothers Against Drunk Driving (informal leader)

Informant interviews with social workers and religious leaders can provide data that describe a community that has well-defined clusters of persons with similar problems such as persons of low income, concerns about adolescent pregnancy, and worries about the health of babies. This data could be difficult to acquire without personal interviews.

Windshield surveys are the motorized equivalent of simple observation. They involve the collection of data that "will help define the community, the trends, stability, and changes that will affect the health of the community" (Stanhope and Knollmueller, 2000).

Briefly Noted

If you do a windshield survey as part of your community assessment, go two times: once during the day when people are at work and children are at school, and a second time in the evening after work is done and school is out.

While driving a car or riding public transportation, the nurse can observe many dimensions of a community's life and environment through the windshield:

- Common characteristics of people on the street
- Neighborhood gathering places
- The rhythm of community life
- Housing quality
- Geographic boundaries.

Windshield surveys can be used by themselves for short and simple assessments. An example of a windshield survey can be found in Table 11-3.

HOW TO Obtain a Quick Assessment of a Community

- One way of getting a quick, initial sense of the community is to do a windshield assessment using a format like the one provided as an example in Table 11-3.
- Nurses interested in doing a windshield assessment need to either take public transportation, have someone else drive while they take notes, or plan to frequently stop and write down what they see.
- The windshield survey example is organized into 15 elements with specific questions to answer that are related to each element.
- Some of the questions will need to be answered by visiting the library to get secondary data.
- Nurses who use this approach will have an initial descriptive assessment of community when they are finished.
- Interventions are planned, based on the survey.

COLLECTION OF REPORTED DATA. Secondary analysis and surveys are two methods of collecting reported data. In **secondary analysis,** the nurse uses previously gathered data, such as minutes from community meetings. This type of analysis is extremely valuable because it saves time and effort. Many sources of data are readily available and useful for secondary analysis, including public documents, health surveys, minutes from meetings, statistical data, and health records.

Surveys report data from a sample of persons. They are equally useful, but they take more time and effort than observational methods and secondary analyses because they require time-consuming and costly data collection. Thus the survey method is not often used by the nurse. However, surveys are necessary for identifying certain community problems (Dever, 1997). For example, a lack of accessible personal health services cannot be documented readily and reliably in any other way.

Assessment Issues

Gaining entry or acceptance into the community is perhaps the biggest challenge in assessment. The nurse is usually an outsider and often represents an established health care system that is neither known nor trusted by community members who may therefore react with indifference or even active hostility to the nurse. In addition, nurses may feel insecure about their skills as a community worker, and the community may refuse to acknowledge its need for those skills. Because the nurse's success largely depends on the way he or she is viewed, entry into the community is critical. Often the nurse can gain entry by taking part in community events, looking and listening with interest, visiting people in formal leadership positions, employing an assessment guide, and using a peer group for support. Keeping appointments, clarifying community members' perceptions of health needs, and respecting an individual's right to choose whether he or she will work with the nurse are often useful techniques.

Maintaining **confidentiality** is important. Nurses must be very careful to protect the identity of community members who provide sensitive or controversial data. In some cases the nurse may consider withholding data; in other situations the nurse may be legally required to disclose data. For example, nurses are required by law to report child abuse.

Identifying Community Problems

The windshield assessment activities and the creation of a composite database will result in a list of community strengths and health problems. Each problem needs to be identified clearly and stated. This process is an important first step to planning. In the planning phase, priorities are established and interventions are identified.

In this chapter a version of a three-part community nursing diagnosis format proposed by Muecke (1984) is used:

1. Risk of _____
2. Among _____
3. Related to _____

"Risk of" identifies a specific problem or health risk faced by the community.

"Among" identifies the specific community client with whom the nurse will be working in relation to the identified problem or risk (see Box 11-1).

"Related to" describes characteristics of the community and its environment that were identified in the composite database of the assessment phase.

Each community has its own unique characteristics. Some of these characteristics are strengths that the nurse can build upon, but other characteristics contribute to the problem identified in the community nursing diagnosis. The characteristics, or factors, related to the identified problem are listed after the "related to" statement as the third part of the community assessment.

An example of a community nursing diagnosis for illustration in this chapter is infant malnutrition. Based on

TABLE 11-3   Windshield Survey Components

Element	Description
Housing and zoning	What is the age of the houses, architecture? Of what materials are they constructed? Are all neighborhood houses similar in age, architecture? How would you characterize their differences? Are they detached or connected to others? Do they have space in front or behind? What is their general condition? Are there signs of disrepair—broken doors, windows, leaks, locks missing? Is there central heating, modern plumbing, air conditioning?
Open space	How much open space is there? What is the quality of the space—green parks or rubble-filled lots? What is the lot size of the houses? Lawns? Flower boxes? Do you see trees on the pavements, a green island in the center of the streets? Is the open space public or private? Used by whom?
Boundaries	What signs are there of where this neighborhood begins and ends? Are the boundaries natural—a river, a different terrain; physical—a highway, railroad; economic— difference in real estate or presence of industrial or commercial units along with residential? Does the neighborhood have an identity, a name? Do you see it displayed? Are there unofficial names?
"Commons"	What are the neighborhood hangouts? For what groups, at what hours (e.g., schoolyard, candy store, bar, restaurant, park, 24-hour drugstore)? Does the "commons" area have a sense of "territoriality," or is it open to the stranger?
Transportation	How do people get in and out of the neighborhood—car, bus, bike, walk, etc.? Are the streets and roads conducive to good transportation and also to community life? Is there a major highway near the neighborhood? Whom does it serve? How frequently is public transportation available?
Service centers	Do you see social agencies, clients, recreation centers, signs of activity at the schools? Are there offices of doctors, dentists; palmists, spiritualists, etc.? Are there parks? Are they in use?
Stores	Where do residents shop—shopping centers, neighborhood stores? How do they travel to shop?
Street people	Whom do you see on the street—an occasional housewife, mother with a baby? Do you see anyone you would not expect—teenagers, unemployed males? Can you spot a welfare worker, an insurance collector, a door-to-door salesperson? Is the dress of those you see representative or unexpected? Along with people, what animals do you see—stray cats, pedigreed pets, "watchdogs"?
Signs of decay	Is this neighborhood on the way up or down? Is it "alive"? How would you decide? Trash, abandoned cars, political posters, neighborhood-meeting posters, real estate signs, abandoned houses, mixed zoning usage?
Race Ethnicity	Are the residents Caucasian, African-American, or of another minority, or is the area integrated? Are there indices of ethnicity—food stores, churches, private schools, information in a language other than English?
Religion	Of what religion are the residents? Do you see evidence of heterogeneity or homogeneity? What denominations are the churches? Do you see evidence of their use other than on Sunday mornings?
Health and morbidity	Do you see evidence of acute or of chronic diseases or conditions? Of accidents, communicable diseases, alcoholism, drug addiction, mental illness, etc.? How far it is to the nearest hospital? Clinic?
Politics	Do you see any political campaign posters? Is there a headquarters present? Do you see evidence of a predominant party affiliation?
Media	Do you see outdoor television antennas? What magazines, newspapers do residents read? Do you see *National Enquirer, Readers'* *Digest,* publications geared toward African-Americans or seniors in the stores? What media seem most important to the residents—radio, television, print?

Modified from Anderson ET, McFarlane J: *Community-as-partner: theory and practice in nursing,* Philadelphia, 1999, JB Lippincott.

assessment data the community diagnosis for infant malnutrition using this format would be the following:
1. Risk of infant malnutrition
2. Among families in Jefferson County
3. Related to:
   • Lack of regular developmental screening
   • No outreach program to identify at-risk infants
   • Families' lack of knowledge about WIC
   • Confusion among community families about WIC program enrollment criteria
   • Community families' lack of infant-related nutritional knowledge.

Frequently, a number of community health diagnoses will be made based on the different problems identified during the assessment phase, and the problems have now been stated in a community-focused nursing diagnosis format.

Planning for Community Health

The planning phase includes:
• Analyzing the community health problems identified in the community nursing diagnoses
• Establishing priorities among them
• Establishing goals and objectives
• Identifying intervention activities that will accomplish the objectives.

Analyzing Problems

Analyzing the problems seeks to clarify the nature of the problem. The nurse identifies:
• The origins and effects of the problem
• The points at which intervention might be undertaken
• The parties that have an interest in the problem and its solution.

Analysis often requires identifying:
1. The direct and indirect factors that contribute to the problem
2. The outcomes of the problem
3. Relationships among the problems (whether one problem causes or is affected by other problems)
4. Factors that contribute to the problem

This is important because the nurse can anticipate that several of the same factors that contribute to a problem and affect the outcomes of a problem also underlie many other problems.

Problem analysis should be undertaken for each identified problem. It often requires organizing a special group composed of the nurse and:
1. Persons whose areas of expertise relate to the problem
2. Individuals whose organizations are capable of intervening
3. Representatives of the community experiencing the problem

Together they can identify the contributing factors to the problem and explain the relationships between each factor and the problem.

This process is seen in Table 11-4 as an example of problem analysis. Factors that contribute to the problem and outcomes of the problem for infant malnutrition are listed in the first column. These factors are from all areas of community life. Social or environmental factors are as appropriate as those oriented to the individual. For example, teenage pregnancy is a social factor, and high unemployment is an environmental factor; both are related to infant malnutrition. In the second column the relationships between each factor and the problem are noted. The third column contains data from the community and the literature that support the relationship, using the suspected infant malnutrition example.

TABLE 11-4   Problem Analysis: Infant Malnutrition

Name of community: Jefferson County
Problem statement: Infant malnutrition in Jefferson County

Factors Contributing to the Problem and Outcomes	Relationship of Factors	Data Supportive to Relationships
1. Inadequate diet	Diets lacking in required nutrients contribute to malnutrition.	All county infants and their mothers seen by PHNs in 1997 were referred to nutritionist because of poor diets.
2. Community norms	Bottle-fed babies are less apt to receive adequate amounts of safe milk containing necessary nutrients.	Area general practitioners and nurses agree that 90% of mothers in county bottle feed.
3. Poverty	Infant formulas are expensive.	60% of new mothers in county are receiving welfare.
4. Disturbed mother-child relationship	Poor mother-child relationship may result in infant's failure to thrive.	Data from nursing charts of 43 child-mothers with infants diagnosed as "failure to thrive."
5. Teenage pregnancy	Teenage mothers are most apt to have inadequate diets prenatally, to bottle feed, to be poor, and to lack parenting skills.	90% of births in 1998 were to women 19 years of age or younger.

Infant malnutrition is thought to be related to inadequate diet, community norms, poverty, disturbed mother-child relationships, and teenage pregnancy.

Problem Priorities

Infant malnutrition represents only one of several community health problems identified by the community assessment. In reality, several community health problems may be identified. They may include lack of clinics, poor housing conditions, a mortality rate from cardiovascular disease that was higher than the national norm and—as expressed by many residents—a desire to quit smoking.

Each problem identified as part of the assessment process must be put through a ranking process to determine its importance. This is known as **problem prioritizing.**

PROBLEM PRIORITY CRITERIA. Criteria that have been helpful in ranking identified problems include the following:
1. Community awareness of the problem
2. Community motivation to resolve or better manage the problem
3. Nurse's ability to influence problem solution
4. Availability of expertise to solve the problem
5. Severity of the outcomes if the problem is unresolved
6. Speed with which the problem can be solved

Using the example of infant malnutrition again, these six criteria are listed in the first column of Table 11-5. Note that

TABLE 11-5   Problem Priority: Infant Malnutrition in Jefferson County

Criteria	Rationale for Rating	Problem Priority
1. Community awareness of the problem	Health service providers, teachers, and a variety of leaders have mentioned problem.	2
2. Community motivation to resolve the problem	Most believe that this problem is not solvable because most of those affected are indigent.	4
3. Nurse's ability to influence problem resolution	Nurses are skilled at raising consciousness and mobilizing support.	3
4. Ready availability of expertise relevant to problem resolution	WIC program and nutritionists are available. A county extension agent is interested.	1
5. Severity of outcomes if problem is left unresolved	Effects of marginal health services are not well documented.	3
6. Quickness with which problem resolution can be achieved	Time to mobilize rural community with no history of social action is lengthy.	6

TABLE 11-6   Problem Priority: All Identified Problems

Criteria	Problem	Rationale for Rating	Problem Priority
1. Community awareness of the problem	Community's desire to quit smoking	Health service providers, teachers, and a variety of leaders have mentioned problem.	2
2. Community motivation to resolve the problem	Poor housing standards	Most believe that this problem is not solvable because most of those affected are indigent.	4
3. Nurse's ability to influence problem resolution	Mortality rate from cardiovascular disease	Nurses are skilled at consciousness raising and mobilizing support.	3
4. Ready availability of expertise relevant to problem resolution	Infant malnutrition in Jefferson County	WIC program and nutritionists are available. A county extension agent is interested.	1
5. Severity of outcomes if problem is left unresolved	Lack of primary care clinics	Effects of marginal health services are not well documented.	3
6. Quickness with which problem resolution can be achieved	Teen pregnancy	Time to mobilize rural community with no history of social action is lengthy.	6

this one problem is only an example to show how to evaluate each problem using the six criteria.

The members of the partnership answer questions related to their ability to influence and/or change the situation, and the nurse and the community agree on the ability to resolve the problem. One example of the difference between the perceptions of the nurse and community members is smoking in public buildings; the community nurse might identify smoking as a public health problem, but community members might view smoking as an issue of individual choice and personal freedom.

This process is repeated separately for each identified problem, and all of the problems are compared. Priorities among the identified problems are established. The problems with the highest priority are the ones selected as the focus for intervention. Table 11-6 shows how all problems in the community were prioritized after each one was separately evaluated.

Establishing Goals and Objectives

Once high-priority problems are identified, relevant goals and objectives are developed. **Goals** are generally broad statements of desired outcomes. **Objectives** are the precise statements indicating the means of achieving desired outcomes.

An example of one of the goals and the specific objectives associated with it for the infant malnutrition problem is depicted in Table 11-7.

The goal is to reduce the incidence and prevalence of infant malnutrition. *The objectives must be precise, behaviorally stated, incremental,* and *measurable.* In this example the specific objectives pertain to:

1. Assessing infant developmental levels
2. Determining Women, Infants, and Children (WIC) Program eligibility
3. Implementing an outreach program

4. Enrolling infants in the WIC program
5. Providing supplemental foods in existing diets

As noted previously, establishing these goals and objectives involves collaboration between the nurse and representatives of the community groups affected by both the problem and the proposed intervention. This often requires a great deal of negotiation among everyone taking part in the planning process. One important advantage offered by the continuous active involvement of people affected by the outcomes is that they have a vested interest in those outcomes and therefore are supportive of and committed to the success of the intervention. Once goals and objectives are chosen, intervention activities to accomplish the objectives can be identified.

Identifying Intervention Activities

Intervention activities, the means by which objectives are met, are:

- The strategies used to meet the objectives
- The ways change will be effected
- The ways the problem cycle will be broken.

Because alternative intervention activities do exist, they must be identified and evaluated. Listing possible interventions and selecting the best set of activities to achieve the goal of documenting and reducing infant malnutrition are depicted in Table 11-8.

To achieve the objective related to assessment of infant developmental levels (see Table 11-7, objective 1), five intervention activities are listed in the second column of Table 11-8. Each is relevant to the first objective (80% of infants seen by the health department, neighborhood health center, and private physicians will have their developmental levels assessed). The first two activities involve WIC program personnel as the principal change agents. The last three involve the nurse, WIC program personnel, and the staff of the health department, neighborhood health center, and private physicians' offices as the change partners.

TABLE 11-7	Goals and Objectives: Infant Malnutrition

Name of community: Jefferson County
Problem/concern: Infant malnutrition
Goal statement: To reduce the incidence and prevalence of infant malnutrition

Present Date	Objectives (number and statement)	Completion Date
2002	1. 80% of infants seen by health department, neighborhood health center and private physicians will have their developmental levels assessed.	2004
2002	2. WIC program eligibility will be determined for 80% of infants seen by health department, neighborhood health center, and private physicians.	2004
2002	3. An outreach program will be implemented to identify at-risk infants not now known to health care providers.	2004
2002	4. WIC program eligibility will be determined for 25% of at-risk infants.	2005
2002	5. 75% of all infants eligible for WIC food supplements will be enrolled in the program.	2004
2002	6. 50% of the mothers of infants enrolled in WIC will demonstrate three ways of incorporating WIC supplements into their infants' diets.	2004

TABLE 11-8   Plan: Intervention Activities to Assess Infants' Developmental Levels

Name of community: Jefferson County
Objective number 1 and statement: 80% of infants seen by health department, neighborhood health center, and private physicians will have their development levels assessed

Present Date	Possible Interventions	Intervention Problems/Resources	Priority Intervention for Best Outcome
1-2002	1. WIC program supplies personnel to assess infant developmental levels.	Personnel and time are insufficient; existing community resources (potential) are ignored.	5
1-2002	2. WIC program provides in-service education to staff on assessment of infant development.	Antipathy between WIC personnel and other health workers is high. The need for education must be assessed first, and enthusiasm for objectives must be created.	4
1-2002	3. CN provides in-service education to staff in assessment of infant development.	The CN cannot do it alone.	3
1-2002	4. CN helps WIC personnel identify in-service educational needs of area health care providers about assessment of infant development.	Most likely to build on existing community strengths; CN skilled in needs assessment and interpersonal techniques is needed to decrease antipathy.	2
1-2002	5. CN helps WIC personnel identify driving and restraining forces relative to implementation of objective.	Without this, change effort is likely to fail.	1

The expected effect of each of the activities is considered in the second column of Table 11-8. The **value,** or the likelihood that the activity will help meet the objective and finally resolve the problem, is noted in the third column.

Clearly it is more valuable in the long term to educate others in how to assess infant development (activity 4) than to do it for them (activity 1).

It is also valuable to analyze the change process necessary to complete the objective (activity 5).

As a result, activities 4 and 5 have higher value scores than activity 1, in which the professional staff alone carries out the intervention.

Implementation for Community Health

Implementation, the fourth phase of the nursing process, involves the work and activities aimed at achieving the goals and objectives. Implementation efforts may be made by the person or group who established the goals and objectives, or they may be shared with or even delegated to others.

Factors Influencing Implementation

Implementation is shaped by:
- The nurse's chosen roles
- The type of health problem selected as the focus for intervention
- The community's readiness to take part in problem solving
- Characteristics of the social change process.

The nurse taking part in community-oriented intervention has knowledge and skills that the other intervenors do not have; the question is how the nurse uses the position, knowledge, and skills.

NURSE'S ROLE. Nurses can act as content experts, helping communities select and attain task-related goals. In the example of infant malnutrition, the nurse can use epidemiological skills to determine the incidence and prevalence of malnutrition. The nurse can serve as a process expert by increasing the community's ability to document the problem rather than by only providing help as an expert in the area.

Content-focused roles often are considered **change agent** roles, whereas process roles are called **change partner** roles. Change agent roles stress gathering and analyzing facts and implementing programs, whereas change partner roles include those of enabler-catalyst, teacher of problem-solving skills, and activist advocate.

THE PROBLEM AND THE NURSE'S ROLE. The role the nurse chooses depends on the nature of the health problem, the community's decision-making ability, and on professional and personal choices. Some health problems clearly require certain intervention roles:
- If a community lacks democratic problem-solving abilities, the nurse may select teacher, facilitator, and advocate roles. Problem-solving skills must be explained and modeled.
- A problem with determining the status of community health, on the other hand, usually requires fact-gatherer and analyst roles.

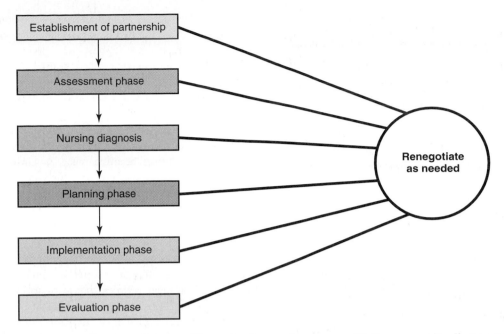

Figure 11-1   Summary flow sheet illustrating the nursing process with the community client as partner.

- Some problems require multiple roles. Managing conflict among the involved health care providers, a common problem, demands process skills.
- Collecting and interpreting the data necessary to document a problem require both interpersonal and analytical skills.
- The community's history of taking part in decision making is a critical factor. In a community skilled in identifying and successfully managing its problems, the nurse may best serve as technical expert or advisor. Different roles may be required if the community lacks problem-solving skills or has a history of unsuccessful change efforts. The nurse may have to focus on developing problem-solving capabilities or on making one successful change so that the community becomes empowered to take on the job of promoting change on its own behalf.

SOCIAL CHANGE PROCESS AND THE NURSE'S ROLE. The nurse's role also depends on the social change process. Not all communities are open to innovation. Ability to change is often related to the extent to which a community adheres to traditional norms. The more traditional the community, the less likely it is to change. Innovation is often directly related to:

- High socioeconomic status
- A perceived need for change
- The presence of liberal, scientific, and democratic values
- A high level of social participation by community residents (Rogers, 1995).

Innovations with the highest adoption rates are seen as better than the other available choices. For example, people living in a community might go to an immunization clinic rather than a private physician if the clinic is nearby and less expensive and if the physician is not always available when needed.

Innovations also are easier to accept when:

- The innovation is shared in ways that fit in with the community's norms, values, and customs
- Information is spread by the best communication mode (mass media for early adopters and face-to-face for late adopters)
- Other communities support the change efforts
- There is identification and use of opinion leaders
- Communication about the innovation is clear and straightforward (Rogers, 1995).

Evaluating the Intervention for Community Health

Simply defined, **evaluation** is the appraisal of the effects of some organized activity or program. An example of evaluation is provided in the Evidence-Based Practice box. Evaluation may involve the design and conduct of evaluation research, or it may involve the more elementary process of assessing progress by contrasting the objectives and the results. This section deals with the basic approach of contrasting objectives and results.

Evaluation begins in the planning phase, when goals and measurable objectives are established and goal-attaining activities are identified. After implementing the intervention, only the accomplishment of objectives and the effects of intervention activities have to be assessed. Nursing progress notes direct the nurse to perform such appraisals concurrently with implementation. In assessing the data recorded there, the nurse is requested to evaluate whether the objectives were met and whether the intervention activities used were effective. Such an evaluation process is oriented to community health because the intervention goals and objectives come from the nurse's and the community's ideas about health.

Figure 11-1 presents a summary of the complete nursing process with a community client.

Evidence-Based Practice

The elderly are often seen as one group, but in reality, researchers divide them into three groups: the young old (65 to 74), middle old (75 to 84), and old old (85 and older). The purpose of the study referenced below was to look at the use of community-focused services among these three groups. Existing data from a regional Area Agency on Aging were used for data analysis. Chi-square statistics and regression analyses were conducted to examine the effects of demographic, socioeconomic, and health status variables on the usage of community-based services.

Overall, case management, congregate meals, home-delivered meals, recreation, and outreach were the most frequently used services. Service usage varied among groups. Differences existed among the young old, middle old, and old old in both the types and the number of services that were used.

APPLICATION IN PRACTICE

Study results support planning efforts to tailor community-focused services to specific elderly cohorts rather than treating the young old, middle old, and old old as a homogenous group requiring the same type and mix of services.

Wallace DC, Hirst PK: Community-based service use among the young, middle, and old old, *Public Health Nurs* 13(4):286, 1996.

Role of Outcomes in the Evaluation Phase

The measurement of outcomes is a particularly important part of the evaluation process. This is one reason for placing emphasis on measurable objectives. The Pew Health Professions Commission (1995) reports the need for improving the health of the entire population and the need to focus on outcomes and evidence-based measures. Outcomes measures answer questions about results of the intervention. Dever (1997) emphasizes outcomes questions about appropriate and effective interventions such as:

- Was the appropriate intervention done ineffectively or effectively?
- Was an inappropriate intervention done ineffectively or effectively?

To answer these and other outcomes questions, Dever emphasizes epidemiology and the correct use of rates and numbers as one means of evaluating intervention outcomes among defined communities. Often data collected over time can also provide important outcomes information about health trends within the community. As indicated previously, epidemiological data and trends do not provide the only measure of success, but they do provide important information about the intervention. Nurses need to consider the collection of this type of outcome data for use as part of the evaluation phase.

PERSONAL SAFETY IN COMMUNITY PRACTICE

Personal safety is a prerequisite for effective community-oriented nursing practice, and it should be a consideration throughout the process. An awareness of the community and common sense are the two best guidelines for judgment. For example, common sense suggests not leaving anything valuable on a car seat or leaving the car unlocked. Similar guidelines apply to the use of public transportation. Calling ahead to schedule meetings will help prevent delays or confusion, and it gives the nurse an opportunity to lay the groundwork for the meeting. If there is no telephone or no access to a neighbor's telephone, a time for any future meetings should be established during the initial visit. Regardless of whether there has been telephone contact, there are rare situations when a meeting may be postponed because the nurse arrives at a location where people are unexpectedly hanging out by the entrance and the nurse has concerns about personal safety.

For nurses who are either just beginning their careers in community health or who are just starting a new position, there are three clear sources of information that will help answer any questions about personal safety:

1. *Other nurses, social workers, or health care providers who are familiar with the dynamics of a given community.* They can provide valuable insights into when to visit, how to get there, and what to expect because they function in the community themselves.
2. *Community members.* The best sources of information about the community are the community members themselves, and one benefit of developing an active partnership with community members is their willingness to share their insight about day-to-day community life.
3. *The nurse's own observations.* Knowledge gained during the data-collection phase of the process should provide a solid basis for an awareness of day-to-day community activity. Nurses with experience practicing in the community generally agree that if they feel uncomfortable in a situation, they should trust their feelings and leave.

Clinical Application

Lily, a nurse in a small city, became aware of the increased incidence of respiratory diseases through contact with families in the community and the local chapter of the American Lung Association. During family visits, Lily noticed that many of the parents were smokers. Because most of the families Lily visited had small children, she became concerned about the effects of secondhand smoke on the health of the infants and children among her family caseload.

Further assessment of this community indicated that the community recognized several problems, including school safety and the risk of water pollution, in addition to the smoking problem that Lily had identified during her family visits. Talks with different community members revealed that they wanted each of these identified problems "fixed," although these same community members also remained uncertain of how to start.

In deciding which of the three identified problems to address first, which criterion would be most important for Lily to consider?

A. *The amount of money available*
B. *The level of community motivation to "fix" one of the three identified problems*
C. *The number of people in the community who expressed a concern about one of the three identified problems*
D. *How much control she would have in the process*

Answer is in the back of the book.

 ## Remember This!

- A community is defined as a locality-based entity, composed of systems of formal organizations reflecting societal institutions, informal groups, and aggregates that are interdependent and whose function or expressed intent is to meet a wide variety of collective needs.
- A community practice setting is insufficient reason for saying that practice is oriented toward the community client. When the location of the practice is in the community but the focus of the practice is the individual or family, then the nursing client remains the individual or family, not the whole community.
- Community-oriented practice is targeted to the community, the population group in which healthful change is sought.
- *Community health* as used in this chapter is defined as the meeting of collective needs through identifying problems and managing interactions within the community itself and between the community and the larger society.
- Most changes aimed at improving community health involve, of necessity, partnerships among community residents and health workers from a variety of disciplines.
- Assessing community health requires gathering existing data, generating missing data, and interpreting the database.
- Five methods of collecting data useful to the nurse are informant interviews, participant observation, secondary analysis of existing data, surveys, and windshield surveys.
- Gaining entry or acceptance into the community is perhaps the biggest challenge in assessment.
- The nurse is usually an outsider and often represents an established health care system that is neither known nor trusted by community members, who may react with indifference or even active hostility.
- The planning phase includes analyzing and establishing priorities among community health problems already identified, establishing goals and objectives, and identifying intervention activities that will accomplish the objectives.
- Once high-priority problems are identified, broad relevant goals and objectives are developed.
- The goal, generally a broad statement of desired outcome, and objectives, the precise statements of the desired outcome, are carefully selected.
- Intervention activities, the means by which objectives are met, are the strategies that clarify what must be done to achieve the objectives, the ways change will be effected, and the way the problem will be interpreted.
- Implementation, the third phase of the nursing process, is transforming a plan for improved community health into achievement of goals and objectives.
- Simply defined, evaluation is the appraisal of the effects of some organized activity or program.

 ## What Would You Do?

1. Observe an occupational health nurse, community or public health nurse, school nurse, family nurse practitioner, or emergency department nurse for several hours. Determine which of the nurse's activities are community oriented, and state the reasons for your judgment.
2. Using your own community as a frame of reference, develop examples illustrating the concepts of community, community client, community health, and partnership for health.
3. Read your local newspaper and identify articles illustrating the concepts of community, community client, community health, and partnership for health.

REFERENCES

Abraham T, Fallon PJ: Caring for the community: development of the advanced practice nurse role, *Clin Nurse Specialist* 11(5):224, 1997.

Aguirre-Molina M, Parra PA: Latino youth and families as active participants in planning change: a community-university partnership. In Zambrana RE (editor): *Understanding Latino families: scholarship, policy, and practice,* Thousand Oaks, Calif, 1995, Sage.

Anderson ET, McFarlane J: *Community-as-partner: theory and practice in nursing,* Philadelphia, 1999, JB Lippincott.

Baker EA, et al: The Latino Health Advocacy Program: a collaborative lay health advisor approach, *Health Educ Behav* 24(4):495, 1997.

Bechtel GA, Garrett C, Grover S: Developing a collaborative community partnership program in medical asepsis with tattoo studios, *Public Health Nurs* 12(5):348, 1995.

Blum HL: *Planning for health,* New York, 1974, Human Sciences Press.

Consensus set of health status indicators for the general assessment of community health status—United States, *MMWR* 40(27):449, 1991.

Courtney R: Community partnership primary care: a new paradigm for primary care, *Public Health Nurs* 12(6):366, 1995.

Dever GEA: *Improving outcomes in public health practice,* Gaithersburg, Md, 1997, Aspen.

Eng E, Parker EA, Harlan C: Lay health advisors: a critical link to community capacity building, *Health Educ Behav* 24(4):413, 1997.

Flick LH, Reese C, Harris A: Aggregate/community-centered undergraduate community health nursing clinical experience, *Public Health Nurs* 13(1):36, 1996.

Freudenberg N, et al: Strengthening individual and community capacity to prevent disease and promote health: in search of relevant theories and principles, *Health Educ Q* 22(3):290, 1995.

Goeppinger J, et al: From research to practice: the effects of the jointly sponsored dissemination of an arthritis self-care nursing intervention, *Appl Nurs Res* 8(3):106, 1995.

Hemstrom MM: Application as scholarship: a community client experience, *Public Health Nurs* 12(5):279, 1995.

Hildebrandt E: Building community participation in health care: a model and example from South Africa, *Image J Nurs Scholarship* 28(2):291, 1998.

Jackson EJ, Parks CP: Recruitment and training issues from selected lay health advisor programs among African Americans: a 20-year perspective, *Health Educ Behav* 24(4):418, 1997.

Kroeger A, et al: Operational aspects of bednet impregnation for community-based malaria control in Nicaragua, Ecuador, Peru, and Columbia, *Trop Med Int Health* 2(6):589, 1997.

Ludwig-Beymer P, et al: Community assessment in a suburban Hispanic community: a description of method, *J Transcult Nurs* 8(1):19, 1996.

McClowry SG, et al: A comprehensive school-based clinic: university and community partnership, *J Soc Pediatr Nurses* 1(1):19, 1996.

Muecke MA: Community health diagnosis in nursing, *Public Health Nurs* 1(1):23, 1984.

Parker EA, et al: Detroit's East Side Village Health Worker Partnership: community-based lay health advisor intervention in an urban area, *Health Educ Behav* 25(1):24, 1998.

Pew Health Professions Commission: *Critical challenges: revitalizing the health professions for the twenty-first century,* San Francisco, 1995, University of California–San Francisco Center for the Health Professions.

Rogers E: *Diffusion of innovations,* ed 4, New York, 1995, Free Press.

Ryan W: *Blaming the victim,* New York, 1976, Vintage Books.

Schulz AJ, et al: "It's a 24-hour thing . . . a living-for-each-other concept": identity, networks, and community in an urban village health worker project, *Health Educ Behav* 24(4):465, 1997.

Shiell A, Hawe P: Health promotion community development and the tyranny of individualism, *Health Econ* 5(3):241, 1996.

Stanhope M, Knollmueller R: *Handbook of community-based and home health nursing practice,* ed 3, St Louis, 2000, Mosby.

U.S. Department of Health and Human Services: *Healthy people 2000: national health promotion and disease preventive objectives,* Washington, DC, 1991, U.S. Department of Health and Human Services.

U.S. Department of Health and Human Services: *Healthy people 2010,* Washington, D.C., 2000, U.S. Department of Health and Human Services.

Wallace DC, Hirst PK: Community-based service use among the young, middle, and old old, *Public Health Nurs* 13(4):286, 1996.

World Health Organization: Community health nursing: report of a WHO expert committee, *Tech Rep Series* no 558, Geneva, Switzerland, 1974, World Health Organization.

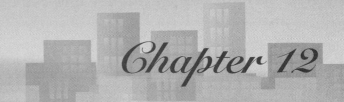

Chapter 12

Case Management

ANN H. CARY

Objectives

After reading this chapter, the student should be able to:
- Distinguish between continuity of care, care management, case management, and advocacy.
- Describe the scope of practice, roles, and functions of a case manager.
- Compare and contrast the nursing process with the process of case management.

- Identify methods to manage conflict and the process of achieving collaboration.
- Define and explain the legal and ethical issues confronting case managers.
- Identify the relationship between advocacy and case management.

Chapter Outline

Concepts of Case Management
    Definitions of Case Management
    Healthy People 2010 and the Case Management
       Process
    Case Management and the Nursing Process
    Characteristics and Roles
    Knowledge and Skill Requirements
    Tools of Case Managers
Community Models of Case Management

Advocacy, Conflict Management, and Collaboration
Skills for Case Managers
    Advocacy
    Conflict Management
    Collaboration
Issues in Case Management
    Legal Issues
    Ethical Issues

Key Terms

advocacy: activities for the purpose of protecting the rights of others while supporting the client's responsibility for self-determination; involves informing, supporting, and affirming a client's self-determination in health care decisions.

affirming: ratifying, asserting, or giving strength to the declarations of self or others.

aggregate: populations or defined groups.

assertiveness: the ability to state one's own needs.

autonomy: freedom of action as chosen by an individual.

beneficence: ethical principle stating that one should do good and prevent or avoid doing harm.

CareMaps tool: a tool developed by Zander showing cause and effect and identifying expected client/family and staff behaviors against a timeline. It has four components: index

of problems with intermediate and outcome criteria, timeline, critical path, and variance record.

care management: a program or process which established systems and monitors the health status of individuals, families, and/or groups. The program or process develops planning and intervention activities as well as targeted evaluation outcomes for the client and program.

case management: includes the activities implemented with individual clients in the system. The case manager builds on the basic functions of the traditional role and adapts new competencies for managing transition from one part of the system to another or to home, wellness and prevention, and multidisciplinary teams. Specialty case management by masters-prepared clinical nurse specialists is an emerging role in this field.

Continued

collaboration: mutual sharing and working together to achieve common goals in such a way that all persons or groups are recognized and growth is enhanced.

conflict management: a process of assisting clients in resolving issues between competing needs and resources.

constituency: a group or body that patronizes, supports, or offers representation.

cooperation: working together or associating with others for common benefit; a common effort.

coordinating: conscious activity of assembling and directing the work efforts of a group of health providers so that they can function harmoniously in the attainment of the objective of client care.

critical paths: a planning technique that focuses on activities, best use of time and resources, and estimated time to complete activities. The technique can be used for planning programs or individual client care as it is related to a specific diagnosis.

demand management: a program that provides to consumers, at the point at which they are deciding how to enter the health care system, information and support to access care. A telephone clinical triage system provides nurses to talk to clients about their presenting problem and provide advice and coordination of care.

disease management: a proactive treatment approach focused on a specific diagnosis that seeks to manage a chronic health condition and minimize acute episodes in a population.

informing: a communication process in which the nurse interprets facts and shares knowledge with clients.

intercessor: one who acts on behalf of the client when the client could act for self.

intermediate criteria: incremental incidents that serve to monitor progress toward outcomes.

justice: ethical principle that claims that equals should be treated equally and those who are unequal should be treated differently according to their differences.

liability: an obligation one has incurred or might incur through any act or failure to act, or responsibility for conduct falling below a certain standard that is the cause of client injury.

mediator: a role in which the nurse acts to assist parties to understand each other's concerns and to determine their conclusion of the issues. The mediator has no authority to decide on behalf of another.

negotiating: working with others in a formal way to achieve agreement on areas of conflict, using principles of communication, conflict resolution, and assertiveness. Negotiation may be relatively informal, as when two staff members negotiate which vacation times each will have. It may also be formal, as when labor and management negotiate a contract in a unionized environment.

outcome criteria: measurable ends to be achieved based on the problems presented by the client's condition of health or illness.

problem-purpose-expansion method: a way to broaden limited thinking that involves restating the problem and expanding the problem statement so that different solutions can be generated.

problem solving: a process of seeking to find solutions to situations that present difficulty or uncertainty.

promoter: an advocacy role in which the nurse partners with the client and promotes the client's rights to make his or her own decision.

supporting: upholding the client in making decisions about care or entering the health care system.

telehealth: an organized health care delivery approach to do triage and provide advice, counseling, and referral for a client's health problem using phones or computers with cameras. The client is usually in the home and the nurse is at an office, health care facility, or phone bank location.

timelines: landmarks of an episode of health or illness care from initial encounter to the transfer of accountability to the client or another health care agency.

use management: a continual process of evaluating the appropriateness, necessity, and efficiency of health service over a period of time. Includes data obtained during preadmission certification, service delivery, and postdischarge periods to determine the extent to which the service meets established guidelines (May, Schraeder, and Britt, 1997).

variance: difference between what is expected and what is occurring with the client.

CONCEPTS OF CASE MANAGEMENT

Case management is a strategy that is used in an overarching process called **care management.** Care management is an enduring process in which a manager establishes systems and monitors the health status, resources, and outcomes for an **aggregate**—a targeted segment of the population or a group. Care management strategies were initially developed by health maintenance organizations (HMOs) in the late 1970s to manage the care of different populations while promoting quality of care and ensuring appropriate use and costs. Care management strategies include **use management, critical paths, disease management, demand management,** and **case management** (Box 12-1). Case management in contrast to the definition of care management is activities implemented with individual clients in the system. The case manager builds on the basic functions of the traditional role and adapts new competencies for managing transition from one part of the system to another or to home, wellness and prevention, and multidisciplinary teams. Specialty case management by masters-prepared clinical nurse specialists is an emerging role in this field.

The case manager is the architect for the target group's health in the care management delivery process. The building blocks that are used by the case manager include:

- Risk analysis
- Data monitoring for health indicators and differences of the group from the norm

- Epidemiologic investigation of causes of these differences
- Multidisciplinary development of action plans and programs
- Identification of case management triggers or events that promote earlier referrals of high-risk clients when prevention can have dramatic results (Qudah and Brannon, 1996).

Definitions of Case Management

A focus on collaboration is seen in the National Case Management Task Force definition: "a collaborative process which assesses, plans, implements, coordinates, monitors and evaluates the options and services to meet an individual's health needs, using communication and available resources to promote quality, cost effective outcomes" (Mullahy, 1998, p. 9). Case management is defined in the public health nursing literature (Kenyon, et al, 1990) as the "ability to establish an appropriate plan of care based on assessment of the client and family and to coordinate the necessary resources and services for the client's benefit" (p. 36). Case management is viewed as only one competency, or skill, that nurses need to provide quality care. Case management is identified as one of the eleven competencies for practice in community health nursing. Knowledge and skills required to achieve this competency include:

- Knowledge of community resources and financing methods
- Written and oral communication and documentation skills
- Negotiation and conflict-resolution skills
- Critical thinking processes to identify and prioritize problems from the provider and client views
- Identification of best resources for the desired outcomes.

Case management practice is complex because of the **coordinating** activities of multiple providers, payers, and

Box 12-1	Additional Definitions of Case Management Strategies

- *Use management* attempts to redirect care and monitors the appropriate use of provider care and treatment services for both acute and community/ambulatory services.
- *Critical paths* are tools that name activities that can be used in a timely sequence to achieve desired outcomes for care. The outcomes are measurable, and the critical path tools strive to reduce differences in client care.
- *Disease management* activities target chronic and costly disease conditions that require long-term care interventions (e.g., diabetes). These strategies address the entire cycle of a disease process typically incorporating primary, secondary, and tertiary care interventions and self-care activities.
- *Demand management* seeks to control use by providing clients with correct information to empower themselves to make healthy choices, use healthy and health-seeking behaviors to improve their health status, and make fewer demands on the health care system (Coleman and Zagor, 1998).

settings throughout a client's continuum of care. Care by many (the client, family, significant others, and community organizations) must be assessed, planned, implemented, adjusted, and based on mutually agreed-upon goals. Although the nurse may be employed and located in one setting, the nurse will be influencing the selection and monitoring of care provided in other settings by formal and informal care providers. With the use of electronic care delivery through telehealth activities, case management activities are now delivered via telephone, e-mail, fax, and video visits in a client's residence. They may also be delivered to a global network of clients located in different countries.

Briefly Noted

Although the activities in case management may differ among providers and clients, the goals are:
- To promote quality services provided to clients
- To reduce institutional care while maintaining quality processes and satisfactory outcomes
- To manage resource use through protocols, evidence-based decision making, guideline use, and disease-management programs
- To control expenses by managing care processes and outcomes

Modified from Flarey DL, Blancett SS (editors): *Handbook of nursing case management: health care delivery in a world of managed care,* Gaithersburg, Md, 1996, Aspen.

A particularly challenging problem is the fragmenting of services, which can result in overuse, underuse, gaps in care, and miscommunication. This may ultimately result in costly client outcomes. Case management in rural settings is more complex because of:
- Fewer organized community-based systems
- Geographic distance to delivery
- Population density
- Finances
- Pace and life-style
- Values
- Social organization differences from the urban setting.

Healthy People 2010 and the Case Management Process

Nurse case managers in their practices have as core values the goals of *Healthy People 2010.* Many of the interventions that nurses use with clients, as well as the design of the health care system and the number of covered lives in those systems, promote further progress in meeting the *Healthy People 2010* objectives. Case management strategies offer opportunities for nurses to help in meeting the objectives for specific population targets listed in *Healthy People 2010* (U.S. Department of Health and Human Services, 2000). The target populations include those who do not have access to health care and those whose life-style or health conditions

TABLE 12-1 The Nursing Process and Case Management

Nursing Process	Case Management Process	Activities
Assessment	Case finding, identifying incentives for clients, screening and intake, determining eligibility, performing assessment	Develop networks with clients; distribute written materials; seek referrals; apply screening tools according to program goals and objectives; use written and on-site screens; apply comprehensive assessment methods (physical, social, emotional, cognitive, economic, and self-care capacity); perform interdisciplinary, family, and client conferences
Diagnosis	Identifying the problem	Determine conclusion based on assessment; use interdisciplinary team
Planning/outcome	Establishing problem priority, planning to address care needs	Validate and prioritize problems with all participants; develop activities, timeframes, and options; gain client's consent to implement; have client choose options
Implementation	Advocating client's interests, arranging delivery of service, monitoring clients during service	Contact providers; negotiate services and price; coordinate service delivery; monitor for changes in client or service status
Evaluation	Reassessing	Examine outcomes against goals; examine needs against service; examine costs; examine satisfaction of client, providers, and case manager

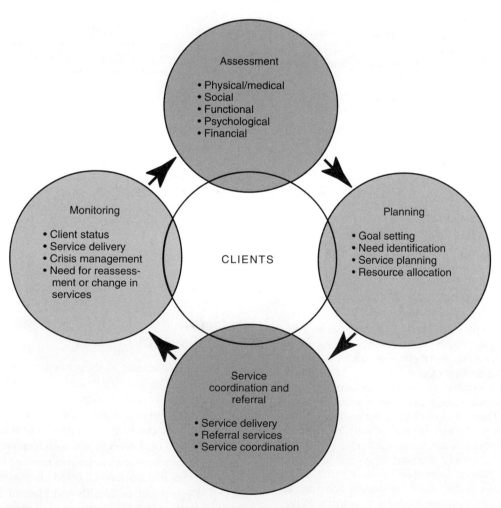

Figure 12-1   Core components of case management. (From Secord LJ: Private case management for older persons and their families, Excelsior, Minn, 1987, Interstudy.)

may limit the quality and length of healthy life; variables include minority race, low income, limited education, gender or sexual orientation, those living in the inner city or rural areas, those without health insurance, and the disabled or those experiencing chronic disease.

This chapter guides the reader through the nature and process of case management for individual and family clients. Case management has had a rich tradition in community health nursing while assuming more recent importance in the acute care literature (Cohen and Cesta, 1993). Nursing has maintained the leadership among health care providers in coordinating resources to achieve health care outcomes based on quality, access, and cost. As health care delivery moves to capitated financing with an emphasis on pursuing the most efficient use of services to manage client outcomes, case management emerges to play a strong role.

Case Management and the Nursing Process

Case management activities with individual clients and families will reveal the larger picture of health services and health status of the community. Through a nurse's case management activities, general community weaknesses in quality and quantity of health services often are discovered. For example, the management of a severely disabled child by a nurse case manager may uncover the absence of respite services or parenting support and education resources in a community.

Briefly Noted

Use the components of the nursing process when implementing the functions of a case manager with clients.

While managing the disability and injury claims at an industry, the nurse may discover that referrals for home health visits and physical therapy are generally underused by the acute care providers in the community (Table 12-1). Secord's illustration of case management (1987) remains an appropriate picture of the process that nurses use (Fig. 12-1).

Characteristics and Roles

Case management can be labor intensive, time consuming, and costly. Because of the increasing number of clients with complex problems in nurses' caseloads, the intensity and duration of activities required to support the case management function may soon exceed the demands that the direct caregiver can meet. Managers and clinicians in community health are exploring methods to make case management more efficient.

Coleman and Hagen (1991) and Cary (1998) have described the roles that case managers assume in the practice setting (Box 12-2). The roles demanded of the nurse as case manager are vividly influenced by the forces at work in the employing agency. Figure 12-2 presents factors that demand the attention of both the nurse and the client during the case management process.

Box 12-2	Case Manager Roles

- Facilitator: supports all parties to work toward mutual goals
- Liaison: provides a formal communication link among all parties concerning the plan of care management
- Coordinator: arranges, regulates, and coordinates needed health care services for clients at all necessary points of services
- Broker: acts as an agent for provider services that are needed by clients to stay within coverage according to budget and cost limits of health care plan
- Educator: educates client, family, and providers about case management process, delivery system, community health resources, and benefit coverage so that informed decisions can be made by all parties
- Negotiator: negotiates the plan of care, services, and payment arrangements with providers; uses effective collaboration and team strategies
- Monitor/reporter: provides information to parties on status of members and situations affecting patient safety, care quality, and patient outcome and on factors that alter costs and liability
- Client advocate: acts as advocate, provides information, and supports benefit changes that assist member, family, primary care provider, and capitated systems
- Standardization monitor: formulates and monitors specific, time-sequenced critical path and CareMap (see text) plans and disease management protocols that guide the type and timing of care to comply with predicted treatment outcomes for specific client and conditions; attempts to reduce variation in resource use; targets deviations from standards so adjustments can occur in a timely manner
- *Systems allocator:* distributes limited health care resources according to a plan or rationale

From Cary AH: Advocacy or allocation, *Nurs Connection* 11(1):1, 1998.

Box 12-3	Knowledge Areas for Case Management

- Knowledge of health care financing and of the finances of the client populations
- Clinical knowledge, skill, and maturity to direct quality-care activities
- Care resources for clients within institutions and communities
- Transition planning for ideal timing and sequencing of care
- Management skills: communication, delegation, persuasion, use of power, consultation, problem solving, conflict management, confrontation, negotiation, management of change, marketing, group development, accountability, authority, advocacy, ethical decision making, and profit management
- Teaching, counseling, and education skills
- Program evaluation
- Performance-improvement techniques
- Peer consulting and evaluating
- Requirements of client eligibility and benefits offered by third-party payers
- Legal issues
- Information systems: clinical and management

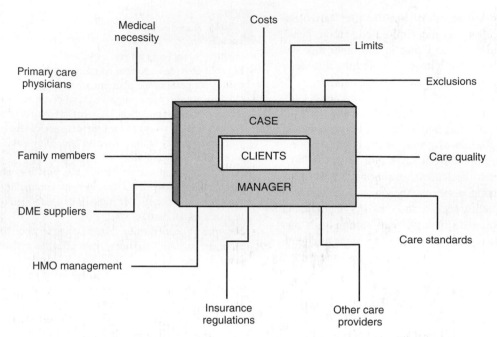

Figure 12-2 **Forces affecting solutions in the case management process.** (From Hicks LL, Stallmeyer JM, Coleman JR: *The role of the nurse in managed care,* Washington, D.C., 1993, American Nurses Publishing.)

Knowledge and Skill Requirements

Adopting the case management role for a nurse does not happen automatically with an agency position. Knowledge and skills that are developed and refined are essential to success. Bower (1992) suggests knowledge areas useful for nurses and the agency desiring to implement quality case management roles (Box 12-3). If a nurse seeks a case manager position, some of the skills and knowledge areas will need to be developed through orientation and mentoring experiences.

Telehealth is a contemporary intervention approach that is used by case managers. **Telehealth** is an organized health care delivery approach to do triage, provide advice, counseling, and referral for a client's health problem using phone or computers with cameras. The client is usually in the home and the nurse is at an office, health care facility, or phone bank location.

HOW TO Learn About Telehealth Interventions for Clients

1. Make it a point to learn how telehealth works in your community.
2. Consider telehealth as an option when considering available resources.
3. Seek continuing education on the art and science of telehealth application.
4. Seek networking opportunities with professional organizations and other case managers about the uses of telehealth.
5. Improve your personal interaction skills that will assist in decision making about the use of telehealth services.

From Wrinn MM: The emerging role of telehealth in health care, *Continuing Care* 17(8):18, 1998.

Tools of Case Managers

Case management plans have evolved with a variety of names and methods (e.g., critical paths, critical pathways, CareMaps, multidisciplinary action plans, nursing care plans, disease management). Regardless of the term used, standards of client care, standards of nursing practice, and standards of practice for case management serve as a core foundation of case management plans. Likewise, in multidisciplinary action plans, core professional standards of each discipline guide the development of the standards process.

Briefly Noted

The five "rights" of case management are right care, right time, right provider, right setting, and right price. How does the nurse judge the effectiveness of case management?

A critical path is a case management tool composed of abbreviated versions of processes that are specific to each discipline (e.g., nursing); it is used to achieve a measurable outcome for a specific client "case" (Zander, Etheredge, and Bower, 1987). *CareMaps* became the second generation of critical paths of care. As described by Zander and McGill (1994), A **CareMaps tool** is a "cause-and-effect grid which identifies expected patient/family and staff behaviors against a time line for a case-type or otherwise defined homogeneous population" (p. 4). The four components of the CareMaps tool are as follows (Box 12-4):

1. Index of problems with intermediate and outcome criteria
2. Timeline
3. Critical path
4. Variance record

Box 12-4 Four Components of CareMaps

- **Outcome criteria** are the measurable ends to be achieved based on the problems presented by the client's condition of health or illness.
- **Intermediate criteria** are incremental incidents that serve to monitor progress toward outcomes.
- **Timelines** are landmarks of an episode of health or illness care from initial encounter to the transfer of accountability to the client or another health care agency. The timeline plan can be in hours, days, weeks, or months.
- **Variance** is the difference between what is expected and what is occurring with the client. Cohen and Cesta (1993) describe variances as operational (broken equipment, staffing mix, delays, lost documentation), health care provider (variance in provider practice, level of expertise/experience), client (client refusal, nonavailability, change in status), and unmet clinical quality indicators.

Adapting the case management care plan is a crucial skill for standardizing the process and outcome of care. It links multiple provider interventions to client responses and offers reasonable predictions for the client's progress. Self-responsibility by clients truly links autonomy and self-determination as the core of case management. As a nurse employed to function as a case manager, ample opportunities exist to develop, test, and revise CareMap prototypes for specific client groups experiencing health deficits.

Disease management is a systematic program of services for all clients with specific conditions such as cancer, depression, asthma, or diabetes. Chronic disease clients are well suited to the benefits of a disease management approach to case management because the goals are to interrupt and prevent the continuing of a disease process using secondary and tertiary prevention techniques such as monitoring prescriptions, providing health education, and modifying health behaviors like diet. Promoting wellness is paramount to success (McClinton, 1998a). For case managers, disease management strategies shift the client-specific, episodic management functions toward holistic case-management functions that are proactive and client based (Ward and Rieve, 1995; Rieve, 1998).

COMMUNITY MODELS OF CASE MANAGEMENT

Carondelet St. Mary's, in Tucson, Arizona, has developed a community nursing network (CNN) in which 15,000 enrollees are distributed among 17 community health centers. Professional nurse case managers help older clients attain healthier life-styles and maintain themselves in the community. Nurses have been successful in delivering services at a cost of less than $5 per month per Medicare enrollee. Through nurse case management services, this nursing health maintenance organization (HMO) has cut the number of inpatient days per 1000 enrollees by one third at

Evidence-Based Practice

An experimental approach to case management was tested to discover the use of child health clinic and immunization services by 98 Medicaid infants from low-income families. The experimental case management condition consisted of a single public health nurse (PHN) providing both case management and preventive child health services. The control condition consisted of multiple nurse providers of child health services to an infant and the segregating of case management delivery from child health services delivery.

Data were collected from health department clinical records to document the PHN interventions, child health clinic visits, immunizations, and demographics. The health districts' protocols for case management of Medicaid infants and child preventive services were followed for the experimental and control groups. However, the infants in the experimental group received "continuous care" by one PHN, whereas the control-group infants received care from multiple PHN providers, or "fragmented care."

Differences between the preventive services obtained by infants receiving the two approaches were significant, although at the time of the study the sample's immunization rate of 62% was considerably below the national objective of 90% for 2-year-old children by the year 2000 (U.S. Department of Health and Human Services, 1995).

APPLICATION IN PRACTICE

Implications for nursing practice are as follows:
1. Case management delivery by a consistent provider who incorporates case management, delivery of preventive services, and home health visits can result in greater use of age-appropriate services by infants and their families.
2. The use of a consistent (singular) case manager can result in fewer nursing efforts (follow-up contacts) required to achieve adequacy of child preventive services.

Erkel EA, et al: Case management and preventive services among infants from low-income families, *Public Health Nurs* 11(5):352, 1994.

---

an average cost of $900 per day and a savings of $300,000 for every 1000 enrollees (American Nurses Association, 1993; American Nurses Foundation, 1993).

Statewide programs in New Jersey use case management methods to promote early identification, selection, evaluation, diagnosis, and treatment of children with potentially physically compromised needs. Local case management units provide coordinated and comprehensive care. Collaboration with existing local and regional agencies serving children supports this process. The nurse case manager performs the following services:
1. *Provides counseling and education to parents and children* on identifying problems and family knowledge level
2. *Develops individual plans including multidisciplinary services* (education, social, medical development, rehabilitation)

3. *Finds appropriate community services*
4. *Acts as a family resource in crises and when service concerns arise*
5. *Facilitates communication between child and family*
6. *Monitors services for outcomes* (Bower, 1992).

Liberty Mutual Insurance Company has used case management principles for more than 30 years in workers' compensation and has expanded services for employees whose conditions were noted as chronic or catastrophic. Box 12-5 lists examples of case-managed conditions. Case managers coordinate all providers, clients, and services to reduce excessive expenses caused by lack of coordination, failure to use quality alternatives, duplication, and fragmentation (Bower, 1992).

HOW TO Ensure High Quality for Clients

1. Provide access to easily understood information for each client
2. Provide access to appropriate specialists
3. Ensure continuity of care for those with chronic and disabling conditions
4. Provide access to emergency services when and where needed
5. Disclose financial incentives that could influence medical decisions and outcomes
6. Prohibit "gag clauses" that state providers cannot inform clients of all possible treatment options
7. Provide antidiscrimination protections
8. Provide internal and external appeals processes to solve grievances of clients

From McClinton DH: Protecting patients, *Continuing Care* 17(7):6, 1998b.

ADVOCACY, CONFLICT MANAGEMENT, AND COLLABORATION SKILLS FOR CASE MANAGERS

Three specific skills essential to the role performance of the case manager will be discussed: *advocacy, conflict management,* and *collaboration.*

Advocacy

For community health nurses, **advocacy** involves differing activities, ranging from self-reflection to lobbying for health policy. Advocacy is essential for practice with clients and their families, communities, organizations, and colleagues on an interdisciplinary team. The functions of advocacy require scientific knowledge, expert communication, facilitating skills, and problem-solving and affirming techniques. As the Code of Ethics for Nurses (American Nurses Association, 1985) states, "the goal of nursing actions is to support and enhance the client's responsibility and self-determination" (p. 1). The nurse advocate has been described in earlier writings

Box 12-5	Examples of Case Management Conditions

- High-risk neonates
- Severe head trauma
- Spinal cord injury
- Ventilator dependency
- Coma
- Multiple fractures
- Acquired immunodeficiency syndrome (AIDS)
- Severe burns
- Cerebrovascular accident (CVA)
- Amputation
- Terminal illness
- Substance abuse
- Transplantation
- Chronic diseases and disabilities

as one who acted on behalf of or interceded for the client. An example of the **intercessor** role is the community health nurse who calls for a well-child appointment for a mother visiting the family planning clinic when the mother is capable of making an appointment on her own. The contemporary goal of advocacy would direct the nurse to move clients toward making the call themselves.

The change over time in the advocacy role to that of **mediator** by the nurse advocate is described as a response to social change, reimbursers, and providers in the health care system. *Mediation* is an activity in which a third party attempts to provide assistance to those who may be experiencing a conflict in obtaining what they desire. The goal of the nurse advocate as mediator is to help parties understand each other on many levels so that agreement on an action is possible. In the instance of a nurse as case manager for an HMO, mediation activities between an elderly client and the payer (HMO) could accomplish the following results: the client may understand the options for community-based skilled nursing care, and the payer may understand the client's desires for a less restrictive environment for care. Although the case manager as mediator does not decide the plan of action (in contrast to the role of arbitrator), he or she facilitates the decision-making processes between the parties so that the desired care can be reimbursed within the range of options available to the client.

In today's practice the nurse advocate makes the client's rights the priority. The goal of **promoter** for the client's autonomy and self-determination may result in a high degree of client independence in decision making. For example, when a group of young pregnant women is the collective "client," or organization, the nurse advocate's role may be to inform the group of the benefits and consequences of breast-feeding their infants. However, if the new mothers decide on formula feeding, the nurse advocate should support the group and continue to provide parenting, infant, and well-child services.

A different perspective of the nurse advocate as promoter holds that the nurse's role as advocate may demand a vari-

Evidence-Based Practice

The study was designed to measure the effect of coping resources on the amount (hours) of help used by disabled elderly individuals in their homes. These resources enable the disabled elderly to continue living in the community and avoid or postpone nursing home placement. Based on a national sample of 4563 community-dwelling elderly who participated in the 1989 National Long-Term Care survey, the research showed that family help and living arrangements, more than income and public programs, kept elderly, disabled individuals in the community. Disabled elderly individuals with a network of family helpers and who lived with a helper received more in-home help than those living alone or without family helpers. The most important coping resources are a combination of family helpers and helpers that reside with the elderly.

APPLICATION IN PRACTICE

Implications for the case manager include the following:
1. The presence of a willing family caregiver provides more hours of care for a disabled elderly client and maintains the client in the community.
2. Even with cash income and third-party payments to obtain paid help, these effects are relatively smaller by comparison.
3. With reduced family network availability, more funding for paid help will be necessary to reduce institutionalization.

Boaz RF, Hu J: Determining the amount of help used by disabled elderly persons at home: the role of coping resources, *J Gerontol B Psychol Sci Soc Sci* 52B(6):S317, 1997.

TABLE 12-2	Nursing Process and Advocacy Process
Nursing Process	**Advocacy Process**
Assessment/diagnosis	Exchange information Gather data Illuminate values
Planning/outcome	Generate alternatives and consequences Prioritize actions
Implementation	Make decisions Support client Assure client Reassure client
Evaluation	Affirm client decisions Evaluate Reformulate

Box 12-6   The Information Exchange

Guidelines for exchanging information in the advocacy process include the nurse's responsibility to do the following:
1. Assess the client's present understanding of the situation.
2. Provide correct information.
3. Communicate with the client's literacy level in mind, making the information as understandable as possible.
4. Use a variety of media and sources to increase the client's comprehension.
5. Discuss other factors that affect the decision, such as financial, legal, and ethical issues.
6. Discuss the possible consequences of a decision.

ety of functions that are influenced by the client's physical, psychologic, social, and environmental abilities. The nurse adapts the advocacy function to the client's dynamic capabilities as the client follows a path to a healthy status. Examples of advocacy in such cases might include promoting a client group's access to onsite physical fitness programs in the occupational setting or supporting parents' and students' concerns about the high fat content of vending machine food in the school system.

Briefly Noted

For clients who have no health coverage or who do not qualify for other programs, pharmaceutical companies may have a program of free supplies of drugs. Call a pharmaceutical company for information on eligibility of your client.

Process of Advocacy

The goal of advocacy is to promote self-determination in a **constituency** or client group. It is often critical in promoting a client's self-determination. Table 12-2 compares the nursing process with the advocacy process. The constituency may be a client, family, peer, group, or community. It is often easier for the nurse to inform, support, and affirm another

person's decision when it matches the nurse's values. However, when clients make decisions within their value systems that are different than the nurse's values, the advocate may feel conflict. Promoting self-determination in others demands a philosophy of free choice. Communication that shows respect, endorses the client's self-determination, and strives to understand and establish the accuracy of clients' knowledge, beliefs, and behaviors is used through both processes. The process of advocacy involves informing, supporting, and affirming.

INFORMING. Knowledge is essential, but not sufficient, to the outcome of decision making. The interpreting of knowledge is affected by the client's values and the meaning the client assigns to the knowledge. **Informing** clients about the nature of their choices, the content of those choices, and the consequences to the client is not a one-way activity. Although the exchange may be initiated at the factual level, it will likely proceed to include the opinions of both parties—the client and the nurse (Box 12-6).

SUPPORTING. Upholding a client's right to make a choice and to act on the choice involves **supporting.** People who become aware of clients' decisions fall into three general groups: supporters, dissenters, and obstructors. *Supporters* approve and support clients' actions. *Dissenters* do not approve and do not support clients. *Obstructors* cause difficulties while clients try to implement their decisions. Cary (1998) points to the need for the nurse advocate to assure clients that they have the right and responsibility to make decisions and reassure them that they do not have to change their decisions.

AFFIRMING. **Affirming** is based on an advocate's belief that a client's decision is consistent with the client's values and goals. The advocate validates that the client's behavior is purposeful and consistent with the choice that was made. The advocate expresses a dedication to the client's wishes, and a purposeful exchange of new information may occur so the client's choice remains viable.

The importance of affirming activities cannot be emphasized strongly enough. The advocate's role in the decision-making process is not to tell the client which option is "correct" or "right." The advocate's role involves:

- Providing the opportunity for information exchange, giving clients the tools that can empower them in making the best decision from their perspective
- Enabling the client to make an "informed decision." This is a powerful tool for building self-confidence. It gives the client the responsibility for selecting the options and experiencing the success and consequences based on current data
- Empowering clients in their decision making when they can recognize events that are beyond their control and can link events that occur by chance with predictable events to make decisions they want.

Nurses can promote client decision making by:

- Using the information exchange process
- Promoting use of the nursing process
- Including written techniques (contracts, lists)
- Using reflection and prioritizing decisions
- Using role playing to "try on" and determine the "fit" of different options and consequences for the client
- Helping clients recognize the progression of activities they experience as they build their "informed decision-making base"
- Empowering clients with skills that can strengthen their autonomy and confidence in the future.

Advocacy is a process that requires a balance between "doing for" and "promoting autonomy." The process is influenced by the client's physical, emotional, and social abilities. The goal of advocacy is to promote the ultimate degree of self-determination possible for the client given the client's current and potential status: for most clients, this goal can be realized.

Systematic Problem Solving

The nursing process—assessment, diagnosis, planning, implementation, and evaluation—constitutes an example of a method of **problem solving** that can be used in the advocacy role. Advocates can be particularly helpful with clients in illuminating values and generating alternatives as described in the following paragraphs.

Box 12-7   Techniques of Generating Alternatives for Problem Solving

BRAINSTORMING

1. The nurse, client, professionals, or significant others generate as many alternatives as possible, without critical evaluation.
2. They examine the list for the critical elements the client seeks to preserve (e.g., environmental preferences, degree of control).
3. They analyze the list for consequences, the probability of chance events occurring, and the effect of the alternatives on self and others.

PROBLEM-PURPOSE-EXPANSION METHOD

1. Restate the problem.
2. Expand the problem statement so that different solutions can be generated. For example, if the problem statement is to convince the insurance company to approve a longer hospital stay, the nurse and client have narrowed their options. If the problem statement is to make the client's convalescence as beneficial and safe as possible, several solutions and options are available:
   - Obtaining skilled nursing facility placement
   - Obtaining home health skilled services
   - Arranging physician home visits
   - Paying for custodial care
   - Paying for private skilled care
   - Obtaining informal caregiving

ILLUMINATING VALUES. People's values affect their behavior, feelings, and goals. The advocate seeks to understand a client's values. The advocate's role is to assist clients in discovering their values, which can be particularly demanding in the information exchange and affirming process. One way to help clients state their values is through a process called clarification. A simple way to do this is to ask questions like:

1. What are 10 things that you enjoy doing?
2. What are the most important things to you in life (family, money, happiness, health, comfort, pleasure, recognition)?
3. How do you spend a typical day?

GENERATING ALTERNATIVES. Clients and advocates may feel limited in their options if they generate solutions before completely analyzing the problems, needs, desires, and consequences. Several techniques can be used to generate alternatives, including brainstorming and a technique known as the **problem-purpose-expansion method** (Box 12-7).

Impact of Advocacy

Clients are part of larger systems: the family, the work environment, and the community. Each system interacts with the client to shape the available options through resources, needs, and desires. Each system also has both confirming and conflicting goals and processes that need to be understood for client self-determination to be successful. For example, the practice of advocacy among minority groups may entail the ability to focus attention on the magnitude of problems caused by diseases affecting minority clients.

Box 12-8 Categories of Behaviors Used in Conflict Management

Competing: an individual pursues personal concerns at another's expense.
Accommodating: an individual neglects personal concerns to satisfy the concerns of another.
Avoiding: an individual pursues neither personal concerns nor another's concerns.
Collaborating: an individual attempts to work with others toward solutions that satisfy the work of both parties.
Compromising: an individual attempts to find a mutually acceptable solution that partially satisfies both parties.

Modified from Thomas KW, Kilmann RH: *Thomas-Kilmann conflict mode instrument,* New York, 1974, Xicom.

Whether the client is an individual, family, group, or community, the advocacy function can promote the interest of self-determination that characterizes progressive societies.

Advocacy is not without opposition. Clients and advocates may find barriers to services, vendors, providers, and resources. A community may experience a shortage in nursing home beds, a child care facility may experience staffing shortages, a family may not have the financial resources to keep a child at home, or a client may find that the school system cannot fund a full-time nurse for its clinic. The reality of scarce resources constitutes a difficult barrier for advocates. However, it is often events such as these that stimulate a community's self-determination to find innovative actions to correct gaps in service.

Conflict Management

Case managers help clients manage conflicting needs and scarce resources. Mutual benefit with limited loss for everyone is a goal of **conflict management.** Techniques for managing conflict include:

- Using a range of active communication skills directed toward learning all parties' needs and desires
- Detecting areas of agreement and disagreement
- Determining abilities to collaborate
- Assisting in discovering alternatives and valuable activities for reaching a goal.

Negotiating is a strategic process used to move conflicting parties toward an outcome. Parties must see the possibility of achieving an agreement and the costs of not achieving an agreement. Preparations must be made as to time, place, and ground rules concerning participants, procedures, and confidentiality. In a conflict situation, parties engage in behaviors that reflect the dimensions of assertiveness and cooperation. **Assertiveness** is the ability to present one's own needs. **Cooperation** is the ability to understand and meet the needs of others. Behaviors seen in conflict management are described in Box 12-8. The importance of the Thomas-Kilmann categories of behaviors noted in this box, although written some time ago, is that one can use a variety of behaviors that can be valuable in a given situation.

Clearly, flexibility in conflict management behavior can encourage an outcome that meets the client's goals. Helping parties navigate the process of reaching a goal requires effective personal relations, knowledge of the situation and alternatives, and a commitment to the process.

Briefly Noted

A client's health care benefit plan may omit treatments and services that, according to evidence, improve health outcomes. Other complementary health services (e.g., acupuncture) may be omitted from the benefit plan because the evidence to determine health outcomes is not available. What should be the case manager's role with the client, benefit plan administrator, and the provider when services are not eligible to a client from his or her health plan? Choose the most appropriate roles from Box 12-2.

Collaboration

In case management the activities of many disciplines are needed for success. Clients, the family, significant others, payers, and community organizations contribute to achieving the goal. **Collaboration** is achieved through a developmental process. It occurs in a sequence, yet it is reciprocal between those involved.

The goal of communication in the collaborative development process is to promote respect, understanding, and accuracy of communication of all team members' points of view. Although communication is an essential component in collaboration, it is not sufficient to result in or maintain collaboration. Although the collaboration model recognizes the contributions inherent in joint decision making, one member of the team should be held accountable for the outcome, and the client and the nurse should be responsible for monitoring the entire process. Box 12-9 lists stages of collaboration.

Teamwork and collaboration clearly demand knowledge and skills about:

- Clients
- Health status
- Resources
- Treatments
- Community providers
- Clients' and families' complex needs
- Intrapersonal, interpersonal, medical, nursing, and social dimensions
- Team member and leadership skills.

It is unlikely that any single professional has the expertise required in all aspects. It is likely, however, that the synergy produced by all involved can result in successful outcomes.

Briefly Noted

Family caregivers may be poorly prepared to assume high-technology care of the client at home. They often receive inadequate information about the client's illness, likely burdens and benefits of caregiving, financial consequences, and the complex and technical details of a plan of treatment.

Box 12-9   Stages of Collaboration

1. Awareness:
   - Make a conscious entry into a group process.
   - Focus on goals of convening together.
   - Generate a definition of collaborative process and determine what it means to team members.
2. Tentative exploration and mutual acknowledgment:
   - Explore options.
   - Disclose professional skills for the desired process.
   - Determine areas in which contributions cannot be made.
   - Disclose personal values reflecting priorities, including time, energy, interest, and resources.
   - Identify roles of each member.
   - Engage in mutual acknowledgment.
   - Clarify each member's potential contributions.
   - Verify the group's strengths and areas needing consultation.
   - Clarify each member's work style, organizational supports, and barriers to collaborative efforts.
3. Trust building:
   - Determine the degree to which reliance on others can be achieved.

- Examine congruence between words and behaviors.
- Set interdependent goals.
- Develop tolerance for ambiguity.
4. Collegiality:
   - Define the relationships of members with each other.
   - Define the responsibilities and tasks of each member.
   - Define entrance and exit conditions.
5. Consensus:
   - Determine the issues for which consensus is required.
   - Determine the process used for clarifying and decision making to reach consensus.
   - Determine the process for reevaluating consensus outcomes.
6. Commitment:
   - Realize the physical, emotional, and material actions directed toward the goal.
   - Clarify procedures for reevaluating commitments in light of goal demands and group standards for deviance.
7. Collaboration:
   - Initiate a process of joint decision making reflecting the synergy that results from combining knowledge and skills.

Modified from Cary A, Androwich I: A collaboration model: a synthesis of literature and a research survey. Paper presented at the Association of Community Health Nursing Educators Spring Institute, Seattle, June 1989; Mueller WJ, Kell B: *Coping with conflict,* Englewood Cliffs, NJ, 1972, Prentice Hall.

Box 12-10   Five General Areas of Risk for Case Managers

1. Liability for managing care (Hinden, et al, 1994)
   - Inappropriate design or implementation of the case management system
   - Failure to obtain all pertinent records on which case management actions are based
   - Failure to have cases evaluated by appropriately experienced and credentialed clinicians
   - Failure to confer directly with the treating provider at the onset of and throughout the client's care
   - Substituting a case manager's clinical judgment for that of the medical provider
   - Requiring the client or his or her provider to accept case management recommendations instead of any other treatment
   - Harassment of clinicians, clients, and family in seeking information and setting unreasonable deadlines for decisions or information
   - Claiming orally or in writing that the case management treatment plan is better than the provider's plan
   - Restricting access to otherwise necessary or appropriate care because of cost
   - Referring clients to treatment furnished by providers that are associated with the case management agency without proper disclosure
   - Connecting case managers' compensation to reduced use and access
2. Negligent referrals (Hyatt, 1994)
   - Referral to a practitioner known to be incompetent
   - Substituting inadequate treatment for an adequate but more costly option

- Curtailing treatment inappropriately when curtailment caused the injury
- Referral to a facility or practitioner inappropriate for the client's needs
3. Experimental treatment and technology (Saue, 1994)
   - Failure to apply the contractual definition of "experimental" treatment found in the client's insurance policy
   - Failure to review sources of information referenced in the client's insurance policy (e.g., Food and Drug Administration [FDA] determination, published medical literature)
   - Failure to review the client's complete medical record
   - Failure to make a timely determination of benefits in light of timeliness of treatment
   - Failure to communicate to the insured client or participant how coverage was determined
   - Improper financial considerations determining the coverage
4. Confidentiality (Scheutzow, 1994)
   - Failure to deny access to sensitive information that is awarded special protection by state law
   - Failure to protect access allowances to computerized medical records
5. Fraud and abuse (Sollins, 1994)
   - Making false statements of claims or causing incorrect claims to be filed
   - Falsifying the adherence to conditions of participation of Medicare and Medicaid
   - Submitting claims for excessive, unnecessary, or poor-quality services
   - Engaging in payment, bribes, kickbacks, or rebates in exchange for referral

---

Box 12-11   Elements That Reduce Risk Exposure

1. Clear documentation of the extent of participation in decision making and reasons for decisions
2. Records demonstrating accurate and complete information on interactions and outcomes
3. Use of reasonable care in selecting referral sources, which may include verifying of provider licensure
4. Written agreements when arrangements are made to modify benefits other than those in the contract
5. Good communication with clients
6. Informing clients of their rights of appeal

ISSUES IN CASE MANAGEMENT

Legal Issues

Liability concerns of case managers exist when three conditions are met:

- The provider had a duty to provide reasonable care
- A breach occurred through an act or omission to act
- The act or omission caused injury or damage to the client.

Case managers must strive to reduce risks, practice wisely within acceptable standards, and limit legal defense costs through professional insurance coverage (Box 12-10).

Legal citings related to case management and managed care include:

- Negligent referrals
- Provider liability
- Payer liability
- Breach of contract
- Bad faith.

As in any scope of nursing practice, proactive risk-management strategies can lower the provider's exposure to legal liability (Box 12-11). Sauc (1994) notes that court cases influence the legal considerations of case managers. When courts find that cost considerations affect medical care decisions, all parties to the decision will be liable for resulting damages.

Ethical Issues

Case managers as nursing professionals are guided in ethical practice by the Code of Ethics for Nursing (American Nurses Association, 1985) and the contract expressed in Nursing's Social Policy Statement (American Nurses Association, 1995, p. 4):

Nursing is a caring-based practice in which processes of diagnosis and treatment are applied to the human experiences of health and illness. Nurses are guided by a philosophy of caring and advocacy. Nurses have a high regard for patient self-determination, independence and informed choice in decision making. Recognizing that responses to illness and disability may limit independence and self-determination, nurses focus on the rights of individuals, families and communities to define their own health-related goals and seek out health care that reflects their values.

Box 12-12   Case Management Program Accreditation Options

In 2000, the American Accreditation HealthCare/Commission (URAC) began implementing accreditation standards for case management programs, which typically exist within managed care or free-standing companies. The accreditation establishes national standards for the structure and process of case management organizations. See the URAC website for the status of accreditation development and implementation.

(To access this and other websites, refer to the WebLinks on this book's website at www.mosby.com/MERLIN.)

This contractual philosophy of nursing practice is ideally suited to preserving the principles of **autonomy, beneficence,** and **justice** in case management processes. Banja (1994) describes how case managers may confront dilemmas in each of these areas.

- Case management may hamper a client's *autonomy* of individual right to choose a provider if a particular provider is not approved by the case management system.
- *Beneficence* can be influenced when excessive attention to cost supersedes or impairs the nurse's duty to provide measures to improve health or relieve suffering.
- *Justice* as an ethical principle for case managers considers equal distribution of health care with reasonable quality. Levels of quality and care among provider groups can be created when quality providers refuse to accept reimbursement allowances.

Maintaining familiarity with ethical issues published in the case management literature can offer specific assistance for practicing case managers. Box 12-12 and Table 12-3 list credentialing and accreditation options.

Clinical Application

During her regularly scheduled blood pressure clinic in a local apartment cluster, Mrs. Barnes, a 45-year-old woman, complained of feeling dizzy and forgetful. She could not remember which of her six medications she had taken during the last few days. Her blood pressure readings on reclining, sitting, and standing revealed gross elevation. The nurse and Mrs. Barnes discussed the danger of her present status and the need to seek medical attention. Mrs. Barnes called her physician from her apartment and agreed to be transported to the emergency department.

While in the emergency department, Mrs. Barnes manifested the progressive signs and symptoms of a cerebrovascular accident (CVA, stroke). During hospitalization, she lost her capacity for expressive language and demonstrated hemiparesis and loss of bladder control. Her cognitive function became intermittently confused, and she was slow to recognize her physician and neighbors who came to visit. The utilization management nurse contacted the case manager from the health department to screen and assess for the continuum of

TABLE 12-3	Credentialing Resources for Case Managers: Individual Certification Options	
Resource	**Contact**	**Certification Options**
National Board for Certification in Continuity of Care	(217) 245-7811	Multidisciplinary, A-CCC (Continuity of Care Certification–Advanced)
Healthcare Quality Certification Board of the National Association for Healthcare Quality	(818) 286-8074	Multidisciplinary, CPHQ (Certified Professional in Health Care Quality)
Rehabilitation Nursing Certification Board	(800) 229-7530	CRRN (Certified Rehabilitation Registered Nurse)
National Academy of Certified Case Managers	(800) 962-2260	Multidisciplinary, CMC (Care Manager Certified)
Commission for Case Manager Certification	(847) 818-0292	Multidisciplinary, CCM (Certified Case Manager)
Certification of Disability Management Specialists Commission	(847) 394-2106	Multidisciplinary, CDMS (Certified Disability Management Specialist)
American Nurses Credentialing Center	(800) 284-2378	Nurses, RNCm (Case Management)
Commission on Disability Examiner Certification (CDEC)	(804) 272-9192	Specialty certification for life care planners
Center for Care Management	(508) 651-2600	Case Management Administrators

(For further information, see the WebLinks on this book's website at www.mosby.com/MERLIN.)

care needs as early as possible because she lived alone and family members resided out of town.

It became apparent that family caregiving in the community could be only intermittent because members lived too far away. Mrs. Barnes had residual functional and cognitive deficits that would demand longer-term care.

As the case manager contracted by the plan, place the following actions in the order of sequence to construct a case management plan:
A. *Discuss with the family their schedule of availability to offer care in the client's home.*
B. *Call the client and introduce yourself as a prelude to working with her.*
C. *Obtain information on the scope of services covered by the benefit plan for your client.*
D. *Arrange a skilled nursing facility site visit for the patient and family.*

Answer is in the back of the book.

 Remember This!

- An important role of the community health nurse is that of client advocate.
- The goal of advocacy is to promote the client's self-determination.
- When performing in the advocacy role, conflicts may emerge regarding the full disclosure of information, territoriality, accountability to multiple parties, legal challenges to client's decisions, and competition for scarce resources.
- The functions of advocacy and allocation can pose dilemmas in practice.
- Skills important in fulfilling the role of client advocate include the helping relationship, assertiveness, and problem solving.

- Problem solving is a systematic approach that includes understanding the values of each party and generating alternative solutions.
- Brainstorming and the problem-purpose-expansion method are two techniques to enhance the effectiveness of problem-solving skills.
- During conflict, negotiations can move conflicting parties toward an outcome.
- Care management is a strategic program to maintain the health of a population enrolled in a health care delivery system.
- Continuity of care is a goal of community health nursing practice. It requires making linkages with services to improve the client's health status.
- As the structure of the health care system moves toward delivering more services in the community, the achievement of continuity of care will present a greater challenge.
- Case management is typically an interdisciplinary process in which the client is the focus of the plan.
- Documenting case management activities and outcomes is essential to community health nursing practice.
- Case management is a systematic process of assessment, planning, service coordination, referral, monitoring, and evaluation that meets the multiple service needs of clients.
- Community health nurses have within their scope of practice advocacy and case management functions.
- Nurses functioning as advocates and case managers need to be aware of the ethical and legal issues confronting their practice.
- Standardization of care for predictable outcomes can be achieved through critical paths, disease management protocols, and multidisciplinary action plans.
- Telehealth application provides new alternatives within resource delivery options but must be customized for clients.

What Would You Do?

1. Observe a typical workday of a community health or public health nurse, noting the types of activities that are done in coordination and case management and the amount of time spent in these areas. Interview several staff members to determine whether they perceive that the amount of their time spent in case management is changing. To what degree are the staff members involved in care management activities?

2. Initiating, monitoring, and evaluating resources are essential components of community and public health nursing practice. Describe a client situation and the case management process that might occur in the following practices:
   a. School nurse in an elementary school and in a high school
   b. Occupational health nurse in a hospital and in a manufacturing plant
   c. Nurse working in a well-child clinic

3. The values and beliefs held by a community health nurse influence the nurse's ability to be an advocate for clients. Discuss your values and beliefs about rationing health care and how they may affect your ability to be a client advocate.

REFERENCES

American Nurses Association: *Code of ethics for nursing,* Washington, D.C., 1985, The Association.

American Nurses Association: *Managed care: cornerstone for health care reform—a fact sheet,* Washington, D.C., 1993, The Association.

American Nurses Foundation: *America's nurses: an untapped natural resource,* Washington, D.C., 1993, The Foundation.

Banja JD: Ethical challenges of managed care, *Case Manager* 5(3):37, 1994.

Boaz RF, Hu J: Determining the amount of help used by disabled elderly persons at home: the role of coping resources, *J Gerontol B Psychol Sci Soc Sci* 52B(6):S317, 1997.

Bower KA: Case management by nurses, Washington, D.C., 1992, American Nurses Association.

Cary AH: Advocacy or allocation, *Nurs Connection* 11(1):1, 1998.

Cary A, Androwich I: A collaboration model: a synthesis of literature and a research survey. Paper presented at the Association of Community Health Nursing Educators Spring Institute, Seattle, June 1989.

Cohen EL, Cesta TG: *Nursing case management: from concept to evaluation,* St Louis, 1993, Mosby.

Coleman JR, Hagen E: Collaborative practice: case managers and home care agency nurses, *Case Manager* 2(4):64, 1991.

Coleman JR, Zagor KB: Effective care management, *Continuing Care* 17(7):23, 1998.

Erkel EA, et al: Case management and preventive services among infants from low-income families, *Public Health Nurs* 11(5):352, 1994.

Flarey DL, Blancett SS: Case management: delivering care in the age of managed care. In Flarey DL, Blancett SS (editors): *Handbook of nursing case management: health care delivery in a world of managed care,* Gaithersburg, Md, 1996, Aspen.

Hicks LL, Stallmeyer JM, Coleman JR: *The role of the nurse in managed care,* Washington, D.C., 1993, American Nurses Publishing.

Hinden RA, et al: Legal hazards on the case management highway, *Case Manager* 5(3):97, 1994.

Hyatt TK: Negligent referral, *Case Manager* 5(3):102, 1994.

Kenyon V, et al: Clinical competencies for community health nursing, *Public Health Nurs* 7(1):33, 1990.

May CA, Schraeder C, Britt T: *Managed care and case management: roles for professional nursing,* Washington, D.C., 1997, American Nurses Publishing.

McClinton DH: Promoting wellness, *Continuing Care* 17(4):6, 1998a.

McClinton DH: Protecting patients, *Continuing Care* 17(7):6, 1998b.

Mueller WJ, Kell B: *Coping with conflict,* Englewood Cliffs, NJ, 1972, Prentice Hall.

Mullahy CM: *The case manager's handbook,* ed 2, Gaithersburg, Md, 1998, Aspen.

Qudah FJ, Brannon M: Population based case management, *Quality Manag Health Care* 5(1):29, 1996.

Rieve J: Disease management concerns, *Case Manager* 9(2):34, 1998.

Saue JM: Legal issues related to case management. In Fisher K, Weisman E (editors): *Case management: guiding patients through the health care maze,* Chicago, 1994, Joint Commission on Accreditation of Healthcare Organizations.

Scheutzow SO: Confidentiality, *Case Manager* 5(3):108, 1994.

Secord LJ: *Private case management for older persons and their families,* Excelsior, Minn, 1987, Interstudy.

Sollins HI: Fraud and abuse, *Case Manager* 5(3):109, 1994.

Thomas KW, Kilmann RH: *Thomas-Kilmann conflict mode instrument,* New York, 1974, Xicom.

U.S. Department of Health and Human Services: *Healthy people 2000: midcourse review and 1995 revisions,* Washington, D.C., 1995, U.S. Department of Health and Human Services.

U.S. Department of Health and Human Services: *Healthy people 2010: national health promotion and disease prevention objectives,* Washington, D.C., 2000, U.S. Department of Health and Human Services.

Ward MD, Rieve J: Disease management: case management's return to patient-centered care, *J Care Management* 1(4):7, 1995.

Wrinn MM: The emerging role of telehealth in health care, *Continuing Care* 17(8):18, 1998.

Zander K, Etheredge ML, Bower KA: *Nursing case management: blueprints for transformation,* Waban, Mass, 1987, Winslow Printing Systems.

Zander K, McGill R: Critical and anticipated recovery paths: only the beginning, *Nurs Manag* 25(8):34, 1994.

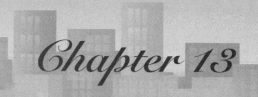

Chapter 13

Disaster Management

SUSAN B. HASSMILLER

OBJECTIVES

After reading this chapter, the student should be able to:
- Define natural and human-made disasters and epidemics.
- Evaluate the effects of disasters on people and their communities.
- Describe the disaster management phases of preparedness, response, and recovery, and explain the nurse's role in each phase.
- Describe the steps to initiate and maintain a disaster clinic.
- Identify how community groups and other organizations such as the American Red Cross can work together to prepare for, respond to, and recover from disasters.

CHAPTER OUTLINE

Disasters
    Defining Disasters
    Healthy People 2010 and Disasters

The Three Stages of Disaster Involvement:
Preparedness, Response, and Recovery
    Preparedness
    Response
    Recovery

KEY TERMS

delayed stress reaction: occurs after a disaster and can include exhaustion and an inability to adjust to post-disaster routines.

disaster: human-made or natural event that causes destruction and devastation that cannot be alleviated without assistance.

disaster medical assistance teams (DMATs): teams of specially trained civilian physicians, nurses, and other health care personnel who are sent to a disaster.

emergency support functions: the 12 functions used in a federally declared disaster; each function is headed by a primary agency.

Federal Response Plan: used in major disasters; has 12 emergency support functions, each headed by a primary agency.

human-made disaster: destruction or devastation caused by humans.

Level I disaster: massive disaster causing severe impact and damage; can involve several states. Typically results in a Presidential disaster declaration.

Level II disaster: moderate disaster that will likely lead to a Presidential disaster declaration.

Level III disaster: minor disaster causing minimal damage; could be declared an emergency or disaster by the President.

mitigation: actions or measures to prevent a disaster from occurring or to reduce the severity of its effects.

natural disaster: destruction or devastation caused by natural events.

preparedness: advance preparation to cope with a disaster.

response: organized actions to deal with a disaster.

recovery: the last stage in a disaster; when agencies join to restore the economic and civic life of the community.

triage: process of separating causalities and allocating treatment based on the victim's potential for survival.

Disasters are events that usually occur suddenly and unexpectedly. They seldom can be fully prevented, nor can they be adequately prepared for by those who will be affected. Accidents, acts of war or terrorism, or environmental mishaps cause disasters. While disasters are inevitable, it is possible to manage the ways people and communities respond. This chapter describes management techniques to be used in the preparedness, response, and recovery phases of disaster. The nursing role is discussed for each phase.

DISASTERS

Disasters can affect a single family or a small group, such as in a single-family fire, whereas floods, earthquakes, tornadoes, hurricanes, war, and acts of terrorism can kill thousands and cause huge economic losses. In a 10-year period, natural disasters cost more than $400 billion (United Nations Office for the Coordination of Humanitarian Affairs, 1998b). Even more devastating have been the three million people who have died in the past 20 years due to earthquakes, volcanic eruptions, landslides, floods, tropical storms, drought, and other natural disasters. In addition to these deaths, another billion people have coped with the injuries, disease, and homelessness that follow disasters (United Nations Office for the Coordination of Humanitarian Affairs, 1998a).

Unfortunately, developing countries experience a disproportionate amount of disasters. These countries are usually poor and have limited resources for dealing effectively and in a timely manner with the effects of the disaster. A person living in a developing country is twelve times more likely to die in a natural disaster than a person living in the United States. This is important since it is projected that by 2050, 80% of the world's population will live in developing countries (United Nations Office for the Coordination of Humanitarian Affairs, 1998a). Often, people who "live on the brink of disaster" every day, physically, emotionally, and/or economically, are among the first to be affected when disaster strikes.

Briefly Noted

Disasters create the most devastation in developing countries, where the death rate is up to twelve times higher than in developed countries. The poor suffer the most because their houses often are less sturdy and they have fewer resources to rebuild.

Population growth and overcrowding in cities has increased the danger of natural disasters since many people occupy areas vulnerable to disasters. Since more people live in "disaster-prone areas" of communities, insurance payments for victims have quadrupled each decade in the United States. It is projected that by 2050, at least 46% of the world's population will live in areas vulnerable to floods, earthquakes, and severe storms. Overcrowding and urban growth have also increased human-made disasters. Over-crowding can lead to community stress and stimulate civil unrest and ensuing riots. In some parts of the world people fight over land rights and access to natural resources such as oil and water.

Disaster recovery efforts are expensive, and costs are growing both because of the number of people involved and the amount of technology that must be restored. People in industrialized countries rely heavily on expensive technology and social and economic systems to meet their needs. When disasters occur, this expensive technology is often damaged.

Defining Disasters

A **disaster** is any human-made or natural event that causes destruction and devastation that cannot be alleviated without assistance. The event does not have to cause injury or death to be considered a disaster. For example, a hurricane may cause millions of dollars in damage without killing or injuring a single person. Box 13-1 lists examples of human-made and natural disasters.

While **natural disasters** cannot be prevented, much can be done to prevent further accidents, death, and destruction after the initial event. A concise, realistic, and well-rehearsed disaster plan is essential. There must also be open, clear, and ongoing communication among involved workers and organizations. In addition, many of the **human-made disasters** listed in Box 13-1 can be prevented (e.g., substance abuse can cause transportation accidents and fires).

Box 13-1	Types of Disasters

NATURAL
- Hurricanes
- Tornadoes
- Hailstorms
- Cyclones
- Blizzards
- Drought
- Floods
- Mudslides
- Avalanches
- Earthquakes
- Volcanic eruptions
- Communicable disease epidemics
- Forest fires (lightning induced)

HUMAN-MADE
- Conventional warfare
- Non-conventional warfare (i.e., nuclear, chemical)
- Transportation accidents
- Structural collapse
- Explosions/bombing
- Fires
- Toxic materials
- Pollution
- Civil unrest (e.g., riots, demonstrations)

The United Nations, an international agency located in Geneva, Switzerland, initiated a campaign to educate people on ways to reduce their risk of injury and death due to natural disasters. This campaign led to a heightened public-private partnering that emphasized **mitigation.** The term *mitigation* refers to actions or measures that can either prevent the occurrence of a disaster or reduce the severity of its effects (American Red Cross, 1998a). Mitigation activities include:

- Awareness and education—community meetings on disaster preparedness
- Disaster relief—building a retaining wall to divert flood water away from a residence
- Advocacy—supporting actions and efforts for effective building codes and careful land use.

Many national, state, and local agencies, such as the Institute for Business and Home Safety, American Red Cross, Centers for Disease Control and Prevention, and local communities of faith, came together during this internationally declared decade for disaster reduction to work proactively to save lives and property.

Healthy People 2010 and Disasters

Since disasters affect the health of people in many ways, they have an effect on almost every *Healthy People 2010* objective. Disasters clearly affect the objectives that relate to unintentional injuries, occupational safety and health, environmental health, and food and drug safety. They also affect the nutrition and exercise objectives but perhaps less so since the energy of those involved is more likely to be devoted to dealing with the emergency situation rather than the health-promotion aspects.

To ensure healthy homes and healthy communities, one objective of the national agenda is to:

8-21 Assure that state health departments establish training, plans, and protocols and conduct multi-institutional exercises to prepare for response to natural and technological disasters.

Community health nurses are often involved in managing and participating in community exercises to prepare for a community disaster.

THE THREE STAGES OF DISASTER INVOLVEMENT: PREPAREDNESS, RESPONSE, AND RECOVERY

Disaster management requires attention to all three stages of a disaster: preparation, response, and recovery. Figure 13-1 explains the disaster management cycle. In disaster **preparedness** the plan must be realistic, yet simple. The reason for this is that, first, no plan will ever exactly fit the disaster as it occurs, and second, all plans must be able to be implemented regardless of which key disaster team members are present at any given time ("Public health responds," 1994). The following section elaborates on all three stages, including the nursing role.

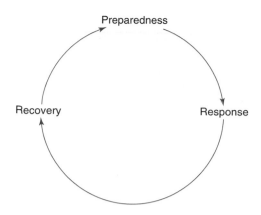

Figure 13-1   Disaster management cycle. (Modified from American Red Cross: *Disasters happen,* Washington, D.C., 1993, American Red Cross.)

Preparedness

Personal Preparedness

Nurses who are disaster victims themselves and are still expected to provide care to others will experience considerable stress (Chubon, 1992). Conflict between family and work-related responsibilities are inevitable. For example, a nurse who is also the mother of a young child will not be effective in her nursing role as long as her child care needs during the disaster are not adequately met. In addition, nurses who are assisting in disaster relief efforts must themselves be physically and mentally healthy. Unhealthy or sick disaster workers are of little service to their families, clients, and other disaster victims. Nurses must make personal and family preparations if they live in an area likely to be affected by a disaster, such as in a major earthquake fault zone, or if a disaster is anticipated, as in a hurricane that can be seen approaching a coast. Once nurses themselves are prepared, they are better able to help others in the community when the disaster does occur.

The American Red Cross (ARC) and the Federal Emergency Management Agency (FEMA), two well known authorities on disaster preparedness, response, and recovery have devised a personal checklist to help individuals and families prepare for disasters before they strike (Federal Emergency Management Agency and American Red Cross, 1992). Box 13-2 has an adapted version of their recommendations entitled *Four Steps to Safety.* Also, the box below lists emergency supplies that should be prepared and stored in a sturdy, easy-to-carry container. Important documents should always be kept in a waterproof container.

HOW TO Assemble Emergency Supplies Needed in Case of Disaster

- Three-day supply of water (one gallon per person per day) and food that won't spoil
- One change of clothing and footwear per person, and one blanket or sleeping bag per person
- A first aid kit that includes the family's prescription medicines

- Emergency tools including a battery-powered radio, flashlight, and plenty of extra batteries
- Candles and matches (kept in a waterproof pouch)
- An extra set of car keys and a credit card, cash, or traveler's checks
- Sanitation supplies, including toilet paper, soap, feminine hygiene items, and plastic garbage bags
- Special items for infant, elderly, or disabled family members
- An extra pair of eyeglasses
- Special items needed for pets (extra food, water, leashes, crates, blankets)

Briefly Noted

Is it reasonable for families to drop off chronically ill members, especially those with Alzheimer's disease, to Red Cross shelters for extended periods of time during the preparedness, response, and recovery phases of disaster?

Professional Preparedness

Professional preparedness requires that nurses know the disaster plans at their workplace and community. Nurses need to read and understand workplace and community disaster plans and participate in disaster drills and community mock disasters. The more adequately prepared nurses are, the more likely they can function in a leadership capacity and assist others to achieve a smoother recovery phase. Personal items that are recommended for any nurse preparing to provide professional help in a disaster include:

- Copy of their nursing license
- Personal equipment (stethoscope and flashlight with extra batteries)
- Cash
- Warm clothing and a heavy jacket (or weather-appropriate clothing)
- Record-keeping materials
- Pocket-sized reference books (Switzer, 1985).

Disaster work is not high tech. To do effective fieldwork, including shelter management, nurses need to be creative and willing to improvise in delivering care. Workers should be certified in first aid and CPR. In addition, the American Red Cross provides a comprehensive program of disaster training for health professionals to enable them to provide assistance both in their own communities and to other stricken communities and countries. The courses give nurses the tools to adapt their existing nursing skills to a disaster setting.

Community Preparedness

The level of community preparedness for a disaster is only as good as the people and organizations in the community make it. Some communities remain vigilant about the possibility that a disaster could hit their community. They remain prepared by having a written disaster plan and by participating in yearly mock disaster drills. Other communities are

Box 13-2 **Four Steps to Safety**

FIND OUT WHAT COULD HAPPEN TO YOU

- Determine what types of disasters are most likely to happen.
- Learn about your community's warning signals.
- Ask about post-disaster pet care (shelters usually will not accept pets).
- Review the disaster plans at your workplace, school, and other places where your family spends time.
- Determine how to help elderly or disabled family members or neighbors.

CREATE A DISASTER PLAN

- Discuss types of disasters that are most likely to happen and review what to do in each case.
- Pick two places to meet: outside your home and outside your neighborhood.
- Choose an out-of-state friend to be your "family contact" to verify location of each family member. After a disaster, it is easier to call long distance than locally.
- Review evacuation plans, including care of pets.
- Identify ahead of time where to go if evacuation is necessary.

COMPLETE THIS CHECKLIST

- Post emergency phone numbers by telephones.
- Teach everyone how and when to call 9-1-1.
- Determine when and how to turn off water, gas, and electricity at the main switches and who will do this.
- Check adequacy of insurance coverage.
- Locate and review use of fire extinguishers.
- Install and maintain smoke detectors.
- Conduct a home hazard hunt and fix potential hazards.
- Stock emergency supplies and assemble a Disaster Supplies Kit.
- Become certified in first aid and CPR.
- Locate all escape routes from your home. Find two ways to get out of each room.
- Find the safe spots in your home for each type of disaster.

PRACTICE AND MAINTAIN YOUR PLAN

- Review your plan every 6 months.
- Conduct fire and emergency evacuation drills.
- Replace stored water every 3 months and stored food every 6 months.
- Test and recharge fire extinguisher according to manufacturer's instructions.
- Test your smoke detectors monthly and change the batteries annually.

Modified from Federal Emergency Management Agency (1998) and The American Red Cross: *Your family disaster plan*, FEMA L-191, ARC 4466, Washington, D.C., 1992, The Authors.

less alert and depend on luck and the fact that they have never been affected before. Likewise, some community organizations are better prepared than others. Specifically, most health care facilities have written disaster plans and require employees to perform mock drills annually. In contrast, businesses typically do not have these requirements.

It is helpful for nurses to review the disaster history of their communities, including how past disasters have affected the community's health care delivery system and how their own organization fits into the plan. Understanding past disasters influences planning for future disasters. For example, disaster history may reveal that the local disaster services committee has not appropriately used the county's community health nurses due to lack of education about their roles. An effective disaster plan relies on the talents, coordination, and cooperation of many different people and organizations. Some key community organizations and professionals involved in disaster work include the clergy, morticians, police, fire and rescue personnel, the mayor and other city officials, and the media. Working cooperatively and with clear role definition before the disaster gives greater assurance that assistance will be delivered smoothly if a disaster hits.

Finally, communities need adequate warning systems, as well as a back-up evacuation plan to remove people from areas of danger even if they hesitate to leave their homes. Individuals must be convinced that pre-disaster warnings are official, serious, and personally relevant before they are motivated to take action. Also, some people mistakenly believe that past experience with a particular type of disaster is preparation enough for the next one. Others may refuse to leave their homes because they are afraid their personal possessions will be lost or destroyed in the disaster and/or from post-disaster looting. It often takes a face-to-face encounter with law-enforcement personnel or others in authority to convince people to leave their homes and retreat to safer quarters.

Role of the Nurse in Disaster Preparedness

Nurses can assist with preparation within the community and in their places of employment. At the place of employment nurses can help initiate or update the disaster plan, provide educational programs and material regarding disasters specific to the area, and organize disaster drills. The nurse can also provide an updated record of vulnerable populations in the community. For example, when calamity strikes, disaster workers must know what kinds of populations they are attempting to assist. If a tornado strikes a retirement village, the needs are much different than if the tornado hits either a church with predominantly young families or a center for the physically challenged. In addition to knowing where special populations exist, the nurse can educate these populations about what impact the disaster might have on them. Individualized strategies should be reviewed, including the availability of specific resources in the event of an emergency.

Finally, the nurse who leads a preparedness effort can help recruit others within the organization who will help if and when a response is required. Although there is no psychological profile of a disaster leader, it is wise to involve persons in this effort who have demonstrated flexibility, decisiveness, stamina, endurance, and emotional stability (Dinerman, 1990). The leader should also possess an intimate knowledge of the institution and a familiarity with the people who work there. Persons with disaster management training, and especially those who have served in "real" disasters, are valuable members of a preparedness team.

There are many roles in communities for nurses. As community advocates, nurses can help maintain a safe environment. Since disasters are both natural and human-made, the nurse working in the community needs to assess for and report environmental health hazards. For example, they should be aware of and report unsafe equipment, faulty structures, and the beginning of disease epidemics such as measles or flu. Nurses need to understand what community resources will be available following a disaster and exactly how the community will work together. A community-wide disaster plan helps nurses know what should occur before, during, and after the response, as well as their role in the plan. Nurses who want more knowledge and involvement in disaster management can become involved in a variety of community organizations that are part of the official response team, such as the American Red Cross, Salvation Army, or Emergency Medical System/Ambulance Corps. The American Red Cross has classes on Disaster Health Services and Disaster Mental Health Services in order to "help participants identify Disaster Health Services preparedness measures that should take place on the local unit level and to become familiar with Red Cross disaster health services policies, regulations, and procedures that apply on locally administered disaster operations" (American Red Cross, 1989, p. 5). The ARC generally requires certification in a Disaster Health Services or a Disaster Mental Health Services course before assigning someone to a disaster site as an ARC representative.

Nurses can work in various ways with official agencies to assist with disasters. Once nurses have had several hours of disaster training, they can do the following:

- Place themselves on a local disaster action team (DAT)
- Act as a liaison with local hospitals
- Determine health-related appropriateness for shelter sites
- Plan with pharmacies, opticians, morticians, and other health personnel ways to provide service for disaster victims
- Plan for and retain needed supplies
- Teach disaster nursing in the community.

It is important to keep nursing and medical protocols and intervention standards, whether they be with the Red Cross or an employing institution, up to date and consistent with local public health standards (American Red Cross, 1989). Finally, nurses can also assist with national and international disaster assignments as well.

Mass Casualty Drills or Mock Disasters

Mass casualty drills or mock disasters are key components of a preparedness plan. Whether the drills are done in a desktop manner or through realistic simulations, the objectives are to:

- Promote confidence
- Develop skills
- Coordinate activities
- Coordinate participants (Lehnhof, 1985).

It is critical that those persons who will be involved in the actual disaster be involved in the drill (Berglin, 1990). The drill leader needs to have special skills in disaster management and

TABLE 13-1	Disaster Preparedness Responsibilities by Agency		
American Red Cross	**Other Voluntary Organizations**	**Business and Labor Organizations**	**Local Government**
Participates with government in developing and testing community disaster plan	Collaborates in developing and maintaining a local Voluntary Organizations Active in Disaster group to identify roles, resources, and plans for disasters	Develops disaster plans for business locations and integrates their plans with the community disaster plan	Coordinates the development of the community plan and conducts evaluation exercises
Designates persons to serve as representatives at government emergency operations centers and command posts	Identifies and trains personnel for disaster response	Develops procedures to facilitate continuity of operations in time of disaster	Trains staff to carry out the plan
Develops and tests local Red Cross disaster plans	Identifies community issues and special populations for consideration in disaster preparedness	Develops plans for assisting business employees after a disaster	Passes legislation to mitigate the effects of potential disasters
Identifies and trains personnel for disaster response	Makes plans to continue to serve regular clients after a disaster	Identifies union and business facilities, resources, and people who may be able to support community disaster plans	Designs measures to warn the population of disaster threats
Collaborates with other voluntary agencies in developing and maintaining a local Voluntary Organizations Active in Disaster group to promote cooperation and coordinate resources and people for disaster work	Identifies facilities, resources, and people to serve in time of disaster	Provides volunteers, financial contributions, and in-kind gifts to Red Cross and other voluntary organizations to support disaster preparedness	Conducts building safety inspections
Works with business and labor organizations to identify resources and people for disaster work Educates the public about hazards and ways to avoid, prepare for, and cope with their effects Acquires material resources needed to ensure effective response	Educates specific client groups on disaster preparedness	Educates employees and union members about disaster preparedness	Develops procedures to facilitate continuity of public safety operations in time of disaster Identifies public facilities, resources, and public employees for disaster work Educates the public about disaster threats in the community and safety procedures

From American Red Cross: *Disasters happen,* ARC pub no 1570, Washington, D.C., 1994, American Red Cross. Used with permission of the American Red Cross.

the ability to coordinate many organizations at one time. Finally, although a successful disaster drill can allow participants to evaluate the rescue plan and make further recommendations, this should not create a misplaced sense of security (Waeckerle, 1991).

Agencies Involved in Disaster Preparedness

Many community agencies contribute to disaster preparedness. Table 13-1 lists the preparedness responsibilities assumed by the American Red Cross, other voluntary organizations, business and labor organizations, and local government.

Briefly Noted

The best time to start thinking about the lessons learned from a recent disaster is during the recovery phase of the disaster cycle.

Response

Levels of Disaster and Agency Involvement

There are many small disasters, such as single-family fires, and other more extensive disasters that do not require the assistance of the Federal Emergency Management Agency (FEMA). In this case, the ARC, along with other organizations such as the Salvation Army, work to assist disaster victims. In cases in which a presidential declaration has been made, the Red Cross works with FEMA personnel to assist with recovery efforts.

The level of the disaster determines the FEMA response. Levels are not determined by the number of casualties per se, but by the amount of resources needed. According to FEMA (1998), there are three levels of **response:**

- A **Level III disaster** is considered a minor disaster. This level involves a minimal level of damage, but could result in a presidential declaration of an emergency or a disaster. A minimal amount of federal involvement may be requested by state and local jurisdictions, in which case the request would be met by existing federal regional resources.
- A **Level II disaster** is considered a moderate disaster. This level will likely result in a major presidential disaster declaration, with moderate federal assistance. Federal regional resources will be fully engaged, and other federal regional offices outside the affected area may be called on to contribute resources.
- A **Level I disaster** is considered a massive disaster. This disaster involves significant damage, with severe impact or multi-state scope. These events result in a presidential disaster declaration, with major federal involvement and full engagement of federal, regional, and national resources. Hurricane George, a catastrophic disaster that devastated parts of the Florida Keys, Mississippi, Louisiana, Alabama, and Florida, as well as several other islands, in 1998, was a Level I disaster.

In any large-scale or major national disaster, not only do official agencies respond, but many concerned citizens, including health professionals, volunteer to help. At times, so many people come to help that role conflict, anger, frustration, and helplessness occur. Because of this, it is best that nurses attach themselves to an official agency with assigned disaster management responsibilities (Alson, Alexander, Leonard, and Stringer, 1993; Switzer, 1985). Table 13-2 lists the responsibilities assumed by the American Red Cross, other voluntary organizations, business and labor organizations, and local government when a disaster strikes.

The Federal Response Plan (FRP)

Once a federal emergency has been declared, the **Federal Response Plan (FRP)** (*Public Law 93-288*) may take effect depending on the specific needs of the disaster. The FRP is "based on the fundamental assumption that a significant disaster or emergency will overwhelm the capability of state and local governments to carry out the extensive emergency operations necessary to save lives and protect property" (Federal Emergency Management Agency, 1993, p. 1). Box 13-3 describes the purpose of the Federal Response Plan.

There are twelve **emergency support functions** (ESFs) in the FRP. Each function is headed by a primary agency. Each primary agency is responsible for coordinating efforts in a particular area with all of its designated support agencies. In all, 26 federal agencies and the American Red Cross must respond if called upon. For example, in a presidentially declared disaster, all ongoing health and medical services fall under the auspices of the U.S. Public Health Service. The U.S. Public Health Service divides its responsibilities among its own agencies as needed. The Centers for Disease Control and Prevention, for instance, may "assist in establishing surveillance systems to monitor the general population and special high-risk population segments; carry out field studies and investigations; monitor injury and disease patterns and injury control measures and precautions" (Federal Emergency Management Agency, 1993, p. ESF 8-10). Sheltering, feeding, performing emergency first aid, providing a disaster welfare information system, and coordinating bulk distribution of emergency relief supplies is the mass care ESF, of which the American Red Cross is the primary agency. Nurses can be involved with any of these response efforts within the local community or, with appropriate training, on a national basis.

The National Disaster Medical System (NDMS) is part of the ESF of Health and Medical Services. In a presidentially declared disaster, including overseas war, the U.S. Public Health Service can activate **disaster medical assistance teams (DMATs)** to an area to supplement local and state medical care needs. DMATs can also be activated by the Assistant Secretary for Health, upon the request of a State Health Officer. Teams of specially trained civilian physicians, nurses, and other health care personnel can be sent to a disaster site within hours of activation. DMATs can provide triage and continuing medical care to victims until they can be evacuated to a national network of hospitals prearranged by the NDMS (Federal Emergency Management Agency, 1993; Delehanty, 1996). In reality, because of the nature of this country's disasters since the initiation of the DMATs, these teams have been used primarily to staff community health outpatient clinics in the affected areas.

How Disasters Affect Communities

Community residents can be affected both physically and emotionally depending on the type, cause, and location of the disaster, its magnitude and extent of damage, its duration, and the amount of warning that was provided. For example, while an earthquake may not cause deaths, it may cause structural damage to buildings. Most injuries and deaths in earthquakes are due to debris falling from or inside of buildings. Fires can also be started by broken gas lines or damaged electrical wires. Landslides can be big problems in hilly areas (Van Arsdale, 2000). The continuous aftershocks from an earthquake can last for weeks and cause intense psychological stress. Also, the longer it takes to clean up and make structural repairs, the longer the psychological effects can last.

TABLE 13-2 Disaster Response Responsibilities by Agency

American Red Cross	Other Voluntary Organizations	Business and Labor Organizations	Local Government
Operates shelters	Provides services that are identified in predisaster planning	Takes action to protect employees and ensure the safety of the facility	Provides for coordination of the overall relief effort
Provides feeding services	Provides regular services to ongoing client groups	Advises public safety forces of hazardous conditions	Advises the public on safety measures such as evacuation
Provides individual and family assistance to meet immediate emergency needs	Identifies unanticipated needs and provides resources to meet those needs	Identifies resources such as union halls, generators, and heavy equipment to support the disaster response	Provides public health services
Services include providing the means to purchase groceries, clothing, and household items	Acts as advocate for their client groups	Provides volunteers, financial contributions, and gifts of goods and services to the relief effort	Provides fire and police protection to the affected area
Provides disaster health services, including mental health support	Coordinates services with all other groups involved with the disaster response		Inspects facilities for safety and health codes
Handles inquiries from concerned family members outside the area	Seeks and accepts donations from those wanting to help		Provides ongoing social services for the community
Coordinates relief activities with other agencies, business, labor, and government			Repairs public buildings, sewage and water systems, streets, and highways
Informs the public of available services			
Seeks and accepts contributions from those wanting to help			

From American Red Cross: *Disasters happen,* ARC pub no 1570, Washington, D.C., 1994, American Red Cross. Used with permission of the American Red Cross.

Box 13-3 Purpose of the Federal Response Plan

- Establishes fundamental assumptions and policies
- Establishes a concept of operations that provides an interagency coordination mechanism to facilitate the immediate delivery of federal response assistance
- Incorporates the coordination mechanisms and structures of other appropriate federal plans and responsibilities into the overall response
- Assigns specific functional responsibilities to appropriate federal departments and agencies
- Identifies actions that participating federal departments and agencies will take in the overall federal response in coordination with the affected state

The bombing of the Alfred P. Murrah Building in Oklahoma City in 1995 created extreme anger and grief, but this act of terrorism also led many to perform extraordinary acts of compassion (Walsh, 1995). Thousands of people helped, from donating blood and money to rescuing victims from the building, to volunteering for the "Compassion Center," a place where family members could go to receive support. One nurse, Rebecca Anderson, paid the ultimate price for her altruism. She was killed by a fall while attempting to rescue survivors inside the gutted building. In this terrorist act, nearly half of the occupants of the Murrah building died, 46% were injured, and only 9% were not harmed. The blast occurred at 9:02 AM, and only four live victims were rescued after 10:30 AM (Anteau and Williams, 1997). Although the worst human-made disaster in American history, the Oklahoma City bombing will also be remembered as the disaster that brought out the soul and character of the American people. Rescue efforts were prompt, and even the injured helped to rescue others.

In 1993, Iowa experienced the worst flood in its history. The flood was especially devastating for the homeless and migrant populations. The flood exacerbated pre-existing health problems and made it difficult for the health care system to meet the crisis level needs of the indigent. Because of the severity of this flood, the entire state was declared a federal disaster area, and subsequently, the Iowa Department of Public Health received a federal grant to develop a strategic plan that would identify the steps to take to better meet the primary health care needs of the migrant and homeless populations during any future environmental disasters. The plan was developed with data gathered during and after the flood and dealt with three critical areas: communication, health care delivery, and community (Washington, 1998).

Individuals react to the same disaster in different ways depending on their age, cultural background, health status, social support structure, and their general adaptability to crisis. Gerrity and Flynn (1997) state that the sequencing of reactions and level of intensity depends to some extent on the characteristics of the disaster such as the suddenness of impact, the duration of the event, and the probability that it could recur. The box below lists common reactions of adults and children to disasters. An extreme sense of urgency is the usual first reaction to a disaster (Chubon, 1992). Victims become obsessed with their personal losses. Other initial reactions include fear, panic, disbelief, reluctance to abandon property, disorientation and numbing, difficulty in making decisions, the need for information, seeking help for self and family, and offering help to other disaster victims (American Red Cross, 1991a). Disturbances in bodily functions, such as gastrointestinal upsets, diarrhea, and nausea and vomiting are also common (Gerrity and Flynn, 1997).

HOW TO Recognize Common Reactions of Children and Adults to Disasters

CHILDREN
- Regressive behaviors (bed wetting, thumb sucking, crying and clinging to parents)
- Fantasies that the disaster never occurred
- Nightmares
- School-related problems, including an inability to concentrate and/or refusal to go back to school

ADULTS
- Extreme sense of urgency
- Panic and fear
- Disbelief
- Disorientation and numbing
- Reluctance to abandon property
- Difficulty in making decisions
- Feeling of a need to help others
- Anger
- Blaming and scapegoating

DELAYED REACTIONS
- Insomnia
- Headaches
- Apathy and depression
- Sense of powerlessness
- Guilt
- Moodiness and irritability
- Jealousy and resentment
- Domestic violence

Anger, especially blaming and scapegoating, is common among victims soon after a disaster (Gerrity and Flynn, 1997). Anger and blaming often arise from an awareness of what has been lost, as well as from physical fatigue, emotional stress, and a continuing change in personal comfort. Often when victims are interviewed on television after a disaster they say that FEMA or the American Red Cross are simply not doing all that they can be doing. Later responses to disaster include difficulty in sleeping, headaches, apathy and depression, moodiness and irritability, anxiety about the future, domestic violence, feelings of being overwhelmed and frustrated, feelings of powerlessness over one's own future, and guilt over not being able to prevent the disaster (American Red Cross, 1991a). Chronic diseases may be exacerbated following a disaster. For example, the emotional stress of being a disaster victim may make it difficult for people with diabetes to gain control over their blood sugar levels.

Jealousy and resentment, even toward fellow victims, is not uncommon. Although typically the poor are the most severely affected disaster victims, a group of nurses in South Carolina, who were themselves disaster victims, became angry after Hurricane Hugo because the poor received more support and attention while they struggled for assistance (Chubon, 1992).

The effects on young children can be especially disruptive. Regressive behaviors such as thumb sucking, bed wetting, crying, and clinging to parents can occur (American Red Cross, 1991b). Children may have nightmares and even fantasize that the disaster really did not occur. Finally, children may have trouble concentrating in school and may refuse to return to school (Gerrity and Flynn, 1997).

An elderly person's reaction to disaster depends a great deal on physical health, strength, mobility, self-sufficiency, and source and amount of income (American Red Cross, 1993). They react deeply to loss of personal possessions because of the high sentimental value attached to the items and the limited time and perhaps money to replace them (Gerrity and Flynn, 1997). Anticipatory guidance may be needed to help the older person move to a nursing home, either temporarily or permanently, or make the adjustment of moving in with an adult child. Relocation will depend on the extent of damage to their home or their compromised health. The elderly may hide the seriousness of their losses because they are afraid of losing their independence (American Red Cross, 1993). Box 13-4 lists other populations who are at risk for severe disruption from a disaster.

Role of the Nurse in Disaster Response
The role of the nurse during a disaster depends a great deal on the nurse's past experience, role in the institution and community preparedness, specialized training, and special interest. The most important attribute for anyone working in a disaster, however, is flexibility ("Public health responds," 1994). If there is one thing certain about disaster, it is that change is a constant (Gaffney, Schodorf, and Jones, 1992).

There may be times when a nurse is the first to arrive on the scene. Should this occur, it is important to remember that

Evidence-Based Practice

The aftermath of a natural disaster presents many challenges to health care workers. Most epidemiological investigations following natural disasters have focused on physiological problems and infectious disease outbreak and containment. However, these investigations tend to neglect the long-term effects of natural disasters on affected populations, specifically, the long-term mental health effects. Two months after Hurricane Andrew struck Dade County, Florida, the Centers for Disease Control and Prevention (CDC) and the State of Florida surveyed the affected community to gauge various mental health indicators. As a result of this survey, a community outreach program for mental health and crisis counseling was initiated. The purpose of this study was to assess the effectiveness of this model for delivering mental health referrals to those experiencing long-term mental health effects as a result of a natural disaster.

The study found that certain households were more likely to experience symptoms of mental health distress. These households included those that had incomes less than $20,000; had trouble affording food; failed to see a doctor due to cost; had poor health; experienced a job change or job loss; had crime or violence in their community after the disaster, and those who reported that their living situation was worsened by the event. The hypothesis was that the community health outreach program would help families more easily find and access mental health services as compared to those who were not visited by an outreach team.

This study found that community health outreach teams were not an effective method of referring patients to mental health services. Of those contacted by the outreach teams, 70% received referrals or instructions on how to receive the mental health care that they needed. However, those households that were contacted by the team were no more likely than those households not contacted to be referred for help. This suggests that the goal of the community outreach team was not met.

APPLICATION IN PRACTICE

The authors of the study cited below suggest that alternatives to the community outreach team approach should be explored since this method is an expensive, labor-intensive intervention with limited benefit. For example, linking victims with familiar neighborhood organizations such as fire departments, schools, and churches might be an option. The long-term mental health needs of an affected community should not be neglected, and even though agreement is lacking on the most efficient, cost-effective model for referring people to necessary services, health care providers in post-disaster areas must continue to strive to ensure that all people receive the care they need.

McDonnell S, Troiano RP, Barker N, Noji E, Hlady WG, Hopkins R: Long-term effects of hurricane Andrew: revisiting mental health indicators, *Disasters* 19(3):235-246, 1995.

Box 13-4	Special Population Groups at Greatest Risk for Disruption From a Disaster

- Persons with disabilities
- Persons living on a low income, including the homeless
- Non-English speaking persons and refugees
- Persons living alone
- Single-parent families
- Persons new to the area
- Institutionalized or chronically mental ill individuals
- Previous disaster victims or victims of traumatic events

1986). Second priority is given to victims whose injuries have systemic complications that are not yet life threatening. Patients considered second in priority should be able to wait up to 45 to 60 minutes for treatment. Last priority is given to victims with local injuries who do not have immediate complications and who can wait several hours for medical attention.

Nurses working as members of an assessment team are responsible for feeding back accurate information to relief managers to facilitate rapid rescue and recovery. Often nurses need to make home visits to gather additional information. Types of information included in initial assessment reports include:

- Geographic extent of disaster's impact
- Population at risk or affected
- Presence of continuing hazards
- Injuries and deaths
- Availability of shelter
- Current level of sanitation
- Status of health care infrastructure (Lillibridge, Noji, and Fredrick, 1993).

These assessments help to match available resources to a population's emergency needs. Also, disaster assessment priorities are related to the type of disaster that has occurred (Lillibridge, Noji, and Fredrick, 1993). For example, sudden-impact disasters, such as tornadoes and earthquakes, are more concerned with ongoing hazards, injuries and deaths, shelter requirements, and potable water. Gradual-onset disasters, such as famines, are most concerned with mortality rates, nutritional status, immunization status, and environmental health.

Lack of or inaccurate information about the scope of the disaster and its initial effects adds to the misuse of resources. For example, after Hurricane Andrew, well-meaning citizens sent thousands of pounds of clothing to South Florida. Much more was sent than could be used. Consequently, a great deal of the clothing eventually had to be burned because there were inadequate on-site personnel to sort and distribute the clothing, and the surplus eventually became a public health nuisance. Local and regional emergency and public health resources can be readjusted as assessment reports continue to come in. The goal of triage is to prioritize needs to help the largest aggregate of imperiled individuals with the most correctable problems (Waeckerle, 1991). Ongoing assessments or surveillance reports are just as important as initial assess-

all life-threatening problems take precedence. Once rescue workers begin to arrive at the scene, immediate plans for triage should begin. **Triage** is the process of separating casualties and allocating treatment based on the victim's potential for survival. Highest priority is always given to victims who have life-threatening injuries yet have a high probability of survival once they are stabilized (Dixon,

ments. Surveillance reports indicate the continuing status of the affected population and the effectiveness of ongoing relief efforts. These reports continue to inform relief managers of needed resources. Nurses involved in ongoing surveillance use the following methods to gather information:

- Interview
- Observation
- Physical examination
- Health and illness screening
- Surveys (sample and special health)
- Records (census, school, vital statistics, and disease reporting) (Switzer, 1985).

Surveillance continues into the recovery phase of a disaster.

Shelter Management

Local Red Cross chapters are typically responsible for shelters. However, in massive disasters the military may set up "tent cities" if large numbers of people need temporary shelter. Nurses, since they are skilled in providing health promotion, disease prevention, and emotional support to aggregates, make ideal shelter managers and team members. While there may be physical health needs, especially among the elderly and chronically ill, many of the problems in shelters revolve around stress. Stress may be intensified by the shock of the disaster itself, loss of personal possessions, fear of the unknown, living in close proximity to total strangers, feelings of helplessness, and even boredom. The box below provides suggestions on how to relieve stress among victims.

HOW TO Relieve Stress Among Victims

- Listen to victims tell and retell their stories and express their feelings about the disaster and their current situation.
- Encourage victims to share their feelings with one another if it seems appropriate to do so.
- Help victims make decisions.
- Delegate tasks (reading, crafts, and playing games with children) to teenagers and others to help combat boredom.
- Provide the basic necessities (food, clothing, safe place to rest).
- Attempt to recover or gain needed items (prescription glasses, medications).
- Provide basic compassion and dignity (privacy when appropriate and if possible).
- Refer to a mental health counselor if needed.

From American Red Cross: *Coping with disaster: emotional health issues for victims,* ARC pub no 4475, 1991a, Washington, D.C., American Red Cross.

The American Red Cross provides specialized training in disaster mental health services to help workers or clients understand "disaster-related stress and grief reactions, develop adaptive coping and problem-solving skills, and return to a predisaster state of equilibrium or seek recommended further treatment" (American Red Cross, 1991c, p. 5). Highly trained mental health counselors are always available in major disasters. These include psychologists, psychiatrists, and psychi-

atric social workers and nurses. They are important members of any disaster team, no matter what the level of disaster, and they should be utilized as often as necessary.

Nurses are also involved in the shelter functions of assessment and referral, assurance of medical needs (prescription glasses, medications), first aid, meal serving, keeping patient records, ensuring emergency communications and transportation, and providing a safe environment (American Red Cross, 1989). The Red Cross provides training for shelter management and expects those trained to follow appropriate protocols.

International Relief Efforts

Disasters occur throughout the world. Countries, especially those involved with political upheavals, suffer not only from natural disasters, but from man-made disasters as well. Civil strife leads to war, famines, and communicable disease outbreaks. Sometimes disaster or relief workers are sent to international calamities at the request of the affected country's government. At other times workers are not welcomed, but instead may go with the support of the United Nations. When workers are not welcomed, their lives may be in danger, even though they go as peacekeeping agents of the Federation of Red Cross and Red Crescent Societies and the International Committee of Red Cross or as health representatives from the World Health Organization. International disaster or relief workers generally have intense training and preparation before embarking on a mission.

Psychological Stress of Disaster Workers

Disaster victims and workers often suffer psychological stress (Gerrity and Flynn, 1997). The degree of worker stress depends on the nature of the disaster, role in the disaster, individual stamina, and environmental factors. Environmental factors include noise, inadequate workspace, physical danger, and stimulus overload, especially exposure to death and trauma. Other sources of stress may emerge when workers do not think they are doing enough to help, from the burden of making life-and-death decisions, and the overall change in the living patterns of the workers (Laube-Morgan, 1992).

Symptoms of early stress and burnout include minor tremors, nausea, loss of concentration, difficulty thinking, and problems with memory (Laube-Morgan, 1992). Suppressing feelings of guilt, powerlessness, anger, and other signs of stress will eventually lead to symptoms such as irritability, fatigue, headaches, and distortions of bodily functions. It is normal to experience stress, but it must be dealt with. It is important to avoid denying the existence of the stress. The box lists strategies for how to deal with stress while working at the disaster.

HOW TO Deal With Stress While Working at a Disaster

- Get enough sleep
- Take time away from the disaster (e.g., take breaks)
- Avoid alcohol
- Eat frequently in small amounts
- Use humor to relieve the tension and provide relief

- Use positive self-talk
- Take time to defuse or debrief
- Stay in touch with people at home
- Keep a journal
- Provide mutual support

Delayed stress reactions, or those that occur once the disaster is over, include exhaustion and an inability to adjust to the slower pace of work or home (American Red Cross, 1991b). Other emotions, while out of the ordinary during normal times, may occur during a disaster. Workers may feel disappointed when their family and friends do not seem interested in what the worker has experienced or when the homecoming simply does not live up to the workers' expectations.

Frustration and conflict may occur if the worker's needs are inconsistent with those of family and co-workers or when the worker leaves the disaster site, when there remains a real or perceived belief that much more could have been done (Gaffney, Schodorf, and Jones, 1992). Issues or problems that once seemed pressing may now seem trivial. Anger may emerge if others present problems that seem trivial compared to those that were faced by the victims who were left behind. Disaster workers may fantasize about returning to the disaster site where they perceive they will be appreciated more than they are at home or the office. Finally, mood swings are common and serve to resolve conflicting feelings. Feelings or actions that persist or that the worker perceives are interfering with daily life should be dealt with by a trained mental health professional (American Red Cross, 1991b).

Recovery

Recovery, the last stage in a disaster takes place when involved agencies join together to restore the economic and civic life of the community (American Red Cross, 1993). For example, the government may lead the rebuilding efforts, while the business community provides economic support. Many religious organizations help with rebuilding efforts as well. The Internal Revenue Service educates victims about how to write off losses, and the Housing and Urban Development Department provides grants for temporary housing. The Centers for Disease Control and Prevention provides continuing surveillance and epidemiological services. Voluntary agencies continue to assess individual and community needs and meet needs as they emerge and as the agencies are able to do so.

Briefly Noted

Much of the destruction caused by natural disasters in the 1990s could have been avoided. In many documented cases, building codes were ignored, warnings were not issued or followed, communities were located in dangerous areas, and plans were forgotten. An "ounce of prevention" or preparedness could have made a big difference (Noji, 1997).

Role of the Nurse in Disaster Recovery

The role of the nurse in the recovery phase is varied, so flexibility remains important. Community clean-up efforts can cause a variety of physical and psychological problems. For example, moving heavy objects can cause back injury, severe fatigue, and even death from heart attacks. In addition, the threat of communicable disease will continue as long as the water supply is threatened and living conditions are crowded (Gaffney, Schodorf, and Jones, 1992). Nurses must continue to teach proper hygiene and make sure immunization records are kept up to date.

The prolonged effects of disasters can intensify both acute and chronic illness. The psychological stress of clean-up and/or moving can lead to feelings of hopelessness, depression, and grief. Recovery can be impeded when the short-term psychological effects of the disaster merge with the long-term results of inadequate living facilities and adverse circumstances (Richman, 1993). For some, stress can precipitate suicide and domestic abuse (Gaffney, Schodorf, and Jones, 1992). And, although the majority of people eventually recover from disasters, mental distress may persist in some vulnerable persons (Goenjian, 1993). Referrals to mental health professionals should continue as long as the need exists.

Nurses need to observe for environmental health hazards during the recovery phase of a disaster. During home visits the nurse may note situations such as a faulty housing structure or the lack of water or electricity. Dangerous objects can be blown into the yard from a tornado or floated in from a flood and need to be removed. Both live and dead animals can pose threats to the health of victims. For example, snakes are often found in and around homes as floodwaters begin to recede. Case finding and referral continue to be key actions during the recovery phase and for some time afterward. The American Red Cross supported the Bombing Recovery Project for 2 years after the Oklahoma City bombing of the Alfred P. Murrah Federal Building (American Red Cross, 1998b). Follow-up home visits were made for all those in need. For many disaster victims, the recovery process will last for years. In the end, all of the nurses and organizations in the world can only provide partnerships with the victims of a disaster. Ultimately, it is up to each individual to recover on his own.

Clinical Application

Paula, a nurse in a mid-size public health department in Lincoln, Nebraska, was asked to serve on her first national disaster assignment when a Level I hurricane hit the Miami, Florida, area. Paula was asked to help manage a shelter in an elementary school cafeteria in Homestead, Florida.

The devastation that Paula saw on her way to the school upset her. Assigned to help with client intake, she patiently listened to the disaster victims, referred many of her most distraught clients to the mental health counselor, and prioritized other needs as they arose. For example, she found that many of her clients had left their medications behind. Other needs included diapers and formulas for infants, prescription eyeglasses, and clothing.

As the days went on, the stress level in Paula's shelter began to intensify. The crowded living conditions and lack of privacy began to take their toll on the residents. By her tenth day Paula began having pounding headaches, and she was having a hard time concentrating. Paula thought she would be fine, but the mental health counselor said she was experiencing a stress reaction.

Which action would likely be the most useful for Paula to take?
A. Share her feelings with the on-site mental health counselor on a regular basis.
B. Call home to share her feelings with family members.
C. Meet the needs of her clients to the best of her ability and accept the fact that stress is a part of the job.

Answer is in the back of the book.

 ## Remember This!

- The number of natural disasters has remained constant over time, but the number of human-made disasters and ensuing deaths continues to rise sharply.
- The number of dollars it takes to recover from a disaster has risen sharply because of the amount of technology that must be restored.
- Professional preparedness entails an awareness and understanding of the disaster plan at work and in the community.
- To counteract a historical lack of use or misuse of nurses in disaster planning, response, and recovery, nurses must get involved in their community's planning efforts.
- Disaster health and disaster mental health training from an official agency such as the American Red Cross will help prepare nurses for the many opportunities that await them in disaster preparedness, response, and recovery.
- The response to a disaster is determined by its assigned level. Levels are not determined by the number of casualties per se, but by the amount of resources needed.
- Helping patients to maintain a safe environment and advocating for environmental safety measures in the community are key nursing roles during all phases of disaster management.
- Becoming knowledgeable about available community resources, especially for vulnerable populations, during the preparedness stage of disaster management will ensure smoother response and recovery stages.
- The Federal Response Plan may be activated if a disaster is so significant that it will overwhelm the capability of state and local governments to carry out the extensive emergency operations needed for community restoration. In all, 26 federal agencies and the Red Cross have specific functions to carry out in such an event.
- People in a community react differently to a disaster depending on the type, cause, and location of the disaster, its magnitude and extent of damage, its duration, and the amount of warning that was provided.

- Individual variables that cause people to react differently include their age, cultural background, health status, social support structure, and their general adaptability to crisis.
- Nurses who are both workers and victims often experience a great deal of stress.
- Disaster shelter nurses are exposed to a wide variety of physical and emotional complaints, including stress. Stress may be instigated by the shock of the disaster, loss of personal possessions, fear of the unknown, living in close proximity to strangers, and boredom.
- The degree of worker stress during disasters depends on the nature of the disaster, the worker's role in the disaster, individual stamina, noise level, adequacy of work space, potential for physical danger, and stimulus overload, especially being exposed to death and trauma.
- Symptoms of worker stress during disasters include minor tremors, nausea, impaired concentration, difficulty thinking and remembering, irritability, fatigue, and other somatic disorders.
- A key attribute in aiding disaster victims is flexibility.
- The recovery stage occurs as all involved agencies pull together to restore the economic and civic life of the community.

 ## What Would You Do?

1. If you thought your community might be a potential target for a hurricane, what steps would you take to adequately prepare for the possible disaster? Whose help would you enlist? Who would you consult for advice? Meet with two classmates and compare your answers in order to develop an action plan.
2. Assume that your community has the potential for a tornado to occur. Identify the population groups who would be most vulnerable. Who are they? What steps would you take in advance to reduce their risk? What community resources are available to help?
3. If you and your classmates witnessed a tornado moving across a small town as you drove to your clinical site, what steps would you take to determine if people were injured? What would you do first? Who else would you involve? Discuss your answers with a classmate to see where you agree and differ.

REFERENCES

Alson R, Alexander D, Leonard RB, Stringer LW: Analysis of medical treatment at a field hospital following hurricane Andrew, 1992, *Ann Emerg Med* 22(11):78-84, 1993.

American Red Cross: *Disaster health services I: Instructor manual,* ARC pub no 3076-1, Washington, D.C., 1989, American Red Cross.

American Red Cross: *Coping with disaster: emotional health issues for victims,* ARC pub no 4475, Washington, D.C., 1991a, American Red Cross.

American Red Cross: *Coping with disaster: returning home from a disaster assignment,* ARC pub no 4473, Washington, D.C., 1991b, American Red Cross.

American Red Cross: *Disaster mental health services,* ARC pub no 3050M, Washington, D.C., 1991c, American Red Cross.

American Red Cross: *Disaster mental health services I,* ARC pub no 3077-1A, Washington, D.C., 1993, American Red Cross.

American Red Cross: The American Red Cross and mitigation, *Disaster Services News Sheet,* Feb 3, Washington, D.C., 1998a, American Red Cross.

American Red Cross: Oklahoma city bombing recovery project. answering the call: Roberta Flynn offers encouragement to victims, *Disaster Services News Sheet,* Feb 27, Washington, D.C., 1998b, American Red Cross.

Anteau CM, Williams LA: The Oklahoma bombing: lessons learned, *Crit Care Nurs Clin North Am* 9(2):231-236, 1997.

Berglin SL: Emergency nurses in community disaster planning, *J Emerg Nurs* 16(4):290-292, 1990.

Chubon SJ: Home care during the aftermath of hurricane Hugo, *Public Health Nurs* 9(2):97-102, 1992.

Delehanty RA: The emergency nurse and disaster medical assistance teams, *J Emerg Nurs* 22(3):184-189, 1996.

Dinerman N: Disaster preparedness: observations and perspectives, *J Emerg Nurs* 16(4):252-254, 1990.

Dixon M: Disaster planning, medical response: organization and preparation, *AAOHN J* 34:580-584, 1986.

Federal Emergency Management Agency: The federal response plan (FRP) FEMA 229, Washington, D.C., April 1993, Federal Emergency Management Agency.

Federal Emergency Management Agency: *Job aid: disaster levels, classifications and conditions,* FEMA 9310.1-JA, Washington, D.C., 1998, Federal Emergency Management Agency.

Federal Emergency Management Agency (1998) and The American Red Cross: *Your family disaster plan,* FEMA L-191, ARC 4466, Washington, D.C., 1992, The Authors.

Gaffney JK, Schodorf L, Jones G: DMATs respond to Andrew and Iniki, *J Emerg Med Serv* 76-79, Nov, 1992.

Gerrity ET, Flynn BW: Mental health consequences of disasters. In Noji EK (editor): *The public health consequences of disasters,* New York, 1997, Oxford University Press.

Goenjian A: A mental health relief program in Armenia after the 1988 earthquake, *Br J Psychiatry* 163:230-239, 1993.

Laube-Morgan J: The professional's psychological response in disaster: implications for practice, *J Psychosoc Nurs* 30(2):17-22, 1992.

Lehnhof DB: Planning mass casualty drills. In Garcia LM (editor): *Disaster nursing: planning, assessment, and intervention,* Rockville, Md, 1985, Aspen.

Lillibridge SR, Noji EK, Fredrick MB: Disaster assessment: the emergency health evaluation of a population affected by a disaster, *Ann Emerg Med* 22(11):72-79, 1993.

McDonnell S, Troiano RP, Barker N, Noji E, Hlady WG, Hopkins R: Long-term effects of hurricane Andrew: revisiting mental health indicators, *Disasters* 19(3):235-246, 1995.

Noji EK (editor): The public health consequences of disasters, New York, 1997, Oxford University Press.

Public health responds to disaster: the Los Angeles earthquake, *The Nation's Health* 1, 6-7 March, 1994.

Richman N: After the flood, *Am J Public Health* 83(11):1522-1524, 1993.

Switzer KH: Functioning in a community health setting. In Garcia LM (editor): *Disaster nursing: planning, assessment, and intervention,* Rockville, Md, 1985, Aspen.

United Nations Office for the Coordination of Humanitarian Affairs. *Natural disasters and sustainable development: linkages and policy options,* 1998a, available online at http://156.106.192.130/dha_ol/programs/idndr/presskit/options.html

United Nations Office for the Coordination of Humanitarian Affairs: *The role of the insurance industry in disaster reduction,* 1998b, available online at http://156.106.192.130/dha_ol/programs/idndr/presskit/role.html

Van Arsdale SK: Earthquake: how will you respond? *Am J Nurs* 100(2):24A-24B, 2000.

Waeckerle JF: Disaster planning and response, *N Engl J Med* (324)12:815-821, 1991.

Walsh KT: The soul and character of America, *US News World Report* 18:10, 1995.

Washington GT: After the flood, *Nurs Health Care Perspect* 19(2):66-71, 1998.

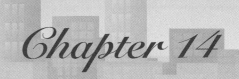

Chapter 14

Program Management

MARCIA STANHOPE

OBJECTIVES

After reading this chapter, the student should be able to:
- Compare the program management process to the nursing process.
- Understand the program planning process and its application to community health nursing.
- Identify the benefits of program planning.
- Understand the components of program evaluation and application to nursing practice.
- Identify an evaluation method.
- Name program evaluation sources.
- Describe types of program evaluation measures.

CHAPTER OUTLINE

Definitions and Goals

Benefits of Program Planning

Planning Process
   Basic Program Planning

Program Evaluation
   Benefits of Program Evaluation
   Evaluation Process
   Formulation of Objectives
   Sources of Program Evaluation
   Aspects of Program Evaluation

KEY TERMS

case register: systematic registration of acute, chronic, and contagious diseases.

community health index: a summary of the health features of a community that enables us to determine health care delivery needs.

evaluation: provision of information through formal means, such as criteria, measurement, and statistics, for making rational judgments about outcomes of care.

evaluation of program effectiveness: examination of the level of client and provider satisfaction with a program.

formative evaluation: an ongoing evaluation instituted for the purpose of assessing the degree to which objectives are met or activities are being conducted.

health program planning: five-step process of formulating a plan, conceptualizing, detailing, evaluating, and implementing.

needs assessment: systematic appraisal of type, depth, and scope of problems as perceived by clients, health providers, or both.

outcome: a change in client health status as a result of care or program implementation.

planning process: a systematic approach to selecting and carrying out a series of actions to achieve a goal.

program: a health care service designed to meet identified health care needs of clients.

program evaluation: collection of methods, skills, and activities necessary to determine whether a service is needed, likely to be used, conducted as planned, and actually helps people.

strategic planning: a process by which client needs, specific provider strengths, and agency and community resources are successfully matched to offer a service to the community.

summative evaluation: a method used to assess program outcomes or as a follow-up of the results of program activities.

Program management consists of assessing, planning, implementing, and evaluating a program. This chapter focuses primarily on planning and evaluation. Although presented in separate discussions, these factors are related and dependent processes that work together to bring about a successful program. This chapter does not deal with implementing programs because the majority of the chapters in the text focus on implementation.

The program management process is like the nursing process. One is applied to a program, whereas the other is applied to clients. The process of program management, like the nursing process, consists of a rational decision-making system designed to help nurses know:

- When to make a decision to develop a program
- Where they want to be at the end of the program
- How to decide what to do to have a successful program
- How to develop a plan to go from where they are to where they want to be
- How to know that they are getting there
- What to measure to know whether what they are doing is appropriate

There is more emphasis on accountability for nursing actions and client outcomes today. The introduction of prospective payment systems, health care reform, and managed care has changed the focus of nursing. Planning for nursing care delivery is necessary today if the nurse is to survive in the field of health care delivery. This chapter examines how nurses can *act* instead of *react* by planning programs that can be evaluated for their effectiveness. These programs may be single health-promotion programs for a client group or an ongoing program to provide health care services to a client group.

DEFINITIONS AND GOALS

A **program** is an organized approach to meet the assessed needs of individuals, families, groups, or communities by reducing or eliminating one or more health problems. Examples of specific programs in community health nursing are home health programs, immunization programs, health-risk screening programs for industrial workers, and family-planning programs. More broadly based group and community programs are the community school health program, the occupational health and safety program, the environmental health program, and community programs directed at specific illnesses through special interest groups (e.g., American Heart Association, American Cancer Society, March of Dimes).

Planning is defined as the selecting and carrying out of a series of actions to achieve stated goals (Kropf, 1995). The goal of planning is to ensure that health care services are acceptable, equal, efficient, and effective. **Evaluation** is defined as the methods used to determine whether a service is needed and likely to be used, whether it is conducted as planned, and whether the service actually helps people in need (Posavac and Carey, 1997). There are two levels of evaluation, which are defined in Box 14-1.

Box 14-1   Two Levels of Evaluation

Formative evaluation: evaluation for the purpose of assessing whether objectives are met or planned activities are completed. This type of evaluation begins with an assessment of the need for a program.

Summative evaluation: evaluation to assess program outcomes or as a follow-up of the results of the program activities.

BENEFITS OF PROGRAM PLANNING

Systematic planning for meeting client needs:

- Benefits clients, nurses, and the employing agencies
- Focuses attention on what the organization and health provider are attempting to do for clients
- Assists in identifying the resources and activities that are needed to meet the objectives of client services
- Reduces role ambiguity (uncertainty) by giving responsibility to specific providers to meet program objectives
- Reduces uncertainty within the program environment
- Increases the abilities of the provider and the agency to cope with the external environment
- Helps the provider and the agency anticipate events
- Allows for quality decision making and better control over the actual program results.

Today this type of planning is referred to as **strategic planning** and involves matching client needs, provider strengths and competencies, and agency resources. Everyone involved with the program can anticipate what will be needed to implement the program, what will occur during implementation, and what the program outcomes will be.

PLANNING PROCESS

Program planning is required by federal, state, and local governments; by charitable organizations; and by the employing agency. Planning programs and planning for the evaluation of programs are two very important activities, whether the program being planned is a national health insurance program such as Medicare, a state health care program such as early childhood developmental screening programs, a local program such as vision screening for elementary school children, or a health education program on diet and exercise for a group of obese clients. Regardless of the type of program, the planning process is the same.

Basic Program Planning

Definition of Problem and Need

The initial and most critical step in **health program planning** is defining the problem and assessing client need. The target population, or client to be served, by any program

---

Box 14-2   **Stages Used in Assessing Client Need**

Preactive: projecting a future need.
Reactive: defining the problem based on past needs identified by the client or the agency.
Inactive: defining the problem based on the existing health status of the population to be served.
Interactive: describing the problem using past and present data to project future population needs.

---

must be identified and involved in designing the program to be developed. Program planners must verify that a current health problem exists and is being ignored or being unsuccessfully treated in a client group. **Needs assessment** is defined as a systematic appraisal of type, depth, and scope of problems as perceived by clients, health providers, or both (Box 14-2).

Needs assessment includes six steps (see the box below). The *client* may be identified as a community or group, as families, or as individuals. The client should be defined by biological and psychosocial characteristics, by geographic location, and by the problems to be addressed. For example, in a community with a large number of preschool children who require immunizations to enter school, the client population may be described as all children between 4 and 6 years of age residing in Central County who have not had up-to-date immunizations.

A health education program may be necessary to alert the population to the existing need. In the example of the need for immunization of preschool children, public service

HOW TO Develop a Program Plan

A. Describe the problem and need.
  1. Assess client need.
    a. Who is the client?
    b. What is the need to be met?
    c. How large is the client population to be served?
    d. Where are they located?
    e. Are there other programs addressing the same need? (describe)
    f. Why is the need not being met?
  2. Establish program boundaries.
    a. Who will be included in the program?
    b. Who will not be included? Why?
    c. What is the program goal?
  3. Program feasibility.
    a. Who agrees that the program is needed (administrators, providers, clients, funders)?
    b. Who does not agree?
  4. Resources (general).
    a. What personnel are needed? What personnel are available?
    b. What facilities are needed? What facilities are available?
    c. What equipment is needed? What equipment is available?
    d. Is money needed? Is money available?
    e. Are resources (printing, paper, medical supplies) being donated?
      (1) Type.
      (2) Amount.
  5. Tools used to assess need.
    a. Census data.
    b. Key informants.
    c. Community forums.
    d. Existing program surveys.
    e. Surveys of client population.
    f. Statistical indicators (e.g., morbidity/mortality data).
B. Name the problem.
  1. List the potential solutions to the problem.
  2. What are the risks of each solution?
  3. What are the consequences?
  4. What are the outcomes to be gained from the solutions?
  5. Draw a decision tree to show the problem-solving process used.
C. Identify objectives and activities for alternatives.
  1. What are the objectives for each solution to meet the program goal?
  2. What activities will be done to conduct each of the alternative solutions listed under B1 and based on objectives?
  3. What are the differences in the resources needed for each of the alternative solutions?
  4. Which of the alternative solutions would be chosen if the resources described under A4 were the only resources available?
D. Evaluate problem solutions.
  1. Which of the alternative solutions is most acceptable to:
    a. The clients
    b. The agency administrator
    c. You
    d. The community
  2. Which of the alternative solutions appears to have the most benefits to:
    a. The clients
    b. The agency administrator
    c. You
    d. The community
  3. Based on costs, which alternative solution would be chosen by:
    a. The clients
    b. The agency administrator
    c. You
    d. The community
E. Choose the program solution.
  1. Based on the data collected, which of the solutions has been chosen?
  2. Why should the agency administrator approve your request? Give your rationale.
  3. When can the program begin? Give the specific date.

announcements on television and radio and in newspapers may be used to alert parents to laws requiring immunizations, to the problems of communicable diseases, and to which communicable diseases, such as smallpox, that have been successfully eradicated by immunization programs. A good example of the use of media is the 1990 outbreak of rubella in Los Angeles. Local and national television was used to bring attention to the problem, to encourage parents to have children immunized, and to encourage other communities to launch campaigns to prevent other outbreaks.

Briefly Noted

The needs to be met for the client population must be identified by both the client and the health provider. If the client population does not recognize the need, the program will usually fail.

The size and location of a client population for a program involves more than counting the number of persons in the community who may be eligible for the program. More specifically, it involves defining the number of persons with the problem who are unserved by existing programs and the number of eligible persons who have and have not taken advantage of existing services. For example, consider again the community need for a preschool immunization program. In planning the program, the estimates of numbers of preschool children in the county may be obtained from census data or birth certificates. The nurse then must determine the number of children unserved and the number of children who have not used services for which they are eligible.

Boundaries for the client population are established by defining the size and location of the client population. The boundaries will stipulate who is included in the health program and who is excluded. If the fictional immunization program were designed to serve only preschool children of low-income families, all other preschool children would be excluded.

What people think about the need for a program, or *program feasibility*, might differ among health providers, agency administrators, policy makers, and potential clients. Collecting data on the opinions and attitudes of all persons directly or indirectly involved with the program's success is necessary to determine the program's feasibility, the need to redefine the problem, or the decision to develop a new program or expand an existing program. For example, policy makers in the 1970s decided that neighborhood health clinics were the answer to providing service for low-income residents. They discovered that their opinions were not the same as those of most health providers or clients who were not supportive of developing neighborhood clinics. The neighborhood health clinics failed because the clients would not use them. If the policy makers had explored the ideas of the clients when planning the program, they might have chosen another type of service to offer.

Before implementing a health program, one must also *identify available resources*. Program resources include personnel, facilities, equipment, and financing. If any one of the four categories of resources is unavailable, the program is likely to be inadequate to meet the needs of the client population.

A number of *needs assessment tools* exist to assist the nurse in the needs assessment process. The major tools used for needs assessment, summarized in Table 14-1, are census data, key informants, community forums, surveys of existing community agencies with similar programs, surveys of residents of the community to be served (client population), and statistical indicators (Rossi and Freeman, 1999).

NAME THE PROBLEM. The need and demand for a program are determined by working with the client. This stage of planning creates options for solving the problem and considers several solutions. Each option for program solution is examined for its uncertainties (risks) and consequences, leading to a set of **outcomes.**

Considering alternative solutions to the problem, some will have more risks or uncertainties than others.

- The nurse must decide between the solution that involves more risk and the solution that is free of risk.
- A "do nothing" decision is always the decision with the least risk to the provider.
- When choosing a solution, the nurse looks at whether the desired outcome can be achieved.
- After careful thought, the nurse rethinks the solutions.
- Information collected with the tool is used to develop these alternative solutions.
- Decision trees are useful graphic aids that will give a picture of the solutions and the consequences and risks of each solution.

Figure 14-1 shows the process of using a decision tree.

In the immunization example, the best consequence would be for families to provide for immunizations. One must consider the value of this action to the parents, the odds that immunizations will be given if a formal clinic is not available, the cost to the parents versus the taxpayer, and the cost to the community. Costs to the community include possible increased incidence of communicable disease or mortality and increased need for more expensive services to treat the diseases if children are not immunized. If the parents provide the immunizations, costs to the taxpayer and to the community are low.

Identify Objectives and Activities for Alternatives

In this phase the nurse, with client input, considers the possibilities of solving a problem using one of the solutions identified. The nurse considers the costs, resources, and program activities needed to choose one of the solutions. For each of the three proposed alternatives in Figure 14-1, the program planner must list activities that would need to be implemented to use each of the alternatives.

To illustrate, consider again the immunization scenario. Using the proposed solution of encouraging the parents to provide the immunizations (the best consequence), examples of activities include developing a script for a health education program and implementing a television program to encourage parents to take children to the physician. If the second, third,

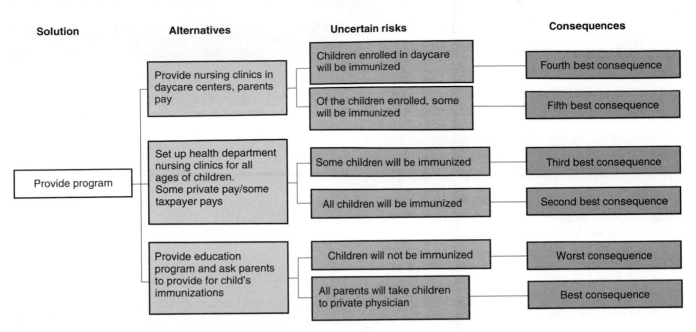

| Solution | Alternatives | Uncertain risks | Consequences |

Figure 14-1   **Ranking of solutions to problem: providing a preschool immunization program to low-income children using a decision tree.**

TABLE 14-1   Summary of Needs Assessment Tools

Name	Definition	Advantages	Disadvantages
Community forum	Community, group, organization, open meeting	Low cost Learn perspectives of large number of persons	Limited data Limited expression of views Discourages less powerful Becomes arena to discuss political issues
Key informant	Knowledgeable leaders identified, selected, and questioned	Provides picture of services needed	Bias of leaders Community characteristics may be incorrectly perceived by informants
Indicators approach	Existing data used to determine problem	Excellent data on problems and location of client groups	Data may be obsolete Growth and change in population may make data outdated
Survey of existing agencies	Estimates of client populations via services used at similar community agencies	Easy method to estimate size of client group Know extent of services offered in existing programs	Records and data may be unreliable All cases of need may not be reported Exaggeration of services may occur
Surveys/census	Measurement of total or sample client population by interview or questionnaire	Direct and accurate data on client population and their problems	Expensive Technically demanding Need many interviews or observations

or fourth best consequence was chosen, offering a clinic 8 hours per day at the health department and providing a mobile clinic to each daycare center for 4 hours each day to provide the immunizations would be possible activities.

For each alternative the nurse lists the resources needed to implement each activity. In the example, personnel could include nurses, volunteers, and clerks; supplies might include handouts, Band-Aids, medications, records, and consent forms; equipment might include syringes, needles, stethoscopes, and blood pressure cuffs; and facilities might include a television studio for a media blitz on the education program and a room with examination tables, chairs, and emergency carts. The costs of each solution must be considered by listing the costs of personnel, supplies, equipment, and facilities for each solution. As indicated, clients should review each solution for acceptance.

Evaluate Problem Solutions

In the evaluation phase of the plan, each alternative is weighed to judge the costs, benefits, and acceptance of the idea to the client, community, and nurse. The information outlined under C in How to Develop a Program Plan on p. 233 would be used to rank the solutions for choice by client and nurse based on cost, benefit, and acceptance. Consideration must be given to the solution that will provide the desired outcomes. Looking at available information through literature reviews or interviews might suggest whether each of the options had been tried before in another place or by someone else. The results from other sources would be helpful in deciding whether a chosen solution would be useful.

Choose the Solution

Clients, nurses, and administrators select the best solution. Providing reasons why a particular solution was chosen will help the nurse get the approval of administration for the plan. Involving clients and administrators throughout the planning process helps to promote acceptance of the plan. Upon approval the plan is implemented.

Briefly Noted

Nurses at all levels of education and preparation can participate in program planning and evaluation.

PROGRAM EVALUATION
Benefits of Program Evaluation

The major benefit of **program evaluation** is that it shows whether the program is meeting its purpose. It should answer the following questions:
- Are the needs for which the program was designed being met?
- Are the problems it was designed to solve being solved?

Quality assurance audits are prime examples of program evaluation in health care delivery. Evaluation data are used to justify continuing programs in community health. Program records—including client evaluations, community indexes, and **case registers**—serve as the major source of information for program evaluation. Surveys, interviews, observations, and diagnostic tests are ways to assess consumer and client response to health programs. Planning for the evaluation process is an important part of program planning. When the planning process begins, program evaluation begins with the needs assessment (formative evaluation).

Evaluation Process

The evaluation process presented by Rossi and Freeman (1999) is explained in this section. It is similar to the steps in the planning process:

Evidence-Based Practice

The purpose of the project in the reference cited below was twofold: (1) to develop a program to prevent diabetes and hypertension among the Chinese population in Chinatown, Hawaii, and (2) to develop a relationship with the Chinese Community Association. This article provides evaluation of the program, which was a collaborative effort between the community, the nurse, and diabetes nurse educators. The authors used several approaches to developing the program: volunteers helped them access the community, the community association identified participants for the program, and surveys of participants were conducted to determine interest. The authors used techniques of community education and health promotion to implement this self-care management program with 200 Chinese residents of the community. Case studies, laboratory diagnostic tests, blood pressure monitoring, and surveys were used to evaluate the outcomes of the program. The evaluation showed the effectiveness of the education, counseling, support, and outreach approaches used in the program to improve blood glucose and blood pressure levels in the population.

APPLICATION IN PRACTICE

The nurse can use this study to find appropriate ways to work with culturally diverse groups and ways to provide culturally sensitive health care programs.

Wang C, Abbott L: Development of a community based diabetes and hypertension prevention program, *Public Health Nurs* 15(6):406, 1998.

1. *Goal setting.* The value and beliefs of the agency, the nurse, and the clients provide the basis for goal setting and should be considered at every step of the evaluation process. In the preschool immunization scenario, the fact that children should not be exposed to early-childhood diseases would lead to a program goal to decrease the incidence of early-childhood diseases in the county where the program is planned.
2. *Determining goal measurement.* In the case of the previous goal, disease incidence would be an appropriate goal measurement.
3. *Identifying goal-attaining activities.* This includes such activities as media presentations urging parents to have their children immunized.
4. *Making the activities operational.* This involves the actual administration of the immunizations.
5. *Measuring the goal effect.* Reviewing the records and summarizing the incidence of early-childhood disease before and after the program is a measure of goal effect.
6. *Evaluating the program.* In this step whether the program goal was achieved is determined.

Keep in mind that only one program goal is used in this example. Most programs have multiple goals (Fig. 14-2).

Formulation of Objectives

The *objectives* identified in the planning process set the stage for conducting the program and provide the method for eval-

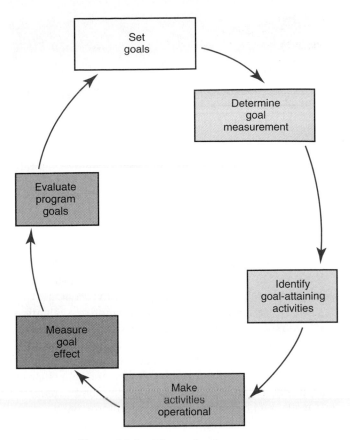

Figure 14-2 The evaluative process.

operational indicator for the previous objective would be a 10% to 25% decrease in the incidence rates of the most frequently occurring childhood vaccine-preventable illnesses in Center County. Such indicators provide a target for persons involved with program implementation. A review of *Healthy People 2010* objectives will give the reader examples of objectives that include all the elements listed above.

Levels of Program Objectives

It is customary for objectives to be stated in levels from general to specific. The first level consists of general and broad objectives that are sometimes called *goals*. Their purpose is to focus on the major reason for the program.

A general program objective (goal) may be to reduce the incidence of low-birth-weight babies in Center County by 2005 by improving access to prenatal care. The specific objectives, or subgoals, describe:

- A measurable behavior
- The circumstances under which the behavior is observed
- The minimal acceptable standard for the performance of the behavior.

A specific objective for this program may be to open a prenatal clinic in each health department within the county by January 2005 to serve the population within each census tract of the county. This specific objective is an action-oriented approach to meeting the goal.

Specific program activities are then planned to meet each specific objective, and resources, such as number of nurses, equipment, supplies, and location are planned for each of the objectives. It is assumed that as each specific objective is met, the general program objective will also be achieved. Remember that several specific objectives are required to meet a general program objective or goal.

Sources of Program Evaluation

Major sources of information for program evaluation are program clients, program records, and community indicators. The program participants, or clients of the service, have a unique and valuable role in program evaluation. Whether the clients, for whom the program was designed, accept the services will determine to a large extent whether the program achieves its purpose. Thus their reactions, feelings, and judgments about the program are important to the evaluation.

To assess the response of participants in a program, the evaluator may use:

- A written survey in the form of a questionnaire
- Attitude scale
- Interviews
- Observations.

Attitude scales are probably used most often, and they are usually phrased in terms of whether the program met its objectives. The client satisfaction survey is an example of an attitude scale often used in the health care delivery system to evaluate the program objectives.

The second major source of information for program evaluation is *program records*, especially clinical records. Clini-

uating the activities of the program. The following discussion helps in the development of clear, concise objectives.

Specifying Objectives (Goals)

If the objectives are too general, program evaluation becomes impossible. The objectives must be specific and stated so that anyone reading them could conduct the program without further instruction. To be truly effective, the program plan should begin with a general program goal and move on to specific objectives that will help meet the program goal. Useful program objectives include:

- A statement of the specific behaviors
- Accomplishments
- Success criteria, or expected result, for the program.

Each program objective requires:

- A strong, action-oriented verb to specify the behavior
- A statement of a single purpose
- A statement of a single result
- A time frame for achieving the expected result.

In this continuing example, a program objective that meets these criteria may be: to decrease (action verb) the incidence of early childhood disease in Center County (result) by providing immunization clinics in all schools (purpose) between August and December of 2005 (time frame).

As objectives are developed, an operational indicator for each objective should be considered so the evaluator knows when and if the objective has been met. For instance, an

cal records provide the evaluator with information about the care given to the client and the results of that care. To determine whether a program goal has been met, one might summarize the data from a group of records. For example, if one overall goal is to reduce the incidence of low-birth-weight babies through prenatal care, records would be reviewed to obtain the number of mothers who received prenatal care and the number of low-birth-weight babies born to them.

A third major source of evaluation is a **community health index.** Health and illness indicators, such as mortality and morbidity data, are probably cited more frequently than any other single index for program evaluation. Incidence and prevalence are valuable indexes used to measure program effectiveness and impact (see Chapter 8 for further discussion of rates and ratios).

An example of a national program based on a needs assessment of the U.S. population is the national health objectives program called *Healthy People 2010* (U.S. Department of Health and Human Services, 2000). *Healthy People 2010* has two overall goals and 467 specific health objectives, which include an action verb, a result, and a time frame (10 years) (see Appendix A.1). Each health status objective reflects targets for specific improvements. See the *Healthy People 2010* box for an example. Many of the objectives focus on interventions designed to reduce or eliminate illness, disability, and premature death among individuals and in communities. Others focus on broader issues such as improving access to quality health care, strengthening public health services and improving the availability and dissemination of health-related information.

Aspects of Program Evaluation

The aspects of program evaluation include the following (Kaluzny and Veney, 1999):

- *Evaluation of relevance:* need for the program
- *Progress:* tracking of program activities to meet program objectives
- *Efficiency:* relationship between program outcomes and the resources spent
- *Effectiveness:* ability to meet program objectives and the results of program efforts
- *Impact:* long-term changes in the client population.

Briefly Noted

Healthy People 2010, the national program to improve the health of all Americans in 10 years, used key informants, census data, statistical indicators, forums, and surveys of existing programs to establish the goals and objectives of the program.

Relevance

Evaluation of *relevance* is an important component of the initial planning phase. As money, providers, facilities, and

Healthy People 2010
Example of a National Health Objective

15-3   Reduce (action verb) deaths caused by unintentional injuries (result) to no more than 20.8 per 100,000 people (target) by the year 2010 (time frame).

supplies for delivering health care services are more closely monitored, the needs assessment done by the nurse will determine whether the program is needed.

Progress

The monitoring of program activities—such as hours of services, number of providers used, number of referrals made, and amount of money spent to meet program objectives—provides an evaluation of the *progress* of the program. This type of evaluation is an example of **formative evaluation** and occurs on an ongoing basis while the program exists. *Progress evaluation* occurs primarily while implementing the program. The nurse who completes a daily or weekly log of clinical activities (e.g., number of clients seen in clinic or visited at home, number of phone contacts, number of referrals made, number of community health-promotion activities) is contributing to progress evaluation of the nursing service.

Efficiency

If the reason for evaluation is to examine the *efficiency* of a program, it may occur on an ongoing basis as formative evaluation or at the end of the program as a **summative evaluation** that looks at the end result of the program. The evaluator may be able to determine whether the program provides better benefits at a lower cost than a similar program or whether the benefits to the clients or number of clients served justify the costs of the program.

Effectiveness and Impact

An **evaluation of program effectiveness** may help the nurse determine both client and provider satisfaction with the program activities, as well as whether the program met its stated objectives. However, if evaluation of *impact* is the goal, long-term effects such as changes in morbidity and mortality must be investigated. Both effectiveness and impact evaluations are usually summative evaluation functions primarily performed as end-of-program activities.

Briefly Noted

The combination of prenatal care programs delivered by nurses and the Women, Infants, and Children (WIC) supplemental nutritional program produces better pregnancy and postnatal outcomes for mothers and babies than traditional medical care.

HOW TO Do a Program Evaluation

A. Program relevance: needs assessment (formative).
  1. Use your answers to all of the questions listed in section A of the box "How To Develop a Program Plan."
  2. Based on needs assessment, was the program necessary?
B. Program progress (formative).
  1. Monitor activities (circle which this reflects: daily, weekly, monthly, annually).
     a. Name the activities provided.
     b. How many hours of service provided?
     c. How many clients have been served?
     d. By how many providers?
     e. What types of clients have been served?
     f. What types of providers were needed?
     g. Where have services been offered (home, clinic, organization)?
     h. How many referrals have been made to community sources?
     i. Which sources have been used to provide support services?
  2. Budget.
     a. How much money has been spent to carry out activities?
     b. Will more/less money be needed to conduct activities as outlined?
     c. Will changes need to be made now to objectives and activities to keep the program going?
     d. What changes do you recommend and why?
C. Program efficiency (formative and summative).
  1. Costs.
     a. How do the costs of this program compare with those of a similar program to meet the same goal?
     b. Do the activities outlined in B1 compare with the activities in a similar program?
     c. Although this program costs more/less than expected, is it needed? Why?
  2. Productivity (may use national or state averages for comparison).
     a. How many clients does each type of staff see per day (public health nurses, community health nurses, nurse practitioners)?
     b. How does this compare with similar programs?
     c. Although the productivity level of this program is low/high, is the program needed? Why?
  3. Benefits.
     a. What are the benefits of the program to the clients served?
     b. What are the benefits to the community?
     c. Are the benefits important enough to continue the program? Why? (Look at cost, productivity, and outcomes of care).
D. Program effectiveness (summative).
  1. Satisfaction.
     a. Is the client satisfied with the program as designed?
     b. Are the providers satisfied with the program outcomes?
     c. Is the community satisfied with the program outcomes?
  2. Goals.
     a. Did the program meet its stated goal?
     b. Are the clients' needs being met?
     c. Was the problem solved for which the program was designed?
E. Impact (summative).
  1. Long-term changes in health status (1 year or more).
     a. Have there been changes in the community's health?
     b. What are the changes seen (e.g., morbidity or mortality rates, teen pregnancy rates, pregnancy outcomes)?
     c. Have there been changes in individuals' health status?
     d. What are the changes seen?
     e. Has the initial problem been solved or has it returned?
     f. Is new or revised programming needed? Why?
     g. Should the program be discontinued? Why?

Clinical Application

The following is a real-life example of the application of the program management process by an undergraduate community health nursing student. This activity resulted in the development and implementation of a nurse-managed clinic for the homeless. This example shows how students as well as providers can make a difference in health care delivery. It also shows that no mystery surrounds the program management process.

Eva was listening to the radio one Sunday afternoon and heard an announcement about the opening of a soup kitchen within the community for the growing homeless population. She was beginning her community health nursing course and wanted to find a creative clinical experience that would benefit herself as well as others. The announcement gave her an idea. Although it mentioned food, clothing, shelter, and social services, nothing was said about health care.

Eva was interested in finding a way to provide nursing and health care services at the soup kitchen. Which of the following should she do?
A. Talk with key leaders to determine their interest in her idea.
B. Review the literature to find out the magnitude of the problem.
C. Survey the community to find out if others were providing services.
D. Discuss the idea with members of the homeless population.
E. Consider potential solutions to the health care problems.
F. Consider where she would get the resources to open a clinic.
G. Talk with church leaders and community health nursing faculty members to seek acceptance for her idea.

Answer is in the back of the book.

 ### Remember This!

• Planning and evaluation are essential elements of program management and vital to the survival of the nursing discipline in health care delivery.

- A program is an organized approach to meet the assessed needs of individuals, families, groups, or communities by reducing or eliminating one or more health problems.
- Planning is defined as selecting and carrying out a series of actions to achieve a stated goal.
- Evaluation is defined as the methods used to determine if a service is needed and will be used, whether a program to meet that need is carried out as planned, and whether the service actually helps the people it intended to help.
- To develop quality programs, planning should include four essential elements: problem diagnosis and assessment of need, identification of problem solutions, analysis and comparison of alternative methods, and selection of the best plan and planning methods.
- The initial and most critical step in planning and evaluating a health program is assessment of need.
- Some of the major tools used in needs assessment are census data, community forums, surveys of existing community agencies, surveys of community residents, and statistical indicators.
- The major benefit of program evaluation is to determine whether a program is fulfilling its stated goals.
- Quality assurance programs are prime examples of program evaluation.
- Plans for implementing and evaluating programs should be developed at the same time.
- Program records and community indices serve as major sources of information for program evaluation.
- Planning programs and planning for their evaluation are two of the most important ways in which nurses can ensure successful program implementation.
- The program management process, like the nursing process, is a rational decision-making process.
- Program planning helps nurses and agencies focus attention on services that clients need.
- Planning helps everyone involved understand their role in providing services to clients.
- The assessment of need process provides an evaluation of the relevance that a new service may have to clients.
- A decision tree is a useful tool to choose the best alternative for solving a problem.
- Setting goals and writing objectives to meet the goals are necessary to evaluate program outcomes.
- *Healthy People 2010* is an example of a national program based on needs assessment that has stated goals and objectives on which the program can be evaluated.

 ## What Would You Do?

1. Choose the definitions that best describe your idea of a program, planning, and evaluation.
2. Apply the program planning process to an identified clinical problem for a client group with whom you are working in the community.
   a. Assess the client need.
   b. Choose tools appropriate to the assessment of needs.
   c. Analyze the overall planning process of arriving at decisions about implementing the program.
   d. Summarize the benefits for program planning that apply to your situation.
3. Given the situation just described, choose three or four of your classmates to work with on the following projects.
   a. Plan for evaluation of the program in activity 2.
   b. Apply the evaluation process to the situation.
   c. Name the measures you will use to gather data for evaluating your program.
   d. Name the sources you will tap to gain information for program evaluation.
   e. Analyze the benefits of program evaluation that apply to your situation.
   f. Talk with a community health nurse or administrator about the application of program planning and evaluation processes at the local agency. Compare their answers to your readings.

REFERENCES

Kaluzny A, Veney J: Evaluating health care programs and services. In Williams S, Torrens P (editors): *Introduction to health services,* New York, 1999, Wiley.

Kropf R: Planning for health services. In Kovner A (editor): *Health care delivery in the United States,* New York, 1995, Springer.

Posavac EJ, Carey RG: *Program evaluation: methods and case studies,* Englewood Cliffs, NJ, 1997, Prentice Hall.

Rossi P, Freeman H: *Evaluation: a systematic approach,* Beverly Hills, Calif, 1999, Sage.

U.S. Department of Health and Human Services: *Healthy people 2010: national health promotion and disease prevention objectives,* Washington, D.C., 2000, U.S. Department of Health and Human Services.

Wang C, Abbott L: Development of a community based diabetes and hypertension prevention program, *Public Health Nurs* 15(6):406, 1998.

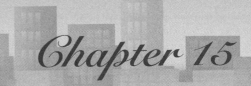

Chapter 15

Managing Quality

JUDITH LUPO WOLD

OBJECTIVES

After reading this chapter, the student should be able to:
- Define quality assurance and explain its role in continuous quality improvement.
- Discuss at least two general and two specific approaches to quality improvement and examine ways to use them in practice.
- Plan a model quality assurance program.

- Identify the purposes for the types of records kept in public health agencies.
- Evaluate a method for documentation of client care in a community setting.
- Examine the ways managed care is changing the way quality is assured in health care.

CHAPTER OUTLINE

KEY TERMS

accountability: being legally, morally, ethically, and socially answerable to someone for something you have done.

accreditation: a credentialing process used to recognize health care agencies or educational programs for provision of quality services and programs.

audit process: a six-step process used to recognize health care agencies or educational programs for provision of quality services and programs.

certification: a mechanism, usually by means of written examination, that provides an indication of professional competence in a specialized area of practice.

charter: a mechanism by which a state governmental agency grants corporate status to institutions with or without rights to award degrees.

concurrent audit: a method of evaluating quality of ongoing care through appraisal of the nursing process.

Continuous Quality Improvement (CQI): an approach to managing quality that emphasizes continual improvement in real time, empowering employees to manage quality themselves, including client and family perceptions of quality, and making changes in organizational systems to enable workers to provide high-quality services.

Continued

KEY TERMS—cont'd

credentialing: a mechanism to produce performance of acceptable quality by individuals or by programs of education and service.

customer: a consumer of products or services.

licensure: legal sanction to practice a profession after attaining the minimum degree of competence to ensure protection of public health and safety.

malpractice litigation: an approach to quality assurance imposed on the health care system by the legal system.

managed care: a health care financing mechanism designed to control costs by influencing the ways, type, and amount of care that clients receive.

outcome: a change in client health status as a result of care or program implementation.

process: the ongoing activities and behavior of health care providers engaged in conducting client care.

Professional Review Organizations (PROs): organizations established by law to monitor delivery of health care to clients of Medicare, Medicaid, and Maternal Child Health Programs and to monitor implementation of prospective reimbursement.

quality: continuously striving for excellence while adhering to set specifications or guidelines.

quality assurance (QA): monitoring of the activities of client care to determine the degree of excellence attained in the implementation of the activities.

retrospective audit: a method of evaluating quality of care through appraisal of the nursing process after the client's discharge from the health care system.

risk management: designed to reduce the liability on the part of an agency or individual by assisting employees to act in accordance with set guidelines and procedures.

sentinel method: uses outcome measures to evaluate quality of care; based on epidemiological principles.

structure: the component in quality improvement that measures the setting and instruments used to provide care.

Total Quality Management (TQM): an approach to managing quality of care through appraisal of the nursing process after the client's discharge from the health care system.

tracer method: a way to evaluate quality of care that measures both process and outcome.

utilization review: review that is directed toward ensuring that care is actually needed and cost is appropriate for the level of care provided.

Health care in most countries is facing enormous pressures. **Managed care** has emerged as one mechanism to influence the ways, type, and amount of care that patients receive. Many hospitals are closing or merging. Hospitals also are looking at ways to treat patients either as outpatients or with shorter hospital stays to increase profits. These changes in hospitals are coming at a time when public health is being redesigned and is providing less primary care to individuals and moving to a more population-based approach. Consumers, insurance companies, and the federal government want good health care outcomes at the lowest cost (Young, 1998). Concern for quality and cost is accompanied by public pressure for better accessibility, more **accountability,** and improved efficiency and effectiveness. Increasingly, health care providers and managers are using the tools, techniques, and approaches to quality management to make decisions about cutting costs while maintaining or improving quality (Maddox, 1998).

This chapter provides an overview of quality management. Commonly used terms are defined, and the general goals of quality management are described. Approaches to commonly used forms of quality management are discussed. Particular attention is paid to quality assurance, the quality management approach of Total Quality Management (TQM), and useful tools for measuring quality. The last section questions how compatible current mandates and priorities for quality are with an overall goal of caring for clients.

HISTORICAL DEVELOPMENTS

Quality management began in nursing with the work of Florence Nightingale, who in 1860 designed a method to collect and present hospital statistics. Nightingale, in her efforts to improve hospital treatment, was also a pioneer in setting standards for nursing care. During the late 1800s, nursing schools were established in the United States. These schools set standards to upgrade nursing care. Licensure for nurses began in 1892, and the first nurse practice acts were established in 1903. By 1903, licensure of nurses was mandatory, and by 1923 all states had either permissive or mandatory laws directing nursing practice. Following World War II, the nursing profession began establishing a scientific method of practice that led to the development of the nursing process. The nursing process with its assessment, planning, and implementation, also added evaluation of nursing activities (Maibusch, 1984). The evaluative steps in the nursing process include quality assurance and quality improvement. Tools to measure quality assurance were developed in the 1950s.

In 1966 the American Nurses Association (ANA) created the Divisions on Practice, and in 1972, the Congress for Nursing Practice developed standards for quality assurance programs. At about the same time in 1973, the Standards for Community Health Nursing Practice were developed. These standards were revised in 1986 and then again in 1999.

In 1972, the Joint Commission on Accreditation of Hospitals (JCAH) included the responsibilities of nursing in its description of standards for nursing services. The JCAH called on the nursing industry to clearly plan, document, and evaluate nursing care. In the mid-1980s JCAH became the Joint Commission on Accreditation of Healthcare Organizations (JCAHO) and began developing quality control standards for hospital and home health nursing. JCAHO currently incorporates continuous quality improvement principles in its standards.

Also in 1972, the Social Security Act (Public Law 92-603) was amended to establish the Professional Standards Review Organization (PSRO) and to mandate the process for review of the delivery of health care to clients of Medicare, Medicaid, and maternal and child health programs. The PSRO program was modified later to become the **Professional Review Organizations** (PROs) by the 1983 Social Security Amendments. PROs monitor implementation of the prospective reimbursement system for Medicare clients. The use and effectiveness of PROs in a managed care environment has yet to be determined.

In response to a growing number of malpractice claims in the United States, the National Health Quality Improvement Act of 1986 was established. When funded in 1989, this Act had two major provisions: (1) it encouraged consumers to become informed about their practitioner's practice record and (2) it created a national clearinghouse of information on provider malpractice records. The Act emphasized structure rather than process or outcome of care (National Association for Healthcare Quality, 1993).

As discussed in Chapter 1, both the ANA (1980) and the American Public Health Association (1981) defined public health nursing and explained the role. The definition and role of public health nursing was revised by the Public Health Nursing Section of the American Public Health Association in March 1996 and is found in Chapter 1. Likewise, in 1999, the ANA revised its definition and standards for public health nursing practice. Just as the ANA and the APHA have developed standards for community health nursing practice, the Association of Community Health Nursing Educators, which was established in 1978, has identified the curriculum content required to prepare community health nursing students for practice (Association of Community Health Nursing Educators, 1991a, 1991b, 1993).

The health care industry began to adopt quality management concepts in 1987 with the National Demonstration Project on Quality Improvement in Health Care. The Joint Commission on the Accreditation of Healthcare Organizations revised their accreditation standards in 1992 and replaced quality assurance requirements with quality assessment and improvement requirements.

QUALITY AND THE CURRENT HEALTH CARE SYSTEM

Both consumers and providers are interested in the quality of health care. Health care providers pride themselves on individual achievement and responsibility for positive client outcomes (Kovner and Jonas, 1998). Maddox (1998) describes four factors that explain why quality management is important for the health care industry.

First, in the past, it has often been accepted that there would be some problems or complications with the production of things or the delivery of services. For example, it was not uncommon for agencies to have a certain number of

charting or medication errors. Likewise, if 20 hospital beds were built, there might be two with errors in their production. What was important was to keep the number of errors within a reasonable range; "good enough" care or products were tolerated.

Second, incentives in health care changed with the prospective payment system in 1984 that reimbursed for health care costs according to conditions listed in a standardized list of diagnostic related groups (DRGs). Before 1984, health care providers were reimbursed on a fee-for-service basis, so the more service provided, the more money received. In contrast, prospective payment set up a fixed rate for payment for procedures and services. That is, removal of the tonsils was reimbursed at the same rate for Joey who stayed in the hospital 3 days due to a post-surgery infection and for Billy who left the next morning. The amount and quality of services provided became much more important. Doing something only "well enough," if this resulted in complications, would cost more. Quality became important.

Third, public expectations for good health care has grown. People want easy access to competent, kind, and cost-effective care. They want everything done that money can buy. However, costs keep growing, and in most countries, there is not an unrestricted budget available for health care in either the public or private sector. Rather, managed care organizations (MCOs) have emerged, and they are designed to deliver and monitor health care services within a set budget (Halverson, Kaluzny, and McLaughlin, 1998). Weiss (1997) states that "in the future, quality will be measured based on the health status of both MCO-enrolled populations and the community or population served as well as individual perceptions of health status" (p. 29). MCOs use many of the traditional public health tools to evaluate their effectiveness.

Likewise, in order to provide quality health care in communities, health departments are examining their place in promoting community-based health care quality (Joint Council Committee on Quality in Public Health, 1996). Nurses are in a perfect position to implement strategies called for in the shift to community-based health status improvement. Community assessments, identification of at-risk individuals, targeted interventions, case management, and management of illnesses across the age and health-care continuum can improve the health of communities and their residents (Weiss, 1997). These are not new strategies for nurses. They are gaining attention because they are cost effective; healthy consumers obviously use fewer health care resources than sick people. Thus everyone—consumers, providers, and those who pay the health care bills—benefits if people stay healthy. An accepted public health principle of including the recipient of care in the planning of care is increasingly being seen as consumers form partnerships in their communities by holding MCOs accountable for the quality of health outcomes for their costs. Partnerships use data-based community assessments to improve health and to ensure that communities do receive quality services (Al-Assaf, 1998; Bushy, 1997; Lasker et al, 1997). Consumers are no longer willing to have care just given to them. Instead, they want to be partners in deciding on their care.

Fourth, not only are consumers and providers concerned about the quality of care, but regulatory groups set standards for agencies and have increased their oversight of agency efficiencies.

Briefly Noted

Managed care has changed the way health care is delivered in the United States. Its focus on outcomes may result in more emphasis on health promotion and disease prevention efforts in order to save on health care expenditures.

DEFINITIONS AND GOALS

What Is Quality?

Quality is a hard term to define. To some extent, quality has to be defined in relation to the product and service under consideration. Also, quality is often determined differently by the provider than by the person receiving the product or service. Davis (1994) defined **quality** as continuous striving for excellence while conforming to set specifications or guidelines. The Institute of Medicine (IOM) defines quality health care as "the extent to which health care services . . . have a net benefit. . . . That benefit is expected to reflect considerations of patient satisfaction and well-being, broad health status and quality of life outcomes, and the processes of patient-provider interaction and decision making" (IOM, 1990, p. 4). The IOM definition includes attention to societal and individual values and urges care to be based on current knowledge. Quality care has four components:

1. Professional performance
2. Efficient use of resources
3. Minimal risk to the client of illness or injury associated with care
4. Patient satisfaction (Davis, 1994, p. 6).

How Does Quality Assurance Relate to Total Quality Management?

"**Quality Assurance (QA)** identifies problems to solve them" or examine what was done wrong (Maddox, 1998, p. 460). **Continuous Quality Improvement (CQI)** builds upon traditional quality assurance by using the analysis methods of the scientific process to look at the work systems and processes of an organization. The box below lists differences between quality assurance and continuous quality improvement. Similarly, Total Quality Management (TQM) is a structured, systematic process for planning within the organization. Traditional approaches to quality, like those used in quality assurance, focus on assessing or measuring performance, ensuring that performance conforms to standards, and taking action to bring about change when care does not meet standards. This definition is too narrow to

meet the needs of many clients, both internal and external to the agency (Donabedian, 1990). Many agencies now also include total quality management strategies in their program of quality evaluation and improvement. It is a process-driven and customer-oriented philosophy of management that embodies leadership, teamwork, employee empowerment, individual responsibility, and continuous improvement of system processes that lead to improved outcomes (Berwick, 1989; Kinney, Freedman, and Cook, 1994). Customer satisfaction is important in TQM. For example, assume that women have to wait a long time in a Women, Infants, and Children's (WIC) program in order to be certified as eligible to receive support. Using CQI, all the steps in the appointment process are considered to see where the system's efficiency and effectiveness have stalled and why the women are waiting for a long time (Davis, 1994).

HOW TO Differentiate Between Quality Assurance and Continuous Quality Improvement

Quality Assurance	Continuous Quality Improvement
1. External determinants	1. Internal determinants
2. Detects errors and deficiencies	2. Determines requirements and expectations
3. Fixes blame and responsibility	3. Identifies process improvement opportunities
4. Post event investigation	4. Prevention
5. QA department responsible	5. All members in organization responsible
6. Inspires fear	6. Inspires hope

APPROACHES TO QUALITY IMPROVEMENT

Two basic approaches exist in quality improvement: general and specific. The general approach involves a large governing or official body's evaluation of the ability of a person or an agency to meet specific criteria or standards. General approaches include licensure of a person or accreditation of a school. Specific quality improvement approaches try to evaluate whether the care given has outcomes that are acceptable to the consumer.

General Approaches

General approaches to quality improvement seek to protect the public by assuring a level of competency among health care professionals. Examples are credentialing, licensure, accreditation, certification, charter, recognition, and academic degrees. While licensure is typically viewed as recognition that a person has met a minimal set of standards in order to practice his/her trade or profession, **credentialing** is defined as "a process by which individuals or institutions or one or more of their programs are designated by a qualified agent as having met minimum standards at a specified time" (Seppanen, 1995, p. 3). Credentialing can be mandatory or voluntary. Mandatory credentialing requires statutory laws. State nurse practice acts are examples of mandatory credentialing. Licensing, certification, and accreditation are examples of credentialing, and certification examinations offered by a professional group are examples of voluntary credentialing.

Licensure is one of the oldest general quality assurance approaches. Individual licensure is a contract between the profession and the state whereby the profession is granted control over who can enter into and who exits from the profession. Licensure controls entry into a profession. Exit is generally punitive for some infraction. The licensing process requires that written regulations define the scope and limits of the professional's practice. Job descriptions based on these regulations set minimum and maximum limits on the functions and responsibilities of the practitioner. All 50 states have mandatory nurse licensure, and nurses take the same computerized examination in all 50 states in order to become licensed to practice nursing.

Briefly Noted

Critics of professional licensure say that licensing is a "market barrier" or a way to keep people out of a particular job market. Supporters say that licensure has protected the public by ensuring at least a beginning level of proficiency.

In contrast, **accreditation,** a voluntary approach to quality control, is used for institutions. Both the National League for Nursing (NLN) and the American Association of Colleges of Nursing (AACN) have established separate affiliates to accredit baccalaureate and higher degree nursing programs (Cary, 1999). The NLN also accredits diploma and associate degree programs, as well as home health programs, through the Community Health Accreditation Program (CHAP). Also, state boards of nursing accredit basic nursing programs so that their graduates are eligible for the licensing examination.

Accreditation is considered to be quasi-voluntary, since accreditation is often linked to governmental regulations that encourage programs to participate in the accrediting process in order to be reimbursed for services. For example, only accredited public health and home health agencies are eligible for reimbursement for Medicare clients. In accreditation, programs do a thorough review of their strengths and limitations in response to a set of criteria that they must address. The program is next reviewed by individuals who are familiar with similar programs; that is, the reviewers may work in comparable programs or agencies. Accreditation processes evaluate an agency's physical structure, organizational structure, personnel qualifications, and the educational qualifications of staff.

Certification, another general and voluntary approach to quality, combines features of licensure and accreditation. Educational achievements, experience, and performance on

an examination determine a person's qualifications for functioning in an identified specialty area, such as community health nursing. The American Nurses Association, through its credentialing program, offers certification in several specialty areas. Other professional groups have established examinations to certify practitioners.

Like accreditation, certification also can be a quasi-voluntary process. For example, to function as a nurse practitioner in some states, one must show proof of educational credentials and take an examination to be "certified" to practice in that state. There are major concerns about certification as a quality assurance mechanism. Certification examinations measure competency by using a written test, and limited clinical performance is measured. Except for occupational health nurses and nurse anesthetists, certification has not been recognized by employers as an achievement beyond basic preparation, so financial rewards are few.

Charter, recognition, and academic degrees are other general approaches to quality assurance. **Charter** is the mechanism by which a state governmental agency grants corporate status to institutions with or without rights to award degrees (e.g., university-based nursing programs). Recognition is defined as a process whereby one agency accepts the credentialing status of and the credentials conferred by another. An example is when state boards of nursing accept nurse practitioner credentials that are awarded by the ANA or by one of the specialty credentialing agencies. Academic degrees are titles awarded by degree-granting institutions to individuals who have completed a predetermined program of studies.

Specific Approaches

Historically, quality assurance programs conducted by healthcare agencies have measured the performance of individuals and their conformance to standards set forth by accrediting agencies. Total quality management and continuous quality improvement are management philosophies and methods that incorporate many tools, including QA, to increase customer satisfaction with quality care. The goal of TQM and CQI is to eliminate errors in the work process before negative outcomes occur rather than waiting until after the fact to correct individual performance; the focus is on problem prevention and continuous improvement.

Total Quality Management

Total Quality Management (TQM) is a philosophy and set of guiding principles that form the operating foundation for organizations that want to continually improve how they work (Lanza, 1997). TQM uses quantitative methods and human resources to improve the services that an organization provides, the processes that it uses, and the degree to which the needs of the customer are met at the present and for the future. Quality improvement is built into every phase of the organization's work, beginning with the planning phase (Maddox, 1998).

In health care, a major group of customers are patients. Health care agencies have only recently begun using TQM, although Donabedian's early discussions of quality that addressed structure, process, and outcome (and will be discussed later in the chapter) have a lot in common with TQM. Applying TQM in health care allows management to look at the contribution of all systems to the outcomes of the organization. TQM emphasizes analyzing how processes can be improved, paying close attention to customers, using multidisciplinary work teams, and evaluating results using data (McLauglin and Kaluzny, 1994).

Deming, a leader in TQM, designed a way to develop organization-wide processes to ensure that high-quality products were produced the first time. He had 14 guidelines for ensuring quality:

1. Create, publish, and distribute to all employees a statement of the organization's aims and purposes. Managers must demonstrate constantly their commitment to this statement (i.e., the organization's purpose and values).
2. Everyone must learn the new philosophy.
3. Understand the purpose of inspection in order to improve processes and reduce costs.
4. End the practice of awarding business on the basis of price tag alone.
5. Improve constantly and forever the system of production and service.
6. Institute training.
7. Teach and institute leadership.
8. Drive out fear. Create trust. Create a climate for innovation.
9. Teams, groups, and staff must continuously work toward the aims and purposes of the company; teams are important in TQM.
10. Eliminate exhortations for the work force.
11a. Eliminate numerical quotes for production. Instead, learn and institute improvement methods.
11b. Eliminate management by objective. Instead, learn the capabilities of processes and how to improve them.
12. Remove barriers that rob people of pride of workmanship.
13. Encourage education and self-improvement for everyone.
14. Take action to accomplish the transformation (Deming, 1986, pp. 23-24).

If an agency uses TQM, it must become "customer driven." **Customers,** defined as "anyone who is affected by the product or process," are the primary focus (Juran, 1989 in Lanza, 1997, p. 97). There are both internal and external customers. Internal customers are employees in other departments or work units, such as environmental health workers, statisticians, or physicians. External customers are those who pay for the service: regulators, accrediting bodies, clients, and families. The internal customer is often overlooked. Employees forget that their professional colleagues are often customers for their services. For example, nurses working in community settings are often customers of the agency's laboratories or data offices. It is easy to take one's co-workers for granted and forget that they deserve efficient, effective service just as do clients, families, and other service recipients. Several key determinants that can lead to customer satisfaction are listed in the box below.

HOW TO Ensure Customer Satisfaction With Services Provided

Tangibles:
- Facility attractiveness
- Employee appearance
- Characteristics of other customers

Reliability:
- Dependability
- Consistency of service delivery

Responsiveness:
- Employee willingness
- Promptness in service delivery

Competence:
- Employee knowledge

Understanding the customer:
- Effort to learn customer needs
- Individualized attention

Access:
- Distance to facility
- Waiting time
- Hours of operation

Courtesy:
- Staff politeness and mannerisms

Communication:
- Ability of employees to explain material in an understandable way
- Openness to questions

Credibility:
- Trustworthiness of staff

Security:
- Physical safety
- Confidentiality

Customer satisfaction for both internal and external users of services can be assessed through the use of focus groups (of clients or employees), surveys (written or telephone), and response cards. Personnel policies that are motivating and provide continuous training and learning opportunities are important parts of a quality improvement program. Deming's eighth point mentions driving out fear, that is, fear of being fired for being innovative or taking risks. In quality improvement, people are not blamed for failures in the system and therefore are supported in looking for problems and seeking ways to improve system performance.

Briefly Noted

Total quality management/continuous quality improvement are concepts that give direction for managing a system of care, whereas quality assurance focuses on the care a client receives within the system.

Evidenced-Based Practice

Client satisfaction as an outcome measure is an important determinant of quality in health care organizations. In the study cited below, the researchers measured client satisfaction with care received from baccalaureate undergraduate student nurses. These students were working in an academic nursing center (ANC) as part of a community health clinical rotation. This academic nursing center is committed to program evaluation, and one facet of their evaluation is client satisfaction. The ANC used the University of North Dakota Survey, a modification of the Group Health Association of American (GHAA) Consumer Satisfaction Survey. This Likert scale (5 = excellent, 1 = poor) survey contained 14 questions that reflected the services provided by the students. Surveys were mailed to a total of 190 clients seen by these students. Clients were in either the child health program, the community health services program, or the expectant family program. One hundred and one (53%) clients responded. Means on each question ranged from 3.9 to 4.7. Only one question resulted in a rating of less than very good to excellent.

APPLICATION IN PRACTICE

The overall ratings revealed a highly satisfied group of clients with no significant difference among those in the child health program, the community health services program, or the expectant family program. Written comments described satisfaction with the amount of time spent in teaching and the inclusion of families in the program. This supports the basic premises of community health nursing to teach and to include families.

Lindsey DL, Henly SJ, Tyree EA: Outcomes in an academic nursing center: client satisfaction with student services, *J Nurs Care Quality* 11(5):30-38, 1997.

Traditional Quality Assurance

Traditional quality assurance programs are compatible with the quality improvement process. In most of health care, the overall goal of quality assurance is to monitor the process and outcomes of client care (Table 15-1). Specific goals are to:

1. Identify problems between provider and client
2. Intervene in problem cases
3. Provide feedback regarding interactions between client and provider
4. Provide documentation of interactions between provider and client.

The specific approaches often are implemented voluntarily by agencies and provider groups interested in the quality of interactions in their setting. However, state and federal governments require mandatory programs within public health agencies. For instance, periodic utilization review, peer reviews (audits), and other quality control measures are required in public health agencies that receive funds from state taxes, Medicaid, Medicare, and other public funding sources. Examples of specific approaches to quality control are agency staff review committees (peer review), utilization review committees, research studies, professional review organization (PRO) monitoring, client satisfaction surveys, risk management, and **malpractice litigation.**

Table 15-1	Traditional Management Model Compared to a Total Quality Management Model

Traditional Management Model	Total Quality Management Model
Legal or professional authority	Collective or managerial responsibility
Specialized accountability	Process accountability
Administrative authority	Participation
Meeting standards	Meeting process and performance expectations
Longer planning horizon	Shorter planning horizon
Quality assurance	Continuous improvement

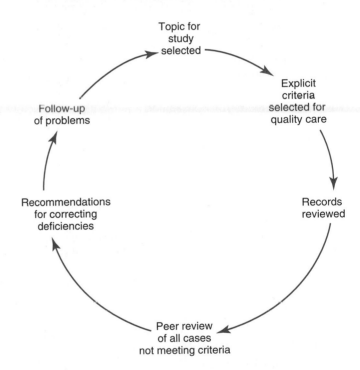

Figure 15-1 The audit process.

Staff Review Committees

Staff review committees are the most common specific approach to quality assurance in the United States. Staff review (or peer review) committees are designed to monitor client-specific aspects of certain levels of care. The audit is the major tool used to determine quality of care.

According to LoGerfo and Brook (1984), the **audit process** (Figure 15-1) consists of six steps:

1. Selection of a topic for study
2. Selection of explicit criteria for quality care
3. Review of records to determine whether criteria are met
4. Peer review of all cases that do not meet criteria
5. Specific recommendations to correct problems

6. Follow-up to determine whether problems have been eliminated.

Two types of audits are used in nursing peer review: concurrent and retrospective. The **concurrent audit** is a process audit that evaluates the quality of ongoing care by looking at the nursing process. Medicare and Medicaid use concurrent audits to evaluate care received by public health and/or home health clients. The advantages of concurrent audits are:

1. Identification of problems at the time care is given
2. Provision of a mechanism for identifying and meeting client needs during care
3. Implementation of measures to fulfill professional responsibilities
4. Provision of a mechanism for communicating on behalf of the client.

The disadvantages of the concurrent audit are:

1. It is time consuming
2. It is more costly to implement than the retrospective audit
3. Because care is ongoing, it does not present the total picture of care that the client ultimately will receive.

The **retrospective audit,** or outcome audit, evaluates quality of care through appraisal of the nursing process after the client's discharge from the health care system. The advantages of the retrospective audit are that it provides:

1. A comparison of actual practice to standards of care
2. Analysis of actual practice findings
3. A total picture of care given
4. More accurate data for planning corrective action.

Disadvantages of the retrospective audit method are:

1. The focus of evaluation is directed away from ongoing care
2. Client problems are identified after discharge, so corrective action can only be used to improve the care of future clients.

Utilization Review

The purpose of **utilization review** is to ensure that care actually is needed and that the cost is appropriate (Davis, 1994). LoGerfo and Brook (1984) described three types of utilization review:

1. Prospective: an assessment of the necessity of care before giving service
2. Concurrent: a review of the necessity of services while care is being given
3. Retrospective: an analysis of the necessity of the services received by the client after the care has been given.

Each of these reviews provides an assessment of the appropriateness of the cost of care. Prospectively, care can be denied and money saved. Concurrently, services can be cut if they are not deemed essential. Retrospectively, payment can be denied to the provider if the care was not necessary.

Utilization review began in the middle of the twentieth century due to concern for increasing health care costs. Insurance companies and professional groups developed the first utilization review committees. These committees became mandatory under the 1965 Medicare Law as a way to control hospital costs (Davis, 1994).

The utilization review process includes development of explicit criteria regarding the need for services and the length of service. Utilization review has been used primarily in hospitals to establish the need for client admission and to determine the length of hospital stay. In community health, especially home health care, utilization review establishes criteria for admission to agency service, the number of visits a client may receive, the eligibility for client services such as a nursing aide or physical therapist, and discharge.

Advantages of utilization review are:

1. Assists clients to avoid unnecessary care
2. May encourage the consideration of alternative care options, such as home health care rather than hospitalization
3. Can provide guidelines for staff and program development
4. Provides for agency accountability to the consumer.

The major disadvantage of utilization review is that not all clients fit the classic picture presented by the criteria used to determine approval or denial of care. For example, an elderly female client was admitted to a home health care agency for care after being discharged from a hospital. The client was paraplegic as a result of a cerebrovascular accident. After several weeks of physical and speech therapy, the client showed little sign of progress. The utilization review committee considered the client's condition to be stable and did not recognize the continued need for management to prevent future complications; therefore, Medicare payment was denied.

Appeal mechanisms have been built into the utilization review process used by Medicare and Medicaid. The appeal allows providers and clients to present additional data that may help to reverse the original decision to deny payment. This is a tedious process and is often difficult to understand and manage for clients.

Risk Management

Risk management committees often are a part of the quality program of a community agency. The goal of risk management is to reduce the liability on the part of the agency and the number of grievances brought against the agency. The risk management committee reviews all risks to which an agency is exposed. It reviews client and personnel safety policies and procedures and determines whether personnel are following the rules. Examples of problems reviewed by a risk management committee are administering an incorrect vaccination dosage, a pediatric client injury caused by a fall from an examining table, or injury to a community health nurse as a result of an accident while making a home visit. Incident reports are reviewed by the risk management committee for appropriate, accurate, and thorough documentation of any problem that occurs relating to clients or personnel. In addition patterns are identified that may require changes in policy or staff development to correct the problem. Grievance procedures are established for both clients and personnel as a part of risk management.

Professional Review Organizations

As mentioned earlier, professional standards review organizations (PSROs) were established in 1972 in an amendment to the Social Security Act (Public Law 92-603) as a publicly mandated utilization and peer review program. This law provided that medical, hospital, and nursing home care under Medicare, Medicaid, and Title V Maternal and Child Health Programs would be reviewed for appropriateness and necessity and such care would be reimbursed accordingly. In 1983 Congress passed the Peer Review Improvement Act (PL 97-248), creating PROs. PROs replaced PSROs and are directed by the federal government to reduce hospital admissions for procedures that can be performed safely and effectively in an ambulatory surgical setting on an outpatient basis, and to reduce inappropriate or unnecessary admissions or invasive procedures by specific practitioners or hospitals. Quality measures include reduction of unnecessary admissions caused by previous substandard care, avoidable complications and deaths, and unnecessary surgery or invasive procedures (Gremaldi and Micheletti, 1985).

Institutions contract with PROs for quality reviews. PROs are local (usually state) organizations that establish criteria for care based on local patterns of practice. They can be for-profit or not-for-profit organizations. They have access to physicians or may include physicians in their membership. PROs must define their operational objectives and are required to consult with nurses and other non-physician health care providers when reviewing the activities of those professionals. PROs monitor access to care and cost of care. Professionals working under the regulation of PROs should develop accurate and complete documentation procedures to ensure compliance with the criteria of the PRO.

There is considerable debate about the limitations and benefits of the federally mandated PRO quality review process. Limitations of the process include jeopardizing professional autonomy because decision making about care includes professionals, consumers, and government representatives. Also, control mechanisms may be developed such that the care provided is determined by cost rather than by professional criteria and judgment. On the positive side, the review system develops standards and uses review processes to increase accountability for the care given (Greenberg & Lezzoni, 1995; Gremaldi and Micheletti, 1985; Lieski, 1985).

In 1985 PRO authority was expanded to include review of services offered by health maintenance organizations and competitive medical plans. In addition, the Medicare Quality Assurance Act was passed to strengthen quality assurance programs and to improve access to care after hospitalization. This act required hospitals receiving Medicare payments to provide to Medicare beneficiaries written discharge plans supervised by registered nurses and social workers.

Evaluative Studies

Evaluative studies for measuring the effectiveness of nursing and health care interventions on client populations increased during the twentieth century. These studies demonstrate the effect of nursing and health care interventions on client populations. Three key models have been used to evaluate quality: Donabedian's structure-process-outcome model, the tracer method, and the sentinel method.

Donabedian's (1981, 1985, 1990) model introduced three major components for evaluating quality care. The first component, **structure,** evaluates the setting and instruments used to provide care. Examples of structure are facilities, equipment, characteristics of the administrative organization, client mix, and the qualifications of health providers. The second component is **process,** or evaluating activities as they relate to standards and expectations of health providers in the management of client care. The third component is **outcome,** the net change (or result) that occurs from health care. The three components or methods may be used separately to evaluate a part of care. To get an overall picture of quality of care, the three components should be used together (Table 15-2).

The **tracer method** measures both process and outcome of care. This method is more effective in evaluating the health care of groups than of individuals. It is also more effective in evaluating care delivered by an institution than by a person (Kessner and Kalk, 1973). The following are the essential characteristics for implementing the tracer method:

- A tracer, or a problem, that has a definite impact on the client's level of functioning
- Well-defined and easily diagnosed characteristics
- Population prevalence high enough to permit adequate data collection
- A known variation resulting from use of effective health care
- Well-defined management techniques in either prevention, diagnosis, treatment, or rehabilitation
- Recognized (documented) effects of non-medical factors on the tracer.

TABLE 15-2 Quality Assurance Measures		
Structure	**Process**	**Outcome**
Internal agency committees	Peer review committees	Internal agency committees
Self-study	Prospective audit	Evaluative studies
Review agency documents	Concurrent audit	Survey health status
	Retrospective audit	
External agency regulatory audit	Client satisfaction survey	Client satisfaction survey
		Malpractice suits

Stevens (1985) provided a classification system for selecting client groups for tracer outcome studies in nursing:

1. A particular disease
2. Similar treatment
3. Similar needs
4. Similar community
5. Similar life-style
6. Similar illness stage.

The tracer method provides nurses with data to show the differences in outcomes as a result of nursing care standards.

The **sentinel method** of quality evaluation is based on epidemiological principles (Rutstein, et al, 1976). This method is an outcome measure for examining specific instances of client care. The characteristics of the sentinel method are:

- Cases of unnecessary disease, disability, complications, and death are counted
- The circumstances surrounding the unnecessary event, or the sentinel, are examined in detail
- A review of morbidity and mortality is used as an index to determine the critical increase in the untimely event, which may reflect changes in quality of care
- Health status indicators, such as changes in social, economic, political, and environmental factors, that may have an effect on health outcomes are reviewed
- Changes in the sentinel indicate potential problems. For example, increases in encephalitis in certain communities may result from increases in mosquito populations.

MODEL QUALITY ASSURANCE PROGRAM

The primary purpose of a quality assurance program is to ensure that the results of an organized activity are consistent with the expectations. All personnel affected by a quality assurance program should be involved in its development and implementation. Although administration and management are responsible for the quality of services, the keys to that quality are the knowledge, skills, and attitudes of the personnel who deliver the service (Porter, 1988).

In 1977 the ANA introduced a model for a quality assurance program. Figure 15-2 depicts the model, which identifies seven basic components of a quality assurance program. According to Gottlieb (1988) quality assurance programs answer the following questions about health care services and nursing care:

- What is being done now?
- Why is it being done?
- Is it being done well?
- Can it be done better?
- Should it be done at all?
- Are there improved ways to deliver the service?
- How much is it costing?
- Should certain activities be abandoned and/or replaced?

The ANA model and Donabedian's framework for evaluating health care programs using the components of structure, process, and outcome can be used in developing a quality assurance program. Outcome is the most important ingredient of a program since it is the key to evaluation of providers and agencies by accrediting bodies, insurance companies, and Medicare and Medicaid through PROs and other accrediting agencies.

Structure

The philosophy and objectives of an agency define the structural standards of the agency. In evaluating the structure of an organization, the evaluator determines whether the agency is adhering to the stated philosophy and objectives. Is the agency providing services to populations across the life span? Are primary, secondary, and/or tertiary preventive services offered? Standards of structure are defined by the licensing or accrediting agency, for example, the NLN standards for accrediting home health agencies (Council of Home Health Agencies/ and Community Health Services, 1986).

Identification of standards and criteria for quality assurance begins with writing the philosophy and objectives of the organization. The philosophy includes values identification, or the beliefs of the agency about humanity, nursing, the community, and health. The beliefs of the community, the population to be served, and the providers of care are equally important to the agency beliefs, and all need to be considered. Objectives define the intended results of nursing care, descriptions of client behaviors, and/or change in health status to be demonstrated on discharge (Rinke and Wilson, 1988). Once objectives are formulated, the required resources are identified to accomplish the objectives. Need for the resources of personnel, supplies and equipment, facilities, and finances are described. Once resources are determined, policies, procedures, and job descriptions are formulated to serve as behavioral guides to the employees of the agency. These documents should reflect the essential nursing and other health provider qualifications needed to implement the services of the agency.

Standards of structure are evaluated internally via a self-study by a committee composed of administrative, management, and staff members. Standards of structure also are evaluated by a utilization review committee often composed of an external advisory group with community representatives for all services offered through an agency, such as a nurse, a physical therapist, a speech pathologist, a physician, a board member, and an administrator from a sister agency. The data from these committees identify the strengths and weaknesses of the agency structure.

Briefly Noted

Know the standards of care for your agency. Keep your eyes open for recurring practices that are not up to the quality standards of your agency. For example: your clients complain daily about long waits for service. Chances are these same practices may be occurring in other areas of the agency. This knowledge will be valuable in the quality improvement process as your agency strives to improve quality.

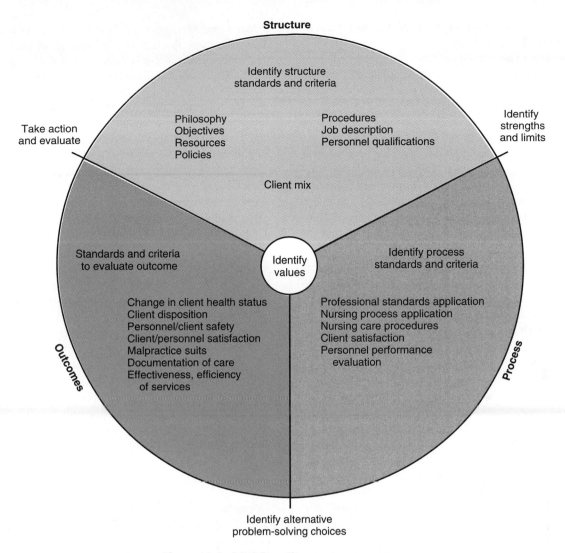

Figure 15-2 Model quality assurance program.

Process

Evaluation of process standards is the specific appraisal of the quality of care being given by agency providers such as nurses. Agencies use various methods to determine criteria for evaluating provider activities: conceptual models, such as a developmental model or Neuman's Systems Model; the standards of care of the provider's professional organization, such as the ANA community health nursing standards; or the nursing process. The activities of the nurse are evaluated to see if they correspond with the nursing care procedures defined by the agency.

The primary approaches used for process evaluation include the peer review committee and the client satisfaction survey. The techniques used for process evaluation are direct observation, questionnaire, interview, written audit, and videotape of client and provider encounters. Once data are collected to evaluate nursing process standards, the peer review committee reviews the data to identify strengths and weaknesses in the quality of care delivered. The peer review committee usually is an internal committee composed of

representatives of the nursing staff who are trained to administer audit instruments and conduct client interviews.

Outcome

It is often challenging to effectively evaluate outcomes or the end result of nursing care. Identifying changes in the client's health status as a result of nursing care provides nursing data that demonstrates the contribution to care made by nurses. Research studies using the tracer method or the sentinel method to identify client outcomes and client satisfaction surveys can be used to measure outcome standards. Outcomes can be measured by looking at client admission data about the client's level of dependence and the acuity of problems, comparing that data to show changes in levels of dependence and activity.

Direct physical observations and interviews are the most common measurement methods used. Rissner (1975) developed a client satisfaction survey to evaluate client attitudes and the content of nursing care in a primary setting. The survey has been adapted for use in home health by Reeder (Meisenheimer, 1989).

Instruments also have been developed to measure general health status indicators in home health (Choi, et al, 1987; Gould, 1985; Padilla and Grant, 1987). The Omaha Visiting Nurses Association Problem Classification System includes nursing diagnosis, protocols of care, and a problem-rating scale to measure nursing care outcomes (Martin, Scheet, and Stegman, 1993). Community health nursing has been involved primarily in evaluating program outcomes to justify program expenditures rather than in evaluating client outcomes.

Outcome evaluation assumes that health care has a positive effect on client status. The major problem with outcome evaluation is determining which nursing care activities are primarily responsible for causing changes in client status (Chernin and Ayer, 1990; Rapheal, 1991). Nurses deal with multiple uncontrolled factors in the clinical area. For example, both environment and family relationships affect client status. It is often difficult to determine whether these factors are the cause of changes in client status or whether nursing interventions have had the most effect. The NLN has published useful guides for developing outcome criteria (Rinke and Wilson, 1988).

Types of problems studied in a quality assurance program include reasons for client death, client injury, personnel and client safety and agency liability, causes of increased costs, denied reimbursement by third-party payers, client complaints, inefficient service, staff noncompliance with standards of structure, lack of resources, unnecessary staff work and overtime, documentation of care, and client health status. See Table 15-2, which summarizes quality assurance measures.

Evaluation, Interpretation, and Action

Interpreting the findings of a quality care evaluation is an essential component of the process. It allows for the identification of discrepancies between the quality care standards of the agency and the actual practice of the nurse or other health providers. These patterns reflect the total agency's functioning over time and generate information for decisions to be made about the strengths and limitations of the agency. Regular intervals for evaluation should be established within the agency, and periodic reports should be written so that the combined results of structure, process, and outcome efforts can be analyzed, and health care delivery patterns and problems identified. These reports should be used to establish an ongoing picture of changes that occur within an agency to justify community nursing services.

Identification and choices of possible courses of action to correct the weaknesses within the agency should involve both the administration and the staff. The courses of action chosen should be based on their significance, economic benefit, and timeliness. For example, if there is a nursing problem in the recording of client health education, the agency administration and staff may analyze the problem to see why it is occurring. Reasons that nurses cite for recording inade-

quacies include a lack of time to do paperwork properly, case overloads that reduce the amount of time spent with clients, and lack of available resources for health education. When such reasons are given, it is not appropriate for managers to deal with the problem by providing a staff development program on the importance of doing and recording health education. Rather, they must assess how to provide the time and resources necessary for the nurses to offer health education to the clients. Economically, it may be more beneficial to provide dictating equipment and clerical assistance so that nurses can dictate notes and other paperwork, giving them more client contact time, or to employ an additional nurse and reduce caseloads.

Taking action is the final step in the quality assurance model. Once the alternative courses of action are chosen to correct problems, actions are implemented to effect a change in the overall operation of the agency. Next, follow-up and evaluation of the actions taken must occur to complete the quality assurance process. Although the performance of nurses is evaluated, remember that the focus of a continuous quality improvement effort is on the process, not the person. It is assumed that nurses and other employees want to provide the best possible care and that problems or variations in a process should not be automatically attributed to their behavior (Laffel and Blumenthal, 1993). Since a key to effective quality improvement is continuous learning, staff development is essential for all employees.

DOCUMENTATION

Documentation is essential to the evaluation of quality care in any organization. The following section focuses on the kinds of documentation that normally occur in a community health agency.

Records

Records are a basic part of the communication structure of organizations. Accurate and complete records are required by law and must be kept by all agencies, governmental and non-governmental. In most states, the state departments of health stipulate the kind and content requirements of records for community health agencies. Records provide complete information about the client, indicate the extent and quality of services provided, resolve legal issues in malpractice suits, and provide information for education and research.

Community Health Agency Records

Community health agencies keep various types of records in order to predict population trends in a community, identify health needs and problems, prepare and justify budgets, and make administrative decisions. The kinds of records that the agency keeps can include reports of accidents, births, census, chronic disease, communicable disease, mortality, life expectancy, morbidity, child and spouse abuse, occupational illness and injury, and environmental health.

Agencies also keep records to maintain administrative contact and control of the organization. These records are clinical, service, and financial. The clinical record is the client health record. The provider service records include information about the numbers of clinic clients seen daily, the immunizations given, home visits made daily, transportation and mileage, the provider's time spent with the client, and the amount and kinds of supplies used. The service record is completed on a daily basis by each provider and is summarized monthly and annually to indicate trends in health care activities and costs relative to personnel time, transportation, maintenance, and supplies. The financial records include salaries, overhead, and transportation costs, and they serve as the basis for the cost accounting system (Pickett and Hanlon, 1990). The provider service records are used to correlate with the agency's financial records. These records are basic to peer review and audit.

As an outgrowth of quality assurance efforts in the health care system, comprehensive methods are being designed to document and measure client progress and client outcome from agency admission through discharge. An example of such a method is the client classification system developed at the Visiting Nurses Association of Omaha, Nebraska (Martin, 1982, Martin, Leak, and Aden, 1992). This comprehensive method for evaluating client care has several components: a classification system for assessing and categorizing client problems, a data base, a nursing problem list, and anticipated outcome criteria for the classified problem. Such schemes are viewed as having the potential to improve the delivery of nursing care, documentation, and the descriptions of client care. Briefly, implementation of comprehensive documentation methods will enhance nursing assessment, planning, implementation and evaluation of client care, and it will allow for the organization of pertinent client information for more effective and efficient nurse productivity and communication.

THE INTERSECTION OF TOTAL QUALITY MANAGEMENT, MANAGED CARE, AND NURSING

One of the fundamental changes that managed care has brought to health care is the shift in who makes the decisions. That is, in many situations the managed care organization, not the health professional, decides what kind or amount of care can be provided. In a simple example, the primary care provider believes that a specific medicine for allergy is the best choice for the client. However, due to its cost, that particular medication is not on the approved medication list for the client's health plan. Thus either the client must personally pay for the medicine or the provider must choose an alternative medication.

TQM, on the other hand, is clear in its need to include all personnel, especially those who play a key role in making decisions for the organization. The central point in TQM is that organizations cannot be transformed if participants are not involved. TQM is participatory and not "top down."

TQM also focuses on the customer whose needs are to be met. This can be the client, family, group, or other health care providers. Clearly, these two areas of focus are consistent with good public health nursing practices. Empowerment is a central concept in TQM. This is the process of allowing people to express their personal power or to take responsibility for their work and be held accountable for the results. An empowered organization encourages individual responsibility, decision making, creativity, and risk taking.

Interestingly, in 1997 the powerful Joint Commission for the Accreditation of Healthcare Organizations (JCAHO) based its new standards on TQM. Since the JCAHO accredits more than 18,000 hospitals, long-term and ambulatory care facilities, home care organizations, and clinical laboratories, its influence is significant (Epstein, 1998). The JCAHO standards specify that staff at all levels will be involved in developing the vision for the organization (Lanza, 1997).

Continuous improvement in quality care begins with top management, but as mentioned, the process is not strictly from the top down. Managers coach their employees and rely on employee participation and teamwork to anticipate possible errors and correct the plan of action before costly errors occur (Deming, 1986). When employees see themselves as valued members of the team, they raise questions and offer suggestions that often lead to better ways of doing things.

There are many aspects of TQM that are compatible both with nursing and with good management practices. For example, TQM focuses on processes rather than people. When things do not work as planned, it is important to look at how the process was designed rather than at ways to blame the people who were involved. "Blaming does not solve the problem, it simply changes the focus of attention" (Lanza, 1997, p. 99).

As nurses integrate quality management techniques into their organizations, it is important to remember that in empowered organizations, managers become facilitators, keepers and distributors of information, and guides. There will be resistance when an organization moves from a hierarchical way of doing business to one that counts on empowered employees at all levels to be involved and accountable. Both managers and employees will resist change. Resistance may take the form of expressing uncertainty or suspicion about the new way. Some people will feel threatened because of the new expectations, and especially about their level of involvement.

McLaughlin and Kaluzny (1997) describe how the Corning-Franklin Health Group uses nurse case managers to manage quality care for the 5% of their cases who use 40% of the funds for hospitalizations. They have an epidemiological and quality management staff who design the most effective strategies for managing their insured clients with such chronic illnesses as AIDS, cancer, and heart surgery. Care is customized to the client and family so that the entire care process is coordinated, including care in the home. This approach saves money for the Health Group and provides greater client and family satisfaction since care is much better organized than it would be without the case manager's assistance.

Healthy People 2010 and Quality Health Care

- Increase the proportion of Federal, Tribal, State, and local health agencies that have made information available to the public in the past year on the Leading Health Indicators, Health Status Indicators, and Priority Data Needs.
- Increase the proportion of population-based *Healthy People 2010* objectives for which national data are available for all population groups identified for the objectives.
- Increase the portion of Leading Health Indicators, Health Status Indicators, and Priority Data Needs for which data—especially for select populations—are available at the Tribal, State, and local levels.
- Increase the proportion of *Healthy People 2010* objectives that are tracked regularly at the national level.
- Increase the proportion of *Healthy People 2010* objectives for which national data are released within 1 year of the end of data collection.
- Data to assess the quality of the health outcomes come from sources like the nurse's documentation.

Healthy People 2010 and Quality Health Care

One of the two goals of *Healthy People 2010* is to increase quality and years of healthy life. This will be accomplished by helping individuals of all ages increase life expectancy and improve their quality of life. According to *Healthy People 2010* there are substantial differences in life expectancy among population groups within the nation. This is influenced by gender, race, and income. Quality of life reflects a sense of happiness and personal satisfaction. Health-related quality of life reflects a personal sense of physical and mental health and the ability to react to one's physical and social environments. Basically all of the objectives are directed toward meeting this goal.

To assess the quality of the outcomes of the objectives related to individuals and communities, several objectives specifically address how the quality assessment will occur. These are listed in the *Healthy People 2010* box above.

Clinical Application

Margaret, a community health nursing student, has been asked to be a member of the health care team designated to monitor the quality of service provided to the clients and community of the health care agency. As a member of this committee she is interested in identifying the current system used to monitor quality. To prepare for her role in planning and implementing a quality assurance program she reads the federal and state regulations to identify those elements that, by law, must be included in the QA program. She finds that Medicare now has specific tools to measure outcomes of client care. She learns that when the Medicare evaluator visits the agency, Margaret will be making home visits with the evaluator to directly observe the physical appearance of the client.

At the first meeting, the student is interested in the relationship between philosophy and objectives of the agency. Does the philosophy reflect beliefs about the clients to be served by the agency, the type of nursing care and services to be delivered, the population or the community to be served and, finally, beliefs about health care versus illness care? Are the objectives of the agency reflective of the stated beliefs in the philosophy? For example, does the philosophy indicate beliefs about client education or research? If so, are there agency objectives that address providing health education or enhancing research related to better client care?

Once the committee establishes from the philosophy and objectives that the agency's goal is to deliver primary health care services to the total population of the community, Margaret is interested in the standards of care used to deliver quality health care. In nursing, are the ANA standards for community health nursing used to evaluate nursing care given? Are the nurses employed by the agency qualified to fulfill their job descriptions through education, experience, or both?

Then the committee looks at the employment criteria of the agency. Do the criteria reflect the beliefs of the agency about nursing and the agency goals? Do the agency's policies and procedures assist the nurse in meeting the stated standards of care?

Given the structure of the agency, how is the process of care evaluated? Does the agency use prospective, concurrent, or retrospective audits to evaluate the process of care given? Are the audits designed to measure the standards of care used by the agency? How are the data used after they are collected? Is there any evidence that the evaluation makes a difference? Has the process of care changed as a result of the evaluation?

After the structure and process elements are identified, the committee members and the student are interested in the outcome elements. What questions should be asked about outcome?

A. *How is health outcome defined by the agency: client satisfaction, change in health status, number of malpractice suits, or number of Medicare payments received?*
B. *How are the data used to make a difference in future quality outcomes?*

Answers are in the back of the book.

Remember This!

- The health care delivery system is the largest employing industry in the United States; society is demanding increased efficiency and effectiveness from the system.
- Quality control is the tool used to ensure effectiveness and efficiency.
- The managed care industry is changing the face of the American health care delivery system and thus how quality will be defined and measured.
- Objective and systematic evaluation of nursing care is a priority within the profession for several reasons, including the effects of cost on health care accessibility, consumer demands for better quality care, and increasing involvement of nurses in public and health agency policy formulation.
- Total quality management/continuous quality improvement is a management philosophy used in health care. It is prevention oriented and process focused.

- The concept of quality includes customer satisfaction.
- Efforts are being made by the public and private sectors to form partnerships to monitor performance of all players in health care delivery for the purpose of improving the health of communities.
- Quality assurance is the monitoring of the activities of care to determine the degree of excellence attained in implementation of the activities.
- Quality assurance has been a concern of the profession since the 1860s, when Florence Nightingale called for a uniform format to gather and disseminate hospital statistics.
- Licensure has been a major issue in nursing since 1892.
- Two major categories of approaches exist in quality assurance and improvement today: general and specific approaches.
- Accreditation is an approach to quality control used for institutions, whereas licensure is used primarily for individuals.
- Certification combines features of both licensing and accreditation.
- Three major models have been used to evaluate quality: Donabedian's structure-process-outcome model, the sentinel model, and the tracer model.
- Seven basic components of a quality assurance program are (1) identifying values; (2) identifying structure, process, and outcome standards and criteria; (3) selecting measurement techniques; (4) interpreting the strengths and weaknesses of the care given; (5) identifying alternative courses of action; (6) choosing specific courses of action; and (7) taking action.
- Records are an integral part of the communication structure of a health care organization. Accurate and complete records are required by law of all agencies, whether governmental or non-governmental.
- Quality assurance and improvement mechanisms in health care delivery are the mechanisms for controlling the system and requesting accountability from individual providers within the system. Records help establish a total picture of the contribution of the agency to the client community.

❓ *What Would You Do?*

1. Write your own definition of TQM/CQI; compare your definition with the one given in the text. Are they the same or different? Give justification for your answer.
2. How does traditional QA fit into the TQM/CQI effort. Explain the relative importance of a continuing QA/QI effort.
3. Interview a nurse who is a coordinator of (or is responsible for) quality assurance and improvement in a local health agency. Ask the following questions and add others you may wish to have answered.
   a. Does the agency subscribe to the TQM/CQI approach to management?
   b. If not, is the agency incorporating elements of the TQM/CQI process as outlined by Deming in his 14 points?
   c. Is a traditional method of QA used to assure quality?
   d. Describe the components of the quality program.
   e. How are records used in your quality effort?
   f. Discuss the approaches and techniques that are used to implement the quality program.
   g. How has the quality program changed in the health agency over the past 20 years?
   h. What influence has the quality program had on decreasing problems attributable to process? to provider accountability?
   i. List and describe the types of records usually kept in a community health agency. Explain the purpose of each type of record.

REFERENCES

Al-Assaf AF: Historical evolution of managed care quality. In Al-Assaf A, Assaf RR (editors): *Managed care quality: a practical guide,* New York, 1998, CRC Press.

American Nurses Association: *A conceptual model of community health nursing,* Kansas City, Mo, 1980, American Nurses Association.

American Public Health Association: The definition and role of public health nursing in the delivery of health care: a statement to the public health nursing section, Washington, D.C., 1981, American Public Health Association.

Association of Community Health Nursing Educators: *Essential components of master's level practice in community health nursing,* Lexington, Ky, 1991a, Association of Community Health Nursing Educators.

Association of Community Health Nursing Educators: *Essentials of baccalaureate education,* Louisville, Ky, 1991b, Association of Community Health Nursing Educators.

Association of Community Health Nursing Educators: *Perspectives on doctoral education in community health nursing,* Lexington, Ky, 1993, Association of Community Health Nursing Educators.

Berwick DM: Continuous improvement as an ideal in healthcare, *N Engl J Med* 320:53, 1989.

Bushy A: Empowering initiatives to improve a community's health status, *J Nurs Care Qual* 11(4):32, 1997.

Cary A: Credentialing in a changing health care environment. In Lancaster J: *Nursing issues in leading and managing change,* St Louis, 1999, Mosby.

Chernin SW, Ayer TS: The outcome audit: assuring quality care, *Caring* 9(2):8-12, 1990.

Choi T, Josten L, Christensen ML, et al: Health specific family coping index for noninstitutional care. In Rinke L (editor): *Outcome measures in home care,* vol 1, New York, 1987, National League for Nursing.

Council of Home Health Agencies and Community Health Services: *Accreditation of home health agencies and community nursing services: criteria and guide for preparing reports,* New York, 1986, National League for Nursing.

Davis ER: *Total quality management for homecare,* Gaithersburg, Md, 1994, Aspen Publishers.

Deming WE: *Out of the crisis,* Cambridge, Ma, 1986, Massachusetts Institute of Technology, Center for Advanced Engineering Study.

Donabedian A: *The criteria and standards of quality,* vol 2, Exploration in quality assessment and monitoring, Ann Arbor, Mi, 1981, Health Administration Press.

Donabedian A: *Explorations in quality assessment and monitoring,* vol 3, Ann Arbor, Mi, 1985, Health Administration Press.

Donabedian A: The seven pillars of quality, *Arch Pathol Lab Med* 114:1115, 1990.

Epstein AM: Rolling down the runway: the challenges ahead for quality report cards, *JAMA* 279(21):1691, 1998.

Gottlieb H: Quality assurance: a blueprint for improved patient care and service, *Home Healthcare Nurs* 6(3):11, 1988.

Gould J: Standardized home health nursing plans: a quality assurance look, *Quality Rev Bull* 11(11):334, 1985.

Greenberg LG, Lezzoni LI: Quality. In Calkins D, Fernandopulle RJ, Marino BS: *Health care policy,* Cambridge, Mass, 1995, Blackwell Science.

Gremaldi PL, Micheletti JA: PRO objectives and quality criteria, *Hospitals* 59:64, 1985.

Halverson PK, Kaluzny AD, McLaughlin CP: *Managed care and public health,* Gaithersburg, Md, 1998, Aspen Publishers.

Institute of Medicine, Lohr KN (editor): *Medicare: a strategy for quality assurance,* vol 1. Washington, D.C., 1990, National Academy Press.

Joint Council Committee on Quality in Public Health: *Promoting quality care for communities: the role of health departments in an era of managed care,* Washington, D.C., 1996, National Association of City and County Health Officials.

Kessner DM, Kalk CE: Assessing health quality: the case for tracers, *N Engl J Med* 288:189, 1973.

Kinney ED, Freedman JA, Cook CA: Quality improvement in community-based, long-term care: theory and reality, *Am J Law Med* 20(1-2):59, 1994.

Kovner A, Jonas S (editors): *Jonas' and Kovner's health care delivery in the United States,* New York, 1998, Springer.

Laffel G, Blumenthal D: The case for using industrial quality management science in health care organizations. In Al-Assaf AF, Schmele JA (editors): *The textbook of total quality in healthcare,* Delray Beach, Fl, 1993, St. Lucie Press.

Lanza ML: Feminist leadership through total quality management, *Health Care Women Internat* 18:95, 1997.

Lasker RD, et al: *Medicine and public health: the power of collaboration,* New York, 1997, The New York Academy of Medicine.

Lieski AM: Standards: the basis of a quality assurance program. In Meisenheimer CG (editor): *A complete guide to effective programs,* Rockville, Md, 1985, Aspen.

LoGerfo J, Brook R: Evaluation of health services and quality of care. In Williams S, Torrens P (editors): *Introduction to health services,* New York, 1984, John Wiley & Sons.

Maddox PJ: Quality management. In Lancaster J (editor): *Nursing issues in leading and managing change,* St Louis, 1998, Mosby.

Maibusch RM: Evolution of quality assurance for nursing in hospitals. In Schrolder PS, Maibusch RM (editors): *Nursing quality assurance,* Rockville, Md, 1984, Aspen.

Martin K: A client classification system adaptable for computerization, *Nurs Outlook* 30:515, 1982.

Martin K, Leak G, Aden C: The Omaha system: a research based model for decision making, *J Nurs Admin* 22:47, 1992.

Martin KS, Scheet NJ, Stegman MR: Home health clients: characteristics, outcomes of care, and nursing interventions, *Am J Public Health* 83(12):1730, 1993.

McLaughlin CP, Kaluzny AD: Defining total quality management/continuous quality improvement. In McLaughlin CP, Kaluzny AD (editors): *Continuous quality improvement in healthcare: theory, implementation and applications,* Gaithersburg, Md, 1994, Aspen.

McLaughlin CP, Kaluzny AD: Total quality management issues in managed care, *J Health Care Finance* 23(1):10, 1997.

Meisenheimer C: *Quality assurance for home health care,* Rockville, Md, 1989, Aspen.

National Association for Healthcare Quality: *Risk management: NAHQ guide to quality management,* Skokie, IL, 1993, NAHQ Press.

Padilla GV, Grant MM: Quality of life as a cancer nursing outcome variable: quality of life index. In Rinke L (editor): *Outcome measures in home care,* vol 1, New York, 1987, National League for Nursing Publications.

Pickett G, Hanlon J: *Public health administration and practice,* St Louis, 1990, Mosby.

Porter A: Assuring quality through staff nurse performance, *Nurs Clin North Am* 23(3):649, 1988.

Rapheal C: Response to "Quality assurance mechanisms in home care—measurement of quality and outcomes in home health care." In National League for Nursing: *Mechanisms of quality in long-term care: service and clinical outcomes,* Pub no 41-2382, New York, 1991, National League for Nursing.

Rinke L, Wilson A: Client oriented project objectives, *Caring* 7(1):25, 1988.

Rissner N: Development of an instrument to measure patient satisfaction with nurses and nursing care in primary care settings, *Nurs Res* 24(1):45, 1975.

Rutstein DD, Berenberg W, Chalmers TC, et al: Measuring the quality of medical care: a clinical method, *N Engl J Med* 294:582, 1976.

Seppanen L: Accreditation: differentiation from regulation, *Issues* 16(2):3-13, 1995.

Stevens BJ: *The nurse as executive,* ed 3, Rockville, Md, 1985, Aspen.

Weiss M: The quality evolution in managed care organizations: shifting the focus to community health, *J Nurs Care Qual* 11(4):27, 1997.

Young G: The privatization of quality assurance in health care. In Halverson PK, Kaluzny AD, McLaughlin CP: *Managed care and public health,* Gaithersburg, MD, 1998, Aspen.

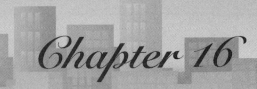

Chapter 16

Working With Groups in the Community

PEGGYE GUESS LASSITER

OBJECTIVES

After reading this chapter, the student should be able to:

- Describe the major group elements of group purpose, member interaction, and cohesion.
- Examine how group members are affected by group norms.
- Explain the usefulness of groups in promoting individual health.

- Evaluate nursing behaviors that assist groups in promoting health for individuals.
- Identify the groups constituting a community and illustrate links between them.
- Describe the role of the nurse in working with established groups to meet community health goals.

CHAPTER OUTLINE

KEY TERMS

avoidance: a passive way to deal with conflict without directly acknowledging that disagreements or differences exist.

cohesion: the amount of attraction among individual group members and between each member and the group.

collaboration: mutual sharing and joint work aimed at gaining a common understanding or reaching a common goal.

communication structure: identifies message pathways and member participation in sending and receiving messages.

conflict: a clash, disagreement, or different viewpoint that occurs when people have different goals, ideas, values, beliefs, needs, or feelings; it can help or hinder the work of a group.

established groups: groups in which membership ties already exist and a structure is already in place.

formal groups: groups that have a defined membership and specific purpose.

group: a collection of interacting individuals who have a common purpose(s).

group culture: formed from a combination of group norms (task, maintenance, and reality norms).

group purpose: the aim or goal that the members seek to attain.

group structure: the particular arrangement of group parts as they combine to make up the group as a whole.

Continued

Working with groups is an important skill for nurses to master. Groups are an effective and powerful way to initiate and implement changes for individuals, families, organizations, and the community. People naturally form groups in their families, in school, and at work, as well as in many social and professional settings. Nurses need to understand group concepts and group process since they will invariably work with groups. Groups form for many reasons. They may form to accomplish a clearly stated purpose or goal, or they may form naturally when people come together because of their shared values, interests, activities, or personal characteristics.

Community groups represent the collective interests, needs, and values of individuals; they provide a link between the individual and the larger social system. Individual attitudes are developed in families and through friendships and associations in school, work, and other settings such as religious, social, or professional organizations. Throughout life, membership in groups influences thoughts, attitudes, values, and behaviors as people interact. Groups serve as channels for communication within any community. Often groups serve as a medium for improving the health and well-being of individuals, families, and communities. Some individual health changes are difficult or impossible to achieve without group support and encouragement. Two notable examples are Alcoholics Anonymous and Weight Watchers, which use group support and encouragement to influence individuals to change their drinking and eating habits.

All nurses have worked with and participated both personally and professionally in groups. As discussed in Chapter 10, nurses often use groups in the community to communicate health information in a cost-effective way to a number of clients who meet together, rather than repeating the information several times to individuals.

Identifying groups, their goals, member characteristics, and their place in the community structure are important first steps toward understanding the community and assessing its health. Nurses often work with community groups to help people identify priority health needs and capabilities and to make valuable changes in their own communities.

GROUP CONCEPTS

In order to work effectively with groups and use them as a way to improve the health of individuals and families in communities, it is necessary to understand core group concepts. These include defining a group, understanding group purpose, membership, cohesion, and task and maintenance functions.

Group Definition

A **group** is a collection of interacting individuals who have a common purpose or purposes. Each member influences and is in turn influenced by every other member. Members believe there is a benefit to be gained from being part of the group. Key group elements are **member interaction** and **group purpose.** Families are one example of a community group. Families have many purposes, including providing psychological support and socialization for their members. Usually, families share kinship bonds, living space, and economic resources. Interactions are diverse and frequent in families.

A group can be formed in response to specific community needs, problems, or opportunities. In one community, residents banded together to form a neighborhood association to protect their health and welfare. This neighborhood of upper-middle-class homes was located in an unincorporated area. For 3 years the residents were threatened with multiple environmental hazards, including a forest fire (fire hydrants had not been installed during the development of the neighborhood), establishment of a small airport near the homes, and construction of an interstate highway adjacent to the homes. To protect their interests, residents formed a neighborhood association and elected officers to represent their interests in a constructive manner. The interaction of this group focused on problem solving.

Other community groups come together because of a mutual attraction among individuals as well as obvious and keenly felt personal needs. Young and single adults often form loosely structured groups for socialization and recreation. Through parties and other social meetings, the young adults establish a pattern for behaving and relating to one another. They select partners; test ideas, attitudes, and behaviors; and establish their identity with a group of people who have similar developmental needs. Their unstated purpose is to practice adult roles.

A fourth example, health-promoting groups, are formed when people meet in community or health care settings to deal with common challenges to their physical and emotional well-being. The purposes of health-promoting groups are to improve members' health and deal with specific threats to health. Chapters of Alcoholics Anonymous, Parents without Partners, and La Leche League are health-promoting groups. Members both give and receive personal support and participate in group problem solving and education. These groups may be one of two types: established groups or selected-membership groups. Both types of groups are discussed later in this chapter. The purpose of a group guides the nature and frequency of interaction.

How do purpose and interaction vary in these four examples? Some groups, such as the neighborhood association and La Leche League, have an obvious purpose that can be easily stated by members. For families, social groupings, and many spontaneously formed groups, the purposes are unstated. However, the purpose can be determined by studying their activities as a group over time.

Group Purpose

Once the need for a particular health change is identified and group work is selected as the most effective way to make it happen, a clear statement of the proposed group's purpose is essential. A clear purpose helps in establishing criteria for member selection. A clear statement of purpose proved valuable in forming a new group in one city's housing development. The local department of social services had received numerous reports of child abuse and neglect. Routine home visits for well-child care documented high stress between parents and their offspring. Some parents requested guidance from the public health nurse in child discipline. The nurse suggested that a parent group be formed, and the following purpose was selected: dealing with kids more effectively in order to have greater child and parent satisfaction. The purpose indicated both the process (to help parents deal with kids) and the desired outcome (satisfaction for parents and children). As potential members were approached, this statement of purpose for the group helped the individuals decide whether they wanted to join.

Briefly Noted

When the purpose for a group is clearly stated and agreed on, the group becomes increasingly attractive for members.

When a group makes a public appeal for members and accepts everyone who wants to join, the membership is self-selected, based on the stated group purpose. In this type of recruitment, publicity must reach those in need of

particular health changes. Prospective members often want to discuss the purpose with leaders or clarify questions concerning the purpose at the first group meeting. Their commitment to the health group is partly based on individual goals and how well the group goal satisfies their personal objectives.

Cohesion

Cohesion is the amount of attraction among members and between each member and the group. Cohesion refers to "all the positive and negative forces that affect whether or not a person remains a member of a group" (Toropainen and Rinne, 1998, p. 106). Individuals in a cohesive group identify themselves as a unit, work toward common goals, endure frustration for the sake of the group, and defend the group against outside criticism. Attraction increases when members feel accepted and liked by others, see similar qualities in each other, and believe they share similar attitudes and values (Figure 16-1). Members' traits that increase group cohesion and productivity include:

1. Compatible personal and group goals
2. Attraction to group goals
3. Attraction to other members
4. An appropriate mix of leading and following skills
5. Good problem-solving skills.

Briefly Noted

Often a group of similar individuals works together better than a group of dissimilar individuals because they are likely to be compatible and have similar goals and aspirations.

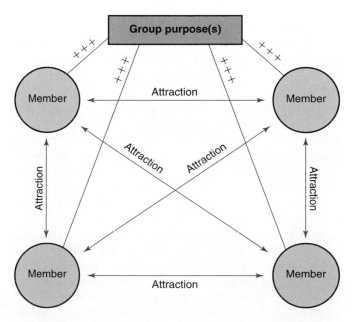

Figure 16-1   Cohesion is the measure of attraction between members and member attraction to group purpose(s).

Anything a member does that deliberately contributes to the group's purpose is termed a **task function.** Members with task-directed traits are attractive to the group. These traits include strong problem-solving skills, access to material resources, and skills in directing. It is equally important for members to affirm and support one another. These **maintenance functions** help members feel accepted and motivated to stay in the group. Maintenance functions also include the ability to help people resolve conflicts and gain social and environmental comfort. Both task and maintenance functions are necessary to group progress. Naturally, those members who provide these maintenance functions are attractive to the group. The presence of an abundance of such traits in the group tends to increase group cohesion.

Other member traits such as those listed below can decrease cohesion and productivity:

- Conflicts between personal and group goals
- Lack of interest in group goals and activities
- Poor problem-solving and communication abilities
- Lack of leadership skills
- Disagreement about types of leadership
- Dislike of other members
- Behaviors and attributes that are poorly understood by others
- Inability or unwillingness to see the point of view that others hold.

Usually, the more alike group members are, the stronger a group's attraction, whereas differences may reduce attractiveness. Members' perceptions of differences can create competition and jealousy. At the same time, personal differences can increase group cohesion if they support complementary functioning or provide contrasting viewpoints necessary for decision making. Clearly, cohesion factors are complex. Many factors influence members' attraction to one another and to the group's goal. High group cohesion increases both group productivity and member satisfaction. Two examples found in everyday nursing practice illustrate factors that influence group cohesion.

A nurse working in the community formed and provided initial leadership for a group of clients who had been treated for burns. Ten residents, all from one town, had been discharged after 3 months in a hospital's burn unit. The stated purpose for the group was to assist members make the difficult transition from hospital to home. Each person had been treated for extensive burns in an intensive care treatment center; each had relied heavily on health workers for physical, social, and emotional rehabilitation; and each had faced the challenge of resuming work and family roles. They shared some similar experiences and hopes for the future but varied in the amount of trauma and stress experienced. They also differed widely in psychological readiness for return to ordinary daily routines. One woman was able to return quickly to her job as cashier in a large supermarket. The strength of her determination to overcome public reaction to her scars, coupled with an ability to "use the right words" and an empathy for others, distinguished her from others in the group. Her behaviors were attractive and inspiring to

group members. As they listened to her, they began to want to return to their previous roles; they wanted to return to a semblance of their former lives. Members' attraction to the common purpose of returning to successful life patterns and managing relations with others provided group cohesion. The members also believed that interaction with others with similar burn experiences could help them reach that goal. This example shows that certain member experiences, such as crises or traumas, may help individuals identify with each other and may increase member attraction.

Being different from the general population yet similar to others in the group may motivate some people to remain in the group. In this instance, others may want to distance themselves from the group because they do not want to be identified as having an aversive characteristic such as disfigurement. Empathy for another's pain, learned only through mutual experience, may provide each individual with a perspective for problem solving or affirming another's view. The nurse in this example helped members use common experiences and learn from their differences. The group was effective.

In contrast, differences created tension in one self-help group for victims of spouse abuse. In this group, nurses met a severe challenge from the group because the nurses had not been abused. The nurses were invited by professional staff to assist the group meet its goal of "learning to manage safety, health, and independence." Victim members of the group thought that the nurses could not understand their intensely personal and devastating injury. They told the nurses this. They isolated the nurses from membership but tolerated their presence. Attraction for the group diminished, and attendance at meetings fell. Discussion of superficial issues occupied group time as the victim members avoided topics of member safety and violence in general. Differences between the nurses and victims hampered group cohesion; the group did not effectively address its goal, and members felt isolated.

When the nurses recognized the reasons for the deterioration of the group, they encouraged all members to describe experiences that threatened their self-respect in their family and work roles. The nurses revealed some of their own struggles as they tried to be self-directed and have control in their own lives. Revealing their vulnerability made the nurses more attractive to the group. The members were able to accept the nurses, whom they now saw as more similar to themselves. They promptly refocused their efforts on the purpose of the group.

Group members began to support one another, to assert individual rights for safety, to locate employment, to make living arrangements apart from their abusers, and to identify changes that they needed to make in how they communicated with others. The clear purpose of maintaining members' safety, combined with the new, broader common goal of asserting their self-respect, contributed to successful group work.

The nature of the group influences members' attraction to the group. Factors affecting attraction include the group's choice of programs, size, type of organization, and position in the community. Attraction to the group is increased when members clearly understand the goals and when they think the group activities are useful to meet their needs.

Group productivity is affected by cohesion. Some cohesion is necessary for people to remain with a group and accomplish the goals. Attractiveness positively influences members' motivation and commitment to work on the group task. Group cohesion may be increased when members understand the experiences of others and can identify common ideas and reactions to various issues. Nurses facilitate this process by pointing out both similarities and differences as well as by helping members redefine differences in ways that make the differences compatible.

Briefly Noted

Group leaders can help group members recognize traits and interests they have in common and how some differences in skills among individuals help to complement the main group purpose.

Norms

Norms are standards that guide, control, and regulate individuals and communities. Group norms set the standards for members' behaviors, attitudes, and even perceptions. All groups have norms and mechanisms to ensure conformity (Sampson and Marthas, 1990). Group norms serve three functions:

1. To ensure movement toward the group's purpose or tasks
2. To maintain the group by supporting members
3. To influence members' perceptions and interpretations of reality.

Even though certain norms keep the group focused on its task, some deviation is permitted as long as members respect central goals and are committed to return to them. This commitment to return to the central goals is the **task norm.** The strength of the task norm determines the group's ability to keep focusing on its goal.

Maintenance norms create group pressures to affirm members and maintain their comfort. Group members seem most productive and at ease when their psychological and social well-being is nurtured. Maintenance behaviors include identifying the social and psychological tensions of members and taking steps to support those members at high-stress times. Maintenance norms can deal with conditions such as temperature, space, seating, an accessible location, food, and scheduling meetings at convenient times. This attention to arrangements may include meeting in places that are easily accessible and comfortable to the participants, providing refreshments, and scheduling meetings at convenient times.

A third important function of group norms relates to members' perceptions of reality. Daily behavior is largely based on the way each aspect of life is understood. Through socializa-

tion, individuals learn how to gather information, assign meaning, and react to situations in a way that satisfies needs. Both decision-making and action taking are influenced by the meanings that the group has of **reality norms.** People look to one another to reinforce, challenge, or correct their ideas of what is real. Groups provide a place to examine the life situations confronting members. As individuals gather information, try to understand the information, make decisions, and consider the facts and their implications, they can act responsibly in relation to themselves, the group, and the community.

Group norms (task, maintenance, and reality norms) combine to form a **group culture.** When nurses work with groups, they can support helpful rules, attitudes, and behaviors. Only when these rules, attitudes, and behaviors become part of the life of the group, independent of the nurse, are they norms. As seen in Figure 16-2, reality norms influence members to see relevant situations in the same way as other members see them. Some members may feel strong normative pressures to support members who are considering change. A person's values are developed first from interaction and influence from family members and other caregivers and then from peers and teachers in school and key people in social groups.

For example, if a group of individuals with diabetes thinks that an uncontrollable diet is harmful, they might try to influence one another to maintain diet control. Nurses in everyday practice would provide accurate information about

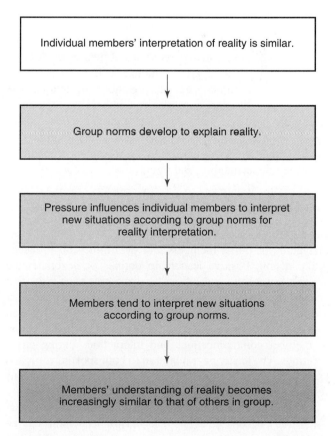

Figure 16-2   Influence of group reality norms on individual members.

diet and the disease process, including cause and effect between food intake and disease. The nurse would also support and reinforce the belief that health through diet control is attainable and desirable.

Briefly Noted

Most of the *Healthy People 2010* objectives can be addressed in health-promotion and disease-prevention groups. In groups, individuals often learn healthier behaviors, examine attitudes and values that are barriers to changing risk-related behaviors, and gain support from others to change high-risk behaviors to healthy life-style choices. For example, groups may support physical activity and fitness, sound nutrition, and safe sexual practices. Through group support, individuals may conquer smoking, drug abuse, or abusive relationships, and they may identify and reduce exposure to environmental hazards and promote safer physical settings for all.

When members of any group have similar backgrounds, their scope of knowledge may be limited. For example, female members in a spouse abuse group may believe that all men are dangerous and cannot be trusted. This belief may come from common childhood and marriage experiences. This stereotypical view of men, reinforced by similar perceptions in other members, can lead to continuing anger, fear of interactions with men, and a hostile or helpless approach to family affairs. Nurses or group members who have known men in loving, helpful, and collaborative ways can describe their different and positive perceptions of men. Such descriptions add information and challenge beliefs to influence members' perceptions and interpretations of reality. The health of the individual improves as members' perceptions of reality are based on more complete data and as cause-and-effect factors are understood. Nurses bring an important perspective to groups in which similar backgrounds of members limit their understanding and interpretation of concerns.

Leadership

Leadership is a complex concept. It consists of behaviors that guide or direct members and determine and influence group action. Positive leadership defines or negotiates the group's purpose(s), selects and helps implement tasks that accomplish the purpose, maintains an environment that affirms and supports members, and balances efforts between task and maintenance. An effective leader pays close attention to member communications and interactions during group meetings. The leader pays attention to both spoken words and body language that provide leaders and members continuous feedback about the participants as well as the group process.

Effective leadership leads to effective group functioning. There may be one designated leader, or leadership can be shared by a few or several group members. Shared leadership can increase productivity, cohesion, and satisfying

Evidence-Based Practice

Story-telling is a process or form of interaction that is used to preserve history and culture and for teaching values, strengthening family and community ties, and communicating practical information about daily living. The study cited below examined the health-promoting functions of storytelling in a group of 28 African-American women. A total of 115 stories were analyzed from four focus groups that took place over a 6-week period.

In this research, six major functions of storytelling were identified: (1) contextual grounding, (2) bonding with others, (3) validating and affirming experiences, (4) venting and catharsis, (5) resisting oppression, and (6) educating others.

APPLICATION IN PRACTICE

It can be seen how storytelling could be used in community groups such as new mothers, adolescents, older adults, or people with a similar health problem (e.g., obesity, diabetes, hypertension) as well as groups such as migrant workers or immigrants from a specific country. As people tell their stories in a group, they have opportunities to describe their pain, struggles, joy, frustrations, and concerns. The groups can provide feedback to help the storyteller realize new ways to think, respond, and behave.

Banks-Wallace J: Emancipatory potential of storytelling in a group, *Image: J Nurs Scholarship* 30(2):17-21, 1998.

interactions among members. A democratic approach to leading is most effective when there are many alternatives, much information is needed, and issues of values and ethics are involved (Sampson and Marthas, 1990).

After initiating or establishing a group, a nurse may stimulate leadership within and among members, often giving up control and encouraging members to lead in a way that best fits the group. Of course, nurses differ in how they lead. In some settings and circumstances, a single leader may be necessary. For example, when members have limited skills or limited time or when group members say they are uncomfortable sharing leadership responsibility, a single leader will work best.

Positive experiences with committees, work teams, and client groups promote self-confidence and appreciation of the leadership skills of others. As one works in groups it becomes clear that getting selected tasks done is only one group outcome. A second, equally valuable result is watching members become more competent and able to share responsibility. Shared leadership limits power seekers and supports group wholeness, flexibility, and freedom.

Leadership behaviors and definitions are listed in the box below. Leaders are able to influence because of their knowledge, ability, access to needed resources, personal attractiveness, status or position in the community or organization, and ability to control sanctions for others.

HOW TO Lead: Useful Behavior

Advise: offer direction based on knowledgeable opinion.
Analyze: review what has occurred to encourage others to examine behavior and its meaning.

Clarify: check out meanings of interaction and communication through questions and restatement.

Confront: present behavior and its effects to the individual and group to challenge existing perceptions.

Evaluate: analyze the effect or outcome of action or the worth of an idea according to some standard.

Initiate: introduce topics, begin work, or change the focus of a group.

Question: bring about analysis of a view or views by questions that support examination.

Reflect behavior: give feedback on how behavior appears to others.

Reflect feelings: name the feelings that may be behind what is said or done.

Suggest: propose or bring an idea to a group.

Summarize: restate discussion or group action briefly, and highlight important points.

Support: give emotionally comforting feedback that helps a person or group continue current actions.

Leadership is typically described as patriarchal, paternal, or democratic; each of these styles has a particular effect on members' interaction, satisfaction, and productivity. Groups may reflect one or a combination of styles.

Patriarchal or paternal leadership occurs when one person has the final authority for group direction and movement. Patriarchal leaders may control members through rewards and threats, often keeping them uninformed about the goals and rationale behind prescribed actions. A paternal leader wins the respect and dependence of followers by parental-like devotion to members' needs. The leader controls group movement and progress through interpersonal power. This leadership style is authoritarian, and group morale and cohesiveness are typically low. These leaders do not teach members how to function independently. Also, issues of authority and control can disrupt productivity if group members challenge the leader's power. These styles are effective for groups such as a disaster team, in which specific tasks must be accomplished in a timely way with high productivity.

Paternal leadership was effective in the following situation. Mary Jones, a public health nurse, asked her neighbors to meet to talk about the threat of drug traffic in the neighborhood. The residents agreed with Mary that several recent drug-related arrests in the area signaled a need for community concern. No one knew what to do, but all believed quick action was necessary. Mary had experience in organizing people, knew of local resources, and thought that information, education, and residents' collaboration with police could substantially control the local drug-traffic problem. She organized the neighborhood group, assigned and monitored their tasks, and praised them as they made progress in achieving the goal of eliminating drug sales in their community.

Democratic leadership is cooperative in nature and promotes and supports members' involvement in all aspects of decision making and planning. Members influence each other as they set goals, plan steps to meet the goals, implement those steps, and evaluate progress.

The following example describes a common experience for nurses. A committee of nurses for a small community health organization met weekly to improve nursing services. Tom initiated a revision of the written standards. Several members of the group felt threatened by Tom's idea. They feared that their daily work would change and that a resulting evaluation using new standards would find them inferior or require them to learn how to do things differently. Jane supported updating the standards. She also recognized the importance of continuing to support and affirm each nurse's worth on the committee. While Tom pushed the committee toward revising the standards, Jane often interrupted to ask members to respond and to make suggestions, noting to the group the excellent contributions that were made. Sara provided a touch of humor whenever group tension became high. Amber added a critical, questioning support to the decision-making process and encouraged members to evaluate each step. In these and other ways, group members shared leadership tasks. Some served predominantly to push the group toward its objective, while others facilitated goal attainment by maintaining member involvement through support. For this group, the chairperson convened the group but did not dominate in leader activities. The members accomplished the tasks of writing and implementing an audit for new nursing standards in a democratic leadership style.

Group Structure

Structure describes the particular arrangement of group parts as they combine to make up the group as a whole. A **communication structure** identifies message pathways and member participation in sending and receiving messages. People who actively send and receive messages and who serve as channels for messages are important in the structure. These "central" individuals influence the group because of their access to and interpretive control over communication flow. Communication and role structures are interrelated.

Role structure describes the expected behaviors of members in relation to each other as the group interacts. Each member has a role that serves a purpose in the life of the group. As seen in Box 16-1, typical group roles are leader, follower, task specialist, maintenance specialist, evaluator, peacemaker, and gatekeeper. Members' roles in the group are described by their predominant actions. Identification of communication patterns helps to determine roles because people occupying particular roles typically use certain kinds of communication.

Group structure emerges from various member influences, including the members' understanding and support of the group purpose. Nurses assess the group structure as it relates to goal accomplishment. Many groups also consider their own structure, assess its usefulness in relation to member comfort and productivity, and then plan for a different division of tasks that is agreeable to the whole.

Evaluator: analyzes the effect or outcome of action or the worth of ideas according to some standard.

Follower: seeks and accepts the authority or direction of others.

Gatekeeper: controls outsiders' access to the group.

Leader: guides and directs group activity.

Maintenance specialist: provides physical and psychological support for group members, thereby holding the group together.

Peacemaker: attempts to reconcile conflict between members or takes action in response to influences that disrupt the group process and threaten its existence.

Task specialist: focuses or directs movement toward the main work of the group.

In the earlier example of nurses working on standards of nursing service, Tom served a role as task specialist, Jane as maintenance specialist, and Amber as evaluator. These members consistently occupied particular roles and were expected by others to maintain their behavior to serve the purposes of the group.

A person occupying a gatekeeper's role controls outsiders' access to the group. Gatekeepers either facilitate or block communication between outsiders and group members. It is important to identify who serves in a gatekeeper role. The gatekeeper usually confronts the nurse after beginning contacts are attempted. An invitation to communicate further with group members is extended only after the nurse and gatekeeper determine mutual benefits and possible risks from continued contact between the nurse and the group.

Tuckman (1965) divided the development of a group function into four stages:

1. Forming
2. Storming
3. Norming
4. Performing.

Forming occurs when the members of the group come together for the first time. No true group has formed. This is the stage where people are gathering and determining their role or relationship to the other people in the group. There is often wariness among members during this stage. Some members may question why others are included in the group. Formal or informal leaders may emerge and be elected or selected. If a formal group leader has been designated, he or she will, at this phase, clarify why people have been asked to join the group and what each is expected to do or contribute.

During the second phase, *storming,* there is chaos as members decide what the task is and what role they are going to play or whether they really want to belong to this group. Conflicts often arise since members may have different agendas, personalities, goals, and backgrounds. This is the phase during which groups are most likely to fail. The leader needs to use guidance and limit setting to help the group resolve conflict and move to a positive way of working together.

The third phase is called *norming.* This is when the group begins to come together and develop cohesion. Group members are now less defensive, and the group begins to develop its identity. This is the time when the group develops the ability to be frank with one another and to express and resolve conflict. The group can now work together to find solutions.

In the last phase, *performing,* the group pursues the goals they have set. The group is now united. When conflict occurs, it is about how to meet the goal rather than about individual agendas and personal turf.

PROMOTING HEALTH THROUGH GROUP WORK

Health behavior is influenced by the groups to which people belong. Individuals live within a social structure of significant others such as family members, friends, co-workers, and acquaintances. The patterns and directions of everyday activities are learned in a family, and these are later reinforced or challenged by new groups. These groups constitute the context in which values, beliefs, and attitudes are formed; individuals usually consider the responses of others in all types of decisions regarding personal welfare.

The following example illustrates the effects of a person's social network on health behavior. Mary was worried about a recently discovered breast lump. She first asked her husband, Lew, to confirm its presence, which he did. He agreed that she should have a diagnostic evaluation, and an appointment was arranged. Mary talked with Lew about the possible consequences of malignancy, and she noted Lew's concern for her safety. She feared radical surgery and its impact on her relationship to Lew, but she did not discuss her fear with him. Mary telephoned two close friends from work and asked them to meet her for coffee. Although they thought it was premature to fret about the lump being malignant, they discussed all they knew about treatment for breast cancer, including the trials, defeats, and successes of three mutual friends who had had surgery for breast cancer. Each of the three breast cancer survivors had reacted differently to her own situation, and Mary's friends retold familiar details. The retelling seemed important to understanding the current situation and helping Mary sort out her feelings. Mary was able to understand her situation better as well as her response to it. These conversations helped Mary face the possible risk involved, recognize the need to follow through with diagnostic procedures, select capable medical providers, and manage her emotional stress.

The responses of Mary's friends and her husband influenced her assessment, decision making, and subsequent behavior. The work done by Mary and her social network in response to her health need was important. It illustrates a common mechanism among individuals and the groups to which they belong. The groups described in this example are Mary's family group, which includes Mary and Lew, and Mary's friendship group, of which those who met for coffee are a subset.

Because of social or emotional isolation, some people do not have access to groups who will support them during a time of health changes. Isolated individuals may have low self-esteem, be mentally ill, or occupy positions of low status in their family or community. They may be disadvantaged, gifted, or deviant, or they may simply live in a rural area or be engaged in solitary work. They may also be new to a community and not yet able to form social ties. These individuals benefit greatly through newly organized groups established for specific purposes.

Choosing Groups for Health Change

Nurses often use groups to help people in a community once they understand the needs of the community and its people. Understanding needs is based on client contacts, expressed concerns from various community spokespersons, health statistics for the area, availability of health resources, and the community's general well-being. These data point to the community's strengths and critical needs. Just as other nursing interventions are based on the assessment of needs and the knowledge of effective treatment, group formation is determined by the assessment of community needs.

Nurses work with existing groups, and they also form new groups. Initiation of change and recruitment of a nurse into the group may come not just from the nurse, but from individuals, the affected group(s), or a related organization. Deciding whether to work in established groups or to begin new ones depends on the clients' needs, the purpose of existing groups, and the membership ties in existing groups.

Established Groups

There are advantages to using **established groups** for individual health change. Membership ties already exist, and the current structure can be used. It is not necessary to find new members because compatible individuals already form a working group. Established groups usually have developed some successful operating methods, and new goals and the approach to achieving them can be built on this history. Members know one another's strengths, limitations, and preferred styles of interaction. Members' comfort levels, which stem from their experience together, enable them to focus on the new goal.

Established groups can influence members. Successful group endeavors have strengthened the ties among members. Their bonds are usually multidimensional because of the length of time they have spent together. Such rich ties support group change efforts for individuals' health.

Before deciding to work with an established group, the nurse needs to decide if introducing a new focus is compatible with group purposes. Sometimes, individual health goals will enhance existing group purposes, and the nurse can bring useful information for health, behavior, and group process.

How can nurses enter existing groups and get members to focus on individual health needs? One nurse employed by an industrial firm noticed the harmful effects of stress on several managers. They had elevated blood pressure, stomach pain, and emotional tension. The nurse learned that the employees with stress were all members of a jogging team that met

weekly for conversation in addition to regular workouts. The other joggers readily agreed to work with their friends on individual stress management, recognizing that their fellow members were having a lot of stress and this was a danger to health. The joggers valued good health, and although jogging was seen as an enjoyable and health-promoting activity, they had never talked about a shared purpose for improved health. In this example, the nurse saw a need for stress reduction. She thought that the individuals at risk could reduce stress if they were supported through a group process from valued friends, and she proposed that a new purpose be added to the jogging team's activities: systematic stress management techniques.

Selected-Membership Groups

At times it is either undesirable or impossible to use existing groups to achieve a new group goal. In these instances, forming a new group is necessary. As mentioned, some groups come together because of common health problems. For example, individuals with diabetes can meet to discuss diet management and physical care and to share in problem-solving remedies; community residents can meet for social support and rehabilitation following treatment for mental illness; or isolated elderly persons can be brought together for socialization and hot meals.

It is important to consider members' attributes when composing a new group. Members are attracted to others from similar backgrounds, with similar experiences, and with common interests and abilities. Selecting members so that common ties or interests balance out dissimilar traits is therefore an important consideration.

Membership ties are influential. Even in newly formed groups, people bring emotional and social ties from previous and parallel group memberships. People are influenced by the interaction in the newly formed group and by their membership in other important groups. Memory serves to keep the norms and role expectations from one group present in people as they move from one group to another. Individual behavior is then influenced not only by the membership, purpose, attraction, norms, leadership, and structure of the group, but also by those processes remembered from other valued group memberships. Consideration of the multiple influences on members helps to determine an appropriate grouping for each situation and its particular dimensions.

It is useful if the membership for **selected-membership groups** contains one or more people who are good communicators and have strong problem-solving skills and others who are comfortable in supportive roles. Many people come to a group with good task and maintenance skills, while others have undeveloped potential for such functions. Support and training for group effectiveness within the unit will help to build cohesion. As members perform increasingly valuable functions for the group, they become more attracted to it and more attractive to others.

Group size influences effectiveness. Typically, 8 to 12 people are considered ideal for group work focused on individual health changes. Groups of up to 25 members may be effective when their focus is on meeting community needs, such as the group discussed previously who formed a neighborhood association. Large groups often divide and assign tasks to smaller subgroups, with the original large groups meeting less frequently for reporting and evaluation.

Establishing membership criteria should be done before members are recruited for the group. Criteria usually cite a mixture of member traits that will give the group a good balance of skills for the processes of decision making and growth.

Beginning Interactions

Once a group forms, members begin to work on the stated purpose. During the early meetings it is necessary to clarify individual and group goals. Members have varying degrees of openness that influence how much they tell about themselves and their backgrounds. Members begin by asking for information about the other members and giving information about themselves. During the early stage, members demonstrate their problem solving and group participation skills. The nurse can support ideas and feelings, invite participation, give information, seek and provide clarification, and suggest structure. Subsequent steps are then planned consistent with the nurse's skill and preference, and according to the group composition and the skills of the members.

In beginning groups, the nurse emphasizes helping members communicate so they feel some degree of satisfaction. This requires close attention to the maintenance tasks of attending, eliciting information, clarifying, and recognizing contributions of members. Attending includes simple responses to people, such as listening carefully to their speech and observing their mood, dress, and informal conversation as they enter the meeting. Attending behavior communicates recognition and acceptance of the person and his or her presentations to the group.

A beginning format that focuses on why members joined the group provides recognition and helps participants recognize similar and different perspectives. Members may be asked to describe what each hopes to accomplish in the group and what their past group experiences have been. Member-to-member exchanges are encouraged, and the leader should facilitate and not talk excessively. People are recognized and supported as they assume leadership functions.

Even in beginning sessions, roles and a structure for the new group begin to take shape. Members practice familiar roles and test their individual abilities. Those approaches to member support, leadership, and decision making that are comfortable and productive become normative ways for the group to work. The work of the group begins while the goals for health change are examined carefully and accepted. During this early period, members' attractions to each other and to the group begin to develop. How to initiate and conduct group work in the community setting is described in the following box.

HOW TO Initiate and Conduct Group Work in the Community Setting

Goal: Community agency group work to address disease prevention

Purpose for Group Members
- Increase awareness of common health risks.
- Use problem solving to make changes for improved health.
- Foster health-promotion behaviors.

Planning and Implementation Steps
- Seek consultation from community agency staff about priority health concerns and interests of the population that the agency serves.
- Determine times when members can meet, where meetings may be held, and standards and procedures related to working within the agency.
- Select a health-related topic. Develop a teaching plan; submit the plan to the designated agency contact for information and approval.
- Market group teaching through a variety of strategies. Make the purpose, benefits to members, time length of meeting, place, and time clear in the recruitment. Group members may be volunteer, referred, or selected through leaders' interviews. Limit membership to 10 to 15 individuals per group.
- Meet with the group at designated times. Stick to a teaching plan; submit any needed revision to the agency contact.
- Record and evaluate process and outcome of group teaching. Keep a meeting journal.
- Keep agency staff informed about progress throughout the group meeting block of time.
- Meet with agency staff for a summary report of the group project, making recommendations for continued teaching and/or other health-focused follow-up for members.
- Write a summary report.

Briefly Noted

Seniors attending a senior center may wish to avoid topics about declining health since their own health may be impaired or they may see family members and friends who are restricted in mobility, in pain, or otherwise dealing with chronic illness. Facing the reality of declining health may be painful.

Conflict

Although **conflict** occurs in all human relations, people often see conflict as the opposite of harmony. Most people try to avoid conflict. This view is an unfortunate one because the tensions created by differences and potential conflict can actually help groups work toward their purposes. Understanding common causes of conflict, conflict management approaches, and conflict resolution models are especially important in light of the dramatic changes occurring both in health care and in communities throughout the world.

Conflict arises whenever people think that their concerns have been or are about to be frustrated (Sitkin and Bies, 1993). Conflict signals that antagonistic points of view must be considered and that one must reexamine beliefs and assumptions underlying relationships. People are generally concerned about security, control of self and others, respect, and access to limited resources. In groups, members express frustrations about trust, closeness and separation, and dependence and independence. These sources of conflict exist to some extent in all interactions and are not unique to groups. Within a group, since members work toward a common purpose, such issues are important.

Responding effectively to conflict encourages personal growth and assists in dealing with group frustrations. Thomas (1992) differentiated two possible positive ways to respond to conflict:

- Assertiveness (attempting to satisfy one's own concerns)
- Cooperation (attempting to satisfy the others' concerns).

Assertive and cooperative behaviors that may also satisfy the frustrated parties include confrontation, competition, compromise, reconciliation, and collaboration. **Avoidance,** coercion, capitulation, and exclusion of members are responses to conflict that fail to satisfy the concerns of frustrated parties.

Resolving group conflict depends on open communication among all parties, diffusion of negative feelings and perceptions, focusing on the issue(s), fair procedures, and a structured approach to the process. In the box below is an outline of the steps in group conflict resolution. These steps list a sequence of behaviors that support and encourage participants to acknowledge and resolve conflicts. Conflict can be overwhelming, especially when members think that expressing controversy is unacceptable or unresolvable. Conflict suppressed over time can build up and finally explode out of proportion to the current frustration. A group that repeatedly avoids expressing conflict becomes fragile, unable to adapt to growth within the group, and helpless to face challenges. Conflict can be destructive if contentious parties do not respect the rights and beliefs of others.

HOW TO Resolve Conflict in Groups

1. Give a full description of concerns and divergent views.
2. Clarify assumptions on the conflict issue.
3. Specify underlying factors, including beliefs, individual desires, and expectations.
4. Identify the real issue(s).
5. Jointly search for a collaborative resolution using problem-solving.
6. Finalize resolution agreement (either a full agreement or a compromise) whereby each party is satisfied on important points.

Conflict-acknowledging and problem-solving approaches that respect others and represent self-concerns are first learned in families and other small groups. These lessons teach people to view conflict as a natural occurrence that supports growth and change. Other individuals learn to avoid conflict or to disregard others in the promotion of self. Examination of conflict and its resolution in supportive groups leads to the following outcomes: improved working relationships, stress reduction, and better coping.

Collaboration can be an effective way to deal with conflict. Collaboration is a process of joint decision-making in which both or all parties are actively involved in the communication. In effective collaboration, participants are skilled communicators who can respond to both verbal and non-verbal cues and who understand and can use group process skills. Participants in successful collaborations recognize stumbling blocks to the group process and actively work to clarify issues or misperceptions, keep the group on topic, and respect the ideas and opinions of others. Collaboration is more likely to be effective when the participants are confident of their skills and contributions and willing to negotiate, disagree and compromise (Lancaster and Lancaster, 1998).

Briefly Noted

Collaboration is often an effective approach to conflict resolution.

Collaboration takes time. Hindrances to collaboration include competitive incentives, people with insufficient problem-solving skills, shortness of time, and lack of trust between parties (Thomas, 1992). Other strategies that are practical, yet not fully collaborative, include restructuring settings, helping concerned parties reframe frustration so it will produce less stress, and increasing competitive incentives. Although some circumstances do warrant these compromise-type responses to conflict, collaboration more completely resolves frustration and differences.

The following example illustrates conflict resolution through collaboration. A small rural church initiated a youth recreation project to intervene in the fast driving behaviors that the youth were exhibiting. The restless youth used a particular road as their speedway. The church enlisted the high school principal and the public health nurse to work with a project group. All supported the development of a local youth center and worked energetically toward the goal.

After 2 months of good cooperation, arguments began erupting at meetings. Conflict about the supervision of the proposed center, its site, and many smaller concerns began to dominate planning time. The group consisted of active, aggressive members; four individuals dominated the discussions and resisted resolution of group differences. After several frustrating meetings, the nurse asked group members to state their concerns and views about the direction and interaction of their work together. Welcoming an opportunity to relieve tension, members described their hopes, misgivings, and frustrated expectations related to the project. Each person elaborated on his or her assumptions about who would do what and how work should proceed. From this full discussion, the real issue became clear to all: there was disagreement related to members' functions in the project. The four dominant individuals wanted to direct the planning, and they were aggravated when their attempts were thwarted. Other members described supportive and task functions but did not want to dominate the leadership functions. The open analysis of role structure clarified to the members that arguments arose from competition for directing roles rather than from true disagreements about the recreation project. Members searched for a collaborative resolution to the issue. They agreed to divide the work into several task areas to be led by separate area directors. Members were relieved that basic agreement about the purpose remained intact. They were now able to modify their role expectations to accommodate all members. They joked together about being a collection of bosses and renewed their productive work.

Strategies for Change

Nurses—who have considerable knowledge about health and health risks for individuals, groups, and communities and skill in problem solving—can lead change in health goals. Change, whether welcome or not, is disruptive. Even though moving from a familiar way of being and interacting with others is uncomfortable (and resisted), all human systems do change over time because of development within the system and adaptation to outside stimuli. A change in one group member affects every other member. The disruption of growth, new opportunities, and threats to security trigger a fertile period for reevaluating, selecting new directions, improving, and maturing. Change creates opportunity for learning that is more than mastery of new information and identification of appropriate adjustment resources.

As discussed throughout this chapter, healthful change requires knowledge, practice of new skills, examination of attitudes and values about the change, and adjustment of roles in one's personal group or network. Helping people accomplish needed changes ideally is done within the small group context.

Basic teaching helps members understand the known association among environment, body response, wellness, and pathological states that are pertinent to desired changes. Together, group members focus on the reality of the problems and ways to understand them. A group reaches its full potential for effecting individual change when members work actively and directly through discussion and other approaches to problem solving. Such group work produces positive individual outcomes for healthful change.

Expectant-parent groups illustrate a type of community group in which teaching is a highly appropriate method. Participants need to understand facts about pregnancy, labor and delivery, self-care, infant care, parenting, and adjusting

to change. They also need to practice these new skills and to examine their attitudes and emotional responses to the anticipated family changes. Specific group learning activities might include demonstration and practice in giving the baby a bath or in calming a crying infant.

With the support of a group, people can often make needed health changes that they are unable to accomplish on their own or with the help of just one individual. Skillful use of group methods can help participants analyze the problem, sustain motivation for change, support people during vulnerable periods, and provide quick interpersonal feedback for success and failure. The discomfort associated with change can be reduced through effective group support and relationships.

Evaluation of Group Progress

Evaluation of individual and group progress toward meeting health goals is important. A Guide for Evaluation of Group Effectiveness is shown in Appendix E.3. Steps to meet the goal are identified early in the planning stage. These small steps may be responses to learning objectives or they may reflect the group's problem-solving plan. These action steps and the indicators of achievement are discussed and written in a group record. Celebration is built into the group's evaluation system to help participants recognize and reinforce each step toward the health goal. Celebration may include concrete rewards such as special foods and drinks, or it may be the personal expression of joy and member-to-member approval. Celebration for group accomplishments marks progress, rewards members, and motivates each person to continue.

BUILDING EFFECTIVE WORK TEAMS

Working effectively in a team is essential in all areas of nursing. A **team** is made up of individuals who are involved in or affected by a problem or who have a goal and who agree to work together to solve it. Specifically, the "team should consist of a small number of people with useful knowledge and skills who are committed to a common purpose or goal for which they hold themselves mutually accountable" (Maddox, 1998, p. 478).

Committees are commonly used by community groups and agencies. However, as shown in the box below, teams are different from committees. In addition, teams may have a different composition in the community as compared to other health care settings. That is, often the team includes both health care workers and community residents. Team effectiveness and the satisfaction of members typically depends on several key factors including the behavior of the members, their skill for producing the work product, the skill of the leader and the members in team building, and their knowledge of group process. Effective teams use group process concepts such as cohesion, purpose, task function, maintenance function, leadership, and conflict resolution.

HOW TO Differentiate Teams From Committees

Team	Committee
Shares leadership roles	Strong, clearly focused leader
Limited members (5-6)	Unlimited members
Members have a range of authority in the organization	Members are at similar levels in the organization
Designed for short-term work	Ongoing
Has defined goals	Has changing goals
Uses a scientific approach for process improvement	May use CQI tools and techniques
Recommends permanent solutions	Recommends quick fixes
Measures performance directly by assessing collective work byproducts	Measures effectiveness indirectly by its influence on others

From Parisi LL: Process empowerment: committee or team, *Nurs Quality Connect* 4(2):5, 1994.

Teams first select members who have the specialized knowledge and skill to produce the desired product. Nurses may want to be involved in the team hiring and personnel selection process. Skill training can occur after hiring if most members come with relevant education and experience for the work. Effective teams need a balance of member behavior types including those who are self-reliant and task oriented, those who are enthusiastic and people oriented, those who are loyal and close in interpersonal relationships, and those who are factual and evaluative in style (Clark, 1994). Once a core team is selected, the leader and members should evaluate the mix of member behavior types and next recruit persons who have the personal styles still needed by the team.

Cohesiveness in the team, as for other groups, is increased by the connections among members. Cohesion and member attraction are built through regular contacts and interactions that strengthen team identity. For example, team identity is increased with cooperation among members and success in meeting goals. Often members are asked to share their experiences and expertise. They are encouraged to work together on parts of their assignments. Negative approaches such as identifying a common enemy or competing with other teams should be used sparingly because they set up win-lose situations (Clark, 1994).

Often the issue that divides team members is the purpose or perceived reason for conducting work. Team purposes need to be stated clearly, understood, and agreed upon by members. If there is a disagreement about the guiding goal and secondary objectives, members will oppose one another, and there will be tension in their communications. As in other groups, team leaders must clearly define and negotiate purposes, objectives, and member roles.

Work projects are divided into the tasks that must be undertaken. Responsibilities of each team member should relate directly to the purpose of the unit's function. The most important criteria in assigning and delegating responsibility are (1) the ability of the team member to carry out the task and (2) the fairness of the assignment.

As tasks are assigned or negotiated among members, differences in interpretation of work purpose are identified. Sometimes the guiding purpose has to be redefined; more often team members refine their understanding of the work goal and adjust role expectations accordingly.

A successful team pays attention to the maintenance needs of members, including their physical, social, and emotional comfort. Members' comfort includes satisfaction with the progress being made toward attaining the work purpose. Members identify more strongly with the team when they think others value their contributions and when they feel that both the leader and other members support their work.

Work teams, like all groups, need effective leadership. While leadership and decision making may be concentrated in one person or more equally shared among all, the pattern and legitimacy of leading should be firmly established and agreed on by the team. Leading patterns may change over the life of the group; at each pattern change the team adjusts expectations about lines of direction, responsibility, and evaluation. Communication must be clear, with messages quickly clarified if they seem vague or contradictory.

Successful teams address in a timely way any differences that are expressed as conflicts. Each member is responsible for supporting factors within and outside the group that facilitate members' performance. Barriers to accomplishing purpose are acknowledged, and the group makes decisions on how to deal with such barriers. Work is monitored by evaluating how the group process helped to accomplish the group's purposes and outcomes related to the stated team purpose. From time to time the team reassesses its purposes, effectiveness in working together, and levels of member satisfaction.

Sometimes teams are ineffective due to the common and chronic problem of inadequate staffing. Effective nursing teams must confront the problem when it occurs. A strong team will point out inadequacies and their consequences for health care, public relations, and inability to expand programs. Strong and effective teams can initiate organizational change to improve health care.

COMMUNITY GROUPS AND THEIR CONTRIBUTION TO COMMUNITY LIFE

An understanding of group concepts provides a starting point for identifying community groups and how they function as components of the community. Because people develop, refine, and change their ideas within the context of the groups to which they belong, groups are vital to community well-being. Groups help identify community problems and are instrumental in managing interactions within the community and between the community and larger society.

Community groups may be informal (e.g., social networks, friendships, neighborhood groups) or formal (e.g., school, church, business groups). **Formal groups** have a defined membership and specific purpose. They may or may not have an official place in the community's organization. In **informal groups,** the ties between members are multiple, and the purposes are unwritten yet understood by members. Informal groups can be identified through interviews with key spokespersons. Information about when and why they gather is learned through interviews or observing gatherings to which the nurse is invited. Informal groups often are recognized in the news when they are distinguished for community action or service. Formal groups usually can be identified in a variety of community media where their meetings are announced and business reported publicly. Membership lists, goals, and mission statements are usually written and available to interested persons. Typically, residents willingly describe the informal and formal groups in their communities once they learn the nurse's purpose for entering and studying their community.

Group communication and member interactions across groups influence the overall harmony and free exchange in the community. Many communities encourage cooperation among groups through interagency councils. In addition, many naturally occurring links among groups exist through family, friendships, and other relationships. Local extended-family groups, club relationships, work, and other acquaintance networks may influence the activities of seemingly separate groups in the larger community.

Nurses can identify goals for the community and for various groups through media reports, from community informants, and from local reports. These goals describe resources and visions for change as perceived by the people living and working in the local community. Data may be organized according to the opinions and behaviors of the groups identified. Such information about community groups and assessment data are used with community representatives to plan interventions. Groups are both units of community analysis and vehicles for change.

The small group can influence and change the larger social community of which it is a part. The social system depends on groups for governing, making policy, identifying community needs, taking steps to alleviate those needs, and evaluating program outcomes. The small group is a mechanism for forming connections among community subsystems, certain subsystems and their counterparts in the larger social structure, and factions within subsystems. Change in the composition and function of strategic small groups may produce change for the wider social system that depends on small groups for direction and guidance (Benne, 1976).

WORKING WITH GROUPS TO ACHIEVE COMMUNITY HEALTH GOALS

Nurses use their understanding of group principles to work with community groups to make needed health changes. The

groupings appropriate for this work include both established, community-sanctioned groups and groups for which nurses select members representing diverse community sectors.

Existing community groups formed for community-wide purposes such as elected executive groups, health-planning groups, better-business clubs, women's action groups, school boards, and neighborhood councils are excellent resources for community health assessment because part of their ongoing purpose is to determine and respond to community needs. In addition, they are already established as part of the community structure. When a group representing one community sector is selected for community health intervention, the total community structure is studied. Data about family ties, experiences with resource centers, and lifelong contacts to other sector groups are evaluated. Groups reflect existing community values, strengths, and normative forces.

How might nurses help established groups work toward community goals? The same interventions recommended for groups formed for individual health change apply to health-focused groups in the community. Such interventions include the following: building cohesion by clarifying goals and individual attraction to groups, building member commitment and participation, keeping the group focused on the goal, sustaining members through recognition and encouragement, maintaining member self-esteem during conflict and confrontation, analyzing forces affecting movement toward the goal, and evaluating progress. Upon joining a group, nurses assess the leadership, communication, and normative structures. This facilitates group planning, problem solving, intervention, and evaluation. The steps used for community health changes are like those used for problem solving in the scientific process or in the nursing process.

One community health nurse, Mrs. Winter, was asked to meet with a neighborhood council to help them study and "do something about" the number of homeless people living on the streets. Community residents knew Mrs. Winter because she worked in a local clinic. They knew she also consulted at a shelter for the homeless in an adjacent community. When the council invited her, they said, "our goal is to be part of the solution rather than part of the problem." Mrs. Winter accepted the invitation to visit. She learned that the neighborhood council had addressed concerns of the neighborhood for 20 years. They had protected zoning guidelines, set up a recreational program for teens, organized an after-school program for latch-key children, and generally represented the area's homeowners. The neighborhood was composed of low-income families who took great pride in their homes. After meeting with the council and listening to their description of the situation, Mrs. Winter agreed to help, and she joined the council.

As the first step in addressing the problem, the council conducted a comprehensive problem analysis of the homeless situation. All known causes and outcomes of homeless persons on the street were identified, and the relationships between each factor and the problem were documented from literature and from the local history. Mrs. Winter brought to the group expertise in health planning and knowledge of the homeless and health risks. She suggested negotiation between the council and the local coalition for the homeless, recognizing that planning would be most relevant if homeless individuals participated. The council was cohesive and committed to the purpose, had developed working operations, and did not need help with group process. They made adjustments in their usual group operation to use the knowledge and health-planning skills of Mrs. Winter.

Interventions for the homeless included establishment of temporary shelter at homes on a rotating basis, provision of daily meals through the city council or churches, and joining the area coalition for the homeless. This example shows how an established, competent group addressed a new goal successfully by building on existing strengths in partnership with the community health nurse.

Community groupings, because of their interactive roles, are logical and natural ways for people to work together for community health change. As the decision-making and problem-solving capabilities of community groups are strengthened, the groups become better representatives for the entire community. Nurses can improve the community's health by working with groups toward that goal.

Healthy People 2010 and Working With Groups

Health promotion in schools, health care centers, and work sites provides a means of targeting interventions for specific groups who may be vulnerable. This increases the success to improve personal and community health. The particular recommendations are presented in the *Healthy People 2010* box.

Clinical Application

Four nursing students in Chicago decided to work with parents at a drop-in family resource center as part of their undergraduate field experience. Parents at the center asked for instruction in how to provide nutritious, low-cost meals at home. The four students recruited three of the center parents who used the drop-in center's programs regularly. The group of students and parents decided to teach economical food planning and preparation through cooking and serving several simple meals and explaining how to plan, select, and prepare them. The meals were planned for three consecutive Mondays at the center.

On the first scheduled Monday everyone in the group worked together successfully. Eight parents attended the class, enjoyed a good economical meal, and were very interested in learning how to plan and prepare it. At the close of the evening three of the students announced they would be unable to come the following Monday. The parents and remaining student on the teaching team felt abandoned and resentful but carried on planning for the next session. They did not talk about their resentment to the offending students even though they were left unfairly "holding the bag."

What went wrong in this example?

Answer is in the back of the book.

Healthy People 2010 and Working With Groups

Healthy People 2010 recommends that community health-promotion programs include the following:

- Involved community participation with representation from at least three of the following community sectors: government, education, business, faith-based organizations, health care, media, voluntary agencies, and the public.
- Community assessment to determine community health problems, resources, and perceptions and priorities for action.
- Measurable objectives that address at least one of the following: health outcomes, risk factors, public awareness, or services and protection.
- Monitoring and evaluation processes to determine whether the objectives are reached.
- Comprehensive, multifaceted, culturally relevant interventions that have multiple targets for change—individuals (e.g., racial and ethnic, age, and socioeconomic groups), organizations (e.g., work sites, schools, and churches), and environments (e.g., local policies and regulations)—and multiple approaches to change, including education, community organization, and regulatory and environmental reforms.

 Remember This!

- Working with groups is an important skill for nurses. Groups are an effective and powerful vehicle for initiating and implementing healthful changes.
- A group is a collection of interacting individuals with a common purpose. Each member influences and is influenced by other group members to varying degrees.
- Group cohesion is enhanced by commonly shared characteristics among members and diminished by differences among members.
- Cohesion is the measure of attraction between members and the group. Cohesion or the lack of it affects the group's function.
- Norms are standards that guide and regulate individuals and communities. These norms are unwritten and often unspoken and ensure group movement toward a goal, maintain the group, and influence group members' perceptions and interpretations of reality.
- Some diversity of member backgrounds usually has a positive influence on a group.
- Leadership is an important and complex group concept. Leadership is described as patriarchal, paternal, or democratic.
- Group structure emerges from various member influences, including members' understanding and support of the group purpose.
- Conflicts in groups may develop from competition for roles or member disagreement about the roles ascribed to them.

- Health behavior is greatly influenced by the groups to which people belong and how much they value membership.
- An understanding of group concepts provides a basis for identifying community groups and their goals, characteristics, and norms. Nurses use their understanding of group principles to work with community groups toward needed health changes.

❓ *What Would You Do?*

1. Consider three groups of which you are a member. What is the stated purpose of each one? Are you aware of unstated but clearly understood purposes? What is the nature of member interaction in each group? How do purpose and interaction differ in the three groups?
2. Observe two working groups in session from the community, a health care agency, or a school. Notice the attractiveness of each group through the eyes of its members.
3. List actions that nurses may take to assist groups in various aspects of their work, such as member selection, purpose clarification, arrangements for comfort in participation, and group problem solving.
4. Observe a nurse working with a health-promotion group. Does the nurse function in the way you anticipated? What nursing behavior facilitated the group process? List the areas of skill and knowledge most likely to be expected of the nurse by the community residents' groups.
5. Identify areas of conflict in a work group to which you belong. Describe how one of these expressed or potential conflicts could be managed. Use the steps for conflict resolution outlined in the How To Resolve Conflict in Groups box on p. 267. What role would you take? Practice conflict-acknowledging and problem-solving behaviors in the next conflict you encounter.

REFERENCES

Benne KD: The current state of planned changing in persons, groups, communities, and societies. In Bennis WG, et al (editors): *The planning of change,* ed 4, New York, 1976, Holt, Rinehart, & Winston.

Clark CC: *The nurse as group leader,* ed 3, New York, 1994, Springer.

Lancaster J, Lancaster M: Communicating to manage change. In Lancaster J (editor): *Issues in leading and managing change in nursing,* St Louis, 1998, Mosby.

Maddox PJ: Quality management in nursing practice. In Lancaster J (editor): *Issues in leading and managing change in nursing,* St Louis, 1998, Mosby.

Parisi LL: Process empowerment: committee or team, *Nurs Quality Connect* 4(2):5, 1994.

Sampson EE, Marthas M: *Group process for the health professions,* ed 3, Albany, NY, 1990, Delmar.

Sitkin SB, Bies RJ: Social accounts in conflict situations: using explanations to manage conflict, *Hum Relations* 46(3):349, 1993.

Thomas KW: Conflict and conflict management: reflections and update, *J Organiz Behav* 13(3):265, 1992.

Toropainen E, Rinne M: What are groups all about? basic principles of group work for health-related physical activity, *Patient Educ Counsel* 33(supp 1):105, 1998.

Tuckman B: Developmental sequence in small groups, *Psychol Bull* 63:384, 1965.

Part 5

Issues and Approaches in Family and Individual Health Care

The family is a major influence on the individual's concept of health and illness. It is within the family that a person's sense of self-esteem and personal competence are developed. The action taken by or for the person with a health problem depends on the sense of self-worth and the family's definition of illness. Environmental, social, cultural, and economic factors, as well as the resources of the community to meet health needs, influence the family's health risks and reaction to health. The goals of the nation for the year 2010 name the individual and the community as the primary targets for changing the overall health of the nation. Through family support the individual may develop the responsibility to participate in activities that will lead to a healthier lifestyle.

Major health problems of individuals can be identified and related to their developmental phase. This factor becomes evident when age-specific morbidity data are reviewed. Community health nurses can influence the actions and reactions to health of all individuals in the community from birth through senescence. The community health nurse can influence the health of children by introducing healthy parenting behaviors, risk factor appraisal, and age-appropriate interventions.

Women and men are faced with many life changes and challenges, some of which are gender specific. Previous lifestyles and increases in stress from social, environmental, and economic constraints often result in risk for major health problems during adulthood.

The community health nurse's primary function with persons of all ages should be to promote quality and quantity of life. As the elderly segment of the population continues to grow, the health care delivery system and nurses must address and plan strategies to cope with increasing longevity, chronic health problems, and technological advances, as well as twenty-first century economic, social, and health issues.

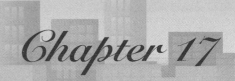

Family nursing is practiced in all settings. The trend in the delivery of health care has been to move health care to community settings; thus family nursing is very pertinent to community health nurses. **Family nursing** is a specialty area that has a strong theory base and is more than just "common sense" or viewing the family as the context for individual health care. Family nursing consists of nurses and families working together to ensure the success of the family and its members in adapting to responses to health and illness. The purpose of this chapter is to present a current overview of families and family nursing, theoretical frameworks, and strategies for assessing and intervening with families in the community.

FAMILY NURSING IN THE COMMUNITY

As the basic social unit of society, within the family is where health care decisions are made. Health care occurs in families who are in the larger community and society. Families are responsible for providing or managing the care of family members. In the current health care system, families are significant members of health care teams since they are the ever-present force over the lifetime of care. Families are more responsible than ever for assisting in the health care of ill family members.

Nurses are responsible for:

- Helping families promote their health
- Meeting family health needs
- Coping with health problems within the context of the existing family structure and community resources
- Collaborating with families to develop useful interventions

Nurses must be knowledgeable about family structures, functions, processes, and roles. In addition, nurses must be aware of and understand their own values and attitudes pertaining to their own families as well as being open to different family structures and cultures.

FAMILY DEMOGRAPHICS

Family demographics is the study of the structure of families and households and the family-related events, such as marriage and divorce, that alter the structure through their number, timing, and sequencing.

An important use of family demography by nurses is to forecast and predict stresses and developmental changes experienced by families and to identify possible solutions to family problems. It is important to note that the structure of families has changed over time. The rapid changes that occurred at the close of the twentieth century, have implications for family relationships and the ability of families to meet the changing needs of their members.

DEFINITION OF FAMILY

The definition of family is critical to the practice of nursing. Family has traditionally been defined using the legal concepts of relationships such as genetic ties, adoption, guardianship, or marriage. Since the 1980s a broader definition of family has been used that moved beyond the traditional blood, marriage, and legal constrictions.

Family refers to two or more individuals who depend on one another for emotional, physical, and/or financial support. The members of the family are self-defined (Hanson, 2001c). Nurses working with families should ask people who they consider to be their family and then include those members in health care planning. The family may range from traditional nuclear and extended family to such "post-modern" family structures as single-parent families, stepfamilies, and same-gender families.

Briefly Noted

Most persons view families and their experiences based on their own family of origin. It is important to be aware of and attempt to understand other family variations.

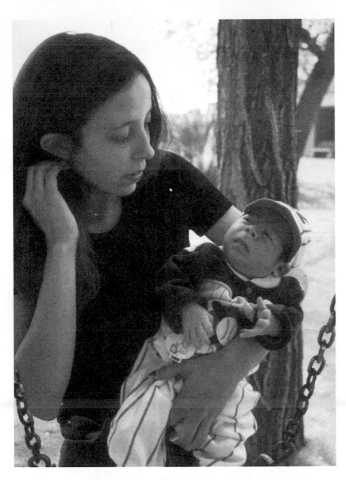

A young single mother with her infant son.

FAMILY FUNCTIONS

Throughout history, a number of functions have traditionally been performed by families (Hanson, 2001b). Six of these **family functions** are summarized in Box 17-1.

Historically, families that performed all of these six functions were considered healthy and good. In contemporary times, the traditional functions of families have been modified and new functions have been added. For example, the financial function of families has changed so that family members do not need each other to stay financially healthy as much as they did in the past. Many married couples are electing to be child-free rather than to reproduce. Families depend on other agencies to provide safety such as law enforcement, while other agencies are involved in the passing of the religious faith (e.g., churches or synagogues). Education (socialization function) is relegated to the schools. Family names are no longer needed to confer status as in the past when names were very important in a community.

The functions that served families have evolved and changed over time. Some have become more important and others less so. Several new functions are more prominent in modern families:

- The relationship function has become important in contemporary families, thus emphasizing how people get along and their level of satisfaction.

Box 17-1   Historical Family Functions

1. Families exist to achieve financial survival. Families are economic units to which all members contribute and from which all members benefit.
2. Families exist to reproduce, thus ensuring survival of the species.
3. Families provide protection from hostile forces.
4. Families pass along the culture, including religious faith.
5. Families educate (socialize) their young.
6. Families confer status in society.

Box 17-2   Family and Household Structures

MARRIED FAMILY

Traditional nuclear family
Dual-career family
- Spouses reside in same household
- Commuter marriage
Husband/father away from family
Stepfamily
- Stepmother family
- Stepfather family
Adoptive family
Foster family
Voluntarily childless family

SINGLE-PARENT FAMILY

Never married
- Voluntary singlehood (with children, either biological or adopted)
- Involuntary singlehood (with children)
Formerly married
- Widow (with children)
- Divorced (with children)
- Custodial parent
- Joint custody of children
- Binuclear family (stepfamily)

MULTIADULT HOUSEHOLD (WITH OR WITHOUT CHILDREN)

Cohabitating couple
Communes
Affiliated family
Extended family
New extended family
Home-sharing individuals
Same-sex partners
Fictive kin (created or imagined)

- The health function has become more evident because it is the basis of a lifetime of physical and mental health or the lack thereof.

FAMILY STRUCTURE

Family structure refers to the characteristics and demographics (gender, age, number) of individual members who make up family units. More specifically, the structure of a family defines the roles and the positions of family members (Box 17-2).

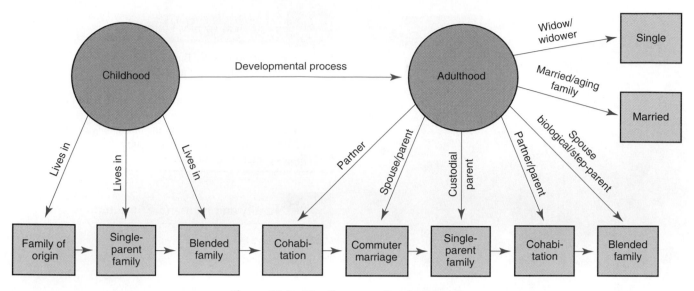

Figure 17-1   Family career of an individual.

Family structures have changed over time. The great speed with which changes in family structure, values, and relationships are happening makes working with families at the beginning of the twenty-first century exciting and challenging. As social norms have become more tolerant of a range of choices in relation to managing one's life, there is no longer a general consensus that the traditional nuclear family model is the only "right" model. There is no "typical family" model. As a consequence, there is a growing number of family and household types. There is an increasing awareness that more variety exists within and among particular family structures. For example, the single-mother household may be represented by the unmarried teenage mother with an infant (unplanned pregnancy), the divorced mother with one or more children; or the career-oriented woman in her late thirties who elects to have a baby and remain single.

An individual may participate in a number of family life-course experiences over a lifetime (Fig. 17-1).

For example, a child may:

- Spend the early, formative years in the family of origin (mother, father, sibling)
- Experience some years in a single-parent family because of divorce
- Participate in a stepfamily relationship when the single parent who has custody remarries
- Experience several additional family types as an adult

As an adult, the individual may:

- Cohabitate while completing a desired education
- Marry and have a commuter-type marriage while developing a career
- Subsequently divorce, and become the custodial parent
- Eventually cohabitate with another partner
- Finally marry another partner who also has children

As this couple ages they will address issues of the aging family, and subsequently the woman may become an elderly single widow. Nurses work with families representing various structures and living arrangements.

Prospects for families for the twenty-first century are numerous. New family structures that currently are experimental will emerge as everyday "natural" families (e.g., families in which the members are not related by blood or marriage, but who provide the services, caring, love, intimacy, and interaction needed by all persons to experience a quality life).

FAMILY HEALTH

Despite the focus on family health within nursing, the meaning of family health lacks consensus and is not precise. The term **family health** is often used interchangeably with the concepts of family functioning, healthy families, or familial health. Hanson (2001c) defines family health as "a dynamic changing relative state of well-being which includes the biological, psychological, sociological, cultural, and spiritual factors of the family system."

This bio/psycho/socio/cultural/spiritual approach refers to individual members as well as the family unit as a whole. An individual's health (wellness-illness continuum) affects the entire family's functioning, and in turn the family's functioning affects the health of individuals. Thus assessment of family health involves simultaneous assessment of individual family members and the family system as a whole.

Healthy Versus Nonhealthy Families

Terms related to healthy versus nonhealthy families have varied in the literature. Health professionals have tended to classify clients and their families into two groups: "good families," who are functioning adequately, and "bad families," who are in need of psychosocial evaluation and intervention (Satariano and Briggs, 1993). The term *family health* implied mental health rather than physical health. Recently the popular term for nonhealthy families is **dysfunctional families**—also called noncompliant, resistant, or unmotivated; these phrases denote families who are not

Box 17-3	Characteristics of Healthy Families

1. The family tends to communicate well and listen to all members.
2. The family affirms and supports all of its members.
3. The family teaches respect for others.
4. The family members have a sense of trust.
5. The family plays together, and humor is present.
6. All family members interact with each other, with a balance in the interactions among the members.
7. The family shares leisure time together.
8. The family has a shared sense of responsibility.
9. The family has traditions and rituals.
10. The family shares a religious core.
11. The family honors the privacy of its members.
12. The family opens its boundaries to admit and seek help with problems.

Modified from Curran D: *Traits of a healthy family,* Minneapolis, 1983, Winston Press (Harper & Row).

functioning well with each other or the world. The label "dysfunctional family" does not allow for family change and intervention and needs to be dropped from the nursing language. Families are neither all good nor all bad; therefore nurses need to view family behavior on a continuum of need for intervention when the family comes in contact with the health care system.

Families with strengths, or **functional families,** are terms often used to refer to healthy families. Research has been conducted about healthy families, but it is clear that the issues examined all relate to those of relational needs. This means that in healthy families, the basic survival needs are met. The traits ascribed to healthy families are based on attachment and are affectionate in nature (Carter and McGoldrick, 1988).

Curran (1983, 1985) reported traits of healthy families as well as family stressors that are useful for nurses to include in their assessment. Box 17-3 shows characteristics of families who are healthy and functioning well in society.

FOUR APPROACHES TO FAMILY NURSING

Central to the practice of family nursing is conceptualizing and approaching the family from four perspectives (Hanson, 2001d). All have legitimate implications for nursing assessment and intervention (Figs. 17-2 and 17-3). Which approach nurses use is determined by many factors, including the health care setting, family circumstances, and nurse resources:

1. *Family as the context,* or structure, has a traditional focus that places the individual first and the family second. The family as context serves as either a resource or a stressor to individual health and illness. A nurse using this focus might ask an individual client, "How has your diagnosis of insulin-dependent diabetes affected your family?" or "Will your need for medication at night be a problem for your family?"
2. *Family as the client.* The family is first, and individuals are second. The family is seen as the *sum* of individual

family members. The focus is concentrated on each individual as he or she affects the family as a whole. From this perspective, a nurse might say to a family member who has just become ill, "Tell me about what has been going on with your own health and how you perceive each family member responding to your mother's recent diagnosis of liver cancer."

3. *Family as a system.* The focus is on the family as client, and the family is viewed as an interacting system in which the whole is more than the sum of its parts. This approach simultaneously focuses on individual members and the family as a whole at the same time. The interactions between family members become the target for nursing interventions (e.g., the direct interactions between the parents, or the indirect interaction between the parents and the child). The systems approach to family always implies that when something happens to one family member, the other members of the family system are affected. Questions nurses ask when approaching a family as system are, "What has changed between you and your spouse since your child's head injury?" or "How do you feel about the fact that your son's long-term rehabilitation will affect the ways in which the members of your family are functioning and getting along with one another?"
4. *Family as a component of society.* The family is seen as one of many institutions in society, along with health, education, religious, or financial institutions. The family is a basic or primary unit of society, as are all the other units, and they are all a part of the larger system of society. The family as a whole interacts with other institutions to receive, exchange, or give services and communicate. Nurses have drawn many of their tenets from this perspective as they focus on the interface between families and community agencies.

Briefly Noted

All families have secrets. Some information gleaned from families may be over-exaggerated, minimized, or withheld from persons outside the family, including health providers.

THEORETICAL FRAMEWORKS FOR FAMILY NURSING

The first and oldest tradition that contributed to the model of **family nursing theory** came from the *family social science tradition* (Hanson and Kaakinen, 2001; Hanson, Kaakinen, and Friedman, 1998). These theories were developed from various family social science disciplines (largely sociology and psychology). Four conceptual approaches have dominated the field of marriage and family within the family social science tradition: structural-functional theory, systems theory, developmental theory, and interactionist theory (Klein and White, 1996; Nye and Berardo, 1981). These

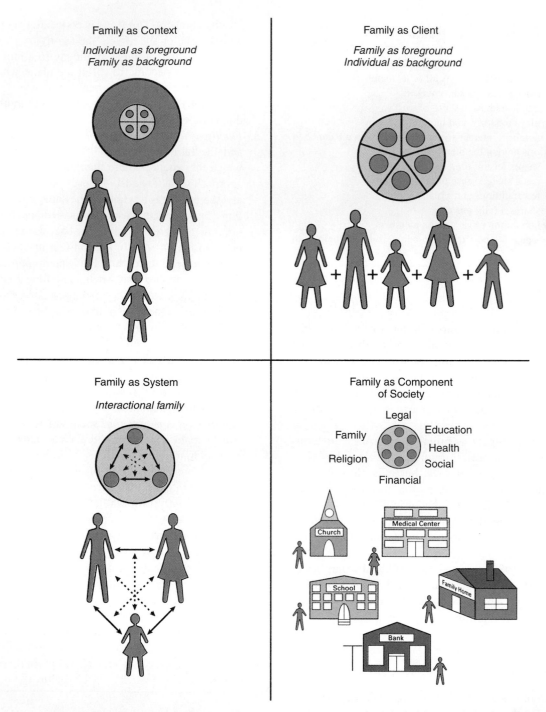

Figure 17-2   Approaches to family nursing. (From Hanson SMH: *Family health care nursing: theory, practice and research,* Philadelphia, 2001, FA Davis.)

approaches are constantly evolving, which makes the knowledge base more user friendly.

The following is a summary of the four major family social theories and what they have contributed to family nursing theory.

Structural-Functional Theory

The *structural-functional framework* from a social science perspective defines families as social systems. Families are examined in terms of their relationship with other major social structures (institutions) such as health care, religion, education, government, and/or the economy. This perspective looks at the arrangement of members within the family, relationships between the members, and the roles and relationships of the members to the whole family (Artinian, 2001; Friedman, 1998). The primary focus is to determine how family patterns are related to other institutions in society and to consider the family in the overall structure of society. Emphasis is placed on the basic functions of fami-

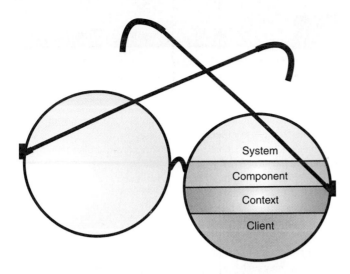

Figure 17-3   Four views of family through a lens. (From Hanson SMH: *Family health care nursing: theory, practice, and research,* Philadelphia, 2001, FA Davis.)

lies. With family structure as the focus, the major concern is how well the structure performs its functions. Individuals or family units receive little attention in this approach. Families are studied from the status-role perspective. Family theorists use this approach to understand the social or family system and its relationship to the overall social system. This approach describes the family as open to outside influences, yet at the same time maintaining its boundaries. The family is seen as passive in adapting to the system rather than as an agent of change. The framework emphasizes a static society structure and neglects change as a structural dynamic. Assumptions of the structural-functional theory are found in Box 17-4.

According to Friedman (1998), nurses refer to this model when they talk about:

- Forms, or type of family such as single-parent families, step-families, nuclear families, or extended families
- Role structure
- Value system
- Communication patterns
- Power structure
- Support networks

This perspective is a useful framework for assessing families and health. Illness of a family member results in alteration of the family structure and function. If a single mother is ill, she cannot carry out her various roles, so grandparents or siblings may have to assume child-care responsibilities. Family power structures and communication patterns are affected with illness of a parent. The family assessment includes determining if changes resulting from the illness influence the family's ability to carry out its functions. Sample assessment questions are, "How did the death alter the family structure?" and "What family roles were changed with the onset of the chronic illness?" Interventions become necessary when a change in the family structure alters the family's ability to function. Examples of interventions using this model include helping families use existing support

- A family is a social system with functional requirements.
- A family is a small group that has basic features common to all small groups.
- Social systems, such as families, accomplish functions that serve the individuals in addition to those that serve society.
- Individuals act within a set of internal norms and values that are learned primarily in the family through socialization.

Box 17-5	**Assumptions of the Systems Approach**

- Family systems are greater than and different from the sum of their parts.
- There are many hierarchies within family systems and logical relationships between subsystems (e.g., mother-child, family-community).
- There are boundaries in the family system that can be open, closed, or random.
- Family systems increase in complexity over time, evolving to allow greater adaptability, tolerance to change, and growth by differentiation.
- Family systems change constantly in response to stresses and strains from within and from outside environments. There are structural similarities in different family systems (isomorphism).
- Change in one part of family systems affects the total system.
- Causality is modified by feedback; therefore causality never exists in the real world.
- Family systems patterns are circular rather than linear; change must be directed toward the cycle.
- Family systems are an organized whole; therefore individuals within the family are interdependent.
- Family systems have homeostasis features to maintain stable patterns that can be adaptive or maladaptive.

structures and helping families modify the way they are organized so that role responsibilities can be distributed.

The major strength of the structure-functional theory to family nursing is its comprehensive approach that views families in the broader community in which they live. The major weakness of this approach is the static picture of the family, which does not allow for dynamic change over time.

Systems Theory

The *systems theory* to understanding families was influenced by theory derived from physics and biology. A system is composed of a set of interacting elements; each system can be identified and is distinct from the environment in which it exists. An open system exchanges energy and matter with the environment (negentropy), whereas a closed system is isolated from its environment (entropy). Systems depend on both positive and negative feedback to maintain a steady state (homeostasis). Seeking therapy when the marital relationship is strained is an example of using negative feedback to maintain a steady state. Assumptions of systems theory are found in Box 17-5.

The family system perspective encourages nurses to view clients as participating members of a family. Nurses using this perspective determine the effects of illness or injury on the entire family system. Emphasis is on the whole rather than on individuals. Nursing assessment of family systems includes assessment of:

- Individual members
- Subsystems
- Boundaries
- Openness
- Inputs and outputs
- Family interactions
- Family processing
- Adaptation or change abilities

Assessment questions include "Who is in the family system?" and "How has one member's critical illness affected the entire family system?" Interventions need to assist individual, subsystem, and whole family functioning. Some nursing strategies using this approach include establishing a mechanism for providing families with information about their family members on a regular basis and discussing ways to provide for a normal family life for family members after someone has become ill.

The major strength of the systems framework is that it views families from both a subsystem and a suprasystem approach. That is, it views the interactions within and among family subsystems as well as the interaction among families and the larger supersystems, such as community, world, and universe. The major weakness of the systems framework is that the focus is on the interaction of the family with other systems rather than on the individual, which is sometimes more important.

Developmental Theory

Individual developmental theory has been core to nursing of people across the life span. This approach looks at the family system over time through different phases that can be predicted with known family transitions based on norms.

Evelyn Duvall (1977) in her classic book, *Marriage and Family Development,* presented a synthesis of developmental concepts. In essence, she took the principles of individual development and applied them to the family as a unit. Her stages of family development are based on the age of the eldest child. Overall family tasks are identified that need to be accomplished for each stage of family development. Developmental concepts include moving to a different level of functioning, implying progress in a single direction. Family disequilibrium and conflicts are described as occurring during transition periods from one stage to another. The family has a predictable natural history designated by stages, beginning with the simple husband-wife pair. The group becomes more complex with the addition of each new child over time. The group again becomes simple and less complex as the younger generation leaves home. Finally the group comes full circle to the original husband-wife pair. At each family life-cycle stage, there are developmental needs

---

Box 17-6	Assumptions of Developmental Theory

- In every family there are both individual and family developmental tasks that need to be accomplished for every stage of the individual/family life cycle that are unique to that particular group.
- Families change and develop in different ways because of internal and environmental stimulation.
- Developmental tasks are goals to work toward rather than specific jobs to be completed at once.
- Each family is unique in its composition and complexity of age-role expectations and positions.
- Individuals and families are a function of their history as well as the current social structure.
- Families have enough in common despite the way they develop over the family life span.
- Families may arrive at similar developmental levels through different processes.

---

of the family and tasks that must be performed. These concepts are further refined by Duvall and Miller (1985).

Developmental theory is an attempt to integrate the small-scale (interactive framework) and large-scale (structural framework) analyses of the other two approaches while viewing the family as an open system in relation to structures in society (Jones and Dimond, 1982). Developmental theory explains and predicts the changes that occur to humans or groups over time. Achievement of family developmental tasks helps individual members to accomplish their tasks. This framework:

- Assists nurses in anticipating clinical problems in families
- Identifies family strengths
- Serves as a guide in assessing the family's developmental stage
- Assesses the extent to which the family is fulfilling the tasks associated with its respective stage
- Assesses the family's developmental history
- Assesses the availability of resources essential for performing developmental tasks

In conducting an assessment of a family using the developmental model, there are several questions that can be asked: Where does this family place on the continuum of the family life cycle? What are the developmental tasks that are not being accomplished? Typical kinds of nursing intervention strategies using this perspective help the family to understand individual and family growth and development stages and deal with the normal transitions between developmental periods (e.g., tasks of the school-age family member versus tasks of the adolescent family member). Assumptions of developmental theory are found in Box 17-6.

The major strength of this approach is that it provides a basis for forecasting what a family will be experiencing at any period in the family life cycle (e.g., role transitions and family structure changes). The major weakness is the fact that the model was developed at a time when the traditional nuclear family was emphasized.

Box 17-7	Assumptions of Interactional Theory

- Complex sets of symbols having common meanings are acquired through living in a symbolic environment.
- Individuals distinguish, evaluate, and assign meaning to symbols.
- Behavior is influenced by meanings of symbols or ideas rather than by instincts, needs, or drives; therefore the meaning an individual assigns to symbols is important to understanding behavior.
- The self continues to change and evolve over time through introspection caused by experience and activity.
- The evolving self has several dimensions: the physical body and characteristics and a complex social self. The "me" is a conventional, habitual self that consists of learned, repetitious responses. The "I" is spontaneous to the individual.
- Individuals are actors as well as reactors; they select and interpret the environment to which they respond.
- Individuals are born into a dynamic society.
- The nature of the infant is determined by the environment and responses to the infant rather than by a predisposition to act in a certain way (this is now being challenged).
- Individuals learn from the culture and become the society.
- Individuals' behavior is a product of their history, which is continually being modified by new information.

Interactional Theory

Interactional theory views families as units of interacting personalities and examines the symbolic communications by which family members relate to one another. Within the family, each member occupies a position to which a number of roles are assigned. Members define their role expectations in each situation through their perceptions of the role demands. Members judge their own behavior by assessing and interpreting the actions of others toward them. The responses of others in the family serve to challenge or reinforce family members' perceptions of the norms of role expectations (Bomar, 1996). Central to the interaction approach is the process of role taking. Every role exists in relation to some other role, and interaction represents a dynamic process of testing perceptions about one another's roles (Stanhope, 1996). The ability to predict other family members' expectations for one's role enables each member to have some knowledge of how to react in the role and indicates how other members will react to performing the role. Assumptions of interactional theory are in Box 17-7.

Assessment of families using the interactional framework emphasizes interaction between and among family members and family communication patterns about health and illness behaviors appropriate for different roles. Nurses intervene using strategies focused on the following (Bomar, 1996):

1. Effectiveness of communication among members
2. Ability to establish communication between nurses and families
3. Clear and concise messages between members

Evidence-Based Practice

STATE OF FAMILY NURSING THEORY

Of the three categories of theory, the family social science theories are the most well developed and informative with respect to how families function, the environment-family interchange, interactions within the family, how the family changes over time, and the family's reaction to health and illness. One striking limitation in using family social science theories as a basis for assessment and intervention in family nursing is that their clinical application is limited, although recent work has made some strides in this direction (Berkey and Hanson, 1991; Danielson, Hamel-Bissell, and Winstead-Fry, 1993; Friedman, 1998; Hanson, 2001b; Vaughan-Cole et al, 1998; Wright and Leahey, 1995). Family therapy theories are the next most developed theories and come from a professional/practice background rather than an academic discipline such as family social science. More family nursing theory, practice, and research is drawing from family therapy theories as the specialty grows more sophisticated. Of all three, theory basis nursing models are the least developed. The major drawback to the nursing models is that they originated using the individual as the focus, and only a few evolved to fit a family or group focus (Berkey and Hanson, 1991).

APPLICATION IN PRACTICE

Currently there is no singular theory or conceptual framework from nursing, family social science, or family therapy that fully describes the relationships and dynamics for family life and family nursing theory. Thus an integrated approach is necessary for the theory, practice, research, and education of family nursing. One theoretical perspective does not give nurses a sufficiently broad knowledge upon which to assess and intervene with families. Therefore nurses must draw upon multiple theories to work effectively with families.

4. Similarities between verbal and nonverbal communication patterns
5. Directions of the interaction

Nurses can center their attention on how family members interact with one another, so this approach is useful in explaining family communication, roles, decision making, and problem solving (Friedman, 1998).

The major strength of this approach is the focus on internal processes within families such as roles, conflict, status, communication, responses to stress, decision-making, and socialization. Processes, rather than end products, of social interactions are the major focus; thus this framework has been used by many nurse scholars. The major weakness is the broadness and lack of agreement about concepts and assumptions of the theory, which has made it difficult to refine. Interactionalists consider families to be comparatively closed units with little relation to the outside society.

FAMILY NURSING PROCESS

The **family nursing process** is a dynamic organized method of critically thinking about the family. It is problem solving with the family to help the family successfully adapt to identified health care needs (Ross, 2001). The family nursing process is the application of the basic nursing process and is grounded in knowledge of family nursing and family theory.

The family nursing process consists of the following steps adapted specifically with family as the focus group (Carnevali and Thomas, 1993):

1. *Collection of a family nursing database (general or focused).* Data collection is focused on both identification of problem areas and strengths of the family. Often this and the following step of diagnostic reasoning become integrated so that assessment and analysis of the data collected occurs concurrently. Nurses make inferences and draw conclusions about the data they collect, which in turn directs more data collection or defines the problem areas.

2. *Diagnostic reasoning and generation of specific family nursing diagnosis.* In this step, nurses make clinical judgments about which problems can be solved by nursing intervention, which problems need to be referred to other professionals, and areas of concern to which the family is successfully adapting on its own without intervention. The problems that require nursing intervention are specifically stated as family nursing diagnoses. The family nursing diagnosis provides direction for the collaboration of the nurse and the family in designing a plan of action. Diagnostic statements for the family as a whole can be derived from any of the common taxonomies that contain statements related to families, such as the North American Nursing Diagnosis Association (NANDA) (Gordon, 2000), *Diagnostic and Statistical Manual of Mental Disorders (DSM-IV)* (American Psychiatric Association, 1994), *International Classification of Disease (ICD)* (American Medical Association, 1997), or the Omaha System (Martin and Scheet, 1992).

3. *Collection of nursing and medical data and generation of data-supported nursing prognosis for each family nursing diagnosis.* The nursing prognosis is a nursing judgment, based on the holistic view of the family and its members, that predicts the probability of the family's ability to respond to the current situation. The predictive, or statement, outlines the most successful course of action on which to focus the interventions.

4. *Treatment planning based on both family nursing diagnosis and prognosis, plus additional data on daily living and family resources and deficiencies, that influences planned nursing actions.* The nurse and family work in a partnership to design and contract for a plan of action based on identified family strengths. The goal of the plan of action is to have the family successfully manage its health care concerns.

5. *Implementation of family-negotiated plans of action.* The specific family and nursing interventions are carried out by the identified family member or provider to achieve the goals upon which they all agreed.

6. *Evaluation of family/family members' responses to plans of action, effects of family diagnosis, prognosis, and pre-vious treatment.* The evaluation phase is based on the family outcomes, not on the effectiveness of the interventions. Modification of family nursing diagnosis and plans occurs as necessary based on an ongoing evaluation.

7. *Termination of the nurse-family partnership included in the plan of action and implemented based on the evaluation.* A more detailed discussion of the family nursing process that demonstrates how to implement the process is presented in the following sections.

Briefly Noted

Assessment is interactive. As you are evaluating families, they are evaluating you.

Collection of Data

The first step in the traditional nursing process is assessment, which is a comprehensive data-collection process. The assessment process is one of the most critical steps in the nursing process because it directs the whole problem-solving process. The selection of the appropriate assessment tool is made by the nurse based on areas of concern identified by the referring source (e.g., the physician) and the theoretical framework the nurse is using.

Purpose of the Family Interview

The purpose of the initial family interview is to identify the health concerns of the family. The central issues often are not the same as the problem for which the family was referred. See the following case study:

The Raggs family is referred to the home health clinic by a physician for medication management after Sam, the 73-year-old husband, was discharged from the hospital with the diagnosis of insulin-dependent diabetes mellitus (IDDM), which he has had for 13 years. The potential area of concern that prompted the referral was the actual administration of insulin. After the initial interview the nurse finds that administration of the medication is not the central issue for Sam and his wife, Rose, but how to manage his nutrition. The inference of the referral source was that the family knew how to manage the dietary aspects of diabetes because Sam had IDDM for 13 years. In this particular case, the focus needs to be on the nutritional management rather than medication administration.

HOW TO Plan for the Assessment Process

Assessment of families requires an organized plan before you see the family. This planning includes the following:

1. Why are you seeing the family?
2. Who will be present during the interview?
3. Where will you see the family and how will the space be arranged?
4. What are you going to be assessing?
5. How are you going to collect the data?
6. What are you going to do with the information you find?

Identifying a Potential Problem Area

Data collection begins with the identification of a potential problem area through a variety of sources, which include the family, the physician, a school nurse, or a case worker. The identification of a problem, actual or potential, triggers the nurse to establish contact with a family. Several examples follow:

1. A family is referred to the home health agency because of the birth of the newest family member. In that district, all births are automatically followed up with a home visit.
2. A family calls the Visiting Nurse Association to request assistance in providing care to a family member who has a terminal illness.
3. The school nurse is asked to conduct a family assessment by a teacher who noticed that a student is frequently absent and has had significant behavior changes in the classroom.
4. A physician requests a family assessment for a child who has failure to thrive.

The initial source of referral has identified an actual or potential family health care problem. The specific problem or the central issue may not have been identified at this point. One of the most important pieces of information provided by the referral source is the focus or the cluster of cues, or symptoms, that lead someone to believe that a problem might exist. The cluster of cues helps to focus the assessment process and selection of the appropriate family assessment tools.

As soon as the referral occurs, the nurse begins the assessment process and data collection. Sources of pre-encounter data collected before the family interview by the nurse include the following:

1. *Referral source.* The information collected from the referral source includes the cues that lead the source to identify that a problem area exists for this family. Demographic information may be obtained from the referral source. Both subjective and objective information is helpful in the assessment process.
2. *Family.* A family may identify a health care concern and seek help. During the initial intake or screening procedure, valuable information can be collected that provides the focus for the assessment interview between the nurse and the family. Information is collected by the nurse during the interaction with the family member on the phone while making arrangements for the initial appointment. This information might include:
   - Family members' views of the problem
   - Surprise that the referral was made
   - Reluctance to set up the meeting
   - Avoidance of setting up the interview
   - Recognition that a referral was made
3. *Previous records.* Previous records may be available for review before the first meeting between the nurse and the family. Often a release of information form is necessary to obtain family or individual records.

Arranging the Meeting With the Family

Before contacting the family to arrange for the initial appointment, the nurse decides the best place to conduct the interview. Often this decision is dictated by the type of agency with which the nurse works (e.g., home health is conducted in the home), or the mental health agency may choose to have the family meet in the neighborhood clinic office.

There are several advantages to conducting the interview in the family home. The everyday environment of the family can be viewed by the nurse during the visit. An important reason to conduct home interviews is to emphasize that the problem is the responsibility of the whole family and not one family member. The family members are likely to feel more relaxed and demonstrate typical family interactions in their own environment. The convenience of conducting the interview in the home may increase the probability of having more family members present. Two important disadvantages of conducting the interview in the home are that (1) the home may be the only sanctuary or safe place for the family or its members to be away from the scrutiny of others, and (2) to conduct an interview in the personal space of the family requires skilled communication ability on the part of the nurse.

Conducting the family interview in the office or clinic allows for easier access to consult with other health care providers about the problem. An advantage of using the clinic may be that the family situation is so intense that a more formal, less personal setting may be necessary for the family to begin discussion of emotionally charged issues. A disadvantage of conducting the family interview in the office is that it may reinforce a possible gap between the nurse and the family's value system, since the nurse does not see the everyday family environment.

HOW TO Set an Appointment With the Family

The assessment process starts immediately upon referral. The following are suggestions that will make the process of arranging a meeting with the family easier:

1. Remember that the assessment is reciprocal and the family will be making judgments about you when you call to make the appointment.
2. Introduce yourself and state the purpose for the contact.
3. Do not apologize for contacting the family. Be clear, direct, and specific about the need for an appointment.
4. Arrange a time that is convenient for the greatest possible number of family members.
5. Confirm place, time, date, and directions.

After the decision is made regarding the location for the family interview, the appointment needs to be arranged with the family. The nurse needs to be confident and organized when making the initial contact. After the introduction, the nurse concisely states the reason for requesting the family visit. All family members are encouraged to attend the interview. Several possible times for the appointment can be offered, which allows the family to select the most convenient time for all members to be present. Often this occurs in the late afternoon or evening.

Family Nursing Diagnosis

The family nursing diagnosis is based on the nurse's determination of the central issue of concern with the family. It is important for the nurse to state the specific family nursing diagnosis because it provides the framework for the remaining steps in the family nursing process. The **family nursing diagnosis** is a public statement of the problem and the specific reason that brings the nurse and family together to solve a family health care need (Ross, 2001). If the family nursing diagnosis is not properly identified, the family and the nurse will collect data, design interventions, and implement plans of care that do not meet the family's needs. A key factor to identifying the correct family nursing diagnosis is asking broad-based questions that allow for concurrent data collection in multiple ways. The importance of identifying the central issue of concern and accurately making the family nursing diagnosis is demonstrated by comparing the following two scenarios:

Scenario #1: The hypothesized central issue for the Raggs family was identified by the referral source: Is insulin being administered correctly by the Raggs family? Based on this central issue, evidence was collected and the family nursing diagnosis identified was the following: Lack of family knowledge related to the administration of insulin secondary to new diagnosis of insulin-dependent diabetes as evidenced by (1) verbal statements of concern about giving the injection, (2) difficulty drawing up the accurate amount of insulin, and (3) questions about the storage of insulin. This nursing diagnosis focuses further data collection and plan for interventions on (1) the psychomotor skills of family members necessary to give the insulin injection, (2) the correct amount of insulin to give according to blood glucose level, and (3) the correct storage and handling of the medication and the equipment.

Based on this family nursing diagnosis, the nurse concluded that the most important area to concentrate on was the ability of the family to administer medication. The data collection process and the nurse's thinking were focused on a single problem, not the whole effect of this health issue on the family. The identification of other family health care needs may occur, but the identification will be delayed, which may cause potential harm.

Scenario #2: The real central issue for the Raggs family identified by the nurse conducting the assessment is as follows: What is the best way to ensure that the Raggs family understands the relationship of insulin-dependent diabetes and the administration of medication? After collecting evidence, the family nursing diagnosis was the following: Lack of family knowledge related to health care management of a family member who has been newly diagnosed with insulin-dependent diabetes.

Asking a broader-based question allows the nurse to view the whole picture of the family dealing with this specific health concern and directs the data-collection process. More evidence was collected in this case scenario because more options for possible interventions were considered concurrently in the data-collection process. Areas of data collection for this nursing diagnosis were (1) administration of medication, (2) nutritional management, (3) blood glucose monitoring, (4) activity and exercise, and (5) knowledge of pathophysiology of diabetes. The nurse was able to collect data looking at the family in a more holistic fashion. The central issue for the family centered around nutritional management, which ultimately affects the administration of medication.

Box 17-8	Helpful Reflective Questions in Family Nursing Diagnosis

- Am I continuing to focus on the central issue?
- Am I sure that I am understanding the information correctly?
- Is everyone involved focused on the central issue?
- Have I collected enough information to be drawing inferences or conclusions?
- Have I made any assumptions that might not be true or valid?

The major difference between the two scenarios was the way in which the nurse framed the question. In the first scenario the nurse asked a question that allowed for only one aspect of the family and the health care concern to be considered at a time. This type of step-by-step problem-solving process is tedious, time consuming, and will likely cause error in the identification of the most pressing family nursing diagnosis. In the second scenario, the nurse asked a question that allowed for critical thinking about several options concurrently.

An important part of defining the family nursing process is continuous reflective questioning, which helps to keep the central issue in focus and allows for modification of the family nursing diagnosis (Alfaro-Lefevre, 1994) (Box 17-8).

The family nursing diagnoses should not be limited to the few that are endorsed by the NANDA (Gordon, 2000). After the family nursing diagnosis has been identified and verified with the family, the next step is the family nursing prognosis.

Family Nursing Prognosis

The **family nursing prognosis** is a realistic statement about the ability of the family to successfully adapt to the nursing diagnosis given the following elements:

- The strengths of the family
- The pattern of family response in similar situations
- The direction of the family health care problem

The prognosis statement represents the nurse's judgment of the family's ability to adapt to the current situation given the evidence collected from the family assessment process. Family nursing prognosis "is a prediction of the possible or probable course of events and outcomes associated with a particular family health status or family situation under various circumstances, treatment options or lack of treatment" (Carnevali and Thomas, 1993, p. 80).

The family prognosis directs the nurse to look for areas where changes can occur based on the types of outcomes and direction of change possible (Carnevali and Thomas, 1993). The treatment plan is based on predicting the areas in which the family can change to achieve successful adaptation.

The areas of change may be focused on the family's response to the situation, the family system process, and the family function most affected or family components, such as:

- Roles
- Communication
- Decision making
- Stress and coping

The nurse predicts the course of events or the pattern of change expected to occur given information known about the family. The types of outcomes that the nurse considers are as follows:

- Preventing a potential problem
- Minimizing the problem
- Stabilizing the problem
- Assisting with a deteriorating problem.

A case example showing the importance of the prognosis statement follows:

Scenario #3: The home hospice nurse has been working with the Brush family for 3 weeks. The Brush family consists of the following members, who all live in the home:

- Dylan (father)
- Myra (mother)
- William (10-year-old son)
- Jessica (7-year-old daughter)
- Beatrice (grandmother, Myra's mother)

Beatrice was diagnosed with terminal liver cancer 4 weeks ago. The Brush family all agreed that Beatrice should live with them and be cared for until her death in their home. Beatrice has other children who live in the same city. The hospice nurse, in collaboration with the Brush family, identified several family nursing diagnoses, but the following family nursing diagnosis is of major importance because it affects the lives of all family members: Family role conflict related to the maternal grandmother moving into her daughter's home after being diagnosed with terminal liver cancer. The daughter showed her role conflict by stating, "Sometimes I do not know who I am—daughter, nurse, mother, or wife."

The prognosis for resolving the role conflict experienced by Myra can be maximized for success by working with the family to spread the caregiver role among the extended family members, negotiating certain tasks and who performs them, and by providing for respite care. One of the strengths of the family is agreement that caring for the dying grandmother in the home is the "right" ethical choice for them. The disruption to the family and their expected roles will be temporary because the grandmother will probably not live for more than 4 months. Home hospice has been contacted and is involved in the care management. The family has strong internal and external support systems. The extended family is willing to be involved in the care of Beatrice.

The prognosis is critical because it serves as the foundation for the interventions or strategies of action that the family and nurse design in response to the identified family nursing diagnosis. The area of change in the case study is family roles and the expected behaviors of each family member. The course of events is short term, but Myra's role conflict may increase as her caregiver role becomes more intense as her mother's health deteriorates. The type of outcome is to mobilize resources to minimize Myra's role conflict.

Planning, Implementing, and Evaluating

After the prognosis statement is made, it is important for the nurse to determine if the family's responses to the problem require nursing intervention or if they should be referred to a different professional. The planning phase is a form of contracting with families. The contract, or plan of action, includes:

- Establishing goals
- Creating plans of action

Box 17-9   Reflective Critical Thinking Process for the Nurse

1. Is this plan being developed in collaboration with the family?
2. Will the proposed approaches enhance family strengths and increase independence of family members?
3. Is this action within the information and skill level of the family members or their own resources?
4. On a scale of one to ten (with ten being the highest), how committed and motivated are family members to adhere to the plan?
5. Are there adequate resources available to carry out the plan?
6. How would family members respond to these questions?
7. Will this action diminish or strengthen the coping ability of the family?

From Friedman MM: *Family nursing: research, theory and practice*, ed 4, Norwalk, Conn, 1998, Appleton & Lange.

- Determining who does what in the plan
- Building the evaluation steps

The written plan of care ensures involvement of each person, involves people in their own care, and increases autonomy and self-esteem of the family members.

Once the nurse determines that the identified central issues are appropriate for nursing, the planning and intervening aspects of the family nursing process help the family members be part of the solution.

The degree of involvement of each family member varies and needs to be negotiated among the family members with the help of the nurse. The types of plans and the implementing and evaluating processes are specific to the family and the family nursing diagnosis. The plan, implementation, and evaluation are designed based on the evidence collected in the assessment and the prognosis statement.

During the planning stage, it is important for the nurse to recognize that the family has the right to make its own health decisions. The role of the nurse is to:

- Offer guidance to the family
- Provide information
- Assist in the planning process

An important part of the planning phase is to determine who does what. The nurse may assist the family by (1) providing direct care, which the family cannot; (2) removing barriers to needed services, which helps the family to function; and (3) improving the capacity of the family to act on its own behalf and assume responsibility (Friedman, 1998) (Box 17-9).

Building the plan of action for the family on family strengths increases the likelihood that the family will achieve the desired outcome. Once the plan has been developed and all individuals involved have approved or committed to the plan, the plan is put into effect. Data collection continues throughout the implementation phase and is part of the formative evaluation process. When a plan is not working well, the nurse and the family should work together to determine the barriers of implementation. Family apathy and indecision are known to be barriers to implementation

<table>
<tr><td>

Box 17-10 **Barriers to Practicing Family Nursing**

- Until the last decade, most practicing nurses had little exposure to family concepts during their undergraduate education and have continued to practice using the individual focus. Family nursing was viewed as "common sense" and not a theory-based nursing approach.
- There has been a lack of good comprehensive family assessment models, instruments, and strategies in nursing.
- Nursing has strong historical ties with the medical model, which views families as structure and not central to individual health care.
- The traditional charting system in health care has been oriented to the individual.
- The medical and nursing diagnosis systems used in health care are disease centered, and diseases are focused on individuals.
- Insurance carriers have traditionally based coverage and reimbursement on the individual, not on the family unit.
- The hours during which health care systems provide services to families are at times of day when family members cannot accompany one another.

</td></tr>
</table>

(Friedman, 1998). Friedman (1998) identified the following nurse-related barriers to implementation:

- Imposing ideas
- Negative labeling
- Overlooking strengths
- Neglecting cultural or gender implications.

Family apathy may occur because of value differences between the nurse and the family, the family may be overcome with a sense of hopelessness, the family may view the problems as too overwhelming, or the family may have a fear of failure. Additional factors to be considered are that the family may be indecisive because they cannot determine which course of action is better, the family may have an unexpressed fear or concern; or the family may have a pattern of making decisions only when faced with a crisis. There are many barriers to family nursing (Box 17-10).

The evaluation process contains both formative (ongoing) and summative (ending) evaluation components. The evaluation is based on the family outcomes and response to the plan, not the success of the interventions. An important part of the plan is the termination of the relationship between the nurse and the family.

Briefly Noted

Too much disclosure during the early contacts between the family and nurse may scare the family away. Slow the process down and take time to build trust.

Termination of the Nurse-Family Relationship

Termination is phasing out the nurse from family involvement. When termination is built into the plan, the family benefits from a smooth transition process. The family is given credit for the outcomes of the plan that they helped design. Strategies often used in the termination component are:

- Decreasing the frequency or length of sessions with the nurse
- Extending invitations to the family for follow-up
- Making referrals when appropriate
- Calling a summative evaluation meeting where the nurse and family put a formal closure to their relationship

When termination occurs suddenly, it is important for the nurse to determine the forces bringing about the closure. The family may be initiating the termination prematurely, which requires a renegotiating process. The insurance or agency requirements may be placing a financial constraint on the amount of time the nurse can work with a family. Regardless of how termination comes about, it is an important aspect in the family nursing process.

FAMILY NURSING ASSESSMENT

Family nursing assessment is the cornerstone for family nursing interventions. By using a systematic process, family problem areas are identified and family strengths are emphasized as the building blocks for interventions. Building the interventions with family-identified problems and strengths allows for equal family and provider commitment to the solutions and ensures more successful interventions. There are some family assessment models available that have been developed by nurses (Hanson, 2001d).

The *Family Assessment Intervention Model* and the *Family Systems Stressor Strength Inventory (FS³I)* measure very specific dimensions of stressors and strengths in the family and give a microscopic view of family health. It is a more extensive and specific model that demands in-depth knowledge of family analysis and is useful for doing family research (Hanson & Kaakinen, 2001).

One family assessment model and approach developed by a nurse—the *Friedman Family Assessment Model and Short Form* (Friedman, 1998)—is presented in Appendix G.2. Genograms and ecomaps are strategies to assess families that provide a clear, concise picture of intergenerational patterns and social supports or direction of family stress (see Chapter 8 in Hanson, 2001d).

Friedman Family Assessment Model

The *Friedman Family Assessment Model* (Friedman, 1998) draws heavily on the structural-functional framework and on developmental and systems theory. The model takes a broad approach to family assessment, which views families as a subsystem of society. The family is viewed as an open social system. The family's structure (organization) and functions (activities and purposes) and the family's relationship to other social systems are the focus of this approach.

This assessment approach is important for family nurses because it enables them to assess the family system as a whole, as part of the whole of society, and as an interaction system. The general assumptions for this model are contained in Box 17-11.

| Box 17-11 | Assumptions Underlying Friedman's Family Assessment Model |

1. The family is a social system with functional requirements.
2. A family is a small group possessing certain generic features common to all small groups.
3. The family as a social system accomplishes functions that serve the individual and society.
4. Individuals act in accordance with a set of internalized norms and values that are learned primarily in the family through socialization.

From Friedman MM: *Family nursing: theory and practice,* ed 4, Norwalk, Conn, 1998, Appleton & Lange.

The guidelines for the Friedman Assessment Model consist of six broad categories of interview questions:

1. Identifying data
2. Developmental family stage and history
3. Environmental data
4. Family structure, including communication, power structures, role structures, and family values
5. Family functions, including affective, socialization, and health care
6. Family coping

Each category has several subcategories. There are both long and short forms of this assessment tool. The short form is presented in Appendix G.2.

In summary, this approach was developed to provide guidelines for family nurses who are interviewing a family to gain an overall view of what is going on in the family. The questions are extensive, and it may not be possible to collect all the data at one visit. All the categories may not be pertinent for every family.

Other Family Assessment Models

Each family nursing assessment model and approach is unique and creates a different database upon which to plan interventions. The Friedman Family Assessment Model is more broad and general. It is particularly useful for viewing families in their communities.

FUTURE IMPLICATIONS FOR FAMILY NURSING

Family nursing practice is an evolving area of nursing and will continue to be a significant aspect of health care in the future, especially with the current focus of health care reform in the United States (Hanson, 2001a). The barriers confronting the practice of family nursing need to be integral aspects addressed in new health care delivery systems.

Most nursing research has focused on the individual rather than family health care (Houck & Kodadek, 2001). Research pertaining to family and mental health is further advanced than family and physical health. Recently nursing has awakened to the connection between family dynamics and health and illness. More family-centered research needs to be conducted by family nurses.

Future Implications for Family Policy

As a profession, nursing is accountable for participating in the development of legislation and family policy. Government actions that have a direct or indirect effect on families are called *family policy.* All government actions, whether at the local, county, state, or national level, affect the family directly or indirectly, in both negative and positive ways. The range of social policy decisions that affect families is vast, such as health care access and coverage, low-income housing, social security, welfare, food stamps, pension plans, affirmative action, and education. Although all government polices affect families, the United States has no overall, official explicit family policy (Gebbie & Gebbie, 2001).

Most government policy indirectly affects families. Much debate has taken place within government regarding the definition of family. An argument often cited for the lack of more explicit family policies is related to the financial burden that would occur if the definition of family was too broad.

The national health promotion and disease prevention objectives outlined in *Healthy People 2000* (U.S. Department of Health and Human Services, 1990), *Healthy People 2010* (U.S. Department of Health and Human Services, 1998), and *Healthy Communities 2000* (American Public Health Association, 1991) have direct and indirect consequences and outcomes that affect families. The Family Leave legislation passed in the 1990s by the U.S. Congress is an example of a type of family policy that has been positive for families. A family member may take a defined amount of leave for family events (e.g., births, deaths) without fear of losing his or her job. Equally important today is the role that families will be assigned in health care reform. Since families are a primary source for health care beliefs and delivery, it is important that the issues of families and their place in health care reform be obvious. "All policies affect families, strengthening or diminishing their ability to sustain themselves and to prepare the next generation" (Elliott, 1993, p. ii).

At the beginning of the twenty-first century, it is natural and wise to look forward and speculate on the future of family nursing, families, and what this might mean for family social policy. A brief discussion is provided for students to ponder and realize that we all have an opportunity to write the script for this new century.

Future of Families

Each family is an unexplored mystery, unique in the ways in which it meets the needs of its members and of society. Healthy and vital families are essential to the world's future because family members are affected by what their families have invested in them or failed to provide for their growth and well-being. Families will continue to survive and serve as the basic social unit of society.

The following projections and trends for the future of families provide an important lens to view the future (Hanson, 2001a):

- Marriage rates remain high in the United States and are among the highest of all developed nations in the world. However, there has been a slight decline in the rate of marriage since World War II, largely because of the trend to postpone marriage and the increase in the rates of cohabitation. Nevertheless, marriages continue to dissolve as a result of abandonment, separation, divorce, or death of a spouse.
- Divorce rates during the 1970s and 1980s increased rapidly. More than 60% of all marriages end in divorce. In recent years, there has been a slight trend downward, possible resulting from the increase in age at first marriage, which lowers the risk of divorce. According to Gelles (1995), divorce will continue to be the typical way the majority of marriages will end.
- Children will increasingly live in below-poverty-level, single-mother households because of lack of support from fathers.
- Birthrates appear to be generally down since the baby boom. Children's overall share of the population has declined since 1970 and will continue to decline in the foreseeable future as fertility rates stay low and baby boomers age. Delays in first marriage often means that couples delay having their first child. The birthrate among women who have never married is rising and will likely continue; unmarried motherhood currently accounts for almost one third of all births in the United States. Fertility rates will likely stay below replacement for the general population, although there is a significant variation in fertility rates across socioeconomic, racial, and ethnic groups.
- The proportion of married women (with or without children) employed in the workforce has increased rapidly in the past 40 years, with the greatest growth among married women with preschool children. The combined effects of the economy and women's movement will continue the upward trend in maternal employment. Mothers in two-parent households carry increasing economic responsibilities.
- The future of families is one of diversity of family forms and structures. There is little evidence that any of the forces will move families back toward the "idyllic nuclear family of the 1950s" (Gelles, 1995). Families and intimate relationships will continue to evolve. For example, continued development exists in single-parent families, gay and lesbian relationships, interracial marriages, and multigenerational families (new extended family). Diversity includes both cohabitation and living as single.
- The future of families will call for increased and changing marital roles. Twenty years ago, it was predicted by many that household equality was quickly approaching. However, it appears that working women simply added a second "shift" to their lifestyles. The home and child care are still considered the province and responsibility of women.

Although more men are involved in housework and child care, more men also have abandoned their families and failed to provide court-ordered child support after divorce. There is reason to predict that role options in families will continue to become more flexible. There is also reason to believe that families will always have a gender-based division of labor.

- Parents face growing concerns about caring for children through more years of education (and living at home) at the same time that their own longer-living parents survive. Middle-age adults find themselves in the "sandwich generation" between prolonged dependency of adult children remaining or returning to the home of origin and elderly parents and grandparents entering into their homes on a somewhat permanent basis. It is estimated that 20% of American children will be raised by their grandparents (Burton, et al, 1995).
- Families will have more complicated family histories and kinship relationships resulting from divorce, remarriage, and serial relationships. Society will need to come up with a whole new vocabulary to relate to the complexity of relationships in modern families.
- The increase in the number of elderly persons accompanied by the decline in the fertility rate and decreased mortality rate has a direct effect on families. The fastest growing population group includes individuals older than 85 years of age who are more likely to be frail, dependent, and have multiple health needs. The availability of kin to provide family care becomes a major issue for families. Families will be managing care of family members from a distance, via phone, e-mail, and fax technology (Kaakinen, 1999; Kinsella, 1996). In the future the old will be cared for by their children in their eighties or grandchildren in their sixties (Dreman, 1997; Kaakinen, 1999).
- Although controversial, genetic technology will be a part of the future. Today there is rapid movement toward a future when knowledge of genetic makeup and its implications for individual futures will radically transform the world. There are social, legal, political, and ethical issues arising for the future from recent discoveries made in genetic research.

Gelles (1995, p. 508) believes that the two major threats and unknowns to families in the future are the following:

- *AIDS.* "The cloud that hangs over the family and intimate relations is not divorce, cohabitation, working mothers, or alternative lifestyles. Today's cloud is AIDS (acquired immunodeficiency syndrome)." The disease was barely recognized 10 years ago and today it has moved way beyond its original gay male culture.
- *Status of American children.* The status of children in families has changed, and the changes have not all been to the advantage of the children. Although some argue that the key change is the absence of fathers, the major structural change is the poverty that affects children in single-parent homes. There is a significant increase in the percentage of children in the United States who live in poverty. The major problems that children face do not come from

Healthy People 2010
Family Implications

The following objectives directly or indirectly name families as the target for the objective:

1-6   Reduce the proportion of families that experience difficulties or delays in obtaining health care or do not receive needed care for one or more family members.

7-7   Increase the proportion of health care organizations that provide patient and family education.

8-18   Increase the proportion of persons who live in homes tested for radon concentrations.

8-19   Increase the number of new homes constructed to be radon resistant.

8-22   Increase the proportion of persons living in pre-1950s housing that have tested for the presence of lead-based paint.

8-23   Reduce the proportion of occupied housing units that are substandard.

9-12   Reduce the proportion of married couples whose ability to conceive or maintain a pregnancy is impaired.

11-1   Increase the proportion of households with access to the Internet at home.

15-4   Reduce the proportion of persons living in homes with firearms that are loaded and unlocked.

15-25   Reduce residential fire deaths.

19-18   Increase food security among U.S. households and in so doing reduce hunger.

29-9   Increase the use of appropriate personal protective eyewear in recreational activities and hazardous situations around the home.

cohabitation, daycare, or the fact that their mothers work. Families are not declining because of divorce, working mothers, and lower fertility. The family is declining because American society continues to ignore the needs of a substantial portion of its children. Many children do not get immunizations, are not fed or clothed, do not get health care, and live in dangerous environments.

Healthy People 2010 and Family Implications

While *Healthy People 2010* emphasizes individual and community issues, some objectives relate specifically to families or homes. These are listed in the *Healthy People 2010* box.

Clinical Application

The idealized family portrayed in the media during the twentieth century consists of a working father, a mother who stays home, and their children. Many families today compare their turbulent, hectic lives with those of the fictionalized past and find their situations wanting.

A. Did the idealized version of the traditional family ever really exist?

B. Some people believe that American families are in decline while others believe that families are healthy. What do you think?

C. What do you think is happening with American families and what do you think the future will bring?

D. What are the implications for the practice of family community nursing?

Answers are in the back of the book.

Remember This!

- Families are the context within which health care decisions are made. Nurses are responsible for assisting families in meeting health care needs.
- Family nursing is practiced in all settings.
- Family nursing is a specialty area that has a strong theoretical base and is more than just common sense.
- Family demographics is the study of structures of families and households as well as events that alter the family, such as marriage, divorce, births, cohabitation, and dual careers.
- Demographic trends affecting the family include the age of individuals when they marry, increase in intraracial marriages with subsequent children, most divorced people remarrying, increase in dual-career marriages, increased number of children from maritally disrupted families, high divorce rate, dramatic increase in cohabitation, increased number of children who spend time in a single-parent family, delay of childbirth, increased number of children born to women who are single or who have never married, and increased number of children who live with grandparents.
- Traditionally, families have been defined as a nuclear family: mother, father, and young children. A variety of family definitions exist, such as a group of two or more, a unique social group, and two or more persons joined together by emotional bonds.
- The six historical functions performed by families are economic survival, reproduction, protection, cultural heritage, socialization of young, and conferring status. Contemporary functions involve relationships and health.
- Family structure refers to the characteristics, gender, age, and number of the individual members who make up the family unit.
- Family health is difficult to define, but it includes the biological, psychological, sociological, cultural, and spiritual factors of the family system.
- There are four approaches to viewing families: family as context, family as client, family as a system, and family as a component of society.
- Structural-functional theory views the family as a social system with members who have specific roles and functions.
- Systems theory describes families as a unit of the whole, composed of members whose interactional patterns are the focus of attention.

- Family developmental theory is one theoretical framework used to study families. This approach emphasizes how families change over time and focuses on interactions and relationships among family members.
- Interactional theory focuses on the family as a unit of interacting personalities and examines the communication processes by which family members relate to one another.
- Nurses should ask clients whom they consider to be family and then include those members in the health care plan.
- The family nursing process is a dynamic, systematic, organized method of critically thinking about the family.
- The purpose of the initial family interview is to identify the health concerns of the family.
- The family nursing diagnosis is based on the nurse's determination of the actual issues of concern within the family.
- An important part of defining the family nursing process is continuous reflective questioning.
- The family prognosis is a realistic statement about the ability of the family to successfully adapt to the nursing diagnosis.
- It is essential in the beginning of the planning step to determine if the family's response to the problem requires nursing intervention or referral to a different professional.
- It is important for the nurse to recognize that the family has the right to make its own health decisions.
- The nurse, in working with families, must evaluate the family outcomes and response to the plan, not the success of the interventions.
- The Friedman Family Assessment Model takes a macroscopic approach to family assessment, which views the family as a subsystem of society.
- The future of family, health care, and nursing is not an exact science. However, all areas are changing and there are many challenges to be understood and overcome in this new century.

What Would You Do?

1. Select six or more health professionals and ask them to define *family*. Analyze the responses for commonalities and differences. Write your definition of family.
2. From the chapter, define *family nursing*. Does this match your definition? Why? Why not? State your definition and explain why yours is different from the one in the chapter.
3. Discuss how family fits into nursing.
4. Form small groups and discuss the implications of family demography and demographic trends for nursing.
5. Develop a typology of the different family structures and household arrangements representative of the community. This information may be available from various sources, such as the health department, schools, other social and welfare agencies, and census data.
6. Identify five barriers to practicing family nursing in a community setting.
7. Describe how a family assessment is different from an individual client assessment.

8. Discuss the importance of family nursing diagnosis and prognosis related to developing a plan of action with a family.
9. Explain why family assessment is the most critical aspect of the family nursing process.
10. What kind of difficulties could you experience when arranging for a family assessment interview?
11. Discuss factors to be considered when determining the place to conduct a family assessment interview. Include pros and cons.
12. How would you select which family assessment tool to use?
13. Break into small groups and discuss the family from the point of view of each of the four family social science theories.

References

Alfaro-LeFevre R: *Applying nursing process: a step-by-step process,* ed 3, Philadelphia, 1994, JB Lippincott.

American Medical Association: International classification of diseases: clinical modifications (ICD-9-CM), vols 1 and 2, rev 9, Dover, Del, 1997, American Medical Association.

American Psychiatric Association: *Diagnostic and statistical manual of mental disorders,* ed 4, Washington, D.C., 1994, American Psychiatric Association.

American Public Health Association: *Healthy communities 2000: model standards: guidelines for community attainment of year 2000 national health objectives,* Washington, D.C., 1991, The Association.

Artinian NT: Family-focused medical-surgical nursing. In Hanson SMH: *Family health care nursing: theory, practice and research,* ed 2, Philadelphia, 2001, FA Davis.

Berkey KM, Hanson SMH: *Pocket guide to family assessment and intervention,* St Louis, 1991, Mosby.

Bomar P: *Nurses and family health promotion: concepts, assessment, and interventions,* ed 2, Philadelphia, 1996, WB Saunders.

Burton LM, Dilworth-Anderson P, Merriwether-deVries C: Context and surrogate parenting among contemporary grandparents. In Hanson SMH, et al (editors): *Single-parent families: diversity, myths, and realities,* New York, 1995, Haworth Press.

Carnevali D, Thomas MD: *Diagnostic reasoning and treatment decision making in nursing,* Philadelphia, 1993, JB Lippincott.

Carter E, McGoldrick M: The family life cycle and family therapy: an overview. In Carter E, McGoldrick M (editors): *The changing family life cycle: a framework for family therapists,* New York, 1988, Gardner Press.

Curran D: *Traits of a healthy family,* Minneapolis, 1983, Winston Press (Harper & Row).

Curran D: *Stress and the healthy family,* Minneapolis, 1985, Winston Press (Harper & Row).

Danielson CB, Hamel-Bissell B, Winstead-Fry P: *Families, health and illness: persectives on coping and intervention,* St Louis, 1993, Mosby.

Dreman S (editor): *The family on the threshold of the 21st century,* Mahwah, NJ, 1997, Lawrence Erlbaum Associates.

Duvall EM: *Marriage and family development,* ed 5, Philadelphia, 1977, JB Lippincott.

Duvall EM, Miller BL: *Marriage and family development,* ed 6, New York, 1985, Harper & Row.

Elliott B: *Vision 2010: families and health care,* Minneapolis, 1993, National Council on Family Relations.

Friedman MM: *Family nursing: research, theory and practice,* ed 4, Norwalk, Conn, 1998, Appleton & Lange.

Gebbie K, Gebbie E: Families, nursing and social policy. In Hanson SMH: *Family health care nursing: theory, practice and research,* ed 2, Philadelphia, 2001, FA Davis.

Gelles RJ: *Sociology: an introduction,* ed 5, New York, 1995, McGraw Hill.

Gordon M: *Manual of nursing diagnosis,* ed 9, St Louis, 2000, Mosby.

Hanson SMH: Families and family nursing in the new millennium. In Hanson SMH: *Family health care nursing: theory, practice and research,* ed 2, Philadelphia, 2001a, FA Davis.

Hanson SMH: *Family health care nursing: theory, practice and research,* ed 2, Philadelphia, 2001b, FA Davis.

Hanson SMH: Family health care nursing: an introduction. In Hanson SMH: *Family health care nursing: theory, practice and research,* ed 2, Philadelphia, 2001c, FA Davis.

Hanson SMH: Family nursing assessment and intervention. In Hanson SMH: *Family health care nursing: theory, practice and research,* ed 2, Philadelphia, 2001d, FA Davis.

Hanson SMH, Kaakinen JR: Nursing of families in the community. In Stanhope M, Lancaster J (editors): *Community health nursing: promoting health of aggregates, families, and individuals,* ed 5, St Louis, 2000, Mosby.

Hanson SMH, Kaakinen JR: Theoretical foundations for family nursing. In Hanson SMH: *Family health care nursing: theory, practice and research,* ed 2, Philadelphia, 2001, FA Davis.

Hanson SMH, Kaakinen JR, Friedman MM: Theoretical approaches to family nursing. In Friedman MM: Family nursing: research, theory, and practice, ed 4, Norwalk, Conn, 1998, Appleton & Lange.

Houck GM, Kodadek S: Research in families and family nursing. In Hanson SMH: *Family health care nursing: theory, practice and research,* ed 2, Philadelphia, 2001, FA Davis.

Jones SL, Dimond SL: Family theory and family therapy models: comparative review with implications for nursing practice, *J Psychosoc Nurs Ment Health Serv* 20(10):12, 1982.

Kaakinen J: An ecological view of elders and their families: needs for the 21st century. In Dempsey C, Butkus R (editors): *All creation is groaning,* Collegeville, Minn, 1999, Liturgical Press.

Kinsella K: Aging and the family: present and future demographic issues. In Blieszner T, Bedford V (editors): *Aging and the family: theory and research,* Westport, Conn, 1996, Praeger.

Klein DM, White JM: *Family theories: an introduction,* Thousand Oaks, Calif, 1996, Sage.

Martin K, Scheet M: *The Omaha system: application for community health nursing,* Philadelphia, 1992, WB Saunders.

McGoldrick M, Gerson R, Shellenberger S: *Genograms: assessment and intervention,* New York, 1999, WW Norton & Company.

Nye FI, Berardo F (editors): *Emerging conceptual frameworks in family analysis,* New York, 1981, Praeger.

Ross BJ: Nursing process and family health care. In Hanson SMH: *Family health care nursing: theory, practice and research,* ed 2, Philadelphia, 2001, FA Davis.

Satariano HJ, Briggs NJ: The good family syndrome. In Wegner GD, Alexander RJ: *Readings in family nursing,* Philadelphia, 1993, JB Lippincott.

Stanhope M: Family theories and development. In Stanhope M, Lancaster J (editors): *Community health nursing: promoting health of aggregates, families, and individuals,* ed 4, St Louis, 1996, Mosby.

U.S. Department of Health and Human Services: *Healthy people 2010 objectives: draft for public comment,* Washington, D.C., 1998, U.S. Government Printing Office.

U.S. Department of Health and Human Services: *Healthy people 2000: national health promotion and disease prevention objectives,* Washington, D.C., 1990, U.S. Department of Health and Human Services.

Vaughan-Cole B, Johnson MA, Malone JA, Walker BL: *Family nursing practice,* Philadelphia, 1998, WB Saunders.

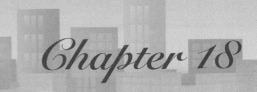

Chapter 18

Family Health Risks

CAROL J. LOVELAND-CHERRY

OBJECTIVES

After reading this chapter, the student should be able to:
- Analyze the various approaches to defining and conceptualizing family health.
- Analyze the major risks to family health.
- Analyze the interrelationship among individual health, family health, and community health.
- Explain the relevance of knowledge about family structures, roles, and functions for the family-focused community health nursing process.
- Explain the application of the nursing process for reducing family health risks and promoting family health.

CHAPTER OUTLINE

KEY TERMS

adaptive model: a model in which assessment focuses on identifying changes that have occurred since original diagnosis.

biologic risk: risk of illness due to a familial component that can be accounted for from either a genetic basis or an established life-style pattern.

clinical model: a model in which assessment focuses on identifying realistic perceptions of health risks for the client.

contracting: engaging in a working agreement that is continuously renegotiable and agreed upon by nurse and client.

economic risk: a situation in which a client's health status may be compromised or at risk due to lack of family resources. The risk is determined by the relationship between the family's resources and the demands on those resources.

empowerment: helping people acquire the skills and information necessary for informed decision making and ensuring that they have the authority to make decisions that affect them.

eudaimonistic model: a model in which health is viewed as maximizing individual and family well-being and potential.

family crisis: a situation whereby the demands of the situation exceed the resources and coping capacity of the family.

family health: a condition including the promotion and maintenance of physical, mental, spiritual, and social health for the family unit and for individual family members.

health-protecting behavior: behavior directed toward decreasing the probability of specific illness or dysfunction in individuals, families, and communities, including active protection against unnecessary stressors.

Continued

KEY TERMS—cont'd

health promotion: strategies designed to increase the physical, social, and emotional health and well-being of individuals, families, and communities.

health risk appraisal: process of identifying and analyzing an individual's prognostic characteristics of health and comparing them with those of a standard age-group, thereby providing a prediction of a person's likelihood of prematurely developing the health problems that have high morbidity and mortality in this country.

health risk reduction: application of selected interventions to control or reduce risk factors and minimize the incidence of associated disease and premature mortality.

health risks: disease precursors whose presence is associated with higher-than-average morbidity and/or mortality. Disease precursors include demographic variables, certain individual behaviors, positive individual and/or family history, and some physiological changes.

home visits: provision of community health nursing care where the individual resides.

life-event risk: normative or non-normative event that can increase the risk for illness and disability.

life-style risk: factors that predispose a family to ill health that are caused by the personal health behaviors of the members.

normative events: events that are generally expected to occur at a particular stage of development or of the life span.

non-normative events: events that are not anticipated to occur with any ability to predict (e.g., loss of a job).

risk: the probability of some event or outcome within a specified period of time.

role-performance model: a model in which health is viewed as the individual's ability to effectively perform roles and the family's ability to effectively meet their functions and developmental tasks.

social risks: family living situations that can be detrimental to a family's health such as living in high-crime neighborhoods, living in communities without adequate recreational or health resources, or living in communities with high noise, contaminants, or other high-stress environments that increase a family's health risk.

transitions: movement from one stage or condition to another.

The importance of the family in promoting the health of individuals and communities is well established (Bomar, 1996; Feetham, et al, 1992; Gilliss, et al, 1989; Nightingale, et al, 1978). Acknowledgment of the family as a client unit has been a basic assumption underlying the practice of community health nursing. The family is both an important environment affecting the health of individuals and a unit whose health is basic to that of the community and larger population. It is within the family that health behavior—including health values, health habits, and health risk perceptions—are developed, organized, and performed. Individuals' health behaviors are affected by and acted out within the family environment, larger community, and society. In turn, the larger community and society are made up of and depend upon the functioning of individuals for continued well-being.

To intervene effectively and appropriately with families to reduce their health risk and thereby promote their health, it is necessary to understand family structure and functioning. However, it is also necessary to go beyond the individual and the family and understand the complex environment in which the family exists. Increasing evidence of the effect of social, biological, economic, and life events on health requires a broader approach to addressing **health risks** for families.

Pender (1996) identifies six categories of **risk** factors:

- Genetics
- Age
- Biologic characteristics
- Personal health habits
- Life-style
- Environment.

In this chapter, health risks in these six categories for families are identified and analyzed, and approaches to reducing these risks are discussed. Options for structuring nursing interventions with families to decrease health risks and to promote health and well-being are explored.

CONCEPTS IN FAMILY HEALTH RISK

Individuals are motivated to participate in behaviors for two reasons. One of these underlying forces is **health promotion,** "behaviors directed toward increasing the level of well-being and actualizing the health potential of individuals, families, communities and society" (Pender, 1996, p. 4). In contrast, **health-protecting behaviors** are those "directed toward decreasing the probability of specific illness or dysfunction in individuals, families, and communities, including active protection against unnecessary stressors" (Pender, 1996, p. 4).

Understanding family health risk requires an examination of several related concepts:

- Family health
- Family health risk
- Risk appraisal
- Risk reduction
- Life events
- Life-style
- Family crisis

Although *health* is a vague term that can be defined from a number of perspectives, it usually is defined by the individual within his or her own culture and value system. Similarly, *illness* is the experience of a disease process.

Family Health

Family theorists refer to *healthy families* but generally do not define *family health.* Based on the various family theoretical perspectives (see Chapter 17), definitions of healthy

TABLE 18-1 Smith's Four Models of Health

Model	View of Health	Assessment	Nursing Goals
Clinical	*Family:* The absence of disease or dysfunction	Includes family health/illness history; family's definition of health and illness; family's value of health, family's knowledge of health promotion and illness prevention/treatment; family practices related to nutrition, sleep/rest, exercise, and recreation; use of alcohol, tobacco, drugs; family processes for determining illness and whether and how professional care will be sought	To promote family's physical, mental, and social health; to provide comfort in the family; to prevent deterioration of the family system
Role performance	*Individual:* Effective performance of roles *Family:* Effective meeting of family functions and developmental tasks	Includes family's current developmental stage/history; family's role structure, socialization patterns, resources for meeting functions and developmental tasks; family's perceptions of family functioning	To promote effective performance of family functions; to promote achievement of developmental tasks; to assist in identifying and mobilizing support systems and resources
Adaptive	*Individual:* Condition of the whole person engaged in effective interaction with physical/social environment *Family:* Condition of the whole family engaged in effective interaction with physical/social environment; family/environment fit	Includes the identification of family coping patterns, social networks, and support systems; family's perceptions of their environment; family's flexibility in altering behaviors, roles, rules, and perceptions when needed	To promote the family's adaptation and health-directed patterning with the environment
Eudaimonistic	*Individual:* Complete development of individual's potential for general well-being and self-realization *Family:* Development of family's well-being and maximum potential	Includes family's values and goals; family interaction patterns of recreation and relaxation; family cohesion; family promotion of autonomy	To clarify the family's values; to assist in identifying and prioritizing the family's goals; to assist the family in implementing plans to meet goals

Modified from Smith JA: *The idea of health: implications for the nursing professional,* New York, 1983, Teachers College Press, Columbia University.

families can be derived within the guidelines of any one of the frameworks. For example, within the perspective of the developmental framework, **family health** can be defined as possessing the abilities and resources to accomplish family developmental tasks. Thus the accomplishment of stage-specific tasks is one indicator of family health.

Another approach to defining family health can be through the use of Smith's (1983) four models of health, which are listed in Table 18-1:

- Clinical model
- Role-performance model
- Adaptive model
- Eudaimonistic model.

The following clinical example applies these models to one family's situation:

The Harris family consists of Mr. and Mrs. Harris, 12-year-old Kevin, and 6-year-old Leisha. Kevin was recently diagnosed with insulin-dependent diabetes mellitus (IDDM), and the family was referred by the endocrinology clinic for community health nursing service to work with the family in adjusting to the diagnosis.

The focus in a **clinical model** approach might be to identify realistic perceptions of health risks for Kevin and to teach the parents how to recognize and deal with symptoms of complications.

Assessment would include:

- Completing a family health/illness history
- Determining Mr. and Mrs. Harris' perceptions and knowledge of diabetes mellitus
- Identifying the family's health care resources

- Recognizing their concerns about caring for a child with a chronic disease

Assessment in the **role-performance model** includes exploring with the family their feelings about their abilities and resources to accomplish developmental tasks.

This family is in the developmental stage of families with school-age children based on the age of the oldest child. Developmental tasks for families in this stage include the following (Duvall and Miller, 1985, p. 217):

- Providing suitable housing and health care for the family
- Meeting family costs and making adjustments when the wife/mother works
- Allocating and monitoring responsibilities for maintaining the home
- Continuing socialization through wider community participation
- Encouraging husband-wife, parent-child, and child-child communication
- Rearing children with appropriate parenting skills in two-parent, one-parent, or reconstituted family households
- Demonstrating interest in children's schooling and in their acquisition of basic skills and knowledge
- Recognizing achievement and growth of individual family members and building solid values and morals in the family

Assessment in the **adaptive model** focuses on:

- Identifying with the family the kinds of changes that have occurred since Kevin's diagnosis
- Identifying the different or new demands that have resulted

The nurse would work with the family members to:

- Help them adapt to having a child with a chronic illness
- Repattern their lives to deal with the related increased and different demands on the family
- Identify appropriate services in the community, such as support groups and summer camps for children with diabetes mellitus

By pointing out the knowledge and skills that the family already has and the ways to adapt them to the changes in the family system, the nurse builds on family competencies.

In the **eudaimonistic model,** the nurse could work with the family in:

- Reassessing family goals and ways to meet them
- Assessing family values and goals, such as socializing and educating children, family recreation, and patterns of interacting
- Informing the family as appropriate about how they could offer support to other families in similar circumstances
- Assisting the family in identifying areas of strength and areas where external community resources may be necessary.

Health Risk

Several factors contribute to the experience of healthy or unhealthy outcomes. Clearly, not everyone exposed to the same event will have the same outcome. The factors that determine or influence whether disease or other unhealthy results occur are called *health risks*. This notion of controlling health risks is central to disease prevention and health promotion. Health risks can be classified into general categories. Califano (1979) identifies four major categories:

- Inherited biological risk
- Environmental risk
- Behavioral risk
- Age-related risk.

Although risk factors can singly influence outcomes, the cumulated risks can work in combination with one another. Their combined effect is more than the sum of the individual effects. For example, a family history of cardiovascular disease is a single risk factor that is affected by smoking, a behavioral risk. This combination of risks is greater for males than females (up to a certain age). Thus the combined effect of a family history, smoking, and being male is greater than the effects of each of the three individual risk factors separately.

Health Risk Appraisal

Health risk appraisal refers to the process of assessing the presence of specific factors within each of the categories that have been identified as being associated with an increased likelihood of an illness, such as cancer, or an unhealthy event, such as an automobile accident. Several techniques have been developed to accomplish health risk appraisal, including computer software programs and paper-and-pencil instruments. The general approach is to determine whether a risk factor is present and to what degree. Based on scientific evidence, each factor is weighted and a total sum score is derived.

Health Risk Reduction

Health risk reduction is based on the assumption that decreasing the number of risks or the magnitude of risk will result in a lower probability of the undesired event (e.g., substance abuse in adolescents). Reduction of health risks can be accomplished through a variety of approaches, usually specific to the theory and research knowledge related to the particular risk. In considering health risk reduction, it is important to note that the characteristics of the specific risk influence individuals' and families' tolerance of the risk (Pender, 1996). Pender (1996) provides examples of the effects of the nature of risks:

1. Voluntarily assumed risks like smoking are tolerated better than those imposed by others.
2. Risks over which scientists debate and are uncertain, like causes of breast cancer, are more feared than risks on which scientists agree.
3. Risks of natural origin like tornadoes or floods are often considered less threatening than those created by humans.

Thus risk reduction is a complex process that requires knowledge of the specific risk and families' perceptions of the nature of the risk.

Life Events

Life events can increase the risk for illness and disability. These events can be categorized as either normative or non-normative. **Normative events** are those that generally are expected to occur at a particular stage of development or of the life span.

Normative events can be identified from the Family Developmental framework. Examples of normative events are:

- A child leaving home to go to college
- Retirement from work
- Starting a first job.

Non-normative events, in contrast, are those that are not anticipated to occur with any ability to predict (e.g., loss of a job). Furthermore, life events and the accumulation of such events can, under certain conditions, result in a **family crisis.**

Briefly Noted

Government priority aimed at funding health risk reduction and health-promotion programs, including assistance programs, would have greater benefit to the population's health than funding for illness activities.

Family Crisis

A crisis exists when the family is not able to cope with the event and becomes *disorganized* or *dysfunctional.* When the demands of the situation exceed the resources of the family,

a family crisis exists. When families experience a crisis or crisis-producing event, they attempt to gather their resources to deal with the demands created by the situation. Burr and colleagues (1994) differentiate between *family resources* and *family coping strategies.* The former are the resources that a family has available to them. The latter are the "active processes and behaviors families actually try to do to help them manage, adapt, or deal with the stressful situation" (Burr, et al, 1994, p. 129). Thus if a family were to experience an unexpected illness in the main wage earner, family resources might include financial assistance from relatives or emotional support. Family coping strategies, in contrast, would include whether the family asked a relative to loan them emergency funds or talked with relatives about the worries they were experiencing. Based on the existing literature, Burr and colleagues developed a three-level classification of coping strategies with seven major categories, 20 subcategories, and 41 sub-subcategories. Although the last level is too extensive to present here, the seven major categories and 20 subcategories are listed in Table 18-2.

MAJOR FAMILY HEALTH RISKS

Risks to families' health arise in several major areas:

- Biologic risk
- Social risk
- Economic risk
- Life-style risk
- Life events leading to crisis

TABLE 18-2	Burr and Klein's Conceptual Framework of Coping Strategies
Highly Abstract Strategies	**Moderately Abstract Strategies**
1. Cognitive	1. Be accepting of the situation and others 2. Gain useful knowledge 3. Change how the situation is viewed or defined (reframe the situation)
2. Emotional	4. Express feelings and affection 5. Avoid or resolve negative feelings and disabling expressions of emotion 6. Be sensitive to others' emotional needs
3. Relationships	7. Increase cohesion (togetherness) 8. Increase adaptability 9. Develop increased trust 10. Increase cooperation 11. Increase tolerance of one another
4. Communication	12. Be open and honest 13. Listen to one another 14. Be sensitive to nonverbal communication
5. Community	15. Seek help and support from others 16. Fulfill expectations in organizations
6. Spiritual	17. Be more involved in religious activities 18. Increase faith or seek help from God
7. Individual development	19. Develop autonomy, independence, and self-sufficiency 20. Keep active in hobbies

From Burr WR, et al: *Reexamining family stress: new theory and research,* Thousand Oaks, Calif, 1994, Sage.

In most instances, no one of these five areas is sufficient to be a single threat to family health; rather a combination of risks from two or more categories is more usual. For example, there may be a family history of cardiovascular disease, but often the health risk is compounded by an unhealthy life-style. An understanding of each of these categories provides the basis for a comprehensive perspective on family health risk assessment and intervention.

Biologic Risk

The family plays an important role in both the development and the management of a disease or condition. Several illnesses have a familial component that can be accounted for either from a genetic basis or from established life-style patterns. These formulated factors contribute to the **biologic risk** for certain conditions. Patterns of cardiovascular disease, for example, often can be traced through many generations of families. Such families are said to be at risk for cardiovascular disease. How or whether cardiovascular disease is found in a family is often influenced by the life-style of the family. Consistent research evidence supports the positive mediating effects on preventing or delaying cardiovascular risks through:

- Diet
- Exercise
- Stress management.

An inclination for hypertension can be managed by:

- Following a low-sodium diet
- Maintaining a normal weight
- Exercising regularly
- Practicing effective stress-management techniques, such as meditation.

Diabetes mellitus is another disease with a strong genetic pattern, and the family plays a major role in the management of the condition. Family patterns of obesity increase the risk in individuals for a number of conditions, including:

- Coronary heart disease
- Hypertension
- Diabetes
- Some types of cancer
- Gallbladder disease (U.S. Department of Health and Human Services, 2000)

Another form of biologic risk experienced by families is being susceptible to certain illnesses. Overall, if a family maintains a level of general health, individual members are less at risk for contracting certain infectious diseases. This protection can be extended by maintaining health practices, such as current immunizations, adequate nutrition, and adequate rest.

Social Risk

The importance of **social risks** to families' health is gaining increased recognition. The following conditions can increase a family's health risk:

- High-crime neighborhoods
- Communities without adequate recreational or health resources
- Communities that have major chemical noise or other contaminants
- Other high-stress environments.

One social stress is discrimination, whether racial, cultural, or other. The psychological burden resulting from discrimination is a stressor in and of itself and also adds to the effects of other stressors. The implication of these examples of risky social situations is that they contribute to the stressors experienced by the families. If adequate resources and coping processes are not available, breakdowns in health can occur.

Economic Risk

The poor are at greater risk for health problems. **Economic risk** is determined by the relationship between family financial resources and demands on those resources. Having adequate financial resources means that a family is able to purchase the necessary commodities related to health. These include:

- Adequate housing
- Clothing
- Food
- Education
- Health/illness care.

The amount of money that a family has available needs to be considered relative to spending and to social factors. A family may have an income well above the poverty level, but because of a devastating illness in a family member, the family may not be able to meet financial demands. Likewise, families from ethnic populations frequently experience discrimination in finding housing; even if they find housing, they may not be welcome and may be harassed, resulting in increased stress.

Unfortunately, not all families have access to health care insurance. For families at the poverty level, programs like Medicaid are available to pay for health and illness care; families in the upper income brackets can either afford to pay for health care out-of-pocket, purchase health insurance, or are in employment situations that have health care benefits. An increasing number of families:

- Have major wage earners in jobs that do not have health benefits
- Do not have a sufficient income to purchase health care
- Earn too much money to qualify for public assistance programs.

Consequently, many families have financial resources that allow them to maintain a subsistence level but limit the quality of their purchasing power. Illness care may be available but not preventive care; food high in fat and calories may be affordable, while fresh fruit and vegetables are not. As an example of the importance of health care and nutrition, a U.S. Department of Agriculture (USDA) study found that for "every $1.00 spent on a pregnant woman in its Women, Infants and Children (WIC) program, $1.77 to $3.13 is saved in Medicaid costs during her child's first 60 days of life" (Greer, 1995, p. 6).

Life-Style Risk

Personal health habits continue to contribute to the major causes of morbidity and mortality in the United States. The pattern of personal health habits and risk behaviors defines individual and family **life-style risk.** The family is the basic unit within which health behavior—including health values, health habits, and health risk perceptions—is developed, organized, and performed. Families maintain major responsibility for:

- Determining what food is purchased and prepared
- Setting sleep patterns
- Planning family activities
- Setting and monitoring norms about health and health risk behaviors
- Determining when a family member is ill
- Determining when health care should be obtained
- Carrying out treatment regimens.

Diet has been identified as an element in 5 of the 10 leading causes of death in the United States (U.S. Department of Health and Human Services, 2000). General guidelines from the USDHHS and the USDA include:

- Eating a variety of foods
- Maintaining healthy weight
- Choosing a diet low in fat and cholesterol
- Including plenty of vegetables, fruits, and grain products
- Using sugars, salt, and sodium only moderately
- Consuming alcohol only in moderation.

Briefly Noted

Adolescents from families that have close, supportive interactions; clearly set and enforced rules; and parents who are involved with their children have decreased risk for alcohol use or misuse. These family patterns can be enhanced through family-focused intervention sessions in the home.

Multiple health benefits of regular physical activity have been identified; regular physical exercise is effective in health promotion, disease prevention, and health maintenance. Among the benefits of regular physical activity are:

- Increased muscle strength, endurance, and flexibility
- Management of weight
- Prevention of colon cancer, stroke, and back injury
- Prevention and management of coronary heart disease, hypertension, diabetes, osteoporosis and depression (U.S. Department of Health and Human Services, 2000).

Families structure time and activities and can be helped to select between those that are sedentary and those that provide moderate, regular physical activity.

Substance use is a major contributor to morbidity and mortality in the United States. Tobacco use has been identified as the single most preventable cause of death; it has been associated with:

- Several types of cancer
- Coronary heart disease
- Low birth weight

- Prematurity
- Sudden infant death syndrome (SIDS)
- Chronic obstructive pulmonary disease.

Furthermore, passive smoking has been linked to disease in nonsmokers and children. Drug use, including alcohol, is a major social and health problem. Alcohol use is a factor in approximately 50% of homicides, suicides, and motor vehicle deaths (U.S. Department of Health and Human Services, 2000). Drug use is associated with:

- Transmission of HIV
- Fetal alcohol syndrome
- Liver disease
- Unwanted pregnancy
- Delinquency
- School failure
- Violence
- Crime.

The literature consistently identifies the effects of family factors in decreasing the risk for substance abuse in children, such as:

- Family closeness
- Families doing activities together
- Behavior modeled in the family.

Although violence and abusive behavior are not limited to families, the amount of intrafamilial violence is thought to be underestimated. The obvious difficulties in collecting sensitive data from families make it difficult to obtain accurate statistics on family violence. Evidence supports the intergenerational nature of violence and abuse; abusers were often abused as children.

Life-Event Risk

Transitions, movement from one stage or condition to another, are times of potential risk for families. Transitions present new situations and demands for families. These experiences often require that families:

- Change behaviors, schedules, and patterns of communication
- Make new decisions
- Reallocate family roles
- Learn new skills
- Identify and learn to use new resources.

The demands that transitions place on families have implications for the health of the family unit and individual family members and can be considered as **life-event risk.**

How well prepared families are to deal with transitions is affected by the nature of the event. If the event is a normative, or anticipated, event, then it is possible for families to identify needed resources, make plans, learn new skills, or otherwise prepare for the event and its consequences. This kind of anticipatory preparation can increase the family's coping processes and lessen stress and negative outcomes. If, on the other hand, the event is non-normative, or unexpected, families have little or no time to prepare and the outcome can be increased stress, crisis, or even dysfunction.

Several normative events have been identified for families. The developmental family framework organizes these events within a staged model and identifies important transition points. The developmental model provides a useful framework for identifying normative events and preparing families to cope successfully with related demands. The developmental tasks associated with each stage define the types of skills families need to acquire (see Chapter 17, p. 282.) The kinds of *normative events* families experience usually are related to:

- The addition or loss of a family member, such as the birth or adoption of a child, the death of a grandparent
- A child moving out of the home to go to school or take a job
- The marriage of a child.

There are health-related responsibilities associated with each of these tasks. For example, the birth or adoption of a child requires that families learn about:

- Human growth and development
- Parenting
- Immunizations
- Management of childhood illnesses
- Normal childhood nutrition
- Safety issues.

Non-normative events present different kinds of issues for families. The nature of unexpected events can be either positive or negative. A job promotion or inheriting a substantial sum of money may be unexpected but are usually positive events. More often non-normative events are unpleasant, such as:

- A major illness
- Divorce
- The death of a child
- Loss of the main family income.

Regardless of whether a life event is normative or non-normative, it is often a source of stress for families.

Burr and colleagues (1994) point out that families develop a series of processes to manage or transform inputs to the system (e.g., energy, time) to outputs (e.g., cohesion, growth, love) known as "rules of transformation." Over time, families develop these patterns in sufficient quantity and variety to handle most changes and challenges. It is when families do not have an adequate variety of rules to allow them to respond to an event that the event then becomes stressful. Rather than proceeding to deal with the situation, they fall into a pattern of trying to figure out what it is they need to do and the usual tasks of the family are not adequately addressed. Rules that were implicit in the family are now reconsidered and redefined.

Furthermore, Burr and colleagues propose three levels of stress:

- *Level I* is change "in the fairly specific patterns of behavior and transformation processes" (e.g., change in who does which household chores)
- *Level II* is change "in processes that are at a higher level of abstraction" (e.g., change in what are defined as family chores)
- *Level III* are changes in highly abstract processes (e.g., family value) (Burr, et al, 1994, pp. 44-45).

There are coping strategies identified to address each level of stress that families go through in sequence, if necessary.

 Evidence-Based Practice

Based on results of a study of 50 families who had experienced a variety of stressors, Burr and colleagues (1994) examined the changes experienced under stress in nine areas of family life:

- Marital satisfaction
- Family rituals and celebrations
- Quality of communication
- Family cohesion
- Functional quality of the executive subsystem
- Quality of the emotional atmosphere
- Management of daily routines and chores
- Contention
- Normal family development versus changed or arrested development.

The results of the study support that families did use the proposed strategies, both the helpful ones and the harmful ones, with significant differences between men and women on 10 of the 80 strategies. Women tended to use a wider range of strategies, and men tended to use more of the harmful strategies. The results supported the sequencing and developmental nature of families' use of strategies in acute stressor situations but not in chronic stressor situations. Thus the pattern was evident in stresses, such as bankruptcy, but not in families with a child with a chronic condition.

APPLICATION IN PRACTICE

Results of this work provide direction for community health nursing intervention with families over the life span. The three levels share similarities with Neuman's (1989) flexible lines of defense (Level I change), normal line of defense (Level II change), and lines of resistance (Level III change). Based on Neuman's model, primary prevention strategies (e.g., parenting classes) would be appropriate for dealing with Level I change; secondary prevention strategies (e.g., crisis intervention) for dealing with Level II change; and tertiary prevention strategies (e.g., family therapy) for dealing with Level III change.

Burr WR, et al: *Reexaming family stress: new theory and research,* Thousand Oaks, Calif, 1994, Sage; Neuman B: *The Neuman systems model,* ed 2, Norwalk, Conn, 1989, Appleton & Lange.

COMMUNITY HEALTH NURSING APPROACHES TO FAMILY HEALTH RISK REDUCTION
Family Health Risk Appraisal

Assessment of *family health risk* requires multiple approaches to address the many components of risk. As in any assessment, the first and most important task is to get to know the family, their strengths, and their needs. This section focuses on appraisal of family health risks within biologic, social, economic, life-style, and life events risk.

Biologic Health Risk

One of the most effective techniques for assessing the patterns of health and illness in families is the use of the family genogram (Bahr, 1990).

A genogram is a schematic representation of a family:

- It depicts the family unit of immediate interest and includes several generations using a series of circles, squares, and connecting lines.
- Basic information on composition of the family, relationships in the family, and patterns of health and illness can be obtained by completing the genogram with the family.

As shown in Figure 18-1, a square indicates a male, a circle indicates a female, and an "X" through either a square or a circle indicates a death.

- Marriage is indicated by a solid horizontal line and offspring by a solid vertical line.
- A broken horizontal line indicates a divorce or separation.
- Dates of birth, marriage, death, and other important events can be indicated where appropriate.
- Major illness or conditions can be listed for each individual.
- Completion of a genogram requires interviews with the family members.

The genogram in Figure 18-1 was completed for the Graham family. Some of the interesting patterns that can be seen from the genogram are the repeated recurrence of hypertension, adult-onset diabetes, cancer, and hypercholesterolemia. Bahr suggests that a family chronology (a timeline of family events over three generations) be completed to extend the genogram.

A more intensive and quantitative assessment of a family's biologic risk can be achieved through the use of a standardized family risk assessment. Because such assessments involve other areas in addition to biologic risk, one will be described later in this section after the description of assessment of other types of risk.

Social Health Risk

Assessment of *social health risk* is less well defined and developed. Information can be assessed through the use of an ecomap on:

- Relationships that the family has with others such as relatives and neighbors
- Their connections with other social units, church, school, work, clubs, and organizations
- The flow of energy, positive or negative.

An ecomap is merely a visual representation of:

- The family's interactions with other groups and organizations, accomplished using a series of circles and lines
- The family of interest represented by a circle in the middle of a page
- Other groups and organizations indicated by other circles
- Flow of energy of other groups and organizations represented by lines drawn between the family circle and the circles representing the groups and organizations
- The direction of the flow of energy (into or out of the family) indicated by an arrowhead at the end of each line
- The intensity of the energy represented by the boldness/darkness of the line.

Thus an ecomap drawn for the Graham family (Fig. 18-2) indicates that much of the family energy goes into work (also a source of stress) for the parents. In contrast, major sources of energy for the Grahams are their immediate and extended families and friends.

Other aspects of social risk include characteristics of the neighborhood and community where the family lives. If the nurse has worked in the general geographic area, he or she already may have done a community assessment and have a working knowledge of the neighborhood and community. It is important, however, for information to be obtained from the family in order to understand their perceptions.

Information about the origins of the family is useful to understand other social resources and stressors. Information about how long the family has lived in their current location and the origin and immigration patterns of their family and ancestors provides insight into the pressures they experience.

Economic Health Risk

Financial information often is considered private by families. It is not necessary to know actual family income except in certain instances when it is necessary to determine whether families are eligible for programs or benefits. It is useful to know whether the family's resources are adequate to meet the demands. In terms of health risk, it is important to understand the resources that families have to obtain health/illness care; adequate shelter, clothing, and food; and access to recreation. Families with limited resources may qualify for programs such as Medicaid, Aid to Dependent Families, WIC, or Maternal Support Systems/Infant Support Systems. Families with wage earners with health/medical benefits and those with sufficient income usually are able to afford adequate health care. Unfortunately, there is a growing number of families whose main wage earner is employed but receives no health/medical benefits.

Life-Style Health Risk

Families are the major source of factors that can promote or inhibit positive life-styles. They regulate time and energy and the boundaries of the system. A number of tools exist for assessing individuals' *life-style risks,* but few are available for assessing family life-style patterns. Although assessment of individual life-style contributes to determining the life-style risk of a family, it is important to look at risks for the family as a unit. Based on the literature in health behavior research, the critical dimensions include the following:

- Value placed on the behavior
- Knowledge of the behavior and its consequences
- Effect of the behavior on the family
- Effect of the behavior on the individual
- Barriers to performing the behavior
- Benefits of the behavior
- Perception of ability to perform the behavior.

In terms of specific behaviors, it is important to assess the frequency, intensity, and regularity of the behavior. It also is important to evaluate the resources available to the family

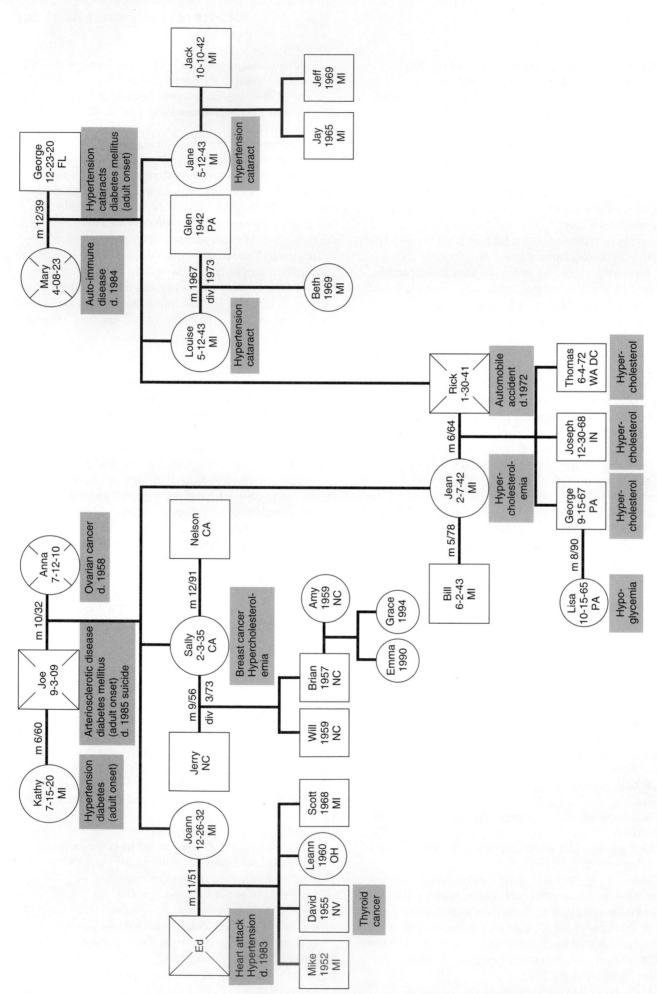

Figure 18-1   Family genogram of the Graham family.

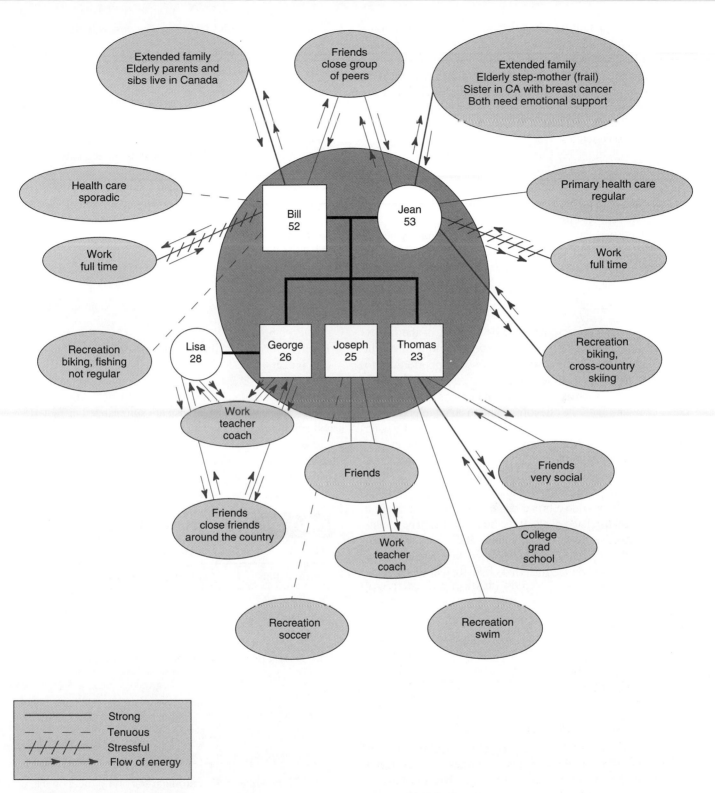

Figure 18-2   Ecomap of the Graham family.

for implementing the behavior. Thus items for assessment of physical activity include:

- The value that a family places on physical activity
- The hours that a family spends in exercise
- The kinds of exercise the family does
- Resources available for exercise.

Life-Event Health Risk

As discussed previously, both normative and non-normative life events pose potential risks to the health of families. Even events that generally are viewed as being positive require changes and can place stress on a family. The normative event of the birth of a child, for instance, requires considerable changes in family structures and roles. Furthermore, family functions are expanded from previous levels, requiring families to add new skills and establish additional resources. These changes in turn can result in strain and, if adequate resources are not available, stress. Therefore to adequately assess the risks associated with life risks, both normative and non-normative events occurring in the family need to be considered.

Home Visits

Community health nurses work with families in a variety of settings including clinics, schools, support groups, and offices. However, an important aspect of community health nursing's role in reducing health risks and promoting the health of populations has been the tradition of providing services to individual families in their homes.

Purpose

Home visits give a more accurate assessment of the family structure, the natural or home environment, and behavior in that environment. Home visits also provide opportunities to identify both barriers and supports for reaching family health-promotion goals such as improving the family's nutrition. The nurse can work with the client firsthand to adapt interventions to meet realistic goals like making a food budget and buying less expensive food. Meeting the family on their home ground also may contribute to the family's sense of control and active participation in meeting their health needs.

Home visiting programs are receiving increased attention and are used to provide a broad range of services to achieve a variety of health-related goals. If the home visit is to be a valuable and effective intervention, careful and systematic planning must occur. The majority of the studies evaluating the home have focused on the maternal-child population (Bradley and Martin, 1994; Kang, et al, 1995; Olds and Kitzman, 1993).

Briefly Noted

A home visit is more than just an alternative setting for service; it is an intervention.

Advantages and Disadvantages

Recently, the effectiveness of providing large portions of health-promotion services in this mode has been critically reexamined by agencies such as health departments and visiting nurses associations (VNAs) (Barnes-Boyd, Norr, and Nacion, 1998; Olds and Kitzman, 1993).

Advantages include:
- Convenience for the client
- Client control of the setting
- Provision of an option for those clients unwilling or unable to travel
- The ability to individualize services
- A natural, relaxed environment for the discussion of concerns and needs

Costs are a major disadvantage. The cost is high for:
- Previsit preparation
- Travel to and from the home
- Time spent with one client
- Postvisit activities.

Many agencies have actively explored alternative modes of providing service to families, particularly group interventions. The important issue is determining which families would most benefit from them and how home visits can most effectively be structured and scheduled. With increasing demands for home health care, the home visit is again becoming a prominent mode for delivery of nursing services.

Building a trusting relationship with the client is the cornerstone of successful home visits. There are five basic helping skills that are fundamental to effective home visits:
- Observing
- Listening
- Questioning
- Probing
- Prompting.

The need for these skills is evident in all phases of the home visit process.

Process

The components of a home visit are summarized in Table 18-3 and are discussed in the following sections.

INITIATION PHASE. Usually, a home visit is initiated as the result of a referral from a health or social agency. However, a family may request services or the nurse may initiate the home

TABLE 18-3 Phases and Activities of a Home Visit

Phase	Activity
I. Initiation phase	Clarify source of referral for visit Clarify purpose for home visit Share information on reason and purpose of home visit with family
II. Previsit phase	Initiate contact with family Establish shared perception of purpose with family Determine family's willingness for home visit Schedule home visit Review referral and/or family record
III. In-home phase	Introduce self and professional identity Interact socially to establish rapport Establish nurse-client relationship Implement nursing process
IV. Termination phase	Review visit with family Plan for future visits
V. Postvisit phase	Record visit Plan for next visit

visit as a result of case-finding activities. The *initiation phase* is the first contact between the nurse and the family. This provides the foundation for an effective therapeutic relationship. Subsequent home visits should be based on need and mutual agreement between the nurse and the family. Frequently, nurses are not sure of the reason for the visit. This carries with it the potential for the visit to be compromised and to come aimlessly or abruptly to a premature halt. Regardless of the reason for making a home visit, it is necessary that the nurse be clear about the purpose for the visit and that this perception or understanding be shared with the family.

PREVISIT PHASE. The *previsit phase* has several components. For the most part, these are best accomplished in order, as presented in the box below.

The possibility exists that the family may refuse a home visit. Less-experienced nurses or students may interpret this as a personal rejection when it is not. Families make decisions about when and which outsiders are allowed entry into their home. The nurse needs to explore the reasons for the refusal; there may be a misunderstanding about the reason

for a visit or there may be a lack of information about services. The contact may be terminated as requested if the nurse determines that either the situation has been resolved or services have been obtained from another source, and if the family understands that services are available and how to contact the agency if desired. However, the nurse should leave open the possibility of future contact. There are instances when the nurse will be mandated to persist in requesting a home visit because of legal obligations, such as follow-up of certain communicable diseases.

How To Prepare for the Home Visit: Previsit Phase

- First, if at all possible, the nurse should contact the family by telephone before the home visit to introduce herself, to identify the reason for the contact, and to schedule the home visit. A first telephone contact should be a maximum of 15 minutes. The nurse should give her name and professional identity, for example, "This is Karen Smith. I'm a community health nurse from the Middle County Health Department."
- The family should be informed of how they came to the attention of the community health nurse, for example, as the result of a referral or a contact from observations or records in the school setting. If a referral has been received, it is important and useful to ascertain whether the family is aware of the referral. This will show a valuing of the client's input and involvement in care.
- A brief summary of the nurse's given information allows the family to know the extent of the nurse's knowledge about the family. For example, the nurse might say, "I understand that your baby was discharged from the hospital yesterday and that you requested some assistance with caring for the child at home."
- A visit that is appropriate for the nurse and the family should be scheduled for as soon as possible. Letting the family know agency hours available for visits, the approximate length of the visit, and the purpose of the visit are helpful to the family in determining when to set the visit. Although the length of the visit may vary, depending on circumstances, approximately 30 minutes to 1 hour is usual depending on the reason for the visit.
- If possible, the visit should be arranged when as many as possible of the family members will be available for the entire visit. It is also important for the nurse to tell the client about any fee for the visit and subsequent visits and possible methods for payment.
- The telephone call can terminate with a review by the nurse of the time, place, and purpose for the visit and a means for the family to contact the nurse in case they need to verify or change the time for the visit or to ask questions. If the family does not have a telephone, another method for setting up the visit can be used. The most obvious is dropping off a note at the family home or sending a letter or postcard informing the family of when and why the home visit will occur with a means for the family to contact the nurse if necessary.

Evidence-Based Practice

The purpose of the multisite field experiment referenced below was to test the effectiveness of hospital and home visit interventions to improve interaction between mothers and preterm infants. The outcomes of a hospital intervention, State Modulation (focused on teaching mothers to read the behavior cues and modulate the states of consciousness of preterm infants during feedings), and the home visit intervention, Nursing Systems for Effective Parenting-Preterm (NSTEP-P), were compared with a hospital program on car seats and standard public health nursing home visits. The sample of 327 mothers and their preterm infants (less than 36 weeks' gestational age at discharge) were randomly assigned to intervention groups based on their education. Highly educated mothers (equal to or more than 13 years of education) were assigned to hospital programs and the less-educated mothers (equal to or less than 12 years of education) were assigned to combinations of hospital and home visit programs. The outcomes were evaluated at 40, 46, and 60 weeks' conceptual age.

APPLICATION IN PRACTICE

The results supported suggest that State Modulation treatment and NSTEP-P are cost-effective treatments for families with healthy preterm infants. State Modulation treatment alone is a powerful intervention for well-educated mothers. State Modulation treatment in combination with NSTEP-P is most effective for mothers with limited formal education. The cost of the two programs, $100 for State Modulation and $550 for combined State Modulation and nine-visit NSTEP-P, were proposed to be cost-effective approaches for promoting positive developmental outcomes for preterm infants via improved mother-infant interactions. The results also support consideration of the use of these interventions by public health nurses with vulnerable populations in the changing health care environment.

Kang R, et al: Preterm infant follow-up project: a multi-site field experiment of hospital and home intervention programs for mothers and preterm infants, *Public Health Nurs* 12(3):171, 1995.

Before visiting the family, it can be useful for the nurse to review the referral or, if not a first visit, the family record. If there is a time lapse between the contact and the visit, a brief telephone call to confirm the time often prevents the nurse from finding no one at home for the visit.

IN-HOME PHASE. The actual visit to the home constitutes the *in-home phase* and affords the nurse the opportunity to assess the family's neighborhood. An issue that may arise either in approaching the family home or once the family has opened the door to the nurse is that of personal safety. Nurses need to examine personal fears and objective threats to determine if safety is indeed an issue. Certain precautions can be taken in known high-risk situations. Agencies may provide escorts for nurses or have them visit in pairs, readily identifiable uniforms may be required, or a sign-out process indicating timing and location of home visits may be used routinely. The nurse needs to use caution; if a reasonable question about the safety of making the visit exists, the visit should not be made.

The nurse needs to be aware that families may feel that they are being "checked up on," are seen as being inadequate or dysfunctional, or that their privacy is being invaded. Nursing services, especially those from health departments, have been identified by the public as being "public services" for needy families or those with insufficient funds to pay for care. These potential areas of concern underlie the needs for sensitivity on the part of the nurse, the need for clarity in information regarding the reason for visits, and the need to establish collaborative, trusting relationships with the family.

Another factor that may affect the nature of the home visit is whether the visit is viewed as "voluntary" or "required" (Byrd, 1995). A "voluntary" home visit (need for a visit by the client) is characterized by:
- Easier entry for the nurse
- Client-controlled interaction
- An informal tone
- Mutual discussion of frequency of future visits.

In contrast, if the client does not feel the need for "required" home visits (often legally mandated):
- Entry is difficult for the nurse
- The interaction is nurse controlled
- There is a more formal, investigatory tone to the visit
- Nurse-client communication is distorted
- There is no mutual discussion of frequency of future visits.

The changing nature of the American family can make it difficult to schedule visits during what have been traditional agency hours. The number of working single-parent or dual-income, two-parent families is increasing, which means that families are busy with more demands on their time. Even if one parent is at home during the usual work day, the ideal is to work with the entire family unit. This often is not possible because of conflict between agency hours and school or work schedules. It may be possible to schedule a visit at the beginning or end of a day to meet with working or school-age members. In some parts of the country, agencies are reconsidering traditional hours and Monday-through-Friday visits.

Families may or may not be able to control interruptions during the visit. Telephones ring, pets join in the visit, people come and go, and televisions are left on. The nurse can ask that televisions be turned off or other disruptive activities be limited during the visit. Families may be so used to the background noises and routine activities that they do not recognize them as being potentially disruptive.

The actual home visit includes several components:
- Once at the family home, the nurse needs to again provide personal and professional identification.
- It is important to tell the client the location of the agency if not known. This is part of the introductory phase.
- Then there should be a brief social period to allow the client to assess the nurse and to establish rapport.
- The next step is a description by the nurse of his or her role, responsibilities, and limitations.
- Another important component is to determine what the client's expectations are for the home visit.
- The major portion of the home visit is concerned with establishing the relationship and implementing the nursing process.
- Assessment, intervention, and evaluation are ongoing.
- It is important that the nurse be realistic about what can be accomplished in a home visit.
- In some situations, one visit may be all that is possible or appropriate. In this instance, needs and resources for meeting needs are explored with the family and it is determined whether further services are desired or indicated.
- If further services are indicated and the current agency is not appropriate, the nurse can assist the family in identifying other services available in the community and can help in initiating any referrals.
- Although it is not unusual to have only one home visit with a family, often multiple visits are made.
- The frequency and intensity of home visits vary with not only the needs of the family but also whether the family is eligible for services and agency policies and priorities.
- It is realistic to expect initial assessment and at least the beginning of building a relationship to occur on a first visit.

What actually occurs in the home visit is largely determined by the reason or focus for the visit. Some reasons for visits are listed in Box 18-1.

TERMINATION PHASE. When the purpose of the visit has been accomplished, the nurse reviews with the family what has occurred and what has been accomplished as the major focus of the *termination phase.* This provides a basis for planning further home visits.
- Ideally, termination of the visit and, ultimately, termination of service begins at the first contact with the establishment of a goal or purpose.
- If communication has been clear to this point, the family and nurse can now plan for future visits, specifically the next visit.

From Keller LO, et al: Population-based public health nursing interventions: a model from practice, *Public Health Nurs* 15(3):207, 1998.

Box 18-1	**Reasons for the Home Visit**

Nursing interventions may include some or all of the 17 categories identified by the Minnesota Department of Health, Section of Public Health Nursing:

1. Advocacy
2. Case management
3. Coalition building
4. Collaboration
5. Community organizing
6. Consultation
7. Counseling
8. Delegated medical treatment and observations
9. Disease investigation
10. Health teaching
11. Outreach/case findings
12. Policy development
13. Provider education
14. Referral and follow-up
15. Screening
16. Social marketing
17. Surveillance

- Planning for future visits is part of another issue: setting goals and planning service.

POSTVISIT PHASE. Even though the nurse has now concluded the home visit and left the client's home, responsibility for the visit is not complete until the interaction has been recorded. A major task of the *postvisit phase* is documenting the visit and services provided.

- Agencies may or may not organize their records by families.
- The basic record may be a "family" folder or record with all members included in one record, or each family member receiving services may have a separate record with other family members' records cross-referenced.
- In reality the concept of a family-focused record often does not occur.
- History and background for the family usually are given to some extent, but often the focus shifts to individual health histories.
- Consequently, nursing diagnoses, goals, and interventions are directed toward individual family members rather than the family unit.
- Record systems and formats vary from agency to agency.
- The nurse needs to become familiar with the particular system used in the agency.

All systems should include:

- A database
- A nursing diagnosis and problem list
- A plan, including specific goals
- Actual actions and interventions
- Evaluation methods.

These are the basic elements needed for legal and clinical purposes. The record format may consist of:

- Narratives
- Flow sheets
- Problem-oriented medical records (POMR)
- Subjective, objective, assessment plan (SOAP)
- A combination of formats.

It is important that recording be current, dated, and signed.

Community health nurses must be sure to use theoretical frameworks that are appropriate to the family-centered nursing process. For example, a nursing diagnosis of "ineffective mothering skill related to lack of knowledge of normal growth and development" is an individual-focused nursing diagnosis. "Inability for family to accomplish stage-appropriate task of providing safe environment for preschooler related to lack of knowledge and resources" is a family-focused nursing diagnosis based on knowledge of the developmental approach to families. At times it may be necessary to present information for a specific family member. However, the emphasis should be on the individual as a member of, and within the structure of, the family.

Contracting With Families

Increasingly, health professionals look at working with clients in a more interactive, collaborative style. This approach is consistent with a more knowledgeable public and the recent self-care movement. **Contracting,** which is an agreement between two or more parties, involves a shift in responsibility and control to a shared effort by client and professional versus that of the professional alone. Contracting is a constructive approach to working with clients and is receiving increasing attention by health professionals as a way of outlining with the family what will happen in each phase of the home visits. The ANA's *Standards of Community Health Nursing Practice* (1986) explicitly states the rights of clients to participate actively in planning their own health care; these same standards designate that "in partnership with the family and individual" the community health nurse:

- Collects, interprets, and analyzes data
- Formulates and validates diagnoses
- Formulates plans and implements interventions
- Evaluates process and revision of the plan.

This active involvement of the client is reflected in several of the existing nursing models, with Orem as an example (1995). Contracting is one strategy aimed at promoting a collaborative working relationship (in this instance, one specifically focused on health risk reduction and health promotion).

Contracting is one way of formally involving the family in the nursing process and explaining their roles. Some nurses are reluctant to use the term "contracting" but discuss it in terms of mutual goal setting. Some of this reluctance may be related to the potential legal terms of a contract, whether formal or informal. There may be concern about possible liability in terms of services agreed upon versus those received and the agreed-upon outcomes. In some cases, the connection between contracting and compliance may be contrary to a philosophy of an interactive partnership between nurse and client.

Thus an important issue is the purpose and/or philosophy that underlies the nurse's use of contracting with families. If contracting is viewed only as another approach to increasing compliance, the basic premises of the concept are violated. Contracting should address the issue of control by the client versus control by the professional.

Purposes

The purpose of the agreement is to enhance and support the clients' active role in health care by defining clients' and professionals' roles in accomplishing health-related goals. The nursing contract is a working agreement that is continuously renegotiable and may or may not be written.

In the instance of family health risk reduction, it is essential that the contract be made with all responsible and appropriate members of the family. Involving only one individual is invalid if the goal is family health risk reduction, which requires a total family system effort and change. Scheduling a visit with all family members present may require extra effort; if meeting with the entire family is not possible, each family member can review a contract, give input, and sign it. This allows for active participation by all family members without the necessity of finding a time when everyone involved can be present.

Process of Contracting

Contracting is a learned skill on the part of both the nurse and the family. All parties involved need to know the purpose and process of contracting. There are three general phases: beginning, working, and termination. The three phases can be further specified into seven sets of activities. The phases and activities are summarized in Table 18-4.

The first activity involves both the family and the nurse in data collection and analysis of the data. An important aspect of this step is obtaining the family's view of the situation and its needs and problems. The nurse can present his or her observations and validate them with the family and also obtain the family's view. It is important that goals be mutually set and realistic.

A pitfall for nurses and clients who are new to contracting is to set overly ambitious goals. The nurse should recognize that there may be discrepancies between professional priorities and those of the client and determine whether negotiation is required.

Because contracting is a process characterized by renegotiation, the goals are not static. Throughout the process, the nurse and family need to continually learn and recognize what each can contribute to meeting health needs. This exploration of resources allows both parties to become aware of their own and each other's strengths and requires a review of the nurse's skills and knowledge, the family's support systems, and available community resources.

Developing a plan to meet the goals involves:
- Specifying activities
- Prioritizing goals
- Selecting a starting point
- Deciding who will be responsible for which activities
- Structuring time limits by setting a deadline for accomplishing or evaluating progress toward accomplishing a goal
- Establishing the frequency of contacts
- Meeting with all parties at the agreed-upon time to evaluate the progress to date in both process and outcome.

Based on the evaluation, the contract can be modified, renegotiated, or terminated.

Advantages and Disadvantages of Contracting

Contracting takes time and effort and may require the family and nurse to reorient their roles. Increased control on the part of the family also means increased responsibility. Some nurses may have difficulty relinquishing the role of the controlling expert professional. Contracts will not always be successful, and contracting is neither appropriate nor possible in some cases. Some clients do not want to have this kind of involvement; they prefer to defer to the "authority" of the professional. Included in this group are individuals who:
- Have minimal cognitive skills
- Are involved in an emergency situation
- Are unwilling to be more active in their care
- Do not see control or authority for health concerns as being within their domain.

Some of these clients may learn to contract; some never will. Although it may not be appropriate in all situations or with all families, contracting can give direction and structure to health risk reduction and health promotion in families.

Enabling and Empowering Families

Help-giving interventions do not always have positive outcomes for clients. If families do not perceive a situation as a problem or need, offers of help may cause resentment. Help

TABLE 18-4	Phases and Activities in Contracting
Phase	**Activity**
I. Beginning phase	Mutual data collection and exploration of needs and problems Mutual establishing of goals Mutual development of a plan
II. Working phase	Mutual division of responsibilities Mutual setting of time limits Mutual implementation of plan Mutual evaluation and renegotiation
III. Termination phase	Mutual termination of contract

giving also may have negative consequences if there is not a match between what is expected and what is offered. Nurses' failure to recognize families' competencies and to define an active role for families can lead to dependency and lack of growth for families. This can be frustrating for both the nurse and the family. For families to become active participants, they need to feel a sense of personal competence and a desire for and willingness to take action. Recently, approaches for helping individuals and families assume an active role in their health care have focused on **empowerment** (Rodwell, 1996). Definitions of empowerment reflect three characteristics of the empowered family seeking help:

• Access and control over needed resources
• Decision-making and problem-solving abilities
• Ability to communicate and obtain needed resources.

The last characteristic refers to the fact that families may need to learn how to:

• Identify sources of help
• Contact agencies
• Ask critical questions
• Negotiate with agencies to have family needs met.

These characteristics generally reflect a process by which people (individuals, families, organizations, or communities) take control of their own lives. The outcomes of empowerment are:

• Positive self-esteem
• The ability to set and reach goals
• A sense of control over life and change processes
• A sense of hope for the future (Rodwell, 1996).

Empowerment requires a viewpoint that often conflicts with the views of many helping professions, including nursing. Empowerment's underlying assumption is one of a partnership between the professional and the client versus one in which the professional is dominant:

• Families are assumed to be either competent or capable of becoming competent.
• This implies that the professional is not an unchallengeable authority who is in control.
• An environment that creates opportunities for competencies to be used is necessary.
• Families need to identify that their actions result in behavior change.

A community health nursing intervention that incorporates the principles of empowerment would be directed toward the building of nurse-family partnerships that emphasize health risk reduction and health promotion. The nurse's approach to the family should be positive and focused on competencies rather than on problems or deficits. The interventions need to be consistent with family cultural norms and the family's perception of the problem. Rather than making decisions for the family, the nurse would support the family in primary decision-making and bolster their self-esteem by recognizing and using family strengths and support networks. Interventions promoting family behaviors increase family competency and decrease the need for outside help, resulting in families seeing themselves as being actively responsible for bringing about desired changes. The goal of an empowering approach is to create a partnership between the nurse and the family characterized by cooperation and shared responsibility.

COMMUNITY RESOURCES

Families have varied and complex needs and problems. The community health nurse often mobilizes several resources in order to effectively and appropriately meet family health-promotion needs. Although the specific resources vary from community to community, general types can be identified. Government resources such as Medicare, Medicaid, Aid to Families of Dependent Children, Supplementary Security Income, Food Stamps, and WIC are available in most communities. These programs primarily provide support for basic needs (e.g., illness/health care, nutritional needs, funds for housing and clothing), and funds are based on eligibility criteria.

In addition to government agencies providing health-related services to families, most communities have voluntary (nongovernmental) programs. Local chapters of such organizations as the American Cancer Society, American Heart Association, American Lung Association, and the Muscular Dystrophy Association provide educational and support services and some direct services to individuals and families regarding specific conditions. These agencies provide primary prevention and health promotion services, as well as screening programs and assistance, once the disease or condition is diagnosed. Local social service agencies (e.g., Catholic Social Services) provide direct services such as counseling to families. Other voluntary organizations provide direct service (e.g., shelters for the homeless or battered individuals, substance abuse counseling and treatment, Meals on Wheels, transportation, clothing, food, furniture).

Health resources in the community may be proprietary, voluntary, or public. In addition to private health care providers, community health nurses should be aware of voluntary and public clinics, screening programs, and health-promotion programs.

Identifying resources in a community requires time and effort. One obvious and valuable source is the telephone book. Often community service organizations, such as the Chamber of Commerce and the local health department, publish community resource listings. Regardless of how the resource is identified, the community health nurse must be familiar with the type of service offered and any requirements or costs involved. If this information is not readily available, the community health nurse can contact the resource directly for more information.

Locating and using these systems often requires skills and patience that many families lack. Community health nurses work with families to identify community resources and act as a client advocate in helping families learn how to use resources. This may involve sharing information with families, rehearsing with families what questions to ask, preparing required materials, making the initial contact, and arranging transportation. The appropriateness and effectiveness of resources should be evaluated with families after referrals.

Clinical Application

The initial referral for community health nursing service to a family provides limited information, and the situation that develops may be much more complex than anticipated. The following example, based on an actual case, illustrates the issues and approaches outlined in this chapter.

A referral was received at the Middle County Health Department indicating that Amy Cress, age 16, had been referred by the school counselor at the local high school for prenatal supervision. Amy was 4 months pregnant, in apparently good health, in the tenth grade, and living at home with her mother, stepfather, and younger sister. The family lived in a rural area outside of a small farming community. The father of the baby also lived in the community and continued to see Amy on a regular basis. The referral information provided the community health nurse with a beginning, but limited, assessment of the family situation.

A. What would you do first as the community health nurse assigned to this family?

B. How would you help this family empower themselves to take responsibility for this situation?

C. After initial contact, how would you extend the assessment to the entire family system?

D. Would you contract with this family? How? On what terms?

Answers are in the back of the book.

 ## Remember This!

- The importance of the family as a major client system for community health nursing in reducing health risks and promoting health of individuals and populations is well documented; the family system is a basic unit within which health behavior—including health values, health habits, and health risk perceptions—is developed, organized, and performed.

- Knowledge of family structure and functioning is fundamental to implementing the nursing process with families in the community. However, community health nurses need to go beyond the individual and family and understand the complex environment in which the family functions to be effective in reducing family health risks. Categories of risk factors that are important to family health are biologic risk, life-style risk, social risk, life-event risk, and economic risk.

- Several factors contribute to the experience of healthy or unhealthy outcomes. Not everyone exposed to the same event will have the same outcome. The factors that influence whether disease or other unhealthy results occur are called health risks. The risks are cumulative; their combined effect is more than the sum of the individual effects.

- An important aspect of community health nursing's role in reducing health risk and promoting the health of populations has been the tradition of providing services to individual families in their homes.

- Home visits afford the opportunity to gain a more accurate assessment of the family structure and behavior in the natural environment. Home visits also provide opportunities to make observations of the home environment and to identify both barriers and supports to reducing health risks and for reaching family health goals.

- Increasingly, health professionals expect to work with clients in a more interactive, collaborative style.

- Contracting, which is an agreement between two or more parties, involves a shift in responsibility and control to a shared effort by client and professional versus that of the professional alone.

- Families have varied and complex needs and problems. The community health nurse often mobilizes several resources to effectively and appropriately meet family health needs.

 ## What Do You Think?

1. Select one of the *Healthy People 2010* objectives and identify how biologic risk, social risk, economic risk, life-style risk, and life-event risk contribute to family health risk for that objective.

2. Select three or four families (hypothetically or from actual situations) representative of different ethnic and socioeconomic backgrounds. Complete a family genogram and ecomap for each family, and identify and compare major health risks.

3. Select one or more agencies in which community health nurses work, and examine the agency's and community health nursing's philosophies and objectives with emphasis on individual care, family care, illness care, risk reduction, and health promotion.

4. Identify three community health problems in your community, and discuss the implications of these problems for the health of families. Identify three health problems common to families in your community, and discuss the implications of the problems for the health and/or health care resources of the community.

REFERENCES

American Nurses Association, Council of Community Health Nurses: *Standards of community health nursing practice,* Kansas City, Mo, 1986, American Nurses Association.

Bahr KS: Student responses to genogram and family chronology, *Family Relations* 39(3):243, 1990.

Barnes-Boyd C, Norr KF, Nacion KW: Evaluation of an inter-agency home visiting program to reduce postneonatal mortality in disadvantaged communities, *Public Health Nurs* 13(3):201, 1998

Belloc NB, Breslow L: Relationship of physical health in a general population survey, *Am J Epidemiol* 93:329, 1972.

Bomar PJ (editor): *Nurses and family health promotion: concepts, assessment, and interventions,* Baltimore, 1996, Williams & Wilkins.

Bradley PJ, Martin J: The impact of home visits on enrollment patterns in pregnancy-related services among low-income women, *Public Health Nurs* 11(6):392, 1994.

Burr WR, et al: *Reexamining family stress: new theory and research,* Thousand Oaks, Calif, 1994, Sage.

Byrd ME: The home visiting process in the contexts of the voluntary vs. required visit: examples from fieldwork, *Public Health Nurs* 12(3):196, 1995.

Califano JA Jr: *Healthy people: the Surgeon General's report on health promotion and disease prevention,* Washington, D.C., 1979, U.S. Government Printing Office.

Duvall EM, Miller BC: *Marriage and family development,* ed 6, New York, 1985, Addison-Wesley.

Feetham SL, et al (editors): *The nursing in families: theory/research/education/practice,* Thousand Oaks, Calif, 1992, Sage.

Gilliss C, et al (editors): *Toward a science of family nursing,* Menlo Park, Calif, 1989, Addison-Wesley.

Greer C: Something is robbing our children of their future, *Parade Magazine,* pp. 4-6, March 5, 1995.

Kang R, et al: Preterm infant follow-up project: a multi-site field experiment of hospital and home intervention programs for mothers and preterm infants, *Public Health Nurs* 12(3):171, 1995.

Keller LO, et al: Population-based public health nursing interventions: a model from practice, *Public Health Nurs* 15(3):207, 1998.

Neuman B: *The Neuman systems model,* ed 2, Norwalk, Conn, 1989, Appleton & Lange.

Nightingale EO, et al: *Perspectives on health promotion and disease prevention in the United States,* Washington, D.C., 1978, Institute of Medicine, National Academy of Sciences.

Olds DL, Kitzman H: Review of research on home visiting for pregnant women and parents of young children, the future of children, *Home Visiting* 3(3):53, 1993.

Orem DE: *Nursing: concepts of practice,* ed 5, St Louis, 1995, Mosby.

Pender NJ: *Health promotion in nursing practice,* ed 3, Stamford, Conn, 1996, Appleton & Lange.

Rodwell CM: An analysis of the concept of empowerment, *J Adv Nurs* 23:305, 1996.

Smith JA: *The idea of health: implications for the nursing professional,* New York, 1983, Teachers College Press, Columbia University.

U.S. Department of Health and Human Services: *Healthy people 2010: national health promotion and disease prevention objectives,* Washington, D.C., 2000, U.S. Department of Health and Human Services.

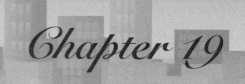

Chapter 19

Health Risks Across the Life Span

MARCIA K. COWAN • SHIRLEEN LEWIS-TRABEAUX
DEMETRIUS J. PORCHE • THOMAS KIPPENBROCK
KATHLEEN FLETCHER • CYNTHIA J. WESTLEY

OBJECTIVES

After reading this chapter, the student should be able to:

- Discuss major health problems of children and adolescents.
- Evaluate the role of the community health nurse with specific at-risk populations in the community.
- Describe ways to promote child and adolescent health within the community.
- Define the term *women's health*.
- Describe the women's health movement in the United States.
- Describe the health status of women in the United States.
- Discuss risk factors and their consequences on men's health.
- Understand how men's life-styles affect their health.
- Define terms commonly used to refer to elders.
- Identify the multidimensional influences on aging and how these affect the health status of an elder.
- List chronic health problems often experienced by elders.
- Describe several community-based models for gerontology nursing practice.

CHAPTER OUTLINE

KEY TERMS

advance directives: written or oral statements by which a competent person makes known treatment preferences and/or designates a surrogate decision maker.

ageism: prejudice toward older people, similar to racism or sexism.

aging: the sum total of all changes that occur in a person with the passing of time.

anorexia: an intense fear of becoming obese and disturbances in body image result in strict dieting and excessive weight loss. Occurs most commonly in females between the ages of 12 and 21 but may occur in older women and men.

anovulation: the lack of production and discharge of an ovum.

assaultive violence: non-fatal and fatal interpersonal violence in which physical force or other means are used by a person with intent of causing harm, injury, or death to another.

attention deficit disorder (ADD): inappropriate degree of inattention, impulsiveness, and hyperactivity for age and development.

basic activities of daily living (ADLs): basic personal care activities that include eating, toileting, dressing, bathing, transferring, walking, and getting outside.

body maintenance: maintaining optimal functioning, performance and capacity to do things.

bulimia: persistent concern with body shape and weight. Recurrent episodes of binge eating followed by extreme methods to prevent weight gain such as purging, fasting, or vigorous exercise.

caregiver burden: the physical, psychological or emotional, social, and financial problems that can be experienced by those who provide care for impaired others.

chronic illness: an illness in which a cure is not expected and nursing activities address function, wellness, and psychosocial issues.

digital rectal examination (DRE): a procedure used to assess the condition of the prostate and rectum; generally used for early detection of cancer.

durable power of attorney: a legal way for a client to designate someone else to make health care decisions when he or she is unable to do so.

five Is: five conditions believed to adversely affect the aging experience are intellectual impairment, immobility, instability, incontinence, and iatrogenic drug reactions.

geriatrics: the study of disease in old age.

gerontological nursing: the specialty of nursing concerned with assessment of the health and functional status of older adults, planning and implementing health care and services to meet the identified needs, and evaluating the effectiveness of such care.

gerontology: the specialized study of the process of growing old.

homeless child syndrome: combination of the effects of homelessness on children resulting in health problems, environmental dangers, and stress.

hormone replacement therapy (HRT): hormone combination of estrogen and progesterone used for post-menopausal women who have not had a hysterectomy.

immunization: a process of protecting an individual from a disease through introduction of a live, killed, or partial component of the invading organism into the individual's system.

instrumental activities of daily living (IADLs): those activities of daily living that help individuals manage their lives, such as cooking, shopping, paying bills, cleaning house, and using the telephone.

living will: a document that allows a client to express wishes regarding the use of medical treatments in the event of a terminal illness.

long-term care: care that is delivered to individuals who are dependent on others for assistance with basic tasks over a sustained period of time.

menopause: permanent cessation of menstruation resulting from loss of ovarian, follicular activity.

men/women death ratio: a statistical comparison of death rates between men and women.

neglect: Failure to act as an ordinary, prudent person; conduct contrary to that of a reasonable person under a specific circumstance.

osteoporosis: condition characterized by increased bone brittleness.

Patient Self-Determination Act: a law that requires providers who receive Medicare and Medicaid payments to give their clients written information regarding their legal options for treatment choices if they become incapacitated.

perimenopausal: the period immediately prior to menopause when endocrinological, biological, and clinical features of approaching menopause commence, continuing for at least the first year after permanent cessation of menstruation.

KEY TERMS—cont'd

prostate cancer: the second most common cancer among men in the United States that is sometimes hard to diagnosis due to lack of symptoms.

respite care: relief time provided by others to a caregiver from responsibilities for care of a family member.

sudden infant death syndrome (SIDS): infant death for which there is no definite cause.

testicular cancer: a commonly found solid malignant mass (tumor) that is found in the testicles of men.

testicular self-examination (TSE): a procedure performed by one's self to assess the condition of the testicles and detect abnormalities.

three D☶: types of intellectual impairment; progressive intellectual impairment (dementia); mood disorder (depression), and acute confusion (delirium).

women's health: women's life span that involves health promotion, maintenance, and restoration.

This chapter examines the health status of individuals across the life span. Emphasis is on the history, health status, leading causes of death and disease, and health risks of four distinct groups: children, women, men, and elders. Strategies in which community health nurses can help meet health needs throughout the life span are emphasized. The pivotal role of individuals in ensuring the family's and community's health is highlighted in the discussion of programs for individual's health services. Factors influencing access to health services, including unequal services, financial and employment issues, gender-power issues, family considerations, health behaviors, and health care providers' attitudes are considered. Health policy, including major legislation affecting health services, and future directions for health are discussed.

CHILDREN'S HEALTH

The future of the United States depends on how the children are cared for. Focusing on the health needs of children increases the chances of future adults who value and practice healthy lifestyles. Community-oriented nurses have two major roles in the area of child and adolescent health:

1. The nurse provides direct services to children and their families: assessment, management of care, education, and counseling (see Appendixes E.2, F.1 through F.7, and G.1 and G.2).
2. Nurses are involved in the assessment of the community and the establishment of programs to ensure a healthy environment for its children.

The roles of the nurse offer the opportunity to teach healthy lifestyles to children and caregivers and to provide family-centered care in the community.

Ongoing growth and development make the pediatric population unique. Physical, cognitive, and emotional changes occur more rapidly during childhood and adolescence than any other time in the life span. Health visits are scheduled at key ages to monitor these changes. Recommendations for well child care are found in Table 19-1. Nursing assessments include growth and health status, development, quality of the parent-child relationship, and family support systems (Box 19-1).

Briefly Noted

One out of seven children in the United States has no health insurance. One third of the uninsured children in the United States are eligible for Medicaid programs.

MAJOR HEALTH PROBLEMS
Injuries and Accidents

Injuries and accidents are the most important cause of preventable disease, disability, and death among children. Injuries cause one half of all childhood and three fourths of all adolescent deaths in the United States. Each year, 20% to 25% of all children will have a serious health problem related to accidents or injuries. Most are preventable. The key to changing behaviors is teaching age-appropriate safety.

Motor vehicle accidents are the leading cause of death among children and teenagers. One fourth of those deaths involve drunk drivers. Two thirds of the children who are killed in motor vehicle accidents are unrestrained. Surveys show that 20% of infants and 40% of children and teens are unrestrained in cars. As many as 80% of children who are using seat belts or car seats are restrained incorrectly (National Center for Injury Prevention and Control, 1998). Motor vehicle accidents include not only automobile collision but also pedestrian injury. Drowning and burns account for most of the other deaths; poisons and falls also contribute heavily. Age-related development is an important issue in identifying risks to children. Table 19-2 lists the three leading injury causes of death by age.

Infants

Infants have the second highest injury rate of all groups of children for the following reasons:

- Small size contributes to the type of injury.
- The small airway may be easily occluded.
- The small body fits through places where the head may be entrapped.
- Infants are handled on high surfaces for the convenience of the caregiver, placing them at great risk for falls.

TABLE 19-1   Guidelines for Well Child Care

	Age												
	Months							Years					
	2	4	6	9	12	15	18	2	3	4-6	7-9	10-13	14-21
Physical exam	+	+	+	+	+	+	+	+	+	+	+	+	+
Height, weight	+	+	+	+	+	+	+	+	+	+	+	+	+
Head circumference	+	+	+	+	+	+	+	+	+				
Blood pressure									+	+	+	+	+
Vision	s	s	s	s	s	s	s	s	+	+	+	+	+
Hearing	s	s	s	s	s	s	s	s	s	+	+	+	+
Developmental	+	+	+	+	+	+	+	+	+	+	+	+	+
LABORATORY TESTS													
Hct/Hb				+						+		+	
Urinalysis										+		+	
Cholesterol screen								c		c		c	c
Lead level					+					+			
Pap smear												∧	∧
Sexually transmitted diseases screening													+
ANTICIPATORY GUIDANCE													
Feeding/nutrition	+	+	+	+	+	+	+	+	+	+	+	+	+
Growth/development	+	+	+	+	+	+	+	+	+	+	+	+	+
Behavior	+	+	+	+	+	+	+	+	+	+	+	+	+
Safety/poisons/injury	+	+	+	+	+	+	+	+	+	+	+	+	+
Sexual behaviors											a	a	a
Substance abuse											a	a	a
Physical activity										a	a	a	a

Modified from American Academy of Pediatrics: *Guidelines for health supervision III: American Academy of Pediatrics guide to clinical preventive services*, Elk Grove Village, Ill, 1997, American Academy of Pediatrics.
a, As appropriate for age; *b*, evoked otoacoustic emissions testing within the first 3 months, preferably before discharge from the nursery; *c*, based on assessment of family risk factors; *s*, subjectively determined by behavioral observations, formal assessment as determined by history; *+*, recommendations will vary according to state guidelines and individual risk; *∧*, annually if sexually active.

TABLE 19-2	Types of Injury Causing Death by Age-Group*		
1 Year	**1 to 4 Years**	**5 to 14 Years**	**15 to 20 Years**
Aspiration	Fires/burns	Pedestrian	Motor vehicle accident
Homicide	Drowning	Motor vehicle accident	Suicide
Motor vehicle accident	Motor vehicle accident	Drowning	Homicide

Based on data from Baker SP, et al: *The injury fact book,* ed 2, New York, 1992, Oxford Press.
*Listed in order of frequency.

Box 19-1	**Nursing Assessment for Child Health**

- Physical assessment
- Nutritional needs
- Elimination patterns
- Sleep behaviors
- Development and behavior
- Safety issues
- Parenting concerns

Box 19-2	**Injury-Prevention Topics**

- Car restraints, seat belts, air bag safety
- Preventing fires, burns
- Poison prevention
- Preventing falls
- Preventing drowning, water safety
- Bicycle safety
- Safe driving practices
- Sports safety
- Pedestrian safety
- Gun control
- Decreasing gang activities
- Substance abuse prevention

- In motor vehicle accidents, the small size of an infant's body increases the risk for being crushed or being propelled into surfaces.
- Immature motor skills do not allow for escape from injury, placing them at risk for drowning, suffocation, and burns.

Toddlers and Preschoolers

This population experiences a large number of falls, poisonings, and motor vehicle accidents. They are active, and their increasing motor skills make supervision difficult. They are inquisitive and have relatively immature logic abilities.

School-Age Children

The school age group has the lowest injury death rate. At this age, it is difficult to judge speed and distance, placing them at risk for pedestrian and bicycle accidents. Universal use of bicycle helmets would prevent 135 to 155 deaths and 39,000 to 45,000 head injuries per year. Peer pressure often inhibits

the use of protective devices such as helmets and limb pads. Sports and athletic injuries are increased in this age group (National Center for Injury Prevention and Control, 1998).

Adolescents

Injury accounts for 75% of all deaths during adolescence. Risk-taking becomes more conscious at this time, especially among males.

- The death and serious injury rates for males are three times higher than for females.
- Adolescents are at the highest risk of any age group for motor vehicle deaths, drowning, and intentional injuries.
- Use of weapons and drug and alcohol abuse play an important role in injuries in this age group (Neinstein and Schack, 1996).
- Youth gangs are more violent than in the past and seem to be increasing in prevalence.
- Suicide is the second leading cause of death among youth between the ages of 15 and 24 (National Center for Injury Prevention and Control, 1998).

Briefly Noted

Most states have enacted laws allowing health care providers to treat adolescents in certain situations without parental consent. These include emergency care, substance abuse, pregnancy, and birth control. All 50 states recognize the mature minors doctrine. This allows youths 15 years of age and older to give informed medical consent if it is apparent that they are capable of understanding the risks and benefits and if the procedure is medically indicated.

Injury and Accident Prevention

The nurse has a responsibility in the prevention of accidents and injuries. The nurse is responsible for identification of risk factors by assessing the characteristics of the child, family, and the environment. Interventions include:

- Anticipatory guidance
- Environmental modification
- Safety education.

Education should focus on age-appropriate interventions based on knowledge of leading causes of death and risk factors. Topics to consider are listed in Box 19-2 (see also Appendix E.2).

Evidence-Based Practice

Data were gathered to determine whether an instructional program for child care could significantly reduce the spread of infectious diseases in the test center. In a test group of 3 to 5 year olds and their teachers, classes were held on germs and handwashing. A similar control group maintained their usual handwashing practices. During 21 weeks, including cold and flu season, the test group had significantly fewer colds than the control group.

Past research suggests that children in center care are 18 times more likely to become ill than children who stay at home. This study demonstrates a way to improve those statistics.

APPLICATION IN PRACTICE

Nurses who are in a position to consult schools and daycare centers can develop educational strategies that are age appropriate and may make a difference in illness in their community.

Niffenegger JP: Proper handwashing promotes wellness in child care, *J Pediatr Health Care* 11:1, 1997.

Box 19-3   Nursing Guide: Home Management of Gastrointestinal Virus in Children

- Education regarding expected course of the illness: gastrointestinal virus is usually self-limited, with vomiting lasting 1 to 2 days and diarrhea lasting up to 7 to 10 days.
- Progressive diet management: NPO for 3 to 4 hours; sips of oral electrolyte solution every 5 to 10 minutes for 2 hours; clear liquids (primarily oral electrolyte solution) for the rest of the day; bland, easily digested foods (BRAT diet: banana, rice, applesauce, toast) for the next 24 to 48 hours.
- Fever management with antipyretic agent if needed (avoid aspirin).
- Monitoring for signs of dehydration and providing instructions on seeking further care: urinates less than usual; parched, dry mouth and mucus membranes; poor skin turgor; sunken eyes with no tears; irritability; lethargy.
- Prevention of spread: instructions on handwashing technique.

Acute Illness

Infection is the most significant cause of illness in infants and children. Infectious diseases, whether bacterial or viral in origin, are usually associated with a variety of symptoms:

- Fever
- Upper respiratory symptoms
- Generalized discomfort and malaise
- Loss of appetite
- Rash
- Vomiting
- Diarrhea.

Young children may experience six to eight episodes of acute infectious illnesses per year. Most are self-limited and can be handled by the family at home with interventions to prevent complications. The nurse may need to identify whether the child can be managed at home based on the severity of symptoms and the family's ability to provide care. The nurse may be involved in developing a home care plan. Also the nurse teaches the family about the illness and prevention of its spread. Nursing interventions for home care of a child with a gastrointestinal virus are shown in Box 19-3. This serves as a model for nursing interventions for an acute illness.

Infectious diseases may be more serious in younger children and infants. Neonates, because of immunological immaturity, are more susceptible to bacterial illness with spread to multiple organ systems, called *sepsis*. Children of all ages are at risk for invasion of the spinal fluid, or meningitis. The morbidity and mortality rates of these forms of infection vary with the age of the child, causative organism, severity of the illness, and the onset of treatment. The nursing role includes:

- Early identification and referral (see a pediatric text for signs and symptoms of sepsis and meningitis)
- Determination of whether the child can be managed at home based on the severity of the symptoms and the family's abilities

- Support of the family during the treatment phase
- Development of a home care plan
- Education of the family about illness and prevention of disease spread.

Preventive measures include:

- Family education in hygiene
- Identification of environmental sources of infection.

Sudden Infant Death Syndrome

Sudden death may occur in infants with a specific disorder such as meningitis or a chronic illness. When no specific cause of death can be determined, the death is labeled **sudden infant death syndrome (SIDS).** Each year, more than 5000 infants die of SIDS in the United States, making it the most common cause of death during the first year of life. Few factors can be used to predict the occurrence. Most deaths occur between 1 and 5 months of age, although it may occur up to 1 year of age. Only a small number of infants who died of SIDS experienced a previous episode of cyanosis or apnea. Cardiorespiratory monitoring has not been shown to decrease the incidence.

SIDS occurs more often in preterm and low-birth-weight infants and possibly in infants with upper respiratory tract infections. SIDS also occurs more often in male infants and in low socioeconomic groups. Maternal cigarette smoking increases the risk three to four times. The risk to younger siblings is unclear at present. Studies show that the prone sleeping position and tight swaddling may increase the risk. The incidence has decreased 38% since the supine sleep position has been promoted. There is no test to identify infants who may die, making this a frustrating clinical problem (Brooks, 1997).

When an infant dies, the family requires tremendous support. The nurse provides empathetic support and assists the family as they progress through the grief process and deal with siblings and other family members. Referral to support groups may be helpful.

Nursing interventions for SIDS include teaching of the following prevention strategies:

- Supine position for healthy infants
- No parental smoking
- Improved access to prenatal and postnatal health care
- Teaching and providing close follow-up care for high-risk groups
- Improved use of baby monitors for selected infants.

Chronic Health Problems

Improved medical technology has increased the number of children surviving with chronic health problems. Examples include Down syndrome, spina bifida, cerebral palsy, asthma, diabetes, congenital heart disease, cancer, hemophilia, bronchopulmonary dysplasia, and acquired immunodeficiency syndrome (AIDS). Despite the differences in the specific diagnoses, the families have complex needs and similar problems. Nurses should assess the following:

- Is the condition stable or life threatening?
- What is the actual health status?
- What is the degree of impairment to the child's ability to develop?
- What type and what frequency of treatments and therapy are required?
- How often are health care visits and hospitalizations required?
- To what degree are the family routines disrupted?

The common issues of chronic health problems include the following:

- All children and adolescents with chronic health problems need routine health care. The issues of pediatric health promotion and health care need to be addressed with this group.
- Ongoing medical care specific to the health problem needs to be provided. Examples include monitoring for complications of the health problem, specific medications, dietary adjustments, and therapies such as speech, physical, or occupational therapy. Ongoing evaluation of the effectiveness of treatment protocols is critical.
- Care is often provided by multiple specialists. This requires coordinating the scheduling of visits, tests, or procedures and the treatment regimen.
- Skilled care procedures are often required and may include suctioning, positioning, medications, feeding techniques, breathing treatments, physical therapy, and use of appliances.
- Equipment needs are often complex and may include monitors, oxygen, ventilators, positioning or ambulation devices, infusion pumps, and suction machines.

Box 19-4	Nursing Guide: Insulin-Dependent Diabetes Mellitus in Children

1. Follow-up care to evaluate child for disease control and to ensure that the family is coping well with management of care
2. Family teaching, including the following:
   - Disease process, complications, insulin action
   - Insulin therapy: technique, storage, dose adjustment
   - Glucose monitoring: technique, frequency of readings, interpretation of results
   - Diet regulation: diet developed to consider family diet, food preferences, and schedules; diet plan; timing meals and snacks; allowing for occasional treats and modifications for "special times"
   - Exercise planning: type, intensity, duration, monitoring, relationship of diet and insulin to exercise, coordination with family patterns and school activity
   - Smoking prevention: additive effects to vascular disease
   - Skin care and hygiene to prevent infections
   - Emergency management of hypoglycemia and hyperglycemia
3. Coordination of specialty services: eye care provider, endocrinologist, nutritionist, primary care provider
4. Referral to support groups, camps for psychosocial needs
5. Referral for qualification for state or federal programs (e.g., Children's Specialty Services)

- Educational needs are often complex. Communication between the family and team of health care providers and teachers is essential to meet the child's health and educational needs.
- Safe transportation to health care services and school must be available. Several barriers exist, including family resources, location, ability to be fitted appropriately in car restraint systems, and the amount and size of supportive equipment.
- Financial resources may not be adequate to meet the needs.
- Behavioral issues include the effect of the condition on the child's behavior as well as other family members.

Chronic health problems may stress family relationships. Nursing interventions in the primary care setting with a child diagnosed with insulin-dependent diabetes mellitus serve as a model for pediatric chronic health problems. Box 19-4 lists nursing care for diabetic children.

Alterations in Behavior

Behavioral problems in the child and adolescent are highly variable and may include:

- Eating disorders
- Attention problems
- Substance abuse
- Elimination problems
- Conduct disorders and delinquency
- Sleep disorders
- School maladaptation.

| Box 19-5 | Nursing Guide: Attention Deficit Disorder |

- *Assessment.* History, physical, parent/family assessment, learning and psychoeducational evaluations.
- *Behavioral modifications.* Home and school: teaching families techniques to support clear expectations, consistent routines, positive reinforcement for appropriate behavior, and time out for negative behaviors.
- *Classroom modifications.* Consult with family and teachers to meet individual needs for remediation or alternate instruction methods if necessary; structure activities to respond to the child's needs.
- *Support.* Referral to family therapy, support groups, or mental health services to assist development of positive coping behaviors.
- *Medications.* Consult with physician to monitor for therapeutic and adverse effects.
- *Follow-up.* Assess at 3- to 6-month intervals when stable. Dynamic process affected by relationships with others. Behaviors will change with age; problem may persist through adulthood.

Modified from Miller KJ, Costellanos FX: Attention deficit/hyperactivity disorders, *Pediatr Rev* 19:11, 1998.

A healthy self-concept is supported by positive interactions with others. Problem behaviors may provide negative feedback, which may generate low self-esteem. A child's coping mechanisms are influenced by the individual developmental level, temperament, previous stress experiences, role models, and support of parents and peers. Maladaptive coping mechanisms present as problem behaviors. Inappropriate behaviors may lead to further physical or developmental problems.

Attention deficit disorder (ADD) interventions are presented as a model for nursing management of a behavior problem (Box 19-5). ADD is a combination of inattention and impulsiveness, and it may include hyperactivity not appropriate for age. ADD frequently includes low self-esteem, labile mood, low frustration tolerance, temper outbursts, and poor academic skills.

- The evaluation is based on symptoms.
- Diagnosis is made by excluding other disorders.
- Symptoms vary with severity of the problem, and interventions range from simple to complex.
- A familial tendency exists; several members of a family may be affected.
- Treatment involves a family focus and includes health professionals and educators (Miller and Costellanos, 1998).

HOMELESS FAMILIES AND CHILDREN

Actual numbers of homeless children and adolescents are difficult to determine. Estimates vary from 200,000 to 800,000 children and adolescents. Families make up the fastest growing segment of the homeless population; 25% to 40% of homeless are families, often a single mother with two or three children (National Center for Health Statistics, 1998). The longer the duration and the amount of disruption of support systems determine the effects of homelessness on health. Children in homeless situations are often not immunized and suffer from poor nutrition. They have limited or no access to health care. Often there is increased exposure to environmental hazards, violence, and substance abuse. The combination of health problems, environmental dangers, and stress is referred to as the **homeless child syndrome** (Redlener, 1991).

Children experience:

- Chronic illness, such as tuberculosis, asthma, anemia, and chronic otitis media
- More frequent hospitalizations
- Behavioral problems such as sleep disorders, withdrawal, aggression, or depression
- Developmental delays as a result of the lack of an appropriate environment to foster development.

The nurse may be involved in outreach programs combining health care workers and community members to take the health care services to the homeless.

- Identifying a consistent team to provide continuity of care on a regular basis is important.
- The family is often removed from its network of neighbors, friends, relatives, and the usual health care providers.
- Emphasis should be placed on preventive and follow-up care and immediate problems.

Services include physical examinations, behavioral and developmental assessments, nutritional support, screening tests, and immunizations (Redlener, 1991).

Briefly Noted

The number of children with health insurance is decreasing. Should insurance companies be required to sell "children only" policies for families who cannot afford the cost of premiums for the entire family?

NUTRITION

Promoting good nutrition and dietary habits is one of the most important parts of maintaining child health. The first 6 years are the most important for developing sound lifetime eating habits. The quality of nutrition has been widely accepted as an important influence on growth and development. It is now becoming recognized for an important role in disease prevention.

Atherosclerosis begins during childhood. Other diseases, such as obesity, diabetes, osteoporosis, and cancer, may have early beginnings also (Forbes, 1997).

Factors Influencing Nutrition

The child and family both provide a range of variables that influence nutritional habits. Ethnic, racial, cultural, and socioeconomic factors influence what the parents eat and how they feed their children. The child brings individual issues to the nutritional arena, such as:

- Slow eating
- Picky patterns

TABLE 19-3 Daily Dietary Guidelines: Childhood and Adolescence

Food Group	1 to 3 Years	4 to 6 Years	7 to 12 Years	Adolescents 13 to 18 Years
Grains	6 servings/day	6 servings/day	6-11 servings/day	6-11 servings/day
	one serving = bread ¼ to ½ slice cereal ¼ cup rice/pasta (cooked) ¼ cup crackers 1 to 2	one serving = bread ½ slice cereal ½ cup rice/pasta ⅓ cup crackers 3 to 4	one serving = bread 1 slice cereal ¾ to 1 cup rice/pasta ½ cup crackers 4 to 5	one serving = bread 1 slice cereal ¾-1 cup rice/pasta ½ cup crackers 4 to 5
Vegetables	2-3 servings/day	2-3 servings/day	2-3 servings/day	3-5 servings/day
	one serving = 1 tablespoons/year of age	one serving = vegetable ¼ cup salad ½ cup	one serving = vegetable ½ cup salad 1 cup vegetable juice ¾ cup	one serving = vegetable ½ cup salad 1 cup vegetable juice ¾ cup
Fruits	2-3 servings/day	2-3 servings/day	2-3 servings/day	2-4 servings/day
	one serving = cooked or canned, ¼ cup fresh, ½ piece 100% juice, ¼ cup	one serving = cooked or canned, ¼ cup fresh, ½ piece 100% juice, ⅓ cup	one serving = cooked or canned, ⅓ cup fresh, 1 piece 100% juice, ½ cup	one serving = cooked or canned, ½ cup fresh, 1 piece 100% juice, ¾ cup
Dairy	2-3 servings/day	2-3 servings/day	2-3 servings/day	2-3 servings/day
	one serving = milk ½ cup cheese ½ oz yogurt/pudding ¼-½ cup	one serving = milk ½ cup cheese ½-¾ oz yogurt/pudding ½ cup	one serving = milk 1 cup cheese 1½ oz yogurt/pudding 1 cup	one serving = milk 1 cup cheese 1½ oz yogurt/pudding 1 cup
Protein	2 servings/day	2 servings/day	2 servings/day	2 servings/day
	one serving = meat, poultry, fish, tofu 1 oz beans, dried cooked ¼ cup egg ½	one serving = meat, poultry, fish, tofu 1 oz beans ⅓ cup egg 1	one serving = meat, poultry, fish, tofu 2-3 oz (½ cup beans, 1 egg, 2 T peanut butter = 1 oz meat)	one serving = meat, poultry, fish, tofu 2-3 oz (½ cup beans, 1 egg, 2 T peanut butter = 1 oz meat)

Modified from Dietz W, Stern L: *American Academy of Pediatrics' guide to your child's nutrition,* New York, 1999, Villard.

- Food preferences
- Allergies
- Acute or chronic health problems
- Changes with acceleration and deceleration of growth.

Parents often have unrealistic expectations of what children should eat. Table 19-3 offers guidelines to daily requirements for all ages.

Nutritional Assessment

Physical growth serves as an excellent measure of adequacy of the diet. Height, weight, and head circumference of children younger than 3 years old are plotted on appropriate growth curves at regular intervals to allow assessment of growth patterns. Good nutritional intake supports physical growth at a steady rate (Fig. 19-1).

A 24-hour diet recall by the parent is a helpful screening tool to assess the amount and variety of food intake. If the recall is fairly typical for the child, the nurse can compare the intake with basic recommendations for the child's age. Nurses should

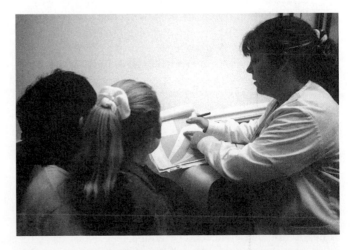

Figure 19-1 A nurse explains the growth patterns on a growth chart to a child and her mother.

ask about the family's and child's concerns regarding diet and look at the family's meal patterns. A key area of nutrition assessment includes the child's and family's exercise. Behavior problems that occur during meals may also be an issue.

Nutrition During Infancy

The first year of life is critical for growth of all major organ systems of the body. Nutrition during this time influences how an infant will grow and thrive. Most of the brain growth that occurs during the life span occurs during infancy. The digestive and renal systems are immature at birth and during early infancy. Certain nutrients are not handled well, and energy needs are high.

Types of Infant Feeding

Breast milk is the preferred method of infant feeding. Breast milk provides appropriate nutrients and antibodies for the infant. Breastfed infants have fewer illnesses and allergies. If breastfeeding is not chosen, commercially prepared formulas are an acceptable alternative. Although evaporated milk with added sugar has been used in the past as a low-cost alternative to breast milk, it is now discouraged. Errors in mixing and the lack of vitamins and minerals have been common problems.

Nutrition During Childhood

The skill and desire to self-feed begins at approximately 1 year of age. The parental role begins to shift at this time to providing a balanced, healthy range of foods as the child assumes more independence. Growth rate and caloric needs decrease during this time. Nurses can best assist parents by offering information on daily needs and healthy food choices. Suggestions for children might include the following:
- Try offering frequent, small meals.
- Offer a balanced diet incorporating variety and foods that the child likes.
- Limit milk intake to the recommendations for age.
- Consider the child's developmental level and safety; avoid nuts, popcorn, grapes, and similar foods to decrease risk of aspiration in young children.
- Encourage children to help with food selection and preparation based on developmental skills.
- Do not give vitamin and iron supplements unless directed otherwise by a physician or nurse practitioner.
- Avoid using food as a punishment or reward.

Adolescent Nutritional Needs

The preadolescent and adolescent years are a time of increased growth that is accompanied by increases in appetite and nutritional requirements. Caloric and protein requirements increase for boys 11 to 18 years of age. Girls have an increased protein need but a decreased caloric need during the same age span. The iron needed by the adolescent is nearly double that needed by adults.

Adolescent nutritional needs are influenced by physical alterations and psychosocial adjustments. Teenagers are often free to eat when and where they choose. Eating habits acquired from the family are abandoned. Most food is consumed away from the home. Fad foods and diets are prominent. Accelerated growth and poor eating habits put the adolescent at risk for poor nutritional health. Adolescents have the most unsatisfactory nutritional status of all age-groups. Deficiencies in iron, vitamins, calcium, riboflavin, and thiamine are most common (Neinstein and Schack, 1996).

Nurses initiate activities that promote improved nutritional status. Such activities include the following:
- Provision of information on good nutrition in individual or group sessions
- Diet assessment
- Educational activities that focus on effects of fad foods and diets
- Supplying the deficient nutrients
- Provision of a daily food guide (see Table 19-3)
- Suggested snacks and quick foods that supply essential nutrients
- Relationship of good nutrition to healthy appearance
- Assessment of risks for eating disorders.

IMMUNIZATIONS

Routine **immunization** of children has been very successful in preventing selected diseases. The ultimate challenge is making sure that children receive immunizations (Fig. 19-2):
- Cost and convenience are two critical issues in determining whether children are immunized.
- Successful programs combine low-cost or free immunizations provided at convenient times and locations.
- Repeatedly urging parents to obtain immunizations for their children is important.
- The goal of immunization is to protect by using immunizing agents to stimulate antibody formation.

Recommendations

Immunization recommendations rapidly change as new information and products are available. Two major organiza-

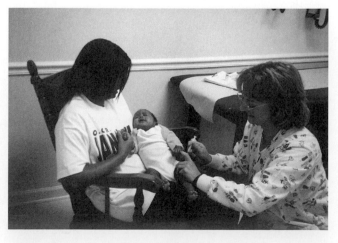

Figure 19-2 An infant receives a regularly scheduled immunization.

tions are responsible for guidelines: the American Academy of Pediatrics (AAP) and the U.S. Public Health Service's Advisory Committee on Immunization Practices (ACIP). Table 19-4 and Table 19-5 list current recommendations. The main goal of the guidelines is to provide flexibility to ensure that the largest number of children will be immunized. All health care providers are urged to access immunization status at every encounter with children and to update immunizations whenever possible. See Appendixes D.1 through D.3 for immunizing agents, contraindications, and side effects.

Contraindications

There are relatively few contraindications to giving immunizations. Minor acute illness is not a contraindication. Immunizations should be deferred with moderate or acute febrile illnesses because the reactions may mask the symptoms of the illness or the side effects of the immunization may be accentuated by the illness.

People of all ages are immunized but those with the following conditions are not routinely immunized and require medical consultation:

- Pregnancy
- Generalized malignancy
- Immunosuppressive therapy or immunodeficiency disease
- Sensitivity to components of the agent
- Recent immune serum globulin, plasma, or blood administration.

WOMEN'S HEALTH

To understand women's health issues, one must first understand the term **women's health.** The American Academy of Nursing's 1996 Expert Panel on Women's Health says that women's health includes their entire life span and involves health promotion, maintenance, and restoration. This term recognizes that the health of women is related to the biological, social, and cultural dimensions of women's lives. Moreover, women's normal life events or rites of passage, such as menstruation, childbirth, and **menopause,** are considered part of normal female development, rather than syndromes or diseases requiring medical treatment only. This broad emphasis on women's health is in contrast to the view of women solely in terms of their reproductive health or their role in parenting children. Box 19-6 offers illness-prevention strategies for women to reflect new emphasis on women's health. Box 19-7 suggests a woman's health program across the adult life span.

HISTORY OF THE WOMEN'S HEALTH MOVEMENT

The *women's health movement* has its origin in the feminist movement. The first wave of feminism began in the United States in the mid-nineteenth century. The second wave of feminism in the 1960s and 1970s gave birth to the women's health movement. At this time, the number of pregnancies continued to decrease, and women continued to earn higher

---

TABLE 19-4   Recommended Immunization Schedules for Children Not Immunized in First Year of Life

Time Interval/Age	Immunizations	Comment
Younger Than 7 Years		
First visit	DTaP, Hib, HBV, MMR	MMR if child is >12 mo; TB testing may be done at the same visit. Hib is not indicated if the child is >60 mo. Pneumococcal vaccine may be indicated if <2 years
Interval After First Visit		
1 mo	DTaP, IPV, HBV, VAR	
2 mo	DTaP, Hib, IPV	Second dose of Hib is not indicated if >15 mo when first dose given
At least 8 mo	DTaP, HBV, IPV	
4 to 6 yrs old	DTaP, IPV, MMR	DTaP not necessary if the fourth dose was given after the fourth birthday; IPV not necessary if the third dose was given after the fourth birthday
7 Years and Older		
First visit	HBV, IPV, MMR, TD, VAR	Varicella is given if there is no history of disease. 13 years and older receive 2 doses, 4 weeks apart
Interval After First Visit		
2 mo	HBV, IPV, MMR, TD	
8 to 14 mo	HBV, IPV, TD	
10 years after last Td	TD	Repeat every 10 years throughout life

Modified from American Academy of Pediatrics: *Red book,* ed 25, Elk Grove Village, Ill, 2000, American Academy of Pediatrics.
DTaP, diphtheria-tetanus toxoid-acellular pertussis; *HBV,* hepatitis B vaccine; *Hib, Haemophilus influenzae* type b conjugate vaccine; *IPV,* inactivated poliomyelitis vaccine; *MMR,* measles-mumps-rubella; *TD,* adult tetanus-diphtheria toxoid; *VAR,* varicella.

TABLE 19-5   Immunization Schedule: Range of Ages for Routine Immunizations

Vaccine	Birth	Age (months)						Age (years)			
		2	4	6	12	15	18	4 to 6	11 to 12	14 to 16	18
HBV	#1 →										
		#2* →		#3			→				
DTaP		#1	#2	#3	#4† →		→	#5	TD →		→
Hib		#1‡	#2‡	#3‡	#4‡ →						
IVP		#1	#2	#3 →			→	#4			
MMR					#1 →		→	#2§ →		→	
VAR					#1 →		→	#2‖			
PNEU		#1	#2	#3	#4 →		→				
MEN											#1¶

Modified from American Academy of Pediatrics: *Red book,* ed 25, Elk Grove Village, Ill, 2000, American Academy of Pediatrics.
HBV, Hepatitis B virus; *DTaP,* diphtheria-tetanus toxoid-acellular pertussis; *Hib, Haemophilus influenzae* type b conjugate vaccine; *IPV,* inactivated poliomyelitis vaccine; *MMR,* measles-mumps-rubella; *VAR,* varicella; *PNEU,* pneumococcal 7-valent conjugate; *MEN,* meningococcal; *TD,* adult tetanus-diphtheria toxoid (used after age 7).
*Thimerosal-free vaccine is recommended under 6 months of age.
†6 months must elapse between DTaP #3 and #4. DTaP/HiB may be combined at 15 months with some products.
‡Hib/HBV combination product is available. See manufacturer's recommendations. Three Hib products are licensed for infant use. Some do not require a dose at 6 months; see manufacturer's recommendations.
§MMR #2 may be given at any visit provided 1 month has elapsed since #1 and both are given after 12 months of age.
‖Varicella vaccine is given at any visit on or after the first birthday if there is no history of disease. Susceptible persons 13 years or older receive 2 doses, 4 weeks apart.
¶Meningococcal vaccine is recommended for college freshmen, particularly those residing in dormitories.

Box 19-6   U.S. Preventive Health Service Recommendations for Primary Prevention Strategies for Women

- Regular dental examinations
- Regular physical examinations, including Pap test and mammography
- Adequate calcium intake
- Regular physical activity, including weight-bearing activities
- Diet with less than 30% fat, limit cholesterol intake, increase intake of high-fiber foods
- Limit alcohol and tobacco use; encourage smoking-cessation programs
- **Hormone replacement therapy** for perimenopausal and postmenopausal women
- Family planning and contraceptive counseling
- Home smoke detectors and security systems
- Daily dental care: floss and brush with fluoride toothpaste
- Set home water temperature at 120° to 130° F
- Appropriate immunizations: pneumococcal, influenza, and tetanus/diphtheria boosters
- Use of lap/shoulder belts
- Sexually transmitted disease prevention: consistent and correct use of barrier protection

From U.S. Preventive Services Task Force: *Guide to clinical preventive services: report of the U.S. Preventive Services Task Force,* Washington, D.C., Philadelphia, 1996, Williams & Wilkins.

Box 19-7   Possible Components of a Comprehensive Women's Health Program

- Comprehensive reproductive and gynecological services, including screenings for breast and cervical cancer and sexually transmitted diseases, preconceptual counseling, and abortion counseling and referral, as well as services for fertility or infertility, late pregnancy, and menopause for women at midlife
- Health promotion that focuses on physical fitness and nutrition; avoidance of cigarettes, alcohol, and other substances; stress management; violence prevention; occupational exposure, including injury prevention; self-image and self-esteem building for adolescents and young adult women
- Parenting classes for young mothers
- Immunizations
- Screening, counseling, and referral for mood disorders, depression, caregiver role strain, and stress-related illnesses, violence, and abuse
- Close monitoring of women at midlife and older for early detection of heart disease; breast, cervical, and colon cancer; diabetes; lung disease; arthritis; and other chronic illnesses

Data from Taylor D, Woods N: Changing women's health, changing nursing practice, *J Obstet Gynecol Neonat Nurs* 25(9):791, 1996.

education. Women's health was considered within the domain of the obstetrician and gynecologist. In the 1960s Congress passed Title VII, which banned sexual discrimination in the workplace, and civil rights for women became an important issue.

Women's health issues focused on women's bodies throughout the 1970s. A women's health conference was held in Boston in 1969 to discuss "Women and Their Bodies." The medicalization of childbirth began to change in 1972 with the formation of the International Childbirth Education Association (ICEA).

The National Women's Health Network (NWHN), established in 1974 to monitor national health care policy, functions as a clearinghouse and advocates for women's health. In 1986 the National Institutes of Health (NIH) developed a health care policy that called for the inclusion of women in clinical research. In 1990 the Office of Research on Women's Health within the NIH was formed. This office has the responsibility to address women's health issues (Geary, 1995).

The women's health movement that was initiated at the grassroots level has now become a national movement. Although the importance of women's health began gaining national recognition during the last two decades, lack of emphasis on women's health needs continues to exist.

Briefly Noted

Women should be actively involved in the planning of women's health programs. Women who are representative of the target population should serve as formal or informal leaders, gatekeepers, or role models.

HEALTH STATUS OF WOMEN

Unfortunately, millions of people, particularly women, do not have access to basic health-related resources. In most countries women live longer than men, but women are generally less healthy. This difference in health is related to poverty. Although women compose half of the world's population, they represent 70% of the people in the world who live in poverty (Craft, 1997b). In the United States, two thirds of all poor adults are women. Of those individuals living below the poverty level, most are single mothers with children.

Although women have made some strides toward financial equality during the last decade, progress has been slow. Worldwide the education of women is the single most important factor in the improvement of the health of women and their families. As women are educated, their socioeconomic status improves and mortality rates decline (Craft, 1997a). Because women's financial stability is closely linked to health outcomes, it is essential to promote policies that support the advancement of women. Nurses can play a vital role as key mobilizers in empowering women, empowering themselves, and working with communities to take control of women's health and ensure that resources are

developed to benefit both genders equally (Conway-Welch et al, 1997).

HOW TO Eat Healthfully and Be Physically Active

1. Set realistic personal goals that focus on personal health and well-being, not weight loss.
2. Measure progress by changes in fitness and energy level, as well as improvements in blood pressure, glucose, and lipids.
3. Make life-style changes that are internally motivated (for self) rather than externally motivated (for spouse, family, or friends).
4. Do not go on a diet; gradually make healthful dietary and life-style choices.
5. Identify weaknesses in dietary practices and physical activity habits and plan strategies for dealing with them.
6. Develop good long-term eating practices such as the following:
   a. Include the daily servings from each food group in the food guide pyramid.
   b. Choose to eat more whole grains, cereals, beans, and soy products, as well as five servings of fruits and vegetables each day.
   c. Avoid one of the pitfalls of overeating by not skipping meals or getting hungry.
   d. Always eat breakfast.
   e. Always have healthful foods available for snacking.
7. Realize that regular physical activity is an absolute requirement to maintain a healthy body weight.
8. Participate in regular physical activity that is enjoyable, convenient, and inexpensive.
9. Find an exercise partner or exercise classmates to help maintain motivation.
10. Find a sport you enjoy and do it regularly.
11. Consider walking, running, dancing, aerobics, soccer, or weight-lifting.
12. Take a break from physical activity at least one day per week.

Modified from Manore M: Running on empty: health consequences of chronic dieting in active women, *American College of Sports Medicine's (ACSM's) Health and Fitness Journal* 2(2):24, 1998.

WOMEN'S HEALTH PROBLEMS: ACUTE AND CHRONIC
Heart Disease

Heart disease is the leading cause of death among women over 50 and the second leading cause of death among women ages 35 to 39 years (National Women's Health Information Center, 1998). Although women are less likely to have heart attacks than men, they are more likely to die from heart attacks. After menopause and by age 75, the incidence of heart disease in women exceeds that of men (Arnstein, Buselli, and Rankin, 1996).

The presentation of heart disease in women is different from men. Men with heart disease initially experience an acute myocardial infarction with few warning signs. Women with heart disease are more likely to report chest pain and other symptoms before experiencing a myocardial infarction. Nearly 90% of women with a myocardial infarction report chest pain. Additionally, women are more likely to present with upper abdominal pain, dyspnea, nausea, and fatigue (Hill and Geraci, 1998; Manson, et al, 1997). Women may delay seeking treatment, expecting that a heart attack involves much more pain than they are experiencing. In addition, women's complaints may not be taken seriously by health care providers, who may attribute symptoms to stress. Thus women may be misdiagnosed until their condition warrants emergency surgery (Hill and Geraci, 1998).

Cessation of smoking is the most important factor in decreasing the morbidity and mortality of heart disease in women.

Cancer

Cancer is the second leading cause of death for women. The most common types of cancer in women are lung, breast, colorectal, ovarian, cervical, and pancreatic. Lung cancer is the leading cause of cancer deaths among women, surpassing breast and colorectal cancer (Baldini and Strauss, 1997; National Women's Health Information Center, 1998). Most lung cancer is preventable by modifying lifestyle, such as through smoking cessation.

Many women identified only a few risks of smoking. Barriers to smoking cessation were closely linked to their difficult life situations. Barriers include:

- Living in highly stressful environments
- Feeling isolated and without social support
- Choosing smoking as an affordable, legal pleasure given limited financial resources.

A comprehensive smoking-cessation program that has other purposes that are meaningful to women's lives, such as dealing with disappointments, handling stress, and obtaining resources, would be more effective than those that focus simply on smoking.

Breast cancer is the second most common cancer in women (Catalano and Satariano, 1998). Carcinoma of the breast accounts for 32% of female cancers (Kuter, 1996).

Risk factors associated with breast cancer are listed in Box 19-8. However, many cases of breast cancer cannot be explained by these established risk factors. Approximately 75% of the women with breast cancer do not have a high-risk profile (Kuter, 1996). Moreover, most risk factors cannot be reduced by lifestyle modifications. The major risk factor is advancing age; risk of breast cancer increases significantly for women over 50 years old.

Although breast cancer occurs most frequently in women of higher socioeconomic status, financially disadvantaged women have the highest mortality rate. The high mortality rate among these women may be related to lack of information about the disease and inadequate health care, which

| Box 19-8 | **Risk Factors Associated With Breast Cancer** |

- Over 50 years of age
- Family history (mother, sister, daughter)
- Genetic predisposition
- Previous breast cancer
- First pregnancy after 30 years of age
- Nulliparity
- Menarche before 12 years of age
- Menopause after 55 years of age
- Proliferative atypical breast hyperplasia
- History of ovarian or endometrial cancer
- Obesity after menopause
- High socioeconomic status

often results in late-stage diagnosis and delayed treatment. Financially disadvantaged women are much less likely to have regular mammograms. Financial concerns such as fear of job loss and making ends meet leave little time for health promotion efforts such as breast self-examination (Catalano and Satariano, 1998; McCance and Jorde, 1998).

Early detection remains the primary factor in survival for women with breast cancer. All women should receive age-appropriate periodic screening and education. This includes a combination of mammography, clinical breast examination, and breast self-examination (BSE) teaching.

The American Cancer Society (ACS) guidelines for mammography are the most widely accepted. ACS recommends that annual mammography begin by age 40 years and consist of annual clinical examination, with a screening mammography performed at 1- to 2-year intervals. States with high rates of mammography screening have demonstrated reduced breast cancer fatality rates, presumably as a result of diagnosing breast cancer at an earlier stage (Cooper et al, 1998). A nurse's recommendation to seek breast cancer screening can be a very powerful motivator. The following nursing considerations apply to mammography:

- Women need to understand the difference between screening and diagnostic mammography. Women with breast signs or symptoms such as a mass, skin changes, and nipple discharge should request diagnostic rather than screening mammography.
- Women need to be informed that the procedure can be uncomfortable or painful.
- If possible, women should schedule mammography when they are not experiencing cyclical breast tenderness or have conditions that increase breast density.
- Women's privacy should be respected.
- Women should not be required to walk or wait in a public area while wearing an examination gown.

Older women have been identified as a group that is less likely to participate in breast cancer screening. Nurses need to target older women for breast cancer teaching and screening.

The incidence of reproductive cancers increases with age. Women over 40 years old are at increased risk for cervical, uterine, and ovarian cancer (Wertheim, Soto-Wright, and

Goodman, 1996). Ovarian cancer causes more deaths than all other forms of gynecological cancer combined.

Symptoms of ovarian cancer usually are not noticeable until the disease has progressed to an advanced stage. Consequently, most women with ovarian cancer are first diagnosed during an advanced stage. A major risk factor for ovarian cancer is family history of breast or ovarian cancer. Other risk factors for ovarian cancer include:

- Nulliparity
- Late first pregnancy
- Infertility
- Late menopause
- High-fat diet
- Higher socioeconomic status
- A family history of ovarian cancer
- Occupational exposure to talc and asbestos.

The periodic pelvic examination is the only reliable screening test available. About one third of gynecological cancers include uterine cancers (cervical and endometrial). Endometrial cancer is the most common malignant disease of the female genital tract. Endometrial cancer occurs most often in postmenopausal women, with the average age at diagnosis of 61 years. A woman's lifetime risk of developing endometrial cancer is 2% to 3% (Wertheim, Soto-Wright, and Goodman, 1996). Risk factors include:

- Nulliparity
- Late menopause
- Early menarche
- Anovulation
- Obesity
- Liver disease
- High socioeconomic status
- Family history of breast cancer.

Symptoms of endometrial cancer include abnormal vaginal bleeding and an enlarged uterus. The Papanicolaou (Pap) test is a poor screening test for endometrial cancer; endometrial biopsy is an accurate diagnostic method for endometrial cancer. There are not enough data, however, to justify screening of the general population of postmenopausal women with endometrial biopsies (Press, 1998).

With early detection, appropriate treatment, and adequate follow-up, cervical cancer is one of the most preventable diseases. Major risk factors for cervical cancer include:

- Cigarette smoking
- Low socioeconomic status
- A history of multiple sexual partners
- Early onset of sexual activity
- Use of oral contraceptives.

Moreover, sexually transmitted viral diseases such as herpes and human papilloma have recently been recognized as playing a possible role in the development of cervical cancer (Wertheim, Soto-Wright, and Goodman, 1996).

Early symptoms of cervical cancer can include vaginal bleeding or discharge, symptoms often associated with douching and sexual intercourse. The principal screening test for cervical cancer is the Pap test. Nurses should refer such women to available community resources that provide these services for financially challenged women or develop programs for these women.

Human Immunodeficiency Virus

HIV is a major health problem and cause of death among women. Women represent the fastest growing groups of individuals with acquired immunodeficiency syndrome (AIDS) in the United States.

Many women are at risk because they are not aware of the modes of HIV transmission and do not acknowledge their risk behaviors (Soet, DiIorio, and Dudley, 1998). The highest HIV seroprevalence rates in women are found in women of childbearing age. Injection drug use or being the sexual partner of an injecting drug user are the main risk factors for women (Kazanjian and Eisenstat, 1996).

Vaginal fungal infections, especially those caused by *Candida albicans,* are frequently the presenting illness in women with AIDS (Minkoff, DeHovitz, and Duerr, 1995). Women with HIV are also prone to cervical neoplasias and pelvic inflammatory disease.

Since women of childbearing age are the largest at-risk group for becoming infected with HIV, attention to issues of perinatal HIV transmission are important. Perinatal transmission is the most common route of HIV infection in children (Minkoff, DeHovitz, and Duerr, 1995). The rate of perinatal HIV transmission can be reduced to as low as 8.3% with prophylactic zidovudine therapy during pregnancy, delivery, and in the infant (Minkoff, DeHovitz, and Duerr, 1995).

Briefly Noted

Women are experiencing an alarming increase in the number of HIV/AIDS cases. The increase in HIV/AIDS cases in women of childbearing age will directly affect the number of HIV/AIDS cases in the pediatric population.

HIV is often a family illness, resulting in extraordinary needs that embrace several domains: physical, psychosocial, spiritual, and economic. The lives of these families are frequently complicated by the death of one or more parents and a child because of HIV illness. In addition, the same circumstances that may have led the mother to become infected with HIV may undermine her ability to provide care for her HIV-infected infant and her other children. Many of these families have other problems:

- Poverty
- Isolation
- Poor education
- Unemployment
- Inadequate housing
- Drug use.

Health care that demonstrates appreciation and respect for HIV-infected families is a challenge.

Women and Weight Control

Obesity is defined as an increase in body weight of 20% or more above the desirable body weight. The number of overweight women in the United States is increasing. Obesity originates in childhood.

Because obesity in women is such a stigma in Western culture, women are at highest risk for suffering adverse social and psychological consequences of obesity. These consequences can include social and financial discrimination.

In the last 20 years, reports of disordered eating have noticeably increased. Many girls and women are dissatisfied with their current shape and weight, but only a small number of these actually develop serious eating disorders. The most common eating disorders seen in women are anorexia nervosa and bulimia. **Anorexia** is defined as fear of gaining weight and disturbances in perception of the body. Excessive weight loss is the most noticeable clue. Individuals with anorexia rarely complain of weight loss because they view themselves as normal or overweight. Many of these women struggle with psychological problems, including depression, obsessive symptoms, and social phobias. **Bulimia** is characterized by persistent concern with body shape and weight, recurrent episodes of binge eating, a loss of control during these binges, and use of extreme methods to prevent weight gain, such as purging, strict dieting, fasting, or vigorous exercise. Unlike anorexia, bulimia is observed across all weight categories, with most women being within a normal weight range. Although bulimia is considered less dangerous medically than anorexia, electrolyte imbalance and dehydration can create serious physical complications, such as cardiac dysrhythmias.

Nurses are in a prime position to include assessment for eating disorders and referral for treatment into their routine clinical practices. The goal of the nurse is to identify not only those women with eating disorders, but also those women at risk for developing eating problems. See the Evidence-Based Practice box for a discussion of a study about overeating. Through a thorough physical and psychosocial assessment, as well as a history of dietary practice, the nurse may be able to identify women with eating disorders and provide appropriate referrals. Community health nurses should promote healthy eating habits and regular physical activity as a weight-control strategy.

Arthritis

Arthritis is the most prevalent chronic condition experienced by women; it is three times as common in women than men (Ross, 1997). In general, the majority of the clients with rheumatoid arthritis are women (Grisso, Ness, and Hendrix, 1997). The rate of arthritis increases significantly with age. Many arthritic diseases exist; the most common form of arthritis is degenerative joint disease, or osteoarthritis. About 25% of women with arthritis experience some limitations in activity because of their condition. Women with arthritis often

 Evidence-Based Practice

The purpose of the study referenced below was to compare eating patterns of women who experience episodes of weight cycling with women of normal weight. A subject was identified as a weight cycler if she reported two cycles of weight loss and regain greater than 10 pounds in the last 2 years.

Semistructured interviews were conducted with 15 women with normal weight and 30 women who were in a previous study of motivational states associated with overeating episodes. The women were between the ages of 21 and 53 years of age, with a weight grouping of normal, overweight, or obese.

This study identified four common themes that emerged from the semistructured interviews: planned overeating; power/control issues; relationships with others; and unpleasant feelings. All of the women reported planning to overeat. The overweight women planned to overeat when alone, whereas the obese women overate with others present. The normal-weight women overate when celebrating special occasions. Personal power or control over their eating was felt by 73% of normal-weight women, 30% of overweight women, and 50% of obese women. Unpleasant feelings related to overeating included anxiety, tension, stress, boredom, tiredness, and loneliness. Obese women reported more boredom, tiredness, and loneliness than overweight and normal-weight women when overeating.

APPLICATION IN PRACTICE

Nurses can use these study findings to plan health-promotion strategies for women who have experienced overeating or to prevent women from experiencing feelings that pose the risk for overeating. Reducing overweight and obesity in women will accomplish the reduction or elimination of a major risk factor for several acute and chronic illnesses. Nurses planning women's health programs should include strategies such as group counseling and peer support programs, encouragement of expression of unpleasant feelings, planned activities to reduce fatigue and occupy their time, and stress-management programs to reduce feelings of anxiety, tension, and stress.

Popkess-Vawter S, Brandau M, Straub J: Triggers of overeating and related intervention strategies for women who weight cycle, *Appl Nurs Res* 11(2):69, 1998.

suffer from chronic, often debilitating, pain. The monetary cost of managing this pain can be devastating to an older woman's limited income (Kington and Smith, 1997; Tindall, 1997). Other areas of concern include obtaining adequate sleep, dealing with medications, maintaining energy, and experiencing depression/anxiety. Nurses can encourage women to prevent progression of osteoarthritis through education on the relationship between obesity and increased "wear and tear" on joints. In addition, women should be cautioned to protect their joints from repeated trauma. Physical therapy may be helpful in reducing pain and disability.

Osteoporosis

Osteoporosis is a major health problem for postmenopausal and elderly women. Osteoporosis causes between 1.3 and 1.5 million spinal, hip, and forearm fractures annually

(Whitmore, 1998). The most common fracture associated with osteoporosis is compression fracture of the vertebrae. Hip fractures are the second most common fractures associated with osteoporosis. The incidence of this type of fracture increases with age.

The first group includes factors that women cannot modify: 50 years and over, being Caucasian or Asian, having a petite or slim bone structure, being menopausal or having experienced an early menopause, and having a family history of osteoporosis (Whitmore, 1998; Woodhead and Moss, 1998). The second group consists of variables that women can modify: inadequate intake of calcium, limited exercise, smoking, and excessive alcohol use. Prevention of osteoporosis includes:

- Maintaining a desirable weight
- Maintaining an adequate intake of dietary calcium, phosphorus, and vitamin D
- Participating in regular weight-bearing exercise.

Prevention efforts for osteoporosis should be targeted at young girls as they develop health promotion behaviors. Women increase bone mass through their twenties, and women with higher bone mass in early adulthood may be able to resist the effects of age-related bone loss (Whitmore, 1998; Woodhead and Moss, 1998). Anorexia and exercise to the point of amenorrhea may be hazardous to women's bones (McGee, 1997). Athletic women should be counseled about preserving bone density. Nursing interventions for adult women include eliciting a careful family, social, and dietary history and teaching preventive behaviors.

For postmenopausal women, nurses should obtain yearly height measures and observe for clinical features of osteoporosis (kyphosis). Nurses can also teach women how to prevent or slow the progression of osteoporosis. Women often consume less than half the recommended daily calcium intake, which predisposes them to osteoporosis (National Women's Health Information Center, 1998).

Urinary Incontinence

Urinary incontinence (UI) is a major women's health issue. *Urinary incontinence* is defined as a condition in which involuntary loss of urine occurs. Urinary incontinence creates a social or hygienic problems for women (Jay and Staskin, 1998). The prevalence of UI in women ranges from 10% to 25% (Jay and Staskin, 1998). Of the people over 65 years of age, 20% are incontinent. It is believed that the incidence of UI is greatly underreported, since many women believe that losing continence is just the normal result of childbearing or growing older. Urine loss may vary from small infrequent amounts to large, frequent amounts.

Individuals typically experience a loss in self-esteem, a sense of guilt, and isolation. UI in elderly persons is the major factor contributing to the family's decision to seek institutional care. In elderly persons, skin breakdown can contribute to the development of pressure ulcers.

Nurses can encourage a number of behaviors that can prevent or minimize UI. Women should be encouraged to maintain adequate hydration (2000 to 3000 ml a day). Constipation can exacerbate incontinence by putting pressure on the bladder and obstructing the urethra. Some fluids increase the urge to urinate; caffeine beverages and citrus juices should be avoided. Obesity can contribute to incontinence; therefore weight reduction may reduce UI. Low estrogen levels can lead to flaccid muscle tissue, causing stress incontinence. **Perimenopausal** and postmenopausal women can be counseled about HRT. Strengthening the sphincter and supporting structures of the bladder (Kegel exercises) should be promoted. Pelvic muscle assessment should become as much a part of preventive health care of women as annual Pap tests and regular mammography. Although several surgical interventions exist for UI, the success rate varies greatly. Comprehensive behavioral and medical management of UI is recommended before referral for surgery (Jay and Staskin, 1998).

Depression

Mental illness patterns vary for women and men. Findings from epidemiology through community-based surveys indicate that women are more likely to experience major depression and phobias. It is possible that 1 in 10 women in a primary care setting may be experiencing major depression (Landau and Milan, 1996). Men have higher rates of antisocial personality disorder and alcohol abuse.

A number of factors that may contribute to the development of depression in women have been identified, including unhappy intimate relationships, history of sexual and physical abuse, reproductive events, multiple roles, ethnic minority status, low self-esteem, poverty, and unemployment. Nursing research has also documented the importance of women's social networks in protecting them from depression and enhancing their self-esteem (Woods et al, 1994). Women may derive great satisfaction from interpersonal relationships, but they are also at greater risk for depression when conflict in these relationships occur.

Research is beginning to document that older women are a high-risk group for depression. Causes of depression in older women are loss of physical health, loss of a spouse from death or divorce, and financial problems.

Nurses should be aware of the signs and symptoms of depression. Depression may be identified in the workplace, adversely affecting the woman's work satisfaction and performance. Prompt referral for professional mental health services should be made if depression is suspected. Women may also benefit from a group support that focuses on developing coping skills for dealing with difficult relationships and role conflict.

MEN'S HEALTH

Males are physiologically more vulnerable than females. More male infants die at birth. More males die of cardiovascular, liver, and chronic pulmonary diseases, as well as cancers and suicide. Males have a shorter predicted life span. Many explanations exist for such differences in gender health outcomes: genetics, risk-taking behaviors, stressors, ignoring warning signs, and many others. Men's health, as a separate and distinct practice of care, is at an early developmental level. Men's health goes beyond care of the prostate, genitalia, sexual dysfunction, and associated diseases. Today's focus is on the entire person, requiring a holistic approach.

HOW MEN DEFINE HEALTH

Although men and women have similar ideas about health, there are some distinct differences. Most people view health as being closely associated with well-being. Both men and women define *health* comprehensively and refer to it as a state or condition of well-being, and they often relate this condition to capacity, performance, and function.

HEALTH STATUS OF MEN IN THE UNITED STATES

Health is related to a sense of self and the physical body, and both are tied to past and future actions. When men are asked about health, they look at physical, mental, and emotional well-being. Also, they believe the state of self has the potential to affect the state of others. Many men believe health is individual. This means one person's idea of health and well-being may differ from another's thoughts of being healthy. Men frequently refer to healthiness as "keeping" or "being in control" and "minding" one's body. Men seem to imagine themselves as having "power over" their relationship to their bodies. Men speak about their bodies as though they "belong" to them in the same way an object belongs to them (Saltonstall, 1993).

The former focus on diseases and treatments is shifting to a new health care focus on identifying health needs and preventing health problems. This preventive focus is a wise one: men have been identified as a high-risk group. They frequently engage in compensatory, aggressive, and risk-taking behavior predisposing them to illness, injury, and even death. Men tend to avoid medical help as long as possible, leading to serious health problems.

Men need to openly express their health care concerns. Health care professionals can help men examine their concerns by encouraging them to discuss non-health problems, as well as health care problems, and by promoting preventive health care. Although some men are apprehensive about intimate interaction with professionals, strategies can be used to reduce men's anxiety. Nurses should remove physical barriers separating themselves from the client, use handouts and other written information to support verbal instructions, and show a genuine interest in men's needs.

In the United States, men's life expectancy for all ages is one of the lowest in developed countries and much lower than women. For American adolescents (15 to 24 years of age) and young adult men (25 to 34 years of age), death rates are more than twice those of men in Japan and the Netherlands. In addition, American men ages 45 to 54 years

rank second highest in death rates among the 13 developed countries; but, interestingly enough, mortality has significantly declined for American men ages 45 to 54 years. The least progress toward decline in death rates is in the men's age group of 25 to 34 years. Accidents, homicides and other violence, cancers, circulatory system diseases, and infectious and parasitic diseases account for most deaths in developed countries. American men rank high in all areas except the last one. The good news is that men's ischemic heart disease is declining in the United States; however, American men's and women's heart disease mortalities are still among the highest in the world (U.S. Congress, Office of Technology Assessment, 1993).

LEADING CAUSES OF MEN'S DEATHS
Heart and Cardiovascular Diseases

For men, heart disease is the leading cause of death. This health statistic is unquestionably significant in young and middle-age men. For young men (25 to 44 years), heart disease is 2.6 times higher than for females; for middle-age men (45 to 64 years), it is 2.5 times higher (Table 19-6) (Report of final mortality statistics, 1997).

Coronary heart disease (CHD) is the leading cause of morbidity and mortality in the United States despite the decline during the last three decades. Table 19-7 describes differences in the types of chest pain.

Cancer

Malignant neoplasms are the second leading cause of death for men of all ages.

Prostate Cancer

The second most common cancer among U.S. men, next to pulmonary neoplasms is **prostate cancer** (Report of final mortality statistics, 1997). The risk for prostate cancer increases with each decade after 50 years of age and is highest among men 75 years and older. In reviewing race and ethnic data, African-American men have the highest reported death percentages, followed by Caucasian men; Hispanic men; American Indian men; and Asian men the lowest (Landis, et al, 1998).

The exact cause of prostate cancer is unknown. Genetics, hormones, diet, environment, and viruses have all been implicated as risk factors. Early diagnosis is essential because treatment is usually unsuccessful unless it is done in the early stages of the disease. One diagnostic problem is the lack of symptoms; thus the cancer may be advanced before detection.

The two most commonly used early diagnosis methods are an annual **digital rectal examination (DRE)** and the *serum prostate-specific antigen (PSA)*. DRE can detect palpable masses. The presence of asymmetry, induration, or a firm nodule is a sign of cancer. Men identify the examination as painful and avoid the procedure; however, the test is inexpensive and results are quick. PSA is a serum protease

TABLE 19-6	Heart and Vascular Disease Death Rates and Death Ratios of Young and Middle-Age Men and Women					
	Young (25 to 44 years)			Middle Age (45 to 64 years)		
	Men	Women	Death Ratio	Men	Women	Death Ratio
Heart disease	29.6	11.5	2.6	286.8	112.7	2.5
Vascular disease	4.5	3.9	1.1	33.2	25.4	1.3

From Report of final mortality statistics, 1995, *Monthly Vital Stat Rep* 45(2suppl), 1997.

TABLE 19-7	Assessing Chest Pain	
	Angina	**Myocardial Infarction**
Onset	Sudden or gradual	Sudden
Duration	Usually 15 min	30 to 120 min
Location	Substernal or anterior chest; however not sharply localized	Same as for angina
Radiation	Back, neck, arms, jaw, abdomen, or fingers	Jaws, neck, back, shoulder, and one or both arms
Quality and intensity	Mild to moderate as tightness, pressure described as squeezing and crushing	Persistent and severe pressure described similarly to angina pain

used to detect nonpalpable and recurrent prostrate lesions. Serial measurements increase over time and are more important than an elevated one-time result (Pobursky, 1995). Other forms of testing include transrectal ultrasounds, x-ray assessment, computerized tomography and magnetic resonance imaging (MRI), and biopsy.

More frequent examinations are recommended for men who are considered at risk. Two factors considered to indicate risk are:

1. Continuing urinary symptoms and a history of blood relatives with prostatic cancer
2. Benign prostatic hypertrophy or a partial prostatectomy. Even though survival rates have improved, it is still necessary to continue to educate men concerning the risks and the need for regular examinations.

Closely related and a precursor to prostate cancer is benign prostatic hyperplasia (BPH). Aging is the major risk factor for BPH. By 60 years of age, more than 50% of men will experience BPH. This rate increases to 90% by 85 years of age. In fact, one in four U.S. men will require treatment of symptomatic BPH by 80 years (Public Health Service, 1994). Symptoms may include:

- Frequency of urination
- Nocturia
- Urgency
- Straining to urinate
- Hesitancy in urination
- Weak or intermittent stream
- Feeling of incomplete emptying.

Prostate enlargement does not necessarily correlate with the severity of the symptoms or the amount of restriction to urine flow. Complications may include urinary retention, renal insufficiency, urinary tract infections, hematuria, or bladder stones.

Testicular Cancer

Testicular cancer is a commonly found solid-tumor malignancy in men 15 to 35 years of age. The etiology of this cancer, testicular germ cell, is unknown. Many possible explanations exist:

- Age
- Endocrine problems
- Genetic disorders
- Socioeconomic factors
- Occupational factors.

The most common presenting symptom is a painless, firm scrotal mass or swelling accidentally discovered. Low back pain may result with retroperitoneal lymph node involvement. It is unfortunate that most men do not practice risk appraisal strategies to detect this cancer. Walker (1993) found 83% of men do not perform **testicular self-examination (TSE).**

Modeling and guided practice should be components of a comprehensive testicular educational program. Instructions are on how to perform a monthly TSE are provided in the How To box on p. 334 and in Figure 19-3. A program may consist of audiovisual aids and pamphlets followed by step-by-step procedures and return demonstrations. These approaches lead to increased frequency of TSE and enhanced comfort levels of the men performing the procedure (Walker, 1993). If tumors are found, the most common form of management is retroperitoneal lymph node dissection and chemotherapy for metastases larger than 3 cm.

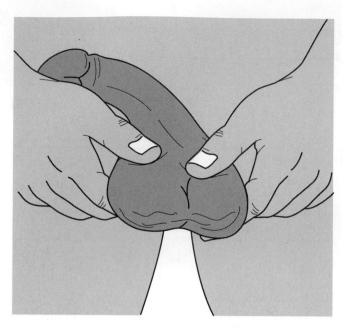

Figure 19-3 Performing a testicular self-examination.

HOW TO Perform a Step-by-Step Monthly Testicular Self-Examination

1. Perform the testicular self-examination during a warm bath or shower.
2. Roll each testicle between your thumb and fingers using warm hands. Testicles should be egg shaped, 4 cm, oblong, similar in size, and have a rubbery texture; the left dangles lower than the right.
3. Check the epididymis for softness and slight tenderness.
4. Check the spermatic cord for firm, smooth tubular structure.

Skin Cancer

The three main types of skin cancers are *basal* and *squamous cell carcinoma* and *malignant melanomas.* When these are combined, skin cancers ranked as the fifth highest new reported cancers among men (Landis, et al, 1998). Men's death rate was much higher than women's death rate in 1995 (Report of final mortality statistics, 1997).

Prolonged sun exposure and high ultraviolet B cause skin cancer. Red-, blond-, or light brown-haired men with light complexions or freckles are the most susceptible. Also, men with a history of long-term occupational or recreational sun exposure such as farmers, construction workers, sailors, swimmers, surfers, and sunbathers are at high risk.

Malignant melanoma is the deadliest form of skin cancer and the incidence is rising worldwide (Fig. 19-4). This cancer can metastasize to the brain, lungs, bones, liver, and other areas of the skin with generally fatal results. With early screening, the 5-year relative survival rate is high (Landis, et al, 1998).

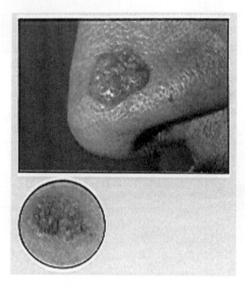

Figure 19-4 Skin cancer.

Prevention includes:
- Decreasing exposure to direct sunlight, especially between the peak hours of 10 AM and 3 PM.
- Wearing protective clothing
- Using a sunblock of at least SPF 15 or higher when outside
- Regularly inspecting and assessing skin.

Early diagnosis and treatment will increase the chances of recovery.

Accidents

The fourth leading cause of men's death for all ages is accidental death.

Fatal Accidents

Men are at higher risk for fatal occupational injuries than women. A breakdown of occupational fatalities by gender is listed in Table 19-8. The **men/women death ratios** differed greatly.

Nonfatal Accidents

Sprains and strains accounted for approximately one half of all work-related injuries in 1992. About one fifth of the nonfatal injuries occurred to the back, caused by overexertion from lifting, pulling, or pushing objects or persons. Again, men accounted for nearly two thirds of these cases. Occupations with the highest back injuries were nonconstruction laborers, truck drivers, and nursing aides or orderlies (U.S. Department of Labor, 1994).

Pulmonary Diseases

Chronic obstructive pulmonary disease is the fifth leading cause of age-adjusted death among men. Men have a 1.5 times greater chance of dying from chronic pulmonary problems than women. It should be noted that the incidence of emphy-

TABLE 19-8	Number and Percent Distribution of Fatal Occupational Injuries by Gender			
	Men (n=5657)		**Women (n=426)**	
	Number	Percent	Number	Percent
Transportation	2263	40	162	38
Assaults and violent acts	1018	18	183	43
Contact with objects and equipment	962	17	21	5
Falls	566	10	30	7
Exposure to harmful substances or environment	566	10	17	4
Fire and exposure	170	3	4	1

From Toscano G, Windau J: *Fatal work injuries: results from 1992 national census,* Report 870, Washington, D.C., 1994, U.S. Department of Labor, Bureau of Labor Statistics.

sema and respiratory system cancer death rates are higher in men than in women (Report of final mortality statistics, 1997).

Smoking is a definite pulmonary disease risk factor. Traditionally, men have used tobacco more than women; however, this trend is changing. Early studies found that men were more likely than women to become regular smokers. More recent data indicate women are more likely than men to have tried smoking. In recent decades the public, and especially men, have received education concerning the dangers of smoking. This has resulted in a decrease in the prevalence of smoking, chiefly in men. Evidence indicates men's cessation rates were higher than women's in middle-age and older smokers during the 1960s and 1970s. In the United States, education is an important factor concerning gender differences in smoking. Men in two categories—ages 19 to 24 years old and those who attended college—are less likely than females in all categories to become smokers.

Briefly Noted

It is clear that tobacco use in any form has detrimental effects on personal health. Current legislation has limited or banned smoking in public places. These policies have been criticized by smokers who cite the "common courtesy approach" as being effective.

Human Immunodeficiency Virus and Acquired Immunodeficiency Syndrome

Acquired immunodeficiency syndrome (AIDS) is a major health concern in the world and United States. Death rates differ widely between men and women for all ages and all races.

The incidence of HIV in the United States during the 1990s had fallen to a level below the peak of the mid-1980s (Karon et al, 1996), but much of the decline reflects trends in Caucasian homosexual men older than 30 years. There is some evidence that the rate is once again increasing. Teenagers and young adults engaging in high-risk sexual behaviors and drug use is the reason the epidemic continues in this age-group.

Homosexual contact was the leading exposure category for young Caucasian, African-American, and Hispanic men with AIDS. In 1995 the incidence of AIDS attributed to homosexual contact was four times higher in African-American men and two times higher in Hispanic men than in Caucasian men. Injection drug use was the second leading exposure category, followed by heterosexual contact (Rosenberg and Biggar, 1998).

AIDS spreads by direct contact with:
- Infected blood or body fluids
- Vaginal secretions
- Semen
- Breast milk.

High-risk groups include sexually active men with multiple partners and intravenous drug users. The risk of HIV and AIDS being introduced through blood and blood products has been greatly reduced. All blood donated in the United States has been tested for the HIV antibody since 1985. Individuals who donate are also screened as to health history and risk behaviors.

The signs and symptoms of AIDS vary from person to person but may include:
- Diarrhea
- Night sweats
- Fever
- Weight loss
- Fatigue
- Persistent cough
- Memory problems.

A person may be asymptomatic or have any one or a combination of symptoms. Treatment is directed at symptom relief.

The occurrence of this disease has created both ethical and financial questions. The cost for care and treatment of AIDS continues to grow, and many male AIDS clients find insurance companies refusing to pay as costs soar. Men have been fired from their jobs, refused medical treatment, and driven out of their communities. Although such discrimination is against the law, it still occurs. Ethical standards of confidentiality, privacy, and treatment have been challenged. The result is that men with HIV and AIDS remain silent about their disease. Many persons in high-risk groups decline to be tested out of fear of potential results. Health care workers both in acute care and community health must maintain confidentiality and demonstrate high ethical standards.

Briefly Noted

If a person with HIV or AIDS knowingly infects another person, it may be considered a criminal offense.

Suicide

Some of the most significant gender health differences occur in the mental health domain. Suicide is five times more likely to occur in men than women. In addition, suicide is the ninth leading cause of death overall for men. High-risk groups are men 15 to 24 years old (the third leading cause) and men 25 to 44 years old (the fourth leading cause) (Report of final mortality statistics, 1997).

Suicide is a significant problem in men, since they are more likely to make a serious attempt to kill themselves rather than to use a suicide attempt as a cry for help. Elderly persons are more likely to use violent and lethal means, and they communicate their intentions less frequently.

Suicide is tragic because it can often be prevented and such a loss causes grief for family members and friends. Nurses in community health often can identify men at risk for suicide. Table 19-9 shows selected suicidal risk factors.

TABLE 19-9   Suicide Risk Factors

Factors	Conditions
Gender	Men use more violent means and have a higher completed suicide rate.
Marital status	Unmarried men have a greater risk than married men.
Employment	Unemployed men are at greater risk.
Previous attempts	Men with more than one attempt have a much higher chance of attempting again. One fourth to one half of completed suicides are by people who have made previous attempts.
Family history	A positive family history increases the risk of suicide.
Medical illness	Men suffering from terminal illness or other medical conditions are at high risk.

Despite the widespread use of telephone crisis lines, school-based intervention programs, and antidepressive medications, high rates of suicide continue. All suicide attempts should be taken seriously. The nurse's goals are to:
- Detect risk factors
- Promote safety
- Prevent self-harm
- Make appropriate referrals
- Help people return to health.

Homicide

Men are prone to engage in dangerous and risky behavior, such as carrying weapons and fighting. Homicides are the tenth leading cause of death in men of all ages. More significantly, for 15- to 24-year-old men, homicides are the second leading cause of death.

Assaultive violence is defined as "nonfatal and fatal interpersonal violence where physical force or other means is used by a person with intent of causing harm, injury, or death to another" (Rosenberg and Mercy, 1991, p. 14).

Multiple causes are attributed to violent behavior. For example, brain dysfunction is associated with irregularities in the limbic system, the part of the brain that regulates emotions and motivation and is associated with violence. Other causes of dysfunction include organic brain disease, psychosis, depression, mental retardation, and brain tumors.

Violence is associated with social, economic, cultural, and environmental factors that especially contribute to assaults among African-American youth (Hammond and Yung, 1993). Poverty and inner-city residency also have been shown to be strongly associated with violent victimization among all adolescents. For African-American males 15 to 24 years, homicide is the leading cause of death. Further, for African-American males 25 to 44 years, it is the second leading death cause in their age bracket (Report of final mortality statistics, 1997).

The Justice Department estimates half the households in the United States have a gun (Maguire and Pastore, 1994). One example of health-related problems of gun ownership is workplace homicides. Gunshot wounds account for more than 80% of workplace homicides, and male workers make up 83% of the victims (Windau and Toscano, 1994).

Violence is a public health emergency. Solutions are complex but are believed to be reachable. First, nurses need to identify signs and symptoms of violent behavior. The practitioner should be concerned about a man who is excessively restless and agitated; he may pace up and down or start pounding on walls, doors, furniture, and other objects. He may appear angry and tense by clenching his teeth, jaw, and fists. His voice may become loud, and he may use profanity. He may become argumentative by refusing to follow directions and making threats. Another sign to watch for includes impulsive behaviors. Alcohol and drug abuse and psychiatric disorders are highly associated with violent behavior. Finally, the most predictive indicator of violence is a history of aggressive behavior and family violence.

Alcohol-Induced Disorders

An evaluation of gender differences reveals the men's age-adjusted death rate for alcohol-induced causes is higher for men than for women (Report of final mortality statistics, 1997).

Chronic liver disease and cirrhosis represent a health hazard associated with alcohol abuse. Age-adjusted gender death rates from alcohol abuse demonstrate striking differences. African-American men have an even higher death rate than African-American women (Report of final mortality statistics, 1997).

Patterns of alcohol, tobacco, and drug usage established during the teen years often persist into adulthood, contributing to a leading cause of mortality and morbidity. Alcohol is closely associated with several negative aspects of society:

- Suicide
- Violent crime
- Birth defects
- Domestic and sexual abuse.

Alcohol is the major cause of all fatal and nonfatal motor vehicle accidents among teenage drivers. Among high school seniors, males drink more (binge drinking) than females in all ethnic groups. In addition to alcohol-related injuries, illnesses, and deaths, drinking can have negative consequences on family, friends, and employment.

Alcohol leads to dependence associated with one's inability to cut down on drinking, including morning drinking, memory losses, and other related medical problems. Almost 50% of separated and divorced men under 45 years of age have been exposed to alcoholism in the family. Also, separated and divorced men are three times more likely than married men to say they have been married to an alcoholic or problem drinker.

Society must remember that alcohol consumption is a major drug problem. Nurses must start educating the younger population about the effects of alcohol. One focal point is the message to "stop underage drinking." Even though alcohol use by persons under 21 years of age is illegal in most states, alcohol is easily accessible. Education is the best prevention at this time and should begin in elementary schools.

MEN'S HEALTH PRACTICES IN EVERYDAY LIFE

Men and women both have unquestionable biological and physiological needs for rest, exercise, and food consumption to maintain health. When asked, men and women differ on the most important needs to maintain health. Women listed food first, then exercise, and then rest. Men rate exercise first, then sleep, and food last. Men emphasized the nutrient quality of food; women focused on the food's calories rather than its nutrient quality. Men perceived **body maintenance** activities as essential to producing health for oneself and

emphasized sports and outdoor activities as influencing better body maintenance. Further, men viewed the body as a medium of action; function and capacity were of major importance (Saltonstall, 1993).

The concept of *body maintenance images* has two components: inner and outer. Inner refers to optimal functioning, performance, and capacity to do things. Outer refers to appearance, movement within social space, and having the potential to be heard and touched. Men discern the inner phenomenon as a function and capacity more than the outer body phenomenon of appearance. Men would rather look at how they went through the day, what they accomplished, and what kind of physical shape they are in so they can perform their tasks and life activities. Less attention is given to having good color and skin tones.

Men need to take an individual conscious look at themselves and develop a plan to stay healthy and free of illness by becoming knowledgeable about health and their own individual bodies. Along with knowledge comes desire to be healthy. In addition, men need to set health-related goals and develop an action plan. With the support of the nursing profession, men can take responsibility in changing and maintaining healthier lifestyles. Table 19-10 summarizes men's biological and psychosocial health care needs.

ELDER HEALTH

The growth of the population ages 65 and older in the United States has steadily increased since the turn of the century. Estimates are that two thirds of a nurse's career today is spent working with elders (Simon, Fletcher, and Francis, 1998). Since most health care for elders is delivered outside of the acute care setting, nurses in community health in particular have been providing nursing care to an increased proportion of elders, which calls for specialized knowledge, skills, and abilities in gerontology.

HEALTH STATUS OF ELDERS

An individual born in 1900 could expect to live to be about 47 years of age. A newborn in 1996 represented about one in every eight Americans (American Association of Retired Persons, 1996). The oldest old (those over age 85) are the fastest growing subgroup of elders. The longer an individual lives, the more likely that person will live even longer. Persons reaching age 65 have an average life expectancy of an additional 18 years. Future growth projections reveal that by the year 2030, when the baby boom generation reaches age 65, there will be about 70 million elders. That number represents more than twice the number of elders in society today.

A closer look at the demographics of elders today reveals a sex ratio of 145 women for every 100 men. Women outlive men by about 7 years, an advantage that is suspected to be biological. Minority populations today represent about 15% of all elders, with projections that the minority composition will double by the year 2030. Most older adults live in a noninstitutional

TABLE 19-10	Men's Health Care Needs	
Need	**Source of Need**	**Description**
Expression	Psychosocial	Desire to communicate with others about health care concerns
Support	Psychosocial	Support from others about certain sex roles and life-styles that influence their physical and mental health
Respect and dignity	Combination of Biological and Psychosocial	Attention from professionals regarding factors that may cause illness or affect a man's expression of illness, including occupational factors, leisure patterns, and interpersonal relationships
Health-seeking knowledge and behaviors	Biological	Information about their body's functions, what is normal and abnormal, what action to take, and the contributions of proper nutrition and exercise Self-care instruction including testicular and genital self-examinations Physical examination and history taking that include sexual and reproductive health and illness across the life span
Holistic medical care and availability	Psychosocial	Adjustment of health care system to men's occupational constraints regarding time and location of source of health care
	Combination of Biological and Psychosocial	Treatment for problems of couples, including interpersonal problems, infertility, family planning, sexual concerns, and sexually transmitted diseases
Parental guidance	Psychosocial	Help with fathering (e.g., being included as a parent in care of children) Help with fathering as a single parent, in particular, with a child of the opposite sex, in addressing the child's sexual development and concerns
Coping	Psychosocial	Recognition that feelings of confusion and uncertainty in a time of rapid social change are normal and may mark onset of healthy adaptation to change
Fiduciary	Biological	Financial ways to obtain health

community setting, and a majority of them live with someone else. About 4% of the elderly live in a nursing home, a likelihood that increases significantly as one ages. Elders as a whole are not an affluent group. Chronological age is an arbitrary way to project health care needs because the state of health differs widely among elders. The age of 65 has been used as a benchmark since 1935, when Franklin Delano Roosevelt used this age in eligibility criteria for Social Security. This seemed to be a reasonable criteria at the time since most individuals did not live long enough to collect Social Security. As life expectancy has grown, consideration has been given to increasing the age at which one might be eligible for Social Security. Although chronological age is limiting, some projections in the area of physical function and prevalence of chronic illness can be made. More than half of elders report having difficulty in carrying out **basic activities of daily living (ADLs)** such as bathing, dressing, eating and **instrumental activities of daily living (IADLs)** such as preparing meals, taking medications, managing money, with a disproportionate share of individuals with disability in the higher age group (Fig. 19-5).

The last few years of an elder's life are often spent in declining physical functioning. A goal for nurses is to help elders maximize functional status and minimize functional

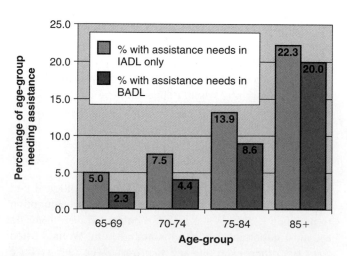

Figure 19-5 Percentage of individuals needing assistance with activities of daily living by age: 1992. (From American Association of Retired Persons: *A profile of older Americans: 1995,* Washington, D.C., 1996, American Association of Retired Persons.)

decline. Health promotion and disease prevention strategies must be emphasized in the elderly.

Briefly Noted

Surveys documenting the functional status rating of an individual by the nurse, the caregiver, and the clients themselves often differs. What factors cause the different perspectives in measuring and noting functional status?

DEFINITIONS RELATED TO ELDER HEALTH

Aging, if defined purely from a physiological perspective, has been described as a process of deterioration of body systems. This definition is obviously inadequate to describe the multidimensional aging process in elders. *Aging* can be more appropriately defined as the sum total of all changes that occur in a person with the passing of time. Influences on how one ages come from several domains that include the physiological processes, as well as psychological, sociological, and spiritual processes. The physiological declines associated with aging have been easier to understand than aging as a process of growth and development.

Myths associated with aging have evolved over time. Some of the common myths involve the perception that all elders:

- Are infirm
- Are senile
- Cannot adapt to change
- Cannot learn new behaviors or skills.

These myths are easily debunked by elders who run marathons, learn to use the internet, and are vibrant members of society. **Ageism** is the term used for prejudice toward older people. Prejudice may be obvious or subtle. Ageism fosters a stereotype of elders that does not allow them to be viewed realistically.

Gerontology is the specialized study of the processes of growing old. **Geriatrics** is the study of disease in old age. **Gerontological nursing** is the specialty of nursing concerned with assessment of the health and functional status of older adults, planning and implementing health care and services to meet the identified needs, and evaluating the effectiveness of such care (Lueckenotte, 1996).

MULTIDIMENSIONAL INFLUENCES ON AGING

The elder experiences aging in many ways: physiologically, psychologically, sociologically, and spiritually. Physiologic changes occur in all body systems with the passing of time. How and when these processes occur between individuals varies widely, as well as the degree of aging within the various body systems in the same individual. Table 19-11 highlights physiological changes with the aging of body systems and the nursing implications of these changes. The effect of

TABLE 19-11   Physiological Aging Changes in Body Systems

Age-Related Change	Implication for Nursing
Skin	
Thinning	Prone to skin breakdown and injury
Atrophy of sweat glands	Increased risk of heat stroke
Decrease in vascularity	Frequent pruritus / Dry skin
Respiratory	
Decreased elasticity of lung tissue	Reduced efficiency of ventilation
Decreased respiratory muscle strength	Prone to atelectasis and infection
Cardiovascular	
Decrease in baroreceptor sensitivity	Prone to orthostatic hypotension and falls
Decrease in number of pacemaker cells	Increased prevalence of dysrhythmias
Gastrointestinal	
Dental enamel thins / Gums recede	Periodontal disease common
Delay in esophageal emptying	Prone to swallowing dysfunction
Decreased muscle tone / Altered peristalsis	Prone to constipation
Genitourinary	
Decreased number of functioning nephrons	Modifications in drug dosing may be required
Reduced bladder tone and capacity	Incontinence more common
Prostate enlargement	May compromise urinary function
Neuromuscular	
Decrease in muscle mass	Decrease in muscle strength
Decrease in bone mass	Osteoporosis increases risk of fracture
Loss of neurons/nerve fibers	Altered sensitivity to pain / Delayed reaction time
Sensory	
Decreased visual acuity, depth	May pose safety issue because of altered perception, adaptation to light changes
Loss of auditory neurons	Hearing loss may cause limitation in activities
Altered taste sensation	May change food preferences and intake
Immune	
Decrease in T cell function	Increased incidence of infection
Appearance of autoantibodies	Increased prevalence of autoimmune disorders

these physiological changes overall result in a diminished physiological reserve, decrease in homeostatic mechanisms, and a decline in immunological response.

No known intrinsic psychological changes occur with aging. The influences of the environment and culture on personal development and maturation are substantial and further limit the ability of the nurse to predict how an individual psychologically ages.

Some known and some disputed changes in brain function over time may influence cognition and behavior. Reaction speed and psychomotor response is somewhat slower, which can be related to the neurological changes with aging. This is demonstrated particularly during timed tests of performance in which speed is an influencing variable. It has also been demonstrated in simulated tests of driving skills where speed of response, perception, and attention slow with age. Typically older individuals can learn and perform as well as younger individuals, although they may be slower and it may take them longer to accomplish a specific task.

Intellectual capacity does not decline with age as was previously thought. An age-associated memory impairment, benign senescent forgetfulness, involves very minor memory loss. This is not progressive and does not cause dysfunction in daily living. Reassurance is important for the older adult and families since anxiety often exacerbates the problem of mild memory impairment. Memory aids (e.g., mnemonics, signs, notes) may help the elder compensate for this type of impairment.

Many external factors affect mental health and aging, particularly those associated with loss and change. Adapting and coping responses of even the most resilient individuals will be challenged when successive losses and changes occur within a relatively short period.

The later years for many elders mark a period of changing social dynamics. Social networks provide the structure for social support. Demographics of marital status and living arrangements of elders reveal the magnitude of social change. Half of all older women in 1995 were widows. Although women are more likely to live alone than men (Fig. 19-6), they frequently have more extensive social networks than men, who rely more dominantly on the spousal support.

Higher socioeconomic status, income, and education tend to be reflected in large and differing social networks (Ebersole and Hess, 1998). Families typically remain involved with aging parents, with estimates that more than 5 million are involved in some type of parent care. Not all individuals do remain in their own home or in the home of another. As one ages, social role and status may change, and elders are more vulnerable to social isolation.

Although most of the multidimensional influences of aging are marked by decline and loss, some have suggested that an increased spiritual awareness and consciousness accompanies aging and that religion is a powerful cultural force in the lives of older clients. Spirituality refers to the need to transcend physical, psychological, and social identities to experience love, hope, and meaning in life. Religious

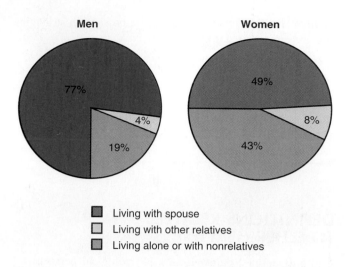

Figure 19-6   **Living arrangements of persons 65 and older: 1995.** (Data from U.S. Census Bureau: *Statistical abstract of the United States, ed 113,* Washington, D.C., 1993, U.S. Government Printing Office.)

affiliations and religious rituals are two aspects of spirituality that can include other activities and relationships. Caring for pets and plants or experiencing nature through a walk in the woods can also foster spiritual growth. Physical and functional impairments and fear of death may challenge one's spiritual integrity. Having a strong sense of spirituality enables individuals who are physically and functionally dependent on others to avoid despair by appreciating that they are still capable of giving and deserving of receiving love, respect, and dignity.

CHRONIC HEALTH CONCERNS OF ELDERS IN THE COMMUNITY

Chronic illnesses occur over a long period with occasional acute exacerbations and remissions. They can affect multiple systems and be expensive and discouraging. The prevalence of chronic disease rises with lengthening of life span and highly technical medical care. Table 19-12 shows the prevalence of chronic conditions for men and women. Not only do chronic conditions cause disability and activity restriction, they often require frequent hospitalizations for exacerbations.

Health care in general is oriented toward acute illness. In **chronic illness,** cure is not expected, so nursing activities need to be more holistic, addressing function, wellness, and psychosocial issues. With chronic illness the focus is on healing (a unique process resulting in a shift in the body/mind/spirit system) rather than curing (elimination of the signs and symptoms of disease). Eliopoulos (1997) lists the following goals for chronic care:

- Maintain or improve self-care capacity
- Manage the disease effectively
- Boost the body's healing abilities
- Prevent complications
- Delay deterioration and decline

TABLE 19-12	Rank Order Prevalence of Chronic Conditions by Gender per 1000 People Ages 70 and Older (1995)	
Condition		**Rate**
Men		
Arthritis		495
Hearing impairment		445
Hypertension		315
Heart disease		300
Vision impairment		179
Orthopedic impairment		144
Women		
Arthritis		633
Hypertension		396
Orthopedic impairment		320
Hearing impairment		318
Heart disease		240
Vision impairment		209

From U.S. Census Bureau: *Statistical abstract of the United States,* ed 113, Washington, D.C., 1993, U.S. Government Printing Office.

- Achieve highest possible quality of life
- Die with comfort, peace, and dignity.

The trajectory model of chronic illness (Corbin and Cherry, 1997) traces a course of illness through phases upward, downward, or plateaued.

HOW TO Evaluate the Phases of Chronic Illness Using the Trajectory Model

The chronic illness may include the following:
- A pretrajectory phase, with certain factors that put an individual at risk
- A trajectory phase when symptoms become noticeable
- Stable and/or unstable phases as the symptoms vary from controlled to reactivated
- Acute and/or episodic phases when symptoms or the development of the illness became more serious or life threatening
- A comeback phase of gradual return to an acceptable level of functioning
- A downward course of decline, deterioration, and an inability to control symptoms, to dying or a shutting down of body processes

Attention is paid to the client's self-concept and self-esteem, as well as to the resources that are needed to manage the disease outside the medical system. Goals for care are structured to:

- Help clients adjust their day-to-day choices
- Maintain the highest level of functional ability possible within the limits of their conditions.

The motivation to make life-style choices necessary to cope with chronic illness stems from the fear of death; disability; pain; and negative effects on work, family, or activity.

Tierney, McPhee, and Papadakis (1996) outline chronic conditions called the **five Is** that can adversely affect the aging experience. These include:
- Intellectual impairment
- Immobility
- Instability
- Incontinence
- Iatrogenic drug reactions.

In addition, Tierney named the **three Ds** of intellectual impairment:
- Dementia (progressive intellectual impairment)
- Depression (mood disorder)
- Delirium (acute confusion).

Immobility is most often caused by degenerative joint disease and results in pain, stiffness, loss of balance, and psychological problems. Fear of falling is a major cause of immobility. This is related to instability, which results in falls in 30% of elders each year.

Urinary incontinence often contributes to institutional care and social isolation. For that reason it is difficult to estimate the numbers of individuals and cost of incontinence. It is important to address continence routinely in the assessment process, identify the type of incontinence, and intervene appropriately.

Iatrogenic drug reactions result from changes in the older individual's absorption, metabolism, and excretion process that lead to altered responses to drugs. Many elderly take numerous medicines, increasing the chance of drug reactions.

Briefly Noted

The average older adult in the community has eleven different prescriptions filled each year. What are some of the hazards of this situation?

One often overlooked concern of elders is that of abuse. *Elder abuse* encompasses physical, psychological, financial, and social abuse or violation of an individual's rights (McKenna, 1997). Abuse consists of the following:
- The willful infliction of physical pain or injury
- Debilitating mental anguish and fear
- Theft or mismanagement of money or resources
- Unreasonable confinement or the depriving of services.

Neglect refers to a lack of services that are necessary for the physical and mental health of an individual by the individual or a caregiver. Elderly persons can make independent choices with which others may disagree. Their right to self-determination can be taken from them if they are declared incompetent. Exploitation is the illegal or improper use of a person or their resources for another's profit or advantage.

During the assessment process, nurses need to be aware of conflicts between injuries and explanation of cause, dependency issues between client and caregiver, and substance abuse by the caregiver. Nearly all 50 states have enacted mandatory reporting laws and have instituted protective service programs. The local social services agency or area agency on aging can help with information on reporting requirements.

The **Patient Self-Determination Act** of 1991 requires those providers receiving Medicare and Medicaid funds to give clients written information regarding their legal options for treatment choices if they become incapacitated. A routine discussion of advance medical directives can help ease the difficult discussions faced by health care professionals, family, and clients. The nurse can assist an individual to complete a values history instrument. These instruments ask questions about specific wishes regarding different medical situations.

This clarifying process then leads to completion of **advance directives** to document these preferences in writing. There are two parts to the advance directives. The **living will** allows the client to express wishes regarding the use of medical treatments in the event of a terminal illness. A **durable power of attorney** is the legal way for the client to designate someone else to make health care decisions when he or she is unable to do so. A Do Not Resuscitate order (DNR) is a specific order from a physician not to use cardiopulmonary resuscitation. State laws vary widely regarding the implementing of these tools, so it is important to consult a knowledgeable source of information. It is also important to involve the family, and especially the designated decision maker or agent, in these discussions so that everyone understands the client's choices.

Briefly Noted

Legislated rights of the elderly include the following:
- Individualized care
- Freedom from discrimination
- Privacy
- Freedom from neglect and abuse
- Control of one's own funds
- Ability to sue
- Freedom from physical and chemical restraint
- Involvement in decision making
- Voting
- Access to community services
- Raise grievances
- Obtain a will
- Enter into contracts
- Practice the religion of one's choice
- Dispose of one's own personal property

Family Caregiving

Eighty-five percent of all elderly live in homes alone, with spouses, or other family or friends. Female spouses represent the largest group of family caregivers of the elderly family

caregivers. *Stress, strain,* and *burnout* are words that are used to reflect the negative effects of the family **caregiver burden.** Issues involve the work itself, past and present relationships, effect on others, and the caregivers' lifestyle and well-being. It is estimated that at least 5 million adults are providing direct care to an elderly relative at any given time, with another 44 to 45 million assuming some type of responsibility for an elder relative. For many families the caregiving experience is a positive, rewarding, and fulfilling one. Nursing intervention can facilitate good health for older persons and their caregivers and contribute to meaningful family relationships during this period. Eliopoulos (1997) uses the acronym TLC to represent these interventions:

T = training in care techniques, safe medication use, recognition of abnormalities, available resources
L = leaving the care situation periodically to obtain respite and relaxation and maintain their normal living needs
C = care for themselves (the caregiver) through adequate sleep, rest, exercise, nutrition, socialization, solitude, support, financial aid, and health management

Briefly Noted

Older adults are at increased risk for infection. Prevention in the community includes encouraging routine handwashing and adapting universal precautions specifically to the practice setting.

COMMUNITY RESOURCES
Strategies for Child Health Care in the Community

Nurses are in a position to work with groups of families or individuals through programs targeting the health care needs of those at risk. Three strategies for common pediatric concerns are identified to model nursing interventions in the community. Strategies include programs based in the home, targeted at the needs of homeless persons, or centered in daycare or school settings. Community resources for children can be found in Box 19-9.

Programs and Services for Women

Changes in the health care delivery system have a profound effect on women. Women are the gatekeepers of their families' health care. They make three fourths of the health care decisions in American households. Additionally, women make more than 61% of physician visits and purchase 59% of prescription drugs (Smith Barney Research, 1997). Because of women's greater involvement with health services, they can play a major role in family health promotion.

Traditional centers of care for women such as Planned Parenthood, feminist women's health centers, and local community health centers can serve as models for women-centered health care delivery. Unfortunately such centers are

Box 19-9	Community Resources for Children's Health Care

- Children's service clinics
- Well-child clinics
- Immunization clinics
- Infectious disease clinics
- Children's specialty services
- Family violence and child abuse centers
- School health programs
- Head Start
- Parents Anonymous
- Crisis hotlines
- Community education classes
- Early intervention/developmental services
- Childbirth education classes
- Breastfeeding support groups
- Parent support groups
- Family planning clinics
- Women, Infants, and Children (WIC) programs
- Medicaid
- Youth employment and training programs

not included in large managed care organizations (MCOs). The women's health service providers authorized by MCOs do not copy these traditional women's health care models. Subsequently, women suffer from the loss of women's centered care (Taylor and Woods, 1996).

Community Care Settings for Elders

Senior centers were developed in the early 1940s to provide social and recreational activities. Now many centers are multipurpose, offering recreation, education, counseling, therapies, hot meals, and case management, as well as health screening and education. Some offer respite care.

Adult day health is for individuals whose mental and/or physical function requires additional health care and supervision. It serves as more of a medical model than the senior center and often individuals return home to their caregivers at night.

Home health can be provided by working in multidisciplinary teams. Nurses provide individual and environmental assessments, direct skilled care and treatment, and short-term guidance and instruction. They work closely with the family and other caregivers to provide necessary communication and continuity of care.

Hospice represents a philosophy of caring for and supporting life to its fullest until death occurs. The hospice team encourages the client and family to jointly make decisions to meet physical, emotional, spiritual, and comfort needs.

Assisted living covers a wide variety of choices from a single shared room to opulent independent living accommodations in a full-service, life care community.

Nursing homes or *long-term care facilities,* as they are often called, house only 4% of the elderly population at a given time; however, 25% of those over 65 years old will

spend some time in a nursing home. Nursing homes provide a safe environment, special diets and activities, routine personal care, and the treatment and management of health care needs for those needing rehabilitation, as well as those needing a permanent supportive residence.

Clinical Application

Using the concepts in this chapter, analyze the following case. Focus on the issues of how men define health, developmental patterns, the health practices of men, and a nursing care plan.

John, a 29-year-old Caucasian man with a wife and three children, was employed as a sales representative in a small, rural community. John's health was excellent except for injuries sustained in a car accident several years ago that required three blood transfusions. After the accident, John returned to work, thinking he was fully recovered. His business success continued, and he was well respected by employers, co-workers, and community leaders.

Years after the accident, John became ill with pneumonia, requiring hospitalization. While he was hospitalized, a blood test discovered HIV. A series of devastating events followed. John and his family decided to keep his condition confidential so he could live the rest of his life as normally as possible.

When John returned to work from the hospital, his co-workers seemed distant and they avoided him. He began to receive threatening telephone calls telling him to leave town, and his car was spray-painted with derogatory words. Clearly, there had been a breach of confidentiality. John later discovered his hospital file was marked "AIDS" in large red letters. Further, he learned nurses refused to care for him while he was hospitalized and he was the focus of dinner conversation throughout the hospital.

John's circumstances worsened, and he felt isolated and rejected. He eventually was fired from work, thereby losing health insurance for himself and his family. His wife divorced him. All his accumulated wealth was depleted. He could not pay his hospital bills; his financial state was compounded by filing for bankruptcy. John was homeless. His symptoms gradually progressed. He had a fever, tachypnea, lymphadenopathy, night sweats, and diarrhea. A friend suggested he visit the clinic. Further, John was reluctant to speak about his disease. He was extremely fatigued and could only whisper. He refused any government services; however, the nurse is able to convince him to enter the homeless shelter across the street for the night. The nurse asks him to return to the clinic in the morning.

Imagine you are the nurse in the health clinic.

A. *What information do you want to collect?*
B. *What nursing diagnoses are relevant based on the collected data?*
C. *What short-term goals are appropriate for the first clinic visit?*
D. *What long-term goal do you want to plan with John?*
E. *What social and health agencies would you consult in planning for John's care?*
F. *What outcome criteria should you use to evaluate the effectiveness of your plans and interventions?*
G. *List issues that may need to be addressed with the wife and children.*

Answers are in the back of the book.

Remember This!

- Good nutrition is essential for healthy growth and development and influences disease prevention in later life. The adolescent population is at greatest risk for poor nutritional health.
- Immunizations are successful in prevention of selected diseases. Barriers to immunizing children are cost and inconvenience.
- The family is critical to the growth and development of the child. Social support is one of the most powerful influences on successful parenting.
- Accidents and injuries are the major cause of health problems in the child and adolescent population. Most are preventable. Nurses have a major role in anticipatory guidance and prevention.
- Nurses are involved in strategies to meet the needs of the pediatric population in the community. Home-based service programs have been successful in providing care for at-risk populations. Children of homeless families are at risk for health problems, environmental dangers, and stress. Community programs to provide health care for the homeless may decrease those risks.
- The women's health movement was pivotal in bringing national recognition to women's health issues.
- Women have a longer life expectancy than men. However, women are more likely to have acute and chronic conditions that require them to use health services more than men.
- Relationships are crucial to the development of female identity.
- Women are known as the gatekeepers of health. Women make three fourths of the health care decisions in American households.
- Women of color are statistically more likely to have poor health outcomes because of a poor understanding of health, lack of access to health care, and life-style practices.
- Smoking is a risk factor for a number of major health problems, including lung cancer, heart disease, osteoporosis, and poor reproductive outcomes.
- The failure to include women in medical research has resulted in a lack of understanding about the distinctive issues surrounding the diagnosis and treatment of the major diseases for women.
- Heart disease is the leading cause of death among women over 50 and the second leading cause of death among women ages 35 to 39.
- Cancer is the second leading cause of death for women.
- In response to the past lack of equality in health-related research and the provision of clinical care, there is now a major national focus on women's health issues.
- Men are physiologically the more vulnerable gender, demonstrated by shorter life spans and a higher infant mortality.
- Life expectancy of men in the United States is one of the lowest in developed countries.
- Men engage in more risk-taking behaviors, such as physical challenges and illegal behaviors, than do women.
- The most significant death rate differences between men and women are for AIDS, suicides, homicides, and accidents.
- Men tend to avoid diagnosis and treatment of illnesses that may result in serious health problems.
- The population 65 and older in the United States is steadily growing, accompanied by an increase in chronic conditions, greater demand for services, and strained health care budgets.
- Most older adults live in the community. The last few years of life often represent functional decline. Nurses strive to help elders maximize functional status and minimize costs through direct care and appropriate referral to community resources.
- Nurses address the chronic health concerns of elders with a focus on maintaining or improving self-care and preventing complications to maintain the highest possible quality of life.
- Assessing the elder incorporates physical, psychological, social, and spiritual domains. Individual and community-focused interventions involve all three levels of prevention through collaborative practice.

What Do You Think?

1. Develop a plan of nursing care for a family who has experienced a SIDS death.
2. Develop a nutritional program for a) mothers who are breastfeeding their infants, b) a group of 5 year olds in a kindergarten class, c) and a group of high school sophomores. What factors do these programs have in common? How do they differ?
3. Design a teaching plan for a middle-age woman that reflects a maximum level of health promotion for her and her family.
4. Analyze mortality and morbidity data in your county and rank the order of the 10 most prevalent health problems for women. Compare these to men's health problems.
5. Interview six men ranging in age from 21 to 70 years and ask them to list what they believe are health risk factors for them, what activities they regularly engage in that promote health, and what changes they believe they should make to promote their own health and reduce any existing risk factors.
6. Using the information gathered in activity 1, design a plan for health promotion for each man who is interviewed, using the man's lifestyle, occupation, interest in social and recreational activities, income level, health risks, limitations in activities, and medical conditions. Review this plan with the man and determine how effectively the plan fits his perception of what he might do to ensure a healthier state.

7. Interview an elder within your family, and ask him or her to list any health problems, how your relative would rate his or her health on a scale of 1 to 10 (with 10 being the highest), and what is included in a typical day's activities. Also, ask the elder to provide a 24-hour dietary recall.
8. Describe what you can do to aid in overcoming the myths and examples of ageism that are pervasive in society.

REFERENCES

Administration on Aging: *Profile of older Americans: 1997,* available online: www.aoa.dhhs.gov

American Association of Retired Persons: *A profile of older Americans: 1995,* Washington, D.C., 1996, American Association of Retired Persons.

Arnstein P, Buselli E, Rankin S: Women and heart attacks: prevention, diagnosis and care, *Nurse Pract* 21(5):57, 1996.

Baldini E, Strauss G: Women and lung cancer: waiting to exhale, *Chest* 112(4):229, 1997.

Brooks JG: Sudden infant death syndrome. In Hoekelman R, et al (editors): *Primary pediatric care,* ed 3, St Louis, 1997, Mosby.

Catalano R, Satariano W: Unemployment and the likelihood of detecting early-stage breast cancer, *Am J Public Health* 88(4):586, 1998.

Conway-Welch C, et al: Women's health and women's health care: recommendations of the 1996 AAN expert panel on women's health, *Nurs Outlook* 45(1):7, 1997.

Cooper G, et al: An ecological study of the effectiveness of mammography in reducing breast cancer mortality, *Am J Public Health* 88(2):281, 1998.

Corbin J, Cherry J: Caring for the aged in the community. In Swanson E, Tripp-Reimer T (editors): *Chronic illness and the older adult,* New York, 1997, Springer.

Craft N: Life span: conception to adolescence (women's health, part 2), *Br Med J* 315(7117):1227, 1997a.

Craft N: Women's health: a global issue, *Br Med J* 315(7116):1154, 1997b.

Dietz W, Stern L: *American Academy of Pediatrics guide to your child's nutrition,* New York, 1999, Villard.

Earls F: Positive effects of prenatal and early childhood interventions, *JAMA* 14:1271, 1998.

Ebersole P, Hess P: *Toward health aging: human needs and nursing response,* ed 5, St Louis, 1998, Mosby.

Eliopoulos C: *Gerontological nursing,* ed 4, Philadelphia, 1994, JB Lippincott.

English A: Understanding legal aspects of care. In Neinstein L: *Adolescent health care; a practical guide,* ed 3, Philadelphia, 1996, Williams & Wilkins.

Forbes GB: Nutrition. In Hoekelman R, et al (editors): Primary pediatric care, ed 3, St Louis, 1997, Mosby.

Geary M: An analysis of the women's health movement and its impact on the delivery of health care within the United States, *Nurse Pract* 20(11):24, 1995.

Grisso J, Ness R, Hendrix S: Update in women's health, *Ann Intern Med* 127(11):1006, 1997.

Hammond W, Yung B: Psychology's role in public health response to assaultive violence among young African-American men, *Am Psychologist* 48:142, 1993.

Hill B, Geraci S: A diagnostic approach to chest pain based on history and ancillary evaluation, *Nurse Pract* 23(4):20, 1998.

Jay J, Staskin D: Urinary incontinence, *Adv Nurse Pract* 6(10):32, 1998.

Karon J, et al: Prevalence of HIV infections in the United States, 1984 to 1992, *JAMA* 276:126, 1996.

Kazanjian P, Eisenstat S: Human immunodeficiency virus. In Noble J (editor): *Textbook of primary care medicine,* ed 2, St Louis, 1996, Mosby.

Kington R, Smith J: Socioeconomic status and racial and ethnic differences in functional status associated with chronic diseases, *Am J Public Health* 87(5):805, 1997.

Kuter I: Breast cancer. In Noble J (editor): *Textbook of primary care medicine,* ed 2, St Louis, 1996, Mosby.

Landau C, Milan F: Depression. In Noble J (editor): *Textbook of primary care medicine,* ed 2, St Louis, 1996, Mosby.

Landis S: Cancer statistics, 1998, *CA Cancer J Clin* 48:6, 1998.

Lueckenotte A: *Gerontological nursing,* St Louis, 1996, Mosby.

Maguire K, Pastore A: *Sourcebook of criminal justice statistics, 1993,* Washington, D.C., 1994, U.S. Department of Justice, Bureau of Justice Statistics.

Manore M: Running on empty: health consequences of chronic dieting in active women, *American College of Sports Medicine's (ACSM's) Health and Fitness Journal* 2(2):24, 1998.

Manson M, et al: Cardiovascular disease in women: a statement for health care professionals from the American Heart Association, *Circulation* 96:2468, 1997.

McCance K, Jorde L: Evaluating the genetic risk of breast cancer, *Nurse Pract* 23(8):14, 1998.

McGee C: Secondary amenorrhea leading to osteoporosis: incidence and prevention, *Nurse Pract* 22(5):38, 1997.

McKenna LS: Elder abuse: preparing to identify and intervene in health care, *Home Care Provider* 2(1):30, 1997.

Miller KJ, Costellanos FX: Attention deficit/hyperactivity disorders, *Pediatr Rev* 19:11, 1998.

Minkoff H, DeHovitz J, Duerr A: *HIV infection in women,* New York, 1995, Raven Press.

National Center for Health Statistics: *FASTATS,* Washington, D.C., 1998, U.S. Government Printing Office.

National Center for Injury Prevention and Control: *Fact sheet,* Nov, 1998, available online: www.cdc.gov/ncipc/duip

National Women's Health Information Center: *Priority women's health issues,* 1998; available online at www.4women.org/owh/pub/womhealthissues/whipriority.htm

Neinstein LS, Schack LE: Nutrition. In Neinstein L: *Adolescent health care; a practical guide,* ed 3, Philadelphia, 1996, Williams & Wilkins.

Pobursky J: Prostate cancer: detection and treatment options, *Today's OR Nurse* 17:5, 1995.

Popkess-Vawter S, Brandau M, Straub J: Triggers of overeating and related intervention strategies for women who weight cycle, *Appl Nurs Res* 11(2):69, 1998.

Press M: Gynecologic cancers, *Cancer* 83(8):1751, 1998.

Public Health Service: *Treating your enlarged prostate,* AHCPR Pub No 94-0583, Rockville, Md, 1994, Public Health Service, Agency for Health Care Policy and Research.

Redlener I: Health care for homeless children: special circumstances. In Green M, Haggerty RJ (editors): *Ambulatory pediatrics,* ed 4, Philadelphia, 1991, WB Saunders.

Report of final mortality statistics, 1995, *Monthly Vital Stat Rep* 45(2suppl), 1997.

Rosenberg P, Biggar R: Trends in HIV incidence among young adults in the United States, *JAMA* 279:1894, 1998.

Ross C: A comparison of osteoarthritis and rheumatoid arthritis: diagnosis and treatment, *Nurse Pract* 22(9):20, 1997.

Saltonstall R: Healthy bodies, social bodies: men's and women's concepts and practices of health in everyday life, *Soc Sci Med* 36:7, 1993.

Simon L, Fletcher K, Francis D: The geriatric resource model of care: a vision for the future. In Abraham I, Fulmer T, Milisen K (editors): Advances in geriatric nursing, *Nurs Clin North Am* 33(3):481, 1998.

Soet J, DiIorio C, Dudley W: Women's self-reported condom use: intra and interpersonal factors, *Women Health* 27(4):19, 1998.

Smith Barney Research: *The new women's movement: women's healthcare,* April, 1997, Author.

Taylor D, Woods N: Changing women's health, changing nursing practice, *J Obstet Gynecol Neonat Nurs* 25(9):791, 1996.

Tierney LM, McPhee SJ, Papadakis MA: *Current medical diagnosis and treatment,* ed 35, East Norwalk, Conn, 1996, Appleton & Lange.

Tindall W: When joints—and cost—become inflamed, *Business and Health* 15(12):47, 1997.

Toscano G, Windau J: *Fatal work injuries: results from 1992 national census,* Report 870, Washington, D.C., 1994, U.S. Department of Labor, Bureau of Labor Statistics.

U.S. Census Bureau: *Statistical abstract of the United States,* ed 113, Washington, D.C., 1993, U.S. Government Printing Office.

U.S. Congress, Office of Technology Assessment: *International health statistics: what the numbers mean for the United States: background paper,* pub no OTA-BP-H-116, Washington, D.C., 1993, U.S. Government Printing Office.

U.S. Department of Health and Human Services: *Healthy people 2010: national health promotion and disease prevention objectives,* Washington, D.C., 2000, U.S. Department of Health and Human Services.

U.S. Department of Labor: *Work injuries and illnesses by selected characteristics,* pub no USDL-94-213, Washington, D.C., 1994, Bureau of Labor Statistics.

U.S. Preventive Services Task Force: *Guide to clinical preventive services: report of the U.S. Preventive Services Task Force,* Washington, D.C., 1996, Philadelphia, 1996, Williams & Wilkins.

Walker R: Modeling and guided practice as components within a comprehensive testicular self-examination educational program for high school males, *J Health Educ* 24:162, 1993.

Wertheim I, Soto-Wright V, Goodman H: Gynecologic cancers. In Noble J (editor): *Textbook of primary care medicine,* ed 2, St Louis, 1996, Mosby.

Whitmore S: Rebuilding bone, *Adv Nurse Pract* 6(9):30, 1998.

Windau J, Toscano G: *Workplace homicides in 1992,* Report 870, Washington D.C., 1994, U.S. Department of Labor, Bureau of Labor Statistics.

Woodhead G, Moss M: Osteoporosis: diagnosis and prevention, *Nurse Pract* 23(11):18, 1998.

Woods NF, et al: Depressed mood and self-esteem in young Asian, black and white women in America, *Health Care Women Int* 15:243, 1994.

Part 6

Vulnerability: Predisposing Factors

As the twenty-first century begins and the complexity of health and social problems increases, community health problems remain more a societal problem than an individual problem. Solutions will require an integrated social and health care approach that begins with a commitment to primary health care. Primary health care involves a partnership between public health and primary care to address the problems of the society as well as those of the individual.

Communities increasingly experience significant problems as a result of conditions that are often expensive and hard to treat: violence against people and property, abuse of substances among people of all groups, and an increasing number of people disenfranchised from society, whose personal resources and access to health and social services are limited. This section presents a discussion of the most common problems seen in communities.

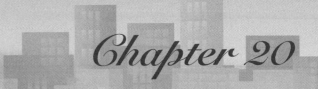

Chapter 20

Vulnerability and Selected Vulnerable Populations

JULIANN G. SEBASTIAN • CHRISTINE DiMARTILE BOLLA

DYAN ARETAKIS • KIM DUPREE JONES

CHERYL PANDOLF SCHENK • MARIE NAPOLITANO

PATRICIA B. HOWARD

OBJECTIVES

After reading this chapter, the student should be able to:

- Define what is meant by vulnerability and describe selected vulnerable groups.
- Discuss the effects of poverty and homelessness on the health and well-being of individuals, families, and communities.
- Describe why pregnant teens, migrant workers, and seriously mentally ill people are considered vulnerable.

- Explain how socioeconomic status, age, health status, biological factors, and life experiences can lead to vulnerability.
- Describe factors to include when assessing for vulnerability.
- Describe community-oriented nursing interventions for vulnerable populations.

CHAPTER OUTLINE

Vulnerability: Definition and Influencing Factors

Conceptual Bases of Vulnerability

Predisposing Factors

Outcomes of Vulnerability

Selected Vulnerable Population Groups
   Poor and Homeless People
   Pregnant Teens
   Migrant Workers
   Severely Mentally Ill Individuals

Public Policies Affecting Vulnerable Populations
   Ways Managed Care Has Affected Vulnerable Populations

Nursing Intervention for Vulnerable Populations
   Assessment of Vulnerable Populations
   Planning and Implementing Care for Vulnerable Populations

KEY TERMS

cumulative risks: the additive effects of multiple risk factors.

deinstitutionalization: effort to move long-term psychiatric patients out of the hospital and back into their own communities.

disadvantaged: lacking adequate resources that other people may take for granted.

disenfranchisement: sense of social isolation; a feeling of isolation from mainstream society.

episodically homeless: moving in and out of homelessness; frequently lacking permanent shelter.

federal poverty level: income level for a certain family size that the federal government uses to define poverty.

Continued

KEY TERMS—cont'd

hidden homeless: people who are usually invisible members of a community since they have no shelter while in that community. An example is migrant workers.

homelessness: the federal government defines a homeless person as one who lacks a fixed, regular, and adequate address or has a primary nighttime residence in a supervised publicly or privately operated shelter for temporary accommodations.

human capital: the combined human potential of the people living in a community.

migrant farm worker: a laborer whose principal employment involves moving from farm to farm, planting or harvesting agriculture, and living in temporary housing.

pesticide exposure: occurs when a person comes into contact with chemical poisons used to eliminate pests or increase crop production by developing healthy crops.

poverty: lacking resources to meet basic living expenses for food, shelter, clothing, transportation, and medical care.

resilience: ability to withstand many forms of stress and deal with several problems simultaneously without developing health problems.

risk: the likelihood that some event or outcome will occur in a given time frame.

severely mentally ill (SMI) individuals: those who have a major psychosis such as schizophrenia or bipolar disorder.

sexual debut: time when sexual activity begins.

vulnerability: results from the interaction of internal and external factors that cause a person to be susceptible to poor health.

vulnerable populations: those with increased risk to develop poor health outcomes.

The old saying, "All men [women] are created equal" is really not true. People have different genetic compositions, social and environmental resources, skills, and access to health services. People with lower incomes and less education are more likely to have shorter lives and more illness, injuries, and exposure to environmental hazards (National Center for Health Statistics, 1998). There are also differences in health status among racial and ethnic groups. However, it is lower socioeconomic status rather than race that contributes to the reduced health status. In general, vulnerable or special populations are those with low income, individuals with disabilities, and members of minority groups. This chapter discusses the concept of vulnerability, some of its causes, and the populations who are most likely to be vulnerable to health risks, as well as nursing interventions for effectively aiding these groups.

VULNERABILITY: DEFINITION AND INFLUENCING FACTORS

Vulnerability is defined as susceptibility to negative events. Vulnerability to poor health does not mean that some people have personal deficiencies. Rather it refers to the interaction effects of many factors over which people have little or no control. It is a result of the interaction of internal and external factors. That is, the person may have some biological limitations that are compounded by pollution, lead-based paint, excessive noise, or other external factors.

Vulnerable populations are those groups who have an increased risk to develop adverse health outcomes (Flaskerud and Winslow, 1998). As discussed in Chapter 8, **risk** is an epidemiological term that means that some people have a higher probability of illness than others. In the epidemiological triangle, the agent, host, and environment interact to produce illness or poor health. The "natural history of disease" model explains how certain aspects of physiology and the environment, including personal habits, social environment, and physical environment, make it more likely that one will develop particular health problems

(Valanis, 1999). For example, a smoker is at risk of developing lung cancer, but not all smokers develop cancer. Some people are more likely, that is, more vulnerable, than others to develop those health problems for which they are at risk.

Vulnerable populations appear to have less control over their health than the general population. Because they are often poor, may live in substandard housing and have limited social and financial resources, they may need to choose between buying food and buying medicine. Interestingly, some members of vulnerable populations do not succumb to the health risks that impinge on them. It is important to learn what factors allow these people to resist, or have **resilience** to, the effects of vulnerability.

Vulnerable populations are often called "special populations." Special populations with whom nurses work in the community include:

- Homeless people
- Pregnant adolescents
- Migrant workers
- People who are severely mentally ill
- Substance abusers
- Members of low-income groups
- Members of certain racial and ethnic groups
- People with disabilities
- Survivors of violence
- People with communicable diseases and those at high risk for these diseases
- People who have tested positive for the human immunodeficiency virus (HIV) or have hepatitis B virus (HBV) or other sexually transmitted diseases (STDs).

Vulnerable individuals and families often belong to more than one of these groups. For example, nurses work with pregnant adolescents who are poor, have been abused, and are substance abusers.

Nurses also work with substance abusers who are HIV or HBV positive, as well as those who are severely mentally ill.

Some of the problems facing vulnerable populations in terms of access to care, quality and appropriateness of care, and health outcomes will be described. Chapters 21 through 24 discuss the four vulnerable populations of substance abusers, survivors of violence, individuals who have a communicable disease, and those with HIV, hepatitis, or a sexually transmitted disease. Later sections in this chapter briefly discuss the special or vulnerable populations of poor and homeless people, those with serious mental illness, pregnant teens, and migrant workers.

CONCEPTUAL BASES OF VULNERABILITY

Vulnerability results from the combined effects of limited resources. Limitations in physical, environmental, and personal resources (or human capital), and biopsychosocial resources (e.g., presence of illness or genetic predispositions) combine to cause vulnerability (Aday, 1993; Rogers, 1997). Poverty, limited social support, and working in a hazardous environment are examples of limitations in physical and environmental resources. People with pre-existing illnesses, such as those with communicable or infectious diseases; or those with chronic illnesses such as cancer, heart disease, or chronic airway disease; have less physical ability to cope with stress than those without such physical problems. **Human capital** refers to all of the strengths, knowledge, and skills that enable a person to live a productive, happy life. People with little education have less human capital because their choices are more limited than those with higher levels of education.

There are many aspects to vulnerability. Vulnerability often comes from a feeling of lack of power, limited control, victimization, disadvantaged status, disenfranchisement, and health risks. Vulnerability can be reversed by obtaining resources to increase resilience. Useful nursing interventions to increase resilience include case finding, health education, care coordination, and policy-making related to improving health for vulnerable populations.

Disenfranchisement refers to a feeling of separation from mainstream society. The person does not seem to have an emotional connection with any group in particular or the larger society. Some groups such as the poor, the homeless, and migrant workers are "invisible" to society as a whole and forgotten in health and social planning. Vulnerable populations are at risk for disenfranchisement since their social supports are generally weak, as are their linkages with formal community organizations such as churches and schools. They may also have few informal sources of support such as family, friends, and neighbors. In many ways, vulnerable groups have limited control over potential and actual health needs. These groups are in the minority and are **disadvantaged,** since typical health planning focuses on the majority. Disadvantage also results from lack of resources that others may take for granted. Vulnerable population groups have limited social and economic resources with which to manage their health care. For example, women may endure domestic violence rather than risk losing a place for themselves and their children to live. Women who are among the working poor are more likely to become homeless when they leave an abusive partner. They may not have adequate financial resources to pay for a place to live when they lose their partner's income.

Vulnerable populations often experience multiple, **cumulative risks,** and they are particularly sensitive to the effects of those risks. Risks come from environmental hazards (e.g., lead exposure from peeling, lead-based paint), social hazards (e.g., crime and violence), personal behavior (e.g., diet and exercise habits), or from biological or genetic makeup (e.g., congenital addiction or compromised immune status). Members of vulnerable populations often have multiple illnesses, with each affecting the others.

PREDISPOSING FACTORS

As will be discussed later in the chapter, social and economic factors predispose people to vulnerability. **Poverty** is a primary cause of vulnerability, and it is a growing problem in the United States (Northam, 1996). Poverty is a relative state. In 1998, the **federal poverty level** for a family of four was $16,450 for all states except Hawaii, Alaska, and the District of Columbia (Superintendent of Documents, 1998). However, many people who earn just a little more than the federal poverty level cannot manage their living expenses, yet they are ineligible for assistance programs.

People who do not have the financial resources to pay for medical care are considered medically indigent. They may be self employed or work in small businesses and are unable to afford health benefits. Some people have inadequate health insurance coverage. This may be because either the deductibles and co-payments associated with the insurance are so high they have to pay for most expenses out-of-pocket or because few conditions or services are covered. In these situations, poverty in its relative sense causes vulnerability because uninsured and underinsured people are less likely to seek preventive health services because of the expense and are more likely to suffer the consequences of preventable illnesses.

In addition to economic status, age is related to vulnerability since people at the extreme ends of the age continuum may be less able physiologically to adapt to stressors. For example, infants of substance-abusing mothers risk being born addicted and having severe physiological problems and developmental delays. Elderly individuals are more likely to develop active infections from communicable diseases such as TB and generally have more difficulty recovering from infectious processes than younger people because of their less-effective immune systems. Elderly people also may be more vulnerable to safety threats and loss of independence due to their age and multiple chronic illnesses. Chapter 21 discusses substance abuse, Chapter 22 discusses violence, and Chapter 23 describes communicable disease risk.

Also, changes in normal physiological status can predispose people to vulnerability. This may result from disease processes, such as in someone with single or multiple chronic diseases. As discussed in Chapter 24, human immunodeficiency virus (HIV) illustrates a pathophysiological situation that increases vulnerability to opportunistic infections.

As has been discussed in several chapters, a person's life experiences, especially those early in life, influence vulnerability or resilience. For example, children who survive disasters may experience difficulties in later life if they do not receive adequate counseling (Yule, 1992). *Internal* locus of control appears to protect children (particularly adolescents) from the negative effects of disaster (Yule, 1992). A person with internal locus of control can control his or her behavior and not depend entirely on external people, events, or forces to control behavior. Vulnerable population groups often develop an *external* locus of control. They may believe that events are outside their control and result from bad luck or fate. An external locus of control makes it more difficult for people to take action or to seek care for health problems. These people may minimize the value of health promotion or illness prevention because they do not think they have control over their health destiny. Another example would be people who have been abused or have experienced chronic stress. They may have used up a lot of the reserves that others would normally have for coping with new forms of stress (Nurius, Furrey, and Berliner, 1992).

OUTCOMES OF VULNERABILITY

Outcomes of vulnerability may be negative, such as a lower health status than the rest of the population, or they may be positive, with effective interventions. Vulnerable populations often have worse health outcomes than other people in terms of morbidity and mortality. These groups have a high prevalence of chronic illnesses such as hypertension and high levels of communicable diseases including tuberculosis, hepatitis B virus (HBV), and sexually transmitted diseases (STDs), as well as upper respiratory infections including influenza. They also have higher mortality rates than the general population due to factors such as poor living conditions, diet, health status, and to crime and violence, including domestic violence.

There is often a cycle to vulnerability. That is, poor health creates stress as individuals and families try to manage health problems with inadequate resources. For example, if someone with AIDS develops one or more opportunistic infections and is either uninsured or underinsured, that person and the family and caregivers will have more difficulty managing than if the individual had adequate insurance. Vulnerable populations often suffer many forms of stress. Sometimes when one problem is solved, another quickly emerges. This can lead to feelings of hopelessness. Hopelessness results from an overwhelming sense of powerlessness and social isolation. For example, substance abusers who feel powerless over their addiction and who have isolated themselves from the people they care about may see no way to change their situation.

SELECTED VULNERABLE POPULATION GROUPS
Poor and Homeless People

Health is influenced by economic status (Adler, et al, 1997; National Center for Health Statistics, 1998). Poverty refers to having insufficient financial resources to meet basic living expenses for food, shelter, clothing, trans-

TABLE 20-1	Poverty Thresholds in 1997*
Size of Family Unit	Income Guidelines
1	$8,350
2	$10,473
3	$12,802
4	$16,400
5	$19,380
6	$21,886
7	$24,802
8	$27,590

From U.S. Census Bureau: *Current population survey, June 1998,* Washington, D.C., 1999, U.S. Government Printing Office.
*Based on size of family and number of related children under 18 years of age.

portation, and health care (Sebastian, 2000). It is estimated that more than 40 million people have incomes below the federal poverty level (National Coalition for the Homeless, 1998). People who live in poverty or in near-poverty have higher rates of chronic illness, higher infant morbidity and mortality, shorter life expectancy, more complex health problems, and more serious complications and physical limitations from chronic disease than their more affluent counterparts. Poor people are more likely to live in environments that present health hazards due to being overcrowded, having inadequate heating or cooling, exposure to rain or snow, inadequate water and plumbing, and the presence of pests (Jargowsky and Band, 1990). They often work at high-risk jobs, eat less-nutritious diets, and are stressed because they do not have the resources to manage unexpected crises and may not even have adequate resources to manage daily life (Erickson, 1996; De la Barra, 1998). Table 20-1 lists the poverty thresholds in the United States.

Poverty—with its limitations in the ability to have nutritious food, safe shelter and good health care—has an especially negative effect on women of childbearing age, teens, and children. At least 20.5% of American's young children live in poverty. Children who are raised in poverty may have difficulty developing resilience and be more likely to be depressed later in life (Adler, et al, 1997). Young children (under 6 years of age) are at highest risk for the harmful effects of poverty due to the effects of inadequate nutrition on brain development (Shore, 1997). Other risk factors found in these vulnerable populations that can limit brain development include maternal depression or substance abuse, exposure to environmental toxins, trauma and abuse, and poor-quality care (National Center for Children in Poverty, 1998).

HOW TO Identify the Risk Factors of Poverty as They Relate to Children's Health

- Higher rates of prematurity, low birth weight, birth defects, and infant mortality
- Greater incidence of chronic disease, traumatic injury and death, nutritional problems, growth retardation, and developmental delays
- More iron-deficiency anemia, elevated lead levels, and infections
- Greater risk for homelessness
- Fewer opportunities for education, income, and occupation

More than 80% of the people in poverty are women, children, and the elderly (Erickson, 1996). These groups are already considered to be high risk for health disruption, and poverty increases their possible risk. Prevalence rates for ulcer disease, asthma, and anemia are higher for women living in poverty. Also, poor women report significantly more HIV risk behaviors than more affluent women (Weinreb, et al, 1998a). For older adults, prevalence rates for chronic illness and their complications, general higher morbidity, poor dental health, and higher mortality are greater than for their younger counterparts (Persson, et al, 1998; Waltzman and Smith, 1997). Older adults are at particular risk if they live alone and are unable to effectively manage their lives. Many older adults are eligible for benefits that would help them, but they are not aware of this. The following reasons have been given for the growing numbers of poor people in the United States:

- Decreased earnings
- Increased unemployment rates in some areas
- Changes in the labor force
- More female heads of households
- Inadequate education and job skills, antipoverty programs, and welfare benefits
- Weak enforcement of child-support statutes
- Decreasing Social Security payments to children
- Increased number of children born to single women.

As the characteristics of most nations have changed from an industrial to a service economy, workers need education and skills in order to be successful in the labor market. Many job opportunities exclude people who do not have a high school education. Manufacturing jobs may be available to people with limited education, but the pay is often low, and the job may not include health care or retirement benefits. Poverty can be grouped into six categories:

1. Acute poverty, which occurs suddenly after a crisis such as job loss or illness
2. Chronic poverty, which persists over many years
3. Absolute poverty, which indicates a lack of food, shelter, and clothing
4. Relative poverty, which indicates less-than-average resources
5. Administrative poverty, which refers to having met a governmentally determined standard for poverty (e.g., the federal poverty level)
6. Subjective poverty, in which the individual has inadequate income for basic necessities within a particular area (Erickson, 1996).

The interaction among multiple socioeconomic stressors makes poor people more susceptible to risk than others with more financial resources who may cope more effectively. For example, the situation below illustrates how living environment and practical problems such as transportation and cost interact to make the poor particularly vulnerable to health problems.

Felicia Delacorte is a 22-year-old single mother of three children whose primary source of income is Aid to Families with Dependent Children. She is worried about the future because she will no longer be eligible for welfare by the end of the year. She has not been able to find a job that will pay enough for her to afford childcare. Her friend Maria said Felicia and her children could stay in Maria's trailer for a short time, but Felicia is afraid that her only choice after that will be a shelter.

Felicia recently took all three children with her to the health department because 15-month-old Hector needed immunizations. Felicia was also concerned about 5-year-old Martina, who had a fever of 100° to 101° F on and off for the past month. Felicia and her friends in the trailer park think that some type of hazardous waste from the chemical plant next door to the park is making their children sick. Now that Martina was not feeling well, Felicia was particularly concerned. However, the health department nurse told her that no appointments were available that day and that she would need to bring Martina back to the clinic on the next day. Felicia left discouraged because it was so difficult for her to get all three children ready and on the bus to go to the health department, not to mention the expense. She thought maybe Martina just had a cold and she would wait a little longer before bringing her back. However, she wanted to take care of Martina's problem before losing her medical card. Felicia is desperate to find a way to manage her money problems and take care of her children.

Briefly Noted

One client's advice to nurses caring for the poor: Treat the poor like everyone else; don't be condescending or make it obvious that someone is poor. Don't act with prejudice; perhaps the person can and wants to pay the bill, but remember that not everyone can pay for his medicine. Provide support in many ways including recommending community agencies like churches, shelters, and food banks that really help. Remember that many poor people do want to maintain their health.

Poverty can lead to **homelessness.** Thirty percent of the homeless in the United States are families, and "85% of those families are headed by women of whom the majority are minorities" (Erickson, 1996, p. 165; Berne, et al, 1991). Homelessness is estimated to be growing by 5% per year (National Coalition for the Homeless, 1998). It is hard to determine the exact number of homeless people or to find them because many sleep in boxcars, on building roofs, in doorways and under freeways or bridges. Some have short intervals of homelessness, other have intermittent episodes, while still others are chronically homeless. Most people do not choose to be homeless. Who would want to be alone, living on the streets, isolated from family and friends? Homelessness is more than not having an address or phone number; it is an isolation from mainstream society. It can mean being totally alone in a time of crisis (Walker, 1998).

Briefly Noted

Who Are America's Homeless?
- Families
- Children
- Single women
- Female heads of household
- Adults who are unemployed, earn low wages, or are migrant workers
- People who abuse alcohol or other substances
- Abandoned children
- Adolescent runaways
- Elderly people with no place to go and no one to care for them
- Persons who are mentally ill
- Vietnam-era veterans

A variety of causes lead to homelessness. As will be discussed later in the chapter, the **deinstitutionalization** of seriously mentally ill people from public psychiatric hospitals has increased the number of homeless people. As these hospitals were downsized, community facilities were no longer available to meet the needs of the patients who were discharged. Other factors include the growing number of people living in poverty, a decrease in the availability of affordable housing, and increased numbers of substance abusers.

Homeless and marginally housed people struggle with heavy demands as they try to manage daily life. Since they have no regular shelter, they must cope with finding a place to sleep at night and to stay during the day, as well as finding food, before even thinking about health care. In fact, many of the health care needs of homeless individuals are related to their regular search for shelter and food. Specifically, many homeless people have problems with their feet due to constant walking and hypothermia because of exposure to the cold. They have a greater incidence of acute and chronic illnesses (Busen and Beech, 1997). Some of the specific health problems accompanying homelessness include hypothermia, infestations, peripheral vascular disease, hypertension, respiratory infections, tuberculosis, AIDS, trauma, and mental illness (White, et al, 1997). Their chronic health problems are intensified because they have no place to store their medications, cannot always find nutritious meals, and cannot balance rest and activity because of vagrancy laws that prohibit loitering in one place for very long (Sebastian, 2000).

Homeless pregnant women are at high risk. They have higher rates of STDs, addiction to drugs and alcohol, poorer nutrition, and a higher incidence of lower-birth-weight babies and less access to prenatal care (Beal and Redlener, 1995).

Like poor children, those who are homeless are at high risk for health problems. Homeless children have more acute illness—including fever, ear infections, diarrhea, and asthma—than their housed counterparts (Weinreb, et al, 1998b). Those who live on the streets in urban areas also suffer more from depression and other mental health problems. These children are likely to have inadequate nutrition, and this can impair growth and development or lead to obesity. Homeless children have higher rates of absenteeism, academic failure, and emotional and behavioral maladjustments. Their stress may be seen in withdrawal, depression, anxiety, aggression, regression, or self-mutilation (David-hizar and Frank, 1992).

In addition to many of the risk factors experienced by homeless children, adolescents who live on the streets also are at risk for contracting serious communicable diseases, including AIDS and hepatitis B. These youth often have histories of running away from home and physical or sexual abuse (Busen and Beech, 1997). Once on the streets, many exchange sex for food, clothing, and shelter, which increases their risk for unintended pregnancy (Rew, 1996). Homeless teens have higher rates of depression, low self-esteem, suicidal thought, and overall poorer health than teens who have shelter (Unger, et al, 1997).

Homeless older adults are an especially vulnerable group. They have typically lived in long-standing poverty, have few supportive relationships, and often become homeless due to a catastrophic event. They typically live 20 years less than middle-class older adults (Hilfiker, 1994). Many have permanent physical deformities due to poor or absent medical care. They may suffer from untreated chronic conditions, tuberculosis, hypertension, arthritis, cardiovascular disease, injuries, malnutrition, poor oral health, and hypothermia (Hilfiker, 1994; Schoenberg and Gilbert, 1998).

Briefly Noted

For homeless people, health care is usually crisis oriented, and those who get care often have a hard time following the prescribed regimen. For example, an insulin-dependent man who lives on the street and sleeps in a shelter has a hard time eating regularly scheduled nutritious meals, taking his insulin on time, and getting adequate exercise and rest.

Homeless people are more likely to have injuries, fractures, and dental problems than people with housing. They also experience problems ranging from violence and trauma associated with life in the streets to difficulty managing dental care because they have no place to store toothbrushes, toothpaste, and other dental supplies. They are not likely to be adequately immunized, and they have more than an average number of upper respiratory infections. Chemical dependency is more common among homeless people than the general population. Women in their childbearing years are more likely than other women to have hypertension, mental illness, injuries, and STDs, and to report being abused.

Pregnant Teens

Births to teenagers make up 12% of all births in the United States (American College of Obstetricians and Gynecologists, 1998). Hispanic/Latino teens currently have the highest rate of births at 107 per 100,000 (Moore, et al, 1997). In fact the United States leads the developed world in the rates of teen pregnancy, teen births, and teen abortions (Hatcher, et al, 1998). Teens tend to view the world differently than older adults. They may fail to appreciate the risks involved in unprotected sex. Most teens report that their pregnancy was unplanned. The earlier the teen begins engaging in sexual activity—the **sexual debut**—the less likely a form of birth control will be used.

Teen pregnancy contributes to a cycle of poverty. Teenagers who are from poor families, or who are homeless or runaways, are more likely to get pregnant (Fullerton, et al, 1997). Those who keep and raise their infants are more likely to remain poor themselves. With the increased social acceptability of out-of-wedlock pregnancy (Pierre and Cox, 1997), many teenage mothers choose to keep and raise their children. This can lead to interrupted education for one or both of the parents, limited job opportunities, the expenses of raising a child, and a long-term cycle of economic problems that affect both the parents and their children. If the teen mother is a single parent, the economic consequences are often more difficult.

Adolescent females (especially those under 14 years of age) are more likely to deliver low-birth-weight infants than are women in their twenties and thirties (Maynard, 1996; U.S. Department of Health and Human Services, 1997). This is thought to result from the combined interaction of physiological variables (Yoos, 1987) and socioeconomic conditions (Trussell, 1988). Being unable to afford prenatal care, not knowing the importance of such care and how to obtain it, and being likely to initiate prenatal care later in pregnancy than older mothers all contribute to the poor pregnancy outcomes of adolescents. Some teens delay seeking prenatal care because they do not recognize signs such as breast tenderness and a late menstrual period as being indicative of possible pregnancy. Others may suspect pregnancy but just hope that if they ignore the signs, the problem will go away. Teens report that they delay getting care because they are afraid to talk with their parents, they lack transportation, or they worry what the staff will think of them (Cartoof, Klerman, and Zazveta, 1991). Other health problems that pregnant adolescents experience include toxemia, pregnancy-induced hypertension, and anemia.

Special issues for nurses to understand when dealing with pregnant teens include recognizing that some teens become pregnant through sexual victimization. They may be afraid to discuss what happened from fear of retaliation from the aggressor. All pregnant teens need counseling that includes information about abortion services, adoption, personal care for the teen and infant, education and the available options, finances, and qualifications for assistance.

Since teens are at risk for low-birth-weight and preterm deliveries, special nursing actions need to be taken. The sooner the teen receives prenatal care, the sooner this risk begins to be reduced. Nutrition is an important issue since teens do not typically eat an especially healthful diet. Snacks account for about one third of the food eaten by a teen. These snacks often are high in fat, sugar, and salt and are limited in vitamins and minerals. The normal growth spurt that occurs during the teen years in addition to the pregnancy increases the need for nutritious food. Nurses often need to help pregnant teens view their prenatal weight gain positively. Many fear getting fat and will not eat the needed foods during pregnancy. Iron deficiency is a concern that needs to be monitored since it can contribute to prematurity, low birth weight, postpartum hemorrhage, maternal headaches, dizziness, and shortness of breath (Story, 1990).

Teen mothers need to be taught how to care for an infant. Parents and the father can also be involved in the teaching. Learning good parenting skills can help reduce the possibility of abuse as the child gets older. The frustrations of 24-hour-a-day care for an infant are great and may seem nearly overwhelming to a teen. Teens may not know how to interact with an infant, and these skills can be taught and practiced with the nurse present and available to role model, coach, and provide feedback. Teens need to be taught to make eye contact with the infant, talk with the infant, and use age-appropriate toys and other devices to stimulate the infant.

Migrant Workers

The number of legal and illegal immigrants in the United States grew during the 1990s (*San Francisco Chronicle,* Oct. 13, 1998), as did the number of migrant workers. The Office of Migrant Health defines a **migrant farm worker** as a person "whose principle employment is in agriculture on a seasonal basis, who has been so employed within the last 24 months and who establishes for the purpose of such employment a temporary abode" (1998, p. 8). Migrant workers face a wide variety of risk factors, including occupational risks associated with hazardous work and poor working conditions, and socioeconomic risks from poverty and homelessness. The nature of occupational risks varies depending on the type of work, but much of it is on farms dealing with pesticides and heavy equipment, with poor protection from rain, cold, and bugs. Others are employed in different types of seasonal labor, such as traveling with a circus, carnival, or the horse-racing circuit, working at racetracks and on horse farms (Ireson and Weaver, 1992). Migrant workers are at increased risk for tuberculosis since they often live in crowded quarters, travel to work on crowded buses, and lack adequate food (Ciesielski, et al, 1994).

Migrant workers are **episodically homeless,** which means that they move in and out of homelessness (Institute of Medicine, 1988, p. 23). Housing is a major problem for migrant workers since many live in trailers, dirt-floor houses, cabins, labor camps, garages, cars, caves, boxes, ditch banks, tents, chicken coops; under trees, bridges, or tarps; in orchards, parks, fields, or yards; or near streets, highways, or railroad tracks. Migrant workers, who live in migrant camp housing while they are working but may not have a reliable place to live at other times, are among the **hidden homeless.** These workers have many of the same problems as those who are chronically homeless (Institute of Medicine, 1988). Some of the barriers that face them in obtaining good health care include:

- Lack of knowledge about services and poor language skills
- Limited income, and work that is interrupted with poor weather
- Lack of services nearby and provided at a time when the workers can use them
- Lack of child care to take advantage of health care services
- Mobility and lack of tracking: migrant workers are on the move, and no agency may have an accurate health care record for them, nor do the migrants have a health record
- Discrimination in that not all providers want to provide care to migrant workers whom they may view as poor, uneducated, transient, and ethnically different.

It is sometimes hard for migrant workers to get good, reliable health care (Ciesielski, et al, 1994) since some do not have citizenship status. Those who are illegal immigrants may have no legal access to health services, depending on the laws in a particular state. As the number of immigrants without access to public education, health care, and economic subsidies increases, the United States is developing a seriously underserved class of people with numerous health and social problems (*San Francisco Chronicle,* Oct 13, 1998).

Since migrant farm workers make up a large portion of the migrant population, the discussion of health problems focuses on this subgroup. They are especially at risk for parasite infections, hepatitis, skin infections, muscle strain/sprain, and upper respiratory infection (Johnsrud, et al, 1997), as well as tuberculosis and HIV disease. Specifically, reported injuries have included fractures or sprains from falls from ladders or equipment; strains and sprains from prolonged stooping, heavy lifting, and carrying; amputations, deaths, and crush injuries from tractors, trucks, or other machinery; pesticide poisoning; electrical injuries; and drowning in ditches. The constant stooping to pick crops, often using poor body mechanics, increases the chances of back problems. Naturally occurring chemicals or applied poisons can irritate the skin (contact dermatitis) or the eyes (allergic or chemical conjunctivitis).

Pesticide exposure is a big problem for migrant farm workers. Organophosphate anticholinesterase pesticides are the largest group of pesticides in current use. They affect normal neuromuscular functioning. Farm workers have both the immediate effects of these chemicals and the residue effect when they work in wet fields that harbor pesticides.

Acute health effects of pesticide exposure include mild psychological and behavioral deficits such as memory loss, difficulty with concentration, and mood changes; abdominal pain, nausea, vomiting, and diarrhea; headache, malaise, skin rashes, and eye irritation. Acute severe poisoning can cause death. Chronic exposure can lead to cancer, blindness, Parkinson's disease, infertility or sterility, liver damage, and polyneuropathy and neurobehavioral problems.

Briefly Noted

Nurses can demonstrate respect to clients of different cultural backgrounds by learning about the cultural norms, values, and traditions of a cultural group. It is helpful to be fluent in a second language; for example, nurses who work in communities with a large Hispanic population will find it useful to be fluent in Spanish. Similarly, nurses who work with people who are deaf should learn at least some basic sign language.

Migrant farm workers face multiple problems. An organized systematic approach is necessary to help them get the kind of care they need, including primary health care to prevent many of the health risks that face them from working in fields, living in inadequate housing, moving often, and for many, not being able to speak the primary language.

Severely Mentally Ill Individuals

Severely mentally ill (SMI) individuals, defined as those people with a major psychosis such as schizophrenia or bipolar disorder, often face many health and socioeconomic problems. These disorders may not become apparent until adolescence or young adulthood. This is a time when people are trying to establish themselves financially. Severe mental illnesses are thought to be due to biological, behavioral, or psychological dysfunction within a person (Neugebauer, 1999). Untreated severe mental illness interferes with a person's ability to function on a daily basis and thus makes it difficult to maintain a job. People with severe mental illness need multiple health and social services, such as antipsychotic medications, counseling and sometimes group therapy, and vocational assistance (Steinwachs, et al, 1992). Current reports estimate that there are at least 10 million people age 18 years and older in the United States with a serious mental illness (Center for Mental Health Services, 1996). In children ages 9 to 17 the estimated rate is between 9% and 13%. Serious mental disorders are persistent and disabling and affect people of all ages, races, and socioeconomic levels. In adults, they are more common in women, people whose family income is less than $20,000, and those who have little or no college education. These disorders include mood disorders and depression, anxiety and phobic disorders, antisocial personality disorders, schizophrenia and schizo-affective disorders, and organic brain syndrome (American Psychological Association, 1994; Worley, 1997).

Some examples of the risk factors for specific age-groups are as follows. Children and adolescents are at risk for acute and chronic mental health problems resulting from neglect, divorce, environmental situations such as crowded living conditions, violence, separation from parents, and lack of consistent caregivers. Since youth are at risk for suicide, they often require crisis intervention and both short- and long-term counseling. Adults have many of the same risk factors as their younger counterparts, especially when they must cope with job insecurity and unstable relationships and when they have multiple role responsibilities.

Throughout the nineteenth and much of the twentieth centuries, SMI individuals in the United States were treated primarily with long-term hospitalization. Public concern about mental hospitals led to the passage of the 1963 Community Mental Health Centers Act, which intended to deinstitutionalize the SMI population and create comprehensive services for them in their own communities. Unfortunately, comprehensive service networks did not develop in every community, and many individuals with severe mental illness were left with fewer and more fragmented services than they needed in order to function effectively. In many cases, people who had lived in mental hospitals for many years had no idea how to manage on their own in the community. Many of these formerly hospitalized people moved onto the streets where they lived as homeless people or lived in shelters or single-room occupancy hotels.

Briefly Noted

Referring clients to community agencies involves much more than simply picking up the phone and making a call or completing a form. The nurse must make certain that the agency to which a client is referred is the right one to meet that client's needs. Nurses can do more harm than good by referring a stressed, discouraged client to an agency from which the client is not really eligible to receive services. The nurse should help the client learn how to get the most from the referral.

Many of the adults with serious mental illness are treated in their communities in primary care settings and emergency departments. These clients benefit most when services for them are provided by one agency that coordinates their care (Provan, 1997). It appears that the links between agencies must be consistent in order for clients to benefit from integration (Provan and Sebastian, 1998). For example, clients benefit more when agencies that coordinate care also participate in some way in the referral process, rather than having two groups of agencies performing these functions separately.

Behavioral managed care organizations currently provide much of the care for SMI individuals, especially as state Medicaid programs are contracting with such groups to provide SMI care (Mechanic, Schlesinger, and McAlpine, 1995). A concern with many of these organizations is that quality of care may suffer as the managed care organizations

limit services to reduce cost (Wells, et al, 1995). Mentally ill individuals often do not have the resources to challenge eligibility rules and may suffer poorer health outcomes from service limitations that do not meet their needs. Young chronically mentally ill individuals without adequate access to care may be incarcerated for behaviors resulting from their mental health problems. Further, SMI individuals may lack routine preventive health care such as screening for common illnesses and education and support for health prevention and illness promotion.

Nurses working with mentally ill people and their families in the community can assist in several ways. Specifically nurses use their clinical skills to observe if symptoms or presenting behaviors are due to physical or psychological problems. Often, medication management is a key nursing role for mentally ill persons who live in the community in their own or a family member's home, in a group home, or in another shared living arrangement.

The nurse also often counsels the patients and their families, assists in arranging and coordinating care, and teaches skills such as more effective communication or conflict-management skills, as well as health promotion and identification of symptoms that require attention.

PUBLIC POLICIES AFFECTING VULNERABLE POPULATIONS

Three pieces of legislation have provided direct and indirect financial subsidies to certain vulnerable groups. The Social Security Act of 1935 created the largest federal support program for elderly and poor Americans in history. This act was intended to ensure a minimal level of support for people at risk of problems resulting from inadequate financial resources. This was accomplished by direct payments to eligible individuals. Later, the Medicare and Medicaid amendments to the Social Security Act of 1965 provided for the health care needs of elderly, poor, and disabled people who might be vulnerable to impoverishment resulting from high medical bills or to poor health status from inadequate access to health care. These acts created third-party health care payers at the federal and state levels. Title XXI of the Social Security Act, enacted in 1998, provides for the State Child Health Insurance Program (CHIP) to provide funds to insure currently uninsured children. In addition to CHIP, new outreach and case finding efforts enroll eligible children in Medicaid. "Taken together, these two approaches will seek to provide health insurance for at least half of the 10 million uninsured children in this country" (Hamburg, 1998, p. 375).

More recently, the Balanced Budget Act of 1997 has influenced the use of resources for providing health services. In an attempt to curb the rapid growth in spending on home health and financial fraud in that industry, the Health Care Financing Administration moved toward prospective payment for home health services. More stringent regulations about which services will be reimbursed, and for how long, may limit access to care for certain vulnerable groups, such as the frail elderly, chronically ill individuals whose care is largely home-based, and people who are HIV positive. The goal is to ensure that care is appropriate, rather than limiting access. Nurses and other health care providers must work even more closely with families to determine the kinds of services needed to foster self-care and the optimal timing of these services. The Balanced Budget Act of 1997 also reduced payments for services for Medicare beneficiaries, resulting in some providers choosing not to treat Medicare beneficiaries. This means that people with major health needs (some chronically ill and the elderly) may have limited access to care.

Ways Managed Care Has Affected Vulnerable Populations

In many areas, the growth of public managed care (i.e., Medicaid and Medicare managed care options) has reduced the personal health services for individuals such as primary care clinics in health departments. The competition for clients in heavy managed care markets has made it more attractive to private clinics and physicians' offices to provide the personal care services that some public health departments formerly provided because they can obtain payment for these services. Some public health departments have eliminated these services and focus on providing population-focused services only, such as communicable disease control, environmental services, and managing public food and water supplies (Aiken and Salmon, 1994). In this way, many public health departments are refocusing on the core functions of public health: assessment, policy development, and assurance.

However, not all private health agencies wish to provide services to vulnerable populations. Aiken and Salmon (1994) explain that vulnerable populations are more expensive to treat, since they have multiple, cumulative risks and require special service delivery considerations (e.g., to help overcome transportation problems or provide culturally competent care). Managed care organizations (MCOs) have strong incentives to control costs by keeping their enrollees healthy. Many MCOs prefer (or must for financial reasons) to care for the healthiest people rather than those who are most vulnerable. One approach that is used to manage care for high-risk populations is to contract their care to specialty organizations (referred to as "carve outs"). These specialty organizations often develop innovative approaches to caring for these high-risk populations. Carve outs are often used to provide mental health care. For example, one school of nursing contracted with its regional Medicaid office to provide a new care delivery program for families with medically fragile children. This is a family program that aims to strengthen families who rear children with high-risk health problems. Nurse practitioners and a clinical nurse specialist provide primary care, urgent care, health education, health coaching, family counseling and support, and case management for families in the program. Most care is provided in the home, although the program staff also works with clients in hospitals, clinics, and physicians' offices in order to facilitate seamless care delivery.

 Evidence-Based Practice

Providing care to children with HIV/AIDS can be an emotionally demanding and complex task. Caring for a child with HIV/AIDS may result in feelings of guilt, anxiety, stress, uncertainty, isolation, and grief. Previous research has shown that social support interventions are effective strategies for mitigating stress. The study referenced below aimed to test the effectiveness of a social-support–boosting intervention on caregivers of children with HIV/AIDS.

Seventy caregivers participated in this two-group, repeated measures, experimental study. Caregivers were divided into experimental and control groups. Within both groups, caregivers were stratified based on whether they were seropositive for HIV/AIDS (biological parents) or seronegative (blood relatives or foster parents). The experimental group received a social-support–boosting intervention, which was a form of modified case management. The intervention consisted of case managers helping participants identify sources of social support in the areas of emotional support, cognitive support, and instrumental support. Participants in the control group received standard care, which consisted of multidisciplinary health care for the child and respite and social services for the caregiver. Data were collected at entry into the study, 6 months after entry, and 12 months after entry.

The researchers found that seronegative caregivers reported significantly higher levels of perceived social support following the intervention, whereas the seropositive caregivers did not exhibit this outcome. The researchers hypothesized that the needs of caregivers who themselves had HIV/AIDS were more complex than those of caregivers who were not also concerned with the effects of HIV/AIDS on themselves.

APPLICATION IN PRACTICE

The researchers recommended that nurses include social-support–boosting interventions for caregivers of children with HIV/AIDS and recognize the need for more individualized and complex nursing interventions with caregivers who are also seropositive for the virus.

Hartsell PS, Hughes CB, Caliandro G, Russo P, Budin, WC, Hartman B, Hernandez OC: The effect of a social support boosting intervention on stress, coping, and social support in caregivers of children with HIV/AIDS, *Nurs Res* 47(2):79-86, 1998.

Healthy People 2010 addresses many issues of vulnerable populations. See the *Healthy People 2010* box for examples of some relevant objectives.

NURSING INTERVENTION FOR VULNERABLE POPULATIONS

The factors that predispose people to vulnerability and the outcomes of vulnerability create a cycle in which the outcomes reinforce the predisposing factors, leading to more negative outcomes. Unless the cycle is broken, it is difficult for vulnerable populations to change their health status. Nurses can identify areas where they can work with vulnerable populations to break the cycle. The nursing process guides nurses in assessing vulnerable individuals, families, groups, and communities; developing nursing diagnoses of their strengths and needs; planning and implementing appropriate therapeutic nursing interventions in partnership with vulnerable clients; and evaluating the effectiveness of interventions.

Assessment of Vulnerable Populations

Nurses who work with vulnerable populations need good assessment skills, current knowledge of available resources, and the ability to plan care based on client needs and receptiveness to help. They also need to be able to show respect for the client. Guidelines for assessing members of vulnerable population groups are listed in the box below.

HOW TO Assess Members of Vulnerable Population Groups

SETTING THE STAGE

- Create a comfortable, non-threatening environment.
- Learn as much as you can about the culture of the clients you work with so that you will understand cultural practices and values that may influence their health care practices.
- Provide culturally competent assessment by understanding the meaning of language and nonverbal behavior in the client's culture.
- Be sensitive to the fact that the individual or family you are assessing may have other priorities that are more important to them. These might include financial or legal problems. You may need to give them some tangible help with their most pressing priority before you will be able to address issues that are more traditionally thought of as health concerns.
- Collaborate with others as appropriate; you should not provide financial or legal advice. However, you should make sure to connect your client with someone who can and will help them.

NURSING HISTORY OF AN INDIVIDUAL OR FAMILY

- You may have only one opportunity to work with a vulnerable person or family. Try to complete a history that will provide all the essential information you need to help the individual or family on that day. This means that you will have to organize in your mind exactly what you need to ask, and no more, and why the data are necessary.
- It will help to use a comprehensive assessment form that has been modified to focus on the special needs of the vulnerable population group with whom you work. However, be flexible. With some clients, it will be both impractical and unethical to cover all questions on a comprehensive form. If you know that you are likely to see the client again, ask the less pressing questions at the next visit.
- Be sure to include questions about social support, economic status, resources for health care, developmental issues, current health problems, medications, and how the person or family manages their health status. Your goal is to obtain information that will enable you to provide family-centered care.
- Does the individual have any condition that compromises his or her immune status, such as AIDS, or is the individual undergoing therapy that would result in immunodeficiency, such as cancer chemotherapy?

PHYSICAL EXAMINATION OR HOME ASSESSMENT

- Again, complete as thorough a physical examination (on an individual) or home assessment as you can. Keep in mind that you should collect only those data for which you have a use.
- Be alert for indications of physical abuse, substance use (e.g., needle marks, nasal abnormalities), or neglect (e.g., underweight, being inadequately clothed).
- You can assess a family's living environment using good observational skills. Does the family live in an insect- or rat-infested environment? Do they have running water, functioning plumbing, electricity, and a telephone?
- Is perishable food (e.g., mayonnaise) left sitting out on tables and countertops? Are bed linens reasonably clean? Is paint peeling on the walls and ceilings? Is ventilation adequate? Is the temperature of the home adequate? Is the family exposed to raw sewage or animal waste? Is the home adjacent to a busy highway, possibly exposing the family to high noise levels and automobile exhaust?

Because members of vulnerable populations often experience multiple stressors, assessment must balance the need to be comprehensive while focusing only on information that the nurse needs and that the client is willing to provide. The nurse should include questions about the client's perceptions of his or her *socioeconomic resources,* including identifying people who can provide support and financial resources. Support from other people may include information, caregiving, emotional support, and help with instrumental activities of daily living such as transportation, shopping, and baby-sitting. Financial resources may include the extent to which the client can pay for health services and medications, as well as questions about eligibility for third-party payment. The nurse should ask the client about the perceived adequacy of both formal and informal support networks.

When possible, assessment should include evaluation of clients' *preventive health needs,* including age-appropriate screening tests, such as immunization status, blood pressure, weight, serum cholesterol, Papanicolaou smears, breast examinations, mammograms, prostate examinations, glaucoma screening, and dental evaluations. It may be necessary to make referrals to have some of these tests done for clients. Assessment should also include preventive screening for physical health problems for which certain vulnerable groups are at a particularly high risk. For example, people who are HIV positive should be evaluated regularly for their T4 cell counts and for common opportunistic infections, including TB and pneumonia. Intravenous (IV) drug users should be evaluated for HBV, including liver palpation and serum antigen tests as necessary. Alcoholic clients should also be asked about symptoms of liver disease and should be evaluated for jaundice and liver enlargement. Severely mentally ill clients should be assessed for the presence of tardive dyskinesia, indicating possible toxicity from their antipsychotic medications.

Vulnerable populations should be assessed for *congenital* and *genetic predisposition* to illness and either receive education and counseling as appropriate or be referred to other health professionals as necessary. For example, pregnant adolescents who are substance abusers should be referred to programs to help them quit using addictive substances during their pregnancies and ideally after delivery of their infants as well. Pregnant women over age 35 should receive amniocentesis testing to determine if genetic abnormalities exist in the fetus.

Assess also for the amount of stress the person or family is experiencing. Does the family have healthy coping skills and healthy family interaction? Are some family members able and willing to care for others? What is the level of mental health in each member? Also, are diet, exercise, rest, and sleep patterns conducive to good health?

Assess the *living environment* and *neighborhood surroundings* of vulnerable families and groups for environmental hazards such as lead-based paint, asbestos, water and air quality, industrial wastes, and the incidence of crime.

Planning and Implementing Care for Vulnerable Populations

Nurses who work in community settings typically have considerable involvement with vulnerable populations. The relationship with the client will depend on the nature of the contact. Some will be seen in clinics while others will be in homes, schools, or at work. Regardless of the setting, several key nursing actions need to be used. These are:
- *Create a trusting environment.* Trust is essential since many of these individuals have previously been disappointed in their interactions with health care and social systems. It is important for the nurse to follow through

and do what is promised. If the nurse does not know the answer to a question, the best reply is " I do not know, but I will try to find out."
- *Show respect, compassion, and concern.* Vulnerable people have been defeated again and again by life's circumstances. They may have reached a point where they question if they even deserve to get care. Nurses must listen carefully since listening is both a way to show respect and a way to gather information to plan care.
- *Don't make assumptions.* Each person and family must be assessed. No two people or groups are alike.
- *Coordinate services and providers.* Obtaining health and social services is not always easy. Often people feel like they are traveling through a maze. In most communities a large number of useful services exist. People who need them simply may not know how to find them. For example, people may need help finding a food bank, or a free clinic or obtaining low-cost or free clothing through churches or in second-hand stores. Clients may need help determining whether they meet the eligibility requirements. If gaps in service are found, nurses can work with others to try to get the needed services established.

HOW TO Provide Comprehensive Care for Vulnerable Populations

When working with vulnerable populations, it is a good idea to arrange to have as many services as possible available in a single location and at convenient times. This "one-stop shopping" approach to care delivery is very helpful for populations experiencing multiple social, economic, and health-related stresses. While it may seem costly to provide comprehensive services in one location, it may save money in the long run by preventing illness.

Nurses who work with vulnerable populations will often find it necessary to coordinate services across multiple agencies for members of these groups. It is helpful to have a strong professional network with people who work in other agencies. Effective professional networks make it easier to coordinate care smoothly and in ways that do not add to clients' stress. Nurses can develop strong networks by participating in community coalitions and attending professional meetings. When making referrals to other agencies, a phone call can be a helpful way to obtain information that the client will need about the visit. When possible, having an interdisciplinary, interagency team plan care for clients at high risk of health problems can be quite effective. It is crucial to obtain the clients' written and informed consent before engaging in this kind of planning due to confidentiality issues.

- *Advocate for accessible health care services.* Vulnerable people have trouble getting access to services. Neighborhood clinics, mobile vans, and home visits can be valuable for them. Coordinating services at a central location is also helpful. These multiple-service centers can provide health care, social services, day care, drug and alcohol recovery programs, and case management.

- *Focus on prevention.* Use every opportunity to teach about preventive health care. Primary prevention may include child and adult immunization and education about nutrition, foot care, safe sex, contraception, and the prevention of injuries or chronic illness. It also includes providing prophylactic antituberculosis drug therapy for HIV-positive people who live in homeless shelters or giving flu vaccines to people who are immunocompromised or over age 65. Secondary prevention would include screening for health problems such as tuberculosis, diabetes, hypertension, foot problems, anemia, drug use, or abuse.

Briefly Noted

People who spend time in homeless shelters, substance-abuse treatment facilities, and prisons often get communicable diseases such as influenza and TB. Nurses who work in these facilities should plan regular influenza vaccination clinics and TB screening clinics. When planning these clinics, nurses should work with local physicians to develop signed protocols and should plan ahead for problems related to the transient nature of the population. For example, nurses should develop a way for homeless individuals to read their TB skin test if necessary and transfer the results back to the facility where the skin test was administered. It is helpful to develop a portable immunization chart, such as a wallet card, that mobile population groups such as the homeless and migrant workers can carry with them.

- *Know when to walk beside the client and when to encourage the client to walk ahead.* At times it is hard to know when to do something for someone and when to teach or encourage them to do for themselves. Nursing actions range from providing encouragement and support to providing information and active intervention. It is important to assess for the presence of strengths and for ability to problem-solve and cope and also to access services. For example, a local hospital might provide free mammograms for women who cannot pay. The nurse would need to decide whether to schedule the appointments for clients or to give them the information and encourage them to do the scheduling.
- *Know what resources are available.* It is important to be familiar with community agencies that offer health and social services to vulnerable populations. The nurse must also follow up after making a referral to be sure the client was able to obtain the needed help. Examples of agencies found in most communities are health departments, community mental health centers, voluntary organizations such as the American Red Cross, missions, shelters, soup kitchens, food banks, nurse-managed or free clinics, social service agencies like the Salvation Army or Travelers' Aid, and church-sponsored health and social services.
- *Develop a personal support network.* Working with vulnerable populations can be challenging, rewarding, and at times exhausting. Nurses need to find sources of support

and strength. This can come from friends, family, colleagues, hobbies, exercise, poetry, music, and so forth.

In addition to the nursing actions described, the box below summarizes goals, interventions, and evaluating outcomes with vulnerable populations.

HOW TO Intervene With Vulnerable Populations

GOALS

- Set reasonable goals that are based on the baseline data you collected. Focus on reducing disparities in health status among vulnerable populations.
- Work toward setting manageable goals with the client. Goals that seem unattainable may be discouraging.
- Set goals collaboratively with the client as a first step toward client empowerment.
- Set family-centered, culturally sensitive goals.

INTERVENTIONS

- Set up outreach and case-finding programs to help increase access to health services by vulnerable populations.
- Do everything you can to minimize the "hassle factor" connected with the interventions you plan. Vulnerable groups do not have the extra energy, money, or time to cope with unnecessary waits, complicated treatment plans, or confusion. As your client's advocate, you should identify what hassles may occur and develop ways to avoid them. For example, this may include providing comprehensive services during a single encounter rather than asking the client to return for multiple visits. Extra visits for more specialized aspects of the client's needs, whether individual or family group, reinforce a perception that health care is fragmented and organized for the professional's convenience rather than the client's.
- Work with clients to ensure that interventions are culturally sensitive and competent.
- Focus on teaching clients skills in health promotion and disease prevention. Also, teach them how to be effective health care consumers. For example, role-play asking questions in a physician's office with a client.
- Help clients learn what to do if they cannot keep an appointment with a health care or social service professional.

EVALUATING OUTCOMES

- It is often difficult for vulnerable clients to return for follow-up care. Help your client develop self-care strategies for evaluating outcomes. For example, teach homeless individuals how to read their own TB skin test, and give them a self-addressed, stamped card they can return by mail with the results.
- Remember to evaluate outcomes in terms of the goals you have mutually agreed on with the client. For example, one outcome for a homeless person receiving isoniazid therapy for TB might be that the person return to the clinic daily for direct observation of compliance with the drug therapy.

As can be seen, many of these nursing actions are a part of case management in which the nurse makes referrals and links clients with other community services. In the case manager role, the nurse often is an advocate for the client or family. The nurse serves as an advocate when referring clients to other agencies, when working with others to develop health programs, and when trying to influence legislation and health policies that affect vulnerable population groups.

HOW TO Use Case Management in Working With Vulnerable Populations

- Know available services and resources
- Find out what is missing; look for creative solutions
- Use your clinical skills
- Develop long term relationships with the families you serve
- Strengthen the family's coping and survival skills and resourcefulness
- Be the road map that guides the family to services, and help them get the services
- Communicate with the family and with the agencies who can help them
- Work to change the environment and the policies that affect your clients.

Clinical Application

Ms. Green, a 46-year-old farm worker pregnant with her fifth child, has come to the clinic requesting treatment for swollen ankles. During your assessment, you learned that she had seen the nurse practitioner at the local health department 2 months ago. The NP gave her some sample vitamins, but Ms. Green lost them. She has not received regular prenatal care and has no plans to do so. Her previous pregnancies were essentially normal, although she said she was "toxic" with her last child. She also said that her middle child was "not quite right." He is in the 7th grade at age 15. Ms. Green is 5' 2", weighs 180 pounds, and has a blood pressure of 160/90, with pitting edema of the ankles and a mild headache.

Ms. Green says that she usually takes chlorpromazine hydrochloride (Thorazine) but has run out of it and cannot afford to have her prescription refilled. She says that she has been in several mental hospitals in the past and that she has been more agitated recently and is having problems managing her daily activities. As her agitation grows, she says that she usually hears voices and this really makes her aggressive.

None of her children live with her, and she has no plans for taking care of the infant. She thinks she will ask the child's father, a racetrack worker, to help her since she usually travels around the country with him.

A. *What additional information do you need to help you adequately assess Ms. Green's health status and current needs?*
B. *What nursing activities are suggested by her historical, physical, and psychological descriptions?*

Answers are in the back of the book.

 Remember This!

- Vulnerable populations are more likely to develop health problems as a result of exposure to risk or to have worse outcomes from those health problems than the population as a whole.
- Vulnerable populations are more sensitive to risk factors than those who are more resilient since they are often exposed to cumulative risk factors. These populations include poor or homeless persons, pregnant adolescents, migrant workers, severely mentally ill individuals, substance abusers, abused individuals, people with communicable diseases, and people with sexually transmitted diseases, including HIV and HBV.
- Factors leading to the growing number of poor people in the United States include reduced earnings, decreased availability of low-cost housing, more households headed by women, inadequate education, lack of marketable skills, welfare reform, and reduced Social Security payments to children.
- Poverty has a direct effect on health and well-being across the life span. Poor people have higher rates of chronic illness and infant morbidity and mortality, shorter life expectancy, and more complex health problems.
- Child poverty rates are twice as high as those for adults. Children who live in single-parent homes are twice as likely to be poor than those who live with both parents.
- The complex health problems of homeless people include the inability to get adequate rest, sleep, exercise, nutrition, and medication; exposure; infectious diseases; acute and chronic illness; infestations; trauma, and mental health problems.
- Health care is increasingly moving into the community. This began with deinstitutionalization of the severely mentally ill population and is continuing today as hospitals reduce inpatient stays. Vulnerable populations need a wide variety of services, and because these are often provided by multiple community agencies, nurses coordinate and manage the service needs of vulnerable groups.
- Socioeconomic problems such as poverty and social isolation, physiological and developmental aspects of age, poor health status, and highly stressful life experiences can predispose people to vulnerability. Vulnerability can become a cycle in which the predisposing factors lead to poor health outcomes, chronic stress, and hopelessness. These outcomes increase vulnerability.
- Nurses assess vulnerable individuals, families, and groups to determine which socioeconomic, physical, biological, psychological, and environmental factors are problematic for clients. They work as partners with vulnerable clients to identify client strengths and needs and to develop intervention strategies designed to break the cycle of vulnerability.

 What Would You Do?

1. Examine health statistics and demographic data in your geographical area to determine which vulnerable groups

predominate in your area. Look through your phone book for examples of agencies that provide services to these vulnerable groups. Make appointments with key individuals in several of these agencies to discuss the nature of their target population, the types of services they provide, and how they reimburse for services. Visit different agencies and share results during class. Based on your findings, identify gaps or overlaps in services provided to vulnerable groups in your community. How could you deal with these gaps and overlaps to help clients receive needed services?

2. Identify nurses in your community who work with vulnerable groups. Invite these nurses to come to class and talk about their experiences. What is their typical day? What are the rewards? What are the challenges? How do they deal with frustration, competing demands, and stress?

3. Discuss welfare reform with your classmates. How does the U.S. welfare system work? Who gets welfare payments? What should be done to improve the system? Is your state a leader in welfare reform?

4. Suppose you are making a home visit to a person whose home is not clean. There is food everywhere and roaches are crawling around the house. What do you do if the person asks you to sit down? What if you are offered food?

REFERENCES

Aday LA: *At risk in America: the health and health care needs of vulnerable populations in the United States,* San Francisco, 1993, Jossey Bass.

Adler NE, Boyce WT, Chesney MA, Folkman S, Syme SLL: Socioeconomic inequalities in health: no easy solution. In Lee PR, Estes CL (editors): *The nation's health,* ed 5, Sudbury, Mass, 1997, Jones & Bartlett.

Aiken LH, Salmon ME: Health care workforce priorities: what nursing should do now, *Inquiry* 31(3):318-329, 1994.

American College of Obstetricians and Gynecologists: *Adolescent pregnancy fact sheet,* Washington, D.C., 1998, American College of Obstetricians and Gynecologists.

American Psychiatric Association: *Diagnostic and statistical manual of mental disorders,* ed 4, Washington D.C., 1994, American Psychiatric Association.

Beal AC, Redlener I: Enhancing perinatal outcome in homeless women: the challenge of providing comprehensive health care, *Semin Perinatol* 19(4):307-313, 1995.

Berne AS, Dato C, Mason DJ, Rafferty M: A nursing model for addressing the health needs of homeless families, *Image J Nurs Scholarship* 22(1):8-13, 1991.

Busen NH, Beech B: A collaborative model for community-based health care screening of homeless adolescents, *J Prof Nurs* 13(5):316-324, 1997.

Cartoof VG, Klerman LV, Zazveta VD: The effect of source of prenatal care on care seeking behavioral and pregnancy outcomes among adolescents, *J Adolesc Health* 12:124-129, 1991.

Center for Mental Health Services: Mental health, United States, 1996. In Manderscheid RW, Sonnenschein MA (editors): DHHS pub no (SMA)96-3098, Washington D.C., 1996, Department of Health and Human Services.

Ciesielski S, Esposito D, Protiva, J, Piehl M: The incidence of tuberculosis among North Carolina migrant farm workers, 1991, *Am J Public Health* 84(11):1836-1838, 1994.

Davidhizar R, Frank B: Understanding the physical and psychosocial stressors of the child who is homeless, *Pediatr Nurs* 18(6):559-562, 1992.

De la Barra X: Poverty: the main cause of ill health in urban children, *Health Educ Behav* 25(1):46-59, 1998.

Erickson GP: To pauperize or empower: public health nursing at the turn of the 20th and 21st centuries, *Public Health Nurs* 13(3):163-169, 1996.

Flaskerud JH, Winslow BJ: Conceptualizing vulnerable populations health-related research, *Nurs Res* 47(2):69-78, 1998.

Fullerton D, Dickson R, Eastwood AJ, Sheldon TA: Preventing unintended teenage pregnancies and reducing their adverse effects, *Quality Health Care* 6(2):102-108, 1997.

Hamburg M: Eliminating racial and ethnic disparities in health: response to the presidential initiative on race, *Public Health Rep* 113(July/August):372-375, 1998.

Hatcher RA, Trussel J, Stewart F, Cates W Jr, Guest F, Kowal D: *Contraceptive technology,* New York, 1998, Ardent Media.

Hilfiker D: *Not all of us are saints: a doctor's journey with the poor,* New York, 1994, Hill & Wang.

Institute of Medicine: *Homelessness, health, and human needs,* Washington, D.C., 1988, National Academy Press.

Ireson C, Weaver D: Marketing nursing beyond the walls, *J Nurs Admin* 22(1):57-60, 1992.

Jargowsky MP, Band MJ: Ghetto poverty: basic questions, In Lynn KE, McGeary M (editors): *Inner city poverty in the United States,* Washington D.C., 1990, National Academy Press.

Johnsrud P, Lobdell S, Stewart B, Timm V, Napolitano M: Migrant outreach van evaluation, unpublished master's thesis, 1997, Oregon Health Sciences University, School of Nursing.

Maynard R (editor): *Kids having kids: a Robin Hood Foundation special report on the cost of adolescent childbearing,* 1996, New York, Robin Hood Foundation.

Mechanic D, Schlesinger M, McAlpine DD: Management of mental health and substance abuse services: state of the art and early results, *Milbank Q* 73:19-55, 1995.

Moore KA, Driscoll AK, Lindberg LD: *A statistical portrait of adolescent sex, contraception and childbearing,* Washington D.C., 1998, National Campaign to Prevent Teen Pregnancy.

Moore KA, et al: *Facts at a glance,* Washington, D.C., 1997, Child Trends; sponsored by the Charles Matt Foundation, Flint, Mich.

National Center for Children in Poverty: *How welfare reform can help or hurt children,* New York, 1998, Columbia University.

National Center for Health Statistics: Health: United States, 1998, Hyattsville, Md, 1998, Public Health Service.

National Coalition for the Homeless: *Why are people homeless?* Fact Sheet #1, Washington, D.C., 1998, National Coalition for the Homeless.

Neugebauer R: Mind matters: the importance of mental disorders in public health's 21st century mission (editorial), *Am J Public Health* 89(9):1309-1311, 1999.

Northam S: Access to health promotion, protection, and disease prevention among impoverished individuals, *Public Health Nurs* 13(5):353-364, 1996.

Nurius PS, Furrey J, Berliner L: Coping capacity among women with abusive partners, *Violence Vict* 7(3):229-243, 1992.

Persson RE, Persson GR, Kiyak HA, Powell LV: Oral health and medical status in dentate low-income adults, *Specialty Care Dent* 18(2):70-77, 1998.

Pierre N, Cox J: Teenage pregnancy and prevention programs, *Curr Opin Pediatr* 9(4):310-316, 1997.

Provan KG: Services integration for vulnerable populations: lessons from community mental health, *Fam Commun Health* 19(4):19-30, 1997.

Provan KG, Sebastian JG: Networks within networks: service link overlap, organizational cliques and client outcomes. *Acad Manag J* 41(4):453-463, 1998.

Rew S: Health risks of homeless adolescents: implications for holistic nursing, *J Holistic Nurs* 14(4):348-359, 1996.

Rogers AC: Vulnerability, health and health care, *J Adv Nurs* 26:65-72, 1997.

Schoenberg NE, Gilbert GH: Dietary implications of oral health decrements among African American and white older adults, *Ethnic Health* 3(102):59-70, 1998.

Sebastian J: Vulnerable populations in the community. In Stanhope M, Lancaster J (editors): *Community and public health nursing: process and practice for promoting health,* ed 5, St Louis, 2000, Mosby.

Shore R: *Rethinking the brain: new insights into early development,* New York, 1997, Families and Work Institute.

Steinwachs DM, Cullum HM, Dorwart RA, et al: Service systems research, *Schizophr Bull* 18:627-668, 1992.

Story M (editor): *Nutrition management of the pregnant adolescent,* Washington D.C., 1990, National Clearinghouse.

Superintendent of Documents: *Federal Register* 63(36), Washington, D.C., 1998, U.S. Government Printing Office.

Trussell J: Teenage pregnancy in the United States, *Fam Plann Perspect* 20(6):262-272, 1988.

Unger JL, Kipke MD, Simon TR, Montgomery SB, Johnson CJ: Homeless youths and young adults in Los Angeles: prevalence of mental health problems and the relationship between mental health and substance abuse disorders, *Am J Psychiatry* 25(3):371-394, 1997.

U.S. Department of Health and Human Services: Secretary Shalala launches new national strategy to prevent teen pregnancy: new state-by-state data show decline in teen birth rates, *Health and Human Services News* 1-3,1997.

Valanis B: *Epidemiology in nursing and health care,* ed 3, East Norwalk, Conn, 1999, Appleton & Lange.

Waitzman NJ, Smith KR: *Separate but equal: the effects of economic segregation on mortality in metropolitan America,* Washington D.C., 1997, U.S. Census Bureau.

Walker C: Homeless people and mental health, *Am J Nurs* 98(11):26-32, 1998.

Weinreb L, Goldberg R, Bassuk E, Perloff J: Determinants of health and service use patterns in homeless and low-income housed children, *Pediatrics* 102(3 pt 1):554-562, 1998a.

Weinreb L, Goldberg R, Bassuk E, Perloff J: Health characteristics and medical service use patterns of sheltered homeless and low income housed mothers, *J Gen Intern Med* 13(6):389-97, 1998b.

Wells KB, Astrachan BM, Tischler GL, et al: Issues and approaches in evaluating managed mental health care, *Milbank Q* 73:57-75, 1995.

White MC, Tulsky JP, Dawson C, Zolopa AR, Moss AR: Association between time homeless and perceived health status among the homeless in San Francisco, *J Community Health* 22(4):271-282, 1997.

Worley NK: *Mental health nursing in the community,* St Louis, 1997, Mosby.

Yoos L: Perspectives on adolescent parenting: effect of adolescent egocentrism on the maternal-child interaction, *J Pediatr Nurs* 2(3):193-200, 1987.

Yule W: Resilience and vulnerability in child survivors of disasters. In Tizard B, Varma V (editors): *Vulnerability and resilience in human development,* London, 1992, Kingsley.

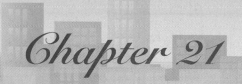

Chapter 21

Substance Abuse in the Community

MARY LYNN MATHRE

OBJECTIVES

After reading this chapter, the student should be able to:

- Differentiate among these terms: *addiction, substance abuse,* and *dependence.*
- Explain the scope of the problem of substance or alcohol, tobacco and other drug (ATOD) abuse and dependence.
- Discuss the differences among the major psychoactive drug categories of depressants, stimulants, marijuana, hallucinogens, and inhalants.

- Describe how nurses can effectively communicate with substance abusers.
- Explain the nursing role in assisting persons with substance abuse problems.
- Examine the effect of substance abuse on the community and on people within the community.

CHAPTER OUTLINE

Scope of the Problem

Definitions

Psychoactive Drugs
  Depressants
  Stimulants
  Marijuana
  Hallucinogens
  Inhalants

The Role of the Nurse in Primary
  Prevention
  Promotion of Healthy Life-Styles and Resiliency
    Factors

Drug Education
Healthy People 2010 and Substance Abuse

The Role of the Nurse in Secondary Prevention
  Assessing for ATOD Problems
  Drug Testing
  High-Risk Groups
  Codependency and Family Involvement

The Role of the Nurse in Tertiary Prevention
  Detoxification
  Addiction Treatment
  Smoking-Cessation Programs
  Support Groups

KEY TERMS

abstinence: withholding or not consuming substances.
addiction: compulsive, uncontrolled psychological or physical dependence on a substance or habit.
alcohol abuse: excessive use of alcohol to the extent that it interferes with effective functioning and affects health.

ATOD: the phenomenon of alcohol, tobacco, and other drug use, abuse, and dependence.
blood alcohol concentration (BAC): determined by the concentration of alcohol in the drink, the rate of drinking, absorption and metabolism, and the person's weight and sex.

Continued

KEY TERMS—cont'd

codependency: an illness in drug and alcohol addiction in which a codependent person is actually addicted to the addict.

denial: a symptom of addiction in which the person may lie about use, minimize use, or use humor to distract from acknowledging the amount of substances being used.

detoxification: gradual withdrawal from an abused substance; best achieved in a treatment setting.

drug addiction: a pattern of abuse characterized by an overwhelming preoccupation with getting and using a drug and its continued use despite adverse effects.

drug dependence: occurs when there is a physiological change in the CNS due to chronic use of a drug.

Employee Assistance Programs (EAPs): services provided at work sites to help employees reduce stress and cope with their own problems as well as those with co-workers.

enabling: shielding or preventing an addict from experiencing the consequences of the illness.

fetal alcohol syndrome (FAS): occurs when a pregnant woman has consumed substantial amounts of alcohol (about

6 drinks/day) and the infant subsequently could be affected in the form of low birth weight and mental retardation, and may have behavioral, facial, limb, genital, cardiac, or neurological impairments.

hallucinogens: drugs capable of producing hallucinations.

inhalants: substances made of organic solvents, volatile nitrites, and nitrous oxide that are inhaled to produce stimulation.

mainstream smoke: smoke inhaled and exhaled by the smoker.

psychoactive drug: alters emotions and often is used in social and recreational settings and for self-medication of physical and emotional discomfort.

sidestream smoke: smoke generated by a smoldering cigarette that affects nonsmokers who breathe the smoke; sometimes called second-hand smoke.

substance abuse: use of chemicals having actual or potential undesirable effects.

tolerance: the need to continually increase the dosage of a drug to achieve the desired results.

withdrawal: physical or psychological symptoms that occur when a drug upon which a person is dependent is removed.

Many forms of morbidity and mortality are linked to substance abuse. Specifically, substance abuse is associated with low-birth-weight babies and those born with congenital abnormalities; accidents, homicides, suicides, and family violence; and chronic diseases such as cancer and cardiovascular and lung disease.

Nurses who work in the community encounter individuals and families who have substance abuse problems. In order to provide effective care, nurses must understand the ways in which alcohol, tobacco, and other drug (**ATOD**) use, abuse, and dependency affect individuals, families, and communities (Allen, 1998).

SCOPE OF THE PROBLEM

Alcohol abuse precipitates between 25% and 40% of admissions to general hospitals, and one in five Medicaid dollars is spent on substance abuse (Institute for Health Policy, 1993; Merrill Fox, and Chang, 1993). More deaths and disabilities annually are attributed to substance abuse than to any other preventable cause. Of the 2 million U.S. deaths each year, one fourth are attributed to tobacco, alcohol, and illicit drug use (Institute for Health Policy, 1993). Cigarette smoking decreased from 42% of the population in 1965 to 29% or 62 million people in 1996 (National Institute on Drug Abuse, 1998c). Also, in 1998, an estimated 13.6 million Americans (6.2% of the population age 12 or older), were current illicit drug users, while 33 million Americans (15.7% of the population) have engaged in binge drinking and 12.4 million Americans (5.9 percent) were heavy drinkers (Office of Applied Studies, 1999). The substance abuser is not only at risk for personal health problems, but also may pose a threat to the health and safety of family members, co-workers, and other members of the commu-

nity. Substance abuse and **addiction** affect all ages, races, sexes, and segments of society.

It is important to remember that substance abuse includes abuse of illegal as well as prescription or over-the-counter (OTC) drugs. Substances of abuse also include alcohol, tobacco, and caffeine. In the current fast-paced societies of the world, people tend to rely on prescription, OTC, and illegal drugs to relieve anxiety, tension, fatigue, and physical and emotional pain.

It is equally important for nurses to be aware that excessive use of substances such as alcohol, tobacco, and other drugs needs to be viewed as a health problem rather than a criminal act or social deviation. In thinking about substance abuse it is important to consider three contributing factors: the drug used; the set (person's expectations about the effects of the drug); and the setting or influence of the physical, social, and cultural environments. This chapter discusses the extent of the problem of substance abuse, defines its various forms, describes the most prevalent types of substance use and abuse and presents nursing interventions to assist with both short- and long-term assistance.

DEFINITIONS

Many terms currently describe alcohol, tobacco, and other drug (ATOD) use, abuse, and dependence. The terms *drug use* and *drug abuse* have limited descriptive utility because the public and government have narrowed the term *drug* to include only illegal drugs, rather than including prescription, OTC, and legal recreational drugs. The more useful term *ATOD* calls attention to the significant drug problems associated with alcohol and tobacco. The term *substance* broadens the scope to include alcohol, tobacco, legal drugs, and even foods. **Substance abuse** is the use of any substance that threatens a person's health or impairs his or her social or economic functioning.

Drug dependence and drug addiction, while often used interchangeably, are not synonymous. **Drug dependence** occurs when there is a physiological change in the central nervous system (CNS) caused by the chronic, regular administration of a drug whereby continued use of the drug is needed to prevent **withdrawal** symptoms (O'Brien, 1996). For example, a person might be given an opiate such as morphine on a regular basis for pain management. To prevent withdrawal symptoms, the morphine should be gradually tapered rather than abruptly stopped.

Drug addiction is a pattern of abuse characterized by an overwhelming preoccupation with getting and using a drug and its continued use despite negative consequences. There is also a tendency to relapse if the drug is removed. Addicts are often both physically and psychologically dependent on a drug, with the psychological component causing intense cravings and subsequent relapse. Anyone can become drug dependent if he or she regularly uses drugs that alter the CNS; however, only 7% to 15% of the drug-using population develop a drug addiction. It is not known why some people develop a drug addiction and others do not.

It is important to remember that alcohol is also a drug. The diseases of both alcoholism and drug addiction are chronic, progressive diseases in which a person's use of a drug or drugs continues despite problems it causes in any area of life—physical, emotional, social, economical, or spiritual.

PSYCHOACTIVE DRUGS

Although any drug can be abused, abuse and addiction problems generally involve the **psychoactive drugs.** Because they can alter emotions, these drugs are used for enjoyment in social and recreational settings and for personal use to self-medicate physical or emotional discomfort. Psychoactive drugs are divided into categories according to their effect on the CNS and the general feelings or experiences the drugs may induce, and people often substitute another drug from the same category if their drug of choice is unavailable. For example, a person who cannot drink alcohol may begin using a benzodiazepine as an alternative because both are CNS depressants.

Depressants

Depressants reduce both a person's energy level and sensitivity to outside stimulation, and, in high doses, induce sleep. Low doses of depressants may produce a feeling of stimulation caused by initial sedation of the inhibitory centers in the brain. In general, depressants decrease heart rate, respirations, muscular coordination, and energy, and dull the senses. Higher doses lead to coma and, if the vital functions shut down, death. Major categories include alcohol, barbiturates, benzodiazepines, and the opioids.

Alcohol

Alcohol (ethyl alcohol or ethanol) is the oldest and most widely used psychoactive drug in the world (Manwell,

Fleming, Barry, and Johnson, 1997). In 1998, approximately 113 million Americans age 12 and older consumed alcohol. This is 52% of the population. The level of alcohol use was strongly associated with illicit drug use. That is, heavy drinkers were likely to use illegal drugs as well. Also, in the same year, 10.4 million current drinkers were between 12 and 20 years old (Office of Applied Studies, 1999). **Alcohol abuse** ranks third following coronary diseases and cancer as the major cause of death in the United States. The life expectancy of a person with alcoholism is reduced by 15 years, and mortality is two and a half times greater than that of persons without alcoholism (Kinney and Leaton, 1995).

Briefly Noted

Alcohol use in moderation can provide mild relaxation and lower the serum cholesterol. The National Institute on Alcohol Abuse and Alcoholism (1995) recommends that men consume no more than two drinks per day and women and persons over age 65 no more than one drink per day.

Alcohol abuse costs billions of dollars in lost productivity, property damage, medical expenses from alcohol-related illnesses, accidents, family disruptions, and violence. Chronic alcohol abuse can have major metabolic and physiological effects on all organ systems. Gastrointestinal (GI) disturbances include inflammation of the GI tract, malabsorption, ulcers, liver problems, and cancers. Cardiovascular disturbances include cardiac dysrhythmias, cardiomyopathy, hypertension, atherosclerosis, and blood dyscrasias. CNS problems include depression, sleep disturbances, memory loss, organic brain syndrome, Wernicke-Korsakoff syndrome, and alcohol withdrawal syndrome. Neuromuscular problems include myopathy and peripheral neuropathy. Males may experience testicular atrophy, sterility, impotence, or gynecomastia; and females who consume alcohol during pregnancy may produce neonates with fetal alcohol syndrome (FAS) or fetal alcohol effects (FAE). Some of the metabolic disturbances include hypokalemia, hypomagnesemia, and ketoacidosis. Also, endocrine disturbances can lead to pancreatitis or diabetes (National Institute on Alcohol Abuse and Alcoholism, 1997).

The **blood alcohol concentration (BAC)** is determined by the concentration of alcohol in the drink, the rate of drinking, the rate of absorption (slower in the presence of food), the rate of metabolism, and a person's weight and sex. The amount of alcohol the liver can metabolize per hour is equal to about ¾ ounce of whiskey, 4 ounces of wine, or 12 ounces of beer. Chronic consumption often leads to tolerance; therefore a person can have a high BAC with minimal CNS effects.

Females cannot consume as much alcohol as males before they have adverse effects. They have less alcohol dehydrogenase activity than men (except for males with chronic alcoholism). This enzyme detoxifies alcohol, and because females have less enzyme, they suffer the long-term effects of alcohol intake at much lower doses in a shorter time span (Talashek, Gerace, and Starr, 1994; Frezza, et al, 1990).

Barbiturates

These drugs are generally known as sleeping pills or "downers." High doses help people sleep, and low doses have a calming effect. Short-acting barbiturates, similar to alcohol in their effects, are frequently abused. These drugs are not as toxic to the body's organ systems as alcohol; however, the tolerance that develops is more dangerous. **Tolerance** (the need for a higher dose to yield the same effect) to the effects on mood develop faster than the physical tolerance to the lethal dose, resulting in a greater risk of accidental overdose. Barbiturates used in combination with alcohol intensify the effects of both and increase the risk of overdose.

Benzodiazepines

These drugs were introduced in the 1960s as a treatment for stress. In 1994, more than 80 million benzodiazepine prescriptions were filled, with 1 in 10 Americans reporting use of a benzodiazepine once a year or more for a medical reason other than insomnia (Gold, et al, 1995). At one time, diazepam (Valium) and chlordiazepoxide (Librium) were used to treat alcoholism, but it soon became apparent that these drugs produced an alcohol-like effect and were addictive. These drugs continue to be used too often for long-term therapy instead of treating the underlying stress. While the benzodiazepines have a relatively safe therapeutic index (difficult to overdose), withdrawal can be life threatening.

Opioids

These drugs (opium, morphine, and codeine) are found naturally in the opium poppy. Opioids are also synthetic drugs—such as heroin (semisynthetic), meperidine, methadone, oxycodone, and propoxyphene—that mimic the effects of the natural opiates. Opiates are highly effective in pain relief. Opioid addicts (approximately 0.1% of opioid users) take prescription opioid analgesics obtained legally (present with false or exaggerated complaints of pain) or illegally (forged prescriptions or diversion).

The United States has approximately 750,000 to 1 million heroin addicts, and more than 2 million people who have tried the drug (O'Brien, 1996). The typical heroin addict is a male from a poor socioeconomic background, and began use between 16 and 19 years of age (Foley, 1993).

Tolerance develops easily with opioids, and tolerance to one opioid extends to other opioids, leading to cross-tolerance. Physical dependence develops quickly, and in less than 2 weeks of continuous use a person can have withdrawal symptoms if the opioid is not tapered. Chronic abuse of the opioids causes few physiological problems except for constipation. The negative consequences primarily result from their illegal status. Heroin is usually consumed intranasally, subcutaneously, intravenously, or by inhalation, and costs $10 to $100 per bag. A "bag" varies in amount and purity.

Stimulants

People use stimulants because these drugs make them feel more alert or energetic by activating or exciting the nervous system. An increase in alertness and energy results as the stimulant causes the nerve fibers to release noradrenaline and other stimulating neurotransmitters. However, these drugs do not give the person more energy; they only make the body expend its own energy sooner and in greater quantities than it normally would.

If used carefully, stimulants are useful and have few negative health effects. The body must be allowed time to replenish itself after use of a stimulant. There is a "down" state following the use of a stimulant during which the person feels sleepy, lazy, mentally fatigued, and possibly depressed. Many persons abusing stimulants soon find themselves in a vicious cycle of avoiding the down feeling by taking another dose, and they become physically dependent on the stimulant in order to function. Common stimulants include nicotine, cocaine, caffeine, and amphetamines.

Nicotine

An estimated 2.1 million people began smoking cigarettes daily in 1997. The rate of initiation among youths ages 12 through 17 increased between 1991 and 1995, from 11.1 to 25.0 per thousand potential new users, and was constant from 1995 to 1997. Current smokers are more likely than non-smokers to be heavy drinkers and illicit drug users (Office of Applied Studies, 1999). The Centers for Disease Control and Prevention (CDC) estimates more than 430,000 deaths per year are caused by complications of cigarette smoking, including 30% of all heart disease deaths, 90% of all lung cancer deaths, and about 90% of all chronic obstructive pulmonary disease deaths (Leshner, 1998). See Figure 21-1 for cigarette smoking mortality. The *Morbidity and Mortality Weekly Report* (Medical-Care Expenditures, 1994) estimated 1993 smoking-related medical costs at $50 billion. Nicotine, the active ingredient in the tobacco plant, is a toxic drug, and smokers quickly develop tolerance to the nicotine. If a person smokes regularly, tolerance to nicotine develops within hours, compared to days with heroin or months with alcohol. Pipes and cigars are less hazardous than cigarettes because the harsher smoke discourages deep inhalation. However, pipes and cigars increase the risk of cancer of the lips, mouth, and throat.

Smoke can be inhaled directly by the smoker (**mainstream smoke),** or it can enter the atmosphere from the lighted end of the cigarette and be inhaled by others in the vicinity (**sidestream smoke).** Sidestream smoke contains greater concentrations of toxic and carcinogenic compounds than mainstream smoke. Diseases and conditions associated

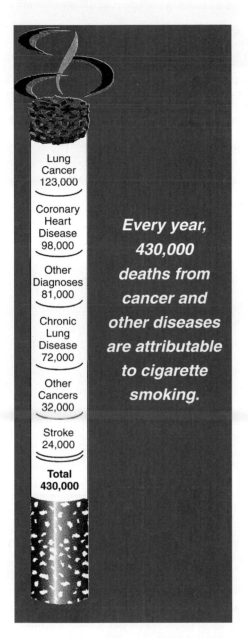

Figure 21-1   Cigarette smoking mortality. (From Centers for Disease Control and Prevention: Cigarette smoking-attributable mortality and years of lives lost–United States, 1984, *MMWR* 46[20]:444-451, 1997.)

with smoking include cancer, cardiovascular and pulmonary problems, and perinatal effects.

Nicotine is also found chewing tobacco, or snuff. Marketed as "smokeless tobacco," a wad is put in the mouth, and the nicotine is absorbed sublingually. Higher doses of nicotine are delivered in the smokeless forms because the nicotine is not destroyed by heat. Nevertheless, this form is less addictive because nicotine enters the bloodstream less directly.

Cocaine

Cocaine was first used by the South American Indians. They cultivated it and chewed a mixture of the coca leaf and

Evidence-Based Practice

Levels of nicotine and cotinine, a metabolite of nicotine, were measured in the urine of a sample of 40 black and 39 white smokers after they were given infusions of deuterium-labeled nicotine and had continued their regular smoking patterns. Both groups were matched for age (mean, 32.5 and 32.3), body weight, and number of cigarettes smoked daily (mean, 14 and 14.7). The total and non-renal clearance of nicotine was not significantly different in comparing the two groups. The total and non-renal clearance of cotinine was significantly lower in blacks than in whites. The intake of nicotine per cigarette smoked was estimated to be 30% higher in blacks than in whites based on cotinine levels during smoking and clearance results. Additional testing showed that cotinine half-life was longer (but not significantly) in blacks than in whites, indicating varying nicotine metabolism rates.

Blacks in the study had both a slower clearance of cotinine and a higher intake of nicotine per cigarette. Previous studies have shown that a genetic trait that may protect an individual from nicotine addiction may be missing in blacks. These results may help explain why blacks have a higher risk for lung cancer and have higher rates of relapse with smoking-cessation strategies.

APPLICATION IN PRACTICE

Since blacks are at higher risk for health disruption from cigarette smoking, careful patient and family history of smoking and lung cancer is recommended. Clear, easy-to-understand explanations of the relationship between smoking and lung cancer should be given.

Perez-Stable EJ, Herrera B, Jacob P, Benowitz NL: Nicotine metabolism and intake in black and white smokers, *JAMA* 280:152-156, 1998.

lime to get a mild stimulant effect similar to coffee. By 1860 cocaine was isolated from the plant as a hydrochloride salt, dissolved in water, and used intravenously or orally when mixed in soft drinks. By the early 1900s the white powder was used intranasally by "snorting" (Weil and Rosen, 1993).

"Freebasing" began in the 1970s, and this involved making the hydrochloride salt a more volatile substance using highly flammable substances such as ether to convert the powder to a crystal that could then be smoked in a pipe. In the early 1980s, smokeable cocaine was introduced. Cocaine was dissolved in water, mixed with baking soda, and then heated to form rocks, or "crack." Approximately 90% of cocaine users have snorted cocaine, 33% have smoked it, and 10% have injected it (Warner, 1993). Intranasal cocaine has been a popular recreational drug among the "rich and famous," but the cheaper crack form, sold in small quantities at $2 to $20, has become popular, particularly among inner-city black populations.

Briefly Noted

More than 400,000 whites use cocaine compared to 200,000 Hispanics and 48,000 blacks (Marwick, 1998). There were an estimated 730,000 new cocaine users in 1997, which is similar to the high first-time use rate of the 1980s (Office of Applied Studies, 1999).

Cocaine produces a feeling of intense euphoria, increased confidence, and a willingness to work for long periods. Smoking cocaine gives intense effects because the drug quickly reaches the brain through the blood vessels in the lungs. Cocaine's interaction with dopamine may be the basis for the addictive patterns. The extreme euphoria seems to be caused by cocaine's effect of dopaminergic stimulation. Chronic administration can lead to neurotransmitter depletion (especially of dopamine), which results in an extreme dysphoria characterized by apathy, sadness, and anhedonia (lack of joy). Thus a cocaine user can get caught up in a dangerous cycle of having an extreme high followed by an extreme low and avoiding that low by consuming more cocaine. Crack addiction develops rapidly and is expensive, with addicts needing between $100 and $1000 per day. Addicts soon learn that their ill health and drug use are related, but overwhelmed by cravings, they may resort to criminal activities such as theft or prostitution to get the drug.

Street cocaine ranges in purity from 5% to 60% and may be cut with other drugs, such as procaine or amphetamine, or any white powder, such as sugar or baby powder. The incidence of cocaine-related emergency room visits increased twelve-fold from 1985 to 1992. Some of this increase is the result of the lack of quality control; however, most is the result of the use of crack. High doses can cause extreme agitation, hyperthermia, hallucinations, cardiac dysrhythmias, pulmonary complications, convulsions, and possibly death (Das and Laddu, 1993; Warner, 1993).

Caffeine

Caffeine is one of the most widely used psychoactive drugs in the world, with a U.S. daily per capita consumption of 211 mg. Caffeine is found in coffee, tea, chocolate, soft drinks, and various medications (Table 21-1). Caffeine in soft drinks and cold coffee drinks is growing as a drug of choice for American youth (Cordes, 1998). Moderate doses of caffeine (from 100 to 300 mg) per day increase mental alertness and probably have little negative effect on health. Note that 5 ounces of brewed coffee has 60 to 180 mg of caffeine, and 5 ounces of brewed tea has 20-90 mg of caffeine. Higher doses can lead to insomnia, irritability, tremulousness, anxiety, cardiac dysrhythmias, and headaches. Regular use of high doses can lead to physical dependence, and the withdrawal symptoms may include headaches, slowness, and occasional depression (Strain, et al, 1994).

Amphetamines

Amphetamines are a class of stimulants similar to cocaine. They cost less, and their effects last longer. They have a

TABLE 21-1   Caffeine Content in Commonly Consumed Substances

Substance	Caffeine content (mg)
Coffee (5 oz)	
Brewed	60-180
Instant	0-120
Decaffeinated	1-5
Chocolate	
Cocoa (5 oz)	2-20
Semisweet (1 oz)	5-35
Tea (5 oz)	
Brewed	20-90
Iced	67-76
Soft drinks (12 oz)	
Colas	40-45
Mountain Dew	53
Orange, ginger ale, root beer	0
Prescription drugs	
Propoxyphene (Darvene)	32.4
Fiorinal	40
Ergotamine (Cafergot)	100
Over-the-counter drugs	
Aqua-ban	100
Anacin	32
Excedrin	65
No Doz	100
Vivarin	200

chemical structure similar to adrenaline and noradrenaline and are used to decrease fatigue, increase mental alertness, suppress appetite, and create a sense of well-being. These drugs are taken orally, intranasally, by injection, or by smoking. When taken intravenously, they quickly induce an intense euphoric feeling (a "rush"). The user may speed for several days (go on a "speed run") and then fall into a deep sleep for 18 or more hours ("crash"). "Ice," a smokeable form of crystallized methamphetamine, was introduced in the late 1980s as an alternative to crack because it can be easily manufactured and the effects last up to 24 hours. Methamphetamine use increased during the 1990s in both rural and urban areas (National Institute on Drug Abuse, 1998a).

Other drugs containing caffeine, ephedrine, or phenylpropanolamine (singly or in combination), referred to as "look-alikes," became popular when amphetamines began to be controlled by prescription. These chemicals are often found in OTC cold remedies as a nasal decongestant and in diet pills (e.g., Dexatrim).

Marijuana

Marijuana (*Cannabis sativa* or *Cannabis indica)* is the most widely used illicit drug in the United States. It is estimated that from 20 to 30 million Americans are regular users, and as many as 60% of those between the ages of 18 and 25 years have tried marijuana at some time. In the last two decades, teens who reported having used marijuana decreased from a high of about 60% in the late 1970s to under 50% by 1997; only 5.8% were daily users in 1997 (Cargo, 1998).

Compared with the other psychoactive drugs, marijuana has little toxicity and is a safe therapeutic agent (Petro, 1997). However, since it is illegal, there is no quality control, and a user may consume contaminated marijuana. Users enjoy a mild euphoria, a relaxed feeling, and an intensity of sensory perceptions. Side effects include dry and reddened eyes, increased appetite, dry mouth, drowsiness, and mild tachycardia. Adverse reactions include anxiety, disorientation, and paranoia.

The greatest physical concern for chronic users is possible damage to the respiratory tract. Both tolerance and physical dependence can occur; however, the withdrawal symptoms are mild. Addiction can occur for some chronic users and is difficult to treat because the progression is subtle.

Briefly Noted

Prior to the marijuana prohibition, cannabis was a popular plant grown for its fiber (hemp), seed (popular birdseed), oil, and medicinal as well as psychoactive properties. During World War II the hemp fiber was so valuable that farmers were required to grow marijuana to ensure a supply. Hemp fiber and seeds do not contain enough active THC to produce any psychoactive effects, and these products are becoming available in the United States.

Prior to the *Marijuana Tax Act of 1937,* tincture of cannabis was listed in the *U.S. Pharmacopoeia* through 1941 for such ailments as migraines, spasticity, and dysmenorrhea, and in the treatment of heroin or cocaine addiction. In 1970 marijuana was placed in the Schedule I category of drugs by the passage of the *Controlled Substances Act* and has not been available for medicinal use. The only legal access was through the U.S. Food and Drug Administration's (FDA's) Compassionate Investigational New Drug Program; this program was closed in 1992 (Mathre, 1997). In 1999, the Institute of Medicine completed an 18-month study to review the usefulness of medical cannabis and concluded that cannabis does have therapeutic value. However, the federal government refuses to remove marijuana from the Schedule I category of drugs.

Hallucinogens

Also called *psychedelics* (mind vision), **hallucinogens** can produce hallucinations. Many of these drugs have been used for centuries in religious ceremonies, healing rituals, to produce euphoria, and as aphrodisiacs. With hallucinogens the user's mood, basic emotional makeup, and expectations (set) along with the immediate surroundings (setting) all influence the mental effects experienced by the user. The physical effects are more constant and produce CNS stimulation.

The two broad chemical families of hallucinogens are the indole hallucinogens and those that resemble adrenalin and amphetamines. The indoles are related to hormones (serotonin) made in the brain by the pineal gland and include such drugs as lysergic acid diethylamide (LSD), psilocybin mushrooms, and morning glory seeds. The second group lacks the chemical structure called the indole ring and includes peyote, mescaline, and MDMA (Ecstasy). Phencyclidine (PCP) is in a class by itself. LSD and PCP will be discussed.

Lysergic Acid Diethylamide

LSD, a highly potent drug, is the best-known hallucinogen. It is administered orally in small tablets, in gelatin chips ("window panes"), or on pieces of paper soaked with the drug or stamped with ink containing LSD. The effects from a dose of 25 to 300 micrograms can last up to 10 to 12 hours (Weil and Rosen, 1993).

The desired effects include euphoria, a heightened sense of awareness, distorted perceptions, and synesthesia (a mixing of senses, e.g., sounds appearing as visual images). Adverse reactions to LSD include depersonalization, hypertension, panic, and psychosis. Another adverse reaction may be a flashback, or a recurrence of the "trip" weeks or months after the LSD has been ingested. Flashbacks can be frightening, especially because of their unpredictability, but will decrease in frequency over time.

Phencyclidine

Phencyclidine (PCP) is a potent anesthetic and analgesic with CNS depressant, stimulant, and hallucinogenic properties. PCP comes as pills or powder and can be sold as mescaline, psilocybin, THC, or other drugs. "Angel dust" is PCP sprinkled on a marijuana joint. The mental effects vary but often include a feeling of disconnection from the body and reality, apathy, disorganized thinking, a drunk-like state, and distortions of time and space perception. Adverse reactions include combative behavior, inability to talk, a rigid robotic attitude, confusion, paranoid thinking, catatonia, coma, and convulsions. Unlike the other hallucinogens, phencyclidine can be addicting.

Inhalants

Teens are the most frequent inhalant users. **Inhalants** do not fit neatly into other categories but include gases and solvents. The three main types of inhalants are organic solvents, volatile nitrites, and nitrous oxide. These substances are inhaled ("huffed") from bottles, aerosol cans, or soaked cloth, or are put into bags or balloons to increase the concentration of the inhaled fumes and decrease the inhalation of other substances in the vapor (e.g, paint particles).

Organic solvents include rubber cement, model airplane glue, paint thinner, and aerosol products such as spray paint, deodorant, and hair spray. The effects are similar to alcohol but have a rapid onset and last a short time. The user initially feels stimulated as the inhibitions are depressed; then a drunk-like state occurs that may include hallucinations. Users may also experience headache, tinnitus, diplopia, abdominal pain, nausea, or vomiting. "Sudden sniffing death" may occur; it appears to be related to acute cardiac dysrhythmia (Dinwiddie, 1994). These drugs are inexpensive and easy to obtain by youth.

Amyl nitrite is the most common of the volatile nitrites and is most often used by urban male homosexuals. It is frequently used during sexual activity to intensify the experience and prolong orgasm. This yellow liquid is packaged in cloth-covered glass capsules that have to be popped (hence the common name of "poppers") to release the drug for inhalation.

Often referred to as laughing gas, nitrous oxide is widely used in dentistry and minor surgery as a tranquilizer to sedate and create an analgesic effect by changing the patient's mood and interpretation of pain. Nitrous oxide is also found in whipping cream aerosol cans ("whippets") and is released by spraying the can upside down. Dangers with administration increase when inhaling directly from pressurized tanks because the gas is very cold and can cause frostbite to the nose, lips, and vocal cords. Also, if nitrous oxide is not mixed with oxygen, the user may die from asphyxiation (Espeland, 1993).

THE ROLE OF THE NURSE IN PRIMARY PREVENTION

Primary prevention for substance abuse or ATOD problems includes (1) promoting healthy life-styles and resiliency factors and (2) education about drugs and guidelines for use. Nurses working in the community are ideally prepared to promote and facilitate healthful alternatives to indiscriminate, careless, and often dangerous drug use practices and to educate about drugs to decrease harm from irresponsible or unsafe drug use.

Promotion of Healthy Life-Styles and Resiliency Factors

Health promotion includes helping people learn interventions for stress, fatigue, or pain other than or in addition to the use of drugs. Teaching assertiveness, decision-making, and conflict-resolution skills helps clients cope more effectively. Nagging health problems such as difficulty sleeping, muscle tension, lack of energy, chronic stress, and mood swings often cause people to use medications, especially the psychoactive drugs. Nurses can help clients understand that medications only mask the problems rather than solve them. Stress reduction, relaxation techniques, healthy eating, exercise, and adequate sleep can reduce stress and support effective coping. Nurses can provide information about healthful habits at community recreational facilities and to community groups.

In addition to decreasing risk factors associated with ATOD problems, it is important to increase protective or resiliency factors. Children from high-risk environments who survive successfully have more resiliency factors than do non-surviving children (Kumpfer and Hopkins, 1993). Strategies to increase resiliency include:

- Helping children develop a sense of responsibility for their own success

- Helping them identify their talents
- Encouraging them to participate in activities to help society rather than believing that their only purpose in life is to "take"
- Providing realistic appraisals and feedback
- Stressing multicultural competence
- Encouraging and valuing education and skills training
- Increasing cooperative solutions to problems rather than competitive or aggressive solutions.

Nursing actions directed at ATOD prevention are described in the box below.

HOW TO Set Up Community-Based Activities Aimed at ATOD Problem Prevention

- Increase involvement and pride in school activities
- Organize student assistant programs (students helping students)
- Organize a Students Against Drunk Driving (SADD) chapter
- Mobilize parent awareness and action groups (e.g., MADD)
- Increase availability of recreation facilities
- Encourage parental commitment to nondrinking parties
- Encourage involvement of religious institutions in conveying nonuse messages and providing activities associated with nonuse
- Curtail media messages that glamorize drug and alcohol use
- Support and reinforce antidrug use peer pressure skills
- Provide general health screenings, including for ATOD use
- Collaborate among community leaders to solve problems related to crime, housing, jobs, and access to health care

Drug Education

With more than 450,000 different drugs and drug combinations available, ATOD problems are much bigger than just abuse of psychoactive drugs. Prescription drugs are estimated to be involved in almost 60% of all drug-related emergency room visits and 70% of all drug-related deaths. Approximately 25% of hospital admissions of older people result from problems related to noncompliance and drug reactions (Larrat, Taubman, and Willey, 1990).

Nurses are experts in medication administration, understand the dangers of indiscriminate drug use, know that drugs cannot "cure" all problems, and are aware that both "good" and "bad" drugs can harm. Nurses can (1) teach clients that no drug is completely safe and any drug can be abused and (2) help persons make informed decisions about their drug use to minimize possible harm. An effective method of drug education is to review the client's prescription medications. The fact that a drug has been prescribed does not guarantee that no risk is involved.

People often mix drugs to regulate how they feel. This is polysubstance use or abuse. For example, a person may drink alcohol when snorting cocaine to "take the edge off"; or some intravenous drug users combine cocaine with heroin (speedball) for similar reasons. Polysubstance use can cause various

Box 21-1	Drug Consumer Safety Guidelines

Before using a drug/medication always ask:

- What chemical is being taken
- How and where the drug works in the body
- What is the correct dosage
- Whether there will be drug interactions
- If there are allergic reactions
- If there will be drug tolerance
- Whether the drug will produce physical dependence*

From Miller M: *Drug consumer safety rules,* Mosier, Ore, 1994, Mothers Against Misuse and Abuse (MAMA).
*Caution: Approximately 10% of the population may suffer from the disease of addiction. For those persons, responsible use of psychoactive drugs is limited secondary to their disease. Individuals should always notify their physician of their addiction if use of psychoactive medicines is being considered in their treatment.

drug interactions that have additive, synergistic, or antagonistic effects. Indiscriminate polysubstance abuse may lead to serious physiological consequences and can be complicated for the health care professional to assess and treat. Nurses in the community need to assess whether clients are mixing a variety of drugs and if so, advise them of possible dangers.

Briefly Noted

Think of the 4 Hs to remember what to ask when assessing drug use patterns:

- How taken (route)
- How much
- How often
- How long.

People need to know what questions to ask regarding their personal drug use and should seek the answers to their questions before using any drug. Encouraging clients to ask questions regarding their drug use can increase their responsibility for personal health as well as increase their awareness that drugs will alter their body chemistry. Box 21-1 has seven questions that can help clients decide if they should take a drug. These questions are useful resources, as are reference books written for the public that discuss drugs, drug interactions, and the interaction of drugs with food and beverages (Griffith, 1998; Rybacki and Long, 1999).

Nurses can teach clients to ask questions about their prescription medications and about the self-administration of OTC and recreational drugs. This does not mean that nurses should encourage other drug use but rather that the potential harm from self-medication can be reduced if clients have the necessary information to make more informed decisions.

Nurses can also help parents learn to role model for their children asking relevant drug-related questions. It can be confusing for youth to be told to "just say no" to drugs, while they see their parents or drug advertisements try to "quick fix" every health complaint with a medication. The simple "just say no" approach does not help young people for several reasons. First, children are naturally curious, and

Box 21-2	The Evolution of Prevention

1960s: Prevention approaches have evolved since the 1960s, when a high level of illegal drug use was well noted in the media. The first response was to use scare tactics. Drugs were only depicted as harmful, and the information was often exaggerated or inaccurate. Information from peers often invalidated these scare tactics and caused distrust of the "experts."

1970s: During the early 1970s, some professionals began using the strategy of giving accurate information to young people. This strategy may have increased usage rates, creating educated drug users. By the late 1970s, the focus was on teaching young people life skills, which included personal self-awareness, independent living, job skills, and communication skills.

1980s: In the early 1980s, healthy alternatives to ATOD use looked at natural highs through recreational experiences. Also in the 1980s, emphasis was placed on changing policies to decrease drug use. These policy changes centered around legislative and law-enforcement efforts. And by the late 1980s the new approach was community involvement, which attempted to bring societal pressure to bear on the problem.

1990s: The strategy for the 1990s was a comprehensive approach that combined all of the previous approaches with the exception of scare tactics.

From National Nurses Society on Addictions: *Prevention of alcohol, tobacco, and other drugs,* 1994, Macro International Inc, and J & E Associates, under contract by the Center for Substance Abuse Prevention.

drug experimentation is often a part of normal development (Shedler and Block, 1990). Second, children from dysfunctional homes often use drugs to get attention or to escape an intolerable environment. And finally, the "just say no" approach does not address the powerful influence of peer pressure (Donaldson, Graham, and Hansen, 1994).

Basic ATOD prevention programs for young people should combine efforts to increase resiliency factors with drug education. Nurses can serve as educators or as advisors to the school systems or community groups to ensure all of these areas are addressed. Role-playing can be an effective method of teaching many of these skills. Box 21-2 provides an historical overview of the prevention approaches.

Healthy People 2010 and Substance Abuse

Substance use and abuse and related health problems are among the most pervasive health problems and social problems today. The nurse will want to address these issues with clients in assessment, direct care, health education/counseling, and referral. The *Healthy People 2010* box lists the objectives directed at substance abuse.

THE ROLE OF THE NURSE IN SECONDARY PREVENTION

To identify substance abuse and plan appropriate interventions, nurses must assess each client individually. When drug abuse, dependence, or addiction is identified, nurses must assist clients to understand the connection between

Healthy People 2010
Substance Abuse

Objectives directed at reducing the use and abuse of substances:

26-9 Increase the age and proportion of adolescents who remain alcohol and drug free.

26-10 Reduce past-month use of illicit substances.

26-11 Reduce the proportion of persons engaging in binge drinking of alcoholic beverages.

26-12 Reduce average annual alcohol consumption.

26-13 Reduce the proportion of adults who exceed guidelines for low-risk drinking.

26-14 Reduce steroid use among adolescents.

26-15 Reduce the proportion of adolescents who use inhalants.

26-16 Increase the proportion of adolescents who disapprove of substance abuse.

26-17 Increase the proportion of adolescents who perceive great risk associated with substance abuse.

27-1 Reduce tobacco use by adults.

27-2 Reduce tobacco use by adolescents.

27-3 Reduce initiation of tobacco use among children and adolescents.

27-4 Increase the average age of first use of tobacco products by adolescents and young adults.

27-5 Increase smoking cessation attempts by adult smokers.

27-6 Increase smoking cessation during pregnancy.

27-7 Increase smoking cessation attempts by adolescent smokers.

27-8 Increase insurance coverage of evidence-based treatment for nicotine dependency.

27-9 Reduce the proportion of children who are regularly exposed to tobacco smoke at home.

27-10 Reduce the proportion of nonsmokers exposed to environmental tobacco smoke.

27-11 Increase smoke-free and tobacco-free environments in schools, including all school facilities, property, vehicles, and school events.

27-12 Increase the proportion of worksites with formal smoking policies that prohibit smoking or limit it to separately ventilated areas.

27-13 Establish laws on smoke-free indoor air that prohibit smoking or limit it to separately ventilated areas in public places and worksites.

their drug use patterns and the negative consequences on their health, their families, and the community.

Assessing for ATOD Problems

All health assessments should check for substance use and abuse and include inquiry about self-medication practices as well as recreational drug use. Screening for ATOD use needs to be done in a safe, private location, paying attention to the person's culture, gender, age and religion (Allen, 1998). After obtaining a medication history, follow-up questions can determine whether any problems exist. For prescription drug use, is the client following the directions correctly? Be especially inquisitive about any prescribed psychoactive drug use: How long has the client been taking the drug? Has the client increased the dosage or frequency above the prescription?

When assessing self-medication and recreational or social drug use patterns, the reason for use should be elicited. Some underlying health problems (i.e., pain, stress, weight, or insomnia) may be relieved by non-pharmaceutical interventions. Ask about the amount, frequency, duration of use, and route of administration of each drug.

To determine if a substance abuse problem exists, find out if the drug use is causing any negative health consequences or problems with relationships, employment, finances, or the legal system. Examples of questions to ask clients to determine if there are socioeconomic problems that accompany the substance abuse are presented in the box below. If the nurse detects a pattern of chronic, regular, and frequent drug use, assess for a history of withdrawal symptoms to determine if there is physical dependence on the drug. **Denial,** a primary symptom of addiction, is often seen in lying about use, minimizing use patterns, blaming or rationalizing, intellectualizing, changing the subject, defensiveness, using anger or humor, and "going with the flow" (agreeing there is a problem, stating behavior will change, but then doing nothing different).

HOW TO Assess Socioeconomic Problems Secondary to Substance Abuse

If the client admits to use of alcohol, tobacco or other drugs, ask the following questions:

1. Do your spouse, parents, or friends worry or complain about your drinking or using drugs?
2. Has a family member gone for help about your drinking or using drugs?
3. Have you neglected family obligations secondary to drinking or using drugs?
4. Have you missed work because of your drinking or using drugs?
5. Does your boss complain about your drinking or using drugs?
6. Do you drink or use drugs before or during work?
7. Have you ever been fired or quit secondary to drinking or using drugs?
8. Have you ever been charged with driving under the influence (DUI) or drunk in public (DIP)?
9. Have you ever had any other legal problems related to drinking or using drugs, such as assault and battery, breaking and entering, or theft?
10. Have you had any accidents while intoxicated, such as falls, burns, or motor vehicle accidents?
11. Have you spent your money on alcohol or other drugs instead of paying your bills (telephone, electricity, rent, etc.)?

Drug Testing

Some employers require pre-employment or random drug testing. This can be done by examining a person's urine, blood, saliva, breath (alcohol), or hair; urine testing is the most common. However, urine testing only indicates past use of certain drugs, not intoxication or the extent of performance impairment. Also, most drug-related problems in the workplace are due to alcohol, and alcohol is not always included in a urine drug screen. Other problems with urine testing include using it as a tool of intimidation, false-positive results, and invasion of privacy; in addition, it is not cost effective.

When is drug testing appropriate? Drug testing after documented impairment can help to substantiate the cause of the impairment and serve as a backup rather than the primary screening method. It is also useful for recovering addicts. Part of their treatment is to abstain from psychoactive drug use; therefore a urine test yielding positive results for a drug indicates a relapse.

Blood, breath, and saliva drug tests can indicate current use and amount. Any of these tests can help determine alcohol intoxication, and they often are used to substantiate suspected impairment. A serum drug screen can be useful when overdose is suspected to determine the specific drug ingested.

Employee assistance programs (EAPs) are useful in work settings; at least 30% of U.S. workers have access to an EAP. Roughly 86% of work sites with 5000 or more employees have EAPs (Callery, 1994). These programs can identify health problems, including those involving substance abuse, among employees and offer counseling or referral to other health care providers. EAP programs also offer services to help employees reduce stress and provide health care or counseling so that they may prevent substance abuse problems from developing. Nurses frequently develop and run these programs.

High-Risk Groups

While people of all age-groups are at risk for ATOD problems, adolescents and elderly persons have particular risk characteristics. *Adolescents* are at risk because of their tendencies to experiment with new things (including drugs), their quest for independence, and their tendency to rebel against parents and other significant adults. Surveys of high school students show that by 12th grade, about 81.7% have used alcohol, 65.4% smoked cigarettes, 49.6% used marijuana, and 8.7% tried cocaine (National Institute on Drug Abuse, 1998b). These figures are probably low since they do not include high school dropouts.

Family-related factors (genetics, family stress, parenting styles, child victimization) seem to have the strongest influence on substance abuse among adolescents. Psychiatric disorders (especially mood disorders) and behavioral problems are also associated with substance abuse among adolescents, leaving peer pressure as a lesser influential factor. The most effective treatment approach for adolescents appears to be the use of family-oriented therapy (Weinberg, et al, 1998).

Elderly persons (65 years of age and older) make up 13% of the U.S. population and are the fastest growing segment of U.S. society, expected to represent 21% by the year 2030. They consume more prescribed and OTC medications than any other age-group. Alcohol and prescription drug misuse affects as many as 17% of people age 60 and older. Problems with alcohol consumption, including interactions with prescribed and OTC drugs, outnumber other substance abuse problems among the elderly (Center for Substance Abuse Treatment, 1998).

Older adults often use prescription drugs and alcohol in order to cope with relocation, possible loss of independence, retirement, illness, death of friends, and reduced achievement. These events lead to feelings of sadness, boredom, anxiety, and loneliness. Also, slowed metabolic turnover of drugs, age-related organ changes, increased drug sensitivities, a tendency to use drugs over long periods of time, and use of multiple drugs all contribute to greater negative consequences for older people.

Alcohol abuse may go undetected since its effects on cognitive abilities may mimic changes associated with normal aging or degenerative brain disease. Also, depression may simply be attributed to the more frequent losses rather than the depressant effects of alcohol, and the elderly person may subsequently receive medical treatment for depression rather than alcoholism.

In addition to the problem of addiction, *intravenous (IV) drug users* are at risk for health complications. IV administration of drugs always carries a greater risk of overdose because the drug goes directly into the bloodstream. With illicit drugs the danger is increased because the exact dosage is unknown, and the drug may be contaminated with other chemicals. Needle sharing is common among addicts, and the spread of human immunodeficiency virus (HIV) through needle sharing is a major public health risk. Hepatitis and other blood-borne diseases can also be transmitted through contaminated needles. Infections and abscesses may result from the use of dirty needles or poor administration techniques. While abstinence is ideal but unrealistic for many addicts, nurses can educate about the use of bleach to clean needles between use and needle-exchange programs to decrease the spread of the virus.

Since the fetus is at risk for negative effects from most drugs, their use during *pregnancy* should be discouraged unless medically necessary. *Healthy People 2000* objectives 14.4 and 14.10 address this issue. **Fetal alcohol syndrome (FAS)** is the third leading cause of birth defects and the leading cause of mental retardation in the United States, with a 1992 estimate of 5.2 cases per 10,000 live births (Cordero, et al, 1994). Despite the increased focus in the health care system on interventions for drug abuse, many pregnant women with drug problems do not receive the help they need. Reasons for not receiving treatment include ignorance, poverty, lack of concern for the fetus, lack of available services, and fear of the consequences including criminal prosecution. Women may conceal their drug use from medical providers, and deliver their babies in out-of-hospital settings, thus further jeopardizing the pregnancy outcome (Kain, Rimar, and Barash, 1993).

Codependency and Family Involvement

Drug addiction is often a family disease. One in four Americans have family problems related to alcohol abuse; 52.9% of individuals 18 years old and older have a family history

Evidence-Based Practice

The study referenced below identified infant and maternal outcomes associated with self-reported illicit drug use during pregnancy to determine if illicit polydrug use prior to pregnancy caused added risk to the mother or infant. Participants were identified from newborn referrals to the local visiting nurses association and unrestricted birth certificates over a 3-month study period in a city outside of Boston. Of 360 mothers contacted, 284 (78.9%) agreed to participate. Data were collected using an interview schedule designed for this study and were analyzed using descriptive statistics and logistic regression. Of the subjects, 26.8% reported using an illicit drug, 22.5% reported marijuana use, and 10.6% reported cocaine use during pregnancy.

Pregnancy users of illicit drugs had a 2.2 greater risk of experiencing premature birth, precipitous labor, low weight gain, placental abruption, and/or vaginal bleeding than nonusers. Infants of the pregnancy users had a 2.8 greater risk of being small for gestational age, having low birth weight, having early gestational age, and/or being shaky or jittery. The use of drugs prior to pregnancy but not during pregnancy was not associated with any negative maternal or fetal outcome.

APPLICATION IN PRACTICE

Nurses can identify women who are illicit drug users and help them receive treatment to ensure future low-risk pregnancies. Specifically, nurses can use three health-promotion activities:

1. Identify drug users before they become pregnant and provide education and drug-treatment services
2. Use every opportunity to encourage drug-dependent pregnant women to receive regular prenatal care
3. If a woman is a drug user at the time the baby is born, teach her parenting skills. The infants of drug-using mothers often are premature, small for gestational age, or have structural deformities that make parenting difficult.

Mahoney DL: Infant and maternal outcomes associated with self-reported illicit drug use during pregnancy, *J Addict Nurs* 10(3):115-122, 1998.

Box 21-3   Brief Interventions Using the FRAMES Acronym

Feedback: Provide the client direct feedback about the potential or actual personal risk or impairment related to drug use.
Responsibility: Emphasize personal responsibility for change.
Advice: Provide clear advice to change risky behavior.
Menu: Provide a menu of options or choices for changing behavior.
Empathy: Provide a warm, reflective, empathic, and understanding approach.
Self-efficacy: Provide encouragement and belief in the client's ability to change.

From Bien TH, Miller WR, Tonigan JS: Brief interventions for alcohol problems: a review, *Addiction* 88:315-336, 1993.

---

behavior. Family members then develop roles that grossly exaggerate normal family roles, and they cling to these roles, even when they are no longer functional. Family members often become enablers. **Enabling** is the act of shielding or preventing the addict from experiencing the consequences of the addiction. As a result the addict does not always understand the cost of the addiction and thus is "enabled" to continue to use.

Although codependency and enabling are related, a person does not have to be codependent to enable. Anyone can be an enabler: a police officer, a boss or co-worker, a drug treatment counselor or a nurse who does not address the negative health consequences of the drug use with the addicted person.

Nurses can help families recognize the problem of addiction and confront the addicted member in a caring manner. Whether or not the addicted family member agrees to treatment, family members need guidance about the resources and services available. This includes identifying treatment options, counseling assistance, financial assistance, support services, and (if necessary) legal services for the family members. Children of ATOD abusers or addicts are themselves at greater risk for developing addiction and must be targeted for primary prevention.

THE ROLE OF THE NURSE IN TERTIARY PREVENTION

Nurses, with their knowledge of community resources, can help addicts and their families and also find ways to improve the quality of care clients receive. Many people with alcoholism and drug addiction become lost in the health care system. If satisfactory care is not provided by one agency or the waiting list is months long, the person may give up rather than seek alternative sources of care. Nurses can offer guidance to the most effective treatment, including brief interventions, as well as long-term treatment. Box 21-3 describes six elements commonly included in brief interventions using the acronym FRAMES.

Strategies used with clients depend on their readiness for change. Understanding the stages of change (Box 21-4) and recognizing which stage a client is in are important factors

---

of alcoholism among first- or second-degree relatives (Dawson and Grant, 1998). People in a close relationship with the addict often develop unhealthy coping mechanisms to continue the relationship. This behavior is known as **codependency,** a stress-induced preoccupation with the addicted person's life, leading to extreme dependence and excessive concern with the addict (Talashek, Gerace, and Starr, 1994).

Strict rules typically develop in a codependent family to maintain the relationships: don't talk, don't feel, don't trust, don't lose control, and don't seek help from outside the family. Codependents try to meet the addict's needs at the expense of their own. Codependency may underlie many of the medical complaints and emotional stress seen by health care providers such as ulcers, skin disorders, migraine headaches, chronic colds, and backaches.

When the addicted person refuses to admit the problem, the family often adapts to emotionally survive the stress of the addict's irrational, inconsistent, and unpredictable

Box 21-4	Stages of Change

Precontemplation: At this stage the individual has no intention to change in the foreseeable future. The person is often unaware of any problem. Resistance to recognizing or modifying a problem is the hallmark of precontemplation.

Contemplation: At this stage the individual is aware that a problem exists and is seriously thinking about overcoming it but has not yet made a commitment to take action. In this stage the nurse can encourage the individual to weigh the pros and cons of the problem and the solution to the problem.

Preparation: Preparation was originally referred to as decision making. At this stage the individual is prepared for action and may make some reduction in the problem behavior but has not yet taken effective action (e.g., cuts down amount of smoking but does not abstain).

Action: At this stage the individual modifies his or her behavior, experiences, or environment to overcome the problem. The action requires considerable time and energy. Modification of the target behavior to an acceptable criterion and significant overt efforts to change are the hallmarks of action.

Maintenance: In this stage the individual works to prevent relapse and consolidate the gains attained during action. Stabilizing behavior change and avoiding relapse are the hallmarks of maintenance.

From Prochaska JO, DiClemente CC, Norcross JC: In search of how people change: applications to addictive behaviors, *Am Psychologist* 47(9):1102-1114, 1992.

in determining which interventions and programs may be most helpful to the client (Center for Substance Abuse Treatment, 1998). Once a person has received treatment, nurses working in the community can coordinate aftercare referrals, follow up, and support the client and family as they adapt to changing roles. Relapses do occur, and nurses can support and encourage clients and families to continue to work toward recovery and an improved quality of life.

Detoxification

Detoxification is the process of clearing toxins or drugs from the person's body and managing the withdrawal symptoms. The time needed varies from a few days to weeks depending on the drug and the degree of dependence; the degree of discomfort from withdrawal also varies. Stimulants or opiates may cause withdrawal symptoms that are uncomfortable but not life threatening and do not require direct medical supervision. Medical management of these withdrawal symptoms increases the comfort level. In contrast, alcohol, benzodiazepines, and barbiturates can produce life-threatening withdrawal symptoms. These clients need close medical supervision during detoxification and should receive medical management of the withdrawal symptoms. For those persons who develop delirium tremens, 15% may not survive despite medical management; therefore close medical management should be initiated as the blood alcohol level begins to fall.

A general rule in detoxification management is to wean the person off the drug by gradually reducing the dosage and

frequency of administration. Thus a person with chronic alcoholism could be safely detoxified by a gradual reduction in alcohol consumption. In practice, however, the switch to another drug, usually a benzodiazepine, may produce a safer withdrawal from alcohol as well as an abrupt end to the intoxication from the drug of choice. For example, chlordiazepoxide (Librium) is commonly used for alcohol detoxification (Haack, 1998). Nurses who work with people during detoxification use a range of skills to assess both physical and mental functioning. Assessment begins with a careful health history that includes all substances, including prescribed medication and OTC drugs, alcohol, and recreational drugs. The nurse would observe for signs of depression, injury to self and others, dehydration, seizures, or the presence of a concurrent illness that may be masked by withdrawal symptoms (Haack, 1998). The signs and symptoms of withdrawal are usually the exact opposite of the direct pharmacologic effect of the drug. That is, if a person uses a drug for sedation, withdrawal causes anxiety and agitation. The nurse needs to teach families what to expect and which signs and symptoms they should report.

Briefly Noted

Because of cost-containment efforts, more primary care providers and drug treatment programs are initiating outpatient or home detoxification for persons requiring medical detoxification for alcohol withdrawal. Nurses can monitor and evaluate the client's health status in the home environment to reduce the risk of medical complications related to alcohol withdrawal as well as to provide encouragement and support for the client to complete the detoxification.

Addiction Treatment

Addiction treatment focuses on the addiction process: helping clients view addiction as a chronic disease and assisting them to make life-style changes to halt the progression of the disease. On any given day, more than 800,000 persons receive addiction treatment in specialized programs (Institute for Health Policy, 1993). Most treatment facilities are multidisciplinary, include a range of programs and approaches, and include the addict, family, culture, and community. Strategies include medical management, education, counseling, vocational rehabilitation, stress management, and support services. The most recommended approach is total **abstinence.** Treatment can be accomplished as an inpatient or outpatient, with the latter more common due to the costs involved. Once a person has completed detoxification, counseling and group interaction are begun. It is important to educate the person about the disease, how drugs affect people physically and psychologically, and what tools and life-style changes may be needed.

For those addicted individuals unwilling or unable to completely abstain from psychoactive drugs, other drugs have been used to assist them in abstaining from their drug of choice. For example, methadone has been used successfully to treat heroin addiction. Methadone, when administered in moderate or high daily doses, produces a cross-tolerance to other narcotics, thereby blocking their effects and decreasing the craving for heroin. Methadone is long acting, effective orally, and inexpensive, and has few known side effects. The oral use of methadone offers a solution to the danger of the spread of AIDS and other blood-borne infections that commonly occur among needle-sharing addicts. Although not recognized as a cure for heroin (or other opiate) addiction, methadone maintenance reduces deviant behavior and introduces addicted persons to the health care system. This may ultimately lead to total abstinence. The disadvantage to using substitute drugs is that the person may become addicted to the substitute.

Smoking-Cessation Programs

Nearly 35 million Americans try to quit smoking each year, and fewer than 10% are able to stop for a year. Smokers receiving interventions compared to those smokers who do not receive interventions have much more success, and interventions involving medications and behavioral treatments appear most promising (Leshner, 1998).

Briefly Noted

Antidepressants can help persons stop smoking. GlaxoWellcome has developed a specific drug, bupropion hydrochloride (Zyban), to help individuals stop smoking. Insurance companies, Medicare, and Medicaid do not pay for smoking-cessation drugs. However, bupropion hydrochloride is the same as the older antidepressant Wellbutrin, which is less expensive and is covered by insurance.

Nicotine-replacement therapy can help smokers withdraw from nicotine while breaking the psychological craving and habit. Four types of nicotine-replacement products are available: nicotine gum and skin patches are available over-the-counter, and nicotine nasal spray and inhalers are available by prescription. These products are about equally effective and can almost double the chances of successfully quitting. Other treatments include smoking-cessation clinics, hypnosis, and acupuncture. The most effective way to get people to stop smoking and prevent relapse involves multiple interventions and continuous reinforcement since most smokers require several attempts at cessation until they are successful. Many resources are available on smoking-cessation programs and support groups. Helping the client develop a plan to stop smoking can increase the likelihood of success.

Support Groups

It is important for nurses who work with people in the community to know what support groups are available. An effective support system is important in helping substance abusers change their patterns of behavior. Support groups can provide information about healthy life-styles, especially managing stress and conflict; emotional support; decision-making and refusal skills; communication and problem-solving techniques; and acceptance and recognition of a person's worth and value (Allen, 1998).

In 1935, Alcoholics Anonymous (AA) began a movement that uses peer support to treat a chronic illness. AA groups have developed throughout the world, and their success has led to the development of other support groups such as Narcotics Anonymous (NA) for persons with narcotic addictions and Pills Anonymous for persons with polydrug addictions. Similar programs have been developed for process addictions, such as Overeaters Anonymous and Gamblers Anonymous. AA and NA help people with addictions develop a daily program of recovery and reinforce the recovery process. The fellowship, support, and encouragement among AA members provide a vital social network for the person recovering from an addiction.

Al-Anon and Alateen are similar self-help programs for spouses, parents, children, or others involved in a painful relationship with an alcoholic (Nar-Anon for those in relationships with persons with narcotic addictions). Al-Anon family groups are available to anyone who has been affected by their involvement with an alcoholic person. Alateen provides a forum for adolescents to discuss family stressors, learn coping skills from one another, and gain support and encouragement from knowledgeable peers. Adult Children of Alcoholics (ACOA) groups are also available in most areas to address the recovery of adults who grew up in alcoholic homes and are still carrying the scars and retaining dysfunctional behaviors.

Clinical Application

Jane Doe, RN, is home health case manager for an agency that provides services to residents of a large, low-income housing facility. She designs care plans and coordinates services. She makes the initial visits to determine the level and frequency of care and acts as supervisor of the volunteers and nurses' aides who perform most of the day-to-day care. Many families are headed by a single mother, and drug dealing is common.

Jane visited Anne, a 26-year-old mother of three who was taking care of her 62-year-old maternal grandfather, Mr. Jones, who was recovering from cardiac bypass surgery. Mr. Jones has smoked two packs of cigarettes per day for 40 years; he had decreased to one pack after surgery. He refused to quit. He had a history of alcohol dependence, reportedly consuming up to a fifth of liquor a day and a history of withdrawal seizures. Four years ago he went through alcohol detoxification, but he refused to stay at the facility for continued treatment, stating he could stay sober on his own. Since that time, he has had several binge episodes, but Anne reports that he has not been drinking since the surgery.

A. What type of interventions can Jane provide for Mr. Jones regarding his smoking?

CHAPTER 21   Substance Abuse in the Community   **379**

B. How can Jane help Anne cope with the potential risk of Mr. Jones continuing to drink when he progresses to more independence?

C. Is it realistic for Anne to stop her grandfather from drinking if he doesn't want to? What else would be helpful to know about his drinking?

Answers are in the back of the book.

 Remember This!

- Substance abuse is a national health problem linked to many kinds of morbidity and mortality.
- Social conditions such as a fast-paced life, excessive stress, and the availability of drugs influence the incidence of substance abuse.
- Important terms to understand when working with individuals, groups, or communities for whom substance abuse is prevalent are *drug dependence, drug addiction, alcoholism, psychoactive drugs, depressants, stimulants, marijuana, hallucinogens,* and *inhalants.*
- Primary prevention for substance abuse includes education about drugs and guidelines for use, as well as the promotion of healthy alternatives to drug use for either recreation or to relieve stress.
- Nurses assume key roles in developing community prevention programs.
- Secondary prevention depends heavily on careful assessment of the client's use of drugs. Such assessment should be part of all basic health assessments.
- High-risk groups include pregnant women, young people, elderly persons, intravenous drug users, and illicit drug users.
- Drug addiction is often a family problem and not only an individual problem.
- Codependency describes a companion illness to the addiction of one person in which the codependent member is addicted to the addicted person.
- Brief interventions can often be highly effective in helping people with substance abuse problems.
- Nurses are in ideal roles to assist with tertiary prevention for both the addicted person and the family.

 What Would You Do?

1. Read your local newspaper for 4 days, and select stories that illustrate the effect of substance abuse on individuals, families, and the community. What interventions would you plan? Who would you involve in your planning for interventions? Are the interventions primary, secondary, or tertiary prevention efforts?
2. For each of the stories in the newspaper related to substance abuse, describe preventive strategies that a community health nurse might have tried before the problem reached such a dire state.
3. Looking at your local community resources directory or the telephone book, identify agencies that might serve as referral sources for individuals or families for whom substance abuse is a problem.
4. Attend an open AA or NA meeting and an Al-Anon meeting. Go alone if possible or with an alcoholic or a drug-addicted friend. As the members introduce themselves, give your first name and state, "I am a visitor." Plan to listen and do not attempt to take notes. Respect the anonymity of the persons present. Discuss your experiences with your classmates.
   a. Pay particular attention to your attitudes toward the participants.
   b. What themes did you hear?
   c. How could nurses be helpful to members of such groups?

REFERENCES

Allen K: Essential concepts of addiction for general nursing practice, *Nurs Clin North Am* 33(1):1-13, 1998.

Bien TH, Miller WR, Tonigan JS: Brief interventions for alcohol problems: a review, *Addiction* 88:315-336, 1993.

Callery YC: Chemical abuse rehabilitation for hospital employees, *Am Assoc Occup Health Nurses J* 42(4):67-75, 1994.

Cargo S: *Increases in teen drug use appear to level off,* NIDA Notes 13(2):10-11, NIH pub no 98-3478, 1998, National Institutes of Health.

Center for Substance Abuse Treatment: Substance abuse among older adults: Treatment Improvement Protocol (TIP) series, no 26, DHHS pub no (SMA) 98-3179, Washington, D.C., 1998, U.S. Government Printing Office.

Cordero JF, Floyd RL, Martin ML, et al: Tracking the prevalence of FAS, *Alcohol Health Res World* 18(1):82-85, 1994.

Cordes H: Generation wired: caffeine is the new drug of choice for kids, *The Nation* 266(15):11-12, 14, 16, 1998.

Das G, Laddu A: Cocaine: friend or foe? *Intern J Clin Pharmacol Ther Toxicol* 31(9):449-455, 1993.

Dawson DA, Grant BF: Family history and gender: their combined effects on *DSM-IV* alcohol dependence and major depression, *J Stud Alcohol* 59(1):97-106, 1998.

Dinwiddie SH: Abuse of inhalants: a review, *Addiction* 89(8):925-939, 1994.

Donaldson SI, Graham JW, Hansen WB: Testing the generalizability of intervening mechanism theories: understanding the effects of adolescent drug use prevention interventions, *J Behav Med* 17(2):195-216, 1994.

Espeland K: Inhalant abuse: assessment guidelines, *J Psychosoc Nurs Ment Health Serv* 31(3):11-14, 1993.

Foley KM: Opioids, *Neurol Clinics* 11(3):503-521, 1993.

Frezza M, di Padova C, Pozzato G, et al: High blood alcohol levels in women: the role of decreased gastric alcohol dehydrogenase activity and first-pass metabolism, *N Engl J Med* 322(2):95-99, 1990.

Gold MS, Miller NS, Stennie K, Populla-Vardi C: Epidemiology of benzodiazepine use and dependence, *Psychiatr Ann* 25(3):146-148, 1995.

Griffith WH: *Complete guide to prescription and nonprescription drugs,* New York, 1998, The Body Press/Perigee.

Haack MR: Treating acute withdrawal from alcohol and other drugs, *Nurs Clin North Am* 33(1):75-92, 1998.

Institute for Health Policy, Brandeis University: *Substance abuse: the nation's number one health problem, key indicators for policy,* Princeton, NJ, 1993, The Robert Wood Johnson Foundation.

Kain ZN, Rimar S, Barash PG: Cocaine abuse and the parturient and effects on the fetus and neonate, *Anesth Analg* 77(4):835-845, 1993.

Kinney J, Leaton G: *Loosening the grip,* ed 5, St Louis, 1995, Mosby.

Kumpfer KL, Hopkins R: Prevention: current research and trends, *Psychiatr Clin North Am* 16(1):11-20, 1993.

Larrat EP, Taubman AH, Willey C: Compliance-related problems in the ambulatory populations, *Am Pharm* NS30(2):18-23, 1990.

Leshner AI: *Addiction research can provide scientific solutions to the problem of cigarette smoking,* NIDA Notes, 13(3):3-4, 1998, NIH pub no 98-3478, National Institutes of Health.

Mahoney DL: Infant and maternal outcomes associated with self-reported illicit drug use during pregnancy, *J Addict Nurs* 10(3):115-122, 1998.

Manwell L, Fleming MF, Barry K, Johnson K: Tobacco, alcohol, and drug use in a primary care sample: 90 day prevalence and associated factors, *J Addict Dis* 17(1):67-81, 1997.

Marwick C: Physician leadership on national drug policy finds addiction treatment works, *JAMA* 279(15):1149-1150, 1998.

Mathre ML (editor): *Cannabis in medical practice: a legal, historical, and pharmacological overview of the therapeutic use of marijuana,* Jefferson, NC, 1997, McFarland & Company.

Medical-care expenditures attributable to cigarette smoking–US, 1993, *MMWR* 43(26):469-472, 1994.

Merrill J, Fox K, Chang H: *The cost of substance abuse to America's health care system,* report 1: Medicaid hospital costs, New York, 1993, Center on Addictions and Substance Abuse at Columbia University.

Miller M: *Drug consumer safety rules,* Mosier, Ore, 1994, Mothers Against Misuse and Abuse (MAMA).

National Institute on Alcohol Abuse and Alcoholism: The physician's guide to helping patients with alcohol problems, NIH pub no 95-3769. Rockville, Md, 1995, National Institutes of Health.

National Institute on Alcohol Abuse and Alcoholism: Alcohol's effect on organ function, *Alcohol Res World* 21(1):3-92, 1997.

National Institute on Drug Abuse: Comparing methamphetamine and cocaine, *NIDA Notes* 13(1):15, NIH pub no 98-3478, 1998a, National Institutes of Health.

National Institute on Drug Abuse: Trends in drug use among 8th, 10th, and 12th graders, *NIDA Notes* 13(2):15, NIH pub no 98-3478, 1998b, National Institutes of Health.

National Institute on Drug Abuse: *Facts about nicotine and tobacco products,* NIDA Notes, 13(3):15, NIH pub no 98-3478, 1998c, National Institutes of Health.

National Nurses Society on Addictions: *Prevention of alcohol, tobacco, and other drugs,* 1994, Macro International Inc, and J & E Associates, under contract by the Center for Substance Abuse Prevention.

O'Brien CP: Drug abuse and drug addiction. In Hardman JG, Limbird LE (editors): *Goodman & Gilman's the pharmacological basis of therapeutics,* ed 9, New York, 1996, McGraw-Hill.

Office of Applied Studies: *Summary of findings from the 1998 National Household Survey on Drug Abuse,* National Clearinghouse for alcohol and drug information, 1999, Rockville, Md.

Perez-Stable EJ, Herrera B, Jacob P, III, Benowitz NL: Nicotine metabolism and intake in black and white smokers, *JAMA* 280(2):152-156, 1998.

Petro DJ: Pharmacology and toxicity of cannabis. In Mathre ML (editor): *Cannabis in medical practice: a legal, historical and pharmacological overview of the therapeutic use of marijuana,* Jefferson, NC, 1997, McFarland & Company.

Prochaska JO, DiClemente CC, Norcross JC: In search of how people change: applications to addictive behaviors, *Am Psychologist* 47(9):1102-1114, 1992.

Rybacki JJ, Long JW: *The essential guide to prescription drugs,* New York, 1999, Harper Perennial.

Shedler J, Block J: Adolescent drug use and psychological health: a longitudinal inquiry, *Am Psychol* 45(5):612-630, 1990.

Strain EC, Mumford GK, Silverman K, Griffiths RR: Caffeine dependence syndrome: evidence from case histories and experimental evaluation, *JAMA* 272(13):1043-1048, 1994.

Substance Abuse and Mental Health Services Administration: *National Household Survey on Drug Abuse advance report no 18,* Rockville, Md, 1996, Substance Abuse and Mental Health Services Administration.

Talashek ML, Gerace LM, Starr KL: The substance abuse pandemic: determinants to guide interventions, *Pub Health Nurs* 11(2):131-139, 1994.

Warner EA: Cocaine abuse, *Ann Intern Med* 119(3):226-235, 1993.

Weil A, Rosen W: *Chocolate to morphine: understanding mind-active drugs,* Boston, 1993, Houghton Mifflin.

Weinberg NZ, Rahdert E, Colliver JD, Glantz MD: Adolescent substance abuse: a review of the past 10 years, *J Am Acad Child Adolesc Psychiatry* 37(3):252-261, 1998.

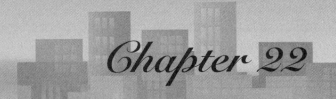

Violence in the Community

JACQUELYN C. CAMPBELL

KÄREN M. LANDENBURGER

OBJECTIVES

After reading this chapter, the student will be able to:

- Describe the problem of violence in American communities and discuss at least three factors in most communities that encourage violence and human abuse.
- Identify common predictors of the onset of child abuse and indicators of its presence.
- Discuss the four general types of child abuse: neglect and physical, emotional, or sexual abuse.
- Discuss the dynamics and signs of female abuse by male partners.
- Examine the growing community health problem of elder abuse.
- Analyze the nursing role in working with survivors of violence.

CHAPTER OUTLINE

KEY TERMS

assault: violent physical attack on a person.

child abuse: maltreatment of children that is either active (physical or sexual) or more passive as in neglect or emotional abuse.

child neglect: physical or emotional failure to meet the child's needs.

elder abuse: a form of violence against older people. May include neglect and failure to provide adequate food, clothing, shelter, and physical or safety needs. Can also include roughness in care or actual violent, aggressive behavior toward the elderly.

emotional neglect: the omission of the basic nurturing, acceptance, and caring essential for healthy development.

emotional abuse: abuse, often verbal, that seeks to control another person through degradation, humiliation, and fear.

homicide: death resulting from injury deliberately inflicted by one person onto another.

incest: sexual abuse among family members.

physical neglect: failure to provide adequate food, proper clothing, shelter, hygiene, or necessary medical care.

physical abuse: the intentional use of force that can cause death, injury, or harm.

rape: sexual intercourse forced on an unwilling person.

sexual abuse: behavior ranging from unwanted sexual touching to rape.

spouse abuse: physical or emotional maltreatment of one's partner.

suicide: killing oneself.

survivors: people who may be injured but are not killed by violence toward them.

violence: non-accidental acts that result in physical or psychological injury to another person.

The word *violence* comes from the Latin *violare,* meaning to violate, injure, or rape. Violence is a violation that has both physical and emotional effects.

The amount of violence in the world has increased in the last two decades. One has only to read newspapers or magazines, listen to the radio, or watch television or movies to know how much violence is reported and also how often violence is shown as entertainment.

Violence is generally defined as those non-accidental acts, interpersonal or intrapersonal, that result in physical or psychological injury to one or more persons. It is thought that violent behavior is predictable and thus is preventable (Rosenberg and Fenley, 1991). Violence-related morbidity increases the costs of health care.

While considerable progress has been made in decreasing deaths from all other causes since 1940, the risk of assault and homicide in the United States remains large. The United States has the fifth highest homicide rate in the world. Of the 26,009 homicides reported in the United States in a year, one-third occurred among persons between the ages of 15 and 24 years. Of these homicides, 71% were related to the use of firearms. Overall homicide rates increased from 1985 to 1991 but decreased from 1991 to 1994 (Trends in Rates, 1996).

Violence is primarily learned behavior rather than an innate aggressive drive. That is, people primarily learn to be violent rather than being born violent. Everyone is capable of violence, yet some societies are totally nonviolent (Counts, Brown, and Campbell, 1992). What conditions in society promote aggression? What conditions in society keep violence in check and encourage nonviolent interactions, especially those involving conflict resolution? In nonviolent societies, several patterns are seen. For example, some cultures discourage any overt expression of violence. In others, families live in kin groupings and intervene to stop any signs of violence, while in other societies, the living arrangements are so close that friends, neighbors, and family would get involved and stop the expression of violence (Counts, Brown, and Campbell, 1992).

Nurses working in the community are ideally positioned to both detect the signs of violence and to initiate, support, or encourage people and communities to engage in alternative behaviors. Violence is a public health concern. Communities across the United States are angry and concerned about rising crime and violence rates. Unfortunately, health care and human service workers have been slow to develop systems for identifying and intervening. As a result, the estimated 4 million victims of violence annually may also experience great physical and emotional pain that might have been avoided or relieved by timely and effective interventions.

This chapter examines violence as a public health problem and discusses ways that nurses can help individuals, families, groups, and the community recognize, cope with, and reduce violence and abuse. Since nurses work with clients in a wide variety of settings, including the home, they are in key positions to detect and intervene in community and family violence. Thus nurses need to understand what factors in society and the community influence violence.

SOCIAL AND COMMUNITY FACTORS INFLUENCING VIOLENCE

Many things within a community can support or minimize violence. Changing social conditions, multiple demands on people, economic conditions, and social institutions influence the level of violence and human abuse. The following discussion of the social conditions of work, schools, media, religion, community structure, and facilities are discussed in relation to how each might influence violent behavior.

Productive and paid work is an expectation, and work can be fulfilling and contribute to a sense of well-being or it can be frustrating, unfulfilling, and stressful and can lead to aggression and violence. Repetitive, boring, non-stimulating, or strenuous, stressful, conflict-filled jobs often frustrate people. During economic downturns, people are often afraid to give up a disliked job. They feel trapped in the undesirable job, but they must work to meet the needs of the family. They may begin to resent those who depend on them. Their frustration and resentment can lead to violence. Unemployment is also associated with violence both within and outside the home. Unemployment also can precipitate aggressive outbursts due to feelings of inadequacy, guilt, boredom, dissatisfaction, and frustration.

Young, minority males have the highest rates of unemployment in the United States. Even in prosperous times, their unemployment rate can be over 50%. This group also has the highest rate of violence. These young men are described as living in a world of oppression, with lack of opportunity and enormous anger. They express their feelings with violence when they feel that they have been pushed out of mainstream society. Most analyses conclude that the different rates of violence between blacks and whites in the United States are related more to economic realities, such as poverty, unemployment, and overcrowding, than to race (Reiss and Roth, 1993-1994).

In recent years, schools have assumed many responsibilities traditionally assigned to the family. Schools teach sexual development, discipline children, and often serve as a place to "dump" children who have no other place to go. Large classes often mean that teachers spend more time and energy monitoring and disciplining children than challenging and stimulating them to learn. In large classes, disruptive behavior is often dealt with by isolating the child. The nonconforming child is simply removed from the classroom because the teacher has no time to help the child learn alternative ways to behave.

Beginning in childhood, people need to be stimulated, to feel loved and valued, and to have some degree of power and some appropriate ways to vent anger. Social institutions can help meet these needs but many, due to the heavy demands made on them or the lack of training of the workers, fail to do so. Schools can teach and be a place to practice nonviolence. Classes can teach adolescents peaceful conflict resolution and about violence in couples, and they can help young children deal with the threat of sexual abuse and other forms of violence (Gelles and Conte, 1990; Webster, 1993).

The media can influence violence. Hitting, kicking, stabbing, and shooting are seen as ways to handle anger and frustration. By the age of 18 years, the average child has seen 1800 murders and countless acts of nonfatal violence on television. Frequent viewing of violent television programs by children has been associated with aggressive behavior (Campbell and Humphreys, 1993). On the other hand, the media can be a powerful force for increasing public awareness of various forms of violence and what can be done to address them (Klein, Campbell, Soler, and Ghez, 1997). Television programs and print articles can increase public awareness about family violence. Abused women and rape victims can benefit when the media describes the effects of this abuse, since this may lessen the stigma of such victimization. The media can also publicize services.

However, the media may serve as a source of frustration to poor persons who see a disproportionate number of "rich and beautiful" people on the shows and in print. Children often see how much is available to others yet they may have few possessions. Such polarization between their reality and what is possible can stimulate the development of abusive patterns. Frustration, unfilled dreams, and unmet wishes are often handled through hurting someone who cannot fight back.

Briefly Noted

It is unfortunate that television and movies entertain by using violence. Consider how many cartoons show incredible violence in their attempt to entertain.

Churches can meet many human needs, including the need for stimulation, a sense of value, belonging, closeness, and worth, as well as for power. Religion generally teaches nonviolent conflict resolution. Church, clergy, and members of church groups often provide positive role models and reinforcement for peaceful behavior. However, a historically contradictory relationship exists between abuse and religion. For example, many religious groups believe in "spare the rod, spoil the child." Also, some faiths victimize people with their disapproval of divorce. Family members may stay together, although they are at emotional or physical war with one another, because of religious commitments (Prince, 1980).

A community's structure can influence the potential for violence. For example, when people live in crowded conditions and are poor, there is more potential for community tensions and violence. High-population-density communities can have a positive or negative influence on violence. Those with a sense of cohesiveness may have a lower crime rate than areas of similar size that lack unity among members. Bonds formed among church groups, clubs, and professional organizations may promote harmony among members. Such groups provide members an opportunity to talk about what causes stress for them rather than to respond with violence. Other high-population communities feel powerlessness,

helplessness, and generally "put down" by the larger society. Lack of jobs and low-paying jobs can lead to feelings of inadequacy, despair, and social alienation. Social alienation and exclusion from opportunities can decrease social cohesion and lead to increased violence. Fear and indifference can cause community residents to withdraw from social contact. Withdrawal can foster crime because many residents either assume someone else will report suspicious behavior or they fear reprisals for such reports (Moore and Harrisson, 1995).

Youths, especially those who are poor and uneducated, try to deal with their feelings of powerlessness by joining or forming gangs. The gang can provide a way to belong. Gang members may become involved in crime against people and in thefts in order to release frustration or as part of their accepted group behavior.

The potential for violence also tends to occur between diverse populations. Differences in age, socioeconomic status, ethnicity, religion, sexual preference, or other cultural characteristics may be the basis for stability. Highly divergent groups may neither accept nor understand one another. They may not communicate effectively. Many such groups become hostile and antagonistic toward one another. Each group may see the other as different and not belonging. The alienated group may become the focal point for the others' frustrations, anger, and fears. Community disintegration leading to a cycle of dishonesty, distrust, and hate can occur when members hold racist attitudes toward one another or when one group believes that they belong to a better social class or group than members of another group.

Communities differ in the resources and facilities they provide to residents. Some are more desirable places to live, work, and raise families. Community facilities can reduce the potential for crime and violence. Recreational facilities such as playgrounds, parks, swimming pools, movie theaters, athletic fields, and tennis courts provide useful outlets for a variety of feelings, including aggression. The presence of such facilities does not guarantee that crime and violence will not occur. Rather these are wholesome resources to be used by residents for pleasure, personal enrichment, and group development.

Spectator sports also allow members of the community to express feelings of competition, enthusiasm, and excitement. However, viewing violent sports can facilitate expressions of aggression and violence in spectators.

Understanding the factors that contribute to violence or the potential for violence helps nurses recognize their presence or absence and intervene accordingly. Nurses can work with community citizens and agencies to correct or improve deficits as well as to inform and educate about the benefits of participating in recreational and other wholesome and cohesive activities.

VIOLENCE AGAINST INDIVIDUALS OR ONESELF

The potential for violence against individuals (e.g., murder, robbery, rape, and assault) or oneself (e.g., suicide) is directly related to the level of violence in the community.

People who live in areas with high rates of crime and violence are more likely to become victims than those in more peaceful areas. The major categories of violence addressed in this chapter include homicide, assault, rape, suicide, family abuse, and violence; including child abuse and neglect or abuse of females and elderly people. The last sections describe nursing interventions designed to recognize and intervene in violence at the individual, family, and community levels.

Homicide

A **homicide** is death resulting from purposeful injury inflicted by another person. Homicide is the eleventh leading cause of death for all Americans, and the number one cause of death for young (age 15 to 34 years) black men and women. However, the black homicide rate has decreased significantly since 1970, whereas the white homicide rate has increased (Bureau of Justice Statistics, 1997). Although the data are not adequate, it also appears that Hispanic-American males have a much higher rate of homicide than non-Hispanic whites. Homicide is increasing the most among adolescents, but even among very young children in the United States, homicide occurs at an alarming rate.

Between 1950 and 1993, the overall annual death rate for children in the United States under the age of 15 years declined considerably. This was primarily due to decreased deaths from unintentional injuries, pneumonia, influenza, cancer, and congenital anomalies. However, during this time period, childhood homicide rates tripled and suicide rates quadrupled. Specifically, for children up to 4 years of age, the U.S. homicide rate was 4.1 per 100,000. For children between the ages of 5 and 15, the U.S. homicide rate was 1.75 per 100,000. This rate is five times higher than for children in 25 other industrialized countries (Rates of Homicide, 1997).

Only 13% to 15% of all homicides in the United States are committed by strangers (Riedel, 1998). Death caused by strangers often is related to the use and sale of illegal substances. The vast majority of homicides, however, are carried out by a friend, acquaintance, or family member during an argument. Therefore prevention of homicide is as much an issue for the public health system as for the criminal justice system (Rosenberg and Fenley, 1991). At least 13% of the homicides in the United States occur within families (Bachman, 1994) and half of these occur between spouses. Husbands made up about 70% of perpetrators in spousal homicides. Self-defense is involved approximately seven times as often when wives kill their husbands (Campbell, 1995; Bachman, 1994). An alarming aspect of family homicide is that small children often witness the murder or find the body of a family member. In most communities there is no automatic follow-up or counseling of these children either by the criminal justice or mental health systems. These children are then at risk for emotional turmoil and for becoming involved in violence themselves.

The underlying dynamics of family homicides vary from those of other murders. Since homicide in families is often preceded by abuse, prevention of family homicide involves working with abusive families. The potential for eventual homicide must always be kept in mind when working with abusive families. Nurses have a "duty to warn" family members of the possibility of homicide when severe abuse is present, just as they warn of the dangers of smoking (Campbell, 1995).

Assault

The death toll from violence is staggering, as are the physical injuries and emotional costs of **assault.** In the United States, it is estimated that at least 100 nonfatal assaults occur for each homicide. Of all simple and aggravated assaults, 33% result in injury (Reiss and Roth, 1993-1994). Youth are the most likely to be involved in an assault. Males are more likely to be the victims of homicide and assault while females are more likely to be victimized by a relative, especially a male partner (Bachman, 1994). Sometimes quick response time and effective emergency transport and treatment can make the difference between an assault and a homicide. Nurses often see assault victims in their homes when they visit clients with head or spinal cord injuries and/or stomas from gunshot wounds to the stomach. In addition to physical care, nurses can help clients deal with the emotional trauma of a violent attack. Victims need to talk about their traumatic experience and try to make some sense of the violence. These survivors may also need to be referred for counseling if anxiety, sleeping problems, or depression persists after the assault.

Rape

Rape is an underreported form of human abuse in the United States. While the number of rapes reported to law enforcement agencies has decreased since 1993, it is thought that only a third of victims report rape and/or sexual assault to a law enforcement agency. In 1992, there were 84 rapes per 100,000 women, the lowest since 1976 (U.S. Department of Justice, 1997). Hospitals, emergency personnel, and police have improved the protocols for use with victims of rape, and forensic nursing is a developing specialty in the care of sexual assault victims (Lynch, 1993). While effective collecting of information leading to prosecution is essential, nurses should also ensure respectful and supportive treatment for all survivors. Be aware that date and marital rape also occur, and that men may be rape victims. A major problem in obtaining statistics on male rape is that the definition of rape used by the Federal Bureau of Investigation to compile the Uniformed Crime Reports is limited to penile-vaginal penetration (Koss and Harvey, 1991). Although much more research on male rape is needed, initial studies suggest that the emotional trauma to a male rape victim is at least as serious as that for a woman.

For reported rapes, cities constitute higher risk areas than do rural areas; and the hours between 8 PM and 2 AM, weekends, and the summer are the most critical times. In about half of rapes the victim and the offender meet on the street, whereas in other cases the rapist either enters the victim's home or somehow entices or forces the victim to accompany him.

Prevention of rape, as in other forms of human abuse, requires a broad-based community focus for educating community residents and groups such as police, health providers, educators, and social workers. There seems to be a correlation between the numbers of rapes and the way communities view violence and how they react to behavior such as corporal punishment in the schools (Donat and D'Emilio, 1997).

A first step in intervening in the incidence and treatment of rape survivors is to change and clarify misconceptions about rape and survivors of rape. Rape is a crime of violence, not a crime of passion. The underlying issues are hostility, power, and control rather than sexual desire. The defining issue is lack of consent. When a woman or man refuses any sexual activity, that refusal means "no" and the victim should not be blamed because of how he or she acts or dresses. People have the right to change their mind, even when they initially were receptive. Pressure in the form of physical contact, threats, or deliberate inducement by drug or alcohol is a violation of the law. Women on college campuses underreport allegations of rape because of issues of confidentiality and because their accusations may be discredited (Koss and Cook, 1998).

During the act of rape, victims or **survivors** are often hit, kicked, stabbed, and severely beaten. This violence traumatizes the person because of the fear for her life, as well as her helplessness, lack of control, and vulnerability. People react to rape differently, depending on their personality, past experiences, background, and the support received after the trauma. Some victims cry, shout, or discuss the experience. Others withdraw and fear discussing the attack. During the immediate and follow-up stages, survivors may blame themselves for what has happened. It has been found that few rape victims seek mental health or crisis services soon after the assault. The intervening life events and responses of others influence whether they will seek this help (Draucker, 1998). When working with rape survivors, nurses need to help them talk about the issues behind any apparent self-blame. Although fault should not be placed on the victim, it is essential to teach mechanisms that enable a survivor to take control, learn assertiveness, and therefore believe that she knows the steps to take to prevent future rapes. Victims need to talk about what happened and to express their feelings and fears in a nonjudgmental atmosphere that nurses can provide.

In any psychological trauma, the right to privacy and confidentiality is essential. Victims also should be informed of health care procedures conducted immediately after the rape and should be linked with proper resources for ease of reporting. Nurses are responsible for providing continuous care once the victim enters the health care system. Because many victims deny the event once the initial crisis has passed, a single-session debriefing should be completed during the initial examination. Physical assessment, examination, and debriefing should be done by trained providers such as forensic nurses or sexual assault nurse examiners (SANEs) (Aiken and Speck, 1995).

In several states nurses perform the physical examination in the emergency department to gather evidence (e.g., hair samples and skin fragments beneath the victim's fingernails) for criminal prosecution (Ledray and Simmelink, 1997). This is an important intervention because physicians may be impatient with the time required for this procedure, and nurses can take advantage of this opportunity to communicate with the person. Nurses can easily be trained to conduct the examination, and their evidence is credible and effective in resultant court proceedings.

Rape is a situational crisis for which advance preparation is rarely possible. Therefore nursing efforts are directed toward helping victims cope with the stress and disruption of their lives caused by the attack. Counseling focuses on the crisis and the fears, feelings, and issues that result. The goal is to help the survivors problem-solve to regroup personal forces. If posttraumatic stress disorder has developed, a referral for professional psychological or psychiatric treatment is indicated.

Many rape survivors need follow-up mental health services to help them cope with the short- and long-term effects of the crisis. The time after a rape is one of disequilibrium and psychological breakdown. Any violence requires that people rethink their attitudes about the safety of the world. Common everyday tasks often overtax the abilities of survivors of violence. Many forget or fail to keep appointments, so nurses must not only make appropriate referrals but also obtain permission from the survivor to remain in telephone contact to assess and support his or her ongoing needs.

Suicide

People are more likely to die from **suicide** than by homicide (Reiss and Roth, 1993-1994), and adolescents between ages 15 and 19 years and adults over 75 years have the greatest risk. In 1994, 31,142 people in the U.S. committed suicide and this was the ninth leading cause of death overall (Regional Variations, 1997) and the sixth leading cause of death among children ages 5 to 14 years. The U.S. suicide rate is twice as high as the rates in 25 other industrialized countries (Rates of Homicide, 1997). Leading risk factors for adolescent suicide are low self-esteem, chronic depression, incest, and sexual and physical abuse (Eggert, et al, 1994; Hernandez, Lodico, and DiClemente, 1993).

Males commit suicide three times more frequently than females, although females attempt suicide more often. The number-one risk factor for actual and attempted suicide in adult women is spouse abuse (Stark and Fitzcraft, 1991). Suicide is four times more frequent among whites than among blacks. Affluent and educated people have higher rates of suicide than do the economically and educationally disadvantaged. Elderly people are more likely to commit suicide than their younger counterparts. Firearms are the leading weapons used in suicide (Regional Variations, 1997).

Several social and environmental factors are associated with suicidal behavior, including lack of a consistent place to live, unemployment, and other economic resources and living in communities in which the social organization and cohesion is low. Various community interventions—including improved suicide surveillance programs, public education, crisis intervention services, and family support programs—may reduce the suicide rate (Regional Variations, 1997).

Nursing care must focus on family, friends, classmates, and co-workers of suicide victims since they may be affected. Survivors often are angry at the dead person and have a hard time dealing with their feelings toward the deceased yet feel guilty for their anger. Survivors may also wonder if they were in any way responsible for the death. They may ask themselves: "should I have seen the signs?" or "Was I as good a friend or relative as I might have been?" They may have difficulty concentrating and may limit their social activities because it is often hard for the survivors and for their friends to talk about the suicide. Nurses can help survivors cope with the trauma of the loss; this may include referral to a counselor or support groups. As Lynch (1993) points out in her discussion of forensic nursing, nurses have excellent skills for dealing effectively with grieving families and friends. Nurses are trained to listen, observe, and convey observations. Regardless of how difficult it may be, nurses are trained to listen to people express their anguish.

FAMILY VIOLENCE AND ABUSE

Family or domestic violence causes significant injury and death. It is estimated that excluding elder abuse, at least 10.5 million Americans are severely assaulted by a family member each year (Straus and Gelles, 1990). Since at least 10% of American families are violent, nurses need to actively access and intervene in abuse or potential abuse situations.

Family violence includes **sexual, emotional,** and **physical abuse.** These three forms tend to occur together as part of a system of coercive control. Often, in family violence, the most powerful person victimizes a less powerful person. Thus approximately 90% of all "spouse abuse" is directed primarily toward wives (although they may physically fight back), whereas approximately 7% to 8% is mutual violence, and 2% to 3% is husband abuse (Campbell and Humphreys, 1993).

Recognizing the battered child or spouse in the emergency room is relatively simple after the fact. It is unfortunate that, by the time medical care is sought, serious physical and emotional damage may have been done. Nurses are in key positions to predict and deal with abusive tendencies and they need to understand factors contributing to the development of abusive behaviors to identify abuse-prone families.

Development of Abusive Patterns

A person's upbringing, living conditions, and level of stress affect the tendency to be violent. Understanding how these factors influence the development of abusive behavior can help the nurse deal with abusive families. Most abusers have a history of abuse in their own upbringing (Straus and Gelles, 1990). As children, abusers were often beaten or saw siblings or a parent being beaten. These children may hate the use of violence, but they have had no experience with other models of family relationships. People who become abusers not only tend to have a history of child abuse, but they often have a hostile personality style and are verbally aggressive. Often, their parents may have set unrealistic goals, and when the children did not perform accordingly, they were criticized, demeaned, punished, and denied affection. These children often were told how to act, what to do, and how to feel. This discourages the development of normal attachment, autonomy, problem-solving skills, and creativity (Briere, et al, 1996). Children raised in this way grow up feeling unloved and worthless. They may want a child of their own so that they will feel assured of someone's love.

To protect themselves from feeling worthless and fear rejection, abused children form a protective shell and many grow increasingly hostile and distrustful of others. Potential abusers often demonstrate a low tolerance for frustration, emotional instability, and the onset of aggressive feelings with minimal provocation. When the needs of abusers are not met by others, they become overly critical. Critical, resentful behavior and unrealistic expectations of others lead to a vicious cycle. The more critical these people become, the more they are rejected and feel alienated from others. Listening for distorted perceptions of children when parents talk about an infant crying because of malicious motives or keeping them up at night "on purpose" (Briere, et al, 1996; Campbell and Humphreys, 1993) is a way to assess for possible violence.

Often a perceived or actual crisis such as unemployment, family mobility, frequent job changes, marital strain, or unplanned pregnancy increases stress and precedes abuse. The crisis reinforces feelings of inadequacy and low self-esteem. Family violence is often associated with stressful life events, crowded living conditions that reduce privacy and increase tension, poverty, and the number of small children in the home.

At the same time, family social isolation or lack of contact and interaction with other people outside the household also is associated with family violence (Briere, et al, 1996). Such isolation reduces social support, decreasing a family's ability to deal with stress. When a family misses clinic or home visit appointments, the nurse must keep in mind that abuse may be present and the absences may reflect social isolation and avoidance.

Types of Family Violence

Family or domestic violence and violence outside the home often occur together. Physical violence is the intentional use of force to cause death, injury, or harm. It includes but is not limited to "scratching, pushing, shoving, throwing, grabbing, biting, choking, shaking, poking, hair-pulling, slapping, punching, hitting, burning, and use of restraints or one's body to harm another person" (American Association of Colleges of Nursing, 1999, p. 3). If child abuse is suspected, also assess for other forms of family violence. When elderly parents report that their (now adult) child was abused or has a history of violence, be aware that the elderly parent may now be at risk for abuse. Physical abuse of women is frequently accompanied by sexual abuse, and many abusers have a history of other acts of violence. Families who are extremely verbally aggressive in conflict resolution (e.g., name calling, belittling, screaming, and yelling) are more likely to be physically abusive. Although the various forms of family violence are discussed separately, they should not be thought of as being separate from one another.

Child Abuse

In 1997, more than 3 million children were reported for child abuse and neglect to child protective service (CPS) agencies in the United States (Wang and Daro, 1998). In 1996, 1,185 children—more than three per day—died from child abuse and neglect, and many of these abusive situations had previously been reported to CPS agencies. There is an association between child abuse and substance abuse in the family. The term *battered child syndrome* originated in 1962 with the work of pediatrician Henry Kempe and his associates, who generated public and professional concern over child maltreatment. Their work led to the passage in 1974 of the Child Abuse Prevention and Treatment Act, which mandated reporting by professionals (including nurses) of child maltreatment.

The presence of **child abuse** signifies ineffective family functioning and has a social stigma attached to it. Children are frequent victims of abuse because they are small and relatively powerless in the family. In many families only one child is abused. The abuser may identify with this child or the child may have certain qualities, such as looking like a relative, being handicapped, or being particularly bright and capable, that provoke the parent.

Abusive parents tend to control their children's behavior and are often insensitive to their needs (Humphreys and Ramsey, 1993). They often are emotionally unstable and have unrealistic expectations of the child's capabilities. It is important for nurses to teach the parents about normal childhood development and behavior but also pay attention to the emotional needs of the parents. The box to the right lists some behavioral indicators of potentially abusive parents.

INDICATORS OF CHILD ABUSE. The primary indicators of physical abuse, physical neglect, sexual abuse, and emotional maltreatment are shown in the box on p. 388. Child abuse includes emotional abuse such as yelling, continually demeaning, or criticizing a child; passive neglect, including malnutrition; and physical attacks such as beating, burning, kicking, or shaking. Extreme criticizing can cause children to feel inadequate, inept, unloved, and worthless. These children learn to hide their feelings and many then act out to get some attention by doing poorly in school, becoming truant, and being hostile and aggressive.

HOW TO Recognize Potentially Abusive Parents

The following characteristics in couples expecting a child constitute warning signs of actual or potential abuse.
1. Denial of the reality of the pregnancy, as evidenced by a refusal to talk about the impending birth or to think of a name for the child
2. An obvious concern or fear that the baby will not meet some predetermined standard: sex, hair color, temperament, or resemblance to family members
3. Failure to follow through on the desire for or seeking of an abortion
4. An initial decision to place the child for adoption and a change of mind
5. Rejection of the mother by the father of the baby
6. Family experiencing stress and numerous crises so that the birth of a child may be the "straw that broke the camel's back"
7. Initial and unresolved negative feelings about having a child
8. Lack of support for the new parents
9. Isolation from friends, neighbors, or family
10. Parental evidence of poor impulse control or fear of losing control
11. Contradictory history
12. Appearance of detachment
13. Appearance of misusing drugs or alcohol
14. Shopping for hospitals or health care providers
15. Unrealistic expectations of the child
16. Abuse of the mother by the father, especially during pregnancy
17. Child is not biological offspring of male stepfather or mother's current boyfriend

Physical symptoms of physical, sexual, or emotional stress may include hyperactivity, withdrawal, overeating, dermatological problems, vague physical complaints, stuttering, enuresis (bladder incontinence), and encoporesis (bowel incontinence). It is ironic that bed-wetting often provokes further abuse, causing a vicious cycle. When a child displays physical symptoms without conditions with a stress component (e.g., asthma) or a clear physiological cause, it is important to assess for abuse.

CHILD NEGLECT. **Child neglect** can be physical or emotional. **Physical neglect** is the failure to provide adequate food, proper clothing, shelter, hygiene, or necessary medical care (Campbell and Humphreys, 1993), and is often associated with extreme poverty. In contrast, **emotional neglect** is the omission of basic nurturing, acceptance, and caring essential for healthy development. This ignoring and nonvaluing form of neglect usually affects self-esteem development and, because it is subtle, is often hard to detect.

SEXUAL ABUSE. Child abuse also includes sexual abuse. Approximately one of four female children and one of ten male children in the United States are sexually abused by age 18. This number may be inaccurate since young children may not always be able to explain the abuse (Kendall-Tackett and Marshall, 1998). The child generally knows the abuser, with between one half and one third of all sexual abuse involving a family member (Russell, 1995b). A child's risk for sexual abuse if done by a caretaker is greatest among stepparents or unrelated caregivers (Gelles, 1998). The long-term effects of sexual abuse include depression, sexual disturbances, and substance abuse (Carlson, et al, 1997).

HOW TO Recognize Signs of Actual or Potential Child Abuse

1. An unexplained injury
   a. Skin: burns, old or recent scars, ecchymosis, soft-tissue swelling, human bites
   b. Fractures: recent or already healed
   c. Subdural hematomas
   d. Trauma to genitalia
   e. Whiplash (caused by shaking small children)
2. Dehydration or malnourishment without obvious cause
3. Provision of inappropriate food or drugs (alcohol, tobacco, medication prescribed for someone else, foods not appropriate for the child's age)
4. Evidence of general poor care: poor hygiene, dirty clothes, unkempt hair, dirty nails
5. Unusually fearful of nurse and others
6. Considered to be a "bad" child
7. Inappropriately dressed for the season or weather conditions
8. Reports or shows evidence of sexual abuse
9. Injuries not mentioned in history
10. Seems to need to take care of the parent and speak for the parent
11. Maternal depression
12. Maladjustment of older siblings

Father-daughter **incest** is the type of incest most often reported (Herman and Hirschman, 1993). Many cases of parental incest go unreported because victims fear punishment, abandonment, rejection, or family disruption if they mention the problem. Incest occurs in all races, religious groups, and socioeconomic classes. Incest is receiving greater attention because of mandatory reporting laws, yet all too often, its incidence remains a family secret.

Because nurses are often involved in helping women deal with the aftermath of incest, it is crucial to understand the typical patterns and the long-term implications. The following is a fairly typical case history:

The daughter involved in paternal incest is usually about 9 years of age at the onset and is often the oldest or only daughter. The father seldom uses physical force; rather he relies on threats, bribes, intimidation, or misrepresentation of moral standards, or he exploits the daughter's need for human affection (Herman and Hirschman, 1993). The victim may have these symptoms: low self-esteem,

depression, headaches, eating and sleeping disorders, menstrual problems, and gastrointestinal distress. There may also be problems in social situations, especially in forming and maintaining close relationships with boys or men; or behavioral problems such as substance abuse and sexual dysfunction (Green, 1996). It is critical when a child describes sexual abuse that the child is believed and the child's safety is made the first priority.

Adolescents who have been sexually abused may display inappropriate sexual activity or truancy or may run away from home. Running away is usually considered a sign of delinquency; some adolescents who run may be using a healthy response to a violent family situation. Therefore assessment of runaway youth should include an inquiry about sexual and physical abuse at home and appropriate intervention.

The effects of any kind of child maltreatment can be lessened if the child has a non-offending parent, another relative, or an adult outside the family to provide stable, ongoing physical and emotional support. Even so, adult survivors of sexual abuse often have significant health problems (Draucker, 1993). Nurses are often the first people to learn about the abuse. A first step for the nurse is to acknowledge that the abuse occurred.

Abuse of Female Partners

Although women do abuse men, by far the greatest proportion of what is called spouse abuse or domestic violence is actually wife abuse. As many as 35% of U.S. adults have seen a man beating his wife or girlfriend (Centers for Disease Control and Prevention, 1998). It is estimated that in the United States at least 20% of adult women, 15% of college women, and 12% of adolescent girls have experienced sexual abuse or assault during their lifetime (Council on Scientific Affairs, 1992). Approximately one of six pregnant women is physically abused during pregnancy; 20% of pregnant teens are abused (McFarlane, Parker, and Soeken, 1994). These women are at risk for spontaneous abortion, premature delivery, low birth weight, substance abuse during pregnancy, and depression (Campbell, 1992; McFarlane, Parker, and Soeken, 1994. Neither the term *wife abuse* nor **spouse abuse** takes into account violence in dating or "living together" relationships or violence in same sex relationships. *Spousal violence* or *partner violence* are more inclusive terms to refer to all kinds of violence between partners. All adults should be assessed for violence in their primary intimate relationships. Although there are no prevalence studies on violence in same-sex relationships, the incidence is estimated to be the same as in heterosexual relationships.

Briefly Noted

When assessing for violence, create an environment where the person feels safe to describe what happened. The survivors may be afraid to discuss what happened if they fear that the abuser will learn about the conversation and harm them (Champion, 1998).

SIGNS OF ABUSE. Battered women often have bruises and lacerations of the face, head, and trunk of the body. Attacks

Evidence-Based Practice

Battered women who live in shelters have disturbed sleep and fatigue that can interfere with their effectiveness in performing daily living activities. The study cited below examined the sleep patterns of 50 ethnically diverse women who spent at least 21 days in a battered women's shelter. The women completed questionnaires to measure sleep and fatigue, participated in an open-ended interview, wore a wrist motion sensor to monitor activity for 2 days, and kept a 2-day diary.

On the sleep questionnaire, scores indicated that 70% of the women had poor sleep and 34% had a sleep efficiency index of 80% or less. Twenty-eight percent of the women went to bed very fatigued and 40% woke up very fatigued. In the interviews, the following sleep behaviors were often cited: waking up often; difficulty initially falling asleep; awaking early in the morning and being unable to go back to sleep; and having unpleasant dreams.

APPLICATION IN PRACTICE

Nurses can advise shelters about the likelihood that the women residents will have sleep difficulties. They can also suggest strategies the shelter can use to help women sleep more productively.

Humphreys JC, Lee KA, Neylan TC, Marmar CR: Sleep patterns of sheltered battered women, *Image: J Nurs Scholarship* 31(2):139-143, 1999.

Evidence-Based Practice

Growing numbers of children are exposed to aggression and violence each year. Children of abused women often see the violence against their mothers. In many parts of the world, children witness and are victims of war violence. A great deal of research has been done to examine the effects on children who are themselves abused. Much less attention has been paid to children who witness violence.

The author of the study referenced below explored how two groups of children who grew up with violence "made sense" of these experiences. Data were collected from 16 refugee children of war and 16 children of battered women. The children were given a choice of being interviewed alone or in small groups. The primary data gathering instrument was an unstructured interview guide made up of open-ended questions designed to encourage the children to tell their stories about their experience with violence.

While each child's story was unique, some common themes emerged. Both groups of children had experienced pain, suffering, and feelings of betrayal. They had used a variety of creative strategies in order to survive, and they showed strength and insight.

APPLICATION IN PRACTICE

It is important for nurses to understand that children who witness violence want to discuss their experiences. Nurses can help them do so and then help them make sense of what has happened to them.

Berman H: Stories of growing up amid violence by refugee children of war and children of battered women living in Canada, *Image: J Nurs Scholarship* 31(1):57-63, 1999.

are often carefully inflicted on parts of the body that can easily be disguised by clothing such as the breasts, abdomen, upper thighs, and back (Campbell and Sheridan, 1989). When a woman has a black eye or bruises about the mouth, the nurse should ask, "Who hit you?" rather than, "What happened to you?" The latter question implies that the nurse is neither knowledgeable nor comfortable with violence, and this may prompt the woman to fabricate a more acceptable cause of her injury.

Abused women often exhibit low self-esteem and have a variety of mental health problems including depression, substance abuse, eating disorders, posttraumatic stress disorder (PTSD), chronic pain, and self-destructive behaviors (Campbell, et al, 1997; Draucker, 1997). They also have many physical health problems such as chronic pain, neurological problems, chronic irritable bowel syndrome, and gynecological problems (Campbell and Lewandowski, 1997).

Many women who are physically abused are also sexually abused. The woman may try to minimize the seriousness of the situation, blame the incident on some unusual stress, or try to change her behavior. The key nursing actions are to assess the seriousness of the situation and to work with the woman to ensure that she and her children are safe. This may include helping her move to a shelter or other protected environment. She may need an order of protection, which is a legal document to keep the abuser away from her. At the least, the nurse can help the woman design a carefully thought-out plan for escape and arrange for a neighbor or an adolescent child to call the police when there is another vio-

lent episode. After the abuse has ended, a period of recovery begins. This includes a normal grief response for the relationship that has ended and a search for meaning in the experience (Landenburger, 1989; Landenburger, 1998). The woman may feel depressed and lonely when the relationship ends, and she will need support.

Abuse of Elderly Persons

Elder Abuse includes emotional, sexual, and physical neglect, as well as physical and sexual violence and financial abuse. The abuse and neglect of elders afflicts between 700,000 and 1 million people yearly (American Nurses Association, 1998). Neglect is a serious form of abuse and accounts for 70% of the cases reported to Adult Protective Services annually (Fulmer, 1999). The elderly are neglected when others fail to provide adequate food, clothing, shelter, and physical care and when physiological, emotional, and safety needs are not met adequately. Roughness in handling elderly people can lead to bruises and bleeding into body tissues because of the fragility of their skin and vascular systems. It is often difficult to determine if the injuries of elderly persons result from abuse, falls, or other natural causes. Careful assessment both through observation and discussion assists in determining the cause of injuries. Elderly people are also abused when caregivers impose unrealistic toileting demands and ignore their special needs, including nutrition, medication, and previous living patterns. Also, some caregivers give elderly people medication to induce confusion or drowsiness so that they will be less troublesome, will need less care, or will allow others to control their financial and personal resources.

The most common form of psychological abuse is rejection or simply ignoring elderly people. This can cause them to feel worthless and useless, and they may regress and become increasingly dependent on others. The caregiver may resent the imposition and demands on their time and life-style. The pattern becomes cyclical: the more regressed the person becomes, the greater the dependence, and the greater the dependence the more the caregiver gets tired, annoyed, and resentful. The box below lists ways to identify signs of potential elder abuse.

HOW TO Recognize Potential or Actual Elder Abuse

- Unexplained or repeated injury
- Fear of the caregiver
- Untreated sores or other skin injuries, such as decubitus ulcers, excoriated perineum, burns
- Overall poor care (e.g., unclean, given inappropriate food)
- Withdrawal and passivity
- Periods of time when elderly person is unsupervised
- Contractures resulting from immobility or restraint
- Unwillingness or inability of caregiver to meet elderly person's needs
- Improper home repair
- Unsafe home situation (e.g., poor heating, ventilation, dangerous clutter)

Modified from Phillips LR: Abuse/neglect of the frail elderly at home: an exploration of theoretical relationships, *J Adv Nurs* 8:379, 1983; Fulmer T: Mistreatment of elders, assessment, diagnosis and intervention, *Nurs Clin North Am* 24(3):707, 1989.

Confused and frail elderly persons are particularly vulnerable to abuse. Persons with Alzheimer's disease and other dementias are at greater risk for physical abuse than other elderly persons. This is often due to the high burden that their care places on the caregiver and the subsequent tiredness and depression of the caregiver (Coyne, Reichman, and Berbig, 1993). Living with and providing care to a confused elderly person is difficult, and 'round-the-clock tasks often exhaust family members. Family stress increases as members struggle to meet their other responsibilities in addition to meeting the needs of the elderly person.

NURSING INTERVENTIONS

Primary prevention begins with a community approach that incorporates strategies from criminal justice, education, social services, community advocacy, and pubic health to prevent violence. Some communities have used:

- School-based curricula that teach children and youth how to cope with anger, stress, and frustration and that also teach communication and mediation skills
- Family programs that teach parents how to deal with their children more effectively
- Preschool programs to develop intellectual and social skills
- Increasing community awareness about violence and its prevention (Trends in Rates, 1996).

Communities must begin by taking a stand against violence and enforcing laws to deal with people who engage in violence. Nurses can be advocates for a nonviolent community and can teach and support members in reporting acts of violence. They can join other groups in teaching residents to protect themselves with good home security such as keeping windows and doors locked, trimming shrubs around their homes, keeping lights on during high-crime periods, installing home security systems, joining neighborhood watch programs, and learning physical defense and handgun safety. Unfortunately, handguns are far more likely to kill family members than intruders. Accidental firearm death is a leading cause of death for young children, and handguns kept in the home are easy to use in moments of extreme anger with other family members or at times of extreme depression.

Nurses in the community can also advocate and teach community residents to advocate for policy changes that would reduce violence. This could include conducting research to document the amount and types of violence in a community in order to support law enforcement or other methods to reduce the level of violence. Nurses see both victims and perpetrators of violence in a variety of health care settings. This gives nurses opportunities to generate information about how to better identify the potential for violence, identify victims of violence, provide interventions to reduce the likelihood of violence, and advocate for changes in laws and law enforcement, as well as treatment and protection options that can be made available.

Identification of risk factors is an important part of primary prevention. Although abuse cannot be predicted with certainty, a variety of factors tend to influence the onset and support continuation of abuse patterns. Since nurses see clients in a variety of settings, often they can identify potential victims of abuse. Figure 22-1 cites several factors to look for when assessing a person or a family's potential for violence.

Primary prevention also includes strengthening individuals and families so they can cope more effectively with the demands in their lives and reduce the destructive elements in the community. Nurses can teach basic parenting skills, including acceptable ways to discipline children. Also support groups can help new parents, families with special children, or abused people themselves. Such groups have a variety of formats, and they can provide information, support, and encouragement. Nurses can help begin such groups or can actually serve as group leaders. Chapter 16 describes the role of the nurse in working with community groups.

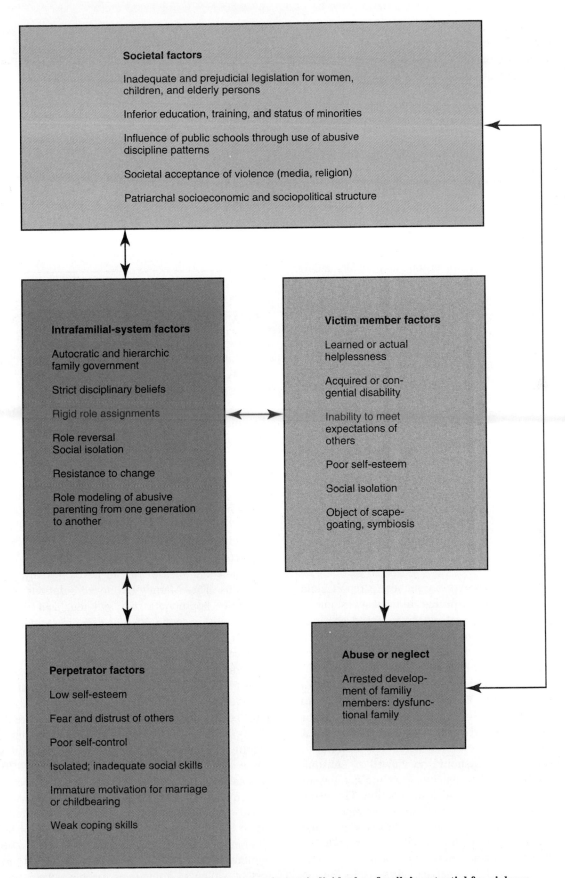

Figure 22-1   Factors to include when assessing an individual or family's potential for violence.

Violence is a family crisis and should be handled using crisis-intervention strategies. When intervening at the secondary prevention level, nurses can help people discuss the problem and seek alternatives for dealing with the tension that led to the abusive situation. Injured persons must be temporarily or permanently placed in a safe location. Secondary preventive measures are most useful when potential abusers recognize their tendency to be abusive and seek help. Children often need 24-hour child protection services or caregivers to care for the child until the acute crisis is resolved. Respite care is important for families with frail elderly members. Telephone crisis lines can be used to provide immediate emergency assistance to families.

Such basic nursing skills as a nonjudgmental attitude, effective communication, compassion, and understanding are important. Some families may need to be coached on ways to have fun and use the available community resources. Safety is, of course, a first priority.

Briefly Noted

Should both women and men entering the health care system be asked about domestic violence and sexual assault experience? Some experts think that men should be asked if they are victims or perpetrators of violence as a secondary prevention activity. If identified early, such behavior may be more amenable to interventions. Others say that since we do not know what interventions are most effective for male perpetrators or victims of violence, it is premature to do routine screening. Also perpetrators of domestic violence or child abuse may become angry if asked about their violent behavior and retaliate against the family member.

It is mandatory in all states for nurses to report child abuse, even when it is only suspected. In most states, nurses are also mandatory reporters of elder abuse and abuse of other physically and cognitively dependent adults as well as felony assaults of anyone. The mandatory reporting laws protect reporters from legal action in cases that are never substantiated. Even so, physicians and nurses are sometimes reluctant to report abuse. They may be more willing to report abuse in a poor family than in a middle-class one, or they may think that an elderly person or child is better off at home than in a nursing home or foster home. Referral to protective service agencies should be viewed as enlisting another source of help, rather than an automatic step toward removal of the victim or criminal justice action. This same attitude can be communicated to families so that reporting is done *with* families rather than without their knowledge and prior input. Absolute honesty about what will be reported to officials, what the family can expect, what the nurse is entering into records, as well as what the nurse is feeling, is essential. The How to box on this page lists ways nurses can help victims of domestic violence.

Box 22-1	**Common Community Services**

- Child protective services
- Child abuse prevention programs
- Adult protective services
- Parents anonymous
- Wife abuse shelter
- Program for children of battered women
- Community support group
- 24-hour hotline
- Legal advocacy or information
- National Hotline (1-800-799-SAFE)
- State coalition against domestic violence
- Batterer treatment
- Victim assistance programs
- Sexual assault programs

HOW TO Assist Survivors of Domestic Violence

- Listen to and believe their stories
- Ask for more details about the abuse than what is initially offered
- Avoid telling the person how you feel
- Don't pressure the person to leave the abuser but do explain options
- Make referrals

Modified from Miles A: When faith is used to justify abuse, *Am J Nurs* 99(5):32-35, 1999.

To further aid the family, nurses must recognize and capitalize on the violent family's strengths, as well as assess and deal with their problems. The nurse can use a nurse-family partnership rather than a paternalistic or authoritarian approach. Families often can develop many of their own solutions. These family-developed solutions may be more culturally appropriate and individualized than those the nurse could generate. Victims of a direct attack need information about their options and resources along with reassurance that abuse is unfortunately rather common and that they are not alone in their dilemma. They also need assurance that their responses are normal and that they do not deserve to be abused. Continued support for their decisions must be coupled with nursing actions to ensure their safety. The emotional investment and sheer amount of energy required to work effectively with abusers and victims of abuse cannot be minimized. Abusers present difficult clinical challenges because of their reluctance to seek help or to remain actively involved in the helping process.

Providing care to victims and referring them for appropriate treatment are important components of tertiary prevention (Champion, 1998). Box 22-1 lists some common community services that may help survivors and perpetrators of violence. Sometimes, people do not seek services early in an abusive situation because they simply do not know what is available to them. Ideally, a program or planned emphasis for abused people begins with a needs

Healthy People 2010
Violence

National goals for reducing violence are:
15-32 Reduce homicides
15-33 Reduce maltreatment and maltreatment fatalities of children
15-34 Reduce the rate of physical assault by current or former intimate partners
15-35 Reduce the annual rate of rape or attempted rate
15-36 Reduce sexual assault other than rape
15-37 Reduce physical assault
15-38 Reduce physical fighting among adolescents
15-39 Reduce weapon carrying by adolescents on school property

assessment to identify potential clients and to determine how to effectively serve this group.

These principles can guide nurses in their work with families experiencing violence:

- Be intolerant of violence
- Acknowledge that violence occurred
- Respect and care for family members
- Make safety the first priority
- Be honest
- Help the family gain strength
- Role-model nonviolent ways to behave and handle conflict

Healthy People 2010 and Violence

While the percent of violent crimes in the nation dropped in the year 2000, if an individual is a victim, it can change the quality of life forever. Violence claims the lives of many and threatens the health and well-being of others. Violence can also change the quality of a family, neighborhood, or community. The national goals for reducing violence are presented in the *Healthy People 2010* box.

Clinical Application

Mrs. Smith, a 75-year-old bedridden woman, consistently became rude and combative when her daughter, Mary, tried to bathe her and change her clothes each morning. During a home visit, Mary told Mrs. Jones, her nurse, that she had gotten so frustrated with her mother on the previous morning that she had hit her. Mary felt terrible about her behavior. She knew that her mother's incontinence made it essential that she be kept clean; her clothes had to be changed every day for her own safety and physical well-being, yet her mother was so difficult.

A. How should Mrs. Jones respond to this disclosure?
B. What specific nursing actions should be taken?
C. What ongoing services does the nurse need to provide?

Answers are in the back of the book.

Remember This!

- Violence and human abuse are not new phenomena, but they are growing community health concerns.
- Nurses are in a position to evaluate and intervene in community and family violence.
- Factors influencing social and community violence include changing social conditions, economic conditions, population density, community facilities, and institutions within a community, such as organized religion, education, the mass-communication media, and work.
- Violence and abuse of family members can happen to any family member: spouse, elderly person, child, pregnant female, or developmentally disabled person.
- People who abuse family members are often abused themselves.
- Child abuse can be physical, emotional, or sexual. Incest is a common and particularly destructive form of child abuse.
- Spouse abuse is usually wife abuse. It involves physical, emotional, and/or sexual abuse within a context of coercive control. It usually increases in severity and frequency and can escalate to homicide of either partner.
- Nurses can identify potential victims of family abuse because they see clients in a variety of settings, such as schools, businesses, homes, and clinics.
- Treatment of family abuse includes primary, secondary, and tertiary prevention, as well as therapeutic intervention.

What Would You Do?

1. For 1 week, keep a log or diary related to violence.
   a. Make a note each time you feel as though you might lose your temper. Consider what it might take to cause you to react in a violent way.
   b. Think back; when was the last time you had a violent outburst? What precipitated it? What were your thoughts? What were your feelings? How might you have handled the situation or those feelings without reacting in a violent way?
   c. During this same week, make note of the episodes of violent behaviors you observe. For example, do parents hit children in the supermarket? What seems to precipitate such outbursts? What alternatives exist for reacting in a less violent way?
2. What resources are available in your community for victims of violence?
   a. Interview a person who works in an agency that serves victims of violence.
   b. What is the role of the agency?
   c. Do its services seem adequate?
   d. Who is eligible?
   e. Is there a waiting list?
   f. What is the fee scale?

3. Cut out all stories about violence in your local newspaper daily for 2 weeks. Note the patterns.
   a. Is the majority of the violence perpetrated by strangers or family members?
   b. How are the victims portrayed?
   c. What kinds of families are involved?
   d. What kinds of stories and families get front-page treatment rather than a few lines in the back of the paper?

REFERENCES

Aiken MM, Speck PM: Sexual assault and multiple trauma: a sexual assault nurse examiner (SANE) challenge, *J Emerg Nurs* 21(5):466-468, 1995.

American Association of Colleges of Nursing: Position statement: violence as a public health problem, Washington, D.C., 1999, American Association of Colleges of Nursing.

American Nurses Association: Culturally competent assessment for family violence, Washington, D.C., 1998, American Nurses Publishing.

Bachman R: *Violence against women: a national crime victimization survey report,* Washington, D.C., 1994, U.S. Department of Justice, Office of Justice Programs, Bureau of Justice Statistics.

Briere J, Berliner L, Bulkley JA, Jenny C, Reid T: *The APSAC handbook on child maltreatment,* Thousand Oaks, Calif, 1996, Sage.

Bureau of Justice Statistics: *Criminal victimization 1996,* Washington, D.C., 1997, U.S. Department of Justice.

Campbell JC: *Assessing dangerousness: potential for further violence of sexual offenders,* Newbury Park, Calif, 1995, Sage.

Campbell JC: "If I can't have you, no one can" homicide in intimate relationships. In Radford J, Russell DEH (editors): *Femicide: the politics of woman killing,* Boston, 1992, Twayne Publishers.

Campbell JC, Humphreys J: *Nursing care of survivors of family violence,* St Louis, 1993, Mosby.

Campbell JC, Kub J, Belknap RA, Templin T: Predictors of depression in battered women, *Violence Against Women* 3(3):271-293, 1997.

Campbell JC, Lewandowski LA: Mental and physical health effects of intimate partner violence on women and children, *Psychiatr Clin North Am* 20:353-374, 1997.

Campbell JC, Sheridan DJ: Clinical articles: emergency nursing interventions with battered women, *J Emerg Nurs* 15(1):12, 1989.

Carlson RB, Furby L, Armstrong J, Shlaes J: A conceptual framework for the long-term psychological effects of traumatic childhood abuse, *Child Maltreatment* 2(3):272-295, 1997.

Centers for Disease Control and Prevention, Office of Women's Health: *Violence and injury,* Atlanta, 1998, Centers for Disease Control and Prevention.

Champion JD: Family violence and mental health, *Nurs Clin North Am* 33(1):201-215, 1998.

Council on Scientific Affairs (AMA): Violence against women, *JAMA* 267(23):3184-3189, 1992.

Counts D, Brown J, Campbell J: Sanctions and sanctuary, Boulder, Colo 1992, Westview Press.

Coyne AC, Reichman WR, Berbig LJ: The relationship between dementia and elder abuse, *Am J Psychiatry* 150(4):643, 1993.

Donat PL, D'Emilio N: A feminist redefinition of rape and sexual assault: historical foundations and change. In LL O'Toole, JR Schiffman (editors): *Gender violence: interdisciplinary perspectives,* New York, 1997, New York University Press.

Draucker CB: Childhood sexual abuse: source of trauma, *Issues Mental Health Nurs* 14:249-262, 1993.

Draucker CB: Impact of violence in the lives of women: restriction and resolve, *Issues Mental Health Nurs* 18:559-586, 1997.

Draucker CB: Narrative therapy for women who have lived with violence, *Arch Psychiatr Nurs* XII (3):162-168, 1998.

Eggert LL, et al: Prevention research program: reconnecting at-risk youth, *Iss Mental Health Nurs* 15(2)107, 1994.

Fulmer T: Our elderly—harmed, exploited, abandoned, *Reflections* 25(3):16-18, 1999.

Gelles RJ: The youngest victims: violence toward children. In Bergen RK (editor): *Issues in intimate violence,* pp. 5-24, Thousand Oaks, Calif, 1998, Sage.

Gelles R, Conte J: Domestic violence and sexual abuse of children: a review of research in the eighties, *J Marriage Fam* 52(4):1045, 1990.

Green AH: Overview of child sexual abuse. In SJ Kaplan (editor): *Family violence: a clinical and legal guide,* Washington, D.C., 1996, American Psychiatric Press.

Herman J, Hirschman L: Father-daughter incest. In Bart PB, Moran EG (editors): *Violence against women: the bloody footprints,* Thousand Oaks, Calif, 1993, Sage.

Hernandez JT, Lodico M, DiClemente RJ: The effects of child abuse and race on risk taking in male adolescents, *J Natl Med Assoc* 85(8):593-597, 1993.

Humphreys J, Ramsey AM: Child abuse. In Campbell J, Humphreys J (editors): *Nursing care of survivors of family violence,* St Louis, 1993, Mosby.

Kempe CH, et al: The battered child syndrome, *JAMA* 181:17, 1962.

Kendall-Tackett K, Marshall R: Sexual victimization of children: incest and child sexual abuse. In Bergen RK (editor): *Issues in intimate violence,* Thousand Oaks, Calif, 1998, Sage.

Klein E, Campbell JC, Soler E, Ghez M: *Ending domestic violence: changing public perceptions/halting the epidemic,* Newbury Park, Calif, 1997, Sage.

Koss MP, Harvey MR: *The rape victim: clinical and community intervention,* ed 2, Newbury Park, Calif, 1991, Sage.

Koss MP, Cook SL: Facing the facts: date and acquaintance rape are significant problems for women. In Bergen RK (editor): *Issues in intimate violence,* Thousand Oaks, Calif, 1998, Sage.

Landenburger K: A process of entrapment in and recovery from an abusive relationship, *Issues Mental Health Nurs* 10:209, 1989.

Landenburger K: Exploration of women's identity: clinical approaches with abused women, Empowering survivors of abuse: health care, battered women and their children, Newbury Hills, Calif, 1998, Sage.

Ledray LE, Simmelink K: Sexual assault: clinical issues: efficacy of SANE evidence collection: a Minnesota study, *J Emerg Nurs* 23(1):75-77, 1997.

Lynch VA: Forensic nursing: diversity in education and practice, *J Psychosoc Nurs* 31(11):7-14, 1993.

McFarlane J, Parker B, Soeken K: Abuse during pregnancy: effects on maternal complications and birthweight in adult and teenage women, *Obstet Gynecol* 84(3):323, 1994.

Miles A: When faith is used to justify abuse, *Am J Nurs* 99(5):32-35, 1999.

Moore R, Harrisson S: In poor health: socioeconomic status and health chances—a review of the literature, *Social Sci Health* 1(4):221-235, 1995.

Phillips LR: Abuse/neglect of the frail elderly at home: an exploration of theoretical relationships, *J Adv Nurs* 8:379, 1983.

Prince J: A systems approach to spouse abuse. In Lancaster J: *Community mental health nursing: an ecological perspective,* St Louis, 1980, Mosby.

Rates of homicide, suicide, and firearm related deaths among children in 26 industrialized countries, *MMWR* 46(5):101-105, 1997.

Regional variations in suicide rates, *MMWR* 46(34):789-793, 1997.

Reiss AJ, Roth JA (editors): Understanding and preventing violence, vol 1-4, Washington, D.C., 1993-1994, National Academy Press.

Riedel M: Counting stranger homicides, *Homicide Studies* 2:206-219, 1998.

Rosenberg ML, Fenley MA (editors): *Violence in America: a public health approach,* New York, 1991, Oxford.

Russell DEH: The prevalence, trauma, and sociocultural cause of incestuous abuse of females: a human rights issue. In K Rolf,

CR Figley, et al (editors): *Beyond trauma: cultural and societal dynamics,* New York, 1995b, Plenum.

Stark E, Fitzcraft A: Spouse abuse. In Rosenberg ML, Finley MA (editors): *Violence in America,* New York, 1991, Oxford.

Straus MA, Gelles RJ: *Physical violence in American families: risk factors and adaptations to violence in 8,145 families,* New Brunswick, NJ, 1990, Transaction.

Trends in rates of homicide—United States, 1985-1994, *MMWR* 45(22):460-464, 1996.

U.S. Department of Health and Human Services: *Healthy people 2000: national health promotion and disease prevention objectives,* Washington, D.C., 1991. U.S. Department of Health and Human Services.

U.S. Department of Justice: Sex offenses and offenders: an analysis of data on rape and sexual assault, Washington, D.C., 1997, NCJ-163392, Bureau of Justice Statistics.

Wang CT, Daro D: *Current trends in child abuse reporting and fatalities: the results of the 1997 Annual Fifty State Survey,* Chicago, 1998, National Committee to Prevent Child Abuse.

Webster DW: The unconvincing case for school-based conflict resolution, *Health Affairs* 12(4):126-141, 1993.

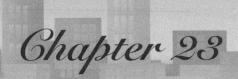

Chapter 23

Communicable Disease: Risk and Prevention

FRANCISCO S. SY
SUSAN C. LONG-MARIN

OBJECTIVES

After reading this chapter, the student should be able to:

- Explain the agent-host-environment triad and how these elements interact to cause infectious diseases.
- Evaluate the factors leading to the emergence or re-emergence of infectious diseases.
- Describe the implications of immunity in terms of active immunity, passive immunity, and herd immunity.

- Define surveillance and discuss the functions and elements of the surveillance system. Describe the risk of food-borne illness and appropriate prevention measures giving special attention to salmonella and *E. coli* 0157:H7.
- Discuss how nurses use the three levels of prevention to control communicable diseases.
- Evaluate the multi-system approach to control of communicable diseases.

CHAPTER OUTLINE

KEY TERMS

acquired immunity: the resistance gained by a host due to past exposure to an infectious agent or a vaccine.

active immunization: administration of an antigen (infectious agent or vaccine) to cause immunity.

common vehicle: transportation of the infectious agent from an infected host to a susceptible host through water, food, milk, blood, serum, or the placenta.

communicable disease: a human or animal disease caused by an infectious agent and resulting from transmission of that agent from an infected person, animal, or inanimate source to a susceptible host. Infectious disease may be communicable or noncommunicable. For example, tetanus is infectious but not communicable.

communicable period: the time or times when an infectious agent may be transferred from an infected source directly or indirectly to a new host.

elimination: removal of a disease from a country or region of the world.

endemic: the constant presence of an infectious disease within a specific geographic area.

environment: everything that is outside the host. The environment can be divided into such categories as physical, biological, social, and cultural.

epidemic: the occurrence of an infectious agent or disease within a specific geographic area in greater numbers than would normally be expected.

epidemiologic triad: host-agent-environment.

eradication: refers to the irreversible termination of all transmission of infection by extermination of the infectious agent worldwide.

herd immunity: resistance of a group or community to an infectious agent.

horizontal transmission: person-to-person transmission through one of these routes: direct/indirect contact, common vehicle, airborne, vector-borne.

host: a living human or animal organism in which an infectious agent can exist under natural conditions.

host resistance: ability of host to withstand infection.

incubation period: the time between first contact with an infectious agent and the first appearance of clinical signs of the resultant disease.

infection and disease: infection results from the invasion of a host by an infectious agent. Such infection may or may not produce clinical signs. if clinical signs are absent, the infection may be referred to as inapparent, subclinical, asymptomatic, or occult. If clinical signs do result from infection, then the host is both infected and diseased. Disease may be referred to as *clinical* or *symptomatic.*

infectious disease: a human or animal disease caused by the entry and development of an infectious agent (bacteria, rickettsia, virus, fungus, or parasite) in the body.

infectiousness: a measure of the potential ability of an infected host to transmit the infection to other hosts.

natural immunity: an innate resistance in a species to an infectious agent.

pandemic: a worldwide outbreak of an epidemic disease.

passive immunization: immunization through the transfer of a specific antibody from an immunized person to a nonimmunized person.

surveillance: gathers the who, when, where, and what; these elements are then used to answer why. Data collection for the purpose of planning, implementing, and evaluating disease prevention and control programs.

universal precautions: designed to protect health care workers from blood and body fluids of persons infected with infectious diseases. Initially designed to respond to the threat of AIDS transmission in health care settings.

vector: a non-human organism, often an insect, that either mechanically or biologically plays a role in the transmission of an infectious agent from source to host.

vertical transmission: infection is passed from parent to offspring through sperm, placenta, breast milk, or contact with the vaginal canal at birth.

In 1900, communicable diseases were the leading causes of death in the United States. By 2000, improved nutrition and sanitation, vaccines, and antibiotics had ended the epidemics that once killed entire populations. In 1900, tuberculosis was the second leading cause of death; in 1995 this disease killed less than 1400 people or was responsible for about 0.06% of all deaths in the United States (National Center for Health Statistics, 1996). As people live longer, chronic diseases— heart disease, cancer, and stroke—have replaced infectious diseases as the leading causes of death. Infectious diseases, however, have not vanished; they are still the number-one cause of death worldwide. Annually, infectious diseases account for 25% of all physician visits, and antibiotics are the second most prescribed type of drug in the United States (Centers for Disease Control and Prevention, 1994a).

New killers are emerging and old familiar diseases are taking on different, more virulent characteristics. For example, the AIDS epidemic that began to spread in developing countries in the 1980s now looks much like many of the plagues from the past. This disease challenges our ability to contain and control infection, and in the United States, AIDS and unintentional injuries are now the leading killers of persons 25 to 44 years of age. In 1996, 10 states had outbreaks of diarrheal disease traced to imported fresh berries due to the organism *Cyclospora cayetanensis,* a coccidian parasite first recognized in humans in 1977 (Centers for Disease Control and Prevention, 1996). Also both in 1996 and again in 2001, the fear that "mad cow disease" (bovine spongiform encephalopathy) could be transferred to humans through beef consumption led to the slaughter of thousands of British and other European cattle and a ban on the international sale of this beef.

This chapter presents an overview of the most common communicable diseases with which nurses deal. Although not all **infectious diseases** are directly communicable from person to person, the terms *infectious* diseases and *communicable* diseases are used interchangeably in this chapter. Diseases are grouped according to descriptive category (by mode of transmission or means of prevention) rather than by individual organism (*E. coli*) or taxonomic group (viral, parasitic).

TRANSMISSION OF COMMUNICABLE DISEASES

Agent, Host, and Environment

Communicable diseases are transmitted by the successful interaction of the infectious agent, host, and environment. These three factors are called the **epidemiologic triad.** Changes in the characteristics of any one of these three factors can cause disease transmission (Benenson, 1995). For example, an antibiotic may remove the agent that causes disease while simultaneously removing some organisms that serve as protective agents. As a result, one agent overruns another, and disease, such as a yeast infection, occurs. HIV performs its deadly work not by directly poisoning the host but by destroying the host's immune reaction to other disease-producing agents.

Four main categories of infectious agents can cause infection or disease:
- Bacteria
- Fungi
- Parasites
- Viruses.

The individual *agent* is described by its ability to cause disease and the nature and the severity of the disease. Human or animal **hosts** can harbor infectious agents. The following characteristics of the host can influence the spread of disease: host resistance, immunity, herd immunity, and infectiousness of the host. **Host resistance** is the ability of the host to withstand infection. This resistance may be due to natural or acquired immunity.

Natural immunity refers to an innate resistance in a species to an infectious agent. For example, opossums rarely contract rabies. **Acquired immunity** is the resistance gained by a host due to previous natural exposure to an infectious agent. Having measles protects against future infection. Both active and passive immunization can induce acquired immunity. **Active immunization** results from the administration of an antigen (infectious agent or vaccine) and the production of an antibody by the host. Specifically, vaccinating children against childhood diseases can induce active immunity. **Passive immunization** refers to the transfer of a specific antibody from an immunized person to a nonimmunized individual. That is, antibody can be transferred from mother to infant or by administration of an antibody-containing preparation (immune globulin or antiserum). Passive immunity from immune globulin is almost immediate but short-lived. It is often induced as a temporary measure until active immunity has time to develop after vaccination. Examples of commonly used immunoglobulins include those for hepatitis A, rabies, and tetanus.

Herd immunity, the immunity of a group or community, is the resistance of a group of people to invasion and spread of an infectious agent. Herd immunity is seen when a large proportion of group members are resistant to a specific infection, and this concept supports increasing immunization coverage for vaccine-preventable diseases. Greater immunization coverage will lead to greater herd immunity, thereby blocking further spread of the disease.

Infectiousness, a measure of the potential ability of an infected host to transmit the infection to other hosts, is concerned with the relative ease with which the infectious agent is transmitted to others. People with measles are extremely infectious; the virus spreads readily on airborne droplets. Thus, daycare centers, Head Start programs, and other places where children come together in groups are prime places for the transmission of the measles virus once one child contracts the disease. In contrast, a person with Lyme disease cannot spread the disease to other people. Unlike measles, which is spread by people, Lyme disease is spread only by infected ticks.

Environment refers to all that is external to the human host, including physical, biological, social, and cultural factors. Environmental factors aid the transmission of an infectious agent from an infected host to other susceptible hosts. Changing environmental factors can reduce communicable disease risk. For example, using mosquito nets and repellents to avoid bug bites, installing sewage systems to prevent fecal contamination of water supplies, and carefully washing utensils after contact with raw meat or eggs to reduce bacterial contamination are all examples of altering the environment to prevent disease.

Modes of Transmission

Infectious diseases can be transmitted horizontally or vertically and by several methods:
- **Vertical transmission:** infection is passed from parent to offspring through sperm, placenta, milk, or contact in the vaginal canal at birth.
  - Examples include transplacental transmission of HIV and syphilis.
- **Horizontal transmission:** person-to-person spread through one or more of the following four routes:
  - Direct/indirect contact: Sexually transmitted diseases are spread by direct sexual contact.
  - **Common vehicle:** transportation from an infected host to a susceptible host via water, food, milk, blood, serum, or plasma. Enterobiasis or pinworm infection is spread through direct contact or by indirect contact with contaminated objects such as toys, clothing, and bedding. Hepatitis A can be transmitted through contaminated food and water, and hepatitis B can be transmitted through contaminated blood products.
  - Airborne: legionellosis and tuberculosis are both spread by an airborne route via contaminated droplets in the air.
  - Vector-borne: **vectors** can be arthropods such as ticks and mosquitos or other invertebrates such as snails that can transmit the infectious agent by biting or depositing the infective material near the host.

It is important to differentiate between **infection and disease.** Exposure to an infectious agent may not always lead to an infection, just as infection does not always cause disease. Infection depends on the amount of the infective dose, infectivity of the infectious agent, and immunocompetence of the host. The relationship between infection and disease can be clearly illustrated by the HIV/AIDS epidemic. *Infection* refers to the entry, development, and multiplication of the infectious agent in the susceptible host. *Disease* is one of the possible outcomes of infection, and it may indicate a physiological dysfunction or pathological reaction. In an example from the sports world, compare the case of Magic Johnson with that of Greg Louganis. Both publicly announced that they had tested positive for HIV, but while Johnson was asymptomatic, Louganis had developed the clinical signs of AIDS. Or in other words, Johnson was infected but not diseased, Louganis was both infected and diseased.

Incubation period and communicable period are not synonymous. **Incubation period** is the time interval between invasion by an infectious agent and the first appearance of signs and symptoms of the disease. The incubation periods of infectious diseases vary from 2 to 4 hours for staphylococcal food poisoning to 10 to 15 years for AIDS. **Communicable period** is the time interval during which an infectious agent may be transferred directly or indirectly from an infected person to another person. The period of communicability for influenza is 3 to 5 days after the clinical onset of symptoms. In contrast, persons infected with hepatitis B are infectious for weeks before the first symptoms appear, and they remain infective during the acute phase and chronic carrier state, which can last for the duration of their lives.

Disease Spectrum

Persons with infectious diseases may exhibit a broad spectrum of disease that ranges from subclinical infection to severe and fatal disease. Those with subclinical or inapparent infections are important from the public health point of view since they are a source of infection, yet they may not be cared for like those with clinical disease. These people should be diagnosed and treated early. Those with clinical disease may have localized or systemic symptoms, and mild to severe illness. The final outcome of a disease can be recovery, death, or something in between, including a carrier state (i.e., the person shows no evidence of the disease but carries it and can pass it along to other people), complications requiring extended treatment or hospital stay, or disability requiring rehabilitation. At the community level, the disease may occur in endemic, epidemic, or pandemic proportion. An **endemic** disease is constantly present in a given geographic area or a population. Pertussis (whooping cough) is endemic in the United States. **Epidemic** refers to a greater-than-normally-expected occurrence of disease in a community or region. While people tend to associate large numbers with epidemics, even one case can be termed *epidemic* if the disease is considered previously eliminated from that area. For example, one or two cases of cholera can be considered an epidemic in the United States. **Pandemic** refers to a worldwide epidemic affecting large populations.

HIV/AIDS can be classified as both epidemic and pandemic since the number of cases is growing rapidly across various regions of the world as well as in the United States.

SURVEILLANCE OF COMMUNICABLE DISEASES

During the first half of the twentieth century, the weekly publication of national morbidity statistics by the U.S. Surgeon General's Office was accompanied by the statement "No health department, state or local, can effectively prevent or control disease without knowledge of when, where, and under what conditions cases are occurring." (Centers for Disease Control and Prevention, 1996). **Surveillance** gathers the *who, when, where* and *what;* these elements are then used to answer *why.* A good surveillance program systematically collects, organizes, and analyzes current, accurate, and complete data for a defined disease condition. This information is promptly provided to those who need it for planning, implementation and evaluation of disease prevention and control programs.

Nurses are involved at different levels of the surveillance system. They collect data, make diagnoses, report cases, and provide feedback information to the general public. Examples of surveillance activities are:

- Investigating sources and contacts in outbreaks of pertussis in school settings or shigellosis in daycare
- Providing TB testing and contact tracing (tracking down close associates of people who tested positive for tuberculosis)
- Collecting and reporting information about notifiable communicable diseases (those that must be reported)
- Providing morbidity and mortality statistics to those who request them, including the media, the public, individuals, or agencies that are planning services or writing grants.

States, rather than federal laws and regulations, mandate disease reporting in the United States. The list of reportable diseases in each state varies. State health departments report cases of selected diseases on a voluntary basis to the Centers for Disease Control and Prevention (CDC) in Atlanta, Georgia. The 52 diseases presently included in the National Notifiable Diseases Surveillance System (NNDSS) at CDC are listed in Box 23-1. The NNDSS data are collated and published weekly in the *Morbidity and Mortality Weekly Report (MMWR),* and this is an excellent source of information for nurses. Final reports are published annually in the *Summary of Notifiable Diseases* (Centers for Disease Control and Prevention, 1996).

EMERGING INFECTIOUS DISEASES

Emerging infectious diseases are those in which the incidence has increased in the past two decades or has the potential to increase in the near future and can include new or known infectious diseases. For example, Hantavirus was first detected in 1993 in the Four Corners area of Arizona and New Mexico when a mysterious and deadly respiratory disease affected young, healthy Native Americans. The disease was

Box 23-1	Nationally Notifiable Infectious Diseases

- AIDS
- Anthrax
- Botulism
- Brucellosis
- Chancroid
- *Chlamydia trachomatis,* genital infections
- Cholera
- Coccidioidomycosis
- Cryptosporidiosis
- Diphtheria
- Encephalitis, California
- Encephalitis, eastern equine
- Encephalitis, St. Louis
- Encephalitis, western equine
- *Escherichia coli* 0157:H7
- Gonorrhea
- *Haemophilus influenzae,* invasive disease
- Hansen disease (Leprosy)
- Hantavirus pulmonary syndrome
- Hemolytic uremic syndrome, post-diarrheal
- Hepatitis A
- Hepatitis B
- Hepatitis, C/non A, non B
- HIV infection, pediatric
- Legionellosis
- Lyme disease
- Malaria
- Measles
- Meningococcal disease
- Mumps
- Pertussis
- Plague
- Poliomyelitis
- Psittacosis
- Rabies, animal
- Rabies, human
- Rocky Mountain spotted fever
- Rubella
- Rubella, congenital syndrome
- Salmonellosis
- Shigellosis
- Streptococcal disease, invasive, Group A
- *Streptococcus pneumoniae,* drug resistant
- Streptococcal toxic-shock syndrome
- Syphilis, congenital
- Syphilis
- Tetanus
- Toxic-shock syndrome
- Trichinosis
- Tuberculosis
- Typhoid fever
- Yellow fever

From Epidemiology Program Office: *National notifiable infectious diseases,* Atlanta, 1998, Centers for Disease Control and Prevention, available online: www.cdc.gov/epo/dphsi/infdis.htm.
NOTE: Although chickenpox is not a nationally notifiable disease, the Council of State and Territorial Epidemiologists (CSTE) recommends reporting of cases of chickenpox via the National Notifiable Diseases Surveillance System (NNDSS).

soon discovered to be a variant of—but to exhibit very different pathology from—a rodent-borne virus previously found only in Europe and Asia. Transmission of Hantavirus apparently occurs when rodent excrement gets into the air. One explanation for the outbreak in the Southwest is that an unseasonably mild winter led to an unusual increase in the rodent population; more people than usual were exposed to a virus that had previously been unrecognized in this country. Infection in Native Americans first brought attention to Hantavirus because of a cluster of cases in a small geographic area, but no evidence suggests that any ethnic group is particularly susceptible to this disease. Hantavirus has now been diagnosed in sites across the United States. The best protection against this virus seems to be avoiding rodent-infested environments.

As seen in Table 23-1 several factors, operating singly or combined, can influence the emergence of these diseases (Centers for Disease Control and Prevention, 1994a). Most of the factors that stimulate the emergence of diseases result from the activities and behavior of the human hosts and from environmental changes such as deforestation, urbanization, and industrialization. The exceptions are microbial adaptation and changes made by the infectious agent such as those likely in the emergence of *Escherichia coli* 0157:H7. The growth in the number of households in which both parents work has increased the number of children in daycare. With this increase in daycare has come an increase in diarrheal diseases such as shigellosis. Changing sexual behavior and illegal drug use influence the spread of HIV/AIDS as well as other sexually transmitted diseases. Before large air-conditioning systems with cooling towers were common, legionellosis was virtually unknown. Since this disease is spread by droplets in the air, large air conditioning systems are an ideal conduit. Immigrants, both legal and illegal, as well as travelers, bring with them a variety of known and potentially unknown diseases. In order to prevent and control emerging diseases, it is important to identify effective ways to educate people so they will be motivated to change their behavior as well as to develop effective drugs and vaccines. Also, current surveillance systems should be strengthened and expanded to improve the detection and tracking of these diseases. Selected emerging infectious diseases, including a brief description of the diseases and symptoms they cause, their modes of transmission, and causes of emergence are listed in Table 23-2.

Briefly Noted

Only discovered in 1983, an infectious agent, *Helicobacter pylori,* is now recognized as the major factor in peptic ulcer disease.

PREVENTION AND CONTROL OF COMMUNICABLE DISEASES

Communicable disease can be prevented and controlled. *Prevention* and *control* programs seek to reduce the prevalence of a disease to a level at which it no longer poses a major public

TABLE 23-1 Factors Contributing to the Emergence of New Infectious Diseases

Category	Specific Examples
Societal events	Economic impoverishment, war or civil conflict, population growth and migration, urban decay
Health care	New medical devices; organ or tissue transplantation, drugs causing immunosuppression, wide-spread use of antibiotics
Food production	Globalization of food supplies, changes in food processing and packaging
Human behavior	Sexual behavior, drug use, travel, diet, outdoor recreation, use of child care facilities
Environmental changes	Deforestation or reforestation, changes in water ecosystems, flood or drought, famine, global warming
Public health infrastructure	Curtailment or reduction in prevention programs, inadequate communicable disease surveillance, lack of trained personnel (epidemiologists, laboratory scientists, vector and rodent-control specialists)
Microbial adaptation and change	Changes in virulence and toxin production, development of drug resistance, microbes as cofactors in chronic diseases

From Centers for Disease Control and Prevention: *Addressing emerging infectious disease threats: a prevention strategy for the US,* Atlanta, 1994, Centers for Disease Control and Prevention.

TABLE 23-2 Examples of Emerging Infectious Diseases

Infectious Agent	Diseases/Symptoms	Mode of Transmission	Causes of Emergence
Borrelia burgdorferi	Lyme disease: rash, fever, arthritis, neurological and cardiac abnormalities	Bite of infective *Ixodes* tick	Increase in deer and human populations in wooded areas
Escherichia coli 0157:H7	Hemorrhagic colitis, thrombocytopenia, hemolytic uremic syndrome	Ingestion of contaminated food, especially undercooked beef and raw milk	Likely caused by a new pathogen
Ebola-Marburg	Fulminant, high mortality, hemorrhagic fever	Direct contact with infected blood, organs, secretions, and semen	Unknown viruses
Legionella pneumophila	Legionnaires' disease: malaise, myalgia, fever, headache, respiratory illness	Air cooling systems, water supplies	Recognition in an epidemic situation
Hantaviruses	Hemorrhagic fever with renal syndrome; pulmonary syndrome	Inhalation of aerosolized rodent urine and feces	Human invasion of virus ecological niche
Human immunodeficiency virus HIV-1	HIV infection, AIDS/HIV disease, severe immune dysfunction, opportunistic infections	Sexual contact with or exposure to blood or tissues of infected persons; perinatal	Urbanization, life-style changes, drug use, international travel, transfusions, transplant
Human papillomavirus	Skin and mucous membrane lesions (warts); strongly linked to cancer of the cervix and penis	Direct sexual contact, contact with contaminated surfaces	Newly recognized; changes in sexual life-style
Cryptosporidium	Cryptosporidiosis, infection of epithelial cells in gastrointestinal and respiratory tracts	Fecal-oral, person-to-person, waterborne	Development near watershed areas; immunosuppression
Pneumocystis carinii	Acute pneumonia	Unknown; possibly airborne or reactivation of latent infection	Immunosuppression

Data from Ledeberg J, Shope RE, Oaks SC: *Emerging infections: microbial threats to health in the U.S.,* Washington, D.C., 1992, National Academy Press; Centers for Disease Control and Prevention: *MMWR* 43(RR-7):1, 1994.

health problem. In some cases, diseases can be eliminated or eradicated. **Elimination** aims to remove a disease from a large geographic area such as a country or region of the world. **Eradication** is the irreversible termination of all transmission of infection by extermination of the infectious agents worldwide (Centers for Disease Control 1993; Last, 1995). The World Health Organization (WHO) officially declared the global eradication of smallpox on May 8, 1980 (Evans, 1985). After the successful eradication of smallpox, the eradication of other communicable diseases became a realistic challenge. Polio appears to have been eliminated from the Americas (Centers for Disease Control and Prevention, 1994b).

Primary, Secondary, and Tertiary Prevention

Prevention of communicable diseases can be attained at three levels: primary, secondary, and tertiary (Last, 1995):

Primary prevention: efforts to reduce the incidence of disease through health promotion and education. Examples:
- Immunizations
- Malaria chemoprophylaxis (taking anti-malarial drugs prior to going to or being in an area in which mosquitoes that carry malaria are prevalent)
- Consistent use of universal precautions by health care workers
- Promotion of safer sex
- Safe water and environment.

Secondary prevention seeks to reduce disease prevalence and disease morbidity through early diagnosis and treatment. Examples:
- Skin testing for tuberculosis
- Serological screening for HIV
- Contact investigation in tuberculosis-control programs
- Partner notification in AIDS and STD programs.

Tertiary prevention tries to reduce complications and disabilities of disease. Examples:
- In *Pneumocystis carinii* pneumonia (PCP) prevention, using chemoprophylaxis for people with AIDS
- Providing footwear and gloves to leprosy patients to prevent trauma to their insensitive and deformed hands and feet.

The Nurse's Role in Controlling Communicable Diseases

Nurses who work in the community can assist in controlling communicable diseases in several ways:
- Education
- Immunization
- Early detection (case finding and contact notification)
- Initiation of appropriate treatment
- Support
- Encouragement
- Referral.

Nurses can educate members of the community about ways to prevent communicable disease, how to detect signs and symptoms of a communicable disease, actions that people can take to reduce the transmission of the disease, and when to seek help. Schools and work sites are good locations to teach about preventing communicable disease. Also, short articles in newspapers or company publications can alert citizens to communicable diseases that are either occurring in the community or that might occur if prevention efforts are not initiated. Nurses working in the community can teach pre-school and school-age children about how important regular and effective hand washing is in preventing colds, viruses, and the flu.

Healthy People 2010 and Communicable Disease

In the twenty-first century, infections and communicable disease remain major causes of illness, disability, and death. New diseases are emerging and old diseases are becoming drug resistant and more difficult to control. Nurses can help! The objectives for the nation related to communicable disease are listed in the *Healthy People 2010* box.

VACCINE-PREVENTABLE DISEASES

Vaccines are one of the most effective methods of preventing and controlling communicable diseases. Diseases such as polio, diphtheria, pertussis, and measles, which previously occurred in epidemic proportions, today are controlled with routine childhood immunizations. However, since these diseases have not been eradicated, children need to continue being immunized against them. In the United States, "no shots, no school" legislation has resulted in the immunization of most children by the time they enter school. However, many infants and toddlers, the group most vulnerable to these potentially severe diseases, do not receive scheduled immunizations even though they are free. Inner city children from minority and ethnic groups are at risk for incomplete immunization. Poor immunization rates may occur when children are seen by several different providers, when families are mobile and their health records do not move to new providers when the family moves, or when parents find the immunization schedule difficult to understand.

Briefly Noted

The vaccine against smallpox, a vaccine that left distinctive scars on the shoulders of people who were immunized, is no longer used because the smallpox virus has been declared totally eradicated from the world's population.

Since many children receive their immunizations at public health departments, nurses can increase immunization coverage of infants and toddlers. Specifically, they can track children known to be at risk for under-immunization and call or send reminders to their parents. They also can help families avoid missed immunization opportunities by checking the immunization status of every young child they encounter whether in the clinic or during a home visit. In addition, they can organize community immunization activities that deliver immunization services; provide answers to

Healthy People 2010
Communicable Disease

The *Healthy People 2010* objectives related to communicable disease are:

14-1   Reduce or eliminate indigenous cases of vaccine-preventable disease.

14-4   Reduce bacterial meningitis in young children.

14-5   Reduce invasive pneumococcal infections.

14-7   Reduce meningococcal disease.

14-8   Reduce Lyme disease.

14-11   Reduce tuberculosis.

14-12   Increase the proportion of all tuberculosis patients who complete curative therapy within 12 months.

14-13   Increase the proportion of contacts and other high-risk persons with latent tuberculosis infection who complete a course of treatment.

14-14   Reduce the average time for a laboratory to confirm and report tuberculosis cases.

14-15   Increase the proportion of international travelers.

14-16   Reduce invasive early onset group B streptococcal disease.

14-17   Reduce hospitalizations caused by peptic ulcer disease in the United States.

14-18   Reduce the number of courses of antibiotics for ear infections for young children.

14-19   Reduce the number of courses of antibiotics prescribed for the sole diagnosis of the common cold.

14-22   Achieve and maintain effective vaccination coverage levels for universally recommended vaccines among young children.

14-23   Maintain vaccination coverage levels for children in licensed day care facilities and children in kindergarten through the first grade.

14-24   Increase the proportion of young children who receive all vaccines that have been recommended for universal administration for at least 5 years.

14-26   Increase the proportion of children who participate in fully operational population-based immunization registries.

14-27   Increase routine vaccination coverage levels of adolescents.

14-29   Increase the proportion of adults who are vaccinated annually against influenza and ever vaccinated against pneumococcal disease.

14-30   Reduce vaccine-associated adverse events.

Evidence-Based Practice

A study of Los Angeles African-American newborns and their families was done to determine how effective parent education and case management might be in developing parent understanding of and demand for immunizations, which in turn might influence providers to not miss opportunities to immunize during child health visits.

Newborns and their families were randomly assigned to a case management or a control group and observed through their first birthday. Families in the case management group were regularly visited and telephoned, educated on the importance and safety of immunizations and encouraged to request immunizations from their providers. After children reached their first birthday, their parents were interviewed and provider records were examined.

Missed opportunities occurred at more than 50% of the visits of all children whose records were examined. Home visits and parent education were only minimally associated with reducing missed opportunities. Missed opportunities occurred more often with private than public providers and at visits for acute illness than well-child visits.

APPLICATION IN PRACTICE

The implications for nursing practice from the study conclusions are:

1. Missed opportunities to immunize are primarily determined by factors controlled by the provider.

2. Immunization history of every child presenting for a child health visit should be assessed and immunization considered if no appropriate contraindications are present.

3. Community health nurses who may contact families for a variety of reasons during and outside child health visits are in an excellent position to assess immunization status and encourage immunization when needed.

Henderson C, et al: Reducing missed opportunities to vaccinate during child health visits: how effective are parent education and case management? *Arch Pediatr Adolesc Med* 152(3):238, 1998.

parents' questions and concerns about immunization; and educate parents about why immunizations are needed, contraindications to immunization, and the importance of completing the immunization schedule on time. It would be ideal if a comprehensive, computer-based information system were available to monitor and track the immunization status of children (DeFriese, et al, 1997).

Routine Childhood Immunization Schedule

Children in the United States are routinely immunized against the following 10 diseases:

- Hepatitis B
- Diphtheria
- Pertussis (whooping cough)
- Tetanus
- Paralytic poliomyelitis (polio)
- *Hemophilus influenzae* type B (Hib)
- Measles
- Mumps
- Rubella
- *Varicella* (chickenpox).

Diphtheria, tetanus, and pertussis (DTaP) are usually given as a combination vaccine, as are measles, mumps, and rubella (MMR). To achieve recommended immunization levels by 2 years of age, most of these immunizations should begin when an infant is 2-3 months of age. Live vaccines such as measles, mumps, and rubella (MMR), and polio should be completed by 15 and 18 months, respectively. *Varicella* may be given at any visit after the first birthday. Other vaccines available for use in special circumstances include those for hepatitis A, influenza, meningococcal meningitis, plague, pneumococcal pneumonia, rabies, and yellow fever.

Measles

Measles is an acute, highly contagious disease that is considered a childhood illness but is often seen in the U.S. in adolescents and young adults. Symptoms include:

- Fever
- Sneezing and coughing
- Conjunctivitis
- Small white spots on the inside of the cheek (Koplik spots)
- Red, blotchy rash beginning several days after respiratory signs.

Measles is caused by the rubeola virus. It is transmitted by

- Inhalation of infected aerosol droplets
- Direct contact with infected nasal or throat secretions
- Direct contact with articles freshly contaminated with nasal or throat secretions.

Measles spreads rapidly since it is very contagious and is actually the most contagious before people realize they are infected. Once a person has measles, the person has lifelong immunity (Benenson, 1995).

Immunization has led to a dramatic decrease in measles cases in the United States. In 1997, only 138 cases were reported to the CDC. This 1997 number represents the lowest number of cases reported since measles became a nationally reportable disease in 1912 and a 55% decrease from the previous record low of 309 cases reported in 1995 (Centers for Disease Control and Prevention, 1998). Of the 138 measles cases reported in 1997, 41% were documented as coming from other countries. Since these imported cases did not result in outbreaks, it appears that vaccination efforts in the United States have successfully increased herd immunity against measles. Groups who remain at risk for measles are those who do not routinely accept immunization such as individuals with religious or philosophic objections, students in schools that do not require two doses of vaccine and infants in areas where immunization coverage is low. The exposure of these groups to an imported case could cause a major outbreak (Centers for Disease Control and Prevention, 1998).

Rubella (German Measles)

The rubella virus causes a mild febrile disease with enlarged lymph nodes and a fine, pink rash that is often difficult to distinguish from measles or scarlet fever. Unlike measles, rubella is only moderately contagious. Transmission is through inhalation of or direct contact with infected droplets from the respiratory secretions of infected persons. Children may show few or no symptoms, while adults often have several days of low-grade fever, headache, malaise, runny nose, and conjunctivitis before the rash appears. Many infections occur without a rash. Infection confers lifelong immunity. Rubella is most common in winter and spring (Benenson, 1995). Since 1991, cases have fallen to all-time lows, with an annual case average of 183 for 1992 through 1996. During this period, most cases have been associated with outbreaks (75%); have been in individuals 15 years of age or older (84%); and have occurred in those of Hispanic ethnicity (87%). The percentage of cases among Hispanics increased from 19% in 1991 to 68% in 1996 (Centers for Disease Control and Prevention, 1997a).

Maternal rubella is linked to certain congenital defects. Congenital rubella syndrome (CRS) occurs in more than 25% of infants born to women who are infected with rubella during the first trimester of pregnancy (Gershon, 1995). Rubella infection, in addition to intrauterine death and spontaneous abortion, can cause anomalies that affect single or multiple organ systems. Defects include cataracts, congenital glaucoma, deafness, microcephaly, mental retardation, cardiac abnormalities, and diabetes mellitus. Twelve cases were reported during 1994-1996. Of the seven indigenous cases born during this period, four were to Hispanic mothers (Centers for Disease Control and Prevention, 1997a).

The CDC maintains a national CRS registry. In 1991, 31 cases of confirmed indigenous CRS were reported, 20 of which occurred in Pennsylvania. A 1991 survey to determine the risk for CRS among babies born to unimmunized Amish mothers in one county in Pennsylvania indicated the rate of CRS was 14 per 1000 live births compared with 0.006 for the total U.S. population. No cases of CRS were reported in 1993 (Centers for Disease Control and Prevention, 1994c). *Healthy People 2000* recommends sustained elimination of both indigenous rubella and CRS.

Preventing rubella and CRS will require many of the same efforts discussed with measles, including the following:

- Attaining and maintaining high rates of immunization among preschoolers
- Early detection and outbreak control
- Taking advantage of opportunities like high school and college entrance to immunize susceptible adolescents
- Extending immunization opportunities to religious groups that traditionally do not seek health care
- Targeting adolescent and young adults who are particularly susceptible because they come from or are exposed to persons from countries that do not routinely vaccinate against rubella. Since there is an increasing number of cases in persons of Hispanic background, immunization efforts should be targeted to this group.

Pertussis

Pertussis (whooping cough) begins as a mild upper respiratory infection that progresses to an irritating cough that within 1 to 2 weeks can become paroxysmal (a series of repeated violent coughs). The repeated coughs occur without intervening breaths and can be followed by a characteristic 'whoop' when the person inspires air. Pertussis is caused by the bacteria *Bordetella pertussis* and is transmitted via an airborne route through contact with infected droplets. It is highly contagious and considered endemic in the United States. Vaccination against pertussis is a part of the routine childhood immunization schedule. Treatment of infected individuals with antibiotics such as erythromycin may shorten the period of communicability but does not relieve symptoms unless given early in the course of the infection. A 2-week treatment with antibiotics is recommended for family members and close contacts of infected individuals regardless of immunization status (Benenson, 1995).

While more children 19 to 35 months of age in the United States were immunized during the 1990s, some parents hesitate to vaccinate their children against pertussis. Their fear of this vaccine is due to the occurrence of minor adverse reactions to the whole-cell pertussis vaccine as well as publicity surrounding infrequent but serious adverse reactions and the inaccurate suggestion that the pertussis vaccine could result in permanent neurologic damage. The licensure in 1996 of an acellular vaccine associated with fewer adverse reactions and which can be administered to young infants may help improve acceptance of pertussis immunization (Marwick, 1996).

While pertussis is still predominantly a disease of young children, the increasing number of cases in adolescents and young adults is a growing problem. Infants are the group most susceptible to pertussis and the most likely to suffer complications. In 1996, 44% of all reported pertussis cases occurred among persons age 10 years or older. Cases in very young children, especially under 6 months, are attributed to their lack of full immunization because of their age. Cases in older children largely result from under-immunization, and cases in adolescents and adults with histories of complete immunization are attributed to waning immunity. While natural infection with pertussis results in permanent immunity, immunization through vaccination does not. Because pertussis in adolescents and adults may be a mild disease without the characteristic signs seen in children, it may go under-diagnosed and under-reported in these age-groups. These individuals then become an important reservoir for the disease, and because pertussis is highly contagious, are responsible for its spread to infants and children as well as other adults. Pertussis vaccines are not labeled for use in individuals older than 6 years; therefore, catching up children who have missed doses and giving booster vaccines to those individuals with waning immunity are not presently options for preventing outbreaks. Routinely giving pertussis booster injections to adults is under discussion (Centers for Disease Control and Prevention, 1997b). Nurses need to encourage parents to immunize their children against pertussis. Since pertussis is highly contagious, nurses working in the community can help limit transmission during outbreaks by teaching family members, classmates, and other close contacts about potential risk, transmission, and treatment.

Influenza

Influenza (the flu) is a viral respiratory infection often indistinguishable from the common cold or other respiratory diseases. Transmission is airborne and through direct contact with infected droplets. Unlike many viruses that do not survive long in the environment, the 'flu' virus appears to survive for many hours in dried mucus. Outbreaks are common in the winter and early spring in areas where people gather indoors such as in schools and nursing homes. Gastrointestinal and respiratory symptoms are common. Because symptoms do not always follow a characteristic pattern, many viral diseases that are not influenza are often called the "flu." The most important factors to note about influenza are its epidemic nature and the mortality that results from its pulmonary complications, especially in the elderly.

There are three types of influenza viruses, A, B, and C. Type A is usually responsible for large epidemics, while outbreaks from type B are more regional, and those from type C are less common and usually only cause mild illness. Influenza viruses often change the nature of their surface appearance or alter their antigenic make-up. Types B and C are fairly stable viruses, but type A is constantly changing. Minor antigenic changes are referred to as antigenic *drift* and are responsible for yearly epidemics and regional outbreaks. Major changes such as the emergence of new subtypes are called antigenic *shift;* these only occur with type A viruses. This antigenic *drift* and *shift* results in epidemic outbreaks every few years and pandemic outbreaks every 10 to 40 years. Mortality rates associated with epidemics may be higher than those in non-epidemic situations (Benenson, 1995).

Influenza vaccines are prepared each year based on the best possible prediction of what type and variant of virus will be most prevalent that year. Because of the changing nature of the virus, immunization is necessary annually and is given in the early fall before the flu season begins. Immunization is highly recommended for the elderly, individuals with chronic respiratory disease, or those with other chronic disease conditions that impair the immune system, as well as health care workers and anyone involved in essential community services. While immunization is recommended for the previously mentioned groups, any individual may benefit from this protection. Flu shots do not always prevent infection, but they do result in milder disease symptoms. Immunization of adults involves one injection. Children under 12 years of age may initially receive two doses 1 to 2 weeks apart and subsequently one dose on a yearly basis. Sensitivity to eggs is a contraindication to immunization, and pregnant women should avoid immunization in the first trimester of pregnancy (Benenson, 1995).

Since adults do not utilize health care services as regularly as children do, different approaches may be required to reach higher immunization coverage rates among adults. Nurses often lead influenza immunization campaigns that target adults by giving shots at polling places during elections or in the parking lots of health departments, churches, and schools conducting "drive-up" clinics. Nurses need to check the immunization history and encourage immunization for both adults and children.

FOOD-BORNE AND WATERBORNE DISEASES

Food-borne illness or "food poisoning" can be categorized as food infection or food intoxication. Food infection such as salmonellosis, hepatitis A, and trichinosis results from bacterial, viral, or parasitic infection of food. Food intoxication results from toxins produced by bacterial growth, chemical contaminants (heavy metals), and a variety of disease-producing substances found naturally in certain foods such as mushrooms and some seafood. Examples of food intoxications are botulism, mercury poisoning, and paralytic shellfish poisoning. Table 23-3 presents some of the most common agents of food intoxication, their incubation period, source, symptoms, and pathology. Although not a hard and fast rule, food infections are associated with incubation periods of 12 hours to several days after ingestion of the infected food, whereas intoxications often emerge within minutes to hours after ingestion. Botulism is a clear exception to this rule, with an incubation period of a week or more in adults. The expression "ptomaine poisoning" is often heard when discussing food-borne illness but does not refer to a specific causal organism.

Briefly Noted

Food irradiation is one option being strongly considered to prevent outbreaks of food-borne disease.

In recent years the following types of outbreaks have occurred due to food-borne diseases:
- Children died after eating undercooked fast-food hamburgers containing a virulent strain of *E. coli*
- Outbreaks occurred across the United States of diarrheal disease from *Cyclospora*–contaminated Guatemalan raspberries
- Outbreaks of hepatitis A occurred in school children who ate tainted frozen strawberries
- *Salmonella* infections were associated with uncooked poultry and eggs.

While the very young, the very old, and the very debilitated, or immunocompromised individuals (resulting from chemotherapy, immunosuppressive drugs, and AIDS) are most susceptible, anyone can acquire food-borne illness regardless of socioeconomic status, race, sex, age, occupation, education, or area of residence. However, some new, susceptible populations are emerging as a result of the increasing older population and the growing numbers of immunocompromised individuals (resulting from chemotherapy, immunosuppressive drugs, and AIDS), as well as the large numbers of children surviving severe illness. Nurses in the community can teach people how to safely prepare and store food (see the

TABLE 23-3 Commonly Encountered Food Intoxications

Causal Agent	Incubation Period	Duration	Clinical Presentation	Associated Food
Staphylococcus aureus	30 min-7 hr	1-2 days	Sudden onset of nausea, cramps, vomiting, and prostration often accompanied by diarrhea; rarely fatal	All foods, especially those most likely to come into contact with foodhandlers' hands that may be contaminated by purulent discharges from infections of the eyes and skin
Clostridium perfringens (strain A)	6-24 hr	1 day or less	Sudden onset of colic and diarrhea, maybe nausea; vomiting and fever unusual; rarely fatal	Inadequately heated meats or stews; food contaminated by soil or feces becomes infective when improper storage or reheating allows multiplication of organism
Vibrio parahaemolyticus	4-96 hr	1-7 days	Watery diarrhea and abdominal cramps; sometimes nausea, vomiting, fever, and headache; rarely fatal	Raw or inadequately cooked seafood; period of time at room temperature usually required for multiplication of organism
Clostridium botulinum	12-36 hr, sometimes days	Slow recovery, may be months	CNS signs; blurred vision; difficulty in swallowing and dry mouth followed by descending symmetrical become flaccid paralysis of an alert person; "floppy baby" w/infant botulism; fatality 15% with antitoxin and respiratory support	Home-canned fruits and vegetables that have not been preserved with adequate heating; infants have infected from ingesting honey

Based on data from Benenson AS (editor): *Control of communicable diseases in man,* ed 16, Washington, D.C., 1995, American Public Health Association.

How To box below). These rules are important for people preparing food at home as well as for commercial food preparation and distribution.

Briefly Noted

Simple changes can be made in food preparation, handling, and storage that will destroy or denature contaminants and prevent their further spread.

HOW TO Safely Prepare Food

- Choose food that has been safely processed.
- Cook food thoroughly.
- Eat cooked food immediately.
- Store cooked food carefully.
- Reheat cooked foods thoroughly.
- Avoid contact between raw foods and cooked foods.
- Wash hands repeatedly.
- Keep all kitchen surfaces meticulously clean.
- Protect foods from insects, rodents, and other animals.
- Use pure water.

From Benenson AS (editor): *Control of communicable diseases in man*, ed 6, Washington, D.C., 1995, American Public Health Association.

Salmonellosis

Salmonellosis is a bacterial disease characterized by sudden onset of headache, abdominal pain, diarrhea, nausea, sometimes vomiting, and almost always fever. Onset typically occurs within 48 hours of eating the contaminated food. The clinical signs of salmonellosis are impossible to distinguish from other causes of gastrointestinal distress. Diarrhea and lack of appetite may last several days, and dehydration may be severe. While morbidity can be significant, death is uncommon except among infants, the elderly, and the debilitated. The rate of infection is highest among infants and small children. It is estimated that only a small proportion of cases are recognized clinically and that only 1% of clinical cases are reported. The number of *Salmonella* infections yearly may be in the millions (Benenson, 1995).

Outbreaks occur commonly in restaurants, hospitals, nursing homes, and children's institutions. The transmission route is eating inadequately cooked food that comes from an infected animal or is contaminated by feces of an infected animal or person. Meat, poultry, and eggs are the foods most often associated with salmonellosis outbreaks. Animals are the common reservoir for the various *Salmonella* serotypes, although infected humans may also be reservoirs. Animals are more likely to be chronic carriers. Reptiles such as iguanas, pet turtles, poultry, cattle, swine, rodents, dogs, and cats have been *Salmonella* carriers. In the community, nurses can teach about person-to-person transmission in daycare and institutional settings and how to prevent salmonellosis and other food-borne and waterborne diseases.

Briefly Noted

When dealing with a communicable disease that has outbreak potential, include family members and close contacts as well as the sick client when developing a treatment and prevention plan.

Escherichia coli 0157:H7

Escherichia coli 0157:H7 belongs to the enterohemorrhagic category of *E. coli* serotypes that can produce a strong cytotoxin that can cause a potentially fatal hemorrhagic colitis. It is estimated that *E. coli* 0157:H7 causes up to 500 deaths annually in the United States. This pathogen was first described in humans in 1992 after two outbreaks of illness were associated with eating undercooked hamburgers from a fast-food restaurant chain. Other less-common outbreaks have been attributed to roast beef, alfalfa sprouts, unpasteurized milk and apple cider, municipal water, and person-to-person transmission in daycare centers (Centers for Disease Control and Prevention, 1994d). Infection with 0157:H7 causes bloody diarrhea, abdominal cramps, and infrequently fever. Children and the elderly are at highest risk for clinical disease and complications. Hemolytic uremic syndrome is seen in 5%-10% of cases and can lead to acute renal failure. The case-fatality rate is 3%-5%.

Hamburger appears to be involved in outbreaks so often because the grinding process exposes pathogens that were on the exterior piece of beef to the interior of the ground meat. Grinding mixes the bacteria from the exterior of the meat so thoroughly throughout the hamburger that searing the surface is no longer sufficient to kill all the bacteria. It is often hard to track the source of the beef's contamination since hamburger is often made of meat ground from several sources. The best protection against this pathogen, as with most food-borne pathogens, is to thoroughly cook food before eating it.

Waterborne Disease Outbreaks and Pathogens

Waterborne pathogens, including viruses, bacteria, and protozoans, usually enter water supplies through animal or human fecal contamination and often cause enteric disease. Hepatitis A virus is the most widely publicized waterborne viral agent. The most important waterborne bacterial diseases are cholera, typhoid fever, and bacillary dysentery. In the past, the most important waterborne protozoans have been *Entamoeba histolytica* (amebic dysentery) and *Giardia lamblia*. Recent outbreaks of cryptosporidiosis in municipal water like that which resulted in diarrheal outbreaks that crippled the city of Milwaukee in 1993 have emphasized the need to safeguard municipal water from pathogens like *Cryptosporidium*. Protozoans are especially problematic for municipal water because they do not respond to traditional chlorine treatment as do enteric and coliform bacteria.

VECTOR-BORNE DISEASES

Vector-borne diseases are transmitted by vectors, usually arthropods, either biologically or mechanically. With biologic transmission, the vector is necessary for the developmental stage of the infectious agent, for example, mosquitoes that carry malaria. Mechanical transmission occurs when an insect simply contacts the infectious agent with its legs or mouth and carries it to the host. An example would be flies and cockroaches that may contaminate food or cooking utensils. Vector-borne diseases commonly encountered in the United States are those associated with ticks such as Lyme disease (*Borrelia burgdorferi*), ehrlichiosis (*Ehrlichia chaffeensis*), and Rocky Mountain spotted fever (*Rickettsii rickettsii*). Nurses who work with immigrant populations or with international travelers may encounter malaria and dengue fever. Both of these diseases are carried by mosquitoes.

Lyme Disease

Lyme disease was first discovered in 1974 when parents in Lyme, Connecticut, noticed a high incidence of juvenile rheumatoid arthritis in their children. It was learned that this arthritis was caused by a tick-borne infection that is now known as Lyme disease. Following are some basic characteristics of Lyme disease:

- Most common vector-borne disease in the United States (Centers for Disease Control and Prevention, 1997c)
- Caused by the spirochete *Borrelia burgdorferi.*
- Transmitted by Ixodid ticks that are associated with white-tailed deer (*Odocoileus virginianus*) and the white-footed mouse (*Peromyscus leucopus*).
- Usually occurs in the summer and has been reported throughout the U.S., but cases are concentrated in northeastern, north-central and Pacific-coast states.
- Key risk factors are whether people spend time in property that is wooded and/or unkempt and if people or dogs come in close contact with deer (Dennis, Fikrig, and Schaffner, 1999).

The clinical spectrum of Lyme disease can be divided into three stages. Stage I is characterized by erythema chronicum migrans, a distinctive skin lesion often called a bull's-eye lesion because it begins as a red area at the site of the tick attachment that spreads outward in a ring-like fashion as the center clears. About 50%-70% of infected people develop this lesion 3 to 30 days after a tick bite. The skin lesion may be accompanied or preceded by fever, fatigue, malaise, headache, muscle pains, and a stiff neck, as well as tender and enlarged lymph nodes and migratory joint pain. Most patients diagnosed in this early stage respond well to 10 to 14 days of oral tetracycline or penicillin.

If not treated during the first stage, Lyme disease can progress to stage II. This stage may include additional skin lesions, headache, neurological, and cardiac abnormalities. Stage III consists of recurrent attacks of arthritis and arthralgia, especially in the knees, that may begin months to years after the initial lesion. The clinical diagnosis of Lyme disease, if the distinctive skin lesion is present, is straightforward. Illness without the lesion is more difficult to diagnose since serological tests are more accurate in stages II and III than in stage I (Steere, 1995).

Rocky Mountain Spotted Fever

Contrary to its name, Rocky Mountain spotted fever (RMSF) is seldom seen in the Rocky Mountains. This disease is most often found in the Southeast, Oklahoma, Kansas, and Missouri. The infectious agent is *Rickettsia rickettsii*. The tick vector varies according to geographic region. The dog tick, *Dermacentor variabilis,* is the vector in the eastern and southern United States. RMSF is not transmitted from person to person. It is thought that one attack confers lifetime immunity.

Clinical signs include sudden onset of moderate to high fever, severe headache, chills, deep muscle pain, and malaise. About 50% of those who get RMSF have a rash on the extremities that begins on the third day and then spreads to most of the body. Cases of a "spotless" RMSF (does not have the rash) may actually be ehrlichiosis, or a more recently recognized tickborne disease caused by organisms of the genus *Ehrlichia*. RMSF and ehrlichiosis responds readily to treatment with tetracycline. Definitive diagnosis can be made with paired serum titers. Since early treatment is important in decreasing morbidity and mortality, treatment needs to be started as soon as clinical signs are present rather than waiting for laboratory confirmation (Benenson, 1995).

Prevention and Control of Tick-Borne Diseases

Vaccines are not currently available for any tick-borne diseases except tularemia and Lyme disease. Nurses need to teach people that the best preventive measures for avoiding tick-borne diseases are wearing protective clothing such as long-sleeve shirts and long pants tucked into socks when outside and searching for ticks afterwards. Ticks require a prolonged period of attachment (6 to 48 hours) before they start blood-feeding on the host. Therefore prompt tick discovery and removal can help prevent transmission of disease. Nurses in the community can instruct people in how to remove a tick:

- Use steady, gentle traction on tweezers applied to the head parts of the tick (Walker and Raoult, 1995).
- Do not squeeze the tick's body during the removal process to avoid infection that could be transmitted from resultant tick feces and tissue juices.
- Tick repellents containing diethyltoluamide (DEET) provide effective protection, but they can cause toxicity in children, including skin irritation, anaphylaxis, and seizures.

ZOONOSES

A zoonosis is an infection transmitted from a vertebrate animal to a human under natural conditions. The agents that cause zoonoses do not need humans to maintain their life cycles; infected humans have simply gotten in their way.

Transmission is by animal bites, inhalation, ingestion, direct contact, and arthropod intermediates. This last transmission route means that some vector-borne diseases may also be zoonoses. Other than vector-borne diseases, some of the more common zoonoses in the United States include:

- Toxoplasmosis (*Toxoplasma gondii*)
- Cat-scratch disease (*Bartonella henselae*)
- Brucellosis (*Brucella* species)
- Listeriosis (*Listeria monocytogenes*)
- Salmonellosis (*Salmonella* serotypes*)
- Rabies (Family *Rhabdoviridae,* genus *Lyssavirus*).

Rabies

Rabies (hydrophobia) is a well-known zoonosis. The term *hydrophobia* comes from the common choking, gagging, and resultant anxiety that may follow a symptomatic patient's attempt to drink. One of the most feared of human diseases, rabies has the highest case fatality rate of any known human infection, essentially 100%. In the 1970s, three cases of presumed recovery from rabies were reported. All had received pre- or post-exposure prophylaxis. Since that time, despite the intensive medical care available in the United States, no survivors have been reported. A significant public health problem worldwide with an estimated 30,000 deaths a year, rabies is rare in humans in the U.S. due to the widespread vaccination of dogs begun in the 1950s. Today the major carriers of rabies in the U.S. are not dogs but wild animals—raccoons, skunks, foxes, and bats. Small rodents, rabbits and hares, and opossums rarely carry rabies. Epidemiological information is useful to determine the potential carriers for a given geographic region. The east coast of the U.S. has in recent years had an epizootic (epidemic) of raccoon rabies.

Nurses in the community can educate residents about how rabies is transmitted. Rabies is transmitted to humans through an animal bite or scratch that passes on virus-carrying saliva. Transmission may also occur if infected saliva comes into contact with a fresh cut or intact mucus membranes. Rabies is found in neural tissue and is not transmitted via blood, urine, or feces. Airborne transmission has been documented in caves with infected bat colonies. Transmission from human to human, while theoretically possible, has been documented in only 6 cases of rabies acquired by receiving corneal transplants harvested from individuals who died of undiagnosed rabies (Fishbein and Bernard, 1995). Current organ donation guidelines prevent this possibility.

The best protection against rabies is vaccinating domestic dogs, cats, cattle, and horses. If a person is bitten, the bite wound should be thoroughly cleaned with soap and water and a physician consulted immediately. Suspect rabies if the bite is from a wild animal or an unprovoked attack from a domestic animal. Even when there is no suspicion of rabies, tetanus or antibiotic prophylaxis may be needed.

No successful treatment exists for rabies once symptoms appear, but if given promptly and as directed, post-exposure prophylaxis (PEP) with human rabies immune globulin and rabies vaccine is effective in preventing the development of the disease. Three products are licensed for use as rabies vaccine in the United States: human diploid cell vaccine (HDCV), rabies vaccine adsorbed (RVA), and purified chick embryo cell (PCEC) culture (RabAvert) (Centers for Disease Control and Prevention, 1998). The vaccine is administered in a series of five 1-ml doses injected into the deltoid muscle. Reactions to the vaccine are fewer and less serious than with previously used vaccines. Individuals who deal frequently with animals such as zookeepers, lab workers, and veterinarians may choose to receive the vaccine as pre-exposure prophylaxis. The decision to administer the vaccine to a bite victim depends on the circumstances of the bite and is made on an individual basis.

Recommendations for providing post-exposure prophylaxis treatment are provided by the Advisory Committee for Recommendations on Immunization Practices available through local public health officials or the CDC. In general, cats and dogs that have bitten someone and have verified rabies vaccinations are confined for 10 days for observation. Treatment is initiated only if signs of rabies are observed during this period. If the animal is known to be or suspected to be rabid, treatment is begun immediately. If the animal is unknown to the victim and escapes, then public health officials should be consulted for help in deciding whether treatment is indicated. With wild animal bites, treatment is begun immediately. With bites from livestock, rodents, and rabbits, treatment is considered on an individual basis. Decisions to treat become more complicated for possible non-bite exposure to saliva from known infected animals, and again public health officials are helpful in making these treatment decisions (Centers for Disease Control, 1991a).

PARASITIC DISEASES

Parasitic diseases are more prevalent in developing countries than the U.S. due to tropical climate and inadequate prevention and control measures. A lack of cheap and effective drugs, poor sanitation, and a scarcity of funding lead to high reinfection rates even when control programs are attempted. Parasites are classified into four groups:
- Helminths
  - Nematodes (roundworms)
  - Cestodes (tapeworms)
  - Trematodes (flukes)
- Protozoa (single celled animals).

Nematodes, cestodes, and trematodes are all referred to as helminths. Table 23-4 lists examples of diseases caused by parasites from these groups.

Nurses working in the community and other health professionals should be aware of the increasing number of parasitic infections in the United States. Several factors that have influenced these increases are:
- International travel
- Immigration of persons from developing countries

TABLE 23-4	Selected Parasite Categories	
Category	**Parasite**	**Disease**
Intestinal nematodes	*Ascaris lumbricoides*	Roundworm
	Trichuris trichiura	Whipworm
	Ancylostoma, Necator	Hookworm
	Enterobius vermicularis	Pinworm
Blood and tissue nematodes	*Wucheria bancrofti*	Filariasis
	Onchocerca volvulus	River blindness
Cestodes	*Taenia solium*	Pork tapeworm
	Taenia saginata	Beef tapeworm
Trematodes	*Schistosoma species*	Schistosomiasis
Protozoans	*Giardia lamblia*	Giardiasis
	Entamoeba histolytica	Amebiasis
	Plasmodium species	Malaria
	Leishmania species	Leishmaniasis
	Trypanosoma species	African sleeping sickness, Chagas' disease
	Toxoplasma gondii	Toxoplasmosis

From Brown H, Neva FA: *Basic clinical parasitology,* ed 5, Norwalk, Conn, 1983, Appleton-Century-Crofts.

- Incidence of AIDS with secondary parasitic opportunistic infections such as *Pneumocystis carinii* pneumonia, cryptosporidiosis, and toxoplasmosis
- Recognition of *Giardia* and *Cryptosporidium* as common infectious agents in daycare centers and waterborne disease outbreaks
- Incidence and recognition of sexually transmitted parasitic enteric infections acquired through oral-anal sex
- Recognition of *Cryptosporidium* species as pathogens in immunocompetent individuals due to improvement in stool examination techniques (Kappus, et al, 1994).

Enterobiasis (pinworm) is the most common helminth infection in the U.S., with an estimated 42 million cases a year. Pinworm infection is most common among children and most prevalent in crowded and institutional settings. Pinworms resemble small pieces of white thread and can be seen with the naked eye. Nurses can teach parents and other caregivers how to detect pinworm infections by pressing cellophane tape to the perianal region of the child early in the morning. The pinworms will stick to the tape. Treatment with oral vermicides has a cure rate of 90%-100%.

A study by state diagnostic laboratories found intestinal parasites in 20% of 216,275 stool specimens examined. The most commonly identified parasites were *Giardia lamblia, Entamoeba histolytica, Trichuris trichiura* (hookworm), and *Ascaris lumbricoides* (roundworm) (Kappus, et al, 1994). The opportunities for widespread indigenous transmission of these intestinal parasites are limited because of improved sanitary conditions in this country. Effective drug treatment is available for these intestinal parasitic infections.

Nurses and other health care workers need to make correct diagnoses and provide appropriate treatment and patient education in order to prevent and control parasitic infections. Diagnosis of parasitic diseases is based on history of travel, characteristic clinical signs and symptoms, and the use of appropriate laboratory tests to confirm the clinical diagnosis. Knowing what specimens to collect, how and when to collect these specimens, and what laboratory techniques to use are all important in interpreting laboratory results. Effective drug treatment is available for most parasitic diseases. High drug cost and drug resistance and toxicity are some of the common therapeutic problems. Measures for prevention and control of parasitic diseases include:

- Early diagnosis and treatment
- Improved personal hygiene
- Safer sex practices
- Community health education
- Vector control
- Improvements in sanitary control of food, water, and waste disposal.

NOSOCOMIAL INFECTIONS

Nosocomial infections are infections that are acquired during hospitalization or developed within a hospital setting. They may involve patients, health care workers, visitors, or anyone who has contact with a hospital. Hospitalized patients are more susceptible than healthy persons because of their underlying illnesses, their exposure to virulent infectious agents from other patients, and their exposure to indigenous hospital flora from the hospital staff. Patients are also subjected to numerous invasive diagnostic and surgical procedures and frequently given multiple broad-spectrum antibiotics and immunosuppressive drugs for treatment of neoplastic or chronic diseases. Studies suggest that at least 5% of patients admitted to hospitals in the U.S. will develop nosocomial infections. These infections extend average hospital stays by 4 days, directly account for 60,000 deaths per year, and add $10 billion dollars to the national health care expenditure (Mandell, Bennett, and Dolin, 1995).

In 1985, in response to concerns about the transmission of HIV infection in health care settings, CDC recommended **universal precautions** for blood and body fluid. Blood and body fluids from *all* patients are handled as if infected with HIV or other blood-borne pathogens. When in a situation where potential contact with blood or other body fluids exists, health care workers must always wash their hands and wear gloves, masks, protective clothing, and other indicated personal protective barriers. Needles and sharp instruments must be used and disposed of properly (Centers for Disease Control, 1989). CDC has recommendations for preventing transmission of HIV and hepatitis B during medical, surgical, and dental procedures (Centers for Disease Control, 1991b).

TUBERCULOSIS

Tuberculosis (TB) is a mycobacterial disease caused by *Mycobacterium tuberculosis.* Following are some basic facts about tuberculosis:

- Most transmission is through exposure to the tubercle bacilli in airborne droplets from persons with pulmonary tuberculosis during talking, coughing, or sneezing.
- Common symptoms are cough, fever, hemoptysis, chest pains, fatigue, and weight loss.
- Incubation period is 4 to 12 weeks.
- The most critical period for development of clinical disease is the first 6 to 12 months after infection.
- About 5% of those initially infected may develop pulmonary tuberculosis or extrapulmonary involvement. In about 95% of those infected, the infection becomes latent and may be reactivated later in life. Reactivation of latent infections is common in the elderly and the immunocompromised; substance abusers; underweight and undernourished persons; and those with diabetes, silicosis, or gastrectomies (Benenson, 1995).

Among adults worldwide, tuberculosis is the leading cause of death from a single infectious agent, and the rate has increased. The increase seems to be due to the growing incidence of tuberculosis among people with AIDS, the homeless, substance abusers, the elderly, immigrants, people in nursing homes and correctional facilities, and the development of multi-drug resistance. Since the peak of the resurgence in 1992, total reported tuberculosis cases in the U.S. have been falling, although cases in foreign-born persons have continued to increase. This overall decline has been attributed to improved prevention and control programs at the state and local levels as a result of increased federal funding to states beginning in the early 1990s (Centers for Disease Control and Prevention, 1997d).

TB screening tests used are skin testing with purified protein derivative (sometimes referred to as "putting on a PPD") and chest radiographs for positive skin reactors with pulmonary symptoms. False-negative skin test reactions due to anergy may occur in persons with immunosuppression caused by drugs or who have diseases such as advanced tuberculosis, AIDS, and measles. Confirmatory tests include stained sputum smears and other body fluids with demonstration of the acid-fast bacilli (for presumptive diagnosis) and culture of the tubercle bacilli for definitive diagnosis.

HOW TO Administer and Read a PPD Test

Since community health nurses usually "put on" the PPD, they need to know the correct procedure for administering this tuberculin skin test and how to interpret the test results.

Applying the PPD Test
- Use intradermal Mantoux test with 0.1 ml of 5 TU PPD tuberculin.
- Read reaction 48-72 hours after injection.
- Measure only induration.
- Record results in millimeters.

Reading the PPD Test

Test is positive if greater than or equal to 5 mm in:
- Persons known or suspected to have HIV infection
- Persons who have a chest radiograph suggestive of previous TB
- Close contacts of a person with infectious TB.

Test is positive if greater than or equal to 10 mm in:
- Persons with certain medical conditions, excluding HIV
- Persons who inject drugs (if HIV negative)
- Foreign-born persons from areas where TB is common
- Medically underserved, low-income populations
- Residents of long-term care facilities
- Children younger than 4 years of age.

Test is positive if greater than or equal to 15 mm in:
- All persons with no risk factors for TB.

From Centers for Disease Control and Prevention: *Screening for TB disease and infection, core curriculum on tuberculosis,* ed 3, 1994.

Patients with tuberculosis should be treated promptly with the appropriate multiple combination of anti-microbial drugs. Effective drug regimens currently used in the United States include isoniazid (INH) combined with rifampin (RIF), with or without pyrazinamide (PZA) for at least 6 months. Treatment failure generally is due to poor compliance to long-term treatment with resulting development of drug resistance (Benenson, 1995). Nurses usually perform tuberculin skin tests and provide patient education on the importance of compliance to long-term therapy. They may also be involved in directly observed therapy (DOT), urine testing to check compliance, and contact investigation of cases in the community.

VIRAL HEPATITIS

Viral hepatitis refers to a group of infections that primarily affect the liver. These infections have similar clinical presentations but different causes and characteristics. Brief profiles of these infections are presented in Table 23-5. Hepatitis A is

TABLE 23-5   Viral Hepatitis Profiles

	Hepatitis A	Hepatitis B	Hepatitis C	Hepatitis D	Hepatitis E	Hepatitis G
Incubation period	Average 30 days, range 15-50 days	Average 75 days, range 40-120 days	Average 45 days, range 14-175 days	Average 28 days, range 14-43 days	Average 40 days, range 15-60 days	Unknown
Mode of transmission	Fecal-oral, waterborne, sexual	Blood-borne, sexual, perinatal	Primarily blood-borne, also sexual and perinatal	Superinfection or co-infection of hepatitis B case	Fecal-oral	Blood-borne, may facilitate other strains of viral hepatitis to progress more rapidly
Incidence	125,00-200,000 cases/year in U.S.	140,000-320,000 cases/year in U.S.	28,000-180,000 cases/year in U.S.	7,500 cases/year in U.S.	Low in U.S.; epidemic outbreaks worldwide	0.3% of all acute viral hepatitis
Chronic carrier state?	No	Yes, 0.1%-15% of cases	Yes, 85% or more of cases	Yes, 70%-80% of cases	No	90%-100% of cases
Diagnosis	Serological tests (anti-HAV), viral isolation	Serological tests (HBsAg), viral isolation	Serological tests (anti-HCV)	Serological tests (anti-HDV), liver biopsy	Serological tests (anti-HEV)	None currently
Sequelae	No chronic infection	Chronic liver disease; liver cancer	Chronic liver disease; liver cancer	Chronic liver disease; liver cancer	No chronic infection	Rare or may not occur
Vaccine availability	Yes: vaccination of preschool children recommended; traveler's to endemic regions	Yes: vaccination of infants recommended; individuals with exposure risks	No	No	No	No
Control and prevention	Personal hygiene; proper sanitation	Preexposure vaccination; reduce exposure risk behaviors	Screening of blood/organ donors; reduce exposure risk behaviors	Preexposure or postexposure prophylaxis for HBV	Protection of water systems from fecal contamination	Unknown

described below and hepatitis B is discussed more fully in Chapter 24.

Following are some facts about hepatitis A:

- The clinical course ranges from mild to severe and often requires prolonged convalescence.
- Onset is usually acute with flu-like aches, diarrhea, fever, nausea, poor appetite, malaise, abdominal discomfort, dark urine, clay-colored stool, and followed in several days by jaundice.
- Transmission is from person to person via the fecal-oral route or through the ingestion of contaminated food or water.
- The virus can survive on a surface for up to a month (Shovein, Damazo, and Hyams, 2000).
- Virus level in the feces appears to peak 1 to 2 weeks before symptoms appear, making individuals highly contagious before they realize they are ill.

Hepatitis A is found worldwide. Every year, over 10 million people worldwide acquire the virus. In developing countries where sanitation is inadequate, epidemics are not common because most adults are immune from childhood infection. In countries with improved sanitation, outbreaks are common in daycare centers that enroll children who wear diapers, among household and sexual contacts of infected individuals and among travelers to countries where hepatitis A is endemic. In the U.S., cases are most common among school children and young adults. Eleven states in the United States between 1987 and 1997 reported a rate of hepatitis A that was about 20% above the national average. They were: Arizona, Alaska, Oregon, New Mexico, Utah, Washington, Oklahoma, South Dakota, Nevada, California, and Idaho. The reason for these high rates has not been determined (Shovein, Damazo, and Hyams, 2000). In many outbreaks an individual is the source of an infection that may become community-wide. In other cases, hepatitis A is spread through food contaminated by an infected food-handler, contaminated produce, or contaminated water. The source of infection may never be identified in as many as 25% of outbreaks.

Nurses can educate other health care providers and patients and remind them that appropriate sanitation and personal hygiene remain the best means of preventing infection. A vaccine for hepatitis A is available and is recommended for those who travel frequently or for long periods of time to countries where the disease is endemic. In cases of exposure through close contact with an infected individual or contaminated food or water, an injection of prophylactic immune globulin (IG) is indicated. IG should be given as soon as possible, but within 2 weeks of exposure (Benenson, 1995).

Clinical Application

One of the biggest problems with tuberculosis prevention and control programs is the required lengthy therapy using multiple drug combinations. Failure to comply with therapy over the entire treatment period may result in treatment failure and the development of drug resistance. The South Carolina Department of Health and Environmental Control, Tuberculosis Control Division, developed an innovative program in collaboration with the American Lung Association, South Carolina Chapter to provide incentives to clients to adhere to their treatment regimens (Pozsik, personal communication, 1995). Incentives are monetary or non-monetary, but are tailored to the wishes of the individual client. Examples of incentives include food, clothing, fish bait, and books. Tuberculosis control nurses personally administer each dose of treatment drugs to the client, and upon completion of an agreed-upon number of treatments, present the client with an incentive item. Each nurse has a regular caseload of clients with whom he or she meets as the treatment schedule demands. Meetings may be at home or at designated meeting places such as parking lots, fishing holes, or fast-food restaurants. The incentive program has been so successful in increasing treatment compliance that several other states have replicated this innovative approach. In addition to direct observation of drug therapy, these nurses also aggressively conduct contact investigation of their clients. This investigation may actually involve observing the client's daily activities to identify possible contacts. The vigorous efforts of these community health nurses assigned to the tuberculosis control unit have paid off in the steady decline of tuberculosis cases in South Carolina over the past 10 years.

A. Discuss with 3 to 5 classmates what the first step would be when developing a directly observed therapy (DOT) program.

B. When developing a proposal to start a DOT program using incentives to encourage clients to follow their treatment regimes, what sort of communicable disease information aside from need should you include?

C. When purchasing incentives (monetary or non-monetary) to encourage clients to follow a treatment plan, remember that the success of incentive programs is often linked with the value the person attaches to the incentive. What would you do first in choosing an incentive?

D. Why would on-site contact investigation be an important part of a tuberculosis-control program?

Answers are in the back of the book.

 Remember This!

- The burden of infectious diseases is high in both human and economic terms. Preventing these diseases must be given high priority in our present health care system.
- The successful interaction of the infectious agent, host, and environment is necessary for disease transmission. Knowledge of the characteristics of each of these three factors is important in understanding the transmission, prevention, and control of these diseases.
- Effective intervention measures at the individual and community levels must be aimed at breaking the chain linking the agent, host, and environment. An integrated approach attacking all three factors simultaneously is an ideal goal to strive for but may not be feasible for all diseases.
- Health care professionals must constantly be aware of vulnerability to threats posed by emerging infectious diseases. Most of the factors causing the emergence of these diseases are influenced by human activities and behavior.

- Communicable diseases are preventable. Preventing infection through primary prevention activities is the most cost-effective public health strategy.
- Health care professionals must always apply infection-control principles and procedures in the work environment. They should practice strictly the universal blood and body fluid precautions strategy to prevent transmission of HIV and other blood-borne pathogens.
- Effective control of communicable diseases requires the use of a multisystem approach focusing on improving host resistance, improving safety of the environment, improving public health systems, and facilitating social and political changes to ensure health for all people.
- Communicable disease prevention and control programs must move beyond providing drug treatment and vaccines. Health promotion and education aimed at changing human behavior must be emphasized.
- Nurses play a key role in all aspects of prevention and control of communicable diseases. Close cooperation with other members of the interdisciplinary health care team must be maintained. Mobilizing community participation is essential to successful implementation of programs.

? *What Would You Do?*

1. Visit a public health department clinic or one that serves a refugee, immigrant, or migrant labor population to observe the infectious diseases commonly seen in these groups. Compare and contrast this visit with a visit to a clinic that serves an inner-city population and a visit to a clinic that serves a rural population.
2. Sit in a clinic waiting room for immunization services and talk with parents about the concerns they may have and the barriers they may perceive in obtaining immunizations for their children.
3. Visit a daycare center. Observe potential situations for the communication of infectious diseases and discuss with the director the steps taken to prevent and control infection, including immunization requirements and procedures for hand washing and food preparation.
4. Find out which reportable diseases are a problem in your community. Note the number of cases that have been reported during the past month, 6 months, and year. Contrast these numbers with national statistics. Discuss with 3 or 4 classmates outbreak procedures that may accompany the reporting of some of these diseases. If possible, go on an outbreak investigation.

REFERENCES

Benenson AS (editor): *Control of communicable diseases in man,* ed 16, Washington, D.C., 1995, American Public Health Association.

Centers for Disease Control: Guidelines for prevention of transmission of HIV and hepatitis B virus to health care and public safety workers, *MMWR* 38(S-6):1, 1989.

Centers for Disease Control: Rabies prevention–United States, 1991, recommendations of the immunization practices advisory committee, *MMWR* 40(RR-3), 1991a.

Centers for Disease Control: Recommendations for preventing transmission of HIV and hepatitis B virus to patients during exposure-prone invasive procedures, *MMWR* 40(RR-8):1, 1991b.

Centers for Disease Control and Prevention: Recommendations of the international task force for disease eradication, *MMWR* 42 (RR-16):1, 1993.

Centers for Disease Control and Prevention: *Addressing emerging infectious disease threats: a prevention strategy for the U.S.,* Atlanta, 1994a, Centers for Disease Control and Prevention.

Centers for Disease Control and Prevention: Certification of poliomyelitis eradication–the Americas, 1994, *MMWR* 43(39):720, 1994b.

Centers for Disease Control and Prevention: *Escherichia coli* 0157:H7 outbreak linked to home-cooked hamburger–California, July 1993, *MMWR* 43(12):214, 1994c.

Centers for Disease Control and Prevention: Expanded tuberculosis surveillance and tuberculosis morbidity–United States, 1993, *MMWR* 43(20):361, 1994d.

Centers for Disease Control and Prevention: Outbreaks of *Cyclospora cayenensis* infection–United States, 1996, *MMWR* 54(25):549, 1996.

Centers for Disease Control and Prevention: Rubella and congenital rubella syndrome–United States, 1994-1997, *MMWR* 46(16):350, 1997a.

Centers for Disease Control and Prevention: Pertussis outbreak–Vermont, 1996, *MMWR* 46(35):822, 1997b.

Centers for Disease Control and Prevention: Lyme disease–United States, 1996, *MMWR* 46(23):531, 1997c.

Centers for Disease Control and Prevention: Tuberculosis morbidity–United States, 1996, *MMWR* 46(30):695, 1997d.

Centers for Disease Control and Prevention: Provisional cases of selected notifiable diseases, United States, weeks ending January 3, 1998, and December 28, 1996 (53rd Week), *MMWR* 46(52&53):1269, 1998.

Dennis DT, Fikrig E, Schaffner W: Now you can prevent Lyme disease, *Patient Care Nurse Pract* 2(6):20-35, 1999.

DeFriese GH, Faherty KM, Freeman VA, Guild PA, Musselman DA, Watson WA, Saarlas K: Developing child immunization registries: the all kids count program. In Isaacs SL, Knickman JR (editors): *To improve health and health care 1997,* San Francisco, 1997, Jossey-Bass.

Evans AS: The eradication of communicable diseases: myth or reality? *Am J Epidemiol* 122(2):199, 1985.

Fishbein DB, Bernard KW: Rabies virus. In Mandell GL, Bennett JE, Dolin R (editors): *Principles and practice of infectious diseases,* ed 4, New York, 1995, Churchill Livingstone.

Gershon A: Rubella virus. In Mandell GL, Bennett JE, Dolin R (editors): *Principles and practice of infectious diseases,* ed 4, New York, 1995, Churchill Livingstone.

Kappus KD, Lundgren RG, Juranek DD, Roberts JM, Spencer HC: Intestinal parasitism in the U.S.: update on a continuing problem, *Am J Trop Med Hyg* 50(6):705, 1994.

Last JM (editor): *A dictionary of epidemiology,* ed 3, New York, 1995, Oxford University Press.

Mandell GL, Bennett JE, Dolin R (editors): *Principles and practice of infectious diseases,* ed 4, New York, 1995, Churchill Livingstone.

Marwick C: Acellular pertussis vaccine is licensed for infants, *JAMA* 276(7):516, 1996.

National Center for Health Statistics: Births and deaths: United States, 1995, Monthly Vital Statistics Report 45(3supp2):21, 1996.

Pozsik C: Personal communication, 1995.

Shovein JT, Damazo RJ, Hyams I: Hepatitis A: how benign is it? *Am J Nurs* 100(3):43-47, 2000.

Steere AC: *Borrelia burgdorferi.* In Mandell GL, Bennett JE, Dolin R, editors: *Principles and practice of infectious diseases,* ed 4, New York, 1995, Churchill Livingstone.

U.S. Department of Health and Human Services: *Healthy people 2010: understanding and improving health,* Washington, D.C., 2000, U.S. Department of Health and Human Services; available online: www.health.gov/healthypeople.

Walker DH, Raoult D: *Rickettsia rickettsii* and other spotted fever group Rickettsiae. In Mandell GL, Bennett, JE Dolin, R (editors): *Principles and practice of infectious diseases,* ed 4, New York, 1995, Churchill Livingstone.

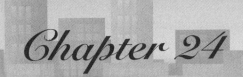

Chapter 24

HIV, Hepatitis, and Sexually Transmitted Diseases

PATTY J. HALE

OBJECTIVES

After reading this chapter, the student should be able to:
- Discuss the clinical signs of HIV, hepatitis, and sexually transmitted diseases.
- Describe the scope of the problem with HIV/AIDS, hepatitis, and sexually transmitted diseases.
- Analyze the behaviors that put people at risk for HIV, hepatitis, and sexually transmitted diseases.
- Describe nursing actions to prevent and care for people who experience these diseases.

CHAPTER OUTLINE

KEY TERMS

acquired immunodeficiency syndrome (AIDS): the final stages of HIV infection, which follow a protracted and debilitating course, characterized by specific opportunistic diseases that have a poor prognosis.

chancroid: a sexually transmitted disease caused by a bacterium, *Haemophilus ducreyi,* that causes a highly infectious ulcer to develop on either the penis, urethra, vulva, or anus.

chlamydia: a sexually transmitted disease caused by the organism *Chlamydia trachomatis,* which causes infection of the urethra and cervix. Infections may be asymptomatic and if untreated, cause severe morbidity.

genital herpes: a virus that attacks the genitals and sacral nerve. Infection is characterized by painful lesions that present as vesicles and progress to ulcerations on the male and female genitals, buttocks, or upper thighs.

Continued

KEY TERMS—cont'd

gonorrhea: a sexually transmitted disease caused by a bacterium, *Neisseria gonorrhoeae,* resulting in dysuria and/or inflammation of the urethra and cervix, or may result in no symptoms.

hepatitis B virus (HBV): a virus that is transmitted through exposure to body fluids. Infection results in a clinical picture that ranges from a self-limited acute infection to fulminant hepatitis or hepatic carcinoma, possibly leading to death.

HIV antibody test: enzyme-linked immunosorbent assay (ELISA) is the test commonly used in screening blood for the antibody to HIV; the Western Blot is used as a confirmatory test.

human immunodeficiency virus (HIV): the virus that causes HIV disease and AIDS.

human papillomavirus (HPV): a sexually transmitted disease that results in genital warts (condyloma acuminata) that grow in the vulva, vagina, cervix, urinary meatus, scrotum, or perianal area. A link exists between HPV infections and cancer.

partner notification: also known as contact tracing; identifying and locating sexual and injectable drug use partners of people who have been diagnosed with a sexually transmitted disease in order to notify them of exposure and encourage them to seek medical treatment.

pelvic inflammatory disease (PID): infection of the female reproductive organs, especially the fallopian tubes and endometrium, resulting in infertility and/or ectopic pregnancy. Acute symptoms and signs include lower abdominal pain, increased vaginal discharge, urinary frequency, vomiting, and fever. PID results from untreated gonorrhea and chlamydia.

sexually transmitted diseases (STDs): communicable diseases such as gonorrhea, chlamydia, and HIV infection that can be passed on during sexual activity.

syphilis: an infectious, chronic STD caused by the bacterium *Treponema pallidum* and characterized by the appearance of lesions or chancres that may involve any tissue. Relapses are frequent, and after the initial chancre and secondary symptoms, syphilis may exist without symptoms for years.

trichomoniasis: a common STD, transmitted by *Trichomonas vaginalis,* that results in infection of the female vulva and vagina and may or may not cause male symptoms. It is curable through effective treatment.

Concerns about sexually transmitted diseases (STDs), human immunodeficiency virus (HIV) infection, and acquired immunodeficiency syndrome (AIDS) have grown dramatically in recent years. These diseases are often acquired through behaviors that can be avoided or changed. For this reason, nursing actions include disease prevention as well as care and treatment. Because of the economic costs associated with the treatment of these diseases, especially HIV, their ease of transmission and serious outcomes, and the effects on families and communities, nurses must understand them and be actively involved in all levels of prevention. This chapter discusses HIV/AIDS, hepatitis, STDs, and the related nursing management.

HUMAN IMMUNODEFICIENCY VIRUS INFECTION

HIV infection and **acquired immunodeficiency syndrome (AIDS)** continue to have a significant effect on society. Considerable effort has been devoted to finding the best ways to reduce the transmission of this devastating disease. While the groups most likely to contract **human immunodeficiency virus (HIV)** are homosexuals and injection drug users, this disease is increasingly affecting women, heterosexuals, and teens. Since 88% of people who have HIV are between the ages of 20 and 49, the economic costs are high. Work productivity is decreased over the duration of the disease, and this is an expensive disease to treat. HIV/AIDS costs in the United States are estimated to be $5 billion (Institute of Medicine, 1997).

Briefly Noted

The Ryan White Comprehensive AIDS Resource Emergency (CARE) Act was passed in 1990 to provide services for persons with HIV infection (CDC, 1997e). This program funds health care in geographical areas with the largest number of AIDS cases. Covered services include emergency services, services for early intervention and care (sometimes including coverage of health insurance), and drug-reimbursement programs for HIV-infected individuals.

HIV infection is caused by a retrovirus, the human immunodeficiency virus, which was discovered in 1983. HIV results in immunological deficiencies that leave the host susceptible to opportunistic infections and cancers. The HIV virus infects mostly lymphoid cells and may remain clinically latent for several months or years, so the person appears symptom free. During this symptom-free period the virus continues to replicate in lymphoid tissue. HIV infects many cells, and the greatest damage is from the infection of the CD4+ T-lymphocyte, the cell that induces nearly every immune response. As CD4+ T-lymphocytes decrease, there are disruptions in immune functioning.

Natural History of HIV

The natural history of HIV includes three stages:

1. The primary infection around 1 month after contracting the virus
2. A period of time where the body shows no symptoms, called clinical latency
3. A final stage of symptomatic disease (Panteleo, et al, 1997).

When HIV enters the body it can cause a flu-like syndrome referred to as a primary infection or acute retroviral syndrome. This may go unrecognized. Initially the body's CD4+ white blood cell count drops for a brief time when the

TABLE 24-1	Clinical Manifestations of AIDS
Disease	**Clinical Signs**
Infections	
Varicella zoster (shingles)	Rash, pain
Isosporiasis, chronic interstitial (>1 mo)	Diarrhea
Coccidioidomycosis	Fever, fatigue, shortness of breath
Histoplasmosis	Fever, chest pain, dyspnea
Recurrent *Salmonella* septicemia	Fever, vasogenic shock
Candidiasis (respiratory or esophageal)	White patches on tongue, difficulty eating
Cryptococcal meningitis	Fever, headache, stiff neck
Pneumocystis carinii pneumonia or recurrent bacterial pneumonia	Shortness of breath, dry cough, fever, fatigue
Toxoplasmosis of brain	Hemiparesis, seizures, aphasia
Cryptosporidium enteritis infection (>1 mo)	Diarrhea, weakness
Mycobacterium tuberculosis infection (pulmonary or extrapulmonary)	Productive, purulent cough; fatigue, weight loss
Mycobacterium avium–complex or other mycobacterium	Septicemia, diarrhea
Cytomegalovirus retinitis or CMV disease	Visual blurring
Herpes simplex virus infection	Chronic vesicles (>1 mo), bronchitis
Pulmonary tuberculosis	Hemoptysis, night sweats
Cancers	
Invasive cervical cancer	Cervical dysplasia
Kaposi's sarcoma	Purple skin lesions, localized edema
Lymphoma (Burkitt's or primary of brain)	Weight loss, fever, night sweats
Syndromes	
Wasting syndrome caused by HIV	Diarrhea, decreased appetite
HIV-related encephalopathy	Decline in cognition, behavior, or coordination
Progressive multifocal leukoencephalopathy	Cognitive dysfunction

virus is most plentiful in the body. The immune system increases antibody production in response to this initial infection, which is a self-limiting illness. The symptoms are lymphadenopathy, myalgias, sore throat, lethargy, rash, and fever (Pantaleo, et al, 1997). At this point an antibody test is usually negative, so the process is often not recognized as HIV. After about 6 weeks to 3 months, HIV antibodies appear in the blood. While most antibodies serve a protective role, HIV antibodies do not.

About 80% to 90% of HIV-infected persons live for about 10 years (Panteleo, et al, 1997). During this prolonged incubation period, clients have a gradual deterioration of the immune system and can transmit the virus to others. AIDS is the last stage on the HIV infection continuum and may result from damage caused by HIV, secondary cancers, or opportunistic organisms. AIDS is defined as a disabling or life-threatening illness caused by HIV, or a CD4+ T-lymphocyte count of less than 200/mL with documented HIV infection.

Many of the opportunistic infections that affect AIDS patients are caused by microorganisms that are normally present in healthy people. These infections do not cause disease in persons with an intact immune system, but the microorganisms leading to infection grow rapidly in people with weakened immune systems such as those with HIV

infection. Opportunistic infections can be caused by bacteria, fungi, viruses, or protozoa. The most common opportunistic diseases are *Pneumocystis carinii* pneumonia and oral candidiasis. Table 24-1 describes diseases commonly associated with AIDS and their clinical symptoms.

Tuberculosis spreads rapidly among immunosuppressed HIV patients. HIV-infected individuals who live in close proximity to one another such as in long-term care facilities, prisons, or drug treatment facilities need to be carefully screened to make sure they are not infectious from tuberculosis before they are admitted to such settings.

Transmission

HIV is transmitted through exposure to blood, semen, vaginal secretions, and breast milk (Levy, 1998). HIV is not transmitted through the following methods:
- Casual contact (hug, handshake, touch)
- Insect bites or stings
- Airborne droplets caused by coughing or sneezing
- Sitting or eating near an infected person
- Touching equipment that has been in contact with an infected person

The modes of transmission are shown in the box on p. 420.

HOW TO Identify Modes of HIV Transmission

HIV can be transmitted by:
- Sexual contact that involves the exchange of body fluids with an infected person.
- Sharing or reusing needles, syringes, or other equipment used to prepare injectable drugs.
- Perinatal transmission from an infected mother to a fetus during pregnancy or delivery or while breast-feeding.
- Transfusions or other exposure to contaminated blood, blood products, organs, or semen.

Potential blood or tissue donors are screened through interviews to assess for a history of high-risk activities and by giving the HIV antibody test. Blood or tissue is not used if donors have a history of high-risk behavior or are HIV seropositive, that is, have antibodies to HIV in their serum. In addition to screening, coagulation factors used to treat hemophilia and other blood disorders are made safe through heat treatments to inactivate the virus. Such screening has significantly reduced the risk of transmission of HIV by blood products and organ donations. It is estimated that the odds of contracting HIV infection through receiving a blood transfusion are 1 in 450,000 units of blood transfused (Levy, 1998).

When a person is infected with STDs, like chlamydia or gonorrhea, the risk of HIV infection increases. Also, HIV may increase their risk for other STDs. This may result from any of the following: open lesions that provide entry of pathogens such as syphilis, when STDs decrease host immune status and hasten the progression of HIV infection, or when HIV changes the natural history of STDs or affects the effectiveness of medications used in treating STDs (Institute of Medicine, 1997).

Distribution and Trends

It is important to understand who is most at risk for HIV and the distribution of the disease across populations. The first reported cases of what was later to be known as AIDS occurred in five homosexual men in Los Angeles in 1981. As of June 1997, the total number of cases in the U.S. was 591,775 (Centers for Disease Control and Prevention, 1997e). It is estimated that between 600,000 and 900,000 people are infected with HIV in the United States, and 13 million people are infected worldwide (Centers for Disease Control and Prevention, 1997d; World Health Organization, 1993). As of June 1997, 62% of all persons reported to have AIDS in the United States had died (Centers for Disease Control and Prevention, 1997d). Table 24-2 shows how AIDS was distributed among persons in the United States in 1996.

Initially the groups with the highest incidence of HIV infection were homosexual and bisexual males, injection drug users and their sexual partners, and hemophiliacs (Centers for Disease Control, 1989). Although homosexual men still make up the largest group infected with HIV in the United States, the number of women contracting HIV through injection drug use and heterosexual transmission is growing. The majority of HIV-infected women are between the ages of 25 and 44 years, and 76% are African American and Hispanic/Latino (Centers for Disease Control and Prevention, 1997d). Sixteen percent of the people with AIDS are women. The occurrence of new cases is highest in women ages 15 to 24 (Wortley and Fleming, 1997).

One percent of those with AIDS are children (Centers for Disease Control and Prevention, 1997d), and they primarily contract the disease by perinatal transmission from an infected mother, blood transfusions, or from hemophilia transmissions. The number of perinatally acquired AIDS cases has decreased due to the effectiveness of the drug

TABLE 24-2 **AIDS Cases and Annual Rates by Race/Ethnicity, Age-Group, and Sex***

	Males		Adults/Adolescents Females		Total		Children (<13 years old)		Total	
Race/ethnicity	Number	Rate	Number	Rate	Number	Rate	Number	Rate	Number	Rate
White, not Hispanic	23,341	29.9	2,888	3.5	26,229	16.2	98	0.3	26,327	13.5
Black, not Hispanic	20,199	177.6	8,147	61.7	28,346	115.3	429	5.7	28,775	89.7
Hispanic	10,337	88.9	2,629	22.7	12,966	55.8	145	1.7	13,111	41.3
Asian/Pacific Islander	480	13.6	81	2.1	561	7.5	1	0.0	562	5.9
American Indian/ Alaska Native	166	23.2	41	5.4	207	14.1	3	0.6	210	0.7
Total†	54,653	51.9	13,820	12.3	68,473	31.4	678	1.3	69,151	25.6

From Centers for Disease Control and Prevention: *HIV/AIDS Surveillance Rep* 8(2):17, 1997.
*Per 100,000 population, reported in 1996, United States.
†Totals include 166 persons whose race/ethnicity is unknown.

zidovudine, which can be given to HIV-infected pregnant women to prevent the transmission from mother to fetus or infant (Centers for Disease Control and Prevention, 1996a). Women who are HIV infected are at risk for infecting their infants, and their own health may be affected. They should be counseled to prevent pregnancy.

The clinical picture of pediatric HIV infection is different from that of adults. The incubation period in infants is shorter, and they may have symptoms during the first year of life. Children also develop different physical signs and symptoms from adults. These include failure to thrive, diarrhea, developmental delays, and bacterial infections such as otitis media and pneumonia. Adolescents are at risk due to their greater likelihood to engage in risky behaviors such as trying drugs or engaging in unprotected sex. In addition, adolescent girls may have sex with older people, which can increase their risk of contracting the disease (Campbell, 1999).

The largest number of reported AIDS cases (45.3%) is in the age-group from 30 to 39 years, and nearly 90% of those with AIDS are between the ages of 20 and 49 years of age (Centers for Disease Control and Prevention, 1997d). Due to the long incubation period, the time when the actual transmission took place likely occurred during adolescence and young adulthood when people may experiment with drugs, sexual behaviors, and other activities that place them at risk.

AIDS disproportionately affects minority groups. African-Americans made up 12.1% of the total U.S. popula-

tion according to the 1990 census, yet they made up 43% of those reported to have AIDS (Centers for Disease Control and Prevention, 1997d). This overrepresentation is associated with low income, urban areas, use of injection drugs, and participation in prostitution (Aral, 1996).

AIDS is more likely to be found in urban areas, however, it is moving into rural areas. Regionally, the Northeast and Southeast sections of the United States and the U.S. territories of Puerto Rico and the Virgin Islands have the highest rates (Centers for Disease Control and Prevention, 1997d). States with an incidence greater than 25 per 100,000 population between July 1996 and June 1997 were Florida, New York, Nevada, South Carolina, Maryland, Georgia, Delaware, Connecticut, New Jersey, California, the District of Columbia, Louisiana, and Texas (Centers for Disease Control and Prevention, 1997d).

Although AIDS is a reportable condition, Table 24-3 shows how the reporting varies among states. As of January 1998,

Evidence-Based Practice

The purpose of the study referenced below was to assess the HIV-related behaviors and mental health of persons who are the closest sources of social support for inner-city women of color. Women who were facing multiple life crises and the person they were closest to were asked about their sexual and drug use history and their psychological well-being, and assessed for depression. The most common HIV risk behaviors among the participants were having sex for money, having sex without a condom, and having multiple sex partners. The women scored higher on a depression scale than did their supportive others. When comparing the homeless women with the drug-dependent women, the women in the drug recovery program were significantly more depressed. Thus, although peer support and social support is often assumed to be associated with health benefits, supportive others may also have a negative impact on health. Several other studies have identified that drug use occurs in social networks where needles and drugs are shared and opposition to drug treatment may be common.

APPLICATION IN PRACTICE

The researchers conclude that there is a need to provide mental health referral for homeless and drug addicted women and their supportive others. Future research needs to identify how supportive networks might be used to promote risk reduction.

Nyamathi A, Flaskerud J, Leake B: HIV-risk behaviors and mental health characteristics among homeless or drug-recovering women and their close sources of social support, *Nurs Res* 46(3):133-137, 1997.

TABLE 24-3 **Reporting Requirements for Human Immunodeficiency Virus (HIV) Infection**

By Name of Infected Person	Anonymous	Not Required
Alabama	Georgia	Alaska
Arizona	Iowa	California
Arkansas	Kansas	Delaware
Colorado	Kentucky	Florida
Connecticut*	Maine	Hawaii
Idaho	Montana	Louisiana
Indiana	New Hampshire	Maryland
Michigan	Oregon	Massachusetts
Minnesota	Rhode Island	New Mexico
Mississippi		New York
Missouri		Pennsylvania
Nebraska		Vermont
Nevada		Washington
New Jersey		District of
North Carolina		Columbia
North Dakota		
Ohio		
Oklahoma		
Oregon*		
South Carolina		
South Dakota		
Tennessee		
Texas*		
Utah		
Virginia		
West Virginia		
Wisconsin		
Wyoming		

From Centers for Disease Control and Prevention: *HIV/AIDS Surveillance Rep* 9(1):32,1997d.
*Connecticut and Texas have confidential HIV infection reporting for pediatric cases only; Oregon has reporting for children younger than 6 years old.

31 states used name-based HIV reporting in addition to the existing name-based AIDS surveillance systems (Centers for Disease Control and Prevention, 1998c). Study of already-diagnosed cases of AIDS does not reveal current HIV infection patterns because of the long interval between infection with HIV and the onset of clinically-apparent disease. Moreover, identification of new cases of AIDS does not distinguish between those recently infected and those infected several years ago. The successful use of several new drugs early in the asymptomatic phase of infection also supports determining early identification of illness in this period. Thus several experts, including the CDC, are calling for mandatory reporting of HIV positive status by name in all 50 states (Gostin, Ward, and Baker, 1997; Centers for Disease Control and Prevention, 1998a). Opponents are concerned about the government's ability to maintain confidential registries and the potential invasions into personal lives, as well as housing, employment, and insurance discrimination.

HIV Testing

The **HIV antibody test** is the most commonly used screening test for determining infection. This test indicates the presence of the antibody to HIV. It does not reveal whether a person has AIDS, nor does it isolate the virus. The most commonly used form of this test is the enzyme-linked immunosorbent assay (EIA) referred to as EIA or ELISA. The EIA effectively screens blood and other donor products. In cases of false-positive results, a confirmatory test, the Western blot, is used to verify the results. False-negative results may also occur after infection before antibodies are produced. This is sometimes referred to as the "window period" and can last from 6 weeks to 3 months.

Testing for HIV infection is done at health department STD clinics and family planning clinics, primary care offices, and freestanding HIV-counseling and HIV-testing sites. Voluntary screening programs for HIV may be either confidential or anonymous: the process for each is unique. With confidential testing, the person's name and address are obtained, and this information is considered privileged. With anonymous testing the client is given an identification number that is attached to all records of the test results. Demographic data such as the person's sex, age, and race may be collected, but there is no record of the client's name and address. An advantage of anonymous testing may be that it increases the number of people who are willing to be tested, because many of those at risk are engaged in illegal activities. The anonymity eliminates their concern about the possibility of arrest or discrimination.

Briefly Noted

Due to impaired immunity, children with HIV infection are more likely to get childhood diseases and have serious effects. Therefore, DPT (diphtheria-pertussis-tetanus), IPV (inactivated polio virus), and MMR (measles-mumps-rubella) vaccines should be given at regularly scheduled times for children infected with HIV. Hib (*Haemophilus influenzae* type B), hepatitis B, pneumococcal, and influenza vaccines may be recommended after medical evaluation.

Caring for AIDS Patients in the Community

AIDS is a chronic disease, and many of these individuals live, work, and go to school in communities. Nurses play key roles not only in providing direct care to AIDS patients but also in teaching them, their families, and significant others about personal care and hygiene, medication administration including pain management, universal precautions to ensure infection control, and healthful life-style behaviors such as adequate rest, good nutrition, stress management, and exercise.

Persons with AIDS have times of illness as well as periods of wellness when they are able to return to school or work. The 1974 Vocational Rehabilitation Act protects employees from termination of employment or other discriminatory action based solely on the presence of the disease. Nurses working in the community can help employers know how to deal effectively with employees who have AIDS. Nurses can sponsor, or encourage employers to sponsor, programs on HIV. They can also teach managers or refer them to appropriate resources to learn how to work with sick or infected workers to reduce the risk of breaching confidentiality or taking wrongful actions such as termination. Revealing a worker's infection to other workers, terminating employment, and isolating an infected worker can lead to litigation. The CDC supports workplace issues through programs offered by its Business and Labor Resource Service.

Children who are HIV infected should attend school because the benefit of attendance far outweighs the risk of transmitting or acquiring infections. None of the cases of HIV infection in the United States have been transmitted in a school setting. An interdisciplinary team made of the child's physician, public health personnel, and parents or guardians need to make decisions about educational and care needs (Centers for Disease Control and Prevention, 1996c).

Individual decisions about risk to the infected child or others should be based on the behavior, neurological development, and physical condition of the child. Attendance may be inadvisable in the presence of cases of childhood infections such as chickenpox or measles within the school, because the immunosuppressed child is at greater risk of suffering complications. Alternative arrangements, such as homebound instruction, can be used if a child cannot control body secretions or displays biting behavior.

As the number of individuals with AIDS has increased, a variety of health care, social, and economic needs have arisen, and a variety of agencies can address these needs. Services available in many communities include client and family counseling, support groups, legal aid, personal care services, housing programs, and community education programs. Each state has established an AIDS hotline. In addition, the federal government and various organizations have established toll-free numbers to meet a variety of needs.

Nurses see AIDS patients in homes, physician offices, clinics, and in hospitals. It is important to remember that this disease often brings with it considerable pain. Pain is assessed both by using a self-report pain-rating scale and also by asking patients how much the pain interferes with their ability to carry on their normal activities. Pain may take a variety of forms. It is important to determine what other symptoms the person has such as fatigue, nausea, or cognitive impairment. Pain can be treated with all three analgesic groups: non-opioids, opioids, and adjuvant analgesics. Non-opioids, including acetaminophen and ibuprofen, can reduce mild to moderate musculoskeletal pain and headaches. If these drugs do not control pain, then opioid analgesics such as morphine, hydromorphone, and fentanyl may need to be added to the treatment regimen. Research is investigating the usefulness of adjuvant analgesics to treat neuropathic pain that may accompany HIV disease. For example, viscous lidocaine can relieve mouth pain and dysphagia (Hughes, 1999).

OTHER SEXUALLY TRANSMITTED DISEASES

The number of new cases (the incidence) of some **sexually transmitted diseases (STDs),** such as syphilis, has been declining recently, while others such as herpes simplex and chlamydia are increasing. It is estimated that actual rates of STDs are twice the reported rate. Since STDs have long-term health effects and eight new STDs have emerged since 1980, it is important to pay attention to their prevention and treatment (Institute of Medicine, 1997).

The common STDs in Table 24-4 are categorized by their biological origin: those caused by protozoa, bacteria, or viruses. Trichomoniasis is a protozoan infection. The bacterial infections include gonorrhea, syphilis, chlamydia, and chancroid. Most of these are curable with antibiotics with the exception of the newly emerging antibiotic-resistant strains of gonorrhea (Stephenson and Lee, 1998).

STDs caused by viruses cannot be cured. These are chronic diseases resulting in years of symptom management and infection control. The viral infections include herpes simplex virus, hepatitis B virus, and human papillomavirus (HPV), also referred to as genital warts. Hepatitis A virus, which may also be transmitted via sexual activity, is discussed in Chapter 23.

Trichomoniasis

Trichomoniasis is a common sexually transmitted disease caused by a unicellular protozoan flagellate, *Trichomonas vaginalis,* that infects the female vulva and vagina but usually does not cause symptoms in males (Krieger, 1995). It is transmitted through sexual contact and is easily diagnosed through microscopic identification of the organism. The symptoms vary but include frothy off-white to green vaginal discharge and pruritus. Trichomoniasis is not a reportable condition in most states. Although considered a benign STD in comparison with other STDs, it is common and recently has been linked with pelvic inflammatory disease, which is a serious condition discussed below (Paisarntantiwong, et al, 1995).

Gonorrhea

Neisseria gonorrhoeae is a gram-negative intracellular diplococcus bacterium that infects the mucous membranes of the genitourinary tract, rectum, and pharynx. It is transmitted through genital-genital contact, oral-genital contact, and anal-genital contact.

Gonorrhea is identified as either uncomplicated or complicated. Uncomplicated gonorrhea refers to limited cervical or urethral infection. Complicated gonorrhea includes salpingitis, epididymitis, systemic gonococcal infection, and gonococcal meningitis. The signs and symptoms of infection in males are purulent and copious urethral discharge and dysuria, although 10% to 20% of males do not appear to have symptoms.

More females than males tend to be asymptomatic; there may be minimal vaginal discharge or dysuria (Hook and Handsfield, 1990). The asymptomatic state is dangerous since people who are unaware of their infection may continue to infect others, whereas those who are symptomatic usually cease sexual activity and seek treatment.

Up to 40% of those infected with gonorrhea are also infected with *Chlamydia trachomatis* (Centers for Disease Control and Prevention, 1998b). Therefore selection of a treatment that is effective against both organisms, such as doxycycline or azithromycin, is recommended (Centers for Disease Control and Prevention, 1998b).

Gonorrhea rates have declined over time due to the testing of asymptomatic women and follow-up with their partners to prevent reinfection. Although the reported number of cases in the U.S. in 1996 was just under 300,000, the CDC estimates the actual number of annual cases to be 600,000 (Centers for Disease Control and Prevention, 1998b). The difference between the actual cases and reported cases occurs because gonorrhea may be unreported by health care providers or clients who are asymptomatic and do not seek treatment, and are therefore not identified. Groups with the highest incidence of gonorrhea are blacks, persons living in the southern United States, and persons 15 to 24 years of age (Division of STD Prevention, 1997).

The number of antibiotic-resistant cases of gonorrhea in the United States has risen at an alarming rate. Penicillin-resistant gonorrhea was first identified in 1976, when 15 cases were reported. Currently certain strains of gonorrhea are resistant to penicillin, tetracycline, and ciprofloxacin (Deguchi, et al, 1997; Centers for Disease Control and Prevention, 1994a). The increase in antibiotic-resistant infections is partially due to the high use of antibiotics as a prophylactic

TABLE 24-4   Summary of Sexually Transmitted Diseases

Disease/Pathogen	Incubation	Signs and Symptoms	Diagnosis	Treatment	Nursing Implications
Protozoan					
Trichomoniasis: *Trichomonas vaginalis*	5-28 Days	Frequently asymptomatic copious, loose yellow or green vaginal discharge; vulvovaginal soreness/irritation; dysuria-internal or external; painful intercourse.	(+) Whiff test; wet-mount visualization of organism and ≥1 PMN per epithelial cell.	One of the following: • Metronidazole 2g PO once; *or* • 500 mg PO bid x 7 days *or* • 250 mg TID x 7 days.	Almost always sexually acquired, so treat partners simultaneously; avoid sex until symptoms gone in both client and partner(s); return for evaluation if symptoms persist; screen for other STDs (gonorrhea, chlamydia, and HIV); medication teaching.
Bacterial					
Chlamydia: *Chlamydia*	3-21 Days	*Male:* NGU; painful urination and urethral discharge; epididymitis *Female:* none or MPC, vaginal discharge. If untreated, progresses to symptoms of PID, diffuse abdominal pain, fever, chills.	Tissue culture; Gram stain of endocervical or urethral discharge: presence of PMNs without gram-negative intracellular diplococci suggests NGU.	One of the following: • Doxycycline 100 mg PO BID x 7 days *or* • Azithromycin 1 g PO x 1 *or* • Erythromycin 500 mg QID x 7 days *or* • Ofloxacin 300 mg PO BID x 7 days *or* • Doxycycline (effective and cheap) *or* • Azithromycin (1-time dose)	Refer partner(s) of past 60 days; counsel client to use condoms and to avoid sex until therapy is complete and symptoms are gone in both client and partners; medication teaching.
Gonorrhea: *Neisseria gonorrhoeae*	3-21 Days	*Male:* urethritis, purulent discharge, painful urination, urinary frequency; epididymitis. *Female:* none or symptoms of PID.	Culture of discharge; Gram stain of urethral discharge, endocervical, or rectal smear	One of the following: • Ceftriaxone 125 mg IM *or* • Ciprofloxacin 500 mg PO x 1 *or* • Ofloxacin 400 mg PO x 1 *or* • Cefixime 400 mg PO x 1 *or* • Azithromycin 1 g PO x 1	Refer partner(s) of past 60 days; return for evaluation if symptoms persist; counsel client to use condoms and to avoid sex until therapy is complete and symptoms are gone in both client and partners; medication teaching.
Syphilis: *Treponema pallidum*	10-90 Days	Primary: usually single, painless. If untreated, heals in a few weeks.	Visualization of pathogen on dark-field microscopic examination; single painless ulcer (chancre) FTA-ABS or MHA-TP VDRL (reactive 14 days after appearance of chancre).	Benzathine penicillin G 2.4 million U IM once. If penicillin allergy, one of the following: • Doxycycline 100 mg PO bid x 2 weeks *or* • Tetracycline 500 mg QID x 14 days For those allergic to penicillin, tetracycline hydrochloride should not be administered to pregnant women or those with neurosyphilis or congenital syphilis.	Counsel to be tested for HIV; screen all partners of past 3 months; re-examine client at 3 and 6 months.

Continued

Disease	Time	Signs/Symptoms	Assessment	Treatment	Nursing Care/Education
	6 Weeks to 6 months	*Secondary:* low-grade fever, malaise, sore throat, headache, adenopathy, and rash.	Clinical signs of secondary syphilis.	Benzathine penicillin G 2.4 million U IM once.	
	Within 1 year of infection	*Early latency:* asymptomatic; infectious lesions may recur.	VDRL: FTA-ABS or MHA-TP	Benzathine penicillin G	
	After 1 year from date of infection	*Late latency:* asymptomatic; noninfectious except to fetus of pregnant women.	Lumbar puncture, CSF cell count, protein level determination and VDRL.	Penicillin G Benzathine 2.4 million U IM weekly x 3 weeks.	
	Late Active: 2-40 years 20-30 years 10-30 years	• Gummas of skin, bone, and mucous membranes, heart, liver • CNS involvement: paresis, optic atrophy • Cardiovascular involvement: aortic aneurysm, aortic value insufficiency.		Penicillins—varying doses depending on diagnoses.	
Charcroid: *Haemophilus ducreyi*	3-7 days	Small irregular papule progressing to deep ulcer that is painful and drains pus or blood on the penis, labia, or vaginal opening; inguinal tenderness, dysuria.	Visual inspection of lesion.	One of the following: • Azithromycin 1 gm PO x 1 *or* • Ceftriaxone 250 mg IM x 1.	Return for exam 3-7 days after treatment begins; partners who had sex within 10 days before client's onset of symptoms should be evaluated; condom use.
Viral Human immunodeficiency virus (HIV)	4 to 6 weeks	Possible: acute mononucleosis-like illness (lymphadenopathy, fever, rash, joint and muscle pain, sore throat).		Prophylactic administration of zidovudine (ZDV) immediately following exposure may prevent seroconversion.	HIV education and counseling.
	Seroconversion: 6 weeks to 3 months	Appearance of HIV antibody.	HIV antibody test: the ELISA, or the Western blot test. New test: OraSure made by SmithKline Beecham—an oral HIV-1 antibody testing system—test results in about 3 days.	Asymptomatic infection with HIV-1 and CD4+ counts ≥500/mm³; treat with ZDV 500-600 mg/day. Treatment can be held in those with asymptomatic infection and CD4+ counts between 500-200/mm³ until symptoms or CD4+ counts <200 develop.	HIV education and counseling, partner referral for evaluation, medication education, assessment and referral.
	AIDS: months to years (average 11 years)	Opportunistic diseases: most commonly *Pneumocystis* pneumonia, oral candidiasis, Kaposi's sarcoma.	CD4+ T-lymphocyte count of less than 200/μL with documented HIV infection, or diagnosis with clinical manifestations of AIDS as defined by the CDC.	Symptomatic infection: start ZDV 20 mg q8h. Alternatives to ZDV: didanosine (ddI), stavudine (d4t), zalcitabine (ddC), and the combination of ZDV and ddI. Additional treatments necessary for opportunistic infections.	

TABLE 24-4   Summary of Sexually Transmitted Diseases—cont'd

Disease/Pathogen	Incubation	Signs and Symptoms	Diagnosis	Treatment	Nursing Implications
Viral—cont'd					
Hepatitis B virus (HBV)	6 weeks to 6 months	Varies greatly from subclinical infection to flu-like symptoms to cirrhosis, fulminant hepatitis; hepatocellular carcinoma.	Serum IgM alpha-HBc.	Hepatitis B immune globulin (HBIG) within 14 days of last exposure; followed by regular three-dose immunization series.	Partner(s) should receive HBIG prophylaxis within 14 days postexposure followed by 3-dose immunization series.
Genital warts; Human papillomavirus (HPV)	4-6 weeks most common; up to 9 months	Often subclinical infection; painless lesions near vaginal opening, anus, shaft of penis, vagina, cervix; lesions are textured, cauliflower appearance; may remain unchanged over time.	Visual inspection for lesions, Papanicolaou smear, colposcopy.	No cure; one third of lesions will disappear without treatment. Patient-applied: topical podofilox 0.5% or imiquimod 5% cream. Provider administered: podophyllin resin 10-25%, trichloracetic acid 80-90%, cryotherapy with liquid nitrogen, laser, or surgical removal.	Warts and surrounding tissues contain HPV, so removal of warts does not completely eradicate virus; examination of partner(s) not necessary since treatment is only symptomatic; condom use may reduce transmission. Medication application of cytotoxic agents
Genital herpes: Herpes simplex virus 2 (HSV-2)	2-20 days; average 6 days	Vesicles, painful ulcerations of penis, vagina, labia, perineum, or anus; lesions last 5-6 weeks and recurrence is common; may be asymptomatic.	Presence of vesicles; viral culture (obtained only when lesions present and before they have scabbed over).	No cure; acyclovir 400 mg PO TID x 7-10 days or Acyclovir 200 mg five times a day for 7-10 days or Valacyclovir 1g PO BID x 7-10 days.	Refer partner(s) for evaluation; teach client about likelihood of recurrent episodes and ability to transmit to others even if asymptomatic; condom use; annual Pap smear.

From Centers for Disease Control and Prevention: 1998 Guidelines for treatment of sexually transmitted diseases, *MMWR* 47:RR-1, 1998b.

CSF, Cerebrospinal fluid; *ELISA,* enzyme-linked immunosorbent assay; *FTA-ABS,* fluorescent treponemal antibody absorption test; *MHA-TP,* microhemagglutination-*Treponema pallidum; MPC,* mucopurulent cervicitis; *NGU,* nongonococcal urethritis; *PID,* pelvic inflammatory disease; *PMN,* polymorphonuclear neutrophil; *VDRL,* Venereal Disease Research Laboratory test for syphilis.

measure by persons with multiple sexual partners (Zenilman, et al, 1988). To ensure proper treatment and cure, those diagnosed with gonorrheal infection should return for health care if symptoms persist, have their partner evaluated for infection, and remain sexually abstinent until antibiotic therapy is completed (Centers for Disease Control and Prevention, 1998b).

The development of **pelvic inflammatory disease (PID)** is a risk for women who remain asymptomatic and do not seek treatment. PID is a serious infection involving the fallopian tubes (salpingitis) and is the most common complication of gonorrhea but may also result from chlamydia infection. Symptoms of PID include fever, abnormal menses, and lower abdominal pain, however PID may not be recognized because the symptoms vary among women. PID can result in ectopic pregnancy and infertility as a result of fallopian-tube scarring and occlusion. It may also cause stillbirths and premature labor. The cost of the complications resulting from PID are estimated at more than $3.5 billion annually (Institute of Medicine, 1997).

Syphilis

Syphilis, caused by *Treponema pallidum,* infects moist mucosal or cutaneous lesions and is spread through direct contact, usually by sexual contact or from mother to fetus. In sexual transmission, tiny breaks in the skin and mucous membranes create a point of entry for the bacteria during sexual contact. The number of reported cases of syphilis was 11,336 in 1996, and the most at-risk groups are blacks and persons between ages 20 and 39 years (Division of STD Prevention, 1997).

Syphilis is divided into early and late stages, and latency or a symptom-free time can occur during either stage. The early stage is the first full year after infection and includes the primary, secondary, and early latent stages. The late stage is the time after this first year and includes late latency and tertiary syphilis. During latency there are no clinical signs of infection, but the person has historical or serological evidence of infection. There is always a possibility of relapse.

The first stage is called primary syphilis. When syphilis is acquired sexually, the bacteria produce infection in the form of a chancre at the site of entry. The lesion begins as a macula, progresses to a papule, and later ulcerates. If left untreated, this chancre persists for 3 to 6 weeks and then heals spontaneously.

In secondary syphilis the organism enters the lymph system and spreads throughout the body. Signs include rash, lymphadenopathy, and mucosal ulceration. Symptoms include sore throat, malaise, headaches, weight loss, variable fever, and muscle and joint pain.

Blindness, congenital damage, cardiovascular damage, or syphilitic psychoses may occur during tertiary syphilis. Another potential outcome of tertiary syphilis is the development of lesions of the bones, skin, and mucous membranes, known as gummas. Tertiary syphilis usually occurs several years after initial infection and is rare in the United

States since antibiotics usually cure the disease in its early stages. Tertiary syphilis is a major problem in developing countries.

Syphilis is transmitted transplacentally and if untreated can cause premature stillbirth, blindness, deafness, facial abnormalities, crippling, or death. Signs include jaundice, skin rash, hepatosplenomegaly, or pseudoparalysis of an extremity. Treatment is penicillin given intravenously or intramuscularly (Centers for Disease Control and Prevention, 1998b).

Chlamydia

Chlamydia infection, from the bacterium *Chlamydia trachomatis,* infects the genitourinary tract and rectum of adults and causes conjunctivitis and pneumonia in neonates. Transmission occurs when mucopurulent discharge from infected sites, such as the cervix or urethra, comes into contact with the mucous membranes of a noninfected person. As with gonorrhea, the infection is often asymptomatic in women and if left untreated can lead to PID. If present, symptoms of chlamydial infection in females are dysuria, urinary frequency, and purulent vaginal discharge. In males the urethra is the most common site of infection, resulting in nongonococcal urethritis (NGU). The symptoms of NGU are dysuria and urethral discharge. Epididymitis is a possible complication.

Chlamydia is the most common reportable infectious disease in the United States, with 4 million infections occurring every year (Centers for Disease Control and Prevention, 1997b). Prevention is key in chlamydia since it can lead to PID, ectopic pregnancy, infertility, and neonatal complications (Centers for Disease Control and Prevention, 1997b).

Chancroid

Chancroid, caused by *Haemophilus ducreyi,* is spread from person to person through sexual contact. Chancroid has an ulcerative lesion that appears on the penis, labia, or clitoris, or at the vaginal orifice. About 1 week after infection, a small papule develops and soon progresses to a painful, deep ulceration. The infection spreads to the inguinal lymph nodes and causes inflammation and tenderness. While one or two lesions typically occur, there may be as many as 10. The number of reported cases of chancroid has decreased from a high of 4986 in 1987 to 386 in 1996. The infection is underreported due to inadequate laboratory testing and unclear definition of what signs confirm diagnosis (Centers for Disease Control, 1992). Although chancroid is not as commonly reported as other STDs in the United States, it is much more prevalent worldwide than gonorrhea or syphilis.

Hepatitis B Virus

The number of new cases of **hepatitis B virus (HBV)** in the United States increased by 37% between 1979 and 1989 (Centers for Disease Control, 1991). Since the use of the

HBV vaccine, the numbers have fallen dramatically—from 10.65 cases per 100,000 persons in 1987 to 4.01 cases per 100,000 in 1996. (Centers for Disease Control and Prevention, 1997g).

The groups with the highest prevalence are users of injection drugs, persons with STDs or multiple sex partners, immigrants and refugees and their descendants who came from areas where there is a high endemic rate of HBV, health care workers, hemodialysis patients, and inmates of long-term correctional institutions.

The HBV is spread through blood and body fluids and, like HIV, is referred to as a blood-borne pathogen. It has the same transmission properties as HIV, and thus individuals should take the same precautions to prevent both HIV and HBV spread. A major difference is that HBV remains alive outside the body for a longer period of time than does HIV and thus has greater infectivity. The virus can survive for at least 1 week dried at room temperature on environmental surfaces, and thus infection-control measures are paramount in preventing transmission from patient to patient (Centers for Disease Control, 1990a; Centers for Disease Control and Prevention, 1997f).

Infection with HBV results in either acute or chronic HBV infection. The acute infection is self-limited, and individuals develop an antibody to the virus and successfully eliminate the virus from the body. They subsequently have lifelong immunity against the virus. Symptoms range from mild (resembling flu) to more severe (includes jaundice, extreme lethargy, nausea, fever, and joint pain). The severe symptoms can necessitate hospitalization. A second possible infection outcome is chronic HBV infection, which occurs in 1% to 6% of infected adults (Centers for Disease Control and Prevention, 1998b). These individuals cannot rid their bodies of the virus and remain lifelong carriers of the hepatitis B surface antigen (HbsAg). As carriers, they can transmit the HBV to others. They may develop hepatic carcinoma or chronic active hepatitis. The signs and symptoms of chronic hepatitis B include anorexia, fatigue, abdominal discomfort, hepatomegaly, and jaundice.

HBV infection can be prevented by immunization, prevention of nosocomial and occupational exposure, and prevention of sexual and injection drug use exposure. Vaccination is recommended for persons with occupational risk, such as health care workers, and for children. The series of vaccines required for protection from HBV consists of three intramuscular injections, with the second and third doses administered 1 and 6 months after the first (Centers for Disease Control, 1991). All pregnant women should be tested for hepatitis B surface antigen (HbsAg), which indicates whether they carry and are able to transmit HBV (Immunization Action Coalition, 1996). If the mother tests positive, newborns require hepatitis B immune globulin in addition to the hepatitis B vaccine at birth, then at 1 and 6 months thereafter (Centers for Disease Control and Prevention, 1996b). Hepatitis B immune globulin is given after exposure to provide passive immunity and thus prevent infection.

In 1992 the Occupational Safety and Health Administration (OSHA) released the standard "Occupational Exposure to Bloodborne Pathogens" (Occupational Safety and Health Administration, 1992), which mandates specific activities to protect workers from HBV and other blood-borne pathogens. Potential exposures for health care workers are needle-stick injuries and mucous membrane splashes. The OSHA standard requires employers to identify the risk of blood exposure to various employees. If the work of employees involves a potential exposure to others' body fluids, employers must offer the HBV vaccine to the employee at the employer's expense and provide annual educational programs on preventing HBV and HIV exposure in the workplace. Employees have the right to refuse the vaccine.

Herpes Simplex Virus 2 (Genital Herpes)

Herpes virus infects genital and nongenital sites. Herpes simplex virus 1 (HSV-1) primarily causes nongenital lesions such as cold sores that may appear on the lip or mouth. Herpes simplex virus 2 (HSV-2) is the primary cause of **genital herpes.** The virus is transmitted through direct exposure and infects the genitalia and surrounding skin. After the initial infection, the virus stays latent in the sacral nerve of the central nervous system and may reactivate periodically with or without visible vesicles.

Briefly Noted

Herpes simplex virus 2 (HSV-2) is the primary cause of genital herpes. This is a chronic disease for which there is no cure at present.

Signs and symptoms of HSV-2 infection include the presence of painful lesions that begin as vesicles and ulcerate and crust within 1 to 4 days. Lesions may occur on the vulva, vagina, upper thighs, buttocks, and penis and have an average duration of 11 days. The vesicles often cause itching and pain and are accompanied by dysuria or rectal pain. Although infectivity is higher with active lesions, some individuals can spread the virus even when they are asymptomatic. Approximately 50% of people experience a prodromal phase. This may include a mild, tingling sensation up to 48 hours before eruption or shooting pains in the buttocks, legs, or hips up to 5 days before eruption (Corey, 1990).

It is estimated that 724,000 people are infected annually with this incurable disease (Fleming, et al, 1997). This disease is of special importance to women and their children since it is linked with the development of cervical cancer. There is also an increased risk of spontaneous abortion and risk of transmission to the newborn during vaginal delivery (Brown, et al, 1997). A pregnant woman who has active lesions at the time of birth should have a cesarean delivery before the rupture of amniotic membranes to avoid fetal contact with the herpetic lesions. Mortality for infected neonates is estimated to be as high as 80%, and neurological damage is a major complication (Martens, 1994).

Human Papillomavirus Infection

Human papillomavirus (HPV), also called genital warts, can infect the genitals, anus, and mouth. HPV is transmitted through direct contact with warts that result from HPV. However, HPV has been detected in semen, and exposure to the virus through body fluids is also possible. Genital warts are most commonly found on the penis and scrotum in men and the vulva, labia, vagina, and cervix in women. The surface of the lesions are often described as having a cauliflower appearance. The warts are usually multiple and vary between 1 and 5 mm in diameter. They may be difficult to visualize, so careful examination is required.

The number of new cases annually of genital HPV infection is estimated to be 500,000 to 1,000,000 (Institute of Medicine, 1997). Between 10% and 20% of American women of childbearing age and between 5% and 19% of women visiting family planning and university student health clinics have genital HPV infection (Aral and Holmes, 1990). As with genital herpes, the actual prevalence is difficult to ascertain because it is not a reported disease, and many infections are subclinical.

Complications of HPV infection are serious for women. There is a link between HPV infection and cervical cancer; it is estimated that 15% of untreated high-grade lesions resulting from HPV develop into cervical cancer (Crum and Nuovo, 1991). HPV infection is increased in both pregnancy and old age due to a decrease in cell-mediated immune functioning. HPV can infect the fetus during pregnancy and lead to laryngeal papilloma that can obstruct the infant's airway.

Briefly Noted

The challenge of HPV prevention is that condoms do not necessarily prevent infection. Warts can grow where barriers, such as condoms, do not cover and skin-to-skin contact can occur.

Because there is no cure for HPV, the treatment goal is to eliminate the lesions. Genital warts spontaneously disappear over time, as do skin warts. However, this condition is worrisome for the client. Also, HPV may lead to the development of cervical neoplasia. Treatment of the lesions is with surgical removal, cytotoxic agents, or immunotherapies.

THE NURSING ROLE IN PREVENTING STDS AND PROVIDING SERVICES

From prevention to treatment, nurses working in the community function as counselors, educators, advocates, case managers, and primary care providers. Strategies include primary, secondary, and tertiary prevention.

Primary Prevention

Primary prevention consists mainly of activities to keep people healthy before the onset of disease. This begins with assessing for risk behavior and providing relevant intervention through education on how to change risky behaviors.

Briefly Noted

Assessing a client's risk of acquiring an STD needs to be done with all sexually active people. This risk assessment needs to include baseline data for clients attending all clinics and those who receive school health, occupational health, public health, and home nursing services.

To assess the risk of acquiring STDs, a sexual and injection drug use history is obtained for clients and their partners. The sexual history provides information about the need for specific diagnostic tests, treatment modalities, partner notification, and risk factors. To assess the risk of acquiring STDs, a sexual and injection drug use history for clients and their partners should be done. It must be made clear to the client that this information is confidential. Most clients feel uneasy disclosing such personal information. This discomfort can be eased by being supportive and open during the interview to facilitate honesty about intimate activities. Direct and simple language should be used when discussing precautions. Discussing sexual behavior is not always comfortable for nurses. They should try to be aware of their own anxiety and/or discomfort and deal with it so that it does not interfere with being able to work with clients. One way for the nurse to address his or her discomfort is by role-playing with colleagues some assessments of sexual and injection drug-using behavior. See the box below for guides to how to improve sexual history taking.

HOW TO Improve Sexual History Taking

- Be supportive and honest.
- Use understandable terms.
- Be candid.
- Ask questions in a non-threatening and non-judgmental manner.
- Acknowledge that many people are uncomfortable talking about personal things.

Identifying the total number of sexual and injection-drug–using partners and the number of contacts with these partners provides information about the client's risk. The chance of exposure decreases as the number of partners decreases, so people in mutually monogamous relationships are at lower risk for acquiring STDs. This information can be obtained by asking, "How many sex (or drug) partners have you had over the past 6 months?" The nurse must avoid assumptions about the sexual partner(s) based on the client's gender, age, race, or any other factor. Stereotypes and assumptions about who people are and what they do are common problems that keep interviewers from asking questions that gather useful information. For example, one should not assume that because a male is homosexual he has more than one partner. Also it is important to remember that the long incubation of HIV and the subclinical phase of many STDs lead some monogamous individuals to assume erroneously that they are not at risk.

Identifying whether the person has sexual contact with men, women, or both can be accomplished by simply asking, "Do you have sex with men, women, or both?" This lets the client know that the nurse is open to hearing about these behaviors; the client is then more likely to share information that is relevant to sexual practices and risk. Women who are exclusively lesbian are at low risk for acquiring STDs, but bisexual women may transmit STDs between male and female partners. Also, men may have sexual contact with other men and not label themselves as homosexual. Therefore education to reduce risk that is aimed at homosexual males will not be heeded by men who do not see themselves as homosexual. In such situations, the nurse might ask, "When was the last time you had sex with another male?"

Some sexual practices, such as unprotected anal or vaginal intercourse, oral-anal contact, and insertion of a finger or fist into the rectum can have greater exposure to and transmission of STDs. The risk is due to possible transmission of enteric organisms or physical trauma during sexual encounters. The nurse might ask "Tell me the kinds of sexual practices in which you engage. This can help tell me what risks you may have and the type of tests we should do." Clients who engage in genital-anal, oral-anal, or oral-genital contact will need throat and rectal cultures for some STDs as well as cervical and urethral cultures.

Drug use is linked to STD transmission in several ways. Sexual enhancers, such as alcohol or other drugs, put people at risk because they can impair judgment about engaging in risky behaviors. Drugs such as crack cocaine or amyl nitrate (also referred to as poppers) may enable multiple orgasms. This increases both the frequency of sexual contacts and the chances of contracting STDs. Addiction to a drug may lead to intense craving of the drug and to trading sex for the drug. For this reason, the nurse must gather information on the type and frequency of drug use and the presence of risk behaviors.

Based on the information obtained in the sexual history and risk assessment, the nurse can identify specific education and counseling needs. Nursing action focuses on contracting with clients to change behavior.

Safer Sex

Sexual abstinence is the best way to prevent STDs. However, for many people, sexual abstinence is undesirable; thus information about making sexual behavior safer must be taught. Safer sexual activities include masturbation on intact skin, dry kissing, touching, fantasy, and vaginal and oral sex using a condom.

Briefly Noted

Most agency protocols recommend the use of latex condoms. Some may be lubricated with nonoxynol-9, a spermicide that may have virucidal properties. The effectiveness of such chemical barriers is still undetermined. For some women, chemical barriers can cause extravasation of the vaginal lining and cervix and lead to breaks in tissue that can facilitate transmission of some STDs (Berer, 1992).

The effective use of condoms can prevent the exchange of body fluids during sexual activity and prevent both pregnancy and STDs. While the failure rate of condoms is about 3.1%, this seems to be related to incorrect use rather than condom failure (Novello et al, 1993). Information about their proper use and how to talk to a partner about them is needed. Condom use may be viewed as inconvenient, messy, or decreasing sensation. Moreover, alcohol use may accompany sexual activity, which also may decrease condom use (Hale, 1996). Nurses can encourage clients to become more skilled in discussing safer sex and learn how to effectively use a condom.

Female condoms can also be a barrier to body fluid contact and therefore protect against pregnancy and STDs. The main advantage of the female condom is that the woman controls its use. Made of polyurethane, it may be used if a latex sensitivity develops to regular male condoms. Symptoms of latex allergy include penile, vaginal, or rectal itching or swelling after use of a male condom or diaphragm. The female condom, which costs about $3, consists of a sheath over two rings, with one closed end that fits over the cervix.

Clients should understand that it is important to know the risk behavior of their sexual partners, including a history of injection drug use and STDs, bisexuality, and any current symptoms. This is because each sexual partner is potentially exposed to all the STDs of the persons that the other partner has been sexually active with.

Drug Use

Injection drug use is risky since pathogens can be injected when needles and syringes are shared. During injection drug use, small quantities of drugs are repeatedly injected. Blood is withdrawn into the syringe and is then injected back into the user's vein. People need to be advised against using injectable drugs and sharing needles, syringes, or other drug paraphernalia. If equipment is shared, it should be in contact with full-strength bleach for 30 seconds, and then rinsed with water several times to prevent injecting bleach (Centers for Disease Control and Prevention, 1994d).

People who inject drugs are difficult to reach for health care services. Effective outreach programs include using community peers, increasing accessibility of drug treatment programs combined with HIV testing and counseling, and long-term repeat contacts after completion of the program (Centers for Disease Control, 1990b).

Community Outreach

Because of the illegal nature of injectable drugs and the poverty associated with HIV, many people at risk do not seek health care. Nurses can take services into the community. Specifically, nurses and other workers can provide information on safer sex, drug treatment programs, and discontinuation of drug use or safer drug use practices (e.g. using new needles and syringes with each injection). Some programs provide sterile needles and syringes, condoms, and information about the location of anonymous test sites.

Community Education

Providing accurate health information to large numbers of people is vital for preventing the spread of STDs. Nurses who work in the community can provide current information about HIV and other STDs. It is best to provide this information in places where people normally gather such as schools, businesses, shelters, soup kitchens, or churches.

Topics to include are:

- Number of people diagnosed with AIDS and STDs, number infected, and modes of transmission
- Ways to prevent infection
- Common symptoms of illness
- Need for a compassionate response to those afflicted
- Available community resources.

Evaluation

Evaluation is based on whether risky behavior is changed to safe behavior and, ultimately, whether illness is prevented. Condom use is evaluated for consistency of use if the client is sexually active. Other behaviors can be evaluated for their implementation, such as abstinence or monogamy. At the community level, behavioral surveys can be done to measure reported condom use and condom sales, and measures of STD incidence and prevalence can be calculated to evaluate the effectiveness of intervention (American Public Health Association, 1991).

Secondary Prevention

Secondary prevention includes screening for STDs to ensure their early identification and treatment, and follow-up with sex and drug-using partners to prevent further spread. In general, client teaching and counseling should include preventing reinfection with a curable STD, managing symptoms, and preventing the infection of others with chronic STDs. Testing and counseling for HIV are discussed later.

People who have engaged in high-risk behavior need to be tested. People with the following behaviors are at risk and should be offered the HIV antibody test:

- A history of STDs
- Multiple sex partners
- Injection drug use
- Those who have intercourse without using a condom; those who have intercourse with someone who has another partner, and those who have had sex with a prostitute

- Males with a history of homosexual or bisexual activity
- People who have been a sexual partner to anyone in one of these groups
- Those who underwent a blood transfusion between January 1978 and March 1985.

If HIV infection is discovered before the onset of symptoms, the disease process can be monitored for changes, such as a decrease in the CD4+ lymphocyte count or viral load. Prophylactic therapy with antibiotics or protease inhibitors can be started early in the infection to delay the onset of symptomatic illness.

HIV Test Counseling

An important part of care is counseling about the HIV antibody test. Clients need to know that the antibody test is not diagnostic for AIDS but is indicative of HIV infection. During counseling the nurse should:

- Assess risk
- Discuss risk behaviors and ways to overcome barriers to change
- Develop a risk-reduction plan
- Establish a follow-up appointment to receive test results and posttest counseling.

Pretest Counseling

During pretest counseling the nurse will

- Conduct the risk assessment
- Provide relevant teaching as described in the primary prevention section of the chapter
- Talk with clients about how they will cope with a positive test
- Assess support systems
- Ask clients to review how they have handled difficult situations in the past can determine how they might cope with learning they are HIV positive.
- Tell the client who will have access to the test results. Although AIDS is reported nationally, the reporting of HIV infection varies among states. States that mandate the reporting of HIV infection are shown in Table 24-3.

Because there is no cure or vaccine available, preventing the transmission of HIV requires a risk assessment of the client's behavior and counseling on how to reduce identified risks. Sexually active individuals with multiple partners must be encouraged to abstain, to enter a mutually monogamous relationship, or to use condoms. Injection drug users should be advised to enter a treatment program or discontinue drug use. If they continue to use drugs, they should be warned not to share needles, syringes, or any other drug paraphernalia.

Posttest Counseling

Persons who have a negative test result are HIV negative, and they should be counseled about risk-reduction activities to prevent any future transmission. They need to understand that the test may not be truly negative, because it does not identify recent infections that may have been acquired several weeks before the test. As noted earlier, seroconversion takes from 6 to 12 weeks. The client needs to know the means of viral transmission and how to avoid infection. The HIV-infected person is responsible to do this:

- Have regular medical evaluations and follow-up care
- Avoid donating blood, plasma, body organs, other tissues, or sperm
- Take precautions against exchanging body fluids during sexual activity
- Inform sexual or injection-drug–using partners of potential exposure to HIV or arrange to have the health department notify them
- Inform health care providers of the HIV infection
- Consider the risk of perinatal transmission and use contraceptives.

The nurse must counsel anyone who is antibody positive about the need for reducing risks and notifying partners. If the client is unwilling or hesitant to notify past partners, nurses can do so. Psychosocial counseling is indicated when positive HIV test results precipitate acute anxiety, depression, or suicidal ideation. Follow-up counseling sessions and telephone calls can monitor the client's status. The client should be told about available counseling services and cautioned to consider carefully who to inform of the test results. Clients should not tell people who have no reason to know. Many individuals have told others about their HIV positive test, only to experience isolation and discrimination. The nurse should help the person explore plans for the future and advise about avoiding stress, drugs, and infections.

Partner Notification

Partner notification, also known as contact tracing, is a public health intervention aimed at controlling STDs. It is done by confidentially identifying and notifying exposed sexual and injection drug-using partners of those found to have reportable STDs. Partner notification programs usually occur in conjunction with reportable disease requirements and are carried out by most health departments.

Individuals diagnosed with a reportable STD are asked to provide the names and locations of their partners so that they can be informed of their exposure and obtain the necessary treatment. Clients may be encouraged to notify their partners and to encourage them to seek treatment. If the client agrees to do so, suggestions on how to tell partners and how to deal with possible reactions may be explored. In some instances, clients may feel more comfortable if the nurse notifies those who are exposed. If clients contact their partners about possible infection, the nurse contacts health care providers or clinics to verify examination of exposed partners.

If the client prefers not to participate in notifying partners, the nurse contacts them—often by a home visit—and counsels them to seek evaluation and treatment. The client is offered literature regarding treatment, risk reduction, and the test site's location and hours of operation. The identity of the infected client who names sexual and injection drug-using partners cannot be revealed. Maintaining confidentiality is critical with all STDs but particularly with HIV, because anti-discrimination laws may not be in place or may be inadequate.

Tertiary Prevention

Tertiary prevention can apply to many of the chronic STDs, such as HSV, HIV, and untreated syphilis. For viral STDs, much of this effort focuses on managing symptoms and psychosocial support regarding future interpersonal relations. Many clients report feeling contaminated, and support groups can help them cope with chronic STDs.

Much of the tertiary prevention focuses on clients with AIDS who return home and are unable to provide care for themselves due to progressing illness. Nurses working in the community can conduct physical assessments and make recommendations to the family about obtaining additional care services or maintaining the client in the home. Case management is important in all phases of HIV infection but is a particularly important activity in this stage to ensure that clients have adequate services to meet their needs. It may be necessary to assist in getting funds for expensive medicines and maintaining infection-control standards, reducing risk behaviors, identifying sources of respite care for caretakers, or referring clients for home or hospice care.

Nurses teach families about managing symptomatic illness by preventing deteriorating conditions such as diarrhea, skin breakdown, and inadequate nutrition. They also teach caregivers about infection control in the home. Caregivers may be afraid of "catching" the disease yet do not want to wear gloves because this may make the patient feel isolated. Universal precautions procedures are taught to caregivers in the home setting. All blood and articles soiled with body fluids must be handled as if they were infectious or contaminated by blood-borne pathogens. Gloves should be worn whenever hands will be expected to touch nonintact skin, mucous membranes, blood, or other fluids. A mask, goggles, and gown should also be worn if there is potential for splashing or spraying of infectious material during any care.

All protective equipment should be worn only once and then disposed of. If the skin or mucous membranes of the caregiver come in contact with body fluids, the skin should be washed with soap and water, and the mucous membranes should be flushed with water as soon as possible after the exposure. Thorough hand washing with soap and water—a major infection-control measure—should be conducted whenever hands become contaminated and whenever gloves or other protective equipment (mask, gown) is removed. Soiled clothing or linen should be washed in a washing machine filled with hot water using bleach as an additive and dried on the hot air cycle of a dryer.

Healthy People 2010 and HIV, Hepatitis, and Sexually Transmitted Diseases

In the United States, HIV, hepatitis and sexually transmitted disease all are significant causes of illness, disability and death. There are 7 different types of Hepatitis and 25 infectious organisms transmitted primarily through sexual activity. All of these diseases are preventable. Select objectives for the nation are listed in the *Healthy People 2010* box.

Healthy People 2010
HIV, Hepatitis, and Sexually Transmitted Diseases

Healthy People 2010 related objectives are:

13-1   Reduce AIDS among adolescents and adults

13-2   Reduce the number of new AIDS cases among adolescent and adult men who have sex with men.

13-3   Reduce the number of new AIDS cases among females and males who inject drugs.

13-4   Reduce the number of new AIDS cases among adolescent and adult men who have sex with men and inject drugs.

13-5   Reduce the number of cases of HIV infection among adolescents and adults.

13-6   Increase the proportion of sexually active persons who use condoms.

13-11   Increase the proportion of adults with tuberculosis (TB) who have been tested for HIV.

13-12   Increase the proportion of adults in publicly funded HIV counseling and testing sites who are screened for common bacterial sexually transmitted diseases (STDs) (chlamydia, gonorrhea, and syphilis) and are immunized against hepatitis B virus.

13-13   Increase the proportion of HIV-infected adolescents and adults who receive testing, treatment, and prophylaxis consistent with current Public Health Service treatment guidelines.

13-14   Reduce deaths from HIV infection.

13-15   Extend the interval of time between an initial diagnosis of HIV infection and AIDS diagnosis in order to increase years of life of an individual infected with HIV.

13-16   Increase years of life of an HIV-infected person by extending the interval of time between an AIDS diagnosis and death.

13-17   Reduce new cases of perinatally acquired HIV infection.

14-2   Reduce chronic hepatitis B virus infections in infants and young children (perinatal infections).

14-3   Reduce hepatitis B.

14-6   Reduce hepatitis A.

14-9   Reduce hepatitis C.

14-10   Increase the proportion of persons with chronic hepatitis C infection identified by state and local health departments.

14-28   Increase hepatitis B vaccine coverage among high-risk groups.

25-1   Reduce the proportion of adolescents and young adults with *Chlamydia trachomatis* infections.

25-2   Reduce gonorrhea.

25-3   Eliminate sustained domestic transmission of primary and secondary syphilis.

25-4   Reduce the proportion of adults with genital herpes infection.

25-5   Reduce the proportion of persons with human papillomavirus (HPV) infection.

25-6   Reduce the proportion of females who have ever required treatment for pelvic inflammatory disease (PID).

25-7   Reduce the proportion of childless females with fertility problems who have had a sexually transmitted disease or who have required treatment for pelvic inflammatory disease (PID).

25-8   Reduce HIV infections in adolescent and young adult females aged 13 to 24 years that are associated with heterosexual contact.

25-10   Reduce neonatal consequences from maternal sexually transmitted diseases, including chlamydial pneumonia, gonococcal and chlamydial ophthalmia neonatorum, laryngeal papillomatosis (from human papillomavirus infection), neonatal herpes, and preterm birth and low birth weight associated with bacterial vaginosis.

25-11   Increase the proportion of adolescents who abstain from sexual intercourse or use condoms if currently sexually active.

25-16   Increase the proportion of sexually active females aged 25 years and under who are screened annually for genital chlamydia infections.

25-17   Increase the proportion of pregnant females screened for sexually transmitted diseases (including HIV infection and bacterial vaginosis) during prenatal health care visits, according to recognized standards.

25-19   Increase the proportion of all sexually active transmitted disease clinic patients who are being treated for bacterial STDs (chlamydia, gonorrhea, and syphilis) and who are offered provider referral services for their sex partners.

Clinical Application

When Yvonne Jacks, a 20-year-old woman, visits the Hopetown City Health Department's maternity clinic, she is 14 weeks pregnant. She is single but has been in a steady relationship for the past 6 months with Phil. She states that she has no other children. The HIV test done as part of the routine prenatal workup is positive. Yvonne reacts with an expression of disbelief about the positive test results. Understanding that this is a common reaction and that Yvonne will not be able to concentrate on all of the questions and information that need to be covered, the nurse prioritizes essential information to obtain and provide during this visit.

A. *What questions does the nurse need to ask regarding controlling the spread of HIV to others?*

B. *What information should the nurse give to Yvonne?*

Answers are in the back of the book.

Remember This!

- Nearly all STDs are preventable because they are transmitted through specific, known behaviors.
- STDs are one of the most serious public health problems in the United States. HIV infection is a major public health problem.
- There is an increased incidence of drug-resistant gonococcal infection.
- STDs are more likely to affect certain groups in greater numbers. Risk factors are being under 25 years of age, being a member of a minority group, living in an urban area, being poor, and using crack cocaine.

- The increasing incidence, morbidity, and mortality of STDs support the need for nurses to provide health education.
- Many STDs do not produce symptoms in clients. Other STDs, such as HPV (genital warts), HIV, and HSV (genital herpes), are associated with cancer.
- Aside from death, the most serious complications caused by STDs are pelvic inflammatory disease, infertility, ectopic pregnancy, neonatal morbidity and mortality, and neoplasia.
- AIDS is the most extreme stage of HIV infection. As more is learned about methods to prevent disease progression, such as effective medications, stress reduction, and proper nutrition, greater emphasis is being placed on early detection and management of HIV infection.
- HIV testing plays an important role in early detection and treatment and provides opportunities for risk assessment and preventive counseling.
- Partner notification, also known as contact tracing, may be done by the infected client or by the health professional. It includes identifying, contacting, and encouraging evaluation and treatment of sexual and injectable-drug–using partners.
- HIV infection has created a new group of people needing health care. This rapidly growing population is placing demands on an already stretched health care system.
- Most of the care that is provided, both home and outpatient care, is done in the community. This reduces direct health care costs but increases the need for support of home and community health services.

? What Would You Do?

1. Identify the number of reported cases of AIDS and the number of reported cases of HIV infection in your community and state (if reportable in your state). How are the cases distributed by age, sex, geographical location, and race?
2. Identify the location or locations of HIV testing services in your community. Are the test results anonymous or confidential? Describe how and to whom the results are reported. Do you agree with how reporting is handled in your state?
3. Identify counseling and home care services that are available for the person with HIV infection within your community. Are they adequate to meet the needs of those infected? How much do these services cost?
4. Form small groups and role-play a nurse-client interaction involving a risk assessment and counseling regarding safer sex and injection drug-using practices.

REFERENCES

American Public Health Association: *Healthy communities 2000 model standards,* ed 3, Washington, D.C., 1991, American Public Health Association.

Aral SO: The social context of syphilis persistence in the southeastern United States, *Sex Transmit Dis* 23(1):9-15, 1996.

Aral SO, Holmes KK: Epidemiology of sexual behavior and sexually transmitted diseases. In Holmes KK, et al (editors): *Sexually transmitted diseases,* New York, 1990, McGraw-Hill.

Berer M: Adverse effects of nonoxynol-9, *Lancet* 340:615-616, 1992.

Brown ZA, Selke S, Zeh J, Kopelman J, Maslow A, et al: The acquisition of herpes simplex virus during pregnancy, *N Engl J Med* 337(8):509-515, 1997.

Campbell C: *Women, families & HIV/AIDS,* Cambridge, 1999, Cambridge University Press.

Centers for Disease Control: Guidelines for effective school health education to prevent the spread of AIDS, *MMWR* 37(S-2):1-14, 1988.

Centers for Disease Control: First 100,000 cases of acquired immunodeficiency syndrome: United States, *MMWR* 38:561, 1989.

Centers for Disease Control: Nosocomial transmission of hepatitis B virus associated with a spring-loaded fingerstick device–California, *MMWR* 39(35):610-613, 1990a.

Centers for Disease Control: Update: reducing HIV transmission in intravenous-drug users not in drug treatment–United States, *MMWR* 39(31):529, 536-538, 1990b.

Centers for Disease Control: Hepatitis B virus: a comprehensive strategy for eliminating transmission in the United States through universal childhood vaccination–ACIP, *MMWR* 40(RR-13):1-25, 1991.

Centers for Disease Control: Chancroid–United States, 1981-1990: evidence for underreporting of cases, *MMWR* 41(SS-3):57-61, 1992.

Centers for Disease Control and Prevention: Decreased susceptibility of *Neisseria gonorrhoeae* to fluoroquinolones–Ohio and Hawaii, 1992-1994, *MMWR* 43(18):325-327, 1994a.

Centers for Disease Control and Prevention: *HIV/AIDS Surveillance Rep* 5(4):3-33, 1994b.

Centers for Disease Control and Prevention: Human immunodeficiency virus transmission in household settings–United States, *MMWR* 43(347):353-356, 1994c.

Centers for Disease Control and Prevention: Knowledge and practices among injecting-drug users of bleach use for equipment disinfection: New York City, 1993, *MMWR* 43(24):439, 445-446, 1994d.

Centers for Disease Control and Prevention: AIDS among children–United States, *MMWR* 45(46):1006-1010, 1996a.

Centers for Disease Control and Prevention: Prevention of perinatal hepatitis B through enhanced case management–Connecticut, 1994-95 and United States, 1994, *MMWR* 45(27):584-587, 1996b.

Centers for Disease Control and Prevention: School-based HIV prevention education–United States, 1994, *MMWR* 45(35):760-765, 1996c.

Centers for Disease Control and Prevention: *CDC, HRSA work to implement CARE act provision. HIV/AIDS prevention,* Atlanta, March, 1997a, Centers for Disease Control and Prevention.

Centers for Disease Control and Prevention: CDC reports first-ever decline in AIDS diagnoses—treatment and prevention advances spur new trend, *HIV/AIDS prevention,* Atlanta, December, 1997b, Centers for Disease Control and Prevention.

Centers for Disease Control and Prevention: *Chlamydia trachomatis* genital infections–United States, 1995, *MMWR* 46(9):193-198, 1997c.

Centers for Disease Control and Prevention: Focus on women and HIV, *HIV/AIDS prevention,* Atlanta, March, 1997d, Centers for Disease Control and Prevention.

Centers for Disease Control and Prevention: *HIV/AIDS Surveillance Rep* 9(1):3-37, 1997e.

Centers for Disease Control and Prevention: Nosocomial hepatitis B virus infection associated with reusable fingerstick blood sampling devices, Ohio and New York City, *MMWR* 46(10):217-221, 1997f.

Centers for Disease Control and Prevention: Summary of notifiable diseases, 1996, *MMWR* 45:53, 1997g.

Centers for Disease Control and Prevention: AIDS among person aged >50 years–United States, 1991-1996, *MMWR* 47(2):21-27, 1998a.

Centers for Disease Control and Prevention: 1998 Guidelines for treatment of sexually transmitted diseases, *MMWR* 47:RR-1, 1998b.

Centers for Disease Control and Prevention: *The role of HIV surveillance as U.S. enters new era in the epidemic,* January, 1998c, available online: http://www.cdc.gov/nchstp/od/surveillance.htm.

Corey L: Genital herpes. In Holmes KK, Mardh PF, Sparling PF, Wiesner PJ (editors): *Sexually transmitted diseases,* New York, 1990, McGraw-Hill.

Crum CP, Nuovo GJ: *Genital papillomaviruses and related neoplasms,* New York, 1991, Raven Press.

Division of STD Prevention: *Sexually transmitted disease surveillance–1996,* Atlanta, 1997, Centers for Disease Control and Prevention.

Deguchi T, Saito I, Tanaka M, Sato K, Deguchi K, et al: Fluoroquinolone treatment failure in gonorrhea, *Sex Transmit Dis* 24(5):247, 1997.

Fleming DT, McQuillan GM, Johnson RE, Nahmias AJ, Aral SO, et al: Herpes simplex virus type 2 in the United States, 1976 to 1994, *N Engl J Med* 337(16):1105-1111, 1997.

Gostin LO, Ward JW, Baker AC: National HIV case reporting for the United States, *N Engl J Med* 337(16): 1162-1167, 1997.

Hale PJ: Women's self-efficacy and sexually transmitted disease preventive behaviors, *Res Nurs Health* 19:101-110, 1996.

Hook E, Handsfield H: Gonococcal infections in the adult. In Holmes KK, Mardh P, Sparling PF, Wiesner PJ (editors): *Sexually transmitted diseases,* New York, 1990, McGraw-Hill.

Hughes AM: HIV related pain, *Am J Nurs* 99(6):20, 1999.

Immunization Action Coalition/Hepatitis B Coalition: *Needle tips,* 6:1, 1996.

Institute of Medicine: *The hidden epidemic: confronting sexually transmitted diseases,* Washington, D.C., 1997, National Academy Press.

Krieger JN: Trichomoniasis in men: old issues and new data, *Sex Transmit Dis* 22(2):83-96, 1995.

Levy JA: *HIV and the pathogenesis of AIDS,* Washington, D.C., 1998, ASM Press.

Martens KA: Sexually transmitted genital tract infection during pregnancy, *Emerg Med Clin North Am* 12(1):91-113, 1994.

Novello AC, Peterson HB, Arrowsmith-Lowe JT, et al: Condom use for the prevention of sexual transmission of HIV infection, *JAMA* 269(22):2840, 1993.

Occupational Safety and Health Administration: *Occupational exposure to bloodborne pathogens,* Standard 1910, 1030, Richmond, Va, 1992, Department of Labor and Industry.

Pantaleo G, Cohen O, Graziosi C, Vaccarezza M, Paolucci S, et al: Immunopathogenesis of human immunodeficiency virus infection. In DeVita VT, Hellman S, Rosenberf SA: AIDS: *Biology, diagnosis, treatment and prevention,* 1997, Lippincott-Raven.

Paisarntantiwong R, Brockmann S, Clarke L, Landesman S, Feldman J: The relationship of vaginal trichomoniasis and pelvic inflammatory disease among women colonized with chlamydia trachomatis, *Sex Transmit Dis* 22(6):344-347, 1995.

Stephenson NL, Lee RT: Creative strategies for updating knowledge on sexually transmitted diseases, *J Contin Educ Nurs* 29(1):32-34, 1998.

World Health Organization: The HIV/AIDS pandemic: 1993 overview, WHO Global Programme on AIDS, pub no WHO/GPA/CNP/EVA/93-1, Geneva, Switzerland, 1993, World Health Organization.

Wortley PM, Fleming PL: AIDS in women in the United States: Recent trends. *JAMA* 278, 911-916, 1997.

Zenilman J, Bonner M, Sharp K, et al: Penicillinase-producing *Neisseria gonorrhoeae* in Dade County, Florida: evidence of core-group transmitters and the impact of illicit antibiotics, *Sex Transmit Dis* 15(1):45, 1988.

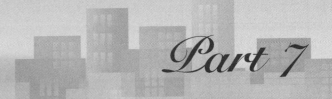

Part 7

Community Health Nurse: Roles and Functions

At one time the role of nurse in the community included primarily visiting clients at home and identifying cases of communicable disease. Over the decades the role has become multifaceted and now involves community-oriented practice. The community health nurse's role is focused on improving the health of individuals and families through the delivery of personal health services with emphasis on primary prevention, health promotion, and health protection. Nurses are able to provide care to individuals, families, and communities in a variety of settings and roles.

With increasing emphasis on the community, community health nurses recognize that addressing community health issues requires meeting the needs of the individuals, families, and groups who are the nucleus of the community. Unlike in the past, when the primary practice setting for the nurse was the hospital, nurses deal with their clients in many settings. Regardless of type of client, practice setting, specialty area of practice, or the functional role of the nurse, the community health nurse advocates for clients in meeting their needs through the health care system.

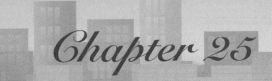

Chapter 25

Community Health Nursing in the Local Health Department

MARY EURE FISHER

OBJECTIVES

After reading this chapter, the student should be able to:
- Define public health, community health nursing, and local community roles.
- Describe the similarities and differences in local health department roles.
- Identify trends in nursing in public health.
- Describe examples of nursing roles.
- Identify educational preparation of nurses and skills essential to practice at different levels.

- Discuss lessons learned from the past that may affect the future of nursing in public health.
- Describe the role of the nurse in a disaster.
- Explore team concepts in public health settings.
- Identify functions of nurses in public health.
- Distinguish the scope and standards of community health nursing from public health and other nursing roles.

CHAPTER OUTLINE

Definitions
History and Trends of Public Health
Roles of Nurses in Public Health
Issues and Trends

Education and Knowledge
   Requirements for Community Health Nurses
   Certification for Community Health Nurses
National Health Objectives
Functions of Nurses in Public Health

KEY TERMS

advocate: one who works to protect the rights of the client while supporting the client's responsibility for self-determination.

assessor: a health professional who uses data in a systematic way to help identify needs, questions to be addressed, abilities, and available resources.

case manager: a nurse who works to enhance continuity and provide appropriate care for clients whose health problems are actually or potentially chronic and complex.

counselor: a health professional who works with people to achieve workable solutions for their problems or conflicts.

disaster responder: a person who works as a member of a team in a disaster to feed back information to relief workers to facilitate paid rescue and recovery.

local public health departments: the agency responsible for implementing and enforcing local, state, and federal public health codes and ordinances and providing essential public health programs to a community.

outreach worker: a health worker who makes a special, focused effort to find people with specific health problems for the purpose of increasing their access to health services.

Continued

KEY TERMS—cont'd

primary caregiver: the health care professional who is primarily responsible for providing for health needs of clients.

public health: organized efforts designed to fulfill society's interest in assuring conditions in which people can be healthy.

public health programs: programs designed with the goal of improving a population's health status.

referral resource: an agency or source in the community with whom nurses communicate and to which clients are sent for assistance.

role model: a person who is an example of professional or personal behavior for others.

"Just as all politics is local, all health is local" (Bunker, et al, 1994, p. 87). Understanding nursing in public health at the local level requires understanding the different responsibilities and characteristics of the local public health department and the nurses who work there. **Local public health departments** have responsibilities that vary depending on the locality, but they are the agencies that are responsible for implementing and enforcing local, state, and federal public health codes and ordinances and providing essential public health programs to a community. The health department's authority is delegated by the state for specific functions (Box 25-1). Because of this delegation of specific duties, local public health agencies vary greatly from state to state, as well as within states, depending on the expectations of local governments.

The *goal* of the local public health department is to safeguard the public's health and to improve the community's health status. Nurses work with a wide range of staff within the health department and the community to meet this goal including physicians, nutritionists, environmental health professionals, paraprofessional home visitors, and other health workers. About two thirds of the nurses in public health do not have baccalaureate degrees but are providing public health services based on skills acquired through experience. Nurses in associate degree programs today are being provided education to function in public health.

DEFINITIONS

Community health nursing focuses on individuals, families, and groups who live, work, go to school, and play. *Community health nursing* is defined as the synthesis of nursing theory and public health theory applied to promoting, preserving, and monitoring the health of populations through the delivery of personal health care services to individuals, families and groups. *Community health nurses* work with these clients while looking at the effect of their health status on the health of the community as a whole. The Institute of Medicine defined **public health** in its 1988 Report as "fulfilling society's interest in assuring conditions in which people can be healthy" (p. 7).

Public health nursing is defined in Chapter 1 and is distinguished from the community health nurse by the emphasis by the public health nurse on the population rather than the individual, family, and group.

Additional knowledge, efforts, and skills are necessary for a nurse to go beyond focusing on the health needs of the individual, family, or group to focusing on the health needs

---

Box 25-1   Public Health Agency Functions

Generally, local public health agencies perform the following functions:

- Provide and disseminate health information
- Provide leadership in health planning
- Provide essential public health and environmental services
- Collect statistics on births
- File a certificate for every birth or death in that area

---

of populations (see Chapter 1). This additional effort distinguishes the public health nurse from the community health nurse and those who are simply practicing in the community setting. Community health nursing practices arise from knowledge gained from the physical and social sciences, psychological and spiritual fields, environmental areas, political arena, economics, and life experience.

Public health programs are often designed with the goal of improving a population's health status. Public health programs include public education, outreach, record keeping, professional education for providers, surveillance, compliance to regulations for some institutions/agencies and school systems, and follow-up of noncompliant populations, such as persons with active, untreated tuberculosis. Public health programs are frequently implemented by the development of partnerships or coalitions with other providers, agencies, and groups in the location being served.

The duties of local health departments vary depending on the state and local public health codes and ordinances and the responsibilities assigned by the state and local governments. Usually the local public health department provides for the administration, regulatory oversight, public health, and environmental services for a geographical area. The majority of local public health agencies will be involved in the following:

- Collecting and analyzing vital statistics
- Providing health education and information to the population served
- Receiving reports, investigating and controlling communicable diseases
- Protecting the environment to reduce the risk to health
- Providing personal health services to particular populations at risk or with limited access to care
- Identifying public health problems for at-risk and high-risk populations

Nurses in public health will be involved in some of these activities depending on the local public health agency and local need.

Public health is not a branch of medicine; it is an organized community approach designed to prevent disease, promote health, and protect populations. It crosses many disciplines and is based on the scientific core of epidemiology (IOM, 1988). Nurses in public health work with multidisciplinary teams of people both within the public health areas and in other human services agencies.

HISTORY AND TRENDS OF PUBLIC HEALTH

A person born today can expect to live 30 years longer than the person born in 1900. Medical care accounts for a minimal number of years of that increase, while public health is responsible for the majority of years through prevention efforts: changes in social policies, community actions, and individual and group behavior changes (U.S. Department of Health and Human Services, 2000).

Historically, nurses working in public health were valued by and important to society and functioned in an autonomous setting. They worked with populations and in settings that were not of interest to other health care disciplines or groups. Much of the public health services were delivered to the poor and to women and children, who did not have political power or voice.

In 1996 nearly 900,000 fewer cases of measles were reported than in 1941 (Turnock, 1997, p. 1). Nurses in public health were a major factor in accomplishing the immunizations that accounted for this dramatic decrease in measles. The general public was not informed about how this immunization activity was accomplished and the resulting effect on improving health and lowering health care cost. Today most of the public do not understand what nurses in public health do, because these nurses have been busy "doing" and not informing the community at large about their public health activities.

Briefly Noted

In this era of managed care a critical question is whether public health will take a position as an advocate for the community or as a part of the medicine marketplace as just another commodity. Once medicine was seen as a "mission-driven, value-laden" profession, but now it is seen as a partner with managed care bargaining for roles and resources and not as a profession serving society for the common good (Citrin, 1998, p. 351). What will be the role of community health nurses in the twenty-first century?

ROLES OF NURSES IN PUBLIC HEALTH

In Virginia (Virginia Department of Health, 1997), a statewide committee looked at the role of nursing in light of the changes in health care. The committee developed a document intended to identify roles within the context of the core public health functions (see Chapter 1) and to identify the educational program needs of staff that would prepare them to function effectively in the changing public health care arena. Essential elements of the nurse's role were identified; they are presented below.

HOW TO Implement the Core Public Health Functions in a Community: Essential Elements of the Public Health Role

- Conduct community assessments
- Prevent and control epidemics
- Provide a safe and healthy environment
- Measure performance, effectiveness, and outcomes of health services
- Promote healthy lifestyles
- Provide laboratory testing
- Provide targeted outreach to vulnerable populations and form partnerships
- Provide personal health care services
- Conduct research and create innovations (in programs)
- Mobilize the community for action

From National Association of City and County Health Officials: *Blueprint for a healthy community: a guide for local health departments,* Washington, D.C., 1994, National Association of City and County Health Officials.

These essential elements are implemented through multidisciplinary public health teams.

In the effort to contain costs and develop leaner, more efficient work-forces at all levels of government, public agencies such as local public health departments have had major changes over the last decade, and more changes will come in the new millennium. These changes may be seen as an opportunity to return to the core values of public health, allowing public health to focus on the prevention of disease, promotion of health, and protection of populations and the environment. In the past several decades public health has moved away from these functions and has provided primary care services.

Driving forces behind these changes are the economy and the increase in managed care providers. To meet local public health needs, primary care responsibility has shifted from the local health department to the development of partnerships with a variety of existing individuals, groups, institutions, and hospitals. These new arrangements give rise to many concerns about the available health care for the uninsured and underinsured. The nurses' role in this latest shift in health care delivery is still being developed for many agencies. The *case management* role is a renewed effort for nurses at the community level rather than having case management done at institutions, such as hospitals.

Evidence-Based Practice

The descriptive study referenced below looked at a health department parenting project to see whether teen mothers' self-esteem, social support, and parenting competence improved while receiving case management services from nurses during the first 18 months of motherhood. A sample of 56 first-time teen mothers participated in the study; 45% were Hispanic. Nurses received special training in assessment of and intervention with teen mothers. The nurses provided assessments, interventions, referrals for medical care, vocational training and finances, and education in prenatal and postnatal care, diet, family planning, child care and child health, and safe-baby environment. The nurses also provided for transportation for mothers to keep appointments and encouraged the teens to stay in school. The nurses used home visits and phone calls to maintain contact with the mothers.

Data were collected at 6, 12, and 18 months using the Rosenberg Self-Esteem Scale, the Inventory of Socially Supportive Behaviors by Barrera, and Parental Sense of Competency Scale by Gibard et al. The study results indicated that mothers need special attention during the first months of parenting to enhance that self-esteem and to encourage better parenting. Social support was found to decrease as the child moved toward 18 months and the parents' competence in caring for the baby slightly increased.

APPLICATION IN PRACTICE

Teen pregnancy is a national concern because it usually results in less education and less future earning power for the teen mother. Early intervention to promote self-esteem and to encourage social support from family, friends, and agencies and competent parenting skills for the mother may make a difference for the health of the baby and the mother's ability to become a happy, healthy, productive adult.

Parenting, competence, social support, and self-esteem in teen mothers case managed by public health nurses, *Public Health Nurs* 15(6):432, 1998.

In 2001 about 44 million American citizens lacked health insurance. These uninsured individuals seek services on a sliding payment scale from such sources as university or public hospital clinics or from a variety of free clinics. Community health nurses can provide direct care and serve as a bridge between these populations and the resource needs for this at-risk group by approaching health care providers on behalf of individuals seeking medical/health services and keeping the needs of this population on the political agenda.

Frequently the indigent and low-income populations lack the knowledge and skills to negotiate the complex medical system made up of physicians and hospitals. This population needs education and training in identifying their problems, approaches to self-care, and illness prevention strategies and lifestyle choices that will affect their health. Community health nurses are skilled in working with this population, which is often defined by other health providers as noncompliant, since this population often faces barriers (such as inad-

equate transportation) to keeping appointments and lacks the knowledge to understand and follow medical instructions.

Although indigent and low-income populations have always benefited from community health nursing services, the populations most acutely in need of services have changed dramatically over the last couple of decades. Of particular concern are the number of young women and their partners who are substance abusers and have risky behaviors, such as hostility and aggression, that put their pregnancy or children at high risk of injury or abuse. Nurses and local public health departments have had to provide innovative, collaborative approaches to prepare their staff to work effectively with this population. As with any profession, ongoing educational resources are essential for nursing staff to develop new skills to meet ever-changing public health challenges.

At the 1998 annual meeting of the Association of State and Territorial Directors of Nursing, Kristine Gebbie, a leader in public health nursing and former national AIDS czar in the Clinton administration, presented a curriculum plan that was developed with help from the Centers for Disease Control and Prevention (CDC), U.S. Public Health Services Health Resources and Services Administration (HRSA) Division of Nursing, and the Preventive Health and Health Promotion Office (PHHPO). The goal is to use a satellite link teleconference approach to retraining and updating nurses in public health for their future job responsibilities.

HOW TO Educate Nurses for Roles in Public Health: Curriculum Objectives for Community Health Nursing

The nurse should be able to do the following:
- Articulate similarities and differences between individual and population-focused nursing practice
- Describe the history and current perspectives of nursing practice in public health
- Demonstrate skills in applying key nursing contributions to public health practice (core functions and essential services) in a community
- Apply principles and skills of population health to his or her practice in the public health agency
- Use current information and communication technology in all public health agencies
- Communicate the benefits of public health and nursing practice

The function of the local nurse in public health varies significantly depending on the education and practice skills of the staff. However, all nursing staff should be able to function at the same level. Nurses in this environment focus on health rather than disease in working with populations. This differs tremendously from nursing practiced in other settings, where the emphasis is usually on illness care and cure. Although community health nurses perform direct hands-on care in many instances, they also perform tasks that one may not be able to see or touch, for example in changing a client's behavior through a health education activity.

Briefly Noted

Many of the epidemics of the future will be defined by social problems such as substance abuse and teen pregnancy.

ISSUES AND TRENDS

Some of the current issues facing nursing services in public health today are:

- Violence in society
- Substance abuse
- Welfare reform effects on families and children
- Multicultural and biracial integration in society
- Lack of health and medical resources for the uninsured and underinsured
- Managed care.

Nurses must keep abreast of the issues that are affecting all of society:

- Assessments need to be changed to include these factors that affect the populations that they serve.
- When childcare is an issue for the welfare mother returning to work, consideration must be given to effects on the individual, family, community, and population.

Nurses in public health must look at the problem and determine what is wrong with the system. An example would be a system that encourages mothers to go to work so that they can be removed from welfare. The following are questions to be considered:

- Do services such as childcare need to be provided so that parents can be successful?
- What will it take to change the system?
- Is the question to be answered by a nurse?

Partnerships and collaboration among groups are much more powerful in making change than the individual client and nurse. These types of problems have not developed in a day and will not be solved overnight. As another example, the depressed, nonfunctional mother in need of counseling is of significant public health concern. The mother's, children's, and family's needs are not being met.

Frequently the presenting problem may not be obvious to the nurse seeing this woman for the first time. Nurses in public health have special preparation to help them identify both the individual client's problem and the effect on the broader community. Some of the problems that may result are:

- Children may carry mental health problems into adulthood. The community mental health services will need to be able to handle this growing population.
- Children may become violent adults, resulting in need for more corrections facilities.
- Mothers may need additional mental health services.
- Children may be absent from school often and may not be able to contribute to society and be productive in the workplace because of lack of skills.

- Mothers may not be able to provide financially and need welfare money.
- Often the problems of the single parent place great burdens on the community.

Briefly Noted

Nurses in public health have to learn to function in an organization that must deal with many changes. Changes occur continually as a result of the many internal and external factors from people, programs, politics, and the unknown, as well as known local, state, and federal actions. Which skills will help the nurse to adapt to changes?

Box 25-2	Societal Level Trends Affecting Public Health Today

- Changes in health care delivery systems
- Changing patterns in the racial and ethnic composition in the U.S. population
- The aging of the population
- Rapid development of information technologies
- Development of numerous and diverse health-related partnerships
- Educational needs and changes within the public health work force
- The antigovernment sentiment
- Polarizing of some factions of the population

From Brownson R, Kreuter M: Future trends affecting public health: challenges and opportunities, *J Public Health Manag Pract* 2(3):49, 1997.

EDUCATION AND KNOWLEDGE
Requirements for Community Health Nurses

The Association of Community Health Nursing Educators states the educational preparation of community health nurses should be at least a baccalaureate degree. Those who have associate degrees are encouraged to seek further degrees because of the increasing complexity of better care delivery in public health.

The Core Public Health Functions Steering Committee of the National Association of City and County Health Officials (1994) identified 10 activities that need to be implemented in a community to meet the public health core functions of assessment, assurance, and policy development:

1. Health status monitoring and surveillance
2. Investigation and control of disease and injuries
3. Protection of environment, workplace, housing, food, and water
4. Laboratory services to support disease control and environmental protection
5. Health education and information
6. Community mobilization for health-related issues

7. Targeted outreach and linkage to personal services
8. Health services quality assurance and accountability
9. Training and education of public health professionals
10. Leadership, policy, planning, and administration.

Many of these core public health functions are provided by nurses who have learned these skills in the work-place while gaining knowledge slowly through years of practice. Rapid changes in public health do not allow sufficient time nor staff to provide as much on-the-job training as is needed to upgrade skills and knowledge of staff. Therefore nurses with baccalaureate or master's preparation will be needed to provide a strong public health system (see Chapter 1).

Certification for Community Health Nurses

Two levels of certification are available for community health nurses. Both are offered through the American Nurses Credentialing Center. Although certification is voluntary, being recognized as competent in a specialty area demonstrates to clients and employers that the nurse has knowledge and skills that are essential to nursing practice. The certified nurse focuses on a holistic approach to care for clients, including the promotion and maintenance of health, health education, case management, and coordination, and the provision of continuity of care. To be eligible to take the certification examination at the generalist level, one must be a registered nurse and licensed in the United States or its territories, have a baccalaureate or higher degree in nursing or related field, have at least 30 contact hours of continuing education applicable to the field in the past 3 years, and have practiced in the community health field a minimum of 1500 hours in the last 3 years. Nurses are examined on such topics as public health science, individual, family and community as client, areas of practice, public health issues/problems, and professional issues. One criterion for the clinical specialist in community health nursing examination is a master's degree. The two certification examinations for community health nurses are based on the scopes and standards for community health nursing practice of the American Nurses Association (1985). These scope and standard statements are currently being reviewed for revision.

NATIONAL HEALTH OBJECTIVES

State and local health departments play a key role in implementing the *Healthy People 2010* objectives. Because the public health departments do not have the resources to accomplish these goals independently, collaboration is essential to quality nursing practice and is encouraged at the local level with existing groups. New partnerships are developed and related to specific goals. For example, to improve pregnancy outcomes, the *Healthy People 2010* objectives were to:

9-1 Increase the proportion of pregnancies that are intended.

9-2 Reduce the proportion of births occurring within 24 months of a previous birth.

9-3 Increase the proportion of females at risk of unintended pregnancy (and their partners) who use contraception.

9-4 Reduce the proportion of females experiencing pregnancy despite use of a reversible contraceptive method.

9-5 Increase the proportion of health care providers who provide emergency contraception.

9-6 Increase male involvement in pregnancy prevention and family planning efforts.

9-7 Reduce pregnancies among adolescent females.

9-8 Increase the proportion of adolescents who have never engaged in sexual intercourse before age 15 years.

9-9 Increase the proportion of adolescents who have never engaged in sexual intercourse.

9-10 Increase the proportion of sexually active, unmarried adolescents aged 15 to 17 years who use contraception that both effectively prevents pregnancy and provides barrier protection against disease.

9-11 Increase the proportion of young adults who have received formal instruction before turning age 18 years on reproductive health issues, including all of the following topics: birth control methods, safer sex to prevent HIV, prevention of sexually transmitted diseases, and abstinence.

9-12 Reduce the proportion of married couples whose ability to conceive or maintain and pregnancy is impaired.

9-13 Increase the proportion of health insurance policies that cover contraceptive supplies and services.

Since the addition of the objective to decrease unintended births, several communities in one state (Virginia Department of Health, 1997) developed new coalitions to address the objectives to include all of the local community players, such as:

- Social services
- Mental health
- Education
- Justice and courts
- Recreation
- Government
- Businesses.

Membership varied from community to community depending on that community's formal and informal structure. The groups joined the coalition for a variety of reasons. For example, businesses see the value of developing a productive work force that will be of importance to them and the community in the future.

The *Healthy People 2010* objectives focus on decreasing deaths from coronary heart diseases, cancers, strokes, chronic obstructive pulmonary disease, injuries, pneumonia/flu, diabetes, suicide, kidney disease, and chronic liver disease, the 10 leading causes of death. Nurses in public health help clients identify unhealthy behaviors and then help them develop strategies to improve their health. Some of the behaviors addressed by nurses are tobacco use, physical activity, and obesity—all of which lead to chronic diseases.

Some *Healthy People 2010* infectious communicable disease areas of focus are:

- Immunizations
- STDs
- HIV/AIDS
- Hepatitis
- Tuberculosis
- Meningitis
- Lyme disease
- Respiratory infections
- Peptic ulcer.

Nurses provide clients with instructions on the use of barrier methods of contraception and information on the hazards of multiple sexual partners, and street drug use to help clients reduce their risk of acquiring a communicable disease. Getting a complete sexual history on all clients coming to the health department for services takes special skills; however, it is essential to determine the behaviors that have brought the client to the local health department. Abstinence as a birth control method can be addressed with all populations. Education of young persons before they become sexually active has helped reduce the incidence of some sexually transmitted diseases in this population.

A 3- or 5-year average is used to compare data to see if trends are changing health behaviors and health status, because the numbers are often extremely small. Data must be comparable with other similar populations in other communities or states to be useful in evaluating public health strategies.

FUNCTIONS OF NURSES IN PUBLIC HEALTH

Nurses in public health play many roles depending on the needs and resources of an area. **Advocate** is one of the many roles of the nurse. As an advocate, the nurse collects data and discusses with clients which services they need, whether an individual, family, or group. The nurse and clients then develop the most effective plan and approach to take, and the nurse helps clients implement the plan so that the clients can become more independent in making decisions and getting the services they need.

Case manager is a major role for nurses in public health. Nurses use the nursing or scientific process of assessing, planning, implementing, and evaluating outcomes to meet clients' needs. Clear and complex communications are frequently an important component of case management. Other health and social agency participants may not be familiar with the home and community living conditions that are known to the nurse. The nurse has seen the living conditions and can tell the story for the client or assist the individual or family with the telling of their story. Case managers assist clients in identifying the services they need the most at the least cost. For example, a nurse may go into the home to visit a new mother and baby. Upon assessment she may find

the mother needs in help in finding a new job, childcare, a pediatrician, and assistance in finding health insurance. The nurse helps the mother in the following ways:

- Assists with prioritizing problems
- Helps make a plan for resolving the problems
- Contacts other agencies on behalf of the mother when needed
- Follows up with the mother to see that the problems are being resolved
- Follows up with the agencies, such as Social Services, to make certain the mother's request to enroll her children in the Child Health Insurance Program has been honored.

Nurses are a **referral resource.** They have to keep up to date on the services that are available to their clients. They know what resources will be acceptable to the client within the social and cultural norms for that group. The nurse educates the client in use of the resources and self-care. Nurses refer to other services in the area, and other services refer to the nurse for care or follow-up. For example, the mother and new baby may be referred to the nurse for postnatal care with postpartum home visit follow-up to hospital care.

Being an **assessor** is a large part of nursing and includes more than simply performing physical assessment. For example, many individuals are limited in their ability to read, write, and communicate clearly. The nurse has to be culturally sensitive and aware of the specific areas of unique problems of clients, such as financial limitations that may in turn limit educational opportunities. Frequently, when individuals go to a physician's office, clinic, or hospital, they are clean and neatly dressed. The assumption is that when they nod affirmatively at the health care provider it means that they understand what has been said. This is frequently not the case, but the client is embarrassed to admit that he or she does not understand what has been said. Some clients may be illiterate, but this should not be confused with low intelligence levels. After assessing the reading level of the client, it is important for the nurse to follow up on the many contacts the individual or family has with medical, social, and legal services to clarify what is understood and to find an answer to any remaining questions. The nurse may check the reading level of materials received from other agencies to determine the ability of the client to understand them. The nurse may need to read materials to the clients. The nurse also asks questions about the materials she has read to the clients to make certain the client understands. She asks clients to explain in their own words the meaning of the materials.

Nurses are a strong **role model** for many of the clients they serve. Some clients may not have had a positive, mature individual to interact with in their family of origin. The nurse becomes an example for the children and family and may encourage them to seek education or employment so that they can improve their social and financial status. The nurse is also an *educator,* teaching to the level of the client so that information received is information that can be used. Patience and repetitions over time are necessary to develop trust and to enable the client to use the relationship with the nurse for more information.

Counselor is another important nursing role. The client frequently cannot define or identify the problem that needs to be handled, much less develop solutions. At-risk populations frequently lack problem-solving skills. For example, a sexually active teenage female is unaware that she has made a decision to be sexually active. Frequently she thinks "things" just happen. Being aware of this is a beginning step in problem identification, and the nurse can then teach about safe contraception. This is an active decision the girl can control. The nurse can help her to set goals and then accomplish these goals.

Nurses are direct **primary caregivers** in many situations both in the clinic and in the community. As primary caregiver the nurse assesses the clients' health and social status. The nurse then helps to define the problems and to marshall the resources available to solve the problems. When visiting a mother and a newborn baby, the nurse's assessment can identify physical and other problems that might have been seen in the hospital in the past, when hospital stays were more than 24 to 48 hours. Teaching before discharge is limited because of the short hospital stays, and many mothers need reinforcement of that teaching after they return to the community. Regardless of the educational, social, or economic level of the family, the nursing assessment is essential for the majority of families. Frequently it may be to reassure the family that everything is normal. When nurses are not providing direct care, they are working to ensure that direct care services are available in the community for at-risk populations, by developing programs that will meet the needs of those populations. The nurse may work in the family planning clinic and see the new mother and baby for teaching parenting skills and performing well child checks as the baby develops.

Currently no **outreach workers** or services in the medical system of care address the multiple needs of high-risk populations. High-risk populations frequently do not understand the medical, social, educational, or judicial system and the professional languages, codes of behavior, or expected outcomes of these services. Clients need a case manager, health educator, advocate, and role model to enable them to benefit from these services and to teach them how to avoid complex and expensive problems in the future. The above roles and many more are filled by the local nurse in public health.

Communicable disease control is an essential and unique role for nurses. Nursing skills are necessary for education and prevention, surveillance, and outbreak investigation. Nurses can identify infected individuals; notify contacts; refer; administer treatments; educate the individual, family, community, professionals, and populations; act as an advocate; and in general be a state-of-the-art resource, which is needed to reduce the individual communicable diseases in the community. For example when a client comes to the health clinic and is diagnosed with tuberculosis it is important to know who the person comes in contact with on a regular basis such as family, work, and friends.

These are examples of the difficult clinical issues that nurses have to face in making ethical and professional decisions. They work for the greater good and must have great patience to work with diverse players in some very complex situations, knowing that not everyone will be satisfied with the outcome.

The nurse's role is unique and essential in many situations because, through his or her access to homes, the nurse has information that usually cannot be gathered in the hospital or clinic setting. The nurse learns to ask intimate questions creatively, to seek information that will facilitate case management, and to provide the clinical and social care needed, including other community resources.

Briefly Noted

Careful attention must be paid to privacy and confidentiality in delivering public health services. The credibility of the nurse and the agency is dependent on the professional handling of the public's health information by each and every staff member.

When a disaster occurs, nurses have multiple roles in assessing, planning, implementing, and evaluating needs and resources for the different populations served. Whether the disaster is local or national, small or large, natural or manmade, nurses are skilled professionals essential to the team. As a health care facility, the local public health department has a disaster plan and a role in the local, regional, and state disaster plans. Local nurses' roles vary from providing education, such as CPR or first aid instruction, to preparing individuals and communities to cope with disasters, to providing professional triage for local shelters. Their presence may be required in other regions of the state or country to provide official public health duties in a time of crisis, such as a hurricane, that requires a lengthy period of recovery. Each local government unit has a local emergency plan, and the public health department is expected to provide planning and staffing for the local area. These local emergency preparedness plans may be multigovernmental, which requires coordination between communities.

In one state an electrical company has a nuclear plant that requires disaster drills that cross political jurisdictions. They are routinely planned and practiced with all the agencies assigned specific roles and responsibilities. These disaster planning and practice sessions are an opportunity for local nurses to get to know other agencies' representatives and to let them know what nursing can offer. Because nurses are out in the communities and have assessment skills, they are essential in evaluating how the disaster was handled and making suggestions about how future events might be managed. Nurses have to be a part of the team *before* an emergency to be most effective as a **disaster responder.** Knowing what type of disaster is likely to occur in a community is essential for planning. Types of disasters vary from place to place, but nurses can help prepare the public based on previous disasters and how they were handled, as well as resources and training from regional, state, and federal agencies. Nurses can help educate the public regarding individual responsibilities and preparations that can be in place both for the person and the community.

Briefly Noted

Nurses in public health must practice confidentiality when they have knowledge about an individual, family, communicable disease outbreak, community-level problem, or any special knowledge obtained in the public health work setting.

Clinical Application

A retirement community in a small town reported to the local health department 24 cases of severe gastrointestinal illness that had occurred among residents and staff of the facility during the past 24 to 36 hours. It was determined that the ill clients became sick within a short, well-defined period, and most recovered within 24 hours without treatment. The communicable disease outbreak team composed of nurses, public health physicians, and an environmental health specialist was called to respond to this possible epidemic.

How should they respond to this situation?
A. *Call the Centers for Disease Control and Prevention and ask for help with surveillance.*
B. *Send all of the retirement community's ill persons to the hospital.*
C. *Evaluate the agent, host, and environment relationships to determine the cause of the problem.*
D. *Close the dining room and find another source to provide food to the residents.*

Answer is in the back of the book.

 Remember This!

- Local public health departments are responsible for implementing and enforcing local, state, and federal public health codes and ordinances while providing essential public health services.
- The goal of the local health department is to safeguard the public's health and improve the community's health status.
- Community health nursing is the practice of promoting and protecting the health of populations using knowledge from nursing and social and public health sciences through the delivery of personal health services to individuals, families, and groups.
- Public health is based on the scientific core of epidemiology.

- Marketing of nursing in public health is essential to inform both professionals and the public about the opportunities and challenges of populations in public health care.
- A driving force behind nursing changes in public health is the economy and the increase in managed care.
- Nurses need ongoing education and training as public health changes nurses' role functions, including advocate, case manager, referral source, counselor, primary care provider, educator, outreach worker, disaster responder, and many more.
- Nurses have an important role in helping with local disasters, including planning, staffing, and evaluating events.

 What Would You Do?

1. What are some of the various roles of nurses in the local health department?
2. How can nurses prepare themselves for change?
3. What can today's nurses learn from the past practice of public health nurses?
4. Describe collaborative partnerships that nurses have developed in communities.
5. What are some external factors that have an effect on nursing in public health?
6. If you were a nurse in a local health department for a day, what would you like to accomplish? Why?
7. How would you determine the most pressing public health issue in your community?

REFERENCES

American Nurses Association: *Statements of community health nursing practice,* Washington, D.C., 1985, American Nurses Publishing.

Brownson R, Kreuter M: Future trends affecting public health: challenges and opportunities, *J Public Health Manag Pract* 2(3):49, 1997.

Bunker JP, et al: Improving health: measuring effects of medical care, *Milbank Q* 72:225, 1994.

Citrin T: Topics for our times: public health—community or commodity? reflections on healthy communities, *Am J Public Health* 88(3):351, 1998.

Institute of Medicine: *The future of public health,* Washington, D.C., 1988, National Academy Press.

National Association of City and County Health Officials: *Blueprint for a healthy community: a guide for local health departments,* Washington, D.C., 1994, National Association of City and County Health Officials.

Turnock BJ: *Public health: what it is and how it works,* Gaithersburg, Md, 1997, Aspen.

U.S. Department of Health and Human Services: *Healthy people 2010,* Washington, D.C., 2000, U.S. Department of Health and Human Services.

Virginia Department of Health: *Healthy Virginia communities,* Richmond, 1997, Virginia Department of Health.

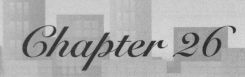

Chapter 26

Community Health Nurse as Parish Nurse

RUTH D. BERRY

OBJECTIVES

After reading this chapter, the student should be able to:
- Describe the heritage of health and healing in faith communities.
- Describe models of the parish nurse.
- Develop awareness of the community health nurse's role as parish nurse in faith communities for health promotion and disease prevention.
- Identify characteristics of the philosophy of parish nursing.
- Help communities of faith include *Healthy People 2010* guidelines in program planning.

- Collaborate with key partners to implement congregational health ministries relevant for the faith community.
- Use models of parish nursing with the nursing process in a faith community.
- Evaluate programs for healthy congregations throughout the life span.
- Examine the legal, ethical, and financial issues related to parish nursing.

CHAPTER OUTLINE

Definitions in Parish Nursing

Heritage and Horizons
  Faith Communities
  Nursing Community
  Health Care Delivery

Parish Nursing Practice
  Characteristics of the Practice
  Scope and Standards of Parish Nursing Practice
  Educational Preparation for a Parish Nurse

Issues in Parish Nursing Practice
  Professional Issues
  Ethical Issues
  Legal Issues
  Financial Issues

National Health Objectives and Faith Communities

Functions of the Parish Nurse

KEY TERMS

congregants: people who gather as part of a faith community of the congregation of a church.

congregational model: parish nurse arrangement in an individual community of faith where the nurse is accountable to the congregation and its governing body.

faith communities: distinct group of people acknowledging specific faith traditions and gathering in churches, cathedrals, synagogues, or mosques.

healing: strengthening the inner spiritual connectedness and choosing healthy life-styles.

health ministries: activities and programs in faith communities directed at improving the health and well-being of individuals, families, and communities across the life span.

holistic care: understanding the body, mind, and spirit relationship of persons in an environment that is always changing.

Continued

holistic health centers: a comprehensive health team that includes family and clergy and encourages personal responsibility for health and preventive health practices.

institutional model: parish nurse arrangement in a larger partnership under contract with hospitals, medical centers, long-term care facilities, or educational institutions.

neighborhood nurse: also known as block nursing, the nurse responds to a defined community or "locality."

parish nurse coordinator: a parish nurse who has completed a certificate program designed to develop the nurse as a coordinator of a parish nursing service.

parish nurses: nurses who respond to health and wellness needs within the faith context of populations of faith communities and are partners with the church in fulfilling the mission of health ministry.

parish nursing: a community-based and population-focused professional nursing practice with faith communities to promote whole person health to its parishioners, usually focused on primary prevention.

partnerships: relationships between individuals, groups or organizations in which the parties are working together to achieve a joint goal. Often used synonymously with coalitions and alliances, although partnerships usually have focused goals, such as jointly providing a specific program. Partnerships generally involve shared power.

pastoral care staff: faith community leaders including clergy, nurses, educational and youth ministry staff.

polity: the policy, governances, expectations, and mission of a specific faith community.

wellness committee: a health cabinet supporting healthy, spiritually fulfilling lives; made up of a nurse and members of the congregation.

Parish nursing has long established roots in the healing and health professions. Historical accounts of nursing document the importance of caring for members of communities. The earliest accounts of concern for others stem from communities of faith. Wholeness in health and being in "right" relationships with one's creator have sustained individuals and groups during times of illness, brokenness, stress, and incurable conditions (Dossey, 1993; Rydholm, 1997; Solari-Twadell, Djupe, and McDermott, 1990). Today parish nurses help individuals, families, and congregations become more aware of the relationship of wholeness in body, mind, and spirit (McDermott, Solari-Twadell, and Mathews, 1998; Schacht, 1992; Schank, Weis, and Matheus, 1996; Solari-Twadell, et al, 1994). Although a current movement focuses on making parish nursing an advanced practice nursing role, nurses with associate degrees and baccalaureate preparation function in these roles. It is important for nurses at all levels to understand this role.

Parish nurses address universal health problems of individuals, families, and groups of all ages. The members of congregations experience:

- Birth
- Death
- Acute and chronic illness
- Stress
- Dependency concerns
- Challenges of life transitions
- Growth and development
- Decisions regarding healthy life-style choices.

Congregational members live in communities that make decisions regarding policies for financing and managing health care and for keeping environments safe and communities healthy for present and future generations.

Parish nursing is gaining prominence as nurses reclaim their traditions of healing, acknowledge gaps in service delivery, and, along with the rise of nursing centers, affirm the independent functions of nursing. In 1998 the American Nurses Association (ANA) accepted parish nursing as the most recognized term for the practice of nurses working with congregations or faith communities. With the Health Ministries Association (HMA), the ANA published the *Scope and Standards of Parish Nursing* (1998). Although most parish nurses are in Protestant congregations, they may be found in most faith communities, including communities that serve diverse cultures. Parish nurses are also serving faith communities in countries such as Korea, Australia, Russia, and Canada (Bondine, 1997; Culp, 1997; Granberg-Michaelson, 1997; McDermott, 1998; Van Loon, 1996).

DEFINITIONS IN PARISH NURSING

Faith communities are congregational communities that gather in churches, cathedrals, synagogues, or mosques and acknowledge common faith traditions. **Parish nursing** is the most commonly used term that denotes the professional advanced nurse practice role in this context. **Parish nurses** respond to health and wellness needs of populations of faith communities and are partners with the church in fulfilling the mission of health ministry. A parish nurse in the church may be referred to as a *congregational health minister, emergency church nurse,* or *health ministries nurse.*

The faith community includes persons throughout the life span: active and less active members, those confined to homes, or those in nursing homes. Often the church's mission also includes individuals and groups in the geographical community who are not designated church members. The services may be extended to those beyond the congregation. The parish nurse emphasizes the nursing discipline's spiritual dimension while incorporating physical, emotional, and social aspects of nursing with individuals, families, and congregational communities.

Health ministries are those activities and programs in faith communities organized around health and healing to promote wholeness in health across the life span. The services may be specifically planned or may be more informal. A professional or a lay person may provide them. These services include:

- Visiting the homebound
- Providing meals for families in crisis or when returning home after hospitalization
- Organizing prayer circles
- Volunteering in community AIDS care groups
- Serving "healthy heart" church suppers
- Holding regular grief support groups

Popular parish nurse models include **congregational** and **institutional models** (Box 26-1).

Within either model, nurses work closely with professional health care members, **pastoral care staff,** and lay volunteers who represent various aspects of the life of the congregational community. To promote **healing,** the nurse builds on strengths to encourage integrating inner spiritual knowledge and healthy life-style choices for optimal wellness. Intentional and compassionate presence of a spiritually mature professional nurse in individual or group situations is vital. In this role, providing such holistic care with congregation populations is important. **Holistic care** is concerned with the body, mind, and spirit relationship in a constantly changing environment (Dossey, 1995). The nurse and members of the congregation assess, plan, implement, and evaluate programs. The process of providing holistic care is enhanced by an active **wellness committee** or health cabinet. These committees are most effective when members represent the broad spectrum of the life of the church. The parish nurse uses all the knowledge and skills of this specialty to give effective services. The outcome is a truly caring congregation that supports healthy, spiritually fulfilling lives. Box 26-2 lists resources for parish nursing.

Briefly Noted

Parish nurses are employed by senior living complexes and nursing homes to offer a spiritual focus to the nursing practice within various levels of living arrangements for elders, in addition to serving one or more congregations in the community.

HERITAGE AND HORIZONS

Faith Communities

In the roots of many faith communities are concerns for justice, mercy, and the need for spiritual and physical healing. The appeal for caring, the healing of diseases, and acknowledging periods of illness and wellness are universal. Throughout a major portion of the twentieth century religion played an important role in the lives of many in this country. An important aspect of living one's spirituality and religion is being a part of a community of faith from birth to death, throughout wellness and illness. Participating as individuals or as families, all benefit from the associations with the supportive faith community or congregation.

Box 26-1	**Parish Nurse Models**

- *Congregational model,* in which the nurse is usually autonomous. The development of a parish nurse/health ministry program arises from the individual community of faith. The nurse is accountable to the congregation and its governing body.
- *Institutional model* includes greater collaboration and partnerships; the nurse may be in a contractual relationship with hospitals, medical centers, long-term care establishments, or educational institutions.

Box 26-2	**Resources for Parish Nursing**

International Parish Nurse Resource Center
205 W. Touhy Avenue, Suite 104
Park Ridge, IL 60068-1174
1-800-556-5368
ann.solari-twadell@advocatehealth.com
(Publication: *Perspectives in Parish Nursing Practice*)

Health Ministries Association
P.O. Box 7187
Atlanta, GA 30357-0187
1-800-280-9919
hmasso@mindspring.com
(Publication: *Connections*)

Interfaith Health Program of the Carter Center
453 Freedom Parkway
Atlanta, GA 30307
(Publication: *Faith & Health*)

See the WebLinks on this book's website at www.mosby.com/ MERLIN/Stanhope/foundations for further information about resources.

Support from members of groups that are meaningful to a person's total well-being aids in recovery and healing (Matthews, et al, 1998; Oman and Reed, 1998; Oxman, Freeman, and Manheimer, 1995). Asking for help and using strengths from earliest faith, traditions, family support, and teachings assist individuals, groups, and communities in interpreting brokenness, disasters, joys, births, deaths, illness, and recovery. Throughout history, health existed at the center of the human interaction with one's Creator.

The integration of faith and health within the caring community results in beneficial outcomes. Persons who encounter assaults with physical and emotional illness and brokenness and who are able to call upon their faith beliefs and religious traditions are able to increase coping skills and realize spiritual growth (see the Research Brief about elderly clients with cancer). These coping skills and spiritual strengths extend beyond the current situation and help with future life challenges and total well being. Foege (1996) identifies three conditions needed for persons to be responsive to life in the future:

- Equity
- Kinship
- Continuity

Evidence-Based Practice

The authors reviewed epidemiological and clinical studies dealing with the relationship among selected religious factors such as frequency of religious attendance, private religious practices, reliance on religious beliefs, and the physical and mental health status in the areas of prevention, coping, and recovery. Studies characteristic of primary, secondary, and tertiary levels of prevention examined involvement in the prevention of illness, coping with current illnesses, and factors to facilitate recovery. A large proportion of the information gathered suggests that religious commitment plays a beneficial role in preventing mental and physical illness, enhances coping with these illnesses, and aids in the recovery from the illness.

APPLICATION IN PRACTICE

The authors contend that although increased studies with special attention directed to religious involvement and health status are needed, the implication for all health care clinicians is that interventions that recognize and involve clients' religious commitments may enhance health care outcomes. Beneficial interventions included incorporating religious orientation in preparing the care plan; praying with clients; encouraging clients to pray alone and with others, to continue attendance to meditations, faith rituals, worship services, and to seek and ask for forgiveness from others in their lives; reading holy writings; and offering referrals to clergy or chaplains. The implications for the parish nurse are to implement the appropriate interventions following assessment of the importance of religious commitment in one's life and supporting other health care professionals in their practice with the individual or family.

Matthews DA, et al: Religious commitment and health status: a review of the research and implications for family medicine, *Arch Fam Med* 7:118, 1998.

Evidence-Based Practice

The authors of the study cited below administered several scales, including an intrinsic and extrinsic religiosity index and a spiritual well-being scale to 100 elderly persons diagnosed with cancer. The mean age was 73 years old. Relationships among spiritual well-being, religiosity, hope, depression, and other mood states were examined to determine whether differences existed in those with high and low intrinsic religiosity and spiritual well-being. Outcomes found consistent positive correlations among intrinsic religiosity, spiritual well-being, hope, and other positive mood states and negative correlations among intrinsic religiosity, depression, and other negative mood states. Those elderly who had high levels of intrinsic religiosity exhibited higher levels of hope and positive moods.

APPLICATION IN PRACTICE

The challenge for professional nursing is to assess and support intrinsic religiosity and promote spiritual well-being in elderly people coping with terminal illnesses.

Fehring RJ, Miller JF, Shaw C: Spiritual well-being, religiosity, hope, depression and other mood states in elderly people coping with cancer, *Oncol Nurs Forum* 24:663, 1997.

These faith beliefs include:
- Equality in the eyes of one's Creator
- Global connectedness
- Traditions that are inherited and handed down to future generations.

Some of the major Protestant faith communities in the late nineteenth and early twentieth centuries used missionaries to develop multipurpose activities in communities, which included education and health activities along with religious messages. Hospitals were built in the United States and abroad, and underserved populations were targeted. As political and economic forces have changed through the years, so health ministries of the churches have altered their approaches. Some churches have identified with community development efforts in helping people empower themselves to meet their needs for:
- Food
- Education
- Clean environments
- Social support
- Primary health care.

Some churches have also recognized and increased their emphasis on:
- Individual responsibility

- The escalating cost of health care
- The need for cost containment
- The increasing numbers of uninsured and underserved
- The ever-increasing dilemma of interpreting the many changes in the health care delivery system.

These efforts have been translated into a variety of positions endorsed by the governing bodies of the faith communities.

The **Holistic Health Centers** of the 1970s emphasized a comprehensive team approach to total health care. The teams in these Centers included family and clergy, who emphasized personal responsibility for health and encouraged preventive health practices. The forming of parish nursing in the early 1980s built on the strengths of the Holistic Health Centers and focused on the team of nurses and clergy, working with individuals with their families. Nurses used their abilities to listen to the spoken and unspoken concerns of individuals and made assessments and judgments based on their knowledge of the health sciences and humanities. As with the early history of the development of public health nursing in this country, parish nurses found that health promotion services were needed in underserved and rural areas. Nurses identified the following:
- Gaps in the delivery of service
- Acknowledged strength within persons to increase healing
- The vital role of families on healthy outcomes
- The community support needed for individuals and families.

Briefly Noted

The International Parish Nurse Resource Center/Advocate Health Care resources are the outgrowth of the early visions of the Rev. Granger Westberg. As a Lutheran clergyman who was involved with the W.K. Kellogg Wholistic Health Cen-

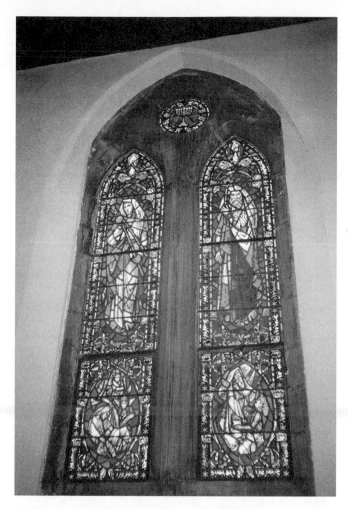

Religious symbols and rituals are a significant part of a faith life-style and practice for many people.

ters, Westberg recognized that nurses were central to the endeavors and that they enhanced minister/doctor communication to promote a "whole person" approach. Westberg suggested placing nurses on the staff of churches and proposed the church as another "health agency" in the community in the mid-1980s (Solari-Twadell, et al, 1990).

Nursing Community

The beginnings of the parish nurse movement coincided with the following:

- Recognition of more independent functions of the nurse
- Articulation and proliferation of advanced practice nursing roles
- The growth of nursing centers
- Technological advances
- DRGs, which resulted in hospitals discharging clients earlier and clients returning to their homes sicker with few, if any, caregivers available
- Caregivers being faced with multiple tasks of coordinating employment, finances, learning new caregiving tasks, and maintaining former and ongoing family responsibilities

- Increased consumer demand for involvement in health care decisions
- Society's emphasis on individual responsibility for health because many diseases were indeed preventable and health care costs had to be cut
- Recognition that fragmented care and inadequate caregiver training and availability were problems for the disenfranchised, underserved, uninsured, economically well situated, and better-educated persons
- Challenges faced by suburban and rural families to seek ways to best meet the multiple demands of young children, teens, and aging parents

These numerous interacting and overlapping forces were burdens for the population. Parish nurse services were one of the responses to assist with coordinating care and fostering continuity of care. The parish nurse services emphasized health promotion and disease prevention and provided the benefits of holistic care through the supportive faith community.

The International Parish Nurse Resource Center's mission is the promotion and development of quality parish nurse programs through research, education, and consultation (International Parish Nurse Resource Center, 1998). To this end, the Center offers resources, catalogs, regular newsletters, and consultation and reference packets with information about the parish nurse role and services offered by the Center. Information about accessing the Center appears in Box 26-2 on p. 451. The Center has also endorsed curricula for the parish nurse and **parish nurse coordinator** (McDermott, Solari-Twadell, and Mathews, 1998).

Community health nurses functioning as parish nurses need to have:

- Leadership skills
- Astute, articulate nonverbal and verbal communication
- Negotiation and collaboration skills.

As with other population groups, the parish nurse attempts to include those persons who are less vocal or visible in the community of faith. If the vision of the congregation extends beyond its immediate membership, then those outside of the immediate faith community who would benefit from the services are also potential recipients. This may be accomplished by including the block nurse or neighborhood nurse in the area surrounding the church.

Health Care Delivery

Community health nursing professionals are aware of the necessity of collaborative practices and formation of **partnerships** to care for groups and individuals throughout the life span. Parish nurses share these and other functions as they serve populations through faith communities.

PARISH NURSING PRACTICE
Characteristics of the Practice

Parish nursing's goal is to develop and sustain health ministries within faith communities. Health ministries promote wholeness in health, emphasize health promotion and disease prevention, and do this within the context of linking healing with the person's faith belief and level of spiritual maturity. The author participated in a 1994 invitational conference that included 26 professionals consisting of nurse educators, practicing parish nurses, and staff of the Parish Nurse Resource Center to discuss and design a document outlining educational guidelines for the rapidly growing new nursing specialty. The final product included five characteristics identified as central to the philosophy of parish nursing (Solari-Twadell, et al, 1994).

- The *spiritual dimension* is central to the practice of parish nursing. Nursing embodies the physical, psychological, social, and spiritual dimensions of clients into professional practice. Although parish nursing *includes* all four, it *focuses* on intentional and compassionate care, which stems from the spiritual dimension of all humankind.
- *The roots of the role balance both knowledge and skills* of nursing, using nursing sciences, the humanities, and theology. The nurse combines nursing functions with pastoral care functions. Visits in the office, home, hospital, or nursing home often involve prayer and may include a reference to scripture, symbols, sacraments, and liturgy of the faith community represented by the nurse. The values and beliefs of the faith community are integral to the supportive care given. Nurses also assist with worship services as appropriate within the faith community.
- *The focus of the specialty is the faith community and its ministry.* The faith community is the source of health and healing partnerships, which result in creative responses to health and health-related concerns. Partnerships may be among individuals, groups, and health care professionals within the congregation. Partnerships may also be among various congregations or community agencies, institutions, or individuals. Partnerships also evolve as the congregation visualizes its health-related mission beyond the walls, stones, and steeples of its own place of worship.
- *Parish nurse services emphasize strengths* of individuals, families, and communities. Parish nurses endorse this fourth characteristic in their practice. As congregations realize the need for care and care for one another, their individual and corporate relationship with their Creator often is enhanced. This provides additional coping strength for future crisis situations within the family and community.
- *Health, spiritual health, and healing* are considered an ongoing, dynamic process. Because spiritual health is central to well-being, influences are evident in the total individual and noted in a healthy congregation. Well-being and illness may occur simultaneously; spiritual healing or well-being can exist in the absence of cure.

Scope and Standards of Parish Nursing Practice

The practice of parish nursing relates to activities of "health promotion within the context of the client's values, beliefs and faith practices." The parish nurse *"client focus . . . is the faith community, including its family and individual mem-*

bers and the community it serves" (Health Ministries Association/American Nurses Association, 1998, p. 3). Nurses encourage individuals, families and entire faith communities to promote health and healing within the context of the faith community to arrive at wellness outcomes. As in other arenas of nursing, the client level is multidimensional. "The clients of a parish nurse represent the total life span of three client levels: the faith community and its families and individuals" (p. 17). Using the nursing process for assessment, program planning, and evaluation, the parish nurses target specified age groups or health-related concerns.

The *Scope and Standards* delineate examples of the parish nurse's independent functions. These functions are in compliance with and reflect current nursing practice, client health promotion needs, professional standards, and the legal scope of professional nursing practice. Nurses function within the nurse practice act of their jurisdiction (state). If dependent functions are practiced, parish nurses must be in compliance with the legal criteria of the jurisdiction's nurse practice act (American Nurses Association, 1998). For example, when influenza vaccine or immunization clinics are offered, appropriate arrangements are made to use nurses from the cooperating agency (health department), or the parish nurse must have a contractual policy agreement with the cooperating agency to provide the immunizations. In addition to a narrative description and glossary of terms, the 1998 document outlines standards of care and standards of professional performance. In keeping with wise use of persons and materials, standards of professional performance elaborate on collaboration and resource use. The parish nurse collaborates with those who "share a commitment to promoting health" and "facilitate a health ministry that maximizes resources to achieve the desired health outcomes for all clients" (American Nurses Association, 1998, pp. 20, 22).

Briefly Noted

The parish nurse benefits from several years of practice experience following the basic undergraduate preparation, because the nature of the position demands a seasoned professional.

Educational Preparation for a Parish Nurse

Adoption of the *Scope and Standards of Parish Nursing Practice* has paralleled the International Parish Nurse Resource Center's efforts on standardizing a basic curriculum for preparation of parish nurses and a curriculum for coordinators of parish nurses. After successful completion of the courses, parish nurses adapt to individual local community needs to gain outcomes congruent with goals established by the congregation and communities they serve.

Before taking the standard basic course recommendations, parish nurses typically must have a baccalaureate degree in nursing and hold a valid license in the state of practice. A basic understanding or introduction to the parish nurse concept, 3 to 5 years experience in professional nurs-

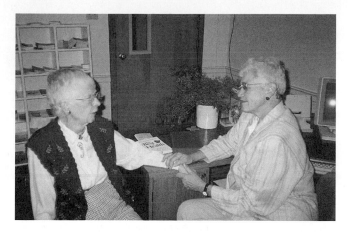

A parish nurse provides support for spiritual and emotional needs as well as physical needs.

ing, and evidence of a mature faith are also required. Varying routes of preparation may be taken. The International Parish Nurse Resource Center offered the earliest orientation courses beginning in 1984. A graduate program in "parish health nurse" preparation at Georgetown University, diverse continuing education offerings, and some undergraduate courses are available.

Several seminars have offered opportunities to raise awareness of the practice and have provided networking and nurturing support for nurses. An intensive continuing education program through Marquette University in Milwaukee has been offered in locations throughout the nation. The annual Westberg Symposium held in Chicago each September offers comprehensive sessions and a forum for nurses to network, gain new knowledge, and stay abreast of current resources and trends in the practice. Although these efforts have been valuable to the parish nurse specialty in its beginning stages, and the need for continuing education networking opportunities are ongoing, the standardizing of basic programs provides similar learning modules and a common knowledge base.

Specialty areas within professional nursing achieve a major milestone in the evolving practice when the standards and scope common to that practice are recognized. Advanced practice opportunities then enrich the specialty. Master's-prepared nurses with specialization in community health nursing, holistic nursing, or mental health nursing and nurse practitioners have found niches in parish nursing. A 1500-member congregation in Florida employs a full-time master's-prepared nurse who is certified in holistic nursing by the American Holistic Nurses' Association. A Kentucky congregation has a collaborative faculty practice agreement with the University of Kentucky College of Nursing. The University of Colorado School of Nursing also has a faculty member who practices in parish nursing. These arrangements provide clinical experiences for doctorate and master's-level community health nursing students (Magilvy and Brown, 1997). A consortium of rural churches pool resources for a parish nurse to facilitate health ministries programs. A Charlotte, North Carolina, hospital system employs a parish nurse coordinator who facilitates differing arrangements with several faith communities of varying backgrounds.

Many parish nurses function in a part-time capacity. Some nurses are responsible for service with several congregations, whereas others engage in parish nursing as part of a full-time commitment in other capacities. Working in several arenas adds distinctive perspectives to a parish nurse service. Depending on the practice model, the nurse has a narrowly defined or a wider realm of responsibility. Parish nurse practices may be integrated into a health care facility or into practices that collaborate with related professional practice areas such as health departments or colleges of nursing. Practices in which several parish nurses are supervised by a coordinator have built-in opportunities for sharing, partnering, and mentoring. Parish nurses may also have regional responsibilities that correspond to intermediate governing areas of the faith community. These regions may be clusters of churches or areas such as districts, synods, presbyteries, or jurisdictions.

Parish nurses accept responsibility for ongoing professional education within nursing and pastoral care arenas. Preparation and continuing education must continue to include the basics and enrichment courses in:

- Nursing
- Theological/pastoral care field
- Public health
- Medicine
- Sociology
- Cultural diversity
- Human growth and development throughout the life span
- Improving collaboration, negotiation, and coordination skills
- Consultation
- Leadership
- Management
- Research skills.

ISSUES IN PARISH NURSING PRACTICE

Every new discipline or care area must be alert to issues of accountability to populations served and to those who entrust the nurse with the responsibility to serve a designated population. This facilitates positive outcomes and avoids conflicts with individual/group rights and state regulations.

Discussions of health promotion plans must include the individual, the family, and the faith community.

Negotiations with the pastoral staff, congregations, institutions, and the wider community may be involved in job description preparation or program planning.

Issues such as privacy, confidentiality, group concerns, access, and record management must be discussed with the pastoral staff or the contracting agency at the outset of any parish nurse agreement.

Professional Issues

Annual and periodic evaluations are required of parish nurse practices and services needed. These evaluations may be self, peer, congregational, and/or institutional. Personnel committees provide guidance and contribute to the evaluation. They also advocate for parish nurse services and raise awareness with the congregational staff members and programs. Professional appraisal is standard in nursing practice. The appraisals guide professional development and program development and planning. Because the scope of parish nursing practice is broad and focuses on the independent practice of the discipline, the nurse must consider a wide variety of issues:

- Position descriptions
- Professional liability
- Professional education
- Experiential preparation
- Collaborative agreements
- Working with lay volunteers and retired professionals.

Abiding by the professional nursing code is understood; however, the nurse must also know the **polity,** expectations, and mission of the particular faith community. The nurse also continually interprets the profession for the faith community.

The nurse must be:

- Knowledgeable about lines of authority and channels of communication in the congregation and in the collaborative institutions
- Well acquainted with the personnel committees of the congregation
- An advocate for well-being to highlight justice issues in local and national legislation
- A contributor of information to policy makers about the implications for health and well-being for the parish and the local and global communities
- An active participant in political activities that contribute to spiritual growth and healthy functioning.

Briefly Noted

Developing a keen sense of the value of the congregation within the geopolitical community and appreciating its associations within the local and wider community are beneficial.

Ethical Issues

Issues evolve from client, faith community, and professional arenas. The nurse's interventions are guided by professional responsibilities that include:

- Code for Nurses (American Nurses Association, 2000)
- Individual and group rights
- Statements of Faith
- Polity of the faith community served.

Professional and therapeutic relationships are maintained at all times; consulting and counseling with minors and individual members of the opposite sex are conducted using professional ethical principles. Policies about these issues are established at the outset of the practice with the pastoral team, the wellness committee, the parish nurse, and the local congregation's governing body.

As in other community health situations, the parish nurse, along with the client:

- Identifies parameters of ethical concerns
- Plans ahead with clients to consider healthy options in making ethical decisions
- Supports clients in their journey to choose alternatives that will strengthen coping skills
- Allows them to grow stronger in faith and health
- Considers the "virtue ethics, such as caring, forgiveness, and compassion, in their decision making" (American Nurses Association, 1998, p. 19).

Communities of faith strive to be caring communities and value the fellowship among its members. However, confidentiality is of utmost importance in parish nursing practice. The parish nurse values client confidentiality while at the same time delicately assisting the client and client's family to "share" concerns with pastoral staff and fellow **congregants.** This sharing gains valuable support to promote optimal healing. The nurse is often the staff member who helps the family to the stage of acceptance of a health concern. How much to share and when to share a concern is indeed a private affair and a part of the important journey of healing. A joyous event for one family may be a devastating event or even a depressing reminder of a past event for another family. The celebrations and joys of a healthy new infant one week may raise guilt and ambivalence for congregational members when, within a brief time, another family's long-awaited child dies at birth.

Briefly Noted

A young couple who has contributed their time, enthusiasm, and skills assisting as church youth group leaders are expecting a first child. What a valuable learning experience for the teens, the parish nurse contends. Having a couple experience healthy life events is indeed beneficial for youth. Upon birth, the infant is diagnosed with Down syndrome. Now the typical celebrations and visions for the future have changed. Instead of parties, what information is to be shared, and with whom, and when? How much privacy is granted? The manner in which the family, other youth leaders, and the nurse work with the team, use the strengths of the congregation, and reflect on the spiritual needs of all concerned are important for healthy outcomes. The learning opportunities are valuable growth experiences for the young teens and for the new parents. Having opportunities to describe one's feelings and dealing with them in supportive groups reaps benefits in the healing process.

Legal Issues

As an advocate of client and group rights, the nurse:

- Identifies and reports neglect, abuse, and illegal behaviors to the appropriate legal sources

- Appropriately refers members to pastoral or community resources if the scope of the problem is beyond the realm of the professional nurse
- Refers to another health care professional if conflict between nurse and client is such that no further progress is possible.

The parish nurse who has a positive relationship that values open dialogue with the pastoral team will be supported in efforts to select the most appropriate community resources for clients.

The nurse must personally and professionally abide by the parameters of the nurse practice act of the jurisdiction and maintain an active license of that state. Additional legal concerns are:

- Institutional contractual agreements
- Records management
- Release of information
- Volunteer liability.

Resources would include the faith community's legal consultant, the faith community's national position statements, and Parish Nurse Resource Center guides (Solari-Twadell, et al, 1994).

Financial Issues

The nurse is called on to partner in finding funds and partnering with potential supporters. The nurse is accountable for money spent and for fundraising whether the position is salaried or voluntary. Educational and promotional materials, equipment, travel time, continuing education, and malpractice insurance are selected areas that must be included in the budget of the parish nurse. If these materials are not budget items, services may be limited; this must be communicated to the faith community.

NATIONAL HEALTH OBJECTIVES AND FAITH COMMUNITIES

The health objectives *Healthy People 2000* and *Healthy People 2010* encourage communities to cooperatively lend support to individuals and families to attain an improved health status that can be passed on to future generations. One of the oldest and strongest partnerships is that established between communities and religious or faith communities. The Carter Center in Atlanta and the Park Ridge Center in Chicago collaborated with health care professionals and leaders of faith traditions to identify roles of faith communities to address national health objectives and approaches to improving overall public health.

Examples of congregational models addressing the specific objectives encouraging *Healthy People 2000* guidelines are increasingly being documented (Berry, 1994; Marty, 1990; Magilvy and Brown, 1997; Weis, Matheus, and Schank, 1997). Additionally, the National Heart, Lung and Blood Institute urges partnerships with faith communities and offers suggestions for program planning (U.S. Department of Health and Human Services, 1998).

A third national level effort to strengthen the potential partnerships between faith communities and health care professionals is the Caucus on Public Health and the Faith Community of the American Public Health Association (APHA). The caucus' first gathering at the 1995 American Public Health Association annual meeting was addressed by then-APHA President Dr. Caswell Evans. Health care professionals of many faiths welcomed the opportunity to voice their interest in holistically supporting their communities and clients.

Wellness committees and parish nurses with the faith community's input may regularly review the various health status objectives, make comparisons between national and specific state objectives, and then assess to what extent the specific congregation or groups of congregations are in need of reducing their risk. Health promotion activities such as regular blood pressure screening and monitoring activities focus on heart disease and stroke prevention and disability.

- Age-appropriate discussion of preventive activities can be held with various groups.
- Signs and symptoms of heart attack and stroke can be noted and described in newsletters and posted in strategic areas.
- The nurse can coordinate healthy low-fat church suppers.
- The nurse can encourage "moms and tots" groups to choose healthy fruit and vegetables as snacks after their faith discussion meetings.
- The nurse can coordinate a series of classes for families of adolescents on stress management and sessions on the use and misuse of alcohol, tobacco, and other drugs.
- The nurse can encourage regular exercise for individuals as a part of ongoing church activities.

Examples of interventions related to selected portions of *Healthy People 2010* objectives that could be addressed by parish nurses are listed in the Box 26-3.

The congregation's health and wellness committee can similarly address other objectives to identify activities in

---

Box 26-3   Healthy People (HP) 2010 Objectives Identified by Parish Nurses

- Blood pressure knowledge and control (Objectives 12-9, 12-10, 12-11, 12-12)
- Overweight prevalence and weight loss practices (Objectives 19-1, 19-2 19-3)
- Vigorous physical activity (Objective 22-3)
- BSE and mammogram (Objective 3-13)
- Home fire safety (Objectives 15-25, 15-26)
- Reduce heart disease and stroke (Objectives 12-1, 12-2, 12-7, 12-8)
- Reduce child abuse (Objective 15-33)
- Maintain ADLs 651 (Objectives 2-2, 2-3)

From Weis D, Matheus R, Schank MJ: Health care delivery in faith communities: the parish nurse model, *Public Health Nurs* 14(6):368, 1997; U.S. Department of Health and Human Services: *Healthy people 2010: national health promotion and disease prevention objectives*, Washington, D.C., 2000, U.S. Department of Health and Human Services.

which to engage individuals, groups, or the congregation as a whole. To promote healthy families, faith communities can address objectives with a maternal and infant health focus (see the How To below). Most advantageous for the faith community would be to engage in partnership activities with other community efforts such as health fairs. Health fairs are effective strategies for health promotion efforts guided by the *Healthy People 2010* framework. Dillon and Sternas (1997) describe steps to successfully plan, implement, and evaluate health fairs that support health promotion and disease prevention efforts. These and similar activities promote increased health of the entire community and include persons of all ages, encourage enthusiastic fellowship and leisure, and reduce duplication of effort.

HOW TO Hold a Health Fair

- A health fair is always based on a community needs assessment for two purposes.
- The purposes of health fairs are always health education and screening of a healthy population.
- Providers do not offer diagnoses but make referrals if an abnormality is found in screening.
- Preparation for the fair should begin 4 months in advance.
- An informal meeting is called of all professionals, volunteers, and community leaders to be involved in the fair to identify topics for the fair.
- The group establishes a theme and clear objectives for the fair.
- A budget, type of exhibits and timelines for meeting the objectives are planned.
- A program date and location are decided.
- The roles and responsibilities of each member of the group is decided.
- Meetings of the planning group are established at the initial meeting.
- A plan for marketing the fair is developed.
- After the fair, follow-up evaluation (2 to 4 weeks after) is done by phone, personal visits to select participants, or a mailed questionnaire to see if the objectives were met.

Dillon DL, Sternas K: Designing a successful health fair to promote individual, family, and community health, *J Comm Health Nurs* 14(1):1, 1997.

Healthy People 2010 categories will incorporate leading health indicators. The 2010 authors hope that use of "leading health indicators" will result in a more precise and accurate way to reflect the intent of *Healthy People 2010*. Communities of faith are among the new health-related partners, which include members such as managed care organizations and business partners. The indicators appear in Chapter 8.

Parish nurses working with groups are pivotal as supportive links to implementing healthy behaviors. The recognition that persons are at greater risk of HIV infection when other sexually transmitted diseases are present is another cue for faith communities to encourage community-based

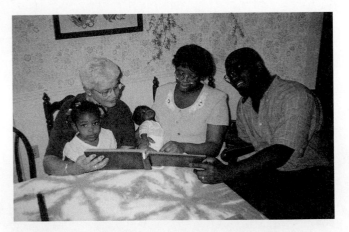

A parish nurse visits with a family of the congregation in their home.

programs to prevent sexually transmitted diseases, especially among adolescents and minorities. As young persons develop values and make life-style choices, their growth in character in a faith community can provide direction, support, and coping skills to select healthy options.

HOW TO Intervene in Maternal and Infant Health

- Visit family immediately after the birth of a new infant to further assess parenting skills and parent/infant bonding, reinforce holistic reflection of life transition, and plan for faith community support as indicated in those areas not addressed by family or other community agencies.
- Augment community prenatal classes or facilitate classes in faith community stressing growth and development of prenatal and postnatal period, family transitions, adequate health monitoring needed by parents, children, and new family members.
- Facilitate expectant parent support group to reinforce positive health during pregnancy, interpret plans negotiated with health care provider, promote spiritual reflection of family life transition to encourage connectedness with Creator and beliefs of faith community; provide emotional, social, community support to family.

FUNCTIONS OF THE PARISH NURSE

Examples of parish nursing interventions have been cited throughout this chapter. This section summarizes and expands some of the usual functions and describes activities. A primary independent function is that of *personal health counseling.* Parish nurses discuss:

- Health risk appraisals
- Spiritual assessments
- Plans for healthier life-styles
- Support and guidance related to numerous acute and chronic actual and potential health problems.

Parish nurses carry out their practice in groups or individually. They make visits to homes, hospitals, and nursing homes. They see persons in the faith community's house of worship. Some nurses have designated offices, whereas others use space that is most conducive to the particular activity or client need.

A second function is that of *health education*. Parish nurses:

- Publish information in congregation news bulletins
- Distribute information
- Have available a variety of resources for the physical, mental, and spiritual health of the congregation
- Hold classes to address identified needs
- Provide individual teaching as needed
- Hold discussions for targeted groups or meetings
- Strive to promote wholeness in health
- Create a fuller understanding of total physical, mental, and spiritual well-being.

As a *liaison* between resources in the faith community and the local community, the parish nurse again:

- Helps clients know what resources are available to solve their problems
- Helps individuals and families choose the appropriate resource match to their problem
- Links clients with the appropriate services.

The parish nurse is also a *facilitator*. The nurse:

- Links congregational needs to the establishment of and referral to support groups
- Facilitates changes in the congregation to increase disability access or to extend meals and services to those who are homebound
- May also work with the volunteer coordinator to train volunteers or ensure that interested persons acquire training to function as lay caregivers to meet congregational needs.

Box 26-4 is an example of how the parish works with other providers and community resources to meet the health needs of a client.

An important function underlying all of the previously mentioned functions is that of *pastoral care*. The nurse:

- Stresses the spiritual dimension of nursing
- Lends support during times of joy and sorrow
- Guides the person through health and illness throughout life
- Helps to identify the spiritual strengths that assist in coping with particular events.

The nurse may use hymns, favorite scripture verses, psalms, pictures, church windows, stories, or other images that are important for the individual or group to hold to the connectedness between faith, health, and well-being.

Healthy activities to be encouraged in congregations are numerous and the nurse often works with the congregation to stretch beyond its immediate borders to augment services in the community that promote health and wellness. Congregations are keenly aware that more than half of the members of mainline churches are part of the growing aging population of our country. Increased numbers of persons who

---

| Box 26-4 | **Parish Nursing as Healing Ministry . . . An Adult Daughter's Reflection** |

What a pleasure to be able to commend (parish nurse's) personal friendship and professional help! Without her support it would have been difficult, if not impossible, for my father to live at home during his last 6 years. But she had, along with his doctor, the sure feeling that it was the right thing for him and that it could be done. When the time came that he needed caregivers around the clock, she skillfully conveyed suggestions in such a way that the caregivers' cultural differences were not a barrier. She helped them grow as caregivers, appreciating their accomplishments, even to having a blackberry-picking "outing" at her home.

My father in his earlier years had been a deacon and had loved visiting shut-ins. It brought him so much happiness that he in turn received his church's caring, healing ministry through his parish nurse. He attended church on Sundays beyond what one would expect of one in his 90s, and almost his last Sunday was the day he celebrated turning 96.

Thank you, [parish nurse], for our "Mission Accomplished"!

With permission, A.F.H.

| Box 26-5 | **A Sampling of Parish Nurse Interventions and Activities** |

- Sharing the joys of a new member in the family; sharing sorrows of losses
- Anticipating changes in health status or in growth and development
- Being present for questions that seem difficult or unacceptable to ask the health care provider
- Explaining and assisting in considering choices when new living and care arrangements must be made
- Listening to the concerns of a youngster anticipating diagnostic procedures
- Praying with the spouse of a dying parishioner
- Helping individuals and families make decisions regarding advance directives in light of faith beliefs
- Helping teens consider options when overwhelmed with serious life issues
- Providing information, support, and prayer regarding advance directives
- Seeking community resources/opportunities for fitness and nutrition classes
- Working with the wellness committee to ensure that fellowship meals meet nutritional and spiritual needs of the elderly
- Offering educational opportunities about health care legislation changes and its influence on the congregation and community
- Accompanying a faith community member to 12-step meeting
- Participating in worship leadership with pastoral staff

From Berry R: A parish nurse. In Office of Resourcing Committees on Preparation for Ministry: *A day in the life of. . . . a kaleidoscope of specialized ministries,* Louisville, Ky, 1994, Presbyterian Church (USA): Distribution Management Service.

are either uninsured or underinsured are in their communities. Thus services offered may include:

- Food pantries
- Daycare for seniors
- Congregate meals
- Preschool and latch-key arrangements
- Tutoring
- Meals on Wheels
- Visiting less-mobile members
- Outreach for vulnerable populations.

Box 26-5 lists several selected activities of parish nurses (Berry, 1994). However the creative implementing of the parish nurse concept by each individual nurse within a unique faith community will result in a wealth of possibilities.

Clinical Application

The nursing process is a method that can be used to begin program planning and evaluation with faith communities. Such an approach can involve congregational members and parish nurses in a dynamic endeavor to jointly learn about the members' individual health status, as well as that of the faith community and the local and broader geographic community. Parish nurse programs are derived in various ways. Initially, the impetus for parish nursing may stem from an unmet health need within the congregation; from visions of a lay or health professions member concerned about caring within the congregation; or from discussions of a committee dealing with health and wellness issues.

Which of the following activities is most likely to increase the interest and involvement of the congregation's members?
A. Writing a contract for parish nurses services
B. Surveying the faith communities' environment
C. Gathering information on leaders and valued activities in the congregation through focus groups of pastoral staff
D. Assessing the needs of the congregational members through a survey
E. Holding a health fair

Answer is in the back of the book.

 Remember This!

- Parish nurse services respond to health, healing, and wholeness within the context of the church. Although the emphasis is on health promotion and disease prevention throughout the life span, the spiritual dimension of nursing is central to the practice.
- The parish nurse partners with the wellness committee and volunteers to plan programs and consider health-related concerns within faith communities.
- To promote a caring faith community, usual functions of the parish nurse include personal health counseling, health teaching, facilitating linkages and referrals to congregation and community resources, advocating and encouraging support resources, and providing pastoral care.

- Parish nurses collaborate to plan, implement, and evaluate health promotion activities considering the faith community's beliefs, rituals, and polity. *Healthy People 2010* guidelines are basic to the partnering for programs.
- Nurses in congregational or institutional models enhance the health ministry programs of the faith communities if carefully chosen partnerships are formed within the congregation, with other congregations, and also with local health and social community agencies.
- Nurses working in the parish nursing specialty must seek to attain adequate educational and skill preparation for the accountability to those served and to those who have entrusted the nurse to serve.
- Nurses are encouraged to consider innovative approaches to creating caring communities. These may be in congregations as parish nurses, among several faith communities in a single locale, or regionally; or in partnership with other community agencies or models such as block nursing.
- To sustain oneself as a parish nurse healer, the nurse takes heed to heal and nurture self while supporting individuals, families, and congregation communities in their healing process.

 What Would You Do?

1. Contact the local council of churches to see if there is a parish nurse in your community. If so, contact the nurse and arrange to spend a day with the nurse.
   a. Interview the nurse regarding the parish nurse role functions.
   b. Ask how the parish nurse standards of practice are integrated into the practice.
2. Discuss with classmates the similarities and differences between parish nursing and other community health nurses. Review the content in this chapter and compare your answers.
3. Choose a *Healthy People 2010* objective to implement in a parish nursing setting. Discuss plans for implementing the objective and evaluating the outcomes. What data did you use to develop a plan for implementing? How did you choose your population?

REFERENCES

American Nurses Association: *Standards of clinical nursing practice,* Washington, D.C., 2000, American Nurses Association.

Berry R: A parish nurse. In Office of Resourcing Committees on Preparation for Ministry: *A day in the life of . . . a kaleidoscope of specialized ministries,* Louisville, Ky, 1994, Presbyterian Church (USA): Distribution Management Service.

Bondine D: Parish nursing, *Perspectives* 21(2):8, 1997.

Culp L: Health ministries: caring for body and soul, *Reg Nurse J* 9(3):8, 1997.

Dillon DL, Sternas K: Designing a successful health fair to promote individual, family, and community health, *J Comm Health Nurs* 14(1):1, 1997.

Dossey BM, et al: *Holistic nursing: a handbook for practice,* ed 2, Gaithersburg, Md, 1995, Aspen.

Dossey L: *Healing words: the power of prayer and the practice of medicine,* New York, 1993, Harper Collins.

Fehring RJ, Miller JR, Shaw C: Spiritual well-being, religiosity, hope, depression and other mood states in elderly people coping with cancer, *Oncol Nurs Forum* 24:663, 1997.

Foege W: A strategy for change, *Faith Health Summer,* 2, 1996.

Granberg-Michaelson K: Staying healthy: the spiritual dimension, *Contact* 155:3, 1997.

Health Ministries Association/American Nurses Association: *Scope and standards of parish nursing practice,* Washington, D.C., 1998, American Nurses Publishing.

International Parish Nurse Resource Center: Role of parish nurse, mission and resources (brochure), Park Ridge, Ill, 1998, International Parish Nurse Resource Center.

Magilvy JK, Brown NJ: Parish nursing: advanced practice nursing model for healthier communities, *Adv Pract Nurs Q* 2:67, 1997.

Marty M: *Healthy people 2000: a role for America's religious communities,* Chicago, 1990, Carter Center and Park Ridge Center.

Matthews DA, et al. Religious commitment and health status: a review of the research and implications for family medicine, *Arch Fam Med* 7(2):118, 1998.

McDermott MA, Solari-Twadell PA, Mathews R: Promoting quality education for the parish nurse and parish nurse coordinate, *Nurs Health Care Perspect* 19(1):4, 1998.

Oman D, Reed D: Religion and mortality among the community-dwelling elderly, *Am J Public Health* 88(10):1469, 1998.

Oxman TE, Freeman DH, Manheimer ED: Lack of social participation or religious strength and comfort as risk factors for death after cardiac surgery in the elderly, *Psychosom Med* 57(1):5, 1995.

Rydholm L: Patient-focused care in parish nursing, *Holist Nurs Pract* 11(3):47, 1997.

Schacht AR: The parish nurse, *Horizons* 5:16, 1992.

Schank MJ, Weis D, Matheus R: Parish nursing: ministry of healing, *Geriatr Nurs* 17(1):11, 1996.

Solari-Twadell A, McDermott MA (editors): *Parish nursing: promoting whole person health within faith communities,* Thousand Oaks, Calif, 1999, Sage.

Solari-Twadell A, et al: *Assuring viability for the future: guideline development for parish nurse education programs,* Park Ridge, Ill, 1994, Lutheran General HealthSystem.

Solari-Twadell PA, Djupe AM, McDermott MA (editors): *Parish nursing: the developing practice,* Park Ridge, Ill, 1990, International Parish Nurse Resource Center.

U.S. Department of Health and Human Services: *Leading indicators for HP 2010:* a report from Health and Human Services working group on sentinel objectives, section one: healthy people 2000 and leading health indicators, Washington, D.C., 1998, U.S. Department of Health and Human Services.

Van Loon A: International faith community nursing, *Internat J Nurs Pract* 2(3):168, 1996.

Weis D, Mathcus R, Schank MJ: Health care delivery in faith communities: the parish nurse model, *Public Health Nurs* 14(6):368, 1997.

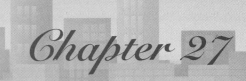

www.mosby.com/MERLIN/Stanhope/foundations

Chapter 27

Community Health Nursing in Home Health and Hospice

LINDA M. SAWYER

OBJECTIVES

After reading this chapter, the student should be able to:
- Define home health and hospice care.
- Analyze the similarities and differences in the types of home health agencies.
- Discuss the educational requirements and competencies for a home health nurse.
- Relate the nursing process and standards of community health nursing practice to the home health setting.
- Identify the roles and functions of the interdisciplinary health care team.
- Examine the regulatory impact on home health care and nursing practice.
- Analyze the reimbursement mechanisms, issues, and trends relative to home health care.

CHAPTER OUTLINE

Definition of Home Health Care

History of Home Health Care

Types of Home Health Care Agencies
Official Agencies
Voluntary and Private Nonprofit Agencies
Combination Agencies
Hospital-Based Agencies
Proprietary Agencies

Scope of Practice
Contracting
Practice Functions of the Home Health Nurse

Standards of Home Health Nursing Practice

Interdisciplinary Approach to Home Health and Hospice Care
Responsibilities of the Disciplines
Hospice Care

Educational Requirements for Home Health Practice
Certification

Accountability and Quality Management
Quality Control Mechanisms
Accreditation
Regulatory Mechanisms

Financial Aspects of Home Health and Hospice Care
Home Health Reimbursement
Hospice Reimbursement

Effects of Legislation on Home Health Care Services

Legal and Ethical Issues

National Health Objectives

Issues for the Twenty-First Century
Access to Health Care
Technology and Telehealth
Pediatric and Maternal-Child Home Care
Family Responsibility, Roles, and Functions
Measuring the Outcomes of Home Health Care

463

KEY TERMS

accreditation: a credentialing process used to recognize health care agencies or educational programs for provision of quality services and programs.

benchmarking: comparing national standards and guidelines to other agencies.

care coordination: linking clients with services.

care planning: home health nurse and clients work together to give adequate service at home.

certification: a mechanism, usually by means of written examination, that provides an indication of professional competence in a specialized area of practice.

client outcome: a change in client health status as a result of care or program implementation.

contracting: any working agreement, continuously renegotiable and agreed upon by nurse and client.

distributive care: health care services that emphasize health promotion, maintenance, and disease prevention.

episodic care: curative and restorative aspect of nursing practice.

family caregiving: assisting the client to meet his or her basic needs and providing direct care such as personal hygiene, meal preparation, medication administration, and treatments.

fiscal intermediaries: insurance companies under contract to the Social Security Administration to pay home care agencies for Medicare-covered services rendered to beneficiaries.

hospice: palliative system of health care for terminally ill people; takes place in the home with family involvement under the direction and supervision of health professionals, especially the visiting nurse. Hospice care takes place in the hospital when severe complications of terminal illness occur or when family becomes exhausted or does not fulfill commitments.

interdisciplinary collaboration: working agreement in which each home health care provider carefully analyzes his or her role in determining the best plan for the client's care.

intermittent care: service for clients who are confined to home and require skilled care for one of the following: speech therapy, physical therapy, or occupational therapy. The amount of time involved could range from 28 or 35 hours per week to full-time service.

Outcomes and Assessment Information Set (OASIS): an instrument to collect client data for doing outcome assessments in home health.

palliative care: alleviating symptoms of, meeting the special needs of, and providing comfort for the dying clients and families by the nurse.

prospective payment system: a mechanism whereby Medicare will pay home health agencies a set amount of money to care for a client who meets the criteria of 1 of 80 home health resource groups (diagnosis based on severity, functional status, and number of services needed).

recertification: in-home health care, the review and certification performed at least every 62 days by the health care team; it demonstrates that the client continues to need a specified plan of care.

regulation: specific statement of law that relates to and clarifies individual pieces of legislation.

reimbursement system: the process by which home health care agencies receive payment, either by the client or three major funding sources: Medicare, Medicaid, and third-party funding sources.

skilled care: care provided to a client that requires the knowledge and skill of a registered nurse.

telehealth: health information sent from one site to another by electronic communication.

This chapter presents an important nursing specialty within community health nursing: home health care and the related subspecialty of hospice nursing. Home health differs from other areas of health care in that health care providers practice in the client's environment. Home is a place where nurses have provided care for more than two centuries in the United States. Nurses provide family care within the community environment.

When working in a client's home, the nurse is a guest and, to be effective, must earn the trust of the family. In this setting nurses have the opportunity to observe family life, a privilege usually reserved for family and friends, including:

- Family dynamics
- Life-style choices
- Communication patterns
- Coping strategies
- Responses to health and illness
- Social, cultural, spiritual, and economic issues (Doherty and Hurley, 1994).

When working with an individual client or family in the home the nurse reaches beyond the boundaries of that household. To provide effective, comprehensive care, nurses will want to:

- Analyze the strength that clients gain from their neighborhoods
- Use the social network to support clients in times when they are vulnerable and in crisis
- Gain the trust of communities by providing for the needs of the clients they serve in that community with caring, honesty, competence, and ethical and cultural sensitivity (Doherty and Hurley, 1994).

The use of home health care continues to expand in response to:

- Increased demands for cost-effectiveness
- Decreased hospital stays
- Consumer preferences
- Technological advances that are becoming user friendly
- Proven quality of service.

DEFINITION OF HOME HEALTH CARE

Home health care in today's society cannot be defined simply as "care at home." It includes an arrangement of disease

Box
27-1 **Definitions of Home Health Care**

Historically home health care was defined as that component of a continuum of comprehensive health care whereby health services are provided to individuals and families in their places of residence for the purpose of promoting, maintaining or restoring health, or of maximizing the level of independence while minimizing the effects of disability and illness, including terminal illness. Services appropriate to the needs of the individual client and family are planned, coordinated, and made available by providers organized for the delivery of home care. The agency employed staff, contractual arrangements, or a combination of the two to deliver service (Warhola, 1980).

A more current definition is the practice of nursing applied to a client with a health condition in the client's place of residence. . . . "Home health nursing is a specialized area of nursing practice with its roots firmly placed in community health nursing" (American Nurses Association, 1999, p. 3). It involves the same primary preventive focus of care of aggregates of the community health nurses and the secondary and tertiary prevention focuses of the care of individuals in collaboration with the family and other caregivers.

A broad spectrum of health and social services offered in the home environment to recovering, disabled, or chronically ill persons (National Association of Home Care, 1997).

---

prevention, health promotion, and episodic illness–related services provided to people in their places of residence (Box 27-1).

The definitions of home health integrate:
- The individual and family client
- Caregivers
- Multidisciplinary health care professionals
- Goals to assist the client to return to an optimum level of health and independence.

Interpretation and actual delivery of home health care vary according to client needs and the provider and payer of these services.

Working with the family in providing care to an individual client is essential. Family is defined by the individual and includes any caregiver or significant person who assists the client in need of care at home. **Family caregiving** includes assisting clients to meet their basic needs and providing direct care such as personal hygiene, meal preparation, medication administration, and treatments. Care provided in the home today by caregivers was historically done only in the hospital by a health care provider. The caregiver is essential in providing the needed maintenance care between the skilled visits of the professional provider.

A client's place of residence has its own uniqueness in terms of the location for providing care, depending on what the person calls home. Home may be a house, apartment, trailer, boarding and care home, shelter, car, makeshift shelter under a bridge, or cardboard box.

Client goals are always related to the principles of health promotion, maintenance, and restoration. By maximizing the level of independence, home health nurses help clients

function at the best possible level and prevent dependence. This assistance includes:
- Providing a combination of direct care and health education
- Enhancing self-care
- Linking the client with community services that provide limited assistance to enable the client to stay at home
- Contributing to the prevention of complications in chronically ill persons
- Helping to minimize the effects of disability and illness.

The development of hospice home care programs has improved the care of terminally ill persons. If the client and family accept the hospice concept, most of their care can be handled comfortably at home instead of in the hospital. Reducing of pain and suffering is possible through the use of medications and other measures that are closely supervised by nurses in the home. In both home health and hospice, nurses continually:
- Assess the client's response to treatment
- Report their findings to the client's physician
- Collaborate to modify the treatment plan as needed.

Services can be tailored to any client need or problem. When the client's level of independence increases, the need for service decreases. Services are coordinated through an agency obligated to maintain quality care and provide for continuity. Thus the range of services provided in home health care is extensive. The strong connections of home health care to community health nursing practice can be seen by briefly tracing the history of this nursing role.

HISTORY OF HOME HEALTH CARE

Home health care began in the United States in the early 1800s. In these early years:
- Nuns and religious sisters cared for the sick in the home.
- The Sisters of Charity of St. Joseph was established in Maryland in 1809.
- The first organized visiting nurse work was done by the Ladies' Benevolent Society of Charleston, South Carolina, founded in 1813.
- The precursor of modern home care, organized visiting nursing, was established in March 1877 when the women's branch of the New York City Mission sent trained nurses into the homes of the poor and the sick.
- The first home health nurse, Frances Root, was a member of the Bellevue Hospital Training School's first class.
- In 1885 Elizabeth Marshall founded the Buffalo District Nursing Association, the first visiting nurses association (VNA) in the United States.
- In 1886 Boston formed the Instructive Visiting Nursing Association. During this same period, Philadelphia's VNA established a pay service.
- By 1890, some 13 years after the first nurse was sent out by the New York City Mission, 21 VNAs existed in the United States, most employing only one nurse each.
- In 1893 the Henry Street Settlement was founded in New York by Lillian Wald.

- In 1909 the Metropolitan Life Insurance Company began offering home nursing services to its millions of industrial policy holders in the United States and Canada. Initially, arrangements were made with Lillian Wald and the Henry Street Settlement to provide these nursing services.
- By 1912 Metropolitan was offering home nursing services from 589 nursing centers.
- Sixteen years later, John Hancock Mutual Life Insurance Company established a similar service for its policy holders.

The number of visiting nurses in the United States increased from 136 in 1902 to 3000 in 1912. With funding from both private and public sources, visiting nurses were employed by some 810 agencies, including VNAs, city and state boards of health and education, private clubs and societies, the tuberculosis leagues, hospitals and dispensaries, business concerns, settlements and day nurseries, churches, and charitable organizations.

In the 1940s, hospitals began to take a more serious interest in home care because of the increased number of chronically ill clients being hospitalized. The Montefiore Hospital Home Care Program in New York began in 1947 and offered comprehensive nursing and social services. Before the enactment of Medicare in 1966, most agencies relied on public contributions and charity for their survival.

Briefly Noted

Throughout its history, home health nurses have epitomized Florence Nightingale's philosophy that nurses are "messengers of health as well as ministers of disease" (Woodham-Smith, 1951).

The community health nurses working in the home:
- Were social reformers, living in immigrant communities and providing nursing clinics, health education, and care for the sick
- Provided for the nutritional needs of their communities as well as clothing, hygiene, and adequate shelter
- Were responsible for developing needed programs and providing necessary services in communities including the following:
  - Prenatal care
  - Postpartum visits to new mothers and babies
  - Hot lunch school programs
  - Preschool clinics
  - Transportation services
  - Summer camp programs
  - Tuberculosis screening
  - Blood typing
  - Immunization for polio
  - "Sick room" equipment programs.

This combination of preventive services and illness care continued until the introduction of Medicare in 1966. Home care reached a turning point with the passage of Medicare,

which introduced regulations for home care practice and for reimbursement mechanisms. In 1967, 1 year after Medicare was enacted, there were 1,753 Medicare-participating home health agencies in the United States. The majority of agencies were either VNAs or programs in public health departments. By 1980 there were 2,924 home health agencies, an increase of about 48%. The Health Care Financing Administration (HCFA) reported 7,747 Medicare-certified home health agencies in 1999, as well as 16,525 non–Medicare-certified home health agencies for a total of 24,272. The growth in certified agencies alone represented a 572% growth in 30 years (National Association of Home Care, 2000). For the first time since 1996 home health services began to decline in 2000. This happened because HCFA reduced the amount of money paid to home health agencies for client services.

The Medicare program emphasized an acute disease–care payment program that influenced the services offered through home health and deleted all emphasis on illness prevention and health promotion. Some home health agencies continued to develop programs to benefit their communities, paying for them through their profits or through contributions. Today, a number of agencies are once again offering a combination of preventive and illness care services as a mechanism to decease the long-term costs of health care.

TYPES OF HOME HEALTH CARE AGENCIES

Since the beginning of organized home care, many organizations have established programs to meet the home care needs of people. Home health agencies are divided into the following five general types based on administrative and organizational structures:
- Official
- Private and voluntary
- Combination
- Hospital-based
- Proprietary.

These types differ in organization and administration but are similar in terms of the standards they must meet for licensure, certification, and accreditation. Figure 27-1 shows the types of home health agencies. Table 27-1 lists the numbers and kinds of home health agencies, and Box 27-2 presents facts concerning home health agencies.

Official Agencies

Official or *public agencies* include those agencies operated by the state, county, city, or other local government units, such as health departments. Most official agencies, in addition to having a home care component, also provide health education and disease prevention programs to people in the community.

Community health nurses employed in this setting provide:
- Well-child clinics
- Immunizations

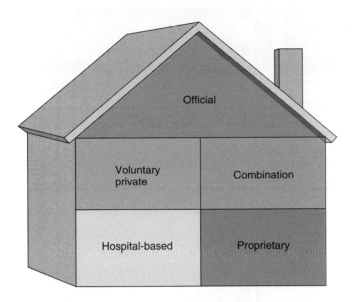

Figure 27-1   Types of home health agencies.

- Health education programs
- Home visits for preventive health care.

Official agencies are funded primarily by tax funds and are nonprofit entities. The home care services provided are reimbursed through Medicare, Medicaid, and private insurance companies. Official agencies offer more comprehensive services for two reasons:

- Their primary objective is health promotion and disease prevention for the community
- They have additional public funding available.

Voluntary and Private Nonprofit Agencies

Voluntary and *private agencies* are grouped together as nonprofit home health agencies. Voluntary agencies are supported by charities such as United Way, as well as by Medicare, Medicaid, other third-party payers, and client payments. The amount of financial assistance the voluntary agency receives depends on the community it serves. Traditionally, VNAs were the principal voluntary type of home health agency. With Medicare in 1966, the private nonprofit agency emerged as an alternative agency to the public-supported program. These agencies included rehabilitation agencies, based in either rehabilitation facilities or skilled facilities.

Boards of directors that represent the communities they serve govern voluntary and private nonprofit agencies. These agencies are nongovernmental organizations and are exempt from federal income tax. Historically, voluntary agencies were responsible for the initial development of nursing in the home, based on the client's need for service rather than the ability to pay.

Combination Agencies

In some communities, to decrease cost and prevent duplicating of services, official and voluntary home health agencies have merged into *combination agencies* to provide home health care. The services remain the same, and the board members come from either one of the two existing agencies or a new board is formed. The nurse may serve in several community health nursing roles, as does the nurse in the official type of agency.

Hospital-Based Agencies

Hospitals are frequently a primary site for health care services. In the 1970s, *hospital based agencies* emerged in response to the recognized need for continuity of care from the acute care setting and because of the high cost of institutionalization.

In 1983 implementation of the prospective payment system and diagnosis-related groups (DRGs) by the federal government caused a fundamental change in the attitudes of hospital personnel toward home care. Cost of care dictated earlier discharge of sicker clients to control profits. Increased liability risks, the desire for better client care, and the potential for several products and services increased the number of hospital-based home care agencies.

Hospital-based agencies differ from other home health care agencies in that the already-established hospital board of directors is responsible for governing the agency. Clients of hospital-based home health care have access to existing inpatient services. Whether the agencies are official, voluntary, private nonprofit, or proprietary depends on the hospital structure. Regardless of the form they take, in most cases these agencies are a source of revenue for the hospital and may compete with community-based agencies. Hospital-based agencies outnumber all other types of Medicare-certified agencies except for proprietary agencies (National Association of Home Care, 1997).

Proprietary Agencies

Agencies that are not eligible for income tax exemption are called *proprietary* (profit-making) agencies. Proprietary agencies can be licensed and certified for Medicare by the state licensing agency. The owner of the agency is responsible for governing. Reimbursement is primarily from third-party payers and individual clients if agencies do not accept

TABLE 27-1 Number of Home Health Agencies by Type

Year	Hospital	Rehabilitation Hospital	Skilled Nursing Facility	Visiting Nurse Association (VNA)	Combination Agency	Public	Proprietary (Nonprofit)	Private	Other	Total
1967	133	0	0	549	93	939	0	0	30	1,753
1980	359	8	9	515	63	1260	186	484	40	2,924
1990	1486	8	101	474	47	985	1884	710	0	5,695
1996	2634	4	191	576	34	1177	4658	695	58	10,027
1997	2698	3	204	553	33	1149	5024	715	65	10,444
1998	2356	2	166	460	35	968	3414	610	69	8,080
1999	2300	1	163	452	35	918	3192	621	65	7,747

From Health Care Financing Administration, Center for Information Systems, Health Standards and Quality Bureau, Washington, D.C., 1999, U.S. Department of Health and Human Services.

Medicare. In recent years the number of Medicare-certified proprietary agencies increased significantly as hospitals began implementing quicker discharge of sicker patients (National Association of Home Care, 1997).

Regardless of the type of home health agency existing in a community, the primary goal should be to provide quality home health care based on the community's health needs. Traditionally, most agencies have remained noncompetitive because of their humanitarian mission. Today competition in home health care is on the rise as a result of the federal government's move to deregulate and deinstitutionalize health care. Competition can potentially be a positive force in developing and maintaining quality home health programs. But home health care is a business and can be profit producing, which requires strong utilization review and quality improvement mechanisms.

The changing environment in home health care has several implications for the community health nurse:

- Clients are discharged from acute care at earlier stages of treatment, thereby needing a highly skilled level of care at home.
- To survive in the competitive arena, agencies must continue to provide quality care and be cost-effective without compromising accountability.
- These home care changes require that home health nurses, as both clinicians and managers, have highly developed administrative and case management skills.

SCOPE OF PRACTICE

A common misconception of home health care is that it is a "custodial" type of nursing. It is important to remember that home health care nursing is part of community health nursing. Thus health promotion and disease prevention activities are fundamental components of practice. Because home health care is often intermittent, a primary objective for the nurse is to facilitate self-care. The American Nurses Association defines *home health* and *home health nursing* as follows:

Home health—The range of health care services provided to a client in his or her place of residence.

Home health nursing—A specialized area of nursing practice with its roots firmly placed in community health nursing. Nursing care is delivered in the residence of the client.

According to Orem (1995, p. 104), "*Self-care* is the practice of activities that individuals initiate and perform on their own behalf in maintaining life, health, and well-being." Home health nurses use this concept for all clients, regardless of the clients' abilities. For example, a client may be recuperating at home after suffering a cerebrovascular accident (CVA, stroke) and be unable to perform activities of daily living (ADLs) without assistance. Such clients can be instructed to perform these activities in a modified form. In this way they have some control over their life and self-care activities and can be taught to prevent possible losses in other self-care areas.

 Evidence-Based Practice

The authors developed a system of nursing interventions, named PREP, and pilot tested the interventions with 22 families. A quasi-experimental design was used, with 11 families randomly assigned to the control group and 11 to the experimental group. The PREP experimental group received care from one of three nurses over a 3- to 6-month period. The control group received standard home health care over the same time period. Effectiveness and acceptability of the intervention were evaluated through interviews at 2, 7, and 12 weeks after admission to PREP or standard home health and by a mailed survey at 8 to 12 months after completion of the study. Six dependent variables were measured: caregiver role strain, rewards of caregiving, caregiver depression, care effectiveness, hospital utilization, and cost for the care receiver.

The PREP system includes 10 key elements identified through previous research: systematic assessment, family focus, local knowledge of the family, cosmopolitan knowledge brought by nurses, blending of both local and cosmopolitan knowledge, family-nurse collaboration, individualized interventions, multiple strategies, therapeutic relationship, and early detection and intervention during difficult transitions. PREP has three goals:

1. Increasing the preparedness and competence of caregivers through highly individualized interventions
2. Enriching caregiving through engaging in or modifying pleasurable and meaningful activities
3. Increasing the predictability in caregiving situations and the family's control over the environment

The PREP system was delivered through expanded home services, a PREP advice line answered by nurses who knew the family, a "keep-in-touch" system of assessment contacts by telephone after home health discharge, completion of PREP with a written summary of the family's strengths and progress, and a discussion with the family about their learning while on PREP.

There were no significant differences on the nine role strain measures, rewards of caregiving, or the two depression scales between the experimental and control groups. The experimental group rated the PREP nurse as significantly more useful than the nurse or physical therapist in the control group. Caregivers in the experimental group perceived greater changes in preparedness for caregiving, enrichment, and predictability. Mean hospital costs were lower in the PREP group, although not significantly, but the number of hospitalizations in each group were equal. Additionally, the PREP system was acceptable to families. This pilot study supports the need for a larger evaluation of the PREP system.

APPLICATION IN PRACTICE

Home health nurses can use this study as a model to develop effective interventions and assess outcomes of interventions. Family-centered interventions may be the most effective in providing for long-term care in the future.

Archbold PG, et al: The PREP system of nursing interventions: a pilot test with families caring for older members, *Res Nurs Health* 18:3, 1995.

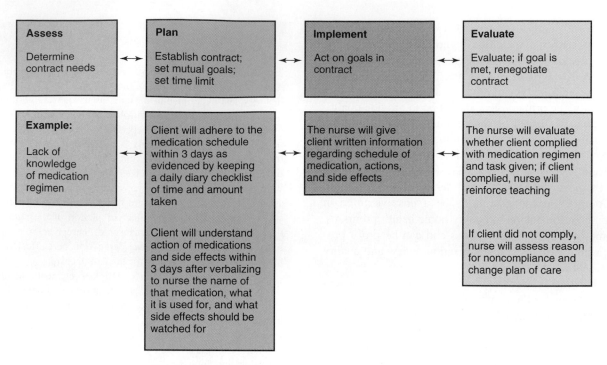

Figure 27-2   **Contracting in relation to the nursing process.**

The primary goals of home health care are to help prevent the occurrence of illness and to promote the client's well-being. In the home care setting, clients possess more control and determine their own health care needs. The effectiveness of service depends on the client's active involvement and understanding of plans established jointly by the client and nurse. The nurse facilitates the development of positive health behaviors for the individual who has had an episode of illness.

Contracting

Contracting is a vital component of all nurse/client relationships. Constantly evolving legislative guidelines, third-party payer requirements, the high risk of liability, and the level of nurse autonomy require that contracting be used in the home care environment.

The process of contracting in home care involves the client, the family, and the nurse. Contracting refers to any working agreement that is continuously renegotiable. The process of contracting is reflected in the client's care plan and clinical notes. Contracting allows the client, family, and nurse to set mutual goals and facilitates the effectiveness of nursing care and the promotion of self-care. Contracting is directly related to use of the nursing process (Fig. 27-2).

As an example, during an initial home visit, the nurse gathers data and determines the plan for actions by establishing the contract with the client and family. Contracts can be formal (written) or informal (verbal), depending on the client's needs. In either case, the process is recorded in the client's chart. The most important aspect of contracting is the client's active participation in developing, implementing, and evaluating the process.

Briefly Noted

To avoid what is often referred to as the "home visit ritual," visits that have no predetermined goal or outcome, the home health nurse must establish both short- and long-term goals with clients and families. The goals provide for continuity of care and state the criteria for evaluating the client's condition and progress toward an optimum level of self-care.

Practice Functions of the Home Health Nurse

Home health nursing involves both *direct* and *indirect* functions. In performing these functions, the home health nurse assumes a variety of roles.

Direct Care

Direct care refers to the actual physical aspects of nursing care, anything requiring physical contact and face-to-face interactions. By serving as a role model, the nurse helps the client and family to develop positive health behaviors. Technical skill competency must be demonstrated by the nurse to receive reimbursement by Medicare and Medicaid. Nursing care is covered by Medicare and other third-party payers as long as the care being delivered is **skilled care.** To determine whether a service performed by the nurse is skilled care, several factors are evaluated and must be adequately documented as shown in the How To Box on p. 471.

HOW TO Determine if the Service Is "Skilled"

- Is the service complex, thereby requiring the knowledge and skill of a registered nurse?
- Does the client's condition warrant skilled intervention?
- Can this service be performed by a nonmedical person?
- Does the instruction of a service to a client involve knowledge, instructions, and demonstrations by a registered nurse?

To adequately answer these questions, the home health nurse must be knowledgeable regarding regulations and be a competent and experienced clinician. Some examples of skilled nursing services include the following:

- Observing and evaluating a client's health status and condition
- Providing direct care in administering treatments, rehabilitative exercises, medications, catheter insertion, colostomy irrigation, and wound care
- Helping the client and family develop positive coping behaviors
- Teaching the client and family to give treatments and medications when indicated
- Teaching the client and family to carry out physician's orders such as treatments, therapeutic diets, or medication administration
- Reporting to physician changes in the client's condition and arranging for medical follow-up as indicated
- Helping client and family identify resources that will help client attain a state of optimal functioning.

Indirect Care

Indirect care activities are those that a nurse does on behalf of clients to improve or coordinate care. These activities include:

- Consulting with other nurses and health providers
- Organizing and participating in client care conferences
- Advocating for clients with the health care system and insurers
- Obtaining results of diagnostic tests
- Documenting care.

Home health care is multidisciplinary care. **Care coordination** of the multidisciplinary team is an essential function of the home health nurse. Team conferences are an ideal time for increasing coordination and continuity of services for optimal client care and use of resources and services.

For example, clients with complex conditions or those with inadequate support in the home are presented to the team, which allows joint **care planning** and problem solving.

Supervision of home health aides is both a direct and an indirect function. The home health nurse may evaluate the home health aide's care either by direct observation in the home or by interviewing clients, caregivers, and the aide. If nursing aide services are provided, then regular supervision of the aide by the nurse at least every 2 weeks is mandated. Regular communication with the client's physician is essential. There is much indirect care in the home health care setting. It may not be directly visible to the client, but it is necessary to provide quality home care.

Although Medicare places an emphasis on episodic, or acute, care because of its limitations on benefits and requirements for skilled care, the home health nurse cannot entirely separate primary, secondary, and tertiary prevention because of their interrelationship. These levels of prevention are categorized into two levels of care: *episodic* and *distributive*.

Briefly Noted

Home health agencies must provide nursing care as their primary service under Medicare.

Episodic Versus Distributive Care

Episodic care refers to the curative and restorative aspect of practice, or secondary and tertiary prevention, and **distributive care** refers to health maintenance and disease prevention, or primary prevention. A clinical example best illustrates the application of these two aspects in home health care.

Mr. Jones, a 70-year-old man discharged from the hospital the previous day, is admitted to home health services for skilled nursing to assess his cardiovascular status after heart surgery for coronary artery disease. Episodic care involves teaching Mr. and Mrs. Jones about medications, exercise, and the signs and symptoms of possible cardiac problems postoperatively. In addition, the home health nurse will provide direct care in assessing Mr. Jones' cardiovascular status, the healing of his incisions, and helping him return to his optimum state of functioning. The Jones family's psychosocial adaptation and needs will also be addressed, in addition to assessing the client's level of self-care and adjustment relative to postcardiac surgery status.

In regard to the distributive aspect, the home health nurse will do additional teaching about ways Mr. Jones can prevent an exacerbation of his condition by maintaining medical follow-up and adapting his life-style to increase his compliance with the programs set up for him.

Nursing Roles in Home Health Care

The roles of clinician, educator, researcher, administrator, and consultant function in home health care. The experienced home health nurse, the nurse manager, or the administrator can fulfill these roles.

Home health nurses in a staff position are *clinicians* who provide direct nursing care to clients and families. They are also *educators* because they teach clients and families the "how to" and "why" of self-care. Nurses also participate in the ongoing education of their colleagues as mentors, both formally, providing in-service education, and informally as team members. Additionally, they may teach classes to community groups regarding health education topics.

The *researcher* role in home health care is increasing in importance as the efficacy, or quality, and cost effectiveness of care becomes mandated by Medicare and other payers. Home health nurses often provide the data required for clinical or administrative changes to occur within their agency of employment. The home health care setting is filled with potential research areas. Research must be a priority in the future if quality and cost effectiveness are to be maintained. A home health administrator can be a nurse who has had advanced education with public health experience; requirements are stipulated by both federal and state rules and regulations. *Consultants* may provide advice and counsel to staff and clients.

Briefly Noted

Disease prevention and health promotion are integral to quality home health care.

STANDARDS OF HOME HEALTH NURSING PRACTICE

The home health nurse practices in accordance with the *Scope and Standards of Home Health Nursing Practice,* developed by the American Nurses Association (American Nurses Association, 1999).

Periodically, the profession revises the scope of practice and standards of specialty practice to reflect the ongoing changes in the health care system and their effect on nursing care.

The Scope and Standards of Home Health Nursing Practice were most recently revised in 1999. These latest Standards have two parts: Standards of Care, which follow the six steps of the Nursing Process, and Standards of Professional Performance. Box 27-3 presents both sets of Standards. The How To box below is related to the first standard of care, assessment.

HOW TO Assess Preferred Learning Style

How does the client decide how to buy a new piece of equipment for an interest or hobby?
- Reads a book or magazine—use written materials
- Watches a television program—use videos
- Talks to expert—verbal teaching
- Goes to store and looks at merchandise—use hands-on demonstrations and practice
- Belongs to a club and talks with others—group teaching

INTERDISCIPLINARY APPROACH TO HOME HEALTH AND HOSPICE CARE

Interdisciplinary collaboration is required in the home health and hospice settings. Its use is mandated for Medicare-certified home care agencies, and it is inherent in the definitions of home health care. Without effective collaboration there would be no continuity of care, and the client's home care program would be fragmented.

The collaborative process for home care directed toward secondary and tertiary prevention activities should begin in

---

Box 27-3	Home Health Nursing Standards of Practice

STANDARDS OF CARE

I. *Assessment:* The home health nurse collects client health data.
II. *Diagnosis:* The home health nurse analyzes the assessment data in determining diagnoses.
III. *Outcome Identification:* The home health nurse identifies expected outcomes customized to the client and client's environment.
IV. *Planning:* The home health nurse develops a plan of care that prescribes interventions to attain expected outcomes.
V. *Implementation:* The home health nurse implements the interventions identified in the plan of care.
VI. *Evaluation:* The home health nurse evaluates the client's progress toward attainment of outcomes.

STANDARDS OF PROFESSIONAL PERFORMANCE

I. *Quality of Care:* The home health nurse systematically evaluates the quality and effectiveness of nursing practice.
II. *Performance Appraisal:* The home health nurse evaluates his or her own nursing practice in relation to professional practice standards, scientific evidence, and relevant statues and regulations.
III. *Education:* The home health nurse acquires and maintains current knowledge and competency in nursing practice.
IV. *Collegiality:* The home health nurse interacts with and contributes to the professional development of peers and other health care practitioners as colleagues.
V. *Ethics:* The home health nurse's decisions and actions on behalf of clients are determined in an ethical manner.
VI. *Collaboration:* The home health nurse collaborates with the client, family, and other health care practitioners in providing client care.
VII. *Research:* The home health nurse uses research finding in practice.
VIII. *Resource Utilization:* The home health nurse assists the client or family in becoming informed consumers about the risks, benefits, and cost in planning and delivering client care.

---

the hospital with the discharge planner and hospital nurse, who identify a client's need for home care and then review their observations and plans with the physician for approval and orders. The discharge planner then contacts the referral intake coordinator of the home care agency, specifying the services requested by the physician. If persons from several disciplines will be involved, the intake coordinator notifies the appropriate staff and monitors the interdisciplinary collaboration. Either the registered nurse or the physical therapist usually functions as the case manager to ensure that care is coordinated.

In home care, as in other health care settings, professionals may experience stress associated with changing roles and overlapping responsibilities. In collaborating, each home health care provider should carefully analyze the roles of all to determine whether overlapping occurs, and then the team should adjust the plan of care accordingly. Professionals in home care are in a unique setting in which they can truly work together to accomplish the client's care goals.

Briefly Noted

A client care conference is convened to discuss issues with a family, develop a consistent team approach, and clarify roles.

In terms of legal accountability and compliance with federal regulations through a Medicare-approved home health agency, it is the physician who must certify the plan of treatment for the client. However, in most instances, other health care professionals evaluate the client's status, report the findings to the physician, and then, in collaboration with the physician, modify the plan of treatment for the client.

Medicare requires documentation of interdisciplinary services. Each professional must document the care provided to demonstrate accountability and provide continuity of care. Interdisciplinary collaboration and coordination through case conferences and contracts made between the caregivers must be documented in the clinical record. Quality improvement mechanisms such as chart audits and peer review verify the appropriate and effective use of collaboration.

Successful interdisciplinary functioning depends on numerous factors, including the knowledge, skills, and attitudes of each team member. Factors necessary for successful interdisciplinary team functioning are shown in Box 27-4. The plan of care should be implemented and reinforced by all involved disciplines. For example, nurses must reinforce the teaching by the physical therapist of the exercise regimen and gait training.

Responsibilities of the Disciplines

The responsibilities and functions of the disciplines in home health care are dictated by Medicare regulations, professional organizations, and state licensing boards. The roles of providers in home health discussed in the following sections may be different from provider roles in other settings. Other specialized services can be provided in home health, such as:

- Enterostomal therapy
- Podiatry
- Pharmaceutical therapy
- Nutrition counseling
- Intravenous therapy
- Respiratory therapy
- Psychiatric or mental health nursing.

Many of these services can be provided on a consultant basis, through either staff education or direct care.

Physician

Each client in the Medicare home care programs must be under the current care of a doctor of medicine, podiatry, or osteopathy to certify that the client has a medical problem. A nurse can make an assessment visit without physician approval but must have the physician's certification if a plan

---

Box 27-4 Factors for Interdisciplinary Functioning

KNOWLEDGE

1. Understand how the group process can be used to achieve group goals.
2. Understand problem solving.
3. Understand role theory.
4. Understand what other professionals do and how they see their roles.
5. Understand the conceptual differences between home care and practice versus institutional care and practices.

SKILL

1. Use principles of group process effectively.
2. Communicate clearly and accurately.
3. Communicate without using profession's jargon.
4. Express self clearly and concisely in writing.

ATTITUDE

1. Feel confident in role as a professional.
2. Trust and respect other professionals.
3. Share tasks with other professionals.
4. Work effectively toward conflict resolution.
5. Be flexible.
6. Be "research-minded."
7. Be timely.

---

of care with follow-up is developed. The physician must certify a plan of treatment for the home health agency before care is provided to the client. The physician must review the plan of treatment in collaboration with home care professionals at least every 62 days, but more often if the client's condition warrants more frequent assessment and changes in care. This process is called **recertification.** Physicians in the community also serve in an advisory capacity to the home health agency by assisting in the development of home care policies and procedures relative to client care.

Physical Therapist

The physical therapist (PT) provides maintenance, preventive, and restorative treatment for clients in the home. PTs must be licensed by the state in which they practice and are graduates of a baccalaureate or master's-level physical therapy program. Like home health nurses, a PT provides direct and indirect care. Direct care activities include:

- Strengthening muscles
- Restoring mobility
- Controlling spasticity
- Gait training
- Teaching active-passive resistive exercises
- Teaching or performing therapeutic exercise
- Providing massage
- Performing transcutaneous electrical nerve stimulation
- Providing heat therapy
- Preforming water therapy
- Providing ultraviolet light therapy
- Performing ultrasound therapy

- Performing postural drainage
- Performing pulmonary exercises.

The therapist is also responsible for teaching the client and family the treatment regimen to promote self-care and responsibility.

Indirect care activities of the PT include consulting with the staff and contributing to client care conferences by sharing skills and expertise. Physical therapy assistants may provide some therapy under the direction of a registered physical therapist. Assistants are high school graduates who have completed an approved assistants' program and have been licensed.

Occupational Therapist

The occupational therapist (OT) helps clients achieve their optimal level of functioning by teaching them to develop and maintain the abilities to perform activities of daily living in their home. Occupational therapists focus most of their treatment on the client's upper extremities by helping to restore muscle strength and mobility for functional skills. Occupational therapists earn baccalaureate degrees. When OTs become registered by the National Occupational Therapy Association, they are subsequently referred to as *OTRs*.

Direct functions of the OT include evaluating the client's level of function and ability by testing muscles and joints. The OT:

- Teaches self-care activities
- Assesses the client's home for safety and the need to modify the home to remove barriers
- Provides adaptive equipment when needed, such as special spoons and other eating utensils for arthritic clients.

Indirect care includes serving as consultants for special client needs regarding self-care activities and adapting the home for the client.

Certified occupational therapy assistants (COTAs) are high school graduates with an approved continuing education certificate from an occupational therapy program. The COTA works under the supervision of the OTR.

Speech Pathologist

The speech pathologist or therapist (ST) is certified by the American Speech, Language, and Hearing Association and is educated at the master's degree level. Speech pathologists work to assist people with communication problems related to speech, language, or hearing. Most clients receive direct care services, such as evaluation of speech and language ability, with specific plans being taught to the client and family for follow-up. The goal of speech therapy is to assist individuals to develop and maintain optimum speech and language ability. Speech pathologists also work with eating and swallowing problems. By serving as a consultant, the speech pathologist can teach other providers of care and families how to encourage development of the best method of communication for clients.

Social Worker

The social worker in home health holds a master's degree in social work (MSW) and has at least 1 year of social work experience. The social worker helps clients and families deal with social, emotional, and environmental factors that affect their well-being. Social workers assist directly by identifying and referring clients to appropriate community resources. Often, after an episode in the hospital, clients return home unable to cope with their present state of functioning and need assistance in reorganizing their lives. The social worker may provide counseling to enhance the client and family's ability to cope with the illness and make difficult decisions about future care. Many indirect care duties are performed by the social worker since consulting and referring constitute the major focus of their practice. Other functions include identifying resources and filling out applications for clients, crisis intervention, and finding equipment for those with limited financial resources. Social work assistants are prepared at the baccalaureate level and function similarly to the social worker, who directly supervises the activities of the assistant.

Homemaker/Home Health Aide

With the beginning of Medicare, the home health aide (HHA) became an important member of the home health care team. The home health nurse or physical therapist directly supervises the HHA. The role of the HHA is to help clients reach their level of independence by temporarily helping with personal hygiene and activities of daily living. Additional duties include light housekeeping, laundry, and meal preparation and shopping. The HHA must be experienced as an aide, be trained, and complete a certification program or a competency evaluation to provide home care services. The HHA implements the plan of care developed by the nurse or other professionals to reinforce teaching.

The role of the homemaker, as different from the HHA, helps with housekeeping chores. The homemaker service is one provided by some home health agencies. Although this service is not reimbursed by Medicare, it is a much-needed program and may be provided by some third-party payers or be paid for by clients on a sliding scale.

Aide supervision is required every 2 weeks except in the absence of skilled care; then a visit is required every 60 days. A therapist may make the visit only when therapy and personal care services are being given.

Hospice Care

Historically, the word **hospice** referred to a place of refuge for travelers. The contemporary meaning refers to palliative care of the very ill and dying, offering both respite and comfort (Gurfolino and Dumas, 1994). Originating in nineteenth-century England, the earliest hospices provided palliative care to terminally ill patients first in hospitals and later extended the services into the homes. In 1970 the hospice movement in the United States gained momentum in response to awakened public interest generated by Dr. Elisabeth Kübler-Ross' book, *Death with Dignity.* Public-sponsored hospices, successful in meeting the special needs of the dying patient, attracted the attention of Congress. After evaluating a limited hospice benefit as a pilot, Congress enacted legislation in 1985 that provided coverage for hospice services under Medicare. Stringent controls and criteria for quality hospice care are imposed both by the HCFA and the Joint Commission for Accreditation of Healthcare Organizations (JCAHO).

As a result of the hospice movement, persons with terminal diseases now have the option of dying at home with support services available. A variety of hospice care models in the United States use institutional services, home care service, or both. In addition to prescribed home care services, core services unique to hospice include the following:

- Volunteers
- Chaplain support
- Respite care
- Financial help with medicines and equipment
- Bereavement support of the family after the client's death.

It should be noted that choosing hospice does not mean a client has chosen to die. It is the goal of hospice to increase the quality of remaining life. The hospice team is usually medically directed and nurse coordinated. Pain management, symptom control, and emotional support are primary areas of expertise they offer. One criterion for hospice care is that death is expected within 6 months. Medicare covers this period, and the hospice usually covers the period after 6 months. Clients who improve during care may be discharged and readmitted when their condition changes. In hospice an on-call nurse is available 24 hours a day to monitor changes in the client's condition. After the death of the client, hospice provides bereavement benefits and attends to family needs for up to 1 year. Although a home care agency may provide hospice services, most hospice agencies are freestanding agencies (Gurfolino and Dumas, 1994).

Hospice care requires a multidisciplinary staff with experience in caring for the terminally ill. The primary goal is to help maintain the client's integrity and comfort. Palliative (providing comfort) rather than curative care is the objective. Nursing actions such as alleviating symptoms and meeting the special needs of the dying clients and families contribute to **palliative care.**

Health care providers who work with the dying often experience unique stress. Staff stress must be identified and appropriately addressed to help in the delivery of quality care and to maintain the care provider's integrity. Some examples of stress experienced by hospice staff include the following:

- Frustration resulting from clients and caregivers not following the plan of care
- Difficulty deciding how or when to set limits on involvement with clients and families
- Difficulty establishing realistic limitations as to what can be provided by hospice.

The hospice nurse needs:

- A firm foundation in home care skills
- Knowledge of community resources
- The ability to function constructively as a team member
- To be comfortable with death and dying
- The mature ability to meet personal emotional needs and the emotional needs of the hospice client and family.

Not all terminal clients choose hospice care, and of those who do, not all are eligible for Medicare or covered by private insurance. If reimbursement becomes the primary admission criterion for hospice care, it will no longer be a real option for all terminal clients. The community health nurse choosing hospice as a specialty area must be prepared to deal with this and other ethical issues. End-of-life care is of great concern to nursing, and many issues are hotly debated by the public (e.g., client choice, available hospice services, reimbursement status, admission criteria, and assisted suicide). The Code for Nurses (American Nurses Association, 2000) should guide nurses in resolving these dilemmas.

EDUCATIONAL REQUIREMENTS FOR HOME HEALTH PRACTICE

Nurses come to home health from a variety of educational and practice settings. Differences in both experience and educational preparation influence the contributions that nurses make to home health care. Home health nurses should be educated to function at a high level of competency so that they can be relied on not only by their professional colleagues but also by the community. Life experience, compassion, and awareness of self are factors that are necessary for the delivery of quality client care and professionalism.

In home health care, the nurse with basic nursing preparation functions in the role of a *generalist* providing skilled nursing and coordinating care for a variety of home health clients. The nurse with a master's degree is prepared for the advanced practice role as *clinical specialist,* nurse practitioner, researcher, administrator, or educator. As home care continues to develop its larger role in community health nursing, the need for specialized nurse clinicians will also increase to meet the highly technological and complex care that has been moved from the hospital into the home setting. In managed care more clinical specialists will be needed to provide case management and to develop programs to meet the needs of the population served by the managed care network. Nurse practitioners can be used to provide primary care to frail elderly and other homebound clients. Educational programs are increasing to prepare nurses for advanced practice roles in home health.

Certification

Home health nurses can seek certification as either a generalist home health nurse or a home health clinical nurse specialist through the American Nurses Credentialing Center. Hospice nurses can be certified by the National Hospice Organization. **Certification** is one means that the profession uses to assure the public of an individual nurse's competence to practice in an area of specialty or in advanced practice. Certification indicates that nurses have met standards set by their peers in the area of practice. Educational and practice requirements, as well as the passing of an examination in the area of specialty, must be met. An associate degree or diploma in nursing is required for certification by the generalist examination. A baccalaureate degree in nursing is required to be recognized as *board certified* in home health and a master's degree for the clinical specialist in home health nursing. Nurses must also demonstrate current practice. Certification is valid for 5 years, and requirements must be met to maintain certification or board certification. National certification is required by some states for advanced practice. In a highly competitive health care environment, certification is expected to become more necessary to assure the public of competence and quality.

ACCOUNTABILITY AND QUALITY MANAGEMENT
Quality Control Mechanisms

Since the beginning of Medicare, home health agencies have monitored the quality of care to their clients as a mandatory requirement for certification as a home health agency. All agencies are accountable to their clients, to their reimbursement sources, to themselves as health care providers, and to professional standards. Quality is demonstrated through evaluations reflecting that appropriate and needed care has been given to clients in a professional manner.

Clinical records are of great importance in assessing quality care. The care and services the client receives and any communication between the physicians and other home health providers must be documented. In the clinical record nurses demonstrate that they are delivering quality care and also identify means to improve the quality of care. It is the legal method by which quality care can be assessed. This documentation also demonstrates the client's ongoing need for services and shows how the multiple disciplines arrange for continuity and comprehensive care.

Evaluation of the agency is required to monitor the cost and quality of care. Standards serve as requirements for the evaluation in accordance with Medicare certification (Health Care Financing Administration, 1999).

Documentation of nursing care is central to home care. The amount of documentation affects the home health nurse more than the nurse in any other setting. As an example, during the initial evaluation visit, the home health nurse assesses the client and family's status. This information becomes a permanent part of the clinical record. Subsequent integrating of health services must be noted. Besides clinical notes of all home visits, progress notes must be sent to the client's physician, including the assessment of the client to verify the application of the plan of care.

Accreditation

Another means of evaluating quality in home health care is **accreditation.** Accreditation is a voluntary process; an agency chooses to participate. The accreditation decision is based on the data in a self-study, the report of the site visit team, and any other relevant information. In the future accreditation may become a requirement for licensure of all home health agencies. Today, home health agencies may be accredited through JCAHO or the Community Health Accreditation Program (CHAP) of the National League for Nursing. Both organizations look at the organizational structure through which care is delivered, the process of care through home visits, and the outcomes of client care focus-

ing on improved health status. Performance improvement must be ongoing in the agency (Box 27-5).

Regulatory Mechanisms

Home health care is carefully regulated. **Regulation** addresses the key aspects of home health care and is an important concern to the home health nurse. The home health nurse is responsible on a daily basis to practice within the guidelines set up by the regulatory agencies. The nurse interprets regulations to colleagues, clients, families, and the community.

The HCFA is accountable for overseeing the Medicare program, federal participation in the Medicaid program, and other health care quality improvement programs. HCFA writes regulations that govern two components of health care: financing and quality improvement (Box 27-6).

Home health regulation is mostly carried out at the state level. State health departments license and certify home health agencies according to state licensing regulations and

---

Box 27-5 **Requirements for Evaluation**

1. The agency must have written policies requiring an overall evaluation of the agency's total program at least once a year by a group of professional personnel, agency staff, and consumers, or by professional people outside the agency working in conjunction with consumers.
2. The evaluation must consist of both an annual policy and an administrative review, and clinical record reviews must be done at least quarterly.
3. The evaluation will assess the extent to which the agency's program is appropriate, adequate, effective, and efficient in promoting client care.
4. Results are reported to and acted upon by those responsible for the agency.
5. A written administrative record of the evaluation is maintained.

Box 27-6 **Medicare Conditions of Participation**

1. Definitions of home health agency terminology
2. Compliance with federal, state, and local laws
3. Organization, services, and administration
4. Group of professional personnel with advisory and evaluation function
5. Acceptance of clients, plan of treatment, and medical supervision
6. Services—skilled nursing, therapies, medical and social work, home health aide
7. Establishment and maintenance of clinical records
8. Evaluation of the agency's total program and behavior
9. Provision of oral and written Clients' Bill of Rights (see Box 27-7)
10. Confidentiality of medical records
11. Disclosure of ownership and management information
12. Compliance with accepted professional standards and principles
13. Qualification to provide outpatient physical or speech pathology services
14. Comprehensive assessment and reporting based on OASIS

the HCFA Conditions of Participation for Home Health Agencies (1997). These conditions of participation serve as the basis to evaluate each aspect of home health agencies.

Under Medicare regulations, a home health agency is defined as one that meets the following criteria:

- Primarily engages in providing skilled nursing and other therapeutic services
- Has policies established by a group of professional personnel, including both physicians and nurses, to govern the services that it provides
- Provides for supervision of services by a physician or registered nurse
- Maintains clinical records on all clients
- Is governed by state or local laws
- Meets the conditions of participation.

Clients are accepted for treatment on the basis of a reasonable expectation that the client's medical, nursing, rehabilitation, and social needs can be met adequately by the agency in the client's place of residence.

Agencies must provide skilled nursing and at least one other service: physical, speech, or occupational therapy; medical, social, or home health aide services. One service must be provided in its entirety by agency employees. The other services may be contracted. Clients are confined to home and require skilled nursing care on an intermittent basis or speech therapy, physical therapy, or a continual need for occupational therapy.

Intermittent care is defined as follows:

- Up to and including 28 hours per week of skilled nursing and home health aide services provided on a less-than-daily basis
- Up to 35 hours per week of the above services provided on a less-than-daily basis, subject to review on a case-by-case basis
- Up to and including full-time service (8 hours per day) needed 7 days per week for temporary periods of up to 21 days.

The state agencies responsible for licensure and certification of home health agencies use these criteria in evaluating whether agencies are conforming to federal regulations. Each criterion has minimum standards to which the program must adhere. Failure to meet these conditions can result in loss of licensure and the closing of the agency.

FINANCIAL ASPECTS OF HOME HEALTH AND HOSPICE CARE

Home Health Reimbursement

The standardized **reimbursement system** for home health care is complicated. Before the federal government became involved, home health care was reimbursed either by clients who could pay for the service or by donations that subsidized care for those who could pay only a portion or not at all. Now Medicare and Medicaid are the principal funding sources for home health care, with private third-party health insurance providing another major source. The conditions for payment under each of these programs appear in Table 27-2.

As of October 2000 the federal government introduced the prospective payment system for reimbursing agencies for home health care of clients. A **prospective payment system** is a mechanism whereby Medicare will pay home health agencies a set amount of money to care for a client who meets the criteria of 1 of 80 home health reserve groups based on severity, functional status, and number of services needed. This new system involves the following:

- Two payments are made to an agency for the client's care.
- The first payment is made when the client is admitted to care based on the HHRB—the Home Health Resource Group (Diagnosis).
- The first payment equal to 60% of the total payment for care is based on the OASIS Start of Care assessment done by the nurse.
- The second payment, or 40% of the total payment, is paid at the end of the episode of care (60 days) and is based on changes in client care as determined by continuous OASIS assessments by the nurse.

This new system makes the nurses' documentation more important to provide the agency sufficient financial resources to provide quality client care.

TABLE 27-2   Comparison of the Two Major Federally Supported Programs for Home Health Care

Medicare (Title XVIII)	Medicaid (Title XIX)
Federal insurance program administered by Social Security Administration	Federal and state assistance program administered by the state
Age 65 and over or disabled	Income-based eligibility
Conditions of participation	Conditions of participation
Homebound status	Not necessarily homebound status
Intermittent service	Intermittent service
Skilled service	Not necessarily skilled service
Restorative program	Custodial and maintenance program
Physician certification	Physician certification
Therapies, medical, or social service	State option—therapist, medical, or social service
Pays rental and purchase of equipment	Pays purchase
Reimbursement by prospective payment	Reimbursement—maximum allowed at state level
Based on national rates	Based on negotiated rate between federal government and state

Hospice Reimbursement

One of the major issues confronting hospice care is the reimbursement structure in the health care delivery system. Initially, many hospices provided free services as a mission of ministering to the dying. Others accepted available payment from third-party payers for billable services. In November 1983, the federal government legislated a Medicare hospice benefit for reimbursement to Medicare hospice-certified agencies (Medicare Program, 1984). Originally, the regulation was to be in effect through September 30, 1986, but additional legislation changed the hospice benefit to a permanent status in April 1986 (Public Law 99-272, 1986).

The hospice reimbursement benefit is optional for the Medicare-eligible client. Hospices may bill for skilled home care services under regular Medicare Part A benefits if the client does not want to use the hospice benefit. Responding to the perceived cost benefit potential of hospice care and the public demand for caring services during end of life, third-party payers are following Medicare's lead in providing hospice service options.

EFFECTS OF LEGISLATION ON HOME HEALTH CARE SERVICES

The federal government plays a significant role in the delivery of home health care services. The information in this section is organized to present an overview of the historical development of the laws affecting home health. Congressional action can change federal legislation regarding home health care. After a law is enacted, the appropriate federal agency develops regulations to implement the law. For updated information concerning amendments, bills presented in Congress, or regulations consult the Federal Register at your local library.

The Social Security Act of 1935 signaled the significant entrance of the federal government into the area of social insurance. The Medicare program was enacted on July 30, 1965, as Title XVIII of the Social Security Act and became effective July 1, 1966. The program offers two coordinated insurance coverages: hospital insurance, referred to as Part A, and supplemental medical insurance, referred to as Part B. Each provides reimbursement for home health services. This legislation established requirements for client eligibility, reimbursement costs, and rules for physician and agency participation. Many changes have been made through the years, including establishment of regional intermediaries for home health agencies by the DHHS and the achievement of more effective administration of the home health benefits.

The Patient Self-Determination Act (U.S. Code, 1990), part of the Omnibus Reconciliation Act of 1990 (Box 27-7), requires all health care agencies to:

- Provide written information to their clients about their rights and their options to refuse treatment
- Sign advance directives in compliance with state's laws
- Include in the clinical record whether the client has signed an advance directive
- Have a copy of the directive or the contents of the directive.

> **Box 27-7   Client's Bill of Rights**
>
> 1. Client has the right to be informed of his or her rights. The home health agency must protect and promote the exercise of these rights.
> 2. The home health agency must provide the client with a written notice of the client's rights before furnishing care to the client or during the initial evaluation visit and before the initiation of treatment.
> 3. The home health agency must maintain documentation showing that it has complied.
> 4. The client has the right to exercise his or her rights as a client of the agency.
> 5. The clients' family or guardian may exercise the client's rights when the client has been judged incompetent.
> 6. The client has the right to have his or her property treated with respect.
> 7. The client has the right to voice grievances regarding treatment or care that is (or fails to be) furnished or regarding the lack of respect for property by anyone who is furnishing services on behalf of the agency and must not be subjected to discrimination or reprisal for doing so.
> 8. The agency must investigate complaints made by a client or the client's family or guardian regarding treatment or care that is (or fails to be) furnished or regarding the lack of respect for the client's property by anyone furnishing services on behalf of the agency, and must document both the existence of the complaint and the resolution of the complaint.
> 9. The agency must inform and distribute information to the client, in advance, concerning the policies on advance directives, including a description of applicable state law.
> 10. The client has the right to confidentiality of clinical records.
> 11. The agency must advise the client of the agency's policies and procedures regarding disclosure of clinical records.
> 12. The client has the right to be advised, before care is initiated, of the extent to which payment for services may be expected from Medicare or other sources and the extent to which payment may be required from the client.
> 13. The client has the right to be advised of the availability of the toll-free home health agency hotline in the state, the purpose of the hotline, and the hours of operation.
>
> From U.S. Congress: *Omnibus reconciliation act of 1990*, Washington, D.C., 1990, U.S. Government Printing Office; U.S. Department of Health and Human Services.

These documents communicate the client's wishes and take the form of either a living will or durable power of attorney for health care.

- The goal of advance directives is to provide a mechanism for clients to make health care decisions while they are able.
- The directives can be changed at any time.
- The durable power of attorney names a person who will make health care decisions when the client is unable, whereas the living will indicates the client's decision to decline or stop treatment.
- States differ in the implementation of advanced directives.

Examples of a living will and a "do not resuscitate" order from the state of Kentucky are presented in Figures 27-3 and 27-4, respectively.

Living Will Directive

My wishes regarding life-prolonging treatment and artificially provided nutrition and hydration to be provided to me if I no longer have decisional capacity, have a terminal condition, or become permanently unconscious have been indicated by checking and initialing the appropriate lines below. By checking and initialing the appropriate lines, I specifically:

Designate _____ as my health care surrogate(s) to make health care decisions for me in accordance with this directive when I no longer have decisional capacity. If _____ refuses or is not able to act for me, I designate _____ as my health care surrogate(s).

Any prior designation is revoked.

If I do not designate a surrogate, the following are my directions to my attending physician. If I have designated a surrogate, my surrogate shall comply with my wishes as indicated below:

_____ Direct that treatment be withheld or withdrawn, and that I be permitted to die naturally with only the administration of medication or the performance of any medical treatment deemed necessary to alleviate pain.

_____ DO NOT authorize that life-prolonging treatment be withheld or withdrawn

_____ Authorize the withholding or withdrawal of artificially provided food, water, or other artificially provided nourishment or fluids.

_____ DO NOT authorize the withholding or withdrawal of artificially provided food, water, or other artificially provided nourishment or fluids.

_____ Authorize my surrogate, designated above, to withhold or withdraw artificially provided nourishment or fluids, or other treatment if the surrogate determines that withholding or withdrawing is in my best interest; but I do not mandate that withholding or withdrawing.

In the absence of my ability to give directions regarding the use of life-prolonging treatment and artificially provided nutrition and hydration, it is my intention that this directive shall be honored by my attending physician, my family, and any surrogate designated pursuant to this directive as the final expression of my legal right to refuse medical or surgical treatment and I accept the consequences of the refusal.

If I have been diagnosed as pregnant and that diagnosis is known to my attending physician, this directive shall have no force or effect during the course of my pregnancy.

I understand the full import of this directive and I am emotionally and mentally competent to make this directive.

Signed this _____ day of _____, 20____.

_____

Signature and address of the grantor.

If our joint presence, the grantor, who is of sound mind and eighteen years of age, or older, voluntarily dated and signed this writing or directed it to be dated and signed for the grantor.

_____

Signature and address of witness.

_____

Signature and address of witness.

OR

STATE OF KENTUCKY

_____ County

Before me, the undersigned authority, came the grantor who is of sound mind and eighteen (18) years of age, or older, and acknowledged that he voluntarily dated and signed this writing or directed it to be signed and dated as above.

Done this _____ day of _____, 20____.

_____

Signature of Notary Public or other

_____

Date commission expires.

Execution of this document restricts withholding and withdrawing of some medical procedures. Consult Kentucky Revised Statutes or your attorney.

Figure 27-3 **Example of a living will directive.**

KENTUCKY EMERGENCY MEDICAL SERVICES PREHOSPITAL DO NOT RESUSCITATE (DNR) ORDER

Patient's Full Legal Name _____

I, the undersigned patient or surrogate who has been designated to make health care decisions in accordance with Kentucky Revised Statutes, hereby direct that in the event of my cardiac or respiratory arrest that this DO NOT RESUSCITATE (DNR) ORDER be honored and that I understand that DNR means that if my heart stops beating or if I stop breathing, no medical procedure to restart breathing or heart function will be instituted by emergency medical services (EMS) personnel.

I understand this decision will NOT prevent emergency medical services personnel from administering other emergency medical care.

I understand that I may revoke this DNR order at any time by physical cancellation, destruction of this form, removal of DNR bracelet, or by expressing a desire to be resuscitated by the EMS personnel. Any attempt to alter or change the content, names, or signatures on the DNR form shall make the DNR form invalid.

I understand that it is my obligation to see that this form, or a standard DNR bracelet, is readily and immediately available to EMS personnel upon their arrival. In the event of my death, the EMS agency which responds shall obtain this form, or the standard DNR bracelet, and it shall become a part of the EMS medical record.

I hereby state that this "Do Not Resuscitate" (DNR) is my authentic wish not to be resuscitated.

_____   _____
Patient/legal surrogate signature   Date

_____
Legal surrogate's relationship to patient

_____   _____
Witness name (print)   Witness signature

This Do Not Resuscitate form has been approved by the Kentucky Board of Medical Licensure. DNR form number (serially numbered).

Figure 27-4 **Example of a "do not resuscitate" order.**

LEGAL AND ETHICAL ISSUES

In any health care system there is the potential for illegal and unethical actions. Much publicity has been given to Medicare fraud and abuse in the last decade. Exploiting the system has been partially caused by the increase in available federal money and the fee-for-service payment system. Examples of such practices include:

- Overuse of home health services when the client does not need them
- Inaccurate billing for services
- Excessive administrative staff
- "Kickbacks" for referrals
- Billing of noncovered medical supplies.

Home health nurses are confronted with multiple issues in everyday practice. **Fiscal intermediaries,** insurance companies, have interpreted the definition of skilled care inconsistently over the years. The home health nurse must abide by established federal regulations when delivering care to clients, even when the needs are greater than what is paid for. However, the new prospective reimbursement system may allow more flexibility in the services offered by the nurse. Frequency of visits poses another issue. Only intermittent visits are reimbursed. If the frequency increases, then full-time skilled services may be required. Continual reassessment of client and family needs is imperative to avoid inappropriate use and overuse of services. Home health nurses must be knowledgeable about which medical supplies are covered. This information is readily available and nurses, as professionals, must work within regulatory guidelines and educate the community as to what is actually covered and what should be.

Several stressors in home health care affect nurses. Documentation is often overwhelming but is an essential part of client care. The home health nurse must justify that care meets reimbursement and legal requirements and is necessary and appropriate. This accountability can be stressful. The role of the home health nurse is complex and continuously expanding, requiring ongoing education and excellent judgment. Home health care may be underused if the hospital orientation or physicians view home care as a burden because of the excess paperwork it entails.

NATIONAL HEALTH OBJECTIVES

Because home health nurses are working with clients and families in the home and community, they are in a position to promote the achievement of some of the key *Healthy People 2010* objectives. The nurse can assess the client's status related to key objectives, identify available resources and gaps to meet client needs, and coordinate care with other providers and community agencies. The *Healthy People 2010* box highlights the objectives the home health nurse can assist the nation in meeting through their client case management activities. Obviously, these objectives relate to the leading causes of death and disability. With appropriate health education and referral to community resources for assistance, numerous lives can be saved or prolonged and chronic disabilities reduced. In this way the nurse can contribute to meeting the national health objectives on a one-to-one client-provider level.

Healthy People 2010
National Health Objectives for the Year 2010

2-4   Increase the proportion of adults aged 18 years and older with arthritis who seek help in coping if they experience personal and emotional problems.

3-1   Reduce the overall cancer death rate.

3-11   Increase the proportion of women who receive a Pap test.

3-12   Increase the proportion of adults who receive a colorectal cancer screening examination.

3-13   Increase the proportion of women aged 40 years and older who have received a mammogram within the preceding 2 years.

4-1   Reduce the rate of new cases of end-stage renal disease (ESRD).

4-2   Reduce deaths from cardiovascular disease in persons with chronic kidney failure.

4-7   Reduce kidney failure due to diabetes.

4-8   Increase the proportion of persons with type 1 or type 2 diabetes and proteinuria who receive recommended medical therapy to reduce progression to chronic renal insufficiency.

5-1   Increase the proportion of persons with diabetes who receive formal diabetes education.

5-2   Prevent diabetes.

5-5   Reduce the diabetes death rate.

5-7   Reduce deaths from cardiovascular disease in persons with diabetes.

5-9   Reduce the frequency of foot ulcers in persons with diabetes.

5-10   Reduce the rate of lower extremity amputations in persons with diabetes.

5-13   Increase the proportion of adults with diabetes who have an annual dilated eye examination.

5-14   Increase the proportion of adults with diabetes who have at least an annual foot examination.

5-15   Increase the proportion of persons with diabetes who have at least an annual dental examination.

5-16   Increase the proportion of persons with diabetes who take aspirin at least 15 times per month.

5-17   Increase the proportion of persons with diabetes who perform self-blood glucose monitoring at least once daily.

6-3   Reduce the proportion of adults with disabilities who report feelings such as sadness, unhappiness, or depression that prevent them from being active.

6-4   Increase the proportion of adults with disabilities who participate in social activities.

6-11   Reduce the proportion of people with disabilities who report not having the assistive devices and technology needed.

6-12   Reduce the proportion of people with disabilities reporting environmental barriers to participation in home, school, work, or community activities.

12-6   Reduce hospitalizations of older adults with heart failure as the principal diagnosis.

12-7   Reduce stroke deaths.

12-8   Increase the proportion of adults who are aware of the early warning symptoms and signs of a stroke.

12-10   Increase the proportion of adults with high blood pressure whose blood pressure is under control.

12-14   Reduce the proportion of adults with high total blood cholesterol levels.

14-5   Reduce invasive pneumococcal infections.

14-19   Reduce the number of courses of antibiotics prescribed for the sole diagnosis of the common cold.

14-20   Reduce antimicrobial use among intensive care unit patients.

15-13   Reduce deaths caused by unintentional injuries.

15-14   Reduce nonfatal unintentional injuries.

15-25   Reduce residential fire deaths.

15-27   Reduce deaths from falls.

15-28   Reduce hip fractures among older adults.

18-1   Reduce the suicide rate.

18-9   Increase the proportion of adults with mental disorders who receive treatment.

24-9   Establish in at least 15 states a surveillance system for tracking asthma death, illness, disability, impact of occupational and environmental factors on asthma, access to medical care, and asthma management.

24-10   Reduce deaths from chronic obstructive pulmonary disease (COPD) among adults.

26-2   Reduce cirrhosis deaths.

From U.S. Department of Health and Human Services: *Healthy people 2010: national health promotion and disease prevention objectives,* Washington, D.C., 2000, U.S. Department of Health and Human Services.

The home health nurse can be instrumental in helping communities to set and meet these objectives by participating in both community planning activities and in the home health agency to identify which of the objectives the agency can work toward to meet their population's needs. The home health nurse can use the protocols developed by the U.S. Preventive Services Task Force in the late 1980s for assessment of clients, care planning, and health education (see Appendix A.2).

Healthy People 2000 was evaluated in 1995 and found that the United States was moving toward the set targets for two thirds of the objectives (U.S. Department of Health and Human Services, 1995). Significant challenges remained for Americans with disabilities, those with low incomes, and minorities who continue to experience disproportionately poorer health outcomes. Several areas that have not been on target include increasing the years of healthy life for persons with chronic conditions, the ability of the elderly to perform self-care activities, and the number of persons experiencing hip fractures. These areas are positively affected by home health nursing practice and need to be highlighted to policy makers and payers of health care.

ISSUES FOR THE TWENTY-FIRST CENTURY

Access to Health Care

Will health care reform and managed care systems improve access to care for the population? Many home health agencies currently use endowment monies, have United Way funds, or have other charitable funds to provide indigent home health care. Some states have programs in which home health agencies agree to contribute a certain percentage of their time to provide indigent care. Nursing is challenged to address access issues through clinical research, public advocacy, and by devising cost-reducing strategies and models of care delivery.

Technology and Telehealth

The Federal Bureau of Labor Statistics (1998) projects that employment in home health care will grow faster in the next decade than in any other health care sector. The main reason for this fast growth is related to technology. The incentives and pressures for early hospital discharge have created a transfer of technology from the hospital to the home care setting. At the same time, some technologies have been simplified and their reliability increased, allowing their safe use in the home. This trend is expected to continue. Examples of current home care technologies are the following:

- Parenteral nutrition
- Chemotherapy
- Intravenous therapy for hydration and antibiotics
- Intrathecal pain management
- Ventilators
- Apnea monitors
- Chest tubes
- Skeletal traction.

The home care nurse must be prepared to evaluate the cost and safety of technology for the home. Clients must be screened and meet specific admission criteria. All clients are not suited for home care, and it is up to the nurse to advocate for clients when home care is appropriate and when it is not appropriate. When appropriate, the nurse will become competent to use these technology skills in the home to maximize their performance, reduce inherent liability risk, increase client rehabilitation, and use research to show that nursing is a vital member of this rapidly developing component of health care.

Telehealth is emerging as a viable and acceptable way to provide health care. **Telehealth** is health information sent from one site to another by electronic communication (Thobaben, 1998). Examples of the uses of telehealth include telephone triage and advice and telemonitoring equipment to measure vital signs, cardiac function, and point-of-care diagnostics.

Pediatric and Maternal-Child Home Care

Pediatric home care has changed tremendously over the past years as children are being treated outside the institutional environment. The family is the key to the successful managing of a child at home. A supportive and stable home environment for children can contribute to healing and maintenance of health. Policymakers in the United States are beginning to appreciate the relationship between home care and pediatrics. Legislation has been proposed to require that private insurance companies cover home care in employee benefit packages. New programs, resources, and options for funding are becoming available for care of children at home.

Specialized programs for the pediatric population are mandatory. Although infants have been treated in the home for years, the focus on high-technology care requires evaluating key issues such as reimbursement, staff competence, and quality improvement. Pediatric needs range from an infant who needs observation and treatment with home phototherapy or a sleep monitor to a child needing ventilator assistance and enteral feeding. Approximately 10 million children are disabled and institutionalized today because of terminal or chronic conditions. Pediatric home care in the future will continue to help parents to care for their children at home if resources and interventions continue to be available.

Although maternal-child home care is not a new concept, there is a revitalized interest in expanding these home care services to reduce maternal and infant mortality and morbidity. The reemerging home care services target high-risk pregnant mothers and provide health education, short-term skilled nursing care, and anticipatory guidance. Recent research has demonstrated long-term positive health outcomes of prenatal and infant home visiting programs by nurses managing pregnancy-induced hypertension, childhood injuries, and subsequent pregnancies among low-income women (Kitzman, et al, 1997). Nursing interventions have reduced the use of welfare, child abuse and neglect, and criminal behavior for low-income, unmarried mothers for up to 15 years after the birth of the first child (Olds, et al, 1997).

Home care of infants focuses on:
- Parent education about infant needs
- Parenting skills
- Instructions to improve growth and development outcomes
- Skilled medical care.

These programs are being shown to be cost effective. Programs to provide skilled home care to addicted mothers and infants include such services as:
- Family counseling
- Medical treatment
- Emotional support
- Methods to improve nutritional state and reduce infant irritability
- Training in improving maternal-infant interaction (Struk, 1994).

Some hospitals are developing programs that allow a nurse to provide continuity of care from hospital to home. A nurse who provides obstetric inpatient care may follow the mother and baby to the home to provide postpartum care. This trend requires that hospital nurses be well-grounded in community health nursing concepts.

Family Responsibility, Roles, and Functions

The family plays an important role in the delivery of home health care. The term *family,* as discussed previously, refers to a caregiver responsible for the client's well-being. Women have been the traditional caregivers for children and the elderly in the United States. Yet women are less available to provide this care without assistance because many are working outside of the home. At issue is whether home health care services should be used as a respite, or relief, type of care. Sometimes a family member is debilitated and unable to help the client without assistance. Should supportive services be paid by the federal government? On the other hand, some family members are capable of providing the needed care but are unwilling to do so. Who should pay for the service and who should provide the needed care? Family responsibility is an issue that is difficult to resolve in this country. Assistance from social support systems helps in coping with the stress of caring for an ill family member. The goal is to maintain the client at home for as long as possible and to provide high-quality care. To do this, resources must be used appropriately and effectively. However, developing a public consensus to resolve these issues has been a problem.

Measuring the Outcomes of Home Health Care

As a method to ensure quality in health care, regulators are mandating that home health agencies measure and report **client outcome** data. Medicare funded a multistate research study to develop the standardized collection tool, the **Out-**

comes and Assessment Information Set (OASIS) to measure quality and client satisfaction with care (U.S. Medicare and Medicaid Programs, 1997). OASIS data are measured and reported to HCFA:
- On admission to home health care
- After an episode of hospitalization
- At the time of recertification
- On discharge from care or death at home.

Data are submitted by each agency to a national databank, and agencies receive both results and comparisons with similar agencies to determine areas needing improvement. The data reported from OASIS determines the payment received by the home health agency for the client's total episode of care. See Appendix B.1 for an example of this assessment.

Accrediting organizations are also mandating the reporting of outcomes as a performance standard. JCAHO (1996) has revised the standards for home health to focus more on performance improvement based on measurable data, including **benchmarking,** or comparing oneself with national standards and guidelines and with other agencies. Clinical guidelines, pathways, and clinical maps are other methods that agencies are using to standardize care and control costs.

These trends will affect the provision of home health care, the viability of agencies, and the role of the home health nurses in the future. Nursing research will be critical to demonstrate the cost effectiveness and the quality of the care provided by professional nurses. The future of home health nursing holds excitement, diversity, and opportunity.

Clinical Application

The home visit is the hallmark of home health nursing. When a nurse enters a client's home, he or she is a guest and must recognize that the services offered can be accepted or rejected. The first visit sets the stage for success or failure. The initial assessment of the client, their support system, and the environment is critical.

A. What strategies would the nurse consider to develop a trusting relationship during the first visit?
B. What would be the most important elements to assess in the home environment?
C. What is necessary for the nurse to include in the client contract?
D. How can the nurse assess preferred learning style?

Answers are in the back of the book.

 Remember This!

- Home health care differs from other areas of health care in that the health care providers practice in the client's environment. This unique characteristic affects several components of nursing practice in the home care setting.

- Family is an integral part of home health care, which includes any caregiver or significant persons who takes the responsibility to assist the client in need of care at home.
- Home care reached a turning point with the arrival of Medicare, which provided regulations for home care practice and reimbursement mechanisms.
- Home health agencies are divided into the following five general types based on the administrative and organizational structures: official, private and voluntary, combination, hospital-based, and proprietary.
- Regardless of the type of home health agency existing in a community, the primary goal should be to provide quality home health care to the community based on the health needs of people.
- Demonstration of professional competency is the foremost requirement for home health care nurses.
- Home health care nursing is a division of community health nursing. Thus health promotion activities are a fundamental component of practice.
- The concept of self-care includes three components: client education, client compliance, and self-help.
- Contracting is a vital component of all nurse-client relationships. Contracting refers to any working agreement, continuously renegotiable, between the nurse, client, and family.
- The home health care nurse practices in accordance with the Scope and Standards of Home Health Nursing Practice developed by the American Nurses Association.
- Interdisciplinary collaboration is a required process in the home health care and hospice settings. Its use is mandated for Medicare-certified home care agencies, and it is inherent in the definition of home health care and hospice.
- In home care and hospice, as in other care settings, professionals experience stress associated with changing roles and overlapping responsibilities. In collaborating, providers should carefully analyze each others' roles to determine whether overlapping occurs and adjust the plan of care as needed.
- Since the advent of Medicare, home health agencies have monitored the quality of care to their clients as a mandatory requirement for certification as a home health agency. All agencies are accountable to clients and families, to their reimbursement sources, to themselves as a health care provider, and to professional standards.
- The home care nurse faces many challenges. Ethical issues (reimbursement criteria and indigent care), role development (high technology and hospice nursing), and opportunities for research (quality of care and cost effectiveness) affect nursing practice in the home.
- The concept of home health care began in the 1800s with an emphasis on health promotion and disease prevention. With the advent of Medicare, the goal became episodic illness care. Today home health is returning to an emphasis on disease prevention and health promotion.
- Hospice care in this country began in the late 1970s.

- With the development of managed care networks, home health agencies will be contracting with a group of health care organizations to provide care or will be purchased by a larger network and provide care only to the network's clients.
- Home care and hospice agencies may be accredited through JCAHO or CHAP.
- The Omnibus Reconciliation Act of 1990 introduced the home care clients' bill of rights and advance directives to empower clients with control over their own health care. This is especially important for hospice clients.

What Would You Do?

1. Make a joint home visit with an experienced home health or hospice nurse to do the following:
   a. Evaluate the process and content of the nurse-client interaction to determine whether the visit was merely ritual or therapeutic and describe the process of the visit.
   b. Compare actual roles and functions with the Scope and Standards of Home Health Nursing Practice.
   c. Assess level of skilled care the clients receive and determine whether the care is needed and appropriate. (Is it within the four criteria described in the section on Family Responsibility, Roles, and Functions? Answer the four questions in relation to the home visit made.)
2. Make a joint home visit with another home health care or hospice professional and assess, as in the preceding activity. Also, attend a client care conference meeting and write a summary of the process of the group.
3. Review a client record and determine what client outcomes were met through home health or hospice care.
4. Review your state's laws governing advance directives. Consider the legal and ethical advantages and disadvantages of having such directives.
5. Interview a nurse and determine how the client's bill of rights has affected practice.

REFERENCES

American Nurses Association: *The scope and standards of practice for home health nursing,* Washington, D.C., 1999, American Nurses Association.

American Nurses Association: *Code for nurses and interpretive statements,* Kansas City, Mo, 1985, American Nurses Association.

Archbold PG, et al: The PREP system of nursing interventions: a pilot test with families caring for older members, *Res Nurs Health* 18:3, 1995.

Bureau of Labor Statistics: *Employment projections: 1999,* Washington, D.C., 1998, U.S. Department of Labor.

Doherty M, Hurley S: Suburban home care, *Nurs Clin North Am* 29(3):483, 1994.

Gurfolino V, Dumas V: Hospice nursing, *Nurs Clin North Am* 29(3):533, 1994.

Health Care Financing Administration: *Conditions of participation for home health agencies,* subpart 1, section 405.1229, Evaluation, Washington, D.C., 1999, U.S. Department of Health and Human Services.

Joint Commission for Accreditation of Healthcare Organizations: *1997-98 Comprehensive accreditation manual for home care,* Oakbrook Terrace, Ill, 1996, Joint Commission for Accreditation of Healthcare Organizations.

Kitzman H, et al: Effects of prenatal and infancy home visitation by nurses on pregnancy outcomes, childhood injuries, and repeated childbearing: a randomized, controlled trial, *JAMA* 278(8):644, 1997.

Medicare Program: Hospice care, *Federal Register* 48:560008-560036, Washington, D.C., 1984, U.S. Government Printing Office.

National Association of Home Care: *A provider's guide to a Medicare home health certification process,* ed 3, Washington, D.C., 1997, National Association of Home Care.

National Association of Home Care: *2000 Basic statistics about home care,* 2000, available online: www.nahc.org/consumer/ ncstats.html.

Olds DL, et al: Long-term effects of home visitation on maternal life course and child abuse and neglect: fifteen year follow-up of randomized trial, *JAMA* 278(8):637, 1997.

Orem DE: *Nursing: concepts of practice,* ed 3, St Louis, 1995, Mosby.

Public Health Law 99-272: *Omnibus Budget Reconciliation Act of 1985,* Medicare and Medicaid Budget Reconciliation Amendments of 1985, CIS-NO: Title IX, December, 1986.

Struk C: Women and children, *Nurs Clin North Am* 29(3):395, 1994.

Thobaben M: Health care technology issues in home care, *Home Care Provider* 3(5):244, 1998.

U.S. Congress: *Omnibus reconciliation act of 1990,* Washington, D.C., 1990, U.S. Government Printing Office.

U.S. Department of Health and Human Services: *Healthy people 2010: national health promotion and disease prevention objectives,* Washington, D.C., 2000, U.S. Department of Health and Human Services.

U.S. Department of Health and Human Services: *Healthy people 2000: midcourse review and 1995 revisions,* Washington, D.C., 1995, U.S. Department of Health and Human Services.

U.S. Medicare and Medicaid programs: revision of conditions of participation for home health agencies and use of Outcome Assessment Information Set (OASIS): proposed rules, *Fed Reg* 62(46):11003-11064, March 10, 1997.

U.S. Preventive Services Task Force: *Guide to clinical preventive services,* Baltimore, Md, 1989, Williams & Wilkins.

Warhola C: *Planning for home health services: a resource handbook,* HRA pub no 80-14017, Washington, D.C., 1980, U.S. Department of Health and Human Services.

Woodham-Smith C: *Lonely crusader,* New York, 1951, McGraw-Hill.

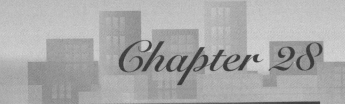

Chapter 28

Community Health Nursing in the Schools

JULIE C. NOVAK

OBJECTIVES

After reading this chapter, the student should be able to:
- Describe the functions of school nurses as generalists and specialists.
- Define the role of the school nurse manager.
- Examine the components of school health.
- Identify health problems of school-age children.
- Plan for school health services.
- Explain the basic requirements for administration of medications in schools.

- Discuss the school health implications of the Individuals with Disabilities Education Act (Public Law 94-142).
- Cite the goals of health education.
- Describe innovative approaches to the planning, organizing, and delivering of school health programs.

CHAPTER OUTLINE

Health Problems of School-Age Children
  Most Common Health Problems
  Nutritional Issues
  Vision and Hearing Problems
  Use of Alcohol, Tobacco, and Other Drugs
  Teenage Sexual Activity and Pregnancy
  Children with HIV/AIDS
  Absenteeism
  Children Living in Poverty
  Children With Disabilities and Chronic Health
    Conditions
  Addressing Children's Health Problems

History of School Nursing
  1900 to 1940
  World War II to the Present

Components of the School Health Program
  Health Services
  Health Education
  Environmental Health

Roles, Functions, and Credentials for School Nurses
  Generalists
  Specialists
  Credentials

Management of the School Health Program
  Education Reform and School Health
  Planning
  Organizing
  Directing
  Quality Control

Innovations in School Health
  School-Based Health Centers
  Family Resource/Service Centers

Employee Health

KEY TERMS

absenteeism: the lack of attending school.

case management: service given to clients that includes the following activities: screening, assessment, care planning, arranging for service delivery, monitoring, reassessment, evaluation, and discharge. Case management is a process that enhances continuity and appropriateness of care. Most often used with clients whose health problems are actually or potentially chronic and complex.

casefinding: careful, systematic observations of people to identify present or potential problems.

Certificates of Immunization Status: document proving that a child has up-to-date immunizations needed to attend school.

Child Find: program that provides early identification of preschool children at risk for school failure because of disabilities such as mental retardation, chronic health conditions, or other special needs. It is funded through the Individuals with Disabilities Education Act.

Child Health Insurance Plan (CHIP): a federally funded insurance program that provides school nurses with options in finding services for children of the working poor who are uninsured and not eligible for Medicaid.

counseling: helping people achieve workable solutions for their problems or conflicts.

Division of Adolescent and School Health (DASH): part of The Centers for Disease Control and Prevention. They define school health according to eight components.

Early and Periodic Screening, Diagnosis, and Treatment (EPSDT) Program: a special screening for preschool children that is funded through Medicaid and gives medical assistance to needy families with dependent children.

exclusion order: document given to an unimmunized student when he or she is not in compliance with the immunization law.

family resource/service centers: school and community resources for families that are consolidated into one agency for the sake of efficiency and reducing costs.

Growing Healthy: a curriculum for elementary grades that is a generalized program aimed at improving students' personal lifestyles.

Head Start: an early childhood education program for children at risk for academic problems because of poverty and lack of sufficient social stimulation.

health education: any combination of learning experiences designed to facilitate adaptations of behavior conducive to health.

Health PACT: health instruction intended to prepare children to communicate with health professionals during visits for health care.

International Classification of Diseases (ICD-9): international classification of disease that contains codes to help record health problems.

individualized education plan (IEP): an evaluation prepared by the school staff for each student that is reviewed and modified at regular intervals during the school year and through the student's school experience.

individualized family service plans (IFSPs): an early intervention program to prepare the infant/toddler/preschooler for school that is developed by an interdisciplinary team along with the parents.

Individuals with Disabilities Education Act (IDEA): a federal law that guarantees a free public education and related services for every disabled child from 5 to 21 years of age.

Know Your Body: a course that focuses on making students aware of their own cardiovascular risk factors through screening activities followed by special instruction related to risk reduction.

new morbidities: illnesses and conditions that are associated with the problems of students living in poverty, students with chronic illnesses or disabilities, and other children with special needs.

nontraditional health care settings: alternative health care delivery systems using various community settings.

pivot management: a plan in which the nurse organizes a school health team using the personnel already in the school system or closely associated with it.

primary health care services: a conceptual framework for providing public health and primary care services; it includes delivering essential, affordable, accessible, and acceptable health care to the community, with an emphasis on disease prevention and health promotion, community involvement, multisectoral cooperation, and appropriate technology.

school-based health centers (SBHCs): facilities that provide physical and/or mental health services to school-age children that are located within or near schools.

school health council: a council composed of teachers, school nurses, parents, students, administrators, and community leaders that plans school health.

school health manager: coordinator of a health program within a school.

school health services: health activities that should include family-centered health promotion and disease-prevention services to be effective.

school nurse clinician: a nurse with basic nursing preparation who works with school children.

school nurse practitioner: registered nurse with certificate or master's-level advanced education in the areas of health assessment, diagnosis, and treatment who is prepared to delivery primary care to school-age children.

screening: the application of a test to people who are as yet asymptomatic for the purpose of classifying them with respect to their likelihood of having a particular disease.

Teen Outreach Program (TOP): focuses on building self-esteem through volunteering.

Teenage Healthy Teaching Modules (THTMs): health education program that has been effective in reducing teen pregnancy and dropout in the experimental groups.

vague, nonspecific health complaints: the first sign of a student who may be having difficulty in school and may drop out.

The school setting is an important place to reach children and their families. Schools have more influence on the lives of young people than any other social setting except the family. The school provides a setting for developing friendships, for socializing, and for reinforcing and introducing norms for behaviors, such as health behaviors.

Nurses who care for children and adolescents in the school setting cover a variety of developmental groups from preschool to college. In 2000, 64 million children through the age of 21 years attended schools and universities in the United States (Centers for Disease Control and Prevention, 2000). This number has decreased since 1990 by about 2 million children. Trends suggest that the school-age population will continue to decline while other age groups increase (e.g., seniors).

The majority of children under 6 (61%) and children age 6 to 17 (76%) have mothers in the workforce. The majority of poor parents of children work outside the home (Children's Defense Fund, 1997), composing the fastest-growing segment among poor children–children of the working poor (Annie Casey Foundation, 1996). Although the majority of children living in poverty are white, a disproportionately high percentage of African-American and Hispanic children also live in poverty. These children and adolescents attend 110,000 public and private schools (U.S. Department of Health and Human Services, 1999). Although the majority of these children can be described as mostly healthy individuals, the stresses of rapid growth and development and society's pressures create health problems.

Nurses who care for children in school settings face many challenges and opportunities as they work with this population. It is unclear how cutting health care and welfare costs will affect health outcomes of school-age children (Children's Defense Fund, 1997). It is clear, however, that innovative partnerships among the schools, university health science centers, managed care agencies, community coalitions, and traditional public health agencies must develop effective, collaborative strategies for meeting the needs of children and youth (Brownson and Kreuter, 1997; Southern Region Educational Board, 1998).

HEALTH PROBLEMS OF SCHOOL-AGE CHILDREN

Nurses who work with the school-age population face a variety of psychosocial, physical, developmental, cultural, and environmental problems, issues, and concerns. School nurses are in a unique position to teach children to manage health problems; to care for those needing assistance; and to provide health education for children, their families and school faculty and staff.

The author acknowledges the contributions of Judith B. Igoe and Sudie Speer to this work.

Most Common Health Problems

The National Health Interview Survey (1997) revealed four major categories of acute conditions of children age 5 through 17 years:
- Respiratory conditions
- Injuries
- Infective and parasitic diseases
- Digestive system conditions

The major problems that interfere with school attendance are:
- Pneumonia
- The effects of homicide on the victims and the community
- Upper respiratory infections
- Malnutrition
- Dental disease
- Chronic illness

Since 1977, acute respiratory diseases consistently accounted for more than 60% of school absences due to illness.

Asthma and chronic bronchitis are the leading chronic conditions limiting children's activity (U.S. Department of Health and Human Services, 1995). There also has been a dramatic increase in the prevalence of asthma over the last decade. Another chronic problem, attention deficit disorder (ADD) and attention deficit–hyperactivity disorder (ADHD) affects 2% to 9.8% of children worldwide, with as many as two thirds of cases lasting into adulthood (Barkley, 1998).

The leading causes of death for preschool-age children ages 1 to 4 in order of frequency are injuries, congenital anomalies, malignant neoplasms, homicide, heart disease, and pneumonia and influenza (Fig. 28-1). For children ages 5 to 14 years, suicide enters the top seven causes of death, ranked at number 6. For leading causes of death among adolescents, refer to Figure 28-2.

Nutritional Issues

The nutritional problems seen in schools have changed over the past two decades. Today fewer children are undernourished; modern problems are related to overconsumption, imbalances in the types and amounts of food, and inactivity. In the third National Health and Nutrition Examination Survey (NHANES III) study, 26% of children reported watching television for more than 4 hours per day. These children had greater body fat and body mass index (Andersen, et al, 1998). Childhood obesity is a serious problem for children ages 2 to 9 years, particularly for females and Hispanic children (Maternal and Child Health Bureau, 1997). Many children consume foods high in sugar, fat, and salt and thus increase their risk of becoming obese and developing diabetes, heart disease, hypertension, and other chronic degenerative diseases later in life (*Guide to Clinical Preventive Services,* 1996). Eating disorders such as anorexia and bulimia are also increasing in the school-age population, which is strongly influenced by the media emphasis on thinness (Gaesser, 1996).

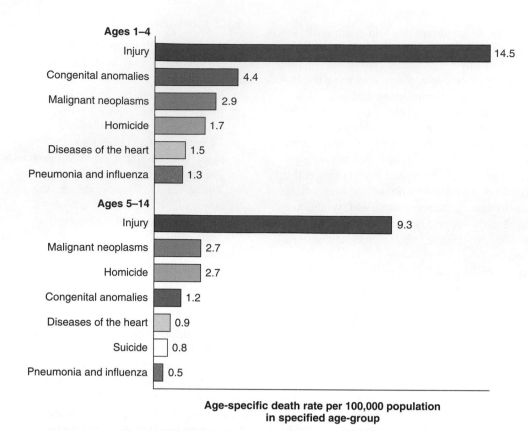

Figure 28-1   Leading causes of death in children ages 1 to 14: 1997. (From U.S. Department of Health and Human Services: *Health, United States,* Washington, D.C., 1999, U.S. Department of Health and Human Services.)

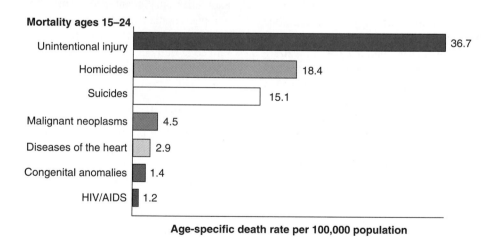

Figure 28-2   Leading causes of death in adolescents and young adults ages 15 to 24: 1997. (From U.S. Department of Health and Human Services: *Health, United States,* Washington, D.C., 1999, U.S. Department of Health and Human Services.)

Vision and Hearing Problems

Many children and adolescents have vision and hearing problems. Sensory motor deficits have increased over the past decade as premature babies weighing less than 1 pound are surviving. The prevalence rate for myopia ranges from 6% to 20%, with the higher rates occurring in children and youth who are neonatal intensive care unit graduates or those 10 to 14 years of age. The National Society for the Prevention of Blindness (NSPB) estimates that 1 in 500 school children in the United States is partially sighted. The NHANES III obtained interview data on hearing loss and audiometric screening outcomes in a national sample of 6,166 children ages 6 to 19 years. Results indicated a prevalence of 14.9% of either low-frequency hearing loss (lfhl) or

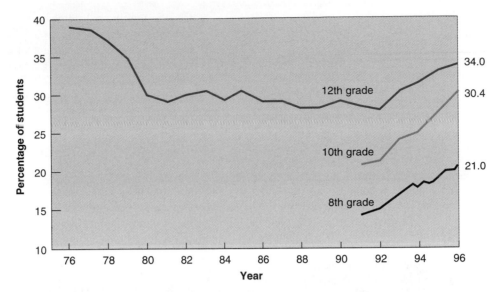

Figure 28-3   Long-term trends in 30-day prevalence of cigarette smoking for eighth-, tenth-, and twelfth-graders: 1976-1996. (From Maternal and Child Health Bureau: Child health USA 96-97, DHHS pub no HRSA-M-DSEA-97-48, Washington, D.C., 1997, U.S. Department of Health and Human Services.)

high-frequency hearing loss (hfhl) in more than 7 million U.S. children (Niskar, et al, 1998). Conductive hearing loss due to otitis media affects 20% to 30% of the preschool and early school-age population. Otitis media is one of the most costly illnesses of children. If untreated, otitis media may result in chronic ear infection, language delay, and hearing loss. Sensory neural hearing loss results from exposure to ototoxic drugs, hyperbilirubinemia, and serious infections such as meningitis (Donowitz, 1996).

Use of Alcohol, Tobacco, and Other Drugs

Tobacco use among teens rose steadily in the 1990s (Fig. 28-3) and is being directly related to the introduction of the Joe Camel media campaign. It is estimated that everyday nearly 3,000 young people take up daily smoking (Centers for Disease Control and Prevention, 2000). As a result, the federal government has tightened restrictions related to tobacco advertising. Tobacco is considered a "gateway drug" to other substances and high-risk behaviors (American Cancer Society, 1996). Increased smoking rates have severe lifelong effects for children because many of those who become addicted during adolescence will continue to smoke for the rest of their lives. If teens remain smoke-free throughout adolescence, it is unlikely that they will use tobacco as adults.

Alcohol is still the most widely abused substance among teenagers, and drug abuse continues. Recent studies, however, show that alcohol and drug use has declined for this age group.

Use of marijuana and cocaine decreased from 1988 to 1996 (U.S. Department of Health and Human Services, 1994; Maternal and Child Health Bureau, 1997). Not only is the use of alcohol and drugs among those 12 to 17 years of age reported to be down, but the awareness of the risks involved in these behaviors also has generally increased. Unfortunately, this profile of declining drug and alcohol use does not hold true for eighth-grade and younger students. Between 1991 and 1996, the proportion using any illegal drug in the previous 12 months more than doubled. Thus education programs must also target the young school-age population (Johnston, O'Malley, and Bachman, 1996).

Teenage Sexual Activity and Pregnancy

Researchers consistently find four factors that predict sexual intercourse at an early age, adolescent pregnancy, and non-marital childbearing among teenagers:
- School failure
- Early behavior problems
- Poverty
- Family problems/family dysfunction

While the teenage pregnancy numbers have been declining since 1990, each year 1 in 10 American girls 15 to 19 years of age becomes pregnant—two times more than in Canada, England, and France (Maternal and Child Health Bureau, 1997), making U.S. rates the highest in the industrialized world, or approximately 1 million adolescent pregnancies per year (Moore, Snyder, and Glei, 1995; Centers for Disease Control and Prevention, 2000).

Children With HIV/AIDS

Almost 12 million cases of sexually transmitted disease occur annually, 3 million in individuals under 25 years of age (Centers for Disease Control and Prevention, 2000). Children under the age of 13 years are exposed to HIV primarily through perinatal transmission before or during birth.

Evidence-Based Practice

This research study sought to determine the effectiveness of a 1-hour on-site educational program concerning HIV/AIDS, universal precautions, and glove use in the classroom setting by teachers, staff and volunteers. This study was planned in collaboration with the school administrators and PTAs to address the problem identified by the World Health Organization of increased susceptibility of persons in schools to risk for potential transmission of the HIV/AIDS virus. Exposure to nose bleeds, cuts, loss of teeth, and injuries from fights make school personnel vulnerable unless proper precautions are used. The study used a pretest, presentation, and posttest design. The study results showed that although school persons were knowledgeable about HIV/AIDS, they had little knowledge of universal precautions and glove use. The 1-hour presentation resulted in increased glove use in risk situations. This study shows that health education programs to address a health problem or risk can make a difference in the school environment.

APPLICATION IN PRACTICE

Involving appropriate administrators, teachers, and parents can help to make programs to address a problem at the aggregate level a success.

Grier E, Hodges H: HIV/AIDS: a challenge in the classroom, *Public Health Nurs* 15(4):257, 1998.

The transmission rate is 25% in untreated HIV-positive mothers. This rate drops to 7% when these women are treated during pregnancy (National Center for Health Statistics, 1997). Adolescents are exposed to HIV primarily through the receipt of blood products and high-risk behaviors. The American School Health Association (ASHA) suggests a broad-based health education approach, addressing the subject of sexually transmitted diseases (STDs) in all grades. Financial resources to provide education regarding AIDS prevention have been substantial. See the Research Brief about the HIV/AIDS educational program.

Absenteeism

Children do not benefit from school when they are not feeling well or are frequently absent from school. For adolescents, pregnancy, alcohol and drug abuse, injuries, suicide, homicide, and sexually transmitted diseases are the most common conditions that lead to school failure and drop out. Students who miss more than 10 days in a 90-day semester (11% of school days) have difficulty keeping up with their grade level. A missed class day is defined here as an absence only when it occurs as the result of an acute or chronic health condition. The absentee rate for girls is slightly higher than for boys, and the rate for Caucasians is somewhat higher than for African-Americans. Children who miss school have a higher rate of visits to the school nurse than other students. Excessive school absence, school failure, and drop-out rates in middle school and high school are often the result of factors such as:

- Chaotic family environments
- Low self-esteem
- Lack of achievement and motivation
- Understaffed and uninviting schools
- Other societal problems

Poor children and adolescents are at highest risk for **absenteeism.**

Children Living in Poverty

Students from poor families are most likely to miss school and therefore need and deserve special attention from the school nurse. These children often have chronic ear infections that will cause conductive hearing loss, language delay in young children, and possibly sensory neural hearing loss if left untreated. Others have repeated upper respiratory infections, allergies, dental decay, skin disorders, and other clinical disorders that will result in extended periods of absenteeism if diagnostic and treatment services are not readily available. These students are:

- Four times as likely to miss school because of their ailments
- Two to three times more likely to have a health condition that limits their school activity
- Twice as likely to have mental health problems
- Without health care because they are uninsured or their parents cannot leave work to take them to a health care provider without risking job loss
- More likely to fail academically due to a lack of parental involvement and adult supervision
- Likely to be homeless and do not attend school regularly

Others live in homes in which English is a second language, and the children do not speak enough English to understand class discussions. Therefore they soon lose interest in attending school.

About 19% of children in the United States are poor; minority youth are often members of this group (U.S. Department of Health and Human Services, 1999). Because poor children often are enrolled in the federally sponsored free breakfast and lunch programs offered at schools, school nurses can discreetly use enrollment rosters for these programs to identify those students who are in special need of school health care and need access to other community health services.

Measures should be taken to reduce physical and emotional health problems and poor health habits among these children and youth. Offering diagnosis and treatment services at school is a cost- and time-effective way to provide access to quality health care. Identifying and intervening in health-related risk factors prevents a cycle of absenteeism and school failure. The **Child Health Insurance Plan (CHIP),** which was passed by Congress in 1997, will provide school nurses with another option in finding services for children of the working poor who were previously uninsured and not eligible for Medicaid.

Children With Disabilities and Chronic Health Conditions

The number of students who have disabilities and chronic health conditions and are enrolled in regular school has increased since the enactment of the Education for All Handicapped Children legislation (Public Law 94-142) in 1975. Over a million more children now have access to a free and appropriate education.

Scientific advances and improved technology make it possible for low-birth-weight babies weighing less than 1 pound to survive, for students with chronic and terminal illnesses to enter remission and live with their diseases, and for severely physically disabled youth to communicate in the school setting. Students in the largest category of those eligible for services under PL 94-142 have specific learning disabilities and are usually in otherwise good health. However, the health problems experienced by those who need nursing care at school have become increasingly complex. Among the treatments and procedures some students require at school are:

- Medications
- Bladder catheterization
- Endotracheal suctioning
- Colostomy
- Ileostomy
- Ureterostomy care
- Nasogastric tube feedings

At the time of the reauthorization of PL 94-142 in 1991, this legislation was retitled the **Individuals With Disabilities Education Act (IDEA).** This federal law guarantees a free public education and related services for every disabled child from 5 to 21 years of age. The IDEA bill PL 101-476 identifies a number of related services, including:

- Health care
- Physical therapy
- Occupational therapy
- Speech therapy
- Psychological services

In addition, each state has its own plan for implementing this legislation, which can be more specific. In a growing number of states, school nursing services are designated as a type of health services that must be available for these students.

Addressing Children's Health Problems

Children and adolescents want and need to address their own problems. Several surveys of school-age youth reveal that they are interested in learning about health and that health topics are most often at the top of their priority lists. In surveys of high school students to determine the health needs with which they wanted help, the top five identified were:

- Acne
- Sex education
- Depression
- Obesity
- Parental disagreements

 Evidence-Based Practice

A survey was conducted of 375 inner-city school children to determine their perception of their neighborhood and to solicit suggestions from the children for improving their city. A qualitative word association format was used to determine the children's perceptions of safety, cleanliness, noise, beauty, friendliness, level of happiness, and helpfulness of the neighborhoods in which they lived. Two survey instruments were used; the Kids Place Survey developed in 1984 was used for older children, and a modified version called the Little Kids Survey was used for kindergarten to second grade.

Using a content analysis process it was determined that the children's response often depended on circumstances such as inner-city residence and the values and meaning they brought to the above words. Most of the children studied found family, home, and school safe environments. Although they find fun and happiness in the neighborhood, they often described them as noisy, dirty, and dangerous. The authors found that these children dealt with violence and potential danger daily. The youth suggested projects to clean up their neighborhoods and remove trash while cutting down the noise.

APPLICATION IN PRACTICE

School health nurses through health education programs can assist students in coping with their environments and in finding ways to improve their environments like block parties for neighborhood clean up, family fun at local parks, and identifying safe places to go in the neighborhood in the event of trouble.

Polivka B, Lovell M, Smith B: A qualitative assessment of inner city elementary school children's perceptions of their neighborhood, *Public Health Nurs* 15(3):171, 1998.

See the Evidence-Based Practice box about a similar survey of elementary school children.

The health problems of school-age children involve social, emotional, behavioral, and technological issues that require a complex range of services delivered by individuals and health care systems in a flexible, coordinated, and collaborative manner. Many practitioners, educators, and policymakers have concluded that the school nurse is a key figure in meeting many of the health care needs of students, especially those who are at high risk.

HISTORY OF SCHOOL NURSING
1900 to 1940

In 1902, Lillian Wald, the founder of the Henry Street Settlement House in New York City, discovered a 12-year-old boy excluded from school because of eczema:

In the early 1900s, I had been downtown only a short time when I met Louis. An open door in a rear tenement revealed a woman standing over a washtub, a fretting baby on her left arm, while with her right hand she rubbed at the butcher's aprons which she washed for a living. Louis, she explained, was "bad." He did not "cure his head," and what would become of him, for they would not take him into the school because of it? Louis, hanging the offending head, said he had been to the dispensary a good many times, but "every time I go to school Teacher tells me to go home." It needed only intelligent application for the dispensary ointments to the affected area, and in September I had the joy of securing the boy's admittance to school for the first time in his life (Woodfill and Beyrer, 1991).

Public health efforts in the early 1900s concentrated on the control of communicable disease. Thousands of immigrants were crowding into the tenement areas of large cities such as New York and Boston. With the tenements came the diseases that resulted from poverty and overcrowding. Having identified this child and many more like him, Lillian Wald and her staff carefully compiled a data-based report that convinced city officials to introduce physicians into schools to examine students and exclude those with contagious diseases. As an isolated event, these daily inspections created more problems than they solved. Follow-up of treatment and **counseling** was definitely needed because students and their families were frequently unable to understand the instructions on the exclusion card.

After 5 years of medical inspections in schools, thousands of children were excluded because of trachoma, and classrooms were empty. "In a single school three hundred children were out at one time" (Rogers, 1905). Lillian Wald proposed to the boards of health and education that a nurse be sent into the schools. As a 1-month demonstration project, Lina L. Rogers visited four schools daily, spending an hour in each.

Between 1903 and 1904, as a result of the successful demonstration project, 39 nurses were recruited by the New York City Health Department, and they were remarkably successful. According to health department records, 98% of students previously excluded from school were retained in classrooms. Improvised dispensaries (clinics) were set up to treat students on-site. Nurses provided the counseling and instruction necessary to overcome parents' fear and indifference.

During home visits, nurses found that many students were out of school for social reasons rather than because of disease, and many were "victims of the temptations of the streets" (Struthers, 1917). Others needed clothing and food before they could come to school, and some were caring for younger children while their mothers worked. In a few instances, these children were providing nursing care to family members who were ill. Steps were taken by the nurses to relieve a number of these social problems, and the children returned to school.

By 1909, municipalities throughout the United States were employing school nurses. Initially, the Visiting Nurses Association provided the nursing service on a demonstration basis. If the project was effective, the tax-supported boards of education or health would take administrative control of the program (Waters, 1909). In 1912, the American Red Cross created a nursing service to meet the school health needs in rural areas (Woodfill and Beyrer, 1991).

The need for school nurses to provide treatment in schools and to focus their efforts almost exclusively on the control of communicable diseases began to diminish

around 1916. Different priorities arose with the onset of World War I. In a time when able-bodied men were needed to defend their country, thousands of recruits were found to be physically unfit to serve because of poor eyesight, hearing loss, advanced dental disease, orthopedic problems, and sexually transmitted diseases. Consequently, the importance of early casefinding and corrective follow-up during childhood became clear to public health officials. School nurses soon shifted their attention from communicable disease control to primary prevention efforts, such as vision and hearing **screening.** It was the first organized large-scale attempt to proactively improve the long-term health status of American children.

By the 1920s, the role of the school nurse had expanded to include the functions of health educator and counselor. The dual role of school nurse-teacher evolved by 1937. A school nurse-teacher group became a section of the newly formed Department of School Health and Physical Education of the National Education Association (NEA). Later a separate department of school nurses was formed, which eventually evolved into the National Association of School Nurses (NASN). Currently, this organization is separate from the NEA, but a close alliance still exists.

World War II to the Present

Over the past 50 years, school nurses have been recognized for their humanitarian, preventive, and educational contributions to child and adolescent health. However, the role of school nurse-teacher has been the subject of continuing debate, and expanded clinical roles for school nurses are emerging. Fortunately, the duties and functions of school nurses are less ambiguous today, largely because of numerous attempts at standardizing the role, as well as state and national certification for the role.

During World War II, the nursing shortage became acute, and the school health program became the responsibility of school personnel other than the school nurse and the few physicians who still worked in the field. Consequently, most school nurses gave up their more labor-intensive roles as health teachers and counselors to take on the role of health consultant/coordinator/liaison between school, home, and community. Ironically, their school assignments doubled and tripled under this arrangement with no extra personnel to help them (e.g., health assistants carry out the screening programs, simple health instructions, and follow-up activities). Consequently, the quality of school health programs deteriorated.

By the end of the 1960s, many working mothers and worried school administrators recognized the educational and economic advantages of offering services at school. Thus the clinical role of the school nurse practitioner appeared. Over the last 25 years, the importance of the health consultant role and school-teacher roles has diminished, and the school nurse practitioner role has become more important. In turn, all school nurses have become more clinically competent while providing more **case management** services.

Success with the **school nurse clinician** role requires administrative support, clerical and paraprofessional assistance, available medical consultation, and a collaborative approach for the planning, coordination, operation, and management of the school health program. In the past, the only dollars available for school health were salaries for school nurses. The strategy today for finding the resources necessary to develop a comprehensive school health program, in which the school nurse clinician is a member of an interdisciplinary team, requires reorganization of schools and community health agencies to include child and adolescent health efforts. Therefore, to be truly effective, school health programs need to include, in addition to the nurse, health, social service, and education personnel who are prepared to deal with the health-related problems of students. These new developments in school health also present new opportunities for nurses to become **school health managers** or health coordinators.

School nurses often have had to try to balance their talents in the two fields of education and nursing. Unfortunately, there has been little power or recognition in either field. However, major changes are under way as the public and policymakers recognize the importance of improving health programs in schools. Here it is possible to increase the health status of all boys and girls and to provide special attention to those who have no other regular source of health care or whose health condition requires special nursing care for them to attend school. The history of school nursing clearly reflects the evolving nature of this role.

COMPONENTS OF THE SCHOOL HEALTH PROGRAM

The components of a comprehensive school health program include:

- An integrated, interdisciplinary approach to school health promotion
- Coordination of activities between the district and state
- Effective communication among faculty, staff, parents, and the community
- The provision of health services and health education
- The promotion and maintenance of a healthy school community environment

Figure 28-4 depicts a model based on Leavell and Clark's three levels of prevention. Figure 28-5 illustrates an integrated, comprehensive school health program. There is tremendous variety from one state to another regarding school health requirements, nurse-to-student ratios, scope of practice, and cost, all of which affect the implementation of any model at the local level.

The Centers for Disease Control and Prevention, **Division of Adolescent and School Health (DASH)** defines school health according to an eight-component model (Fig. 28-6):

1. Health services
2. Health education
3. Healthful school environment
4. Physical education

5. Counseling, psychological, and social services
6. Food services
7. Family and community involvement
8. Site health promotion for faculty and staff

The eight-component model is heavily weighted toward health education. Currently, the rising demand for clinical services at school suggests that additional resources will be required in the future. The important point is the principle of "local control" and the fact that local school districts prefer to develop and define their own programs. Models and definitions of school health should be considered by local policy makers when developing school health programs.

Health Services

School health services generally include:

- Health screenings
- Basic care for minor health problems
- Administration medications
- Assessment of immunization status
- Casefinding for the early identification of problems
- Case management
- Health counseling
- Nursing care of students with special health needs
- In some districts, primary care

All of these activities should be family-centered and should promote health and prevent disease. School nurses are generally the persons responsible for this component of school health. These nurses may or may not have medical and psychological referral sources for children who need them, depending on the size of the school health program and its level of development.

Screening

The school nurse's responsibility in the screening process is to work with families and other team members to do the following:

- Establish what screening will be done
- Develop a plan for the screening and a data management system
- Teach paraprofessionals and others (including students and volunteers) how to conduct the screenings
- Determine the appropriate resources for additional diagnostic work-up for children with signs and symptoms
- Refer students in need of further evaluation to other school and community resources
- Collaborate with others in implementing and evaluating treatment plans

Health promotion and secondary prevention screenings may include:

- Vision
- Hearing
- Pediculosis
- Scoliosis
- Dental
- Cardiovascular risk factor analysis
- Comprehensive surveys of personal health habits known as behavioral risk surveys

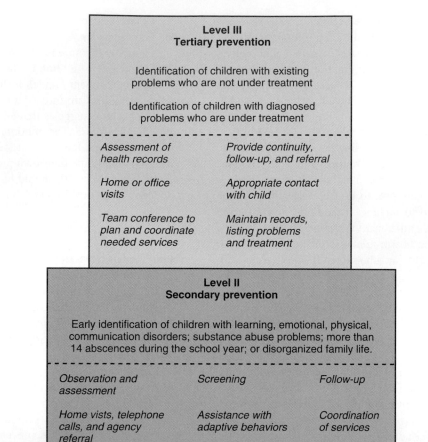

Level III
Tertiary prevention

Identification of children with existing problems who are not under treatment

Identification of children with diagnosed problems who are under treatment

Assessment of health records

Provide continuity, follow-up, and referral

Home or office visits

Appropriate contact with child

Team conference to plan and coordinate needed services

Maintain records, listing problems and treatment

Level II
Secondary prevention

Early identification of children with learning, emotional, physical, communication disorders; substance abuse problems; more than 14 abscences during the school year; or disorganized family life.

Observation and assessment

Screening

Follow-up

Home vists, telephone calls, and agency referral

Assistance with adaptive behaviors

Coordination of services

Level I
Primary prevention

Health promotion

Identification of children and youths at risk

Improvement in the physical environment of the school

Continuous assessment of the emotional climate of the school

Control of communicable diseases

Assistance with developmental crises

Student counseling

Teacher workshops in growth and development of children, first aid, CPR, mental health concepts, values clarification, etc.

Health education

Promotion of parental involvement

Teacher's health appraisal of children

Exercise programs

Anticipatory guidance

Use of all teachable moments

Stress reduction programs

Immunizations

Figure 28-4   School health program based on Leavell and Clark's three levels of prevention. Methods selected to achieve levels of prevention are in italics.

These screenings usually take place as close to the beginning of the school year as possible to reveal problems that may interfere with learning. Table 28-1 lists recommended screenings for school-age youth.

Special screening packages for preschool children are also available in school. One such program is the **Early and Periodic Screening, Diagnosis, and Treatment (EPSDT) Program.** This program is funded through Medicaid. All states have an EPSDT program that offers early screening,

diagnosis, treatment, and periodic follow-up services to children and youth who meet the financial eligibility requirements of Medicaid and who are under 21 years of age.

Two other preschool programs include a number of health screening activities. **Head Start** is an early childhood education program for children who are at risk for academic problems because of poverty and lack of sufficient social stimulation. **Child Find,** funded through the IDEA legislation (Public Law 101-476) provides early identification of

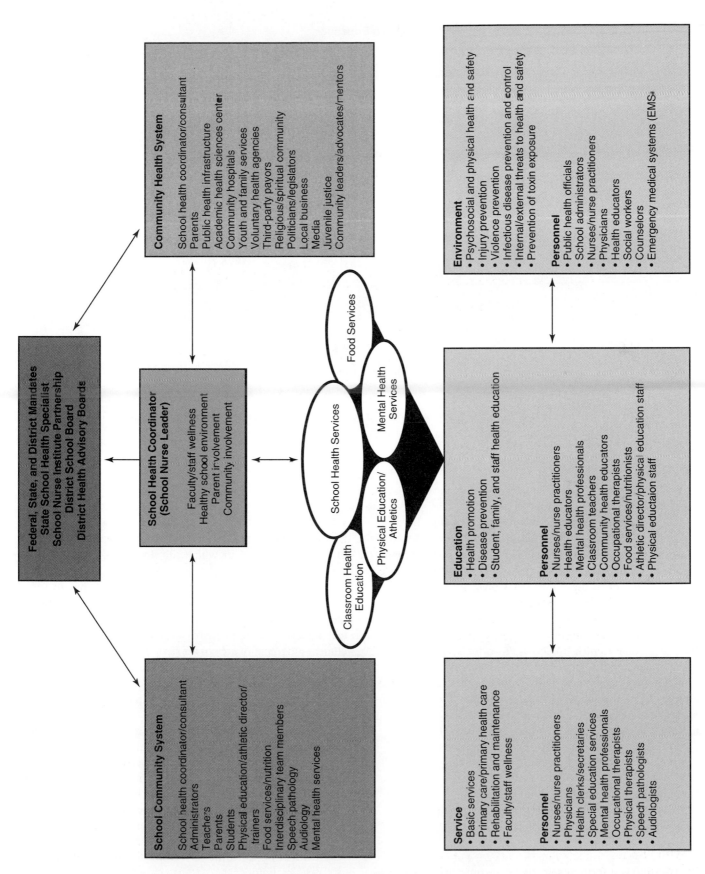

Figure 28-5 **Organization of a school health program.** (Courtesy Julie C. Novak, University of Virginia, 1998; Purdue University, 2001. Robert E. Novak, Illustrator.)

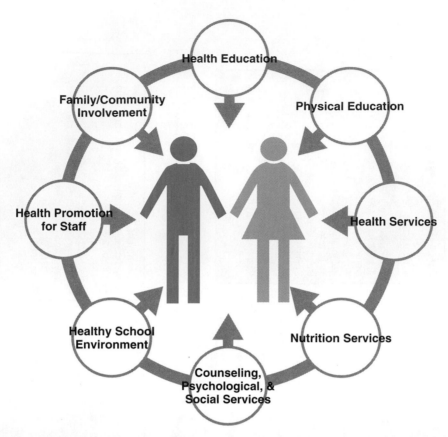

Figure 28-6 Eight-component model for school health. (From Centers for Disease Control and Prevention, Division of Adolescent and School Health: *School Health Programs: An Investment in Our Nation's Future At-A-Glance, 1999,* Washington, D.C., Centers for Disease Control and Prevention, available online: http://www.cdc.gov/nccdphp/ dash/ataglanc1999.htm.)

preschool children who are at risk for school failure because of mental retardation, other disabilities, chronic health conditions, or special health needs. Currently, school administrators, including school health personnel, face the challenge of combining all of these preschool programs into a more consolidated screening package to control costs and avoid unnecessary duplication. Although the EPSDT, Head Start, and Child Find programs offer services only to selected children, a national trend is underway to offer early childhood education and health screenings to all students.

In addition to the traditional school health screenings, the complexity of the school population makes it necessary to deliver more complex clinical services at school. Consequently, selective screening has become available for:
- Pregnancy
- Emotional disorders
- Sexually transmitted diseases
- Psychosocial and behavioral counseling
- Health promotion and disease prevention services
- Standard medical treatments

Casefinding

Casefinding is a form of selective screening that involves a search for certain students whose behavior, family circum-

stances, or health status place them at particular risk for ill health, absenteeism, and poor school performance. Instead of mass screening, in which all students in a variety of grades are involved, casefinding efforts begin by identifying risk factors and then locating students whose behavior suggests they are at risk for certain problems and in need of further assessment and possible referral. Therefore casefinding techniques are more intensive efforts and usually require the clinical judgment of school nurses to determine whether further assessment and diagnosis is necessary. Casefinding is carried out by practicing careful, systematic observation of all children with whom nurses come in contact, looking for anomalies or suspected symptoms.

Because the frequency rates for absenteeism, visits to the school nurse's office, injuries, referrals to the principal's office, and the practice of various personal health habits vary a great deal from school to school, the first step in casefinding is to establish rates for each school building and for the district as a whole. This is done by:
- Keeping track of the students seen by the nurse
- Reviewing screening results and absenteeism records
- Collecting information from teachers and school administrators
- Having students complete personal life-style inventories

TABLE 28-1	Screening and Counseling for School-Age Youth

Ages 7-12	Ages 13-18
Leading causes of death	
Motor vehicle accidents	Motor vehicle accidents
Injuries (non–motor vehicle)	Homicide
Congenital anomalies	Suicide
	Injuries (non–motor vehicle)
	Heart disease
	Malignant neoplasms
Recommended screening	
History	
	Dietary intake
	Physical activity
	Tobacco/alcohol/drug use
	Sexual practices
Physical examination	
Height and weight	Height and weight
Blood pressure	Blood pressure
	Complete skin examination
	Clinical testicular examination
Laboratory/diagnostic procedures	
Tuberculin skin test (PPD)	Rubella antibodies
	VDRL/RPR
	Chlamydia testing
	Gonorrhea culture
	Counseling and testing for HIV
	PPD
	Hearing
	Papanicolaou (Pap) smear
Client and parent counseling	
Diet and exercise	
Fat (especially saturated fat), cholesterol, sweets and between-meal snacks, sodium	Fat (especially saturated fat), cholesterol, sodium, iron, calcium
Caloric balance	Caloric balance
Selection of exercise program	Selection of exercise program
Injury prevention	
Safety belts	Safety belts
Smoke detector	Safety helmets
Storage of firearms, drugs, toxic chemicals, matches	Violent behavior
Bicycle safety helmets	Firearms
	Smoke detectors
	Driving/other dangerous activities while under the influence
Substance use	
	Tobacco: cessation/primary prevention
	Alcohol and other drugs: cessation/primary prevention
	Treatment for abuse
Dental health	
Regular tooth brushing and dental visits	Regular tooth brushing, flossing, and dental visits
Other primary preventive measures	
Skin protection from ultraviolet light	Skin protection from ultraviolet light
	Discussion of hemoglobin testing
High-Risk Practices	
	Sharing/using unsterilized needles and syringes
	Sexual practices
	Sexual development and behavior
	Sexually transmitted diseases: partner selection, condoms
	Unintended pregnancy and contraceptive options
Remain Alert For	
Vision disorders	Depressive symptoms
Diminished hearing	Suicide risk factors
Dental decay, malalignment, mouth breathing	Abnormal bereavement
Signs of child abuse or neglect	Tooth decay, malalignment, gingivitis
Abnormal bereavement	Signs of child abuse or neglect

From U.S. Preventive Services Task Force: *Guide to clinical preventive services*, ed 2, Baltimore, 1992 and 1996, Williams & Wilkins.

HOW TO Identify Students Who Are at Risk for Ill Health, Poor School Performance, and Absenteeism

1 Absent more than 10% of school days.
2. Frequently sent to the principal's or nurse's office for illness.
3. Frequently sent to the principal's office for "acting out" in the classroom.
4. Appear chronically ill to the teacher.
5. Have subtle, as well as obvious, physical defects that cause problems functioning at school.
6. Have subtle, as well as obvious, emotional problems.
7. Frequently seek out the nurse with vague, nonspecific health complaints.
8. Have been seriously injured or have a history of repeated injuries.
9. Genetically predisposed to certain conditions, such as sickle cell disease.

Once the overall frequency rates for student behavior in these instances have been established, it becomes possible to determine whether the behaviors of certain students are the same or different from the rest of their classmates. Within most schools there are school administrators with experience in setting up surveillance systems who can help the school nurse in gathering this type of information and learning how to interpret it if a school health supervisor is not available. In 29 states **school nurse consultants** are located in the state departments of health and education who are also available to help.

The most likely place to begin casefinding efforts is with:

• Assessment of children who have physical or mental disabilities
• Recent psychosocial trauma such as parents separating or divorcing
• A move from a rural, mountain, urban, or suburban setting into a totally different social environment

School nurses are especially concerned with detecting children who are victims of maltreatment (e.g., neglect or physical or sexual abuse). The nurse's responsibility in working with children suspected of being abused is to provide a non-threatening environment—a comfortable, compassionate, safe haven where the child is supported, encouraged, and protected. It is also the nurse's responsibility, and in some states a requirement, to report the problem to appropriate authorities, such as to the Child Protective Services (CPS) usually located in the local welfare offices.

Assessment of Immunization Status

Legally, entry into school requires that students have current, completed immunizations unless exempted for religious or medical reasons. Consequently, up-to-date **Certificates of Immunization Status** must be presented to school personnel for admission. This usually applies to preschool students as well as to boys and girls who are older. Each of the following

vaccines are required: polio, measles, mumps, rubella, and diphtheria/tetanus, and for preschoolers the addition of pertussis, *Haemophilus influenzae,* and hepatitis B. Hepatitis A and varicella are also recommended but not required. Because of the measles epidemic of 1989-1991, an MMR booster is required at school entry.

The school should have a procedure for assessment and documentation of immunization status.

1. A secretary, health aide or parent volunteer who has received necessary instructions from the school nurse conducts a primary review of the child's health record to determine the immunization status.
2. The information collected from the school is shared with the local county health department.
3. Those children not in compliance with the immunization law are cited with an **exclusion order** by the health department.
4. This information is then routed back to the school, where administrators refuse to admit the unimmunized students.
5. If students do not return to school in a reasonable length of time (3 to 4 days), follow-up measures are taken to investigate the truancy.

Often families have no access to immunization services because of poverty. Consequently, some schools have reintroduced school-based immunization clinics to alleviate the problem. This alternative is both efficient and economical.

Managing Minor Complaints

Each school building should have first-aid supplies and equipment in accordance with accepted first-aid guidelines. Local district policies, as well as state and federal occupational health (OSHA) regulations, need to be followed. A clinic area should be available for:

• The delivery of first aid and emergency care
• Daily care for common complaints including abdominal pain, headaches, earaches, fatigue
• Nonspecific complaints
• Dermatologic problems such as pediculosis and scabies

Increasingly nurses have begun to involve teachers and students in the responsibilities associated with first aid. Often first-aid kits are located in the classrooms, and nurses work with school personnel and students to enable them to deal directly with minor injuries. American Red Cross classes are an excellent means of preparing persons to do first aid. This approach is especially important if the nurse is not in the building on a full-time basis.

All school nurses need physical assessment skills and equipment to diagnose, treat, or refer students with common health complaints. This type of information needs to be recorded on the student's health record at school and, to provide continuity of care, on written referrals prepared and sent with the student if another health care provider, such as at the private physician, is to see the student. It is also important for the nurse to receive feedback from the other community health care provider; a system of communication must be developed for collaborating. Although this is more complicated in larger communities, the place to begin is to identify the students' health care providers. This is handled by having parents complete emergency cards that not only specify where the parent may be located during the day but also the name of their health care provider and the health facility or managed care system they use.

Innovative school nurses develop partnerships with university health science centers and other community agencies to enhance care delivery through collaborative projects and consultation to foster community support. These community and university leaders may serve on school health advisory boards and may sponsor educational programs, newsletters, and events such as health fairs.

Administration of Medications

The administration of medications has rapidly become the number one reason why students visit the school health office. In a 6-month period, more than 18,000 visits were made to the school health offices in five middle schools in Albemarle County, Virginia. Fifty percent, or 9,000 visits, were for the purpose of receiving a medication (Albemarle County School Health Advisory Board, 1997). States vary in their interpretation of the school nurse role, relationship, and responsibility to unlicensed personnel who may be handing out medications. The respective state board of nursing, state department of health, and school board are the agencies responsible for writing medication administration policies. In many schools, nonnursing personnel have this responsibility. In these cases instruction is needed, and manuals do exist for teaching purposes (Virginia Department of Health, 1997).

Medication policies are essential in schools today. However, these policies should not serve as a barrier to gaining access to the classroom and to learning. Some students with chronic disease such as asthma are in special self-management programs to help them learn how to function independently. School nurses need to support this approach by individualizing overall medication policies as appropriate.

HOW TO Develop a School-Based Medication Administration Policy: Five Basic Requirements

1. Medications are given only with parents' written permission.
2. Medications requiring a prescription are given only on the written authorization of a physician or nurse practitioner.
3. Medications requiring a prescription must be contained in an individual, pharmacy-labeled bottle for each student.
4. Medications must be recorded by the school personnel who administer them. This record states the student's name, medication, dosage, time, and the person administering the medication.
5. Medications must be stored in a secure, locked, clean container or cabinet.

Improper use of medication is also a problem in the school population. The National Council on Patient Information and Education (1995) found that, in any 2-week period, about 15 million people in the United States under the age of 18 take medicines prescribed or recommended by a physician. Of those, 50% either stop treatment too soon, do not take enough medication, take too much, or refuse to take any at all. When children use medicines improperly, acute illnesses needlessly continue or recur, treatable chronic diseases remain uncontrolled, and lives may be lost. Many of these medications are administered in the school setting; thus school nurses play a vital role in prevention of improper medication use.

Counseling

Counselors must recognize the importance of all children having a stable relationship with at least one adult, a safe environment, adequate health care, and quality life skills (Abu-Nasr, 1997). The ability to counsel students or others skillfully is an art. The counselor's responsibility is to:

- Provide information
- Listen objectively
- Be supportive, caring, and trustworthy

Effective counselors do not make decisions for their clients; rather they help clients arrive at the decisions that best suit them. Counseling therefore differs from teaching and interviewing. For example, **teaching** is giving information; **interviewing** is obtaining information from someone; **counseling** is helping people arrive at workable solutions to their problems or conflicts. See Table 28-1 for recommended counseling topics for school-age youth.

Students usually require counseling when they are unable to make decisions about personal concerns that affect their lives, for example, taking medication and changing lifestyle habits.

Briefly Noted

Counseling of students with high-risk social behaviors that may result in unintended pregnancy, sexually transmitted diseases, and HIV infection in school districts is considered highly controversial. The health professionals attempting to cope with these issues are viewed negatively and accused of encouraging the very problems they are attempting to resolve.

If the nurse lacks the ability to counsel or to recognize that counseling is needed, the student may be unable to fully realize the extent of the problem or to find alternatives to solve the problem. Students' peers can be used as counselors. However, students who act as peer counselors must be trained for the role. After providing students who are acting as peer counselors with technical advice, school nurses also should encourage them to use their personal experiences, to role-play, and to be available and accessible to other students.

Students with **vague, nonspecific health complaints** who visit the health room frequently should be of special concern to school nurses. This may be the first warning sign of a student who is not doing well in school and who is at risk for eventually dropping out. Children at risk of becoming school dropouts develop a type of maladaptive response to stress (vague health complaints) during the early school years. This behavior continues into adulthood, thereby affecting work and school performance. These students can be helped to manage their problems more effectively with the right assistance and counseling from the school nurse. This involves making sure the child is not physically ill and developing plans to increase the student's self-esteem, improve his or her problem-solving skills, and reduce stress levels.

Case Management

As a *case manager,* the school nurse performs a number of general activities. Parents need to be contacted to seek permission to discuss their child's health problem with the family physician or nurse practitioner. The nurse also will need to inform teachers and administrators accurately about the nature and prognosis of the health problem and the specific treatments required during the school day. Situations occurring at school that either interfere with the treatment plan or exacerbate the health condition need to be identified, communicated to the parties involved, and managed. Problems that arise from the student's health condition that influence learning also need to be recognized and handled. This usually involves obtaining and conveying information between health and school personnel. The school nurse is usually the person who bridges this gap through the process of case management.

Primary Care

A few examples of the type of **primary health care services** and health promotion activities now available in most schools are school-wide campaigns to:

- Improve diet and exercise
- Provide individual and small-group counseling to reduce stress and improve self-image
- Offer social skills training and cognitive therapies to prevent substance abuse and delay the onset of sexual activity
- Provide contraceptive education

The American School Health Association also recommends fitness screening, school breakfast and lunch programs, physical education, and mental health programs. Detailed handbooks are available to assist school nurses and other school health personnel in developing these programs. If school or pediatric nurse practitioners are available, students will have the opportunity for comprehensive health assessments in the school setting.

An increasing number of boys and girls today need to obtain additional primary care services in their schools. This type of care includes a comprehensive health history, a physical examination, simple laboratory tests, and diagnosis and treatment of minor health problems. A 24-hour-a-day, 7-day-a-week, year-round referral system also must be in place in case students' problems require additional medical attention, or they become ill when school is closed. The National Health Interview Survey found that 4.5 million (14%) students 10 to 18 years of age are from poor and minority households. These students are the ones who are least likely to have health insurance and access to primary care.

Increasingly, **school nurse practitioners** are becoming involved in more specialized forms of primary care. For example, some nurses serve as sports trainers, offering evaluations and special interventions to reduce the number of sports injuries. Other nurses who are primary care providers work with students experiencing emotional disorders or with students who are medically fragile and technology-dependent, such as a ventilator-dependent child. Still other school nurse practitioners deliver primary care in special settings, such as the diagnostic center for a school system.

Health Services for Students With Special Needs

According to the IDEA bill (Public Law 101-476), students eligible for service must have a comprehensive interdisciplinary evaluation followed by the preparation of an **individualized education plan (IEP).**

This plan is reviewed and modified at regular intervals during the school year and throughout the student's school experience. Parent conferences always occur in conjunction with the evaluation and preparation of the IEP. Students frequently join their parents and school staff for these meetings. For students whose health status significantly interferes with their ability to learn, a health care plan is a component of the IEP.

The health component of the IEP includes the following types of information:

- Specific notes of any special preparations and supervision that may be required in caring for the student
- Health counseling that is necessary for the student to function in the class
- Any changes in the school environment that are necessary, such as the removal of architectural barriers
- Safety measures
- Measures required to relieve pain and discomfort (e.g., suctioning, skin care)
- Special diet
- Medications
- Special assistance with activities of daily living
- Special adaptations of school health activities (e.g., screenings, health education, casefinding)

School staff members often need education and supervision by the school nurse to competently manage health care plans and the special health needs of students.

Health Education

During the past decade, **health education** has been closely identified with the health promotion movement. Basically, health promotion is a social concept or campaign, as well as a set of health education activities intended to develop healthy lifestyles among Americans. Health education efforts must relate to the values and beliefs of students and their families. Because the potential exists for health education to infringe on the constitutional rights of individuals, health education at school is best developed locally, by committee, and should be open for public inspection and parents' approval.

The health education component should include:

- Instructional efforts that foster wellness, such as health classes and courses to prevent the spread of infectious diseases such as AIDS
- Education for students with chronic health problems who need to learn more about their diseases, self-care, and how to effectively use the health care system

Three goals for the health education component of school health are as follows:

1. To teach all children about their bodies and how to keep them healthy
2. To instill lifelong healthy habits and the knowledge to make responsible decisions concerning health, the health of their families, and the health of their communities
3. To teach students how to use the health care system wisely and effectively.

Briefly Noted

A number of quality health education curricula are available today. Five programs are particularly well known. The **Growing Healthy** curriculum for elementary grades is a generalized program aimed at improving students' personal lifestyles. At the high-school level, the **Teen Outreach Program (TOP)**, which focuses on building self esteem through volunteering, has been effective in reducing teen pregnancy and drop-out in the experimental groups. **Teenage Healthy Teaching Modules (THTM)** have also been widely used. A more targeted type of health instruction is the **Know Your Body** course, which focuses on making students aware of their own cardiovascular risk factors through screening activities followed by special instruction related to risk reduction. The **Health PACT** course is a type of health instruction that is designed as consumer health affairs lessons. It is intended to prepare children to communicate effectively with health professionals during visits for health care.

Environmental Health

Another important component of the school health program is *environmental health,* which involves physical and psychosocial factors, such as infectious agent control and the physical and psychosocial environment of children. Evaluating the need to improve the psychosocial environment in schools today is complex. Instilling a sense of pride in students; assessing stressors of teachers, parents, and students; and evaluating the attitudes of the rest of the school team for signs of apathy, powerlessness, and hostility is essential (Comer, 1992). With the increase of violent acts in the school setting over the past decade, it is important for all school per-

sonnel and families to realize that 40% of American households with children ages 3 to 17 have guns; 7% have handguns, 17% have rifles and shotguns, and 18% have both. Children who have access to guns are six times more likely to commit violent acts and six times more likely to commit suicide (Center to Prevent Handgun Violence, 1998).

The physical environment in schools also needs to be evaluated. School nurses should work closely with local public health officials so that this area of school health is not overlooked. Safety programs are most important. For example often nurses actively involve students in identifying areas in the school in which injuries are most frequent and in planning intervention strategies to reduce the risks in areas such as playgrounds and school stairwells. Incident reports need to be completed by school personnel when injuries occur, and school health personnel should review this information regularly to improve conditions. Asbestos, lead poisoning, and toxic substances in the chemistry and art classrooms are areas of concern to school administrators.

Nurses must be well informed and have a close working relationship with the environmental health personnel at the local health department and nearby universities so that they can be a useful resource to the school community. Often the nurse will be involved in surveying areas for risks, collecting information from students and parents, and providing school administrators, parents, and students with current solutions to complex problems. Web-based educational materials and CDROM environmental health programs are excellent resources for the entire school community.

ROLES, FUNCTIONS, AND CREDENTIALS FOR SCHOOL NURSES
Generalists

The majority of the registered professional nurses now employed in school health are generalists prepared at the baccalaureate level who function in the consultant/coordinator role. The newer role for school nurses is as school health manager or coordinator. The functions associated with this role include the following:

- Policy-making activities to ensure a more comprehensive and integrated school health program
- Case management functions to help families find the help they need
- Program management duties so that a system of formal school health activities and protocols develops as an integral part of both the private and public community health system
- Health promotion and health protection responsibilities, including health education in the curriculum; health screening, follow-up, and referral for potential child health problems; and participation in activities that will make the school environment safe for children (e.g., adequate lunch programs, asbestos monitoring, violence prevention).

Because children's health problems are becoming more complex, knowledge of nursing, pediatrics, adolescent health, and public health is essential. These nurses must be prepared to identify health-related situations that place the student at risk and that other school personnel might fail to recognize. In addition, school nurses must be very familiar with community resources and how to gain access to them. Effective communication skills are necessary because this nurse serves as a vital link between the school and community health agencies.

Specialists

For nurses who plan to *specialize* in school nursing, a graduate degree in nursing is recommended. Several tracks are available which focus on primary care, case/care management, and health services delivery. When there is a need to reduce costs, there is a tendency to combine clinical and management roles so that the nurse can provide direct care and supervise the school health program.

The most common clinical roles in the schools include: the school nurse practitioner (SNP), pediatric nurse practitioner (PNP) or clinical specialist in community health, mental health, rehabilitation, and/or developmental disabilities. Only 500 certified SNPs are available and employed in schools, whereas approximately 1000 certified PNPs care for children in the school setting. With school health legislation developing in most states, more school health nurse specialists are needed.

Credentials

In addition to their nurses' license, school nurses often elect to become certified as a school nurse, school or pediatric nurse practitioner, community health nurse, or other type of clinical nurse specialist through professional nursing associations and certifying bodies. In some states, the State Department of Education offers an additional state certification or credentialing program for school nurses. School nurse certification may be obtained through testing offered by the National Association of School Nurses (NASN) or the American Nurses Credentialing Center (ANCC). In some states it may not be possible to be employed in a school system or to receive federal reimbursement for school nursing care for students with disabilities without being certified. Currently, school nurses are promoting credentialing as a way to upgrade the overall quality of school nursing.

MANAGEMENT OF THE SCHOOL HEALTH PROGRAM

A school health program requires good management to operate smoothly and effectively. Essential steps toward reaching this goal include the following: planning, organizing, directing, and controlling the quality of the program through outcome evaluation. Planning for school health should be a joint project involving members of a **school health council.** To ensure broad-based representation, this council should be composed of teachers, school nurses, parents, students, administrators, and community leaders. Members of this team:

- Set the direction for the program
- Make certain that the mission of the school health program is consistent with the goals of the school district and the rest of the community health system
- Plan and set goals for the school health program
- Develop and implement strategies to meet these goals
- Evaluate the program in view of these goals and makes changes as necessary

A school health council is a valuable support mechanism for the proper development, revision, implementation, and evaluation of the school health program. Although traditionally school health councils have been merely advisory bodies, currently these groups strongly influence policy. This has occurred with increased community participation, partnerships, and increased parental involvement.

Education Reform and School Health

In 1990 the National Governor's Association established the following goals for education by the year 2000:

- All children will start school ready to learn.
- The high school graduation rate will increase to at least 90% for all groups.
- All students will leave grades 4, 8, and 12 having demonstrated competency over challenging subject matter in English, mathematics, science, history, and geography.
- U.S. students will be first in the world in mathematics and science achievement.
- Every adult will be literate and possess the knowledge and skills necessary to compete in a global economy and to exercise the rights and responsibilities of citizenship.
- Every school in America will be free of drugs and violence and will offer a disciplined environment conducive to learning (U.S. Department of Education, 1990).

This action and the need for major reform within education are due to many concerns, including:

- Declining academic achievement scores of American youth
- Rising dropout rates, particularly in minority communities (Figs. 26-7, 26-8, and 26-9)
- Increased violence and drug abuse threatening the integrity of school communities
- Minority, disabled, or special needs children who do not have equal opportunities for learning

All of these factors threaten the ability of students to learn and become productive adults. The nurse can address the concerns by offering physical care, mental health counseling, and other types of support to the child in the school setting. The *Healthy People 2010* objectives address many of these issues with suggestions for implementing programs to resolve these issues. These are listed in the *Healthy People 2010* box. The section in this chapter on primary care gives suggestions for implementing strategies to address these issues.

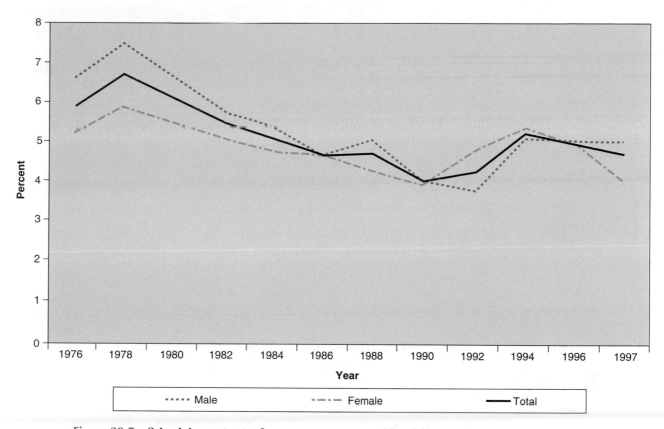

Figure 28-7   School dropout rates for young persons ages 15 to 24 by gender, October 1976-1997. (From U.S. Department of Education, National Center for Education Statistics: *Dropout Rates in the United States, 1997,* Washington, D.C., 1999, U.S. Department of Education, National Center for Education Statistics.)

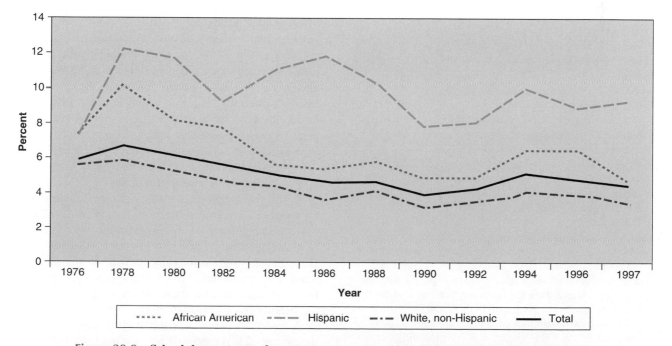

Figure 28-8   School dropout rates for young persons ages 15 to 24 by event, October 1976-1997. (From U.S. Department of Education, National Center for Education Statistics: *Dropout Rates in the United States, 1997,* Washington, D.C., 1999, U.S. Department of Education, National Center for Education Statistics.)

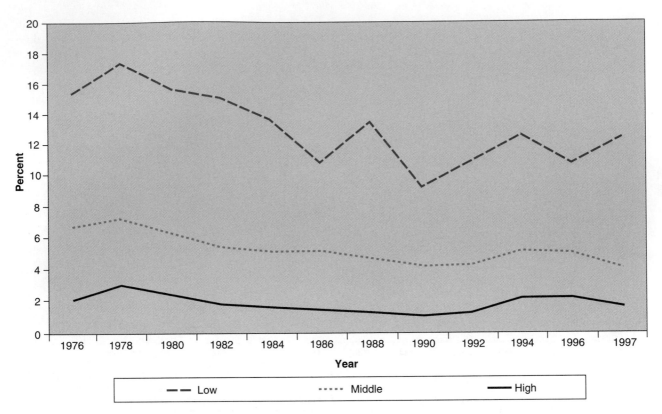

Figure 28-9   School dropout rates for young persons ages 15 to 24 by family income, October 1976-1997. (From U.S. Department of Education, National Center for Education Statistics: *Dropout Rates in the United States, 1997,* Washington, D.C., 1999, U.S. Department of Education, National Center for Education Statistics.)

Healthy People 2010 and
The Schools

The objectives for the nation include:
7-1 Increase high school completion.
7-2 Increase the proportion of middle, junior high, and senior high schools that provide comprehensive school health education to prevent health problems in the following areas: unintentional injury; violence; suicide; tobacco use and addiction; alcohol or other drug use; unintended pregnancy, HIV/AIDS, and STD infection; unhealthy dietary patterns; inadequate physical activity; and environmental health.
7-3 Increase the proportion of college and university students who receive information from their institution or each of the six priority health-risk behavior areas.

Dropping out of school is associated with poor health and other negative consequences. Health education and health promotion activities educate the youth of the nation about the importance of health and encourage a lifelong commitment to prevention. The importance of providing school health services is great. It is known that a child's physical and mental health is linked to abilities to achieve academically and socially.

Planning

Many school nurses are the managers or coordinators of school health programs. School health requires a unique type of management known as **pivot management.** Under this plan, nurses organize a school health team using the personnel already in the school system or closely associated with it: teachers, students, parents, administrators, psychologists, health educators, social workers, speech pathologists, audiologists, counselors, secretarial staff, and maintenance personnel. With the help of a school health council, this team develops:

- A comprehensive school health plan
- A budget for school administrators
- A design for program goals, strategies, and activities so that health services, health education, and environmental components of the program are coordinated with one another

If the health program for students with disabilities is separated from the general school health program, special care must be taken to link these efforts to avoid unnecessary duplication and fragmentation.

A *needs assessment* is the starting point for program development. It is used to determine the problems requiring attention and the way to best meet these needs. Box 28-1 provides an outline of specific areas covered in a needs assessments for school health.

Box 28-1   School Health Needs Assessment

STUDENT HEALTH

- Absenteeism: frequency and nature
- Health problems presented at school (e.g., illness and the nature, frequency, and location of injuries)
- Resolution of health problems: frequency
- Chronic health conditions, handicapping conditions
- Health status of students:
  - a. Immunization level
  - b. Dental
  - c. Vision
  - d. Hearing
  - e. Emotional disorders
  - f. Physical/sexual abuse
  - g. Prevalence of positive health behavior (e.g., nutrition, exercise, safety, and avoidance of substance abuse)
- Change in health status of students

RESOURCES

- Community resources available
- Use of community resources (overuse as well as underuse)
- Health care/education available in regular curriculum (e.g., physical education, home economics, special education, science, and health education)
- Health services available through current school health programs

EMPLOYEE HEALTH

- Health state of school personnel: absenteeism and nature of disability claims

---

All areas of school health must be considered when planning is done, and decisions must reflect innovative and economical ways of combining health services with health education and environmental health. Unfortunately, school health programs may be fragmented, with decisions about the health education curriculum made in one department, health services planned and implemented from another office, and the environmental health component attended to in yet another department.

Traditionally, health services have been limited to screening and first aid. However, the beginning of school-based health centers (SBHCs), the increased numbers of uninsured students, and the admission of students with complex health care needs have affected the development of much more complex school health services. In fact, care now being delivered in schools closely resembles the activities of traditional primary care facilities, including on-site diagnostic and treatment services and sophisticated nursing care for students with complex health problems. Rehabilitative services also may be available. Consequently, public health codes governing primary care facilities often apply to SBHCs. By maintaining a close working relationship with the local public health authorities, the school nurse is aware of local health regulations.

Next, school health planners must decide who will provide the health instruction. Ideally, sufficient numbers of school-employed health educators will teach the classes.

More realistically, these same health educators, who are in very short supply, develop the health education curriculum and work with school nurses, teachers, and other community health professionals to implement the program.

Well-organized school health programs must have clear, relevant, written policies and procedures. To be effective, these regulations must address the problems of students living in poverty, students with chronic illnesses or disabilities, and other children with special needs. The **"new morbidities"** affecting school-age children cannot be managed completely by the health care system alone because many problems have psychosocial, political, and physical features. External environmental and sociopolitical forces that lead to these problems must be considered to have an effective school health program.

Organizing

School nurses face a tremendous challenge daily in managing their time. Therefore it is important to have a written plan that sets the direction, priorities, and schedule for the school health program. The nurse must organize the day in such a way that low priorities do not keep her from getting to the high-priority problems. For example, many school nurses have discovered that an open-door policy fosters continual interruptions throughout the day. Consequently, school nurses in many school systems now have an appointment system for seeing students and for parent-teacher conferences. Sick-call times are often established as another way of cutting down on the number of unnecessary interruptions.

It is important for school nurses to organize an epidemiological database that profiles the health status of the student body both individually and as an aggregate. This is accomplished by using a systematic recording system for the problems that nurses see and the care they provide. Well-organized school health programs have policy and procedure manuals that explain the recording system to be used in a particular school system. Software packages for computerized school health records are used, and school nurses include personal computers in their budget requests. School and community health data systems used by school health personnel frequently use the **International Classification of Disease (ICD-9)** codes in recording student health problems.

Although schools traditionally have employed their own school health personnel or contracted with the public health agency for these services, new partnerships and organizational arrangements are emerging. School nurses in California and New York are forming their own school health companies and contracting directly with schools. University health sciences centers and community hospitals have also begun to contract with schools to develop partnerships and to administer school health programs.

Directing

At the local level, a school nurse supervisor/coordinator usually oversees the health services program and provides supervision for other school nurses. As the health needs of students become increasingly complex and the level of care delivered in school becomes more sophisticated, the school health program needs to be managed by a health professional who knows the clinical aspects of care.

School health managers/coordinators require certain skills to be effective. Among the most frequently cited skills of effective managers are:

- Communicating through effective verbal and listening skills
- Managing time and stress
- Managing individual decisions
- Recognizing problems
- Defining problems
- Solving problems
- Motivating and influencing others
- Delegating
- Setting goals
- Articulating a vision
- Having self-awareness
- Team building
- Managing conflict

The school nurse's role is expanding rapidly in the area of supervision of school health assistants or unlicensed personnel. As the number of children and the complexity of their health needs continues to rise, the need for assessments and care in the school setting increases. This makes it essential that school nurses have available to them a way to train and credential school health assistants to support the school health program and to work with children with special needs.

Quality Control

Outcome evaluation is a critical component of school health programs. Fortunately, practice standards for the school nurse and school nurse practitioner exist, and these serve as useful guides in determining effectiveness (Joint Task Force, 1990). Program evaluation is important to determine effectiveness. School nurses are beginning to use outcome measures as well as process evaluations. For example, the number of referred students who now wear glasses should be noted in an evaluation (outcome measures) as should the number of students screened (process variables). Outcome measures of the effectiveness of a particular school health activity also must reflect what impact the activity had on the child's academic performance.

INNOVATIONS IN SCHOOL HEALTH
School-Based Health Centers

School-based health centers (SBHCs) were established as a result of several demonstration projects conducted during the past two decades. These projects demonstrated that the school can be an effective site for primary care services because most children and youth attend school and have access to this facility. The projects also demonstrated that nurse practitioners with appropriate physician consultation and collaboration

provide excellent health care, reduce unnecessary referrals, and cut down on the time away from school. This is particularly true if a student's only other access to care is a public clinic where the waiting time is extensive.

SBHCs change the school nurse responsibilities in several ways. In some instances the school nurse takes on the responsibility for providing the care as a school nurse practitioner or pediatric nurse practitioner. In other settings the school nurse acts as the manager for the center and designs the programs and activities necessary for its operation. In other settings, nurses serve as team members for the center and their responsibility is triage and case management. However, it should be pointed out that the delivery of individual personal health services is but one aspect of the total school health program.

Family Resource/Service Centers

In Florida, Kentucky, New Jersey, Minnesota, and numerous other states the idea of **family resource/service centers** is attracting attention. Within this organizational structure, a number of school and community resources for families are consolidated into one agency for the sake of efficiency and reducing costs. Various public agencies, including the school, pool their child and adolescent health and childcare resources and reduce their overhead and management expenses by offering a one-stop shopping arrangement. An extension of the school health program logically belongs within these centers.

Family resource centers may be either geographically located in the school or linked to the school in some other way. In addition to student services, education and employment opportunities for parents are offered.

EMPLOYEE HEALTH

Another key aspect of some school health programs is that the program should meet some of the health needs of the teaching staff and other employees of the school system. Currently a number of school districts have wellness programs for employees, as well as medical services (e.g., physical examinations, smoking cessation programs, counseling for drug and alcohol abuse) and in-house evaluations for workmen's compensation claims. These services are often highly valued by the school board and school administrators because of the potential for health care cost containment and reduction in absences. School nurses have offered a variety of consumer health education programs, such as an adult version of the **Health PACT** course, in an effort to enhance teacher satisfaction with the health care system and to improve their use of their health care benefits.

Clinical Application

The school board and the school-based council of James County has agreed to develop a school health program. Such a program was necessary because an assessment of the school environment found an unhealthy environment with a high rate of absenteeism.

A. *A school health program involves which of the following?*
   1. *Health services*
   2. *Health education*
   3. *Environmental health*
B. *How could the school health nurse best address the problem of absenteeism?*
   1. *Keep track of the students seen by the nurse in the school clinic*
   2. *Collect information from teachers and administrators*
   3. *Set up a surveillance system for casefinding*

Answers are in the back of the book.

Remember This!

- The health problems of school-age youth vary substantially between the younger years and the adolescent years.
- Health problems are major risk factors for absenteeism and academic failure.
- Children and adolescents who are poor are at high risk for absenteeism and school failure.
- The three core components of school health are health services, health education, and promotion of a healthy environment.
- School health services generally include health screenings, basic care for minor complaints, administration of medications, surveillance of immunization status, casefinding for the early identification of problems, and nursing care of students with special needs.
- Historically, reducing absenteeism has been the single most important reason for school nursing services. With the current emphasis on education reform and academic performance, reducing absenteeism continues to be a top priority for school nurses.
- The role of the school nurse includes the functions of health education and counseling, as well as the delivery of clinical care to students with disabilities. Coordination of the overall school health program and case management of individual student health problems are other responsibilities of the nurse.
- School health activities are family centered and are intended to promote health and reduce the incidence of disease.
- Although health screenings are an integral component of school health services, nurses must prepare other school personnel, students, and volunteers for this work.
- Administration of medications and clinical care of students with disabilities in school is increasing in frequency. Nevertheless, the risks associated with these practices can be managed successfully as long as there are well-developed policies and procedures.
- School health education involves health promotion instruction for all students to develop their positive personal health habits; self-help classes for students with special health needs; and consumer education for all so that the next generation will be prepared to use the health care system effectively.

- The school environment requires attention, and certain measures are necessary if the climate at school is to be both physically and psychologically healthy.
- Schools are **nontraditional health care settings.** Consequently, it is important to establish health policies, procedures, and plans to provide direction for the school health program.
- Planning and operation of the school health program involves parents, community health professionals, and school personnel.

What Would You Do?

1. Visit a school. Observe the activities and interactions of students as a group both inside and outside the classroom. What are the advantages and disadvantages of learning collectively as opposed to being tutored? What are the implications for health teaching and counseling?
2. Interview a school nurse, school nurse practitioner, or community health nurse clinical specialist for school-age youth working in schools. How do they explain their roles in the school? What are the rewards? What are the frustrations?
3. Visit a school with a school nurse. Observe how the nurse works with individual children with disabilities and with boys and girls who are at high risk for academic failure because of chronic illness, poverty, and family problems. Inquire about any special procedures and precautions they observe in caring for these students. Look at the record-keeping system. Ask to review an individual education plan (IEP) and an **individualized family service plan (IFSP).** Find out whether the school nurse is involved with the school district's preschool program. Does the school also have a program for those infants and toddlers from birth to 3 years of age who have disabilities? How is the nurse involved with this effort?
4. Find a journal or textbook for school teachers. Review the table of contents to determine the areas of interest and importance to them. Select and read one of these articles/chapters. Compare and contrast the school teacher's approach to problem solving with the way nurses solve problems. What benefits and constraints could these differences present when nurses and teachers try to work together?
5. Attend a school board meeting. In preparation for this activity find out whether the board members are appointed or elected. Also find out something about the board members: their names, occupations, special concerns about education. At the time of the meeting, review the agenda, notice the amount of preparatory work the board members must do before meetings, and observe the interactions between the board, school administrators, and members of the audience. What are the chief concerns expressed at this meeting? How will this affect the school health program and school nurses?

6. Find a group of children or adolescents. Ask them to draw you a picture of (or explain) the nature of the health program at their school. What services are provided? What health classes are taught? What activities go on at school to keep it a safe and healthy environment for students? Ask the students to identify one change in the school health program that they would like to make.

7. Contact a parent who is a member of the Parent-Teachers Organization (PTO). Discover the purpose and functions of this organization. Find out whether the PTO is involved in school health locally or nationally. Also discover whether the PTO represents all parents. Are parents who are poor or from minority groups involved?

8. Is there a state school nurse consultant in your state? Find out by contacting the state Department of Health and the state Department of Education/Instruction. If a nurse consultant is available, find out the answers to these questions:

   a. How many school nurses are in your state?

   b. Is a current statewide policy/procedure manual for school health available to guide the practice of all school health personnel, especially those people working in districts too small to develop their own? How is this manual developed?

   c. What is the major school health concern right now in your state and the nurse consultant's strategy for addressing this issue?

   d. Where are the school health programs in your state that work well? What are the ingredients in these school systems that make these programs successful?

REFERENCES

Abu-Nasr D: Volunteer vision turns into reality, *Ann Arbor News,* April 27, 1997, pp A-1, A-11.

Albemarle County School Health Advisory Board: *Visits to the middle school health office: a data analysis,* Charlottesville, Va, 1997, Albemarle County School Board.

American Cancer Society: *Research progress report, cancer facts and figures,* Atlanta, 1996, American Cancer Society.

Andersen RE, et al: Relationship of physical activity and television watching with body weight and level of fatness among children, *JAMA* 279(12):938, 1998.

Annie Casey Foundation: *Kids count data book: 1996,* Baltimore, 1996, Annie Casey Foundation.

Barkley RA: *ADHA: a handbook for diagnosis and treatment,* New York, 1998, Guilford Press.

Brownson RC, Kreuter MW: Future trends affecting public health, *JPH Management Pract* 3(2):49, 1997.

Center to Prevent Handgun Violence: *Guns in American schools 1998,* available online: www.handgun-control.org/protecting/D1/dlgunsch.htm

Centers for Disease Control and Prevention. *School health programs: an investment in our future,* Atlanta, 2000, Centers for Disease Control and Prevention.

Children's Defense Fund: *The state of America's children yearbook 1997,* Washington, D.C., 1997, Children's Defense Fund.

Comer JP: Environmental health: the psychosocial climate. In Wallace, et al: Principles and practices of student health, Oakland, 1992, Third Party Publishing.

Donowitz L: *Infection control in the child care center and preschool,* ed 3, Baltimore, 1996, Williams & Wilkins.

Gaesser GA: *Big fat lies: the truth about your weight and your health,* New York, 1996, Fawcett Columbine.

Grier E, Hodges H: HIV/AIDS: a challenge in the classroom, *Public Health Nurs* 15(4):257, 1998.

Guide to clinical preventive services: report of the U.S. Preventive Services Task Force, Baltimore, 1996, Williams & Wilkins.

Johnston L, O'Malley P, Bachman J: *News release, the rise in drug use among American teens continues,* Ann Arbor, 1996, University of Michigan Institute for Social Research.

Joint Task Force for the Management of Children With Special Health Needs of the American Federation of Teachers, The Council for Exceptional Children, National Association of School Nurses, National Education Association: *Guidelines for the delineation of roles and responsibilities for the safe delivery of specialized health care in the educational setting,* Scarborough, Me, 1990, National Association of School Nurses.

Maternal and Child Health Bureau: Child health USA 96-97, DHHS pub no HRSA-M-DSEA-97-48, Washington, D.C., 1997, U.S. Department of Health and Human Services.

Moore K, Snyder N, Glei D: *Facts at a glance,* Flint, Mich, 1995, Charles Mott Foundation.

National Center for Health Statistics: *Current estimates from the National Health Interview Survey: vital and health statistics,* series 10, Washington, D.C., 1997, National Center for Health Statistics.

Niskar AS, et al: Prevalence of hearing loss 6-19 years of age, *JAMA* 279(14):1071, 1998.

Polivka B, Lovell M, Smith B: A qualitative assessment of inner city elementary school children's perceptions of their neighborhood, *Public Health Nurs* 15(3):171, 1998.

Rogers L: The nurse in the public school, *Am J Nurs* 5:763, 1905.

Southern Region Educational Board: *Developing a school health nursing curriculum,* 1998, Fuld trust grant.

Struthers LR: *The school nurse,* New York, 1917, GP Putnam's Sons.

U.S. Department of Education: *National goals for education,* Washington, D.C., 1990, U.S. Department of Education.

U.S. Department of Health and Human Services: *Health, United States, 1993,* USDHHS pub no (PHS) 73-1232, Washington, D.C., 1994, U.S. Department of Health and Human Services.

U.S. Department of Health and Human Services: *Health, United States, 1998,* USDHHS pub no (PHS) 78-1232, Washington, D.C., 1999, U.S. Department of Health and Human Services.

U.S. Department of Health and Human Services: *Healthy people 2000 midcourse review 1995,* Washington, D.C., 1995, U.S. Department of Health and Human Services.

U.S. Department of Health and Human Services: *National health interview surveys,* Washington, D.C., 1997, National Center for Health Statistics.

U.S. Preventive Services Task Force: *Guide to clinical preventive services,* ed 2, Baltimore, 1992 and 1996, Williams & Wilkins.

Virginia Department of Health: School health data, Richmond, Va, 1997, Virginia Department of Health.

Waters Y: *Visiting nursing in the United States,* New York, 1909, Charities Publications Committee.

Woodfill M, Beyrer M: *The role of the nurse in the school setting: an historical view as reflected in the literature,* Kent, Ohio, 1991, American School Health Association.

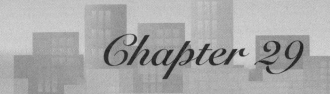

Chapter 29

Community Health Nursing in Occupational Health

BONNIE ROGERS

OBJECTIVES

After reading this chapter, the student should be able to:
- Describe the nursing role in occupational health.
- Describe current trends in the American workforce.
- Describe examples of work-related illness and injuries.
- Use the epidemiological model to explain work-health interactions.

- Cite at least three host factors associated with increased risk from an adverse response to hazardous workplace exposure.
- Explain one example each of biological, chemical, environmental/mechanical, physical, and psychosocial workplace hazards.
- Complete an occupational health history.
- Describe functions of OSHA and NIOSH.
- Describe an effective disaster plan.

CHAPTER OUTLINE

Definition and Scope of Occupational Health Nursing

History and Evolution of Occupational Health Nursing

Professional Roles and Professionalism in Occupational Health Nursing

Workers as a Population Aggregate
  Characteristics of the Workforce
  Characteristics of Work
  Work-Health Interactions

Application of the Epidemiologic Model
  Host
  Agent
  Environment

Organizational and Public Efforts to Promote Worker Health and Safety
  On-Site Occupational Health and Safety Programs

Nursing Care of Working Populations
  Worker Assessment
  Workplace Assessment

Healthy People 2010 Related to Occupational Health

Legislation Related to Occupational Health

Disaster Planning and Management

KEY TERMS

agent: causative factor invading a host through an environment favorable to produce disease, such as a biological or chemical agent.

environment: all those factors internal and external to the client that influence and are influenced by the host and agent-host interactions.

Continued

Hazard Communication Standard: the "right-to-know" standard that requires all manufacturing firms to inventory toxic agents, label them, develop information sheets, and educate employees about these agents.

host: human or animal that provides adequate living conditions for any given infectious agent.

National Institute for Occupational Safety and Health (NIOSH): the branch of the U.S. Public Health Service that is responsible for investigating workplace illnesses, accidents, and hazards.

occupational health hazards: dangerous processes, conditions, or materials within a work environment that can result in harm to an employee.

occupational health history: questions added to a health assessment that provide data necessary to rule out or confirm job-induced symptoms or illnesses.

Occupational Safety and Health Administration (OSHA): federal agency charged with improving worker health and safety by establishing standards and regulations and by educating workers.

work-health interactions: influence of work on health shown by statistics on illnesses, injuries, and deaths associated with employment.

worker's compensation: compensation given to an employee for an injury that occurred while the employee was working.

work site walk-through: an assessment of the workplace conducted by the nurse.

In America, work is viewed as important to one's life experiences, and most adults spend about one third of their time at work (Rogers, 1994). Work—when fulfilling, fairly compensated, healthy, and safe—can help build long and contented lives and strengthen families and communities. Although some workers may never face more than minor adverse health effects from exposures at work, such as occasional eye strain resulting from poor office lighting, every single industry grapples with serious hazards (U.S. Department of Health and Human Services and National Institute for Occupational Safety and Health, 1996). No work is completely risk-free, and all health care professionals should have some basic knowledge about workforce populations, work and related hazards, and methods to control hazards and improve health.

There have been many substantial changes in:
- The nature of work
- Workplace risks
- The work environment
- Workforce composition and demographics
- Health care delivery mechanisms.

An analysis of these trends suggests that work-health interactions will continue to grow in importance, affecting:
- How work is done
- How hazards are controlled or minimized
- How health care is managed and integrated into workplace health delivery strategies.

As a result, significant developments are occurring in occupational health and safety programs designed to prevent and control work-related illness and injury and to create environments that foster and support health-promoting activities. Occupational health nurses have performed critical roles in planning and delivering work site health and safety services. In addition, the continuing increase of health care costs and the concern about health care quality have prompted the including of primary care and management of non–work-related health problems in the health services programs. In

some settings, family services are also provided. This chapter describes the nurse's role with the working population.

DEFINITION AND SCOPE OF OCCUPATIONAL HEALTH NURSING

Adapted from the American Association of Occupational Health Nurses (American Association of Occupational Health Nurses, 1999), *occupational health nursing* is defined as:

The specialty practice that focuses on the promotion, prevention, and restoration of health within the context of a safe and healthy environment. It involves the prevention of adverse health effects from occupational and environmental hazards. It provides for and delivers occupational and environmental health and safety services to workers, worker populations, and community groups. It is an autonomous specialty, and nurses make independent nursing judgments in providing health care.

Occupational health nurses work in traditional manufacturing, industry, service, health care facilities, construction sites, and government settings. Their scope of practice is broad and includes:
- Worker/workplace assessment and surveillance
- Primary care
- Case management
- Counseling
- Health promotion/protection
- Administration and management
- Research
- Legal-ethical monitoring
- Community orientation.

The knowledge in occupational health and safety is applied to the workforce aggregate.

HISTORY AND EVOLUTION OF OCCUPATIONAL HEALTH NURSING

Ada Mayo Stewart, hired in 1885 by the Vermont Marble Company in Rutland, Vermont, is often considered the first industrial nurse. Riding a bicycle, Miss Stewart visited sick

The author wishes to thank June Thompson for her contribution to this chapter.

employees in their homes, provided emergency care, taught mothers how to care for their children, and taught healthy living habits (Felton, 1985). In the early days of occupational health nursing, the nurse's work was family centered and holistic. Nursing care for workers in industry began in 1888 and was called *industrial nursing*. A group of coal miners hired Betty Moulder, a graduate of the Blockley Hospital School of Nursing in Philadelphia (now Philadelphia General Hospital) to take care of their ailing co-workers and families (American Association of Occupational Health Nurses, 1976).

Employee health services grew rapidly during the early 1900s as companies recognized that the provision of work site health services led to a more productive workforce. At that time, workplace accidents were seen as an inevitable part of having a job. However, the public did not support this attitude, and a system for **worker's compensation** arose that remains today (McGrath, 1995).

Industrial nursing grew rapidly during the first half of the twentieth century. Educational courses and professional societies were established. By World War II there were approximately 4000 industrial nurses (Brown, 1981). The American Association of Industrial Nursing (AAIN), now called the American Association of Occupational Health Nurses, was established as the first national nursing organization in 1942. The aim of the AAIN was to improve industrial nursing education and practice and to promote interdisciplinary collaborative efforts (Rogers, 1994).

Passage of several laws in the 1960s and 1970s to protect workers' safety and health led to an increased need for occupational health nurses. In particular, the passing of the landmark *Occupational Safety and Health Act* in 1970, which created the Occupational Safety and Health Administration (OSHA) and the *National Institute for Occupational Safety and Health* (NIOSH), discussed later in this chapter, created a large need for nurses at the work site to meet the demands of the many standards being implemented. The Act focused primarily on education and research. In 1988, the first occupational health nurse was hired by OSHA to provide technical assistance in standards development, field consultation, and occupational health nursing expertise. In 1993 the Office of Occupational Health Nursing was established within the agency.

PROFESSIONAL ROLES AND PROFESSIONALISM IN OCCUPATIONAL HEALTH NURSING

As American industry has shifted from agrarian (agriculture) to industrial to highly technological processes, the role of the occupational health nurse has continued to change. The focus on work-related health problems now includes the spectrum of human responses to multiple, complex interactions of biopsychosocial factors that occur in community, home, and work environments. The customary role of the occupational health nurse has extended beyond emergency treatment and prevention of illness and injury. The interdisciplinary nature of occupational health nursing has become

more critical as occupational health and safety problems require more complex solutions. The occupational health nurse frequently collaborates closely with multiple disciplines, industry management, and representatives of labor.

Occupational health nurses constitute the largest group of occupational health professionals. The occupational health nursing role is unique in that the nurse adapts to an agency's needs as well as to the needs of specific groups of workers.

The professional organization for occupational health nurses is the American Association of Occupational Health Nurses (AAOHN). The AAOHN's mission is comprehensive. It supports the work of the occupational health nurse and advances the specialty. The AAOHN also does the following:
- Promotes the health and safety of workers
- Defines the scope of practice and sets the standards of occupational health nursing practice
- Develops the Code of Ethics for occupational health nurses with interpretive statements
- Promotes and provides continuing education in the specialty
- Advances the profession through supporting research
- Responds to and influences public policy issues related to occupational health and safety.

The AAOHN describes 10 job roles for occupational health nurses: *clinician, case manager, coordinator, manager, nurse practitioner, corporate director, health promotion specialist, educator, consultant,* and *researcher* (American Association of Occupational Health Nurses, 1997). The majority of occupational health nurses work as solo clinicians, but increasingly, additional roles are being included in the specialty practice. In many companies, the occupational health nurse has assumed expanded responsibilities in job analysis, safety, and benefits management. Many occupational health nurses also work as independent contractors or have their own businesses providing occupational health and safety services to industry, as well as consultation. With the current changes in health care delivery and the movement toward managed care, occupational health nurses will need increased skills in primary care, health promotion, and disease prevention. Occupational health nurses devote much attention to keeping workers and, in some cases, their families healthy and free from illness and work site injuries. Specializing in the field is often a requirement.

Academic education in occupational health and safety is generally at the graduate level however many AND and BSN nurses work in occupational health (Morris, 1994). Certification in occupational health nursing is provided by the American Board for Occupational Health Nurses (ABOHN) for AND and BSN graduates and is met through experience, continuing education, professional activities, and examination.

WORKERS AS A POPULATION AGGREGATE

The population of the United States is expected to increase from approximately 272 million people in 1999 to an estimated 297 million people by the year 2010 (U.S.

Census Bureau, 1996). By 2010 the U.S. population will be older, with a median age of more than 37 years, compared to 29 years in 1975. This will be reflected in the workforce with a decrease in the number of young job seekers. It is estimated that by the year 2010 28% of the workforce will be between the ages of 35 and 54.

There are more than 138 million civilian wage and salary workers over 16 years of age in the United States, employed in about 6.3 million different work sites (Bureau of Labor Statistics, 1999). More than 91% of those who are able to work outside of the home do so for some portion of their lives (Bureau of Labor Statistics, 1999). Neither of these statistics indicates the full number of individuals who have potentially been exposed to work-related health hazards. Although some individuals may currently be unemployed or retired, they continue to bear the health risks of past occupational exposures. The number of affected individuals may be even larger as work-related illnesses are found among spouses, children, and neighbors of exposed workers.

Americans are employed in diverse industries that range in size from one to tens of thousands of employees. Types of industries include:

- Traditional manufacturing (e.g., automotive and appliances)
- Service industries (e.g., banking, health care, and restaurants)
- Agriculture
- Construction
- Newer high-technology firms, such as computer chip manufacturers.

Approximately 95% of business organizations are considered small, employing fewer than 500 people (Bureau of Labor Statistics, 1997). Although some industries are noted for the high degree of hazards associated with their work (e.g., manufacturing, mines, construction, and agriculture), no work site is free of occupational health and safety hazards. The larger the company, the more likely it is to sponsor health and safety programs for employees. Smaller companies are more apt to rely on the external community to meet their needs for health and safety services.

Characteristics of the Workforce

The U.S. workplace and workforce is rapidly changing (U.S. Department of Health and Human Services–National Institute for Occupational Safety and Health, 1996):

- Jobs in the economy continue to shift from manufacturing to service.
- Longer hours, compressed work weeks, shift work, reduced job security, and part-time and temporary work are realities of the modern workplace.
- New chemicals, materials, processes, and equipment are developed and marketed at an ever-increasing pace.
- As the U.S. workforce grows to approximately 160 million by the year 2008, it will become older and more racially diverse.

- By the year 2008, minorities will represent 30% of the workforce, and women will represent approximately 48% of the workforce (Fig. 29-1).

These changes will present new challenges to protecting worker safety and health.

In an era in which the demand for workers is expected to outstrip the available supply, businesses must be concerned about strategies to increase:

- Health status
- Employment longevity
- Satisfaction of workers.

For example, although nearly 60% of all women are employed (representing 48% of the workforce), it is predicted that women will account for a majority of the increase in the labor force over the next decade (Bureau of Labor Statistics, 1999). These workers tend to be married, with children and aging parents for whom they are responsible. This aggregate of workers presents new issues for individual and family health promotion, such as childcare and elder care, that can be addressed in the work environment.

Characteristics of Work

There has been a dramatic shift in the types of jobs held by workers. Following the evolution from an agrarian (agriculture) economy to a manufacturing society and then to a highly technological workplace, the greatest proportion of paid employment is now in the following occupations:

- Service (e.g., health care, information processing, banking, and insurance)
- Professional technical positions (e.g., managers and computer specialists)
- Clerical work (e.g., word processors and secretaries).

During the 1996 to 2000 period, service-providing industries accounted for virtually all of the job growth. The 10 fastest-growing occupations include six health-related and four computer-related occupations (Bureau of Labor Statistics, 1998) (Box 29-1).

This change in the nature of work has been accompanied by many new occupational hazards such as:

- Complex chemicals
- Nonergonomic workstation design (the adaptation of the workplace or work equipment to meet the employee's health and safety needs)
- Job stress.

In addition, the emerging of a global economy with free trade and multinational corporations presents new challenges for health and safety programs that are culturally relevant.

Work-Health Interactions

The influence of work on health, or **work-health interactions,** is shown by statistics on illnesses, injuries, and deaths associated with employment. Each day (in 1998), an average of 137 individuals died from work-related diseases, and an additional 16 died from injuries on the job. Every 5 seconds a worker was injured, and every 10 seconds a worker was

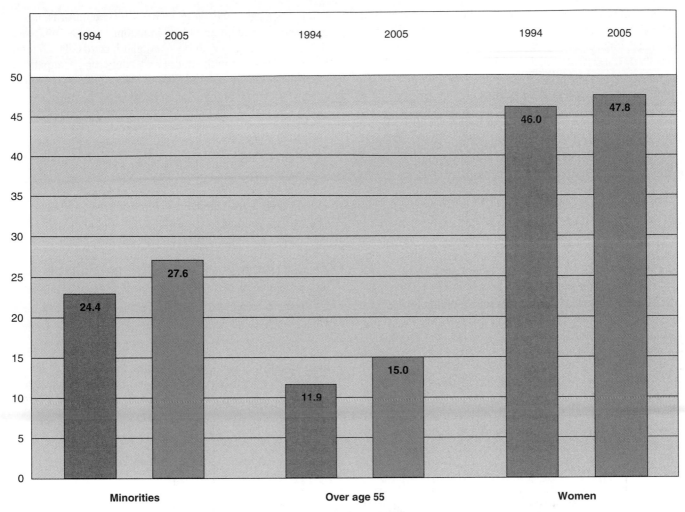

Figure 29-1   Projected changes in civilian labor force 1994 to 2005. (From Fullerton H: The 2005 labor force: growing, but slowly, *Monthly Labor Rev* 118[11]:29, 1995.)

| Box 29-1 | **The 10 Occupations With the Fastest Employment Growth** |

1. Database administrators, computer support specialists, and all other computer scientists
2. Computer engineers
3. Systems analysts
4. Personal and home care aides
5. Physical and corrective therapy assistants and aides
6. Home health aides
7. Medical assistants
8. Desktop publishing specialists
9. Physical therapists
10. Occupational therapy assistants and aides

From Bureau of Labor Statistics: *Employment projections: 1998,* Washington, D.C., 1998, U.S. Government Printing Office.

---

temporarily or permanently disabled (Bureau of Labor Statistics, 1998). Over the past few years, the incidence and severity of work-related injuries have increased. Employers reported 5.7 million work injuries and 430,000 newly reported cases of occupational illnesses in 1997. In 1997 2.9 million reported work-related illnesses and injuries resulted in lost time from work. Of these, approximately 82,000 were severe enough to result in temporary or permanent disabilities that prevented the workers from returning to their usual jobs (Bureau of Labor Statistics, 1998). That same year, occupational injuries alone cost $132 billion in lost wages and lost productivity, administrative expenses, health care, and other costs. This figure does not include the cost of occupational diseases.

These figures are often described as the "tip of the iceberg" because many work-related health problems go unreported. But even the recorded statistics are significant in describing the amount of human suffering, financial loss, and decreased productivity associated with workplace hazards.

The high number of work injuries and illnesses can be drastically reduced. In fact, significant progress has been made in improving worker protection since Congress passed the 1970 Occupational Safety and Health Act. This progress has been largely based on actions—sometimes voluntary, sometimes regulatory—directed by the science and knowledge generated from occupational safety and health research (Klinger and Jones, 1994). For example, vinyl chloride-induced liver cancers and brown lung disease (byssinosis) from cotton dust exposure have been almost eliminated. Reproductive disorders associated with certain glycol ethers have been recognized and controlled (Katz, 1994). Fatal work injuries have declined substantially through the years (Workplace Injury/Illness Rates, 1993). Notably, since 1970, fatal injury rates in coal miners have been reduced by more than 75%, and there has been a general downward trend in the prevalence of coal miner's pneumoconiosis.

The U.S. workplace is rapidly changing and becoming more diverse. Major changes are occurring:
- In the way work is organized
- With increased shiftwork
- With reduced job security
- In part-time and temporary work
- As new chemicals, materials, processes, and equipment (such as latex gloves in health care, or fermentation processes in biotechnology) continue to be developed and marketed at an ever-accelerating pace.

APPLICATION OF THE EPIDEMIOLOGIC MODEL

The epidemiologic triad can be used to understand the relationship between work and health (Fig. 29-2) (Campos-Outcalt, 1994).

With a focus on the health and safety of the employed population, the *host* is described as any susceptible human

being. Because of the nature of work-related hazards, nurses must assume that all employed individuals and groups are at risk of being exposed to occupational hazards. The *agents,* factors associated with illness and injury, are occupational exposures that are classified as *biological, chemical, ergonomic, physical,* or *psychosocial* (Box 29-2).

The third element, the **environment,** includes all external conditions that influence the interaction of the host and agents. These may be workplace conditions such as:
- Temperature extremes
- Crowding
- Shiftwork
- Inflexible management styles (Callahan, 1994).

The basic principle of epidemiology is that health status interventions for restoring and promoting health are the result of complex interactions among these three elements. To understand these interactions and to design effective nursing strategies for dealing with them in a proactive manner, nurses must look at how each element influences the others.

Host

Each worker represents a **host** within the worker population group. Certain host factors are associated with increased risk of adverse response to the hazards of the workplace. These include:
- Age
- Gender

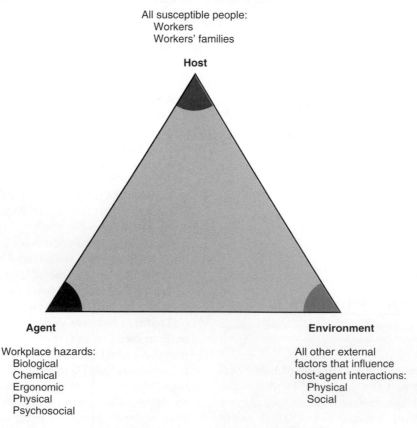

Figure 29-2　The epidemiologic triad.

- Health status
- Work practices
- Ethnicity
- Life-style factors (Barratt, 1994; Girgis, 1994; Jeffrey et al, 1993).

For example, the population group at greatest risk for experiencing work-related accidents with subsequent injuries are men (18 to 30 years old) with less than 6 months experience on the current job. The host factors of age, gender, and work experience combine to increase this group's risk of injury because of characteristics such as:

- Risk taking
- Lack of knowledge
- Lack of familiarity with the new job.

Older workers may be at increased risk in the workplace because of:

- Diminished sensory abilities
- The effects of chronic illnesses
- Delayed reaction times (Stine and Brown, 1996).

A third population group that may be very susceptible to workplace exposure is women in their child-bearing years (Bellow and Rudolph, 1993; Stellman, 1994):

- The hormonal changes during these years
- The increased stress of new roles and additional responsibilities
- Transplacental exposures.

These are host factors that may influence this group's response to potential toxins.

In addition to these host factors, there may be other, less well-understood individual differences in responses to occupational hazard exposures. Even if employers maintain exposure levels below the level recommended by occupational health and safety standards, 15% to 20% of the population may have health reactions to the "safe" low-level exposures (Levy and Wegman, 1995). This group has been

---

| **Box 29-2** | **Categories of Work-Related Hazards** |

Biological and infectious hazards. Infectious/biological agents, such as bacteria, viruses, fungi, or parasites, that may be transmitted via contact with infected patients or contaminated body secretions/fluids to other individuals

Chemical hazards. Various forms of chemicals, including medications, solutions, gases, vapors, aerosols, and particulate matter, that are potentially toxic or irritating to the body system

Environmental and mechanical hazards. Factors encountered in the work environment that cause or potentiate accidents, injuries, strain, or discomfort (e.g., unsafe/inadequate equipment or lifting devices, slippery floors, work station deficiencies)

Physical hazards. Agents within the work environment, such as radiation, electricity, extreme temperatures, and noise, that can cause tissue trauma

Psychosocial hazards. Factors and situations encountered or associated with one's job or work environment that create or potentiate stress, emotional strain, and/or interpersonal problems

From Rogers B: *Occupational health nursing: concepts and practice,* Philadelphia, 1994, WB Saunders.

---

termed *hypersusceptible.* A number of host factors appear to be associated with this hypersusceptibility:

- Light skin
- Malnutrition
- Compromised immune system
- Glucose 6-phosphate dehydrogenase deficiency
- Serum alpha 1-antitrypsin deficiency
- Chronic obstructive pulmonary disease
- Sickle cell trait
- Hypertension.

Individuals who have known hypersusceptibility to chemicals that are respiratory irritants, hemolytic chemicals, organic isocyanates, and carbon disulfide may also be hypersusceptible to other agents in the work environment (Levy and Wegman, 1995). Although this has prompted some industries to consider preplacement screening for such risk factors, the associations between these individual health markers and hypersusceptible response are unclear.

Agent

Work-related hazards, or **agents** (see Box 29-2), present potential and actual risks to the health and safety of workers in the millions of business establishments in the United States. Any work site commonly presents multiple and interacting exposures from all five categories of agents. Table 29-1 lists some of the more common workplace exposures, their known health effects, and the types of jobs associated with these hazards.

Biological Agents

Biological agents are living organisms whose excretions or parts are capable of causing human disease, usually by an infectious process. Biological hazards are common in workplaces such as health care facilities and clinical laboratories where employees are potentially exposed to a variety of infectious agents, including viruses, fungi, and bacteria. Of particular concern in occupational health are infectious diseases transmitted by humans (e.g., from client to worker or from worker to worker) in a variety of work settings (U.S. Department of Health and Human Services–National Institute for Occupational Safety and Health, 1996). Blood-borne and airborne pathogens represent a significant class of exposures for the U.S. health care workers.

Transmission of tuberculosis (TB) within health care settings (especially multidrug-resistant TB) has reemerged as a major public health problem. Since 1989, outbreaks of this type of TB have been reported in hospitals and some workers have developed active drug-resistant TB. In addition, among workers in health care, social service, and corrections facilities who work with populations at increased risk of TB, hundreds have experienced tuberculin skin test conversions. Reliable data are lacking on the extent of possible work-related TB transmission among other groups of workers at risk for exposure.

Many workers in these settings are employed as maintenance workers, security guards, aides, or cleaning people, who tend not to be well-protected from inadvertent exposures which include contaminated bed linen in the laundry, soiled equipment,

TABLE 29-1 Selected Job Categories, Exposures, and Associated Work-Related Diseases and Conditions

Job Categories	Exposures	Work-Related Diseases and Conditions
All workers	Workplace stress	Hypertension, mood disorders, cardiovascular disease
Agricultural workers	Pesticides, infectious agents, gases, sunlight	Pesticide poisoning, "farmer's lung," skin cancer
Anesthetists	Anesthetic gases	Reproductive effects, cancer
Automobile workers	Asbestos, plastics, lead, solvents	Asbestosis dermatitis
Butchers	Vinyl plastic fumes	Meat wrapper's asthma
Caisson workers	Pressurized work environments	"Caisson disease," "the bends"
Carpenters	Wood dust, wood preservatives, adhesives	Nasopharyngeal cancer, dermatitis
Cement workers	Cement dust, metals	Dermatitis, bronchitis
Ceramic workers	Talc, clays	Pneumoconiosis
Demolition workers	Asbestos, wood dust	Asbestosis
Drug manufacturers	Hormones, nitroglycerin, etc.	Reproductive effects
Dry cleaners	Solvents	Liver disease, dermatitis
Dye workers	Dyestuffs, metals, solvents	Bladder cancer, dermatitis
Embalmers	Formaldehyde, infectious agents	Dermatitis
Felt makers	Mercury, polycyclic hydrocarbons	Mercury poisoning
Foundry workers	Silica, molten metals	Silicosis
Glass workers	Heat, solvents, metal powders	Cataracts
Hospital workers	Infectious agents, cleansers, radiation	Infections, latex allergies, unintentional injuries
Insulators	Asbestos, fibrous glass	Asbestosis, lung cancer, mesothelioma
Jackhammer operators	Vibration	Raynaud's phenomenon
Lathe operators	Metal dusts, cutting oils	Lung disease, cancer
Office computer workers	Repetitive wrist motion on computers and eye strain	Tendonitis, carpal tunnel syndrome, tenosynovitis

and trash containing contaminated dressing or specimens (Centers for Disease Control and Prevention, 1996).

Chemical Agents

More than 300 billion pounds of *chemical agents* are produced annually in the United States. Of the approximately 2 million known chemicals in existence, less than 0.1% have been adequately studied for their effects on humans. Of those chemicals that have been linked to carcinogens, approximately half test positive as animal carcinogens. Most chemicals have not been studied epidemiologically to determine the effects of exposure on humans (Levy and Wegman, 1995). As a consequence of general environmental contamination with chemicals from work, home, and community activities, a variety of chemicals are found in the body tissues of the general population (Stine and Brown, 1996).

Briefly Noted

Only 0.1% of the nearly 2 million known chemicals produced have been tested for their effect on humans.

In many workplaces, significant exposure to a daily, low-level dose of chemicals may be below the exposure standards but may still carry a potentially chronic and perhaps cumulative assault on workers' health. Predicting human responses to such exposures is further complicated because several chemicals are often combined to create a new chemical agent. Human effects may be associated with the interaction of these agents rather than with a single chemical. Another concern about occupational exposure to chemicals is reproductive health effects. Workplace reproductive hazards have become important legal and scientific issues. Toxicity to male and female reproductive systems has been demonstrated from exposure to common agents such as lead, mercury, cadmium, nickel, and zinc, as well as in antineoplastic drugs. Because data for predicting human responses to many chemical agents are inadequate, workers should be assessed for all potential exposures and cautioned to work preventively with these agents. High-risk or vulnerable workers should be carefully screened and monitored for optimal health protection, such as those workers with latex allergy, which is a widely recognized health hazard (NIOSH, 1997a).

Environmental and Mechanical Agents

Environmental and *mechanical agents* are those that can potentially cause injury or illness and are related to the work process or cause musculoskeletal or other strains that can produce negative health effects when certain tasks are performed repeatedly. Examples are repetitive motions, poor workstation-worker fit, and lifting heavy loads. Carpal tunnel syndrome, tendonitis, and tenosynovitis are the most frequently seen occupational diseases observed in workers who are chronically exposed to repetitive motion. The most frequently reported upper-extremity musculoskeletal disorders affect the hand/wrist region.

Back pain and injury is one of the most common and significant musculoskeletal problems in the world (National Institute for Occupational Safety and Health, 1997b; Jorgensen, Hein, and Gyntelberg, 1994; Larese and Fiorit, 1994). In 1995, back injuries and disorders accounted for 38% of all nonfatal occupational injuries and illnesses involving days away from work in the United States. Although the exact costs of back disorders are unknown, the estimates are staggering. As many as 30% of American workers are employed in jobs that routinely require them to perform activities that may increase risk of developing low back disorders. Injuries and illnesses related to this category of agents have been termed *cumulative trauma,* which composes the largest category of work-related illness and disability claims in the United States. The most productive strategy in preventing these exposures appears to be redesigning the workplace and the work machinery or processes.

Physical Agents

Physical agents are those that produce adverse health effects through the transfer of physical energy. Commonly encountered physical agents in the workplace include:
- Temperature extremes
- Vibration
- Noise
- Radiation
- Lighting (Payling, 1994; Platt, 1993).

For example, vibration, which accompanies the use of power tools and vehicles such as trucks, affects:
- Internal organs
- Supportive ligaments
- The upper torso
- The shoulder-girdle structure.

Localized effects are seen with handheld power tools; the most common is Raynaud's phenomenon. The control of worker exposure to these agents is usually accomplished through engineering strategies such as eliminating or containing the offending agent. In addition, workers must use preventive actions, such as practicing safe work habits and wearing personal protective equipment when needed. Examples of safe work habits include taking appropriate breaks from environments with temperature extremes and not eating or smoking in radiation-contaminated areas. Personal protective equipment includes:
- Hearing protection
- Eye guards
- Protective clothing
- Devices for monitoring exposures to agents such as radiation.

This class of agents is considered one of the most easily controlled.

Psychosocial Agents

Psychosocial agents are conditions that create a threat to the psychological and/or social well-being of individuals and groups (Rogers, 1994). A psychosocial response to the work environment occurs as an employee acts selectively toward his environment in an attempt to achieve a harmonious relationship. When such a human attempt at adaptation to the environment fails, an adverse psychosocial response may occur. Work-related stress or burn-out is fast becoming a significant problem for many individuals (Fielding, 1994). Responses to negative interpersonal relationships, particularly those with authority figures in the workplace, are often the cause of vague health symptoms and increased absenteeism. Epidemiologic work in mental health has pointed to environmental variables such as these in the incidence of mental illness and emotional disorder.

The psychosocial environment includes characteristics of the work itself, as well as the interpersonal relationships required in the work setting and shiftwork. An estimated 11.5 million Americans do some form of shiftwork that has the potential to lead to a variety of psychological and physical problems including:
- Exhaustion
- Depression
- Anxiety
- Gastrointestinal disturbance.

Strategies to minimize the adverse effects of shiftwork such as rotating shifts clockwise are beneficial. Job characteristics associated with an increased risk of heart disease among clerical and blue-collar workers are:
- Low autonomy
- Poor job satisfaction
- Limited control over the pace of work.

Interpersonal relationships among employees and co-workers or bosses and managers are often sources of conflict and stress. Another aspect is *organizational culture.* This refers to the norms and patterns of behavior that are sanctioned within a particular organization. Such norms and pat-

Evidence-Based Practice

The authors of this study were interested in how organizations and the psychosocial environment of work affect morbidity and mortality, especially related to heart disease. The authors investigated previously established risk factors for heart disease in a sample of 2682 men from Kuopio, Finland.

Baseline assessments were completed of biological, behavioral, and psychosocial factors related to each participant, as well as an assessment of the prevalence of current illnesses and an evaluation of each person's work environment, income, and education.

The study concluded that there were risks of mortality from a number of causes for men in low-income jobs that were high in demand but provided few resources to complete the job. Mortality also increased in all low-income jobs that had lots of resources regardless of the job demands. However, men in the first group—those with high-demand, low-income jobs with few resources—were at greater risk for heart disease than other workers.

The authors believe that, considering all factors related to the individual and the workplace, the results over time of the effects of poor working conditions and low income lead to feelings of hopelessness, depression, poor behavior, psychologic risk profiles, higher levels of morbidity, and increased mortality risk.

APPLICATION IN PRACTICE

Because the low-income worker is at greater risk for mortality, occupational nurses can be aware of the organization of the workplace, the job demands, and the work environment on the population of low-income workers. Increasing the skills of the workers, creating a democratic work environment, and focusing on job satisfaction and economic rewards for enhancing worker skills are a few recommended interventions. Health education and counseling directed to the population, spending quality family time, and encouraging hobbies and recreational events can help.

Lynch J, et al: Workplace conditions, socioeconomic status and the risk of mortality and acute myocardial infarction: the Kuopio ischemic heart disease risk factor study, *Am J Public Health* 87(4):617, 1997.

terns set guidelines for the types of work behaviors that will enable employees to succeed within a particular firm. Examples include:

- Following organizational norms for working overtime
- Expressing constructive dissatisfaction with management
- Making work a top priority.

These factors and the employee's response to them must be assessed if strategies for influencing the health and safety of workers are to be effective.

Nonfatal violence in the health care worker's workplace is a serious problem that seems to be underreported. Much of the study of health care worker violence has been in psychiatric settings; however, reports in other areas such as the emergency department have been reported. Risk factors associated with this type of violence must be identified and strategies implemented to reduce the risk (Poster and Ryan, 1994).

Environment

Environmental factors influence the occurrence of host-agent interactions and may direct the course and outcome of those interactions. The physical environment involves the geological and atmospheric structure of an area and the source of such elements as water, temperature, and radiation, which may serve as positive or negative stressors. Although aspects of the physical environment (e.g., heat, odor, or ventilation) may influence the host-agent interaction, the social and psychological environment can be of equal importance (Hodgson and Storey, 1994).

New environmental problems continue to arise, such as an increase in industrial wastes and toxins and indoor and outdoor environmental pollution, which present opportunities for significant health threats to the working and general population. The social aspects of the environment encompass the economic and political forces affecting society and its health. This includes factors such as:

- Sanitation and hygiene practices
- Housing conditions
- Level and delivery of health care services
- Development and enforcement of health-related codes (e.g., occupational health and safety, pollution)
- Employment conditions
- Population crowding
- Literacy
- Ethnic customs
- Extent of support for health-related research
- Equal access to health care.

In addition, addictive behaviors such as alcohol and substance abuse and various forms of psychosocial stress may be an outgrowth of negative social environments. Consider an employee who is working with a potentially toxic liquid. Providing education about safe work practices and fitting the employee with protective clothing may not be adequate if the work must occur in a very hot and humid environment. As the worker becomes uncomfortable in the hot clothing, his or her protection may be compromised by rolling up a sleeve, taking off a glove, or wiping his face with a contaminated piece of clothing. If the psychosocial norms in the workplace condone such work practices (e.g., "Everyone does it when it's too hot"), the interventions that address only the host and agent will be ineffective.

The epidemiologic triad can be used as the basis for planning interventions to restore and promote the health of workers. These efforts are influenced by society and organization activities related to occupational health and safety (Rabinowitz, et al, 1994; Snyder, et al, 1994).

ORGANIZATIONAL AND PUBLIC EFFORTS TO PROMOTE WORKER HEALTH AND SAFETY

Promotion of worker health and safety is the goal of occupational health and safety programs (Porro, et al, 1993). These programs are offered primarily by the employer at the workplace, but the range of services and the models for delivering them have been changing dramatically over the past few years. In addition to specific services, legislation at the federal and state levels has had a significant effect on efforts to provide a healthy and safe environment for all workers. Under the Occupational Safety and Health Act and increased public concern about worker health and safety, there have recently been citations of companies that do not meet minimal occupational health and safety standards. Criminal charges have been filed against business owners when preventable work-related deaths occurred. These events have redirected an emphasis on preventive occupational health and safety programming.

Unless a company has OSHA-regulated exposures, business firms are not required to provide occupational health and safety services that meet any specified standards. With few exceptions, there is no legal request for specific services or level of personnel provided by employers to protect worker health and safety. Therefore the range of services offered and the qualifications of the providers of occupational health and safety vary widely across industries. An important stimulus for health and safety programs is avoiding cost that can be attributed to the effectiveness of prevention services, as well as the need to support occupational health and safety and health promotion at the work site.

On-Site Occupational Health and Safety Programs

Optimally, on-site occupational health and safety services are provided by a team of occupational health and safety professionals. The core members of this team are:
- The occupational health nurse
- Occupational physician
- Industrial hygienist
- Safety professional.

The largest group of health care professionals in business settings are occupational health nurses; therefore the most frequently seen model is that of the one-nurse unit. This nurse collaborates with a community physician or occupational medicine physician who provides consultation and accepts referrals where medical intervention is needed. The collaboration may occur primarily through telephone contact, or the physician may be under contract with the company to spend a certain amount of time on-site each week. As companies become larger, they are likely to hire:
- Additional nurses
- Safety professionals
- Industrial hygienists
- Physicians part-time or on a consultant basis
- Employee assistance counselors
- Social workers
- Health educators
- Physical fitness specialists
- Toxicologists
- Ergonomists.

> **Box 29-3 Scope of Services Provided Through an Occupational Health and Safety Program**
>
> Health/medical surveillance
> Workplace monitoring/surveillance
> Health assessments
> Preplacement
> - Periodic, mandatory, voluntary
> - Transfer
> - Retirement/termination
> - Executive
> - Return to work
> Health promotion
> Health screening
> Employee assistance programs
> Case management
> Primary health care for workers and dependents
> Worker safety and health education related to occupational hazards
> Job task analysis and design
> Prenatal and postnatal care and support groups
> Safety audits and accident prevention
> Workers' compensation management
> Risk management, loss control
> Emergency preparedness
> Preretirement counseling
> Integrated health benefits programs

The services provided by on-site occupational health programs range from those focused only on work-related health and safety problems to a wide scope of services that includes primary care (Box 29-3).

In industries that have exposures regulated by law, certain programs are required, such as respiratory protection or hearing conservation. The ability of a company to offer additional programs depends on:
- Employee needs
- Management's attitudes and understanding about health and safety
- Acceptance by the workers
- The economic status of the firm.

A significant increase in the number of health promotion and employee assistance programs offered in industry has occurred over the past few years. Health promotion programs focus on lifestyle choices that cause risks to health, e.g., job stress, obesity, smoking, stress responses, or lack of exercise (Paskett, et al, 1994; Rigotti, et al, 1994). Employee assistance programs are designed to address personal problems (e.g., marital/family issues, substance abuse, or financial difficulties) that affect the employee's productivity. Because such efforts are cost effective for businesses, they should continue to increase.

Similar types of occupational health and safety programs are available on a contractual basis from community-based providers. These may be offered by free-standing industrial clinics, health maintenance organizations, hospitals, emergency clinics, and other health care organizations. In addition, consultants in each discipline work in the private sector (self-employed, in group practice, or in insurance companies) and in the public sector (in local and state health departments or departments of labor and industry). These services may be provided on site, delivered elsewhere in the community, or offered through a mobile van that visits companies. These multiple resources have increased the options for companies that need occupational health and safety services and have also broadened the employment opportunities for health and safety professionals.

NURSING CARE OF WORKING POPULATIONS

The nurse is often the first health care provider seen by an individual with a work-related health problem. Consequently, nurses are in key positions to intervene with working populations at all levels of prevention.

Worker Assessment

The initial step of assessment involves the traditional history and physical assessment, emphasizing exposure to occupational hazards and individual characteristics that may predispose the client to increased health risk of certain jobs. The **occupational health history** is an indispensable component of the health assessment of individuals (Rogers, 1994) (see Appendix G.5). Since work is a part of life for most people, including an occupational health history into all routine nursing assessments is essential. Many workers in the United States do not have access to health care services in their workplaces. Yet it is not unusual to find health care providers in the community who have little or no knowledge about workplaces or expertise in occupationally related illnesses and injuries. Because of the large number of small businesses that do not have the resources for maintaining on-site health care, injured and ill workers are first seen in the public and private health care sector (e.g., in clinics, emergency rooms, physicians' offices, hospitals, HMOs, and ambulatory care centers). Nurses are often the first-line assessors of these individuals and perhaps the only contact for education about self-protection from workplace hazards. The identifying of workplace exposures as sources of health problems may influence the client's course of illness and rehabilitation and also prevent similar illnesses among others with potential for exposure.

Including occupational health data into client assessments begins with recognizing the possible relationship between health and occupational factors (Rabinowitz, et al, 1994). The next step is to integrate into the history-taking procedure some routine assessment questions that will provide the data necessary to confirm or rule out occupationally induced symptoms. Symptoms of hazardous workplace exposures may be indicated by vague complaints involving any body system. These complaints are often similar to common medical problems. Three points that occupational health histories should include are:

- A list of current and past jobs the client has held, including specific job titles
- Questions about current and past exposures to specific agents and relationships between the symptoms and activities at work
- Other factors that may enhance the client's susceptibility to occupational agents (e.g., smoking history, underlying illness, previous injury, or handicapping condition).

Questions about the employee's occupational history can be included in existing assessment tools. The more complete the data collected, the more likely the nurse is to notice the influence of work-health interactions. All employees should be questioned about their employment history. To describe only a current status of "retired" or "housewife" may lead to the omission of needed data. The nurse should be aware that not all workers are well-informed about the materials with which they work or about potential hazards. For this reason the nurse must develop basic knowledge about the types of jobs held by clients and the possible hazards associated with them. Because there is an increased likelihood that multiple exposures from other environments such as home and yard may interact with workplace exposures, the nurse should extend the questioning to include this information.

Identifying work-related health problems does not require an extensive knowledge of occupational agents and their effects. A systematic approach for evaluating the potential for workplace exposures is the most effective intervention for detecting and preventing occupational health risks. Figure 29-3 shows one short assessment tool that can be incorporated into routine history taking. Similar questions can be included in the assessment of workers' spouses and dependents, who may have indirect exposure to occupational hazards.

During these health assessments, the nurse has the opportunity to teach about workplace hazards and preventive measures the worker can use. At the same time, the nurse is obtaining information that will be valuable in optimizing work-job fit. Such assessments may be done:

- As preplacement examinations before the client begins a job
- On a periodic basis during employment
- With the onset of a work-related health problem or exposure
- When an employee is being transferred to another job with different requirements and exposures
- At termination
- At retirement.

The goal of these assessments is to identify agent and host factors that could place the employee at risk and to determine prevention steps that can be taken to eliminate or minimize the exposure and potential health problem.

Briefly Noted

There is an acceptable level of risk in any job.

I.   Present Job

A.   What is your job title? _____

B.   What do you do for a living? _____

C.   How long have you had this job? _____

D.   Describe the specific tasks of this job: _____
_____

E.   What product or service is produced by the company where you work:? _____
_____

F.   Are you exposed to any of the following on your present job?

Metals	Radiation	Stress
Vapors, gases	Vibration	Others: _____
Dusts	Loud noise	
Solvents	Extreme heat or cold	

G.   Do you feel you have any health problems that may be associated with your work?
If yes, describe: _____
_____

H.   How would you describe your satisfaction with your job? _____
_____

I.   Have any of your co-workers complained of illness or injuries that they associate with their jobs?
If yes, describe: _____
_____

II.   All Past Work

Starting with your first job, please provide the following information:

Job title	Years held	Description of work	Exposures	Injuries/Illnesses	Personal protection equipment used

III.   Other Exposures

A.   Do you have any hobbies which involve exposure to chemicals, metals or any of the other agents mentioned before? If yes, describe: _____

B.   Are any other members of your household exposed to any of the substances listed above? If yes, describe:
_____

C.   Do you live near any factories, dump sites, or other sources of pollution? If yes, describe: _____
_____

Figure 29-3   Occupational health history form.

When the health data from such assessments are considered collectively, the nurse may determine some patterns in risk factors associated with the occurrence of work-related injuries and illnesses in a total population of workers. For example, a nurse practitioner in a clinic noted a dramatic increase in the number of bladder cancer cases among her clients. When she looked at factors in common among these individuals, she determined that they all worked at a company that used benzidine dyes, which are known bladder carcinogens. She worked with the union and the company to assess the environmental exposure to the employees. This nursing intervention led to a safer work environment and a decrease in bladder cancer among this population group. Such an approach can be used at the company, industry, and community levels. The initial collection of data and the questioning about workplace exposures are vital steps for any intervention.

Workplace Assessment

The nurse may conduct a similar assessment of the workplace itself. The purpose of this assessment, known as a **work site walk-through** or survey, is to know:

- About the work processes and the materials
- The requirements of various jobs
- The presence of actual or potential hazards
- The work practices of employees (American Association of Occupational Health Nurses, 1997).

Figure 29-4 shows a brief outline that can be used to guide a work site assessment.

More complex surveys are performed by industrial hygienists and safety professionals when the purpose of the walk-through is environmental monitoring or a safety audit. However, most occupational health nurses have developed expertise in these areas and include such tasks as part of their functions. For any health care provider who assesses workers, this information makes up an important database. For the on-site health care provider, work site walk-throughs assist the professional in developing rapport and establishing credibility with the employees.

A work site survey begins with an understanding of the type of work that occurs in the workplace. All business organizations are classified by the U.S. Department of Commerce with a numerical code, the Standard Industrial Classification (SIC) Code. This code, usually a two- to four-digit number, indicates a company's product and, therefore, the possible types of **occupational health hazards** that may be associated with the processes and materials used by its employees. SIC codes are used to collect and report data on businesses. For example, illness and injury rates of one company are compared to the rates of other companies of similar size with the same SIC code to determine whether the company is having an excess of illness or injury.

All OSHA and workers' compensation data are reported by the SIC code. In addition, by knowing the SIC code of a company, a health care professional can access reference books that describe the usual processes, materials, and by-products of that kind of company. A simple drawing of the work processes and work areas shows information by jobs or locations in the workplace. These preliminary data provide clues about what hazards may be present and an understanding of the types of jobs and health requirements that may be involved in a particular industry. A description of the work environment is next and provides an overall picture of general appearances, physical layout, and safety of the environment. Are safety signs posted and readable where needed? Is there clutter or dampness on the floor that could cause slips or falls?

How To Assess a Worker and the Workplace

Assessing the worker for a work-related problem is a critical practice element. You need to do the following:

- Complete general and occupational health history taking with emphasis on workplace exposure assessment, job hazard analysis, and list of previous jobs.
- Conduct a health assessment to identify agent and host factors that interact to place workers at risk.
- Identify patterns of risk associated with illness/injury.

Assessing the work environment is necessary to determine workplace exposures that create worker health risk. You need to do the following:

- Understand the work being done
- Evaluate the work-related hazards
- Understand the work process
- Gather data about incidence/prevalence of work-related illness/injuries and related hazards
- Examine control strategies in place for eliminating exposures

A description of the employee group is vital to understanding the demographics and the work distribution in the company. Knowing about shiftwork and productivity can be helpful in pinpointing potential stressors. Human resources management and corporate commitment to health and safety are necessary to develop a support culture for effective and efficient programming. Assessing the status of policies and procedures, as well as opportunities for input into improving service, are important to establish the organization's strength in occupational health and safety management. Gathering data about the incidence and prevalence of work-related illnesses and injuries, and the cost patterns for these conditions, provides useful epidemiologic trend data. It also targets high-cost areas. The types of occupational safety and health services and programs are important to know. This will show whether required programs are being offered and whether they include health-promotion and disease-prevention strategies.

Finally, examining control strategies that are effective in eliminating or reducing exposure is important in determining risk reduction. Engineering controls can reduce worker exposure by modifying the exposure source, such as putting needles in a puncture-proof container.

Work practice controls include good hygiene, waste disposal, and housekeeping. Administrative controls reduce

Name of company: _____   Date: _____
Address: _____
Telephone: _____
Parent company (if any): _____
Location of corporate offices: _____
SIC code: _____

The Work:

Major products: _____
Major processes and operations, raw materials, by products: _____
_____
Type of jobs: _____
_____
Potential exposures: _____
_____

Work Environment
General conditions: _____
Safety signs: _____
Physical environment: _____

Worker Population
Employees
Total number: _____   Number in production: _____   Others: _____
% Fulltime: _____   % Men: _____   % Women: _____
% First shift: _____   % Second shift: _____   % Third shift: _____
Age distribution: _____
% Unionized: _____   Names of Unions: _____

Human Resources Management
Corporate commitment to health
Personnel
Policies/procedures
Input/surveys/committees
Recordkeeping

Health Data
Work related illnesses, injuries, deaths per annum: _____
OSHA recordable: _____   Workers' Compensation: _____
Other: _____   Most frequent complaints: _____
Average number of monthly calls to the health unit: _____
Absenteeism rate: _____

Occupation Health and Safety Services	**Control Strategies**
Examinations	Engineering
Employee assistance	Work practice
Treatment of illness/injury	Administrative
Health Education	Personal protective equipment
Physical fitness, health promotion activities	
Mandatory programs	
Safety audits	
Environmental monitoring	
Health risk appraisal	
Screenings	
Health promotion	

Figure 29-4   **Work site assessment guide.**

exposure through job rotation, workplace monitoring, and employee training and education. Personal protective control is the last resort and requires the worker to actively engage in strategies for protection such as use of gloves, masks, and gowns to prevent blood/body fluid exposure (Rogers, 1994).

Briefly Noted

Both corporate culture and cost-effective programs are key factors in influencing the development of occupational health services.

The more information that can be collected before the walk-through, the more efficient will be the process of the survey. After the survey is conducted, the nurse can use the information with the aggregate health data to evaluate the effectiveness of the occupational health and safety program and to plan future programs.

HEALTHY PEOPLE 2010 RELATED TO OCCUPATIONAL HEALTH

In an attempt to meet the goal of increasing the quality and years of healthy life for Americans, health education and health protection strategies are proposed to address the needs of large population groups such as the American Workforce.

Healthy People 2010 identifies the national health objectives to reduce risk of occupational illnesses and to promote safety. These are listed in the *Healthy People 2010* box.

LEGISLATION RELATED TO OCCUPATIONAL HEALTH

The occupational health and safety services provided by an employer are influenced by specific legislation at federal and state levels. Although the relationship between work and health has been known since the second century (Ramazzini, 1713), public policy that effectively controlled occupational hazards was not enacted until the 1960s. The Mine Safety and Health Act of 1968 was the first legislation that specifically required certain prevention programs for workers. This was followed by the Occupational Safety and Health Act of 1970, which established two agencies to carry out the Act's purpose of ensuring "safe and healthful working conditions for working men and women" (Public Law 91-596, 1970).

Within the context of the OSH Act, the **Occupational Safety and Health Administration (OSHA),** a federal agency within the U.S. Department of Labor, was created to develop and enforce workplace safety and health regulations. OSHA sets the standards that regulate workers' exposure to potentially toxic substances, enforcing these at the federal, regional, and state levels. Specific standards and information about compliance can be obtained from federal, regional, and state OSHA offices.

Healthy People 2010
Occupational Health Nursing

7-5	Increase the proportion of work sites that offer a comprehensive employee health promotion program to their employees.
7-6	Increase the proportion of employees who participate in employer-sponsored health promotion activities.
20-1	Reduce deaths from work-related injuries.
20-2	Reduce work-related injuries resulting in medical treatment, lost time from work, or restricted work activity.
20-3	Reduce the rate of injury and illness cases involving days away from work due to overexertion or repetitive motion.
20-4	Reduce pneumoconiosis deaths.
20-5	Reduce deaths from work-related homicides.
20-6	Reduce work-related assault.
20-7	Reduce the number of persons who have elevated blood lead concentrations from work exposures.
20-8	Reduce occupational skin diseases or disorders among full-time workers.
20-9	Increase the proportion of work sites employing 50 or more persons that provide programs to prevent or reduce employee stress.
20-10	Reduce occupational needle-stick injuries among health care workers.
20-11	Reduce new cases of work-related noise-induced hearing loss.

The **National Institute for Occupational Safety and Health (NIOSH)** was established by the Occupational Safety and Health Act of 1970 and is part of the Centers for Disease Control and Prevention (CDC). The NIOSH agency identifies, monitors, and educates about the incidence, prevalence, and prevention of work-related illnesses and injuries and examines potential hazards of new work technologies and practices (U.S. Department of Health and Human Services–National Institute for Occupational Safety and Health, 1999). Although NIOSH and OSHA were both created by the same act of Congress, they have discrete functions (Box 29-4).

Briefly Noted

NIOSH publications, many of which are free, are available by writing or faxing a request to: NIOSH Publications, Mail Stop C-13, 4676 Columbia Parkway, Cincinnati, OH 45226-1998. See this book's website at www.mosby.com/MERLIN/Stanhope/foundations for additional contact information.

One of the most far-reaching OSHA standards is the **Hazard Communication Standard.** Also known as the federal "right-to-know" law, this standard is based on the premise that working environments cannot eliminate all potentially toxic agents; therefore an important line of defense is an

> ### Box 29-4 Functions of Federal Agencies Involved in Occupational Health and Safety
>
> **Occupational Safety and Health Administration (OSHA)**
> - Determine and set standards for hazardous exposures in the workplace.
> - Enforce the occupational health standards (including the right of entry for inspection).
> - Educate employers about occupational health and safety.
> - Develop and maintain a database of work-related injuries, illnesses, and deaths.
> - Monitor compliance with occupational health and safety standards.
>
> **National Institute for Occupational Safety and Health (NIOSH)**
> - Conduct research and review of research findings to recommend permissible exposure levels for occupational hazards to OSHA.
> - Identify and research occupational health and safety hazards.
> - Educate occupational health and safety professionals.
> - Distribute research findings relevant to occupational health and safety.
>
> From U.S. Department of Health and Human Services–National Institute for Occupational Safety and Health: *National occupational research agenda,* pub no 99-108, Washington, D.C., 1999, U.S. Government Printing Office.

educated workforce. The Hazard Communication Standard, which took effect in 1983, required that all manufacturing firms inventory their toxic agents, label them, and develop information sheets, called *Material Safety Data Sheets (MSDSs),* for each agent. In addition, the employer must have in place a Hazard Communication Program that provides workers with education about these agents. This education must include agent identification, toxic effects, and protective measures. In 1988, this standard was extended to all employers covered by the Occupational Safety and Health Act. Similar right-to-know legislation exists at many state and local levels. The next legislative approach will focus on the *right-to-act standards* and guidelines that protect workers' rights to use the information from right-to-know efforts to change unsafe or unhealthy working conditions.

Workers' compensation acts are important state laws that govern financial compensation of employees who suffer work-related health problems. These acts vary by state; each state sets rules for the reimbursement of employees with occupational health problems for medical expenses and lost work time associated with the illness or injury. Workers' compensation claims and the experience-based insurance premiums paid by industry have been important motivators for increasing the health and safety of the workplace.

DISASTER PLANNING AND MANAGEMENT

Although disaster planning and management have been functions of occupational health and safety programs, this is an area of new legislation that affects businesses and health professionals. The legislation of the *Superfund Amendment and Reauthorization Act* (SARA) requires that written disaster plans of industries be shared with key resources in the community, such as fire departments and emergency rooms. Public concern about disasters, such as the methyl isocyanate leak in Bhopal, India, or the community exposure to chemicals at Times Beach, Missouri, has mandated more attention to disaster planning.

The goals of a disaster plan are to prevent or minimize injuries and deaths of workers and residents, minimize property damage, provide effective triage, and facilitate necessary business activities. A disaster plan requires the cooperation of different personnel within the company and community. The nurse is often a key person on the disaster planning team, along with safety professionals, physicians, industrial hygienists, the fire chief, and company management. The potential for disaster (e.g., explosions, fires, and leaks) must be identified; this is best achieved by completing an exhaustive chemical and hazard inventory of the workplace. The Material Safety Data Sheets and plant blueprints are critical for correctly identifying substances and work areas that may be hazardous. Work site surveys are the first step to completing this inventory.

Effective disaster plans are designed by those with knowledge of the work processes and materials, the workers and workplace, and the resources in the community. Specific steps must be detailed for actions to be put in place by specific individuals in the event of a disaster:

- The written plan must be shared with all who will be involved.
- Employees should be prepared in first aid, CPR, and fire brigade procedures.
- Plans must be clear, specific, and comprehensive (i.e., covering all shifts and all work areas) and must include activities to be conducted within the work site and those that require community resources.
- Transportation plans, fire response, and emergency response services should be coordinated with the agencies that would be involved in actual disaster.
- The disaster plan, emergency and safety equipment, and the first response team's abilities should be tested at least annually with a drill.
- Practice results should be carefully evaluated, with changes made as needed.
- Hospitals and other emergency services, such as fire departments, should be involved in developing the disaster plan and should receive a copy of the plan and a current hazard inventory.
- The occupational health nurse or another company representative should provide emergency health care providers with updated clinical information on exposures and appropriate treatment.
- It should never be assumed that local services will have current information on substances used in industry.
- Representatives of these agencies should visit the work site and accompany the nurse on a work site walkthrough so that they are familiar with the operations.

In disaster planning, the nurse often assumes or is assigned to:
- Coordinating the planning and implementing efforts
- Working with appropriate key people within the company and in the community to develop a workable, comprehensive plan
- Providing ongoing communication to keep the plan current
- Planning the drills
- Educating the employees, management, and community providers
- Assessing the equipment and services that may be used in a disaster.

In the event of a disaster, the nurse should play a key role in coordinating the response. Principles of triage may be used as the response team determines the extent of the disaster and the ability of the company and community to respond. Postdisaster nursing interventions are also critical. Examples include identifying of ongoing disaster-related health needs of workers and community residents, collecting epidemiologic data, and assessing the cause and the necessary steps to prevent a recurrence.

Clinical Application

When an insurance company renovated its claims processing office area, all typewriters were replaced with video display terminals (VDTs) and associated hardware for handling all future work by computer. The company's occupational health nurse noticed an increase in visits to the health unit for complaints of headaches, stiff neck muscles, and visual disturbances. These health problems have been associated with VDT operation.

To conduct a complete investigation of this problem, the nurse assessed the workers, the new agent (the VDTs), previously existing potential agents, and the work environment. Interventions focused on designing a program to resolve the health hazard by changing the work process, if possible. In the present example, the first level of intervention was design of the workstation, the component used by the VDT operations in doing their work. Minimizing the possible hazards of the agent involved recommendations for desks, chairs, and lighting designs that would accommodate the individual worker and allow shielding of the VDT. The nursing interventions included strengthening the resistance of the host by prescribing appropriate rest breaks, eye exercises, and relaxation strategies. Recognizing that previous cervical neck injury or impaired vision may increase the risk of adverse effects from VDT work, the nurse would include assessment for these factors in employees' preplacement and periodic health examinations.

For the environmental concerns, the nurse educated the manager about the health risks of paced, externally controlled work expectations and recommended alternatives.

This case is an example of which of the following?
A. The application of the occupational health history
B. A work site assessment or walk-through
C. A work-health interaction
D. The use of the epidemiologic triad in exploring occupational health problems

Answer is in the back of the book.

 Remember This!

- Occupational health nursing is an autonomous practice specialty.
- The scope of occupational health nursing practice is broad, including worker/workplace assessment and surveillance, case management, health promotion, primary care, management/administration, business and finance skills, and research.
- The workforce and workplace are changing dramatically, requiring new knowledge and new occupational health services.
- The type of work has shifted from primarily manufacturing to service and technological jobs.
- Workplace hazards include exposure to biological, chemical, environmental/mechanical, physical, and psychosocial agents.
- Each day an average of 137 people die from work-related disease and an additional 16 die from on-the-job injuries.
- The Occupational Safety and Health Act of 1970 states that workers must have a safe and healthful work environment.
- The interdisciplinary occupational health team usually consists of the occupational health nurse, occupational medicine physician, industrial hygienist, and safety specialist.
- Work-related health problems must be investigated and control strategies implemented to reduce exposure.
- Control strategies include engineering, work practice, administration, and personal protective equipment.
- The Occupational Safety and Health Administration enforces workplace safety and health standards.
- The National Institute for Occupational Safety and Health is the research agency that provides grants to investigate the causes of workplace illness and injuries.
- Worker's Compensation Acts are important laws that govern financial compensation of employees who suffer work-related health problems.
- The occupational health nurse should play a key role in disaster planning and coordination.
- Academic education in occupational health nursing is generally at the graduate level, however there are many AND and BSN nurses who work in occupational health.

 What Would You Do?

1. Arrange to visit a local industry to observe work processes and discuss working conditions. See if you can identify the work-related hazards and make recommendations for eliminating them.
2. Interview the occupational health nurse in an industry setting and ask questions about scope of practice, job functions, and contributions to the business.
3. Contact the American Association of Occupational Health Nurses and ask what the most pressing trends are in the specialty.

4. Obtain a proposed standard for the Occupational Safety and Health Administration, critique it, and submit your comments.
5. Attend a worker's compensation hearing, analyze the problem, and critique the outcome.

REFERENCES

American Association of Occupational Health Nurses: *Guidelines for developing job descriptions in occupational and environmental health nursing,* Atlanta, 1997, American Association of Occupational Health Nurses.

American Association of Occupational Health Nurses: *Standards for occupational health nursing practice,* Atlanta, 1999, American Association of Occupational Health Nurses.

American Association of Occupational Health Nurses: *The nurse in industry,* New York, 1976, American Association of Occupational Health Nurses.

Barratt A: Worksite cholesterol screening and dietary intervention: the Staff Healthy Heart Project, Steering Committee, *Am J Public Health* 84(5):779, 1994.

Bellow J, Rudolph L: The initial impact of a workplace lead-poisoning project, *Am J Public Health* 83(3):406, 1993.

Brown M: *Occupational health nursing,* New York, 1981, MacMillan.

Bureau of Labor Statistics: *Employment projections: 1997,* Washington, D.C., 1997, U.S. Department of Labor.

Bureau of Labor Statistics: *Employment projections: 1998,* Washington, D.C., 1998, U.S. Department of Labor.

Bureau of Labor Statistics: *Employment projections: 1999,* Washington, D.C., 1999, U.S. Department of Labor.

Callahan E: Quality in occupational health care: management's view, *J Occupat Med* 36(4):410, 1994.

Campos-Outcalt D: Occupational health epidemiology and objectives for the year 2000: primary care, *Clin Office Pract* 21(20):213, 1994.

Centers for Disease Control and Prevention: Tuberculosis morbidity–United States, 1995, *MMWR* 45(18):365, 1996.

Felton J: The genesis of American occupational health nursing, part 1, *Occupat Health Nurs* 33:615, 1985.

Fielding J, Weaver SM: A comparison of hospital- and community-based mental health nurses: perceptions of their work environment and psychological health, *J Adv Nurs* 19:1196, 1994.

Girgis A: A workplace intervention for increasing outdoor workers' use of solar protection, *Am J Public Health* 84(1):77, 1994.

Hodgson M, Storey E: Patients and the sick building syndrome, *J Allergy Clin Immunol* 94(2 Pt 2):335, 1994.

Jeffrey RW, et al: The Healthy Worker Project: a work-site intervention for weight control and smoking cessation, *Am J Public Health* 83(3):395, 1993.

Jorgensen S, Hein HO, Gyntelberg F: Heavy lifting at work and risk of genital prolapse and herniated lumbar disc in assistant nurses, *Occupat Med* 44(1):47, 1994.

Katz E, et al: Exposure assessment in epidemiologic studies of birth defects by industrial hygienic review of maternal interviews, *Am J Indust Med* 26(1):1, 1994.

Klinger C, Jones M: The OSHA standard setting process . . . role of the occupational health nurse, *AAOHN J* 42(8):374, 1994.

Larese F, Fiorit A: Musculoskeletal disorders in hospital nurses: a comparison between two hospitals, *Ergonomics* 37:1205, 1994.

Levy BS, Wegman DH: *Occupational health: recognizing and preventing occupational disease,* Boston, 1995, Little, Brown.

McGrath B: Fifty years of industrial nursing, *Public Health Nurse* 37:119, 1995.

Morris S: Academic occupational safety and health training programs, *Occupat Med* 9(2):189, 1994.

National Institute for Occupational Safety and Health: *Latex allergy,* pub no 97-135, Washington, D.C., 1997a, U.S. Government Printing Office, available online: www.cdc.gov/noish/latexfs.html.

National Institute for Occupational Safety and Health: Musculoskeletal disorders (MSDs) and workplace factors, Washington, D.C., 1997b, U.S. Government Printing Office, available online: www.cdc.gov/noish/ergtx11.html.

Paskett ED, et al: Breast cancer screening education in the workplace, *J Cancer Educ* 9(2):101, 1994.

Payling K: A hazard we can no longer ignore: effects of excessive noise on wellbeing, *Prof Nurse* 9(6):418, 1994.

Platt J: Radon: its impact on the community and the role of the nurse, *AAOHN J* 41(11):547, 1993.

Porro S, et al: The utility of health education among lead workers: the experience of one program, *Am J Indust Med* 23(3):473, 1993.

Poster E, Ryan J: A multiregional study of nurses' beliefs and attitudes about work safety and patient assault, *Hosp Community Psychiatry* 45(11):1104, 1994.

Public Law 91-596. *Occupational Health and Safety Act,* U.S. Congress, Washington, D.C., 1970, U.S. Government Printing Office.

Rabinowitz S, et al: Teaching interpersonal skills to occupational and environmental health professionals, *Psychol Rep* 74(3 Pt 2):1299, 1994.

Ramazzini B: *De Morbis Artificum* [Diseases of Workers], 1713. Translated by W.C. Wright, Chicago, 1940, University of Chicago Press.

Rigotti N, et al: Do businesses comply with a no-smoking law? Assessing the self-enforcement approach, *Prevent Med* 23(2):223, 1994.

Rogers B: *Occupational health nursing: concepts and practice,* Philadelphia, 1994, WB Saunders.

Snyder M, et al: Environmental and occupational health education: a survey of community health nurses' need for educational programs, *AAOHN J* 42(7):325, 1994.

Stellman J: Where women work and the hazards they may face on the job, *J Occupat Med* 36(8):814, 1994.

Stine D, Brown T: *Principles of toxicology,* Boca Raton, Fla, 1996, Lewis.

U.S. Census Bureau: *Resident population of the United States: middle series projections, 2006-2010, by age and sex,* Washington, D.C., 1996, U.S. Government Printing Office.

U.S. Department of Health and Human Services and National Institute for Occupational Safety and Health: *National occupational research agenda,* pub no 99-108, Washington, D.C., 1999, U.S. Government Printing Office.

U.S. Department of Health and Human Services–National Institute for Occupational Safety and Health: *National occupational research agenda,* Cincinnati, 1996, NIOSH Publications Dissemination.

Workplace injury/illness rates for 1991 show a 10-year record drop in incidence, *Occupat Health Safety* 62(1):8, 1993.

Appendixes

Appendix A

International and National Agendas for Health Care Delivery

A.1 National Health Objectives 2010

1. Access to Quality Health Services

Goal: Improve access to comprehensive, high-quality health care services.

Clinical Preventive Care

1-1 Persons with health insurance
1-2 Health insurance coverage for clinical preventive services
1-3 Counseling about health behaviors

Primary Care

1-4 Source of ongoing care
1-5 Usual primary care provider
1-6 Difficulties or delays in obtaining needed health care
1-7 Core competencies in health provider training
1-8 Racial and ethnic representation in health professions
1-9 Hospitalization for ambulatory-care-sensitive conditions

Emergency Services

1-10 Delay or difficulty in getting emergency care
1-11 Rapid prehospital emergency care
1-12 Single toll-free number for poison control centers
1-13 Trauma care systems
1-14 Special needs of children

Long-Term Care and Rehabilitative Services

1-15 Long-term care services
1-16 Pressure ulcers among nursing home residents

2. Arthritis, Osteoporosis, and Chronic Back Conditions

Goal: Prevent illness and disability related to arthritis and other rheumatic conditions, osteoporosis, and chronic back conditions.

Arthritis and Other Rheumatic Conditions

2-1 Mean number of days without severe pain
2-2 Activity limitations due to arthritis
2-3 Personal care limitations
2-4 Help in coping

2-5 Employment rate
2-6 Racial differences in total knee replacement
2-7 Seeing a health care provider
2-8 Arthritis education

Osteoporosis

2-9 Cases of osteoporosis
2-10 Hospitalization for vertebral fractures

Chronic Back Conditions

2-11 Activity limitations due to chronic back conditions

3. Cancer

Goal: Reduce the number of new cancer cases as well as the illness, disability, and death caused by cancer.

3-1 Overall cancer deaths
3-2 Lung cancer deaths
3-3 Breast cancer deaths
3-4 Cervical cancer deaths
3-5 Colorectal cancer deaths
3-6 Oropharyngeal cancer deaths
3-7 Prostate cancer deaths
3-8 Melanoma deaths
3-9 Sun exposure and skin cancer
3-10 Provider counseling about cancer prevention
3-11 Pap tests
3-12 Colorectal cancer screening
3-13 Mammograms
3-14 Statewide cancer registries
3-15 Cancer survival

4. Chronic Kidney Disease

Goal: Reduce new cases of chronic kidney disease and its complications, disability, death, and economic costs.

4-1 End-stage renal disease
4-2 Cardiovascular disease deaths in persons with chronic kidney failure

4-3   Counseling for chronic kidney failure care
4-4   Use of arteriovenous fistulas
4-5   Registration for kidney transplantation
4-6   Waiting time for kidney transplantation
4-7   Kidney failure due to diabetes
4-8   Medical therapy for persons with diabetes and proteinuria

5. Diabetes

Goal: Through prevention programs, reduce the disease and economic burden of diabetes, and improve the quality of life for all persons who have or are at risk for diabetes.

5-1   Diabetes education
5-2   New cases of diabetes
5-3   Overall cases of diagnosed diabetes
5-4   Diagnosis of diabetes
5-5   Diabetes deaths
5-6   Diabetes-related deaths
5-7   Cardiovascular disease deaths in persons with diabetes
5-8   Gestational diabetes
5-9   Foot ulcers
5-10   Lower extremity amputations
5-11   Annual urinary microalbumin measurement
5-12   Annual glycosylated hemoglobin measurement
5-13   Annual dilated eye examinations
5-14   Annual foot examinations
5-15   Annual dental examinations
5-16   Aspirin therapy
5-17   Self-blood-glucose-monitoring

6. Disability and Secondary Conditions

Goal: Promote the health of people with disabilities, prevent secondary conditions, and eliminate disparities between people with and without disabilities in the U.S. population.

6-1   Standard definition of people with disabilities in data sets
6-2   Feelings and depression among children with disabilities
6-3   Feelings and depression interfering with activities among adults with disabilities
6-4   Social participation among adults with disabilities
6-5   Sufficient emotional support among adults with disabilities
6-6   Satisfaction with life among adults with disabilities
6-7   Congregate care of children and adults with disabilities
6-8   Employment parity
6-9   Inclusion of children and youth with disabilities in regular education programs
6-10   Accessibility of health and wellness programs
6-11   Assistive devices and technology
6-12   Environmental barriers affecting participation in activities
6-13   Surveillance and health promotion programs

7. Educational and Community-Based Programs

Goal: Increase the quality, availability, and effectiveness of educational and community-based programs designed to prevent disease and improve health and quality of life.

School Setting

7-1   High school completion
7-2   School health education
7-3   Health-risk behavior information for college and university students
7-4   School nurse-to-student ratio

Worksite Setting

7-5   Worksite health promotion programs
7-6   Participation in employer-sponsored health promotion activities

Health Care Setting

7-7   Patient and family education
7-8   Satisfaction with patient education
7-9   Health care organization sponsorship of community health promotion activities

Community Setting and Select Populations

7-10   Community health promotion programs
7-11   Culturally appropriate and linguistically competent community health promotion programs
7-12   Older adult participation in community health promotion activities

8. Environmental Health

Goal: Promote health for all through a healthy environment.

Outdoor Air Quality

8-1   Harmful air pollutants
8-2   Alternative modes of transportation
8-3   Cleaner alternative fuels
8-4   Airborne toxins

Water Quality

8-5   Safe drinking water
8-6   Waterborne disease outbreaks
8-7   Water conservation
8-8   Surface water health risks
8-9   Beach closings
8-10   Fish contamination

Toxics and Waste

8-11   Elevated blood lead levels in children
8-12   Risks posed by hazardous sites
8-13   Pesticide exposures
8-14   Toxic pollutants
8-15   Recycled municipal solid waste

Healthy Homes and Healthy Communities

8-16   Indoor allergens
8-17   Office building air quality
8-18   Homes tested for radon
8-19   Radon-resistant new home construction
8-20   School policies to protect against environmental hazards
8-21   Disaster preparedness plans and protocols
8-22   Lead-based paint testing
8-23   Substandard housing

Infrastructure and Surveillance

8-24   Exposure to pesticides
8-25   Exposure to heavy metals and other toxic chemicals
8-26   Information systems used for environmental health
8-27   Monitoring environmentally related diseases
8-28   Local agencies using surveillance data for vector control

Global Environmental Health

8-29   Global burden of disease
8-30   Water quality in the U.S.-Mexico border region

9. Family Planning

Goal: Improve pregnancy planning and spacing and prevent unintended pregnancy.

9-1   Intended pregnancy
9-2   Birth spacing
9-3   Contraceptive use
9-4   Contraceptive failure
9-5   Emergency contraception
9-6   Male involvement in pregnancy prevention
9-7   Adolescent pregnancy
9-8   Abstinence before age 15 years
9-9   Abstinence among adolescents aged 15 to 17 years
9-10   Pregnancy prevention and sexually transmitted disease (STD) protection
9-11   Pregnancy prevention education
9-12   Problems in becoming pregnant and maintaining a pregnancy
9-13   Insurance coverage for contraceptive supplies and services

10. Food Safety

Goal: Reduce foodborne illnesses.

10-1   Foodborne infections
10-2   Outbreaks of foodborne infections
10-3   Antimicrobial resistance of Salmonella species
10-4   Food allergy deaths
10-5   Consumer food safety practices
10-6   Safe food preparation practices in retail establishments
10-7   Organophosphate pesticide exposure

11. Health Communication

Goal: Use communication strategically to improve health.

11-1   Households with Internet access
11-2   Health literacy
11-3   Research and evaluation of communication programs
11-4   Quality of Internet health information sources
11-5   Centers for excellence
11-6   Satisfaction with health care providers' communication skills

12. Heart Disease and Stroke

Goal: Improve cardiovascular health and quality of life through the prevention, detection, and treatment of risk fac-

tors; early identification and treatment of heart attacks and strokes; and prevention of recurrent cardiovascular events.

Heart Disease

12-1   Coronary heart disease (CHD) deaths
12-2   Knowledge of symptoms of heart attack and importance of calling 911
12-3   Artery-opening therapy
12-4   Bystander response to cardiac arrest
12-5   Out-of-hospital emergency care
12-6   Heart failure hospitalizations

Stroke

12-7   Stroke deaths
12-8   Knowledge of early warning symptoms of stroke

Blood Pressure

12-9   High blood pressure
12-10   High blood pressure control
12-11   Action to help control blood pressure
12-12   Blood pressure monitoring

Cholesterol

12-13   Mean total blood cholesterol levels
12-14   High blood cholesterol levels
12-15   Blood cholesterol screening
12-16   LDL-cholesterol level in CHD patients

13. HIV

Goal: Prevent HIV infection and its related illness and death.

13-1   New AIDS cases
13-2   AIDS among men who have sex with men
13-3   AIDS among persons who inject drugs
13-4   AIDS among men who have sex with men and who inject drugs
13-5   New HIV cases
13-6   Condom use
13-7   Knowledge of serostatus
13-8   HIV counseling and education for persons in substance abuse treatment
13-9   HIV/AIDS, STD, and TB education in State prisons
13-10   HIV counseling and testing in State prisons
13-11   HIV testing in TB patients
13-12   Screening for STDs and immunization for hepatitis B
13-13   Treatment according to guidelines
13-14   HIV-infection deaths
13-15   Interval between HIV infection and AIDS diagnosis
13-16   Interval between AIDS diagnosis and death from AIDS
13-17   Perinatally acquired HIV infection

14. Immunization and Infectious Diseases

Goal: Prevent disease, disability, and death from infectious diseases, including vaccine-preventable diseases.

Diseases Preventable Through Universal Vaccination

14-1 Vaccine-preventable diseases
14-2 Hepatitis B in infants and young children
14-3 Hepatitis B in adults and high-risk groups
14-4 Bacterial meningitis in young children
14-5 Invasive pneumococcal infections

Diseases Preventable Through Targeted Vaccination

14-6 Hepatitis A
14-7 Meningococcal disease
14-8 Lyme disease

Infectious Diseases and Emerging Antimicrobial Resistance

14-9 Hepatitis C
14-10 Identification of persons with chronic hepatitis C
14-11 Tuberculosis
14-12 Curative therapy for tuberculosis
14-13 Treatment for high-risk persons with latent tuberculosis infection
14-14 Timely laboratory confirmation of tuberculosis cases
14-15 Prevention services for international travelers
14-16 Invasive early onset group B streptococcal disease
14-17 Peptic ulcer hospitalizations
14-18 Antibiotics prescribed for ear infections
14-19 Antibiotics prescribed for common cold
14-20 Hospital-acquired infections
14-21 Antimicrobial use in intensive care units

Vaccination Coverage and Strategies

14-22 Universally recommended vaccination of children aged 19 to 35 months
14-23 Vaccination coverage for children in day care, kindergarten, and first grade
14-24 Fully immunized young children and adolescents
14-25 Providers who measure childhood vaccination coverage levels
14-26 Children participating in population-based immunization registries
14-27 Vaccination coverage among adolescents
14-28 Hepatitis B vaccination among high-risk groups
14-29 Influenza and pneumococcal vaccination of high-risk adults

Vaccine Safety

14-30 Adverse events from vaccinations
14-31 Active surveillance for vaccine safety

15. Injury and Violence Prevention

Goal: Reduce injuries, disabilities, and deaths due to unintentional injuries and violence.

Injury Prevention

15-1 Nonfatal head injuries
15-2 Nonfatal spinal cord injuries
15-3 Firearm-related deaths
15-4 Proper firearm storage in homes
15-5 Nonfatal firearm-related injuries
15-6 Child fatality review
15-7 Nonfatal poisonings
15-8 Deaths from poisoning
15-9 Deaths from suffocation
15-10 Emergency department surveillance systems
15-11 Hospital discharge surveillance systems
15-12 Emergency department visits

Unintentional Injury Prevention

15-13 Deaths from unintentional injuries
15-14 Nonfatal unintentional injuries
15-15 Deaths from motor vehicle crashes
15-16 Pedestrian deaths
15-17 Nonfatal motor vehicle injuries
15-18 Nonfatal pedestrian injuries
15-19 Safety belts
15-20 Child restraints
15-21 Motorcycle helmet use
15-22 Graduated driver licensing
15-23 Bicycle helmet use
15-24 Bicycle helmet laws
15-25 Residential fire deaths
15-26 Functioning smoke alarms in residences
15-27 Deaths from falls
15-28 Hip fractures
15-29 Drownings
15-30 Dog bite injuries
15-31 Injury protection in school sports

Violence and Abuse Prevention

15-32 Homicides
15-33 Maltreatment and maltreatment fatalities of children
15-34 Physical assault by intimate partners
15-35 Rape or attempted rape
15-36 Sexual assault other than rape
15-37 Physical assaults
15-38 Physical fighting among adolescents
15-39 Weapon carrying by adolescents on school property

16. Maternal, Infant, and Child Health

Goal: Improve the health and well-being of women, infants, children, and families.

Fetal, Infant, Child, and Adolescent Deaths

16-1 Fetal and infant deaths
16-2 Child deaths
16-3 Adolescent and young adult deaths

Maternal Deaths and Illnesses

16-4 Maternal deaths
16-5 Maternal illness and complications due to pregnancy

Prenatal Care

16-6 Prenatal care
16-7 Childbirth classes

Obstetrical Care

16-8 Very low birth weight infants born at level III hospitals
16-9 Cesarean births

Risk Factors

16-10 Low birth weight and very low birth weight
16-11 Preterm births
16-12 Weight gain during pregnancy
16-13 Infants put to sleep on their backs

Developmental Disabilities and Neural Tube Defects

16-14 Developmental disabilities
16-15 Spina bifida and other neural tube defects
16-16 Optimum folic acid levels

Prenatal Substance Exposure

16-17 Prenatal substance exposure
16-18 Fetal alcohol syndrome

Breastfeeding, Newborn Screening, and Service Systems

16-19 Breastfeeding
16-20 Newborn bloodspot screening
16-21 Sepsis among children with sickle cell disease
16-22 Medical homes for children with special health care needs
16-23 Service systems for children with special health care needs

17. Medical Product Safety

Goal: Ensure the safe and effective use of medical products.

17-1 Monitoring of adverse medical events
17-2 Linked, automated information systems
17-3 Provider review of medications taken by patients
17-4 Receipt of useful information about prescriptions from pharmacies
17-5 Receipt of oral counseling about medications from prescribers and dispensers
17-6 Blood donations

18. Mental Health and Mental Illness

Goal: Improve mental health and ensure access to appropriate, quality mental health services.

Mental Health Status Improvement

18-1 Suicide
18-2 Adolescent suicide attempts
18-3 Serious mental illness (SMI) among homeless adults
18-4 Employment of persons with SMI
18-5 Eating disorder relapses

Treatment Expansion

18-6 Primary care screening and assessment
18-7 Treatment for children with mental health problems
18-8 Juvenile justice facility screening
18-9 Treatment for adults with mental disorders
18-10 Treatment for co-occurring disorders
18-11 Adult jail diversion programs

State Activities

18-12 State tracking of consumer satisfaction
18-13 State plans addressing cultural competence
18-14 State plans addressing elderly persons

19. Nutrition and Overweight

Goal: Promote health and reduce chronic disease associated with diet and weight.

Weight Status and Growth

19-1 Healthy weight in adults
19-2 Obesity in adults
19-3 Overweight or obesity in children and adolescents
19-4 Growth retardation in children

Food and Nutrient Consumption

19-5 Fruit intake
19-6 Vegetable intake
19-7 Grain product intake
19-8 Saturated fat intake
19-9 Total fat intake
19-10 Sodium intake
19-11 Calcium intake

Iron Deficiency and Anemia

19-12 Iron deficiency in young children and in females of childbearing age
19-13 Anemia in low-income pregnant females
19-14 Iron deficiency in pregnant females

Schools, Worksites, and Nutrition Counseling

19-15 Meals and snacks at school
19-16 Worksite promotion of nutrition education and weight management
19-17 Nutrition counseling for medical conditions

Food Security

19-18 Food security

20. Occupational Safety and Health

Goal: Promote the health and safety of people at work through prevention and early intervention.

20-1 Work-related injury deaths
20-2 Work-related injuries
20-3 Overexertion or repetitive motion
20-4 Pneumoconiosis deaths
20-5 Work-related homicides
20-6 Work-related assaults
20-7 Elevated blood lead levels from work exposure
20-8 Occupational skin diseases or disorders
20-9 Worksite stress reduction programs
20-10 Needlestick injuries
20-11 Work-related, noise-induced hearing loss

21. Oral Health

Goal: Prevent and control oral and craniofacial diseases, conditions, and injuries and improve access to related services.

21-1 Dental caries experience
21-2 Untreated dental decay
21-3 No permanent tooth loss
21-4 Complete tooth loss

21-5   Periodontal diseases
21-6   Early detection of oral and pharyngeal cancers
21-7   Annual examinations for oral and pharyngeal cancers
21-8   Dental sealants
21-9   Community water fluoridation
21-10   Use of oral health care system
21-11   Use of oral health care system by residents in long-term care facilities
21-12   Dental services for low-income children
21-13   School-based health centers with oral health component
21-14   Health centers with oral health service components
21-15   Referral for cleft lip or palate
21-16   Oral and craniofacial State-based surveillance system
21-17   Tribal, State, and local dental programs

22. Physical Fitness and Activity

Goal: Improve health, fitness, and quality of life through daily physical activity.

Physical Activity in Adults

22-1   No leisure-time physical activity
22-2   Moderate physical activity
22-3   Vigorous physical activity

Muscular Strength/Endurance and Flexibility

22-4   Muscular strength and endurance
22-5   Flexibility

Physical Activity in Children and Adolescents

22-6   Moderate physical activity in adolescents
22-7   Vigorous physical activity in adolescents
22-8   Physical education requirement in schools
22-9   Daily physical education in schools
22-10   Physical activity in physical education class
22-11   Television viewing

Access

22-12   School physical activity facilities
22-13   Worksite physical activity and fitness
22-14   Community walking
22-15   Community bicycling

23. Public Health Infrastructure

Goal: Ensure that Federal, Tribal, State, and local health agencies have the infrastructure to provide essential public health services effectively.

Data and Information Systems

23-1   Public health employee access to the Internet
23-2   Public access to information and surveillance data
23-3   Use of geocoding in health data systems
23-4   Data for all population groups
23-5   Data for Leading Health Indicators, Health Status Indicators, and Priority Data Needs at Tribal, State, and local levels
23-6   National tracking of Healthy People 2010 objectives
23-7   Timely release of data on objectives

Workforce

23-8   Competencies for public health workers
23-9   Training in essential public health services
23-10   Continuing education and training by public health agencies

Public Health Organizations

23-11   Performance standards for essential public health services
23-12   Health improvement plans
23-13   Access to public health laboratory services
23-14   Access to epidemiology services
23-15   Model statutes related to essential public health services

Resources

23-16   Data on public health expenditures

Prevention Research

23-17   Population-based prevention research

24. Respiratory Diseases

Goal: Promote respiratory health through better prevention, detection, treatment, and education efforts.

Asthma

24 1   Deaths from asthma
24-2   Hospitalizations for asthma
24-3   Hospital emergency department visits for asthma
24-4   Activity limitations
24-5   School or work days lost
24-6   Patient education
24-7   Appropriate asthma care
24-8   Surveillance systems

Chronic Obstructive Pulmonary Disease (COPD)

24-9   Activity limitations due to chronic lung and breathing problems
24-10   Deaths from COPD

Obstructive Sleep Apnea (OSA)

24-11   Medical evaluation and followup
24-12   Vehicular crashes related to excessive sleepiness

25. Sexually Transmitted Diseases

Goal: Promote responsible sexual behaviors, strengthen community capacity, and increase access to quality services to prevent sexually transmitted diseases (STDs) and their complications.

Bacterial STD Illness and Disability

25-1   Chlamydia
25-2   Gonorrhea
25-3   Primary and secondary syphilis

Viral STD Illness and Disability

25-4   Genital herpes
25-5   Human papillomavirus infection

STD Complications Affecting Females

25-6   Pelvic inflammatory disease (PID)
25-7   Fertility problems
25-8   Heterosexually transmitted HIV infection in women

STD Complications Affecting the Fetus and Newborn

25-9   Congenital syphilis
25-10   Neonatal STDs

Personal Behaviors

25-11   Responsible adolescent sexual behavior
25-12   Responsible sexual behavior messages on television

Community Protection Infrastructure

25-13   Hepatitis B vaccine services in STD clinics
25-14   Screening in youth detention facilities and jails
25-15   Contracts to treat nonplan managed care partners of STD patients

Personal Health Services

25-16   Annual screening for genital chlamydia
25-17   Screening of pregnant women
25-18   Compliance with recognized STD treatment standards
25-19   Provider referral services for sex partners

26. Substance Abuse

Goal: Reduce substance abuse to protect the health, safety, and quality of life for all, especially children.

Adverse Consequences of Substance Use and Abuse

26-1   Motor vehicle crash deaths and injuries
26-2   Cirrhosis deaths
26-3   Drug-induced deaths
26-4   Drug-related hospital emergency department visits
26-5   Alcohol-related hospital emergency department visits
26-6   Adolescents riding with a driver who has been drinking
26-7   Alcohol- and drug-related violence
26-8   Lost productivity

Substance Use and Abuse

26-9   Substance-free youth
26-10   Adolescent and adult use of illicit substances
26-11   Binge drinking
26-12   Average annual alcohol consumption
26-13   Low-risk drinking among adults
26-14   Steroid use among adolescents
26-15   Inhalant use among adolescents

Risk of Substance Use and Abuse

26-16   Peer disapproval of substance abuse
26-17   Perception of risk associated with substance abuse

Treatment for Substance Abuse

26-18   Treatment gap for illicit drugs
26-19   Treatment in correctional institutions
26-20   Treatment for injection drug use
26-21   Treatment gap for problem alcohol use

State and Local Efforts

26-22   Hospital emergency department referrals
26-23   Community partnerships and coalitions
26-24   Administrative license revocation laws
26-25   Blood alcohol concentration (BAC) levels for motor vehicle drivers

27. Tobacco Use

Goal: Reduce illness, disability, and death related to tobacco use and exposure to secondhand smoke.

Tobacco Use in Population Groups

27-1   Adult tobacco use
27-2   Adolescent tobacco use
27-3   Initiation of tobacco use
27-4   Age at first tobacco use

Cessation and Treatment

27-5   Smoking cessation by adults
27-6   Smoking cessation during pregnancy
27-7   Smoking cessation by adolescents
27-8   Insurance coverage of cessation treatment

Exposure to Secondhand Smoke

27-9   Exposure to tobacco smoke at home among children
27-10   Exposure to environmental tobacco smoke
27-11   Smoke-free and tobacco-free schools
27-12   Worksite smoking policies
27-13   Smoke-free indoor air laws

Social and Environmental Changes

27-14   Enforcement of illegal tobacco sales to minors laws
27-15   Retail license suspension for sales to minors
27-16   Tobacco advertising and promotion targeting adolescents and young adults
27-17   Adolescent disapproval of smoking
27-18   Tobacco control programs
27-19   Preemptive tobacco control laws
27-20   Tobacco product regulation
27-21   Tobacco tax

28. Vision and Hearing

Goal: Improve the visual and hearing health of the Nation through prevention, early detection, treatment, and rehabilitation.

Vision

28-1   Dilated eye examinations
28-2   Vision screening for children
28-3   Impairment due to refractive errors
28-4   Impairment in children and adolescents
28-5   Impairment due to diabetic retinopathy
28-6   Impairment due to glaucoma
28-7   Impairment due to cataract
28-8   Occupational eye injury
28-9   Protective eyewear
28-10   Vision rehabilitation services and devices

Hearing

28-11 Newborn hearing screening, evaluation, and intervention
28-12 Otitis media
28-13 Rehabilitation for hearing impairment
28-14 Hearing examination
28-15 Evaluation and treatment referrals
28-16 Hearing protection

28-17 Noise-induced hearing loss in children
28-18 Noise-induced hearing loss in adults

From U.S. Department of Health and Human Services: Healthy people 2010: understanding and improving health, Washington, D.C., 2000, U.S. Department of Health and Human Services; available online at http://www.health.gov/healthypeople/document/html/uih/uih__6.htm.

A.2 Schedule of Clinical Preventive Services

1. BIRTH TO 10 YEARS

Interventions Considered and Recommended for the Periodic Health Examination

Leading Causes of Death

Conditions originating in perinatal period
Congenital anomalies
Sudden infant death syndrome (SIDS)
Unintentional injuries (non-motor vehicle)
Motor vehicle injuries

Interventions for the General Population

Screening
Height and weight
Blood pressure
Vision screen
Hemoglobinopathy screen (birth)*
Phenylalanine level (birth)†
T_4 and/or TSH (birth)‡

Counseling

INJURY PREVENTION

Child safety car seats (age <5 yr)
Lap-shoulder belts (age ≥5 yr)
Bicycle helmet; avoid bicycling near traffic
Smoke detector, flame-retardant sleepwear
Hot water heater temperature <120°-130° F
Window/stair guards, pool fence
Safe storage of drugs, toxic substances, firearms and matches

Syrup of ipecac, poison control phone number
CPR training for parents/caretakers

DIET AND EXERCISE

Breast-feeding, iron-enriched formula and foods (infants and toddlers)
Limit fat and cholesterol; maintain caloric balance; emphasize grains, fruits, vegetables (age ≥2 yr)
Regular physical activity§

SUBSTANCE USE

Effects of passive smoking§
Anti-tobacco message§

DENTAL HEALTH

Regular visits to dental care provider§
Floss, brush with fluoride toothpaste daily§
Advice about baby bottle tooth decay§

Immunizations

Diphtheria-tetanus-pertussis (DTP)‖
Oral poliovirus (OPV)¶
Measles-mumps-rubella (MMR)#
H. influenzae type b (Hib) conjugate**
Hepatitis B††
Varicella§§

Chemoprophylaxis

Ocular prophylaxis (birth)

---

*Whether screening should be universal or targeted to high-risk groups will depend on the proportion of high-risk individuals in the screening area, and other considerations (See Chapter 43).
†If done during first 24 hr of life, repeat by age 2 wk.
‡Optimally between day 2 and 6, but in all cases before newborn nursery discharge.

§The ability of the clinician counseling to influence this behavior is unproven.
‖2, 4, 6, and 12-18 mo; once between ages 4-6 yr (DTaP may be used at 15 mo and older).
¶2, 4, 6-18 months; once between ages 4-6 yr.
#12-15 mo and 4-6 yr.
**2, 4, 6 and 12-15 mo; no dose needed at 6 mo if PRP-OMP vaccine is used for first 2 doses.
††Birth, 1 mo, 6 mo; or 0-2 mo. 1-2 mo later, and 6-18 mo. if not done in infancy: current visit, and 1 and 6 mo later.
§§12-18 mo; or any child without history of chickenpox or previous immunization. Include information on risk in adulthood, duration of immunity, and potential need for booster doses.

Interventions for High-Risk Populations

Population	Potential Interventions
Preterm or low birth weight	Hemoglobin/hematocrit (HR1)
Infants of mothers at risk for HIV	HIV testing (HR2)
Low income; immigrants	Hemoglobin/hematocrit (HR1); PPD (HR3)
TB contacts	PPD (HR3)
Native American/Alaska Native	Hemoglobin/hematocrit (HR1); PPD (HR3); hepatitis A vaccine (HR4); pneumococcal vaccine (HR5)
Travelers to developing countries	Hepatitis A vaccine (HR4)
Residents of long-term care facilities	PPD (HR3); hepatitis A vaccine (HR4); influenza vaccine (HR6)
Certain chronic medical conditions	PPD (HR3); pneumococcal vaccine (HR5); influenza vaccine (HR6)
Increased individual or community lead exposure	Blood lead level (HR7)
Inadequate water fluoridation	Daily fluoride supplement (HR8)
Family history of skin cancer; nevi; fair skin, eyes, hair	Avoid excess/midday sun, use protective clothing* (HR9)

From U.S. Preventive Services Task Force: *Guide to clinical preventive services,* ed 2, Baltimore, 1996, Williams & Wilkins.
*The ability of clinician counseling to influence this behavior is unproven.

High Risk Definitions

HR1 = Infants age 6-12 months who are living in poverty, black, Native American or Alaska Native, immigrants from developing countries, preterm and low-birth-weight infants, infants whose principal dietary intake is unfortified cow's milk.

HR2 = Infants born to high-risk mothers whose HIV status is unknown. Women at high risk include: past or present injection drug use; persons who exchange sex for money or drugs, and their sex partners; injection drug-using, bisexual, or HIV-positive sex partners currently or in past; persons seeking treatment for STDs; blood transfusion during 1978-1985.

HR3 = Persons infected with HIV, close contacts of persons with known or suspected TB, persons with medical risk factors associated with TB, immigrants from countries with high TB prevalence, medically underserved low-income populations (including homeless), residents of long-term care facilities.

HR4 = Persons ≥2 yr living in or traveling to areas where the disease is endemic and where periodic outbreaks occur (e.g., countries with high or intermediate endemicity; certain Alaska Native, Pacific Island, Native American, and religious communities). Consider for institutionalized children aged ≥2 yr. Clinicians should also consider local epidemiology.

HR5 = Immunocompetent persons ≥2 yr with certain medical conditions, including chronic cardiac or pulmonary disease, diabetes mellitus, and anatomic asplenia. Immunocompetent persons ≥2 yr living in high-risk environments or social settings (e.g., certain Native American and Alaska Native populations).

HR6 = Annual vaccination of children >6 mo who are residents of chronic care facilities or who have chronic cardiopulmonary disorders, metabolic diseases (including diabetes mellitus), hemoglobinopathies, immunosuppression, or renal dysfunction.

HR7 = Children about age 12 mo who (1) live in communities in which the prevalence of lead levels requiring individual intervention, including residential lead hazard control or chelation, is high or undefined; (2) live in or frequently visit a home built before 1950 with dilapidated paint or with recent or ongoing renovation or remodeling; (3) have close contract with a person who has an elevated lead level; (4) live near lead industry or heavy traffic; (5) live with someone whose job or hobby involves lead exposure; (6) use lead-based pottery; or (7) take traditional ethnic remedies that contain lead.

HR8 = Children living in areas with inadequate water fluoridation (<0.6 ppm).

HR9 = Persons with a family history of skin cancer, a large number of moles, atypical moles, poor tanning ability, or light skin, hair, and eye color.

2. AGES 11-24 YEARS

Interventions Considered and Recommended for the Periodic Health Examination

Leading Causes of Death

Motor vehicle/other unintentional injuries
Homicide
Suicide
Malignant neoplasms
Heart diseases

Interventions for the General Population

Screening
Height and weight
Blood pressure*
Papanicolaou (Pap) test† (females)
Chlamydia screen‡ (females <20 yr)
Rubella serology or vaccination history‖ (females >12 yr)
Assess for problem drinking

Counseling

INJURY PREVENTION
Lap/shoulder belts
Bicycle/motorcycle/ATV helmets§
Smoke detector§
Safe storage/removal of firearms§

SUBSTANCE USE
Avoid tobacco use
Avoid underage drinking and illicit drug use§
Avoid alcohol/drug use while driving, swimming, boating, etc.§

SEXUAL BEHAVIOR
STD prevention: abstinence; avoid high-risk behavior§; condoms/female barrier with spermicide§
Unintended pregnancy: contraception

DIET AND EXERCISE
Limit fat and cholesterol; maintain caloric balance; emphasize grains, fruits, vegetables
Adequate calcium intake (females)
Regular physical activity§

DENTAL HEALTH
Regular visits to dental care provider§
Floss, brush with fluoride toothpaste daily§

Immunizations

Tetanus-diphtheria (Td) boosters (11-16 yr)
Hepatitis B¶
MMR (11-12 yr)#
Varicella (11-12 yr)**
Rubella (females >12 yr)‖

Chemoprophylaxis

Multivitamin with folic acid (females planning/capable of pregnancy)

---

*Periodic BP for persons aged ≥21 yr.
†If sexually active at present or in the past: q ≤3 yr. If sexual history is unreliable, begin Pap tests at age 18 yr.
‡If sexually active.
§The ability of clinician counseling to influence this behavior is unproven.

‖Serologic testing documented vaccination history, and routine vaccination against rubella (preferably with MMR) are equally acceptable alternatives.
¶If not previously immunized: current visit. 1 and 6 mo later.
#If susceptible to chickenpox.
**Excluding those who have had varicella.

Interventions for High-Risk Populations

Population	Potential Interventions
High-risk sexual behavior	RPR/VDRL (HR1); screen for gonorrhea (female) (HR2), HIV (HR3), chlamydia (female) (HR4); hepatitis A vaccine (HR5)
Injection or street drug use	RPR/VDRL (HR1); HIV screen (HR3); hepatitis A vaccine (HR5); PPD (HR6); advice to reduce infection risk (HR7)
TB contacts; immigrants; low income	PPD (HR6)
Native Americans/Alaska Natives	Hepatitis A vaccine (HR5); PPD (HR6); pneumococcal vaccine (HR8)
Travelers to developing countries	Hepatitis A vaccine (HR5)
Certain chronic medical conditions	PPD (HR6); pneumococcal vaccine (HR8); influenza vaccine (HR9)
Settings where adolescents and young adults congregate	Second MMR (HR10)
Susceptible to varicella, measles, mumps	Varicella vaccine (HR11); MMR (HR12)
Blood transfusion between 1975-1985	HIV screen (HR3)
Institutionalized persons; health care/lab workers	Hepatitis A vaccine (HR5); PPD (HR6); influenza vaccine (HR9)
Family history of skin cancer; nevi; fair skin, eyes, hair	Avoid excess/midday sun, use protective clothing* (HR13)
Prior pregnancy with neural tube defect	Folic acid 4.0 mg (HR14)
Inadequate water fluoridation	Daily fluoride supplement (HR15)

From U.S. Preventive Services Task Force: *Guide to clinical preventive services,* ed 2, Baltimore, 1996, Williams & Wilkins.
*The ability of clinician counseling to influence this behavior is unproven.

High-Risk Definitions

HR1 = Persons who exchange sex for money or drugs, and their sex partners; persons with other STDs (including HIV); and sexual contacts of persons with active syphilis. Clinicians should also consider local epidemiology.

HR2 = Females who have: two or more sex partners in the last year; a sex partner with multiple sexual contacts; exchanged sex for money or drugs; or a history of repeated episodes of gonorrhea. Clinicians should also consider local epidemiology.

HR3 = Males who had sex with males after 1975; past or present injection drug use; persons who exchange sex for money or drugs, and their sex partners; injection drug-using, bisexual, or HIV-positive sex partner currently or in the past; blood transfusion during 1978-1985; persons seeking treatment for STDs. Clinicians should also consider local epidemiology.

HR4 = Sexually active females with multiple risk factors including: history of prior STD; new or multiple sex partners; age under 25; nonuse or inconsistent use of barrier contraceptives; cervical ectopy. Clinicians should consider local epidemiology of the disease in identifying other high-risk groups.

HR5 = Persons living in, traveling to, or working in areas where the disease is endemic and where periodic outbreaks occur (e.g., countries with high or intermediate endemicity; certain Alaska Native, Pacific Island, Native American, and religious communities); men who have sex with men; injection or street drug users. Vaccine may be considered for institutionalized persons and workers in these institutions, military personnel, and day-care, hospital, and laboratory workers. Clinicians should also consider local epidemiology.

HR6 = HIV positive, close contacts of persons with known or suspected TB, health care workers, persons with medical risk factors associated with TB, immigrants from countries with high TB prevalence, medically underserved low-income populations (including homeless), alcoholics, injection drug users, and residents of long-term facilities.

HR7 = Persons who continue to inject drugs.

HR8 = Immunocompetent persons with certain medical conditions, including chronic cardiac or pulmonary disease, diabetes mellitus, and anatomic asplenia. Immunocompetent persons who live in high-risk environments or social settings (e.g., certain Native American and Alaska Native populations).

HR9 = Annual vaccination of: residents of chronic care facilities; persons with chronic cardiopulmonary disorders, metabolic diseases (including diabetes mellitus), hemoglobinopathies, immunosuppression, or renal dysfunction; and health care providers for high-risk patients.

HR10 = Adolescents and young adults in settings where such individuals congregate (e.g., high schools and colleges), if they have not previously received a second dose.

HR11 = Healthy persons aged ≥13 yr without a history of chickenpox or previous immunization. Consider serologic testing for presumed susceptible persons aged ≥13 yr.

HR12 = Persons born after 1956 who lack evidence of immunity to measles or mumps (e.g., documented receipt of live vaccine on or after the first birthday, laboratory evidence of immunity, or a history of physician-diagnosed measles or mumps).

HR13 = Persons with a family or personal history of skin cancer, a large number of moles, atypical moles, poor tanning ability, or light skin, hair, and eye color.

HR14 = Women with prior pregnancy affected by neural tube defect who are planning pregnancy.

HR15 = Persons aged <17 yr living in areas with inadequate water fluoridation (<0.6 ppm).

3. AGES 25-64 YEARS

Interventions Considered and Recommended for the Periodic Health Examination

Leading Causes of Death

Malignant neoplasms
Heart diseases
Motor vehicle and other unintentional injuries
Human immunodeficiency virus (HIV) infection
Suicide and homicide

Interventions for the General Population

Screening

Blood pressure
Height and weight
Total blood cholesterol (men age 35-64, women age 45-64)
Papanicolaou (Pap) test (women)*
Fecal occult blood test† and/or sigmoidoscopy (≥50 yr)
Mammogram ± clinical breast exam‡ (women 50-69 yr)
Assess for problem drinking
Rubella serology or vaccination history§ (women of childbearing age)

Counseling

SUBSTANCE USE
Tobacco cessation
Avoid alcohol/drug use while driving, swimming, boating, etc.‖

---

*Women who are or have been sexually active and who have a cervix: q ≤3 yr.
†Annually.
‡Mammogram q 1-2 yr, or mammogram q 1-2 with annual clinical breast examination.
§Serologic testing, documented vaccination history, and routine vaccination (preferably with MMR) are equally acceptable.
‖The ability of clinician counseling to influence this behavior is unproven.

DIET AND EXERCISE

Limit fat and cholesterol; maintain caloric balance; emphasize grains, fruits, vegetables

Adequate calcium intake (women)

Regular physical activity‖

INJURY PREVENTION

Lap/shoulder belts

Motorcycle/bicycle/ATV helmets‖

Smoke detector

Safe storage/removal of firearms‖

SEXUAL BEHAVIOR

STD prevention: avoid high-risk behavior‖ condoms/female barrier with spermicide

Unintended pregnancy: contraception

DENTAL HEALTH

Regular visits to dental care provider‖

Floss, brush with fluoride toothpaste daily‖

Immunizations

Tetanus-diphtheria (Td) boosters

Rubella§ (women of childbearing age)

Chemoprophylaxis

Multivitamin with folic acid (women planning or capable of pregnancy)

Discuss hormone prophylaxis (peri- and postmenopausal women)

Interventions for High-Risk Populations

Population	Potential Interventions
High-risk sexual behavior	RPR/VDRL (HR1); screen for gonorrhea (female) HR2), HIV (HR3), chlamydia (female) (HR4); hepatitis B vaccine (HR5); hepatitis A vaccine (HR6)
Injection or street drug use	RPR/VDRL (HR1); HIV screen (HR3); hepatitis B vaccine (HR5); hepatitis A vaccine (HR6); PPD (HR7); advice to reduce infection risk (HR8)
Low income; TB contacts; immigrants, alcoholics	PPD (HR7)
Native Americans/Alaska Natives	Hepatitis A vaccine (HR6); PPD (HR7); pneumococcal vaccine (HR9)
Travelers to developing countries	Hepatitis B vaccine (HR5); hepatitis A vaccine (HR6)
Certain chronic medical conditions	PPD (HR7); pneumococcal vaccine (HR9); influenza vaccine (HR10)
Blood product recipients	HIV screen (HR3); hepatitis B vaccine (HR5)
Susceptible to measles, mumps, or varicella	MMR (HR11); varicella vaccine (HR12)
Institutionalized persons	Hepatitis A vaccine (HR6); PPD (HR7); pneumococcal vaccine (HR9); influenza vaccine (HR10)
Health care/lab workers	Hepatitis B vaccine (HR5); hepatitis A vaccine (HR6); PPD (HR7); influenza vaccine (HR10)
Family history of skin cancer: fair skin, eyes, hair	Avoid excess/midday sun, use protective clothing* (HR13)
Previous pregnancy with neural tube defect	Folic acid 4.0 mg (HR14)

From U.S. Preventive Services Task Force: *Guide to clinical preventive services,* ed 2, Baltimore, 1996, Williams & Wilkins.
*The ability of clinician counseling to influence this behavior is unproven.

High-Risk Definitions

HR1 = Persons who exchange sex for money or drugs, and their sex partners; persons with other STDs (including HIV); and sexual contacts of persons with active syphilis. Clinicians should also consider local epidemiology.

HR2 = Women who exchange sex for money or drugs, or who have had repeated episodes of gonorrhea. Clinicians should also consider local epidemiology.

HR3 = Men who had sex with men after 1975; past or present injection drug use; persons who exchange sex for money or drugs, and their sex partners; injection drug-us-

ing, bisexual, or HIV-positive sex partner currently or in the past; blood transfusion during 1978-1985; persons seeking treatment for STDs. Clinicians should also consider local epidemiology.

HR4 = Sexually active women with multiple risk factors including: history of STD; new or multiple sex partners; nonuse or inconsistent use of barrier contraceptives; cervical ectopy. Clinicians should also consider local epidemiology.

HR5 = Blood product recipients (including hemodialysis patients), persons with frequent occupational exposure to blood or blood products, men who have sex with men, injection drug users and their sex partners, persons with multiple recent sex partners, persons with other STDs (including HIV), travelers to countries with endemic hepatitis B.

HR6 = Persons living in, traveling to, or working in areas where the disease is endemic and where periodic outbreaks occur (e.g., countries with high or intermediate endemicity; certain Alaska Native, Pacific Island, Native American, and religious communities); men who have sex with men; injection or street drug users. Consider for institutionalized persons and workers in these institutions, military personnel, and day-care, hospital, and laboratory workers. Clinicians should also consider local epidemiology.

HR7 = HIV positive, close contacts of persons with known or suspected TB, health care workers, persons with medical risk factors associated with TB, immigrants from countries with high TB prevalence, medically underserved low-income populations (including homeless), alcoholics, injection drug users, and residents of long-term care facilities.

HR8 = Persons who continue to inject drugs.

HR9 = Immunocompetent institutionalized persons aged ≥50 yr and immunocompetent persons with certain medical conditions, including chronic cardiac or pulmonary disease, diabetes mellitus, and anatomic asplenia. Immunocompetent persons who live in high-risk environments or social settings (e.g., certain Native American and Alaska Native populations).

HR10 = Annual vaccination of residents of chronic care facilities; persons with chronic cardiopulmonary disorders, metabolic diseases (including diabetes mellitus), hemoglobinopathies, immunosuppression or renal dysfunction; and health care providers for high-risk patients.

HR11 = Persons born after 1956 who lack evidence of immunity to measles or mumps (e.g., documented receipts of live vaccine on or after the first birthday, laboratory evidence of immunity, or a history of physician-diagnosed measles or mumps).

HR12 = Healthy adults without a history of chickenpox or previous immunization. Consider serologic testing for presumed susceptible adults.

HR13 = Persons with a family or personal history of skin cancer, a large number of moles, atypical moles, poor tanning ability, or light skin, hair, and eye color.

HR14 = Women with previous pregnancy affected by neural tube defect who are planning pregnancy.

4. AGE 65 AND OLDER

Interventions Considered and Recommended for the Periodic Health Examination

Leading Causes of Death

Heart diseases
Malignant neoplasms (lung, colorectal, breast)

Cerebrovascular disease
Chronic obstructive pulmonary disease
Pneumonia and influenza

Interventions for the General Population

Screening

Blood pressure
Height and weight
Fecal occult blood test* and/or sigmoidoscopy
Mammogram ± clinical breast exam† (women ≤69 yr)
Papanicolaou (Pap) test (women)‡
Vision screening
Assess for hearing impairment
Assess for problem drinking

Counseling

SUBSTANCE USE
Tobacco cessation
Avoid alcohol/drug use while driving swimming, boating, etc.§
DIET AND EXERCISE
Limit fat and cholesterol; maintain caloric balance; emphasize grains, fruits, vegetables
Adequate calcium intake (women)
Regular physical activity§
INJURY PREVENTION
Lap/shoulder belts
Motorcycle and bicycle helmets§
Fall prevention§
Safe storage/removal of firearms§
Smoke detector§
Set hot water heater to <120°-130° F§
CPR training for household members
DENTAL HEALTH
Regular visits to dental care provider§
Floss, brush with fluoride toothpaste daily§
SEXUAL BEHAVIOR
STD prevention: avoid high-risk sexual behavior§; use condoms

Immunizations

Pneumococcal vaccine
Influenza*
Tetanus-diphtheria (Td) boosters

Chemoprophylaxis

Discuss hormone prophylaxis (peri- and postmenopausal women)

---

*Annually.
†Mammogram q 1-2 yr. or mammogram q1-2 yr with annual clinical breast exam.
‡All women who are or have been sexually active and who have a cervix. Consider discontinuation of testing after age 65 yr if previous regular screening with consistently normal results.
§The ability of clinician counseling to influence this behavior is unproven.

Interventions for High-Risk Populations

Population	Potential Interventions
Institutionalized persons	PPD (HR1); hepatitis A vaccine (HR2); amantadine/rimantadine (HR4)
Chronic medical conditions; TB contacts; low income; immigrants; alcoholics	PPD (HR1)
Persons ≥75 yr; or ≥70 yr with risk factors for falls	Fall-prevention intervention (HR5)
Cardiovascular disease risk factors	Consider cholesterol screening (HR6)
Family history of skin cancer; nevi; fair skin, eyes, hair	Avoid excess/midday sun, use protective clothing* (HR7)
Native Americans/Alaska Natives	PPD (HR1); hepatitis A vaccine (HR2)
Travelers to developing countries	Hepatitis A vaccine (HR2); hepatitis B vaccine (HR8)
Blood product recipients	HIV screen (HR3); hepatitis B vaccine (HR8)
High-risk sexual behavior	Hepatitis A vaccine (HR2); HIV screen (HR3); hepatitis B vaccine (HR8); RPR/VDRL (HR9)
Injection or street drug use	PPD (HR1); hepatitis A vaccine (HR2); HIV screen (HR3); hepatitis B vaccine (HR8); RPR/VDRL (HR9); advice or reduce infection risk (HR10)
Health care/lab workers	PPD (HR1); hepatitis A vaccine (HR2); amantadine/rimantadine (HR4); hepatitis B vaccine (HR8)
Persons susceptible to varicella	Varicella vaccine (HR11)

From U.S. Preventive Services Task Force: *Guide to clinical preventive services,* ed 2, Baltimore, 1996, Williams & Wilkins.
*The ability of clinician counseling to influence this behavior is unproven.

High-Risk Definitions

HR1 = HIV positive, close contacts of persons with known or suspected TB, health care workers, persons with medical risk factors associated with TB, immigrants from countries with high TB prevalence, medically underserved low-income populations (including homeless), alcoholics, injection drug users, and residents of long-term care facilities.

HR2 = Persons living in, traveling to, or working in areas where the disease is endemic and where periodic outbreaks occur (e.g., countries with high or intermediate endemicity; certain Alaska Native, Pacific Island, Native American, and religious communities); men who have sex with men; injection or street drug users. Consider for institutionalized persons and workers in these institutions, and day-care, hospital, and laboratory workers. Clinicians should also consider local epidemiology.

HR3 = Men who had sex with men after 1975; past or present injection drug use; persons who exchange sex for money or drugs, and their sex partners; injection drug-using, bisexual, or HIV-positive sex partner currently or in the past; blood transfusion during 1978-1985; persons seeking treatment for STDs. Clinicians should also consider local epidemiology.

HR4 = Consider for persons who have not received influenza vaccine or are vaccinated late; when the vaccine may be ineffective due to major antigenic changes in the virus; for unvaccinated persons who provide home care for high-risk persons; to supplement protection provided by vaccine in persons who are expected to have a poor antibody response; and for high-risk persons in whom the vaccine is contraindicated.

HR5 = Persons aged 75 years and older; or aged 70-74 with one or more additional risk factors including: use of certain psychoactive and cardiac medications (e.g., benzodiazepines, antihypertensives); use of 4 prescription medications; impaired cognition, strength, balance, or gait. Intensive individualized home-based multifactorial fall prevention intervention is recommended in settings where adequate resources are available to deliver such services.

HR6 = Although evidence is insufficient to recommend routine screening in elderly persons, clinicians should consider cholesterol screening on a case-by-case basis for persons ages 65-75 with additional risk factors (e.g., smoking, diabetes, or hypertension).

HR7 = Persons with a family or personal history of skin cancer, a large number of moles, atypical moles, poor tanning ability, or light skin, hair, and eye color.

HR8 = Blood product recipients (including hemodialysis patients), persons with frequent occupational exposure to blood or blood products, men who have sex with men, injection drug users and their sex partners, persons with multiple recent sex partners, persons with other STDs (including HIV), travelers to countries with endemic hepatitis B.

HR9 = Persons who exchange sex for money or drugs and their sex partners; persons with other STDs (including HIV); and sexual contacts of persons with active syphilis. Clinicians should also consider local epidemiology.

HR10 = Persons who continue to inject drugs.

HR11 = Healthy adults without a history of chickenpox or previous immunization. Consider serologic testing for presumed susceptible adults.

5. PREGNANT WOMEN*

Interventions Considered and Recommended for the Periodic Health Examination

Interventions for the General Population

Screening

FIRST VISIT

Blood pressure

Hemoglobin/hematocrit

Hepatitis B surface antigen (HbsAg)

RPR/VDRL

Chlamydia screen (<25 yr)

Rubella serology or vaccination history

D(Rh) typing, antibody screen

Offer CVS (<13 wk)† or amniocentesis (15-18 wk)† (age ≥35 yr)

---

*See Appendixes A.2-2 and A.2-3 for other preventive services recommended for women of this age group.

†Women with access to counseling and follow-up services, reliable standardized laboratories, skilled high-resolution ultrasound, and, for those receiving serum marker testing, amniocentesis capabilities.

Offer hemoglobinopathy screening

Assess for problem or risk drinking

Offer HIV screening‡

FOLLOW-UP VISITS

Blood pressure

Urine culture (12-16 wk)

Offer amniocentesis (15-18 wk)† (age ≥35 yr)

Offer multiple marker testing† (15-18 wk)

Offer serum α-fetoprotein† (16-18 wk)

Counseling

Tobacco cessation; effects of passive smoking

Alcohol/other drug use

Nutrition, including adequate calcium intake

Encourage breastfeeding

Lap/shoulder belts

Infant safety car seats

STD prevention: avoid high-risk sexual behavior; use condoms

Chemoprophylaxis

Multivitamin with folic acid§

---

‡Universal screening is recommended for areas (states, counties, or cities) with an increased prevalence of HIV infection among pregnant women. In low-prevalence areas, the choice between universal and targeted screening may depend on other considerations.

§Beginning at least 1 mo before conception and continuing through the first trimester.

Interventions for High-Risk Populations

Population	Potential Interventions
High-risk sexual behavior	Screen for chlamydia (1st visit) (HR1), gonorrhea (1st visit) (HR2), HIV (1st visit) (HR3); HbsAg (3rd trimester) (HR4); RPR/VDRL (3rd trimester) (HR5)
Blood transfusion 1978-1985	HIV screen (1st visit) (HR3)
Injection drug use	HIV screen (HR3); HbsAg (3rd trimester) (HR4); advice to reduce infection risk (HR6)
Unsensitized D-negative women	D(Rh) antibody testing (24-28 wk) (HR7)
Risk factors for Down syndrome	Offer CVS* (1st trimester), amniocentesis* (15-18 wk) (HR8)
Prior pregnancy with neural tube defect	Offer amniocentesis* (15-18 wk), folic acid 4.0 mg† (HR9)

From U.S. Preventive Services Task Force: *Guide to clinical preventive services,* ed 2 Baltimore, 1996, Williams & Wilkins.

*Women with access to counseling and follow-up services, reliable standardized laboratories, skilled high-resolution ultrasound, and, for those receiving serum marker testing, amniocentesis capabilities.

†Beginning at least 1 mo before conception and continuing through the first trimester.

High-Risk Definitions

HR1 = Women with history of STD or new or multiple sex partners. Clinicians should also consider local epidemiology. Chlamydia screen should be repeated in 3rd trimester if at continued risk.

HR2 = Women under age 25 with two or more sex partners in the last year, or whose sex partner has multiple sexual contacts; women who exchange sex for money or drugs; and women with a history of repeated episodes of gonorrhea. Clinicians should also consider local epidemiology. Gonorrhea screen should be repeated in the 3rd trimester if at continued risk.

HR3 = In areas where universal screening is not performed due to low prevalence of HIV infection, pregnant women with the following individual risk factors should be screened: past or present injection drug use; women who exchange sex for money or drugs; injection drug-using, bisexual, or HIV-positive sex partner currently or in the past; blood transfusion during 1978-1985; persons seeking treatment for STDs.

HR4 = Women who are initially HbsAg negative who are at high risk due to injection drug use, suspected exposure to hepatitis B during pregnancy, multiple sex partners.

HR5 = Women who exchange sex for money or drugs,

women with other STDs (including HIV), and sexual contacts of persons with active syphilis. Clinicians should also consider local epidemiology.

HR6 = Women who continue to inject drugs.

HR7 = Unsensitized D-negative women.

HR8 = Prior pregnancy affected by Down syndrome, advanced maternal age (≥35 yr), known carriage of chromosome rearrangement.

HR9 = Women with previous pregnancy affected by neural tube defect.

6. CONDITIONS FOR WHICH CLINICIANS SHOULD REMAIN ALERT

Population	Condition
Infants and young children (<3 yr)	Symptoms and signs of hearing impairment
Infants and children	Signs of ocular misalignment
Children	Evidence of early childhood caries, mismatching of upper and lower dental arches, dental crowding or malalignment, premature loss of primary posterior teeth (baby molars) obvious mouth breathing
Adolescents	Large spinal curvatures
Adolescents, young adults, persons at increased risk for depression	Depressive symptoms
General population	Various presentations of family violence
General population	Symptoms and signs of drug abuse
General population	Obvious signs of untreated tooth decay or mottling, inflamed or cyanotic gingiva, loose teeth, and severe halitosis
General population, particularly those with established risk factors	Skin lesions with malignant features
Persons who use tobacco, older persons who drink alcohol regularly	Symptoms and signs of oral cancer and premalignancy
Persons with established risk factors for suicide	Evidence of suicidal ideation
Older persons	Changes in functional performance
Older persons, postpartum women, persons with Down syndrome	Subtle or nonspecific symptoms and signs of thyroid dysfunction
Older persons, smokers, diabetic persons	Symptoms of peripheral arterial disease

Modified from U.S. Preventive Services Task Force: *Guide to clinical preventive services,* ed 2, Baltimore, 1996, Williams & Wilkins.

A.3   Declaration of Alma Ata

The International Conference on Primary Health Care, meeting in Alma Ata this twelfth day of September in the year nineteen hundred and seventy-eight, expressing the need for urgent action of all governments, all health and development workers, and the world community to protect and promote the health of all the people of the world, hereby makes the following Declaration:

I

The Conference strongly reaffirms that health, which is a state of complete physical, mental, and social well-being, and not merely the absence of disease or infirmity, is a fun-

damental human right and that the attainment of the highest possible level of health is a most important worldwide social goal, whose realization requires the action of many other social and economic sectors in addition to the health sector.

II

The existing gross inequality in the health status of the people, particularly between developed and developing countries and within countries, is politically, socially, and economically unacceptable and is therefore of common concern to all countries.

III

Economic and social development, based on a new international economic order, is of basic importance to the fullest attainment of health for all and to the reduction of the gap between the health status of developing and developed countries. The promotion and protection of the health of the people are essential to sustained economic and social development and contribute to a better quality of life and to world peace.

IV

The people have the right and duty to participate individually and collectively in the planning and implementation of their health care.

V

Governments have a responsibility for the health of their people, which can be fulfilled only by the provision of adequate health and social measures. In the coming decades a main social target of governments, international organizations, and the whole world community should be the attainment by all peoples of the world by the year 2000 of a level of health that will permit them to lead a socially and economically productive life. Primary health care is the key to attaining this target as part of development in the spirit of social justice.

VI

Primary health care is essential health care based on practical, scientifically sound, and socially acceptable methods and technology made universally accessible to individuals and families in the community through their full participation and at a cost that the community and country can afford to maintain at every stage of their development in the spirit of self-reliance and self-determination. It forms an integral part both of the country's health system, of which primary health care is the central function and main focus, and of the overall social and economic development of the community. It is the first level of contact for individuals, the family, and the community with the national health system bringing health care as close as possible to where people live and work, and it constitutes the first element of a continuing health care process.

VII

Primary Health Care

1. Reflects and evolves from the economic conditions and sociocultural and political characteristics of the country and its communities and is based on the application of the relevant results of social, biomedical, and health services research and public health experience;

2. Addresses the main health problems in the community, providing promotive, preventive, curative, and rehabilitative services accordingly;

3. Includes at least education concerning prevailing health problems and the methods of preventing and controlling them; promotion of food supply and proper nutrition; an adequate supply of safe water and basic sanitation; maternal and child health care, including family planning; immunization against the major infectious diseases; prevention and control of locally endemic diseases; appropriate treatment of common diseases and injuries; and provision of essential drugs;

4. Involves, in addition to health sector, all related sectors and aspects of national and community development, in particular agriculture, animal husbandry, food industry, education, housing, public works, communication, and other sectors; and demands the coordinated efforts of all those sectors;

5. Requires and promotes maximum community and individual self-reliance and participation in the planning, organization, operation, and control of primary health care making fullest use of local, national and other available resources; and to this end, develops through appropriate education the ability of communities to participate;

6. Should be sustained by integrated, functional, and mutually supportive referral levels, on health workers, including physicians, nurses, midwives, auxiliaries, and community workers, as applicable, as well as on traditional practitioners as needed, suitably trained socially and technically to work as a health team and to respond to the expressed health needs of the community; and

7. Relies, at local and referral levels, on health workers, including physicians, nurses, midwives, auxiliaries, and community workers, as applicable, as well as on traditional practitioners as needed, suitably trained socially and technically to work as a health team and to respond to the expressed health needs of the community.

VIII

All governments should formulate national policies, strategies, and plans of action to launch and sustain primary health care as part of a comprehensive national health system and in coordination with other sectors. To this end, it will be necessary to exercise political will, to mobilize the country's resources, and to use available external resources rationally.

IX

All countries should cooperate in a spirit of partnership and service to ensure primary health care for all people because the attainment of health by people in any one country directly concerns and benefits every other country. In this context the joint WHO-UNICEF report* on primary health care constitutes a solid basis for the further development and operation of Primary Health Care through the world.

X

An acceptable level of health for all the people of the world by the year 2000 can be attained through a fuller and better

use of the world's resources, a considerable part of which is now spent on armaments and military conflicts. A genuine policy of independence, peace, détente, and disarmament could and should release additional resources that could well be devoted to peaceful aims and in particular to the acceleration of social and economic development of which primary health care, as an essential part, should be allotted its proper share.

*From World Health Organization: *Primary health care: report of the International Conference on Primary Health Care,* Alma-Ata, USSR, Sept 6-12, 1978, Geneva, 1978, WHO.

Appendix B

Community Assets and Resources

START OF CARE ASSESSMENT FOR _____

DEMOGRAPHICS AND PATIENT HISTORY

1. (M0080) Discipline of Person Completing Assessment:

① RN
② PT
③ SLP/ST
④ OT

> **USE BLUE OR BLACK PEN**
> **FILL-IN EACH OVAL COMPLETELY**
> ☑ Wrong! ☒ Wrong! ● Right!!!

2. (M0100) This Assessment is Currently Being Completed for the Following Reason:

Start/Resumption of Care

① **Start of care--further visits planned**
② **Start of care--no further visits planned**
③ **Resumption of care (after inpatient stay)**

> **Follow-Up**
> Recertification (follow-up) reassessment [Go to *M0150*]
> Other follow-up [Go to *M0150*]
> **Transfer to an Inpatient Facility**
> Transferred to an inpatient facility--patient not discharged from agency [Go to M0830]
> Transferred to an inpatient facility--patient discharged from agency [Go to M0830]
> **Discharge from Agency--Not to an Inpatient Facility**
> Death at home [Go to *M0906*]
> Discharge from agency [Go to *M0150*]
> Discharge from agency--no visits completed after start/resumption of care assessment [Go to *M0830*]

3. (M0140) Race/Ethnicity (as identified by patient):

① American Indian or Alaska Native
② Asian
③ Black or African-American
④ Hispanic or Latino
⑤ Native Hawaiian or Pacific Islander
⑥ White
Ⓤ UK-Unknown

4. (M0150) Current Payment Sources for Home Care: (Mark all that apply.)

○ 0 - None; no charge for current services
○ 1 - Medicare (traditional fee-for-service)
○ 2 - Medicare (HMO/managed care)
○ 3 - Medicaid (traditional fee-for-service)
○ 4 - Medicaid (HMO/managed care)
○ 5 - Workers' compensation
○ 6 - Title programs (e.g., Title III, V, or XX)
○ 7 - Other government (e.g., CHAMPUS, VA, etc.)
○ 8 - Private insurance
○ 9 - Private HMO/managed care
○ 10 - Self-pay
○ 11 - Other (specify)_____
○ UK - Unknown

5. (M0160) Financial Factors limiting the ability of the patient/family to meet basic health needs: **(Mark all that apply.)**

⓪ None
① Unable to afford medicine or medical supplies
② Unable to afford medical expenses that are not covered by insurance/Medicare (e.g., copayments)
③ Unable to afford rent/utility bills
④ Unable to afford food
⑤ Other (specify)_____

6. (M0170) From which of the following **Inpatient Facilities** was the patient discharged <u>during the past 14 days</u>?
(Mark all that apply.)

① Hospital
② Rehabilitation facility
③ Nursing home
④ Other (specify)_____
Ⓝ NA-Patient was not discharged from an inpatient facility
  ↓ **[If NA, go to *M0200* (Question 9)]**

7. (M0180) Inpatient Discharge Date

     Ⓤ UK-Unknown

Month	Day	Year
○ Jan		
○ Feb		
○ Mar	⓪ ⓪	⓪ ⓪ ⓪ ⓪
○ Apr	① ①	① ① ① ①
○ May	② ②	② ② ② ②
○ Jun	③ ③	③ ③ ③ ③
○ Jul	④ ④	④ ④ ④ ④
○ Aug	⑤ ⑤	⑤ ⑤ ⑤ ⑤
○ Sep	⑥ ⑥	⑥ ⑥ ⑥ ⑥
○ Oct	⑦ ⑦	⑦ ⑦ ⑦ ⑦
○ Nov	⑧ ⑧	⑧ ⑧ ⑧ ⑧
○ Dec	⑨ ⑨	⑨ ⑨ ⑨ ⑨

8. (M0190) Inpatient Diagnoses and ICD code categories (three digits required; five digits optional) <u>for only those conditions treated during an inpatient facility stay within the last 14 days</u> (no surgical or V-codes):

Inpatient Facility Diagnosis

a. _____

b. _____

a. ICD-9 Code   b. ICD-9 Code

⓪ ⓪ ⓪ ⓪ ⓪	⓪ ⓪ ⓪ ⓪ ⓪
① ① ① ① ①	① ① ① ① ①
② ② ② ② ②	② ② ② ② ②
③ ③ ③ ③ ③	③ ③ ③ ③ ③
④ ④ ④ ④ ④	④ ④ ④ ④ ④
⑤ ⑤ ⑤ ⑤ ⑤	⑤ ⑤ ⑤ ⑤ ⑤
⑥ ⑥ ⑥ ⑥ ⑥	⑥ ⑥ ⑥ ⑥ ⑥
⑦ ⑦ ⑦ ⑦ ⑦	⑦ ⑦ ⑦ ⑦ ⑦
⑧ ⑧ ⑧ ⑧ ⑧	⑧ ⑧ ⑧ ⑧ ⑧
⑨ ⑨ ⑨ ⑨ ⑨	⑨ ⑨ ⑨ ⑨ ⑨

9. (M0200) Medical or Treatment Regimen Change Within Past 14 Days: Has this patient experienced a change in medical or treatment regimen (e.g., medication, treatment, or service change due to new or additional diagnosis, etc.) within the last 14 days?

    ⓪ No
        ⬇ [If No, go to *M0220* (Question 11)]
    ① Yes

10. (M0210) List the patient's **Medical Diagnoses** and ICD code categories (three digits required; five digits optional) <u>for those conditions requiring changed medical or treatment regimen</u> (no surgical or V-codes):

Changed Medical Regimen Diagnosis

a. _____

b. _____

c. _____

d. _____

a. ICD-9 Code   b. ICD-9 Code   c. ICD-9 Code   d. ICD-9 Code

⓪ ⓪ ⓪ ⓪ ⓪	⓪ ⓪ ⓪ ⓪ ⓪	⓪ ⓪ ⓪ ⓪ ⓪	⓪ ⓪ ⓪ ⓪ ⓪
① ① ① ① ①	① ① ① ① ①	① ① ① ① ①	① ① ① ① ①
② ② ② ② ②	② ② ② ② ②	② ② ② ② ②	② ② ② ② ②
③ ③ ③ ③ ③	③ ③ ③ ③ ③	③ ③ ③ ③ ③	③ ③ ③ ③ ③
④ ④ ④ ④ ④	④ ④ ④ ④ ④	④ ④ ④ ④ ④	④ ④ ④ ④ ④
⑤ ⑤ ⑤ ⑤ ⑤	⑤ ⑤ ⑤ ⑤ ⑤	⑤ ⑤ ⑤ ⑤ ⑤	⑤ ⑤ ⑤ ⑤ ⑤
⑥ ⑥ ⑥ ⑥ ⑥	⑥ ⑥ ⑥ ⑥ ⑥	⑥ ⑥ ⑥ ⑥ ⑥	⑥ ⑥ ⑥ ⑥ ⑥
⑦ ⑦ ⑦ ⑦ ⑦	⑦ ⑦ ⑦ ⑦ ⑦	⑦ ⑦ ⑦ ⑦ ⑦	⑦ ⑦ ⑦ ⑦ ⑦
⑧ ⑧ ⑧ ⑧ ⑧	⑧ ⑧ ⑧ ⑧ ⑧	⑧ ⑧ ⑧ ⑧ ⑧	⑧ ⑧ ⑧ ⑧ ⑧
⑨ ⑨ ⑨ ⑨ ⑨	⑨ ⑨ ⑨ ⑨ ⑨	⑨ ⑨ ⑨ ⑨ ⑨	⑨ ⑨ ⑨ ⑨ ⑨

11. (M0220) Conditions Prior to Medical or Treatment Regimen Change or Inpatient Stay Within Past 14 Days: If this patient experienced an inpatient facility discharge or change in medical or treatment regimen within the past 14 days, indicate any conditions which existed prior to the inpatient stay or change in medical or treatment regimen. **(Mark all that apply.)**

- ① Urinary incontinence
- ② Indwelling/suprapubic catheter
- ③ Intractable pain
- ④ Impaired decision-making
- ⑤ Disruptive or socially inappropriate behavior
- ⑥ Memory loss to the extent that supervision required
- ⑦ None of the above
- Ⓝ NA-No inpatient facility discharge and no change in medical or treatment regimen in past 14 days
- Ⓤ UK-Unknown

12. (M0230/M0240) Diagnoses and Severity Index: List each medical diagnosis or problem for which the patient is receiving home care and ICD code category (three digits required; five digits optional - no surgical or V-codes) and rate them using the following severity index. (Choose one value that represents the most severe rating appropriate for each diagnosis.)

Severity Rating Index

0 = Asymptomatic, no treatment needed at this time
1 = Symptoms well controlled with current therapy
2 = Symptoms controlled with difficulty, affecting daily functioning; patient needs ongoing monitoring
3 = Symptoms poorly controlled, patient needs frequent adjustment in treatment and dose monitoring
4 = Symptoms poorly controlled, history of rehospitalizations

(M0230) Primary Diagnosis	**Severity Rating**
_____	⓪ ① ② ③ ④

(M0240) Other Diagnoses

a. _____	⓪ ① ② ③ ④
b. _____	⓪ ① ② ③ ④
c. _____	⓪ ① ② ③ ④
d. _____	⓪ ① ② ③ ④
e. _____	⓪ ① ② ③ ④

Primary	Other				
ICD-9 Code	a. ICD-9 Code	b. ICD-9 Code	c. ICD-9 Code	d. ICD-9 Code	e. ICD-9 Code

13. (M0250) Therapies the patient receives at home: **(Mark all that apply.)**

- ① Intravenous or infusion therapy (excludes TPN)
- ② Parenteral nutrition (TPN or lipids)
- ③ Enteral nutrition (nasogastric, gastrostomy, jejunostomy, or any other artificial entry into the alimentary canal)
- ④ None of the above

14. (M0260) Overall Prognosis: BEST description of patient's overall prognosis for recovery from this episode of illness.

- ⓪ Poor: little or no recovery is expected and/or further decline is imminent
- ① Good/Fair: partial to full recovery is expected
- Ⓤ UK-Unknown

15. **(M0270) Rehabilitative Prognosis:** BEST description of patient's prognosis for <u>functional status</u>.

    ⓪ Guarded: minimal improvement in functional status is expected; decline is possible
    ① Good: marked improvement in functional status is expected
    Ⓤ UK-Unknown

16. **(M0280) Life Expectancy:** (Physician documentation is not required.)

    ⓪ Life expectancy is greater than 6 months
    ① Life expectancy is 6 months or fewer

17. **(M0290) High Risk Factors** characterizing this patient: **(Mark all that apply.)**

    ① Heavy smoking
    ② Obesity
    ③ Alcohol dependency
    ④ Drug dependency
    ⑤ None of the above
    Ⓤ UK-Unknown

LIVING ARRANGEMENTS

18. **(M0300) Current Residence:**

    ① Patient's owned or rented residence (house, apartment, or mobile home owned or rented by patient/couple/ significant other)
    ② Family member's residence
    ③ Boarding home or rented room
    ④ Board and care or assisted living facility
    ⑤ Other (specify)_____

19. **(M0340) Patient Lives With: (Mark all that apply.)**

    ① Lives alone
    ② With spouse or significant other
    ③ With other family member
    ④ With a friend
    ⑤ With paid help (other than home care agency staff)
    ⑥ With other than above

20. **(M0310) Structural Barriers** in the patient's environment limiting independent mobility: **(Mark all that apply.)**

    ⓪ None
    ① Stairs inside home which <u>must</u> be used by the patient (e.g., to get to toileting, sleeping, eating areas)
    ② Stairs inside home which are used optionally (e.g., to get to laundry facilities)
    ③ Stairs leading from inside house to outside
    ④ Narrow or obstructed doorways

21. **(M0320) Safety Hazards** found in the patient's current place of residence: **(Mark all that apply.)**

    ○ 0 - None
    ○ 1 - Inadequate floor, roof, or windows
    ○ 2 - Inadequate lighting
    ○ 3 - Unsafe gas/electric appliance
    ○ 4 - Inadequate heating
    ○ 5 - Inadequate cooling
    ○ 6 - Lack of fire safety devices
    ○ 7 - Unsafe floor coverings
    ○ 8 - Inadequate stair railings
    ○ 9 - Improperly stored hazardous materials
    ○ 10 - Lead-based paint
    ○ 11 - Other (specify) _____

22. **(M0330) Sanitation Hazards** found in the patient's current place of residence: **(Mark all that apply.)**

    ○ 0 - None
    ○ 1 - No running water
    ○ 2 - Contaminated water
    ○ 3 - No toileting facilities
    ○ 4 - Outdoor toileting facilities only
    ○ 5 - Inadequate sewage disposal
    ○ 6 - Inadequate/improper food storage
    ○ 7 - No food refrigeration
    ○ 8 - No cooking facilities
    ○ 9 - Insects/rodents present
    ○ 10 - No scheduled trash pickup
    ○ 11 - Cluttered/soiled living area
    ○ 12 - Other (specify) _____

SUPPORTIVE ASSISTANCE

23. **(M0350) Assisting Person(s) Other than Home Care Agency Staff: (Mark all that apply.)**

    ① Relatives, friends, or neighbors living outside the home
    ② Person residing in the home (EXCLUDING paid help)
    ③ Paid help
    ④ None of the above
        ↓ **[If None of the above, go to *M0390* (Question 27)]**
    Ⓤ UK-Unknown
        ↓ **[If Unknown, go to *M0390* (Question 27)]**

24. **(M0360) Primary Caregiver** taking <u>lead</u> responsibility for providing or managing the patient's care, providing the most frequent assistance, etc. (other than home care agency staff):

    ⓪ No one person
        ↓ **[If No one person, go to *M0390* (Question 27)]**
    ① Spouse or significant other
    ② Daughter or son
    ③ Other family member
    ④ Friend or neighbor or community or church member
    ⑤ Paid help
    Ⓤ UK-Unknown
        ↓ **[If Unknown, go to *M0390* (Question 27)]**

0065

25. **(M0370) How Often** does the patient receive assistance from the primary caregiver?

  ① Several times during day and night
  ② Several times during day
  ③ Once daily
  ④ Three or more times per week
  ⑤ One to two times per week
  ○ Less often than weekly
  Ⓤ UK-Unknown

26. **(M0380) Type of Primary Caregiver Assistance: (Mark all that apply.)**

  ① ADL assistance (e.g., bathing, dressing, toileting, bowel/bladder, eating/feeding)
  ② IADL assistance (e.g., meds, meals, housekeeping, laundry, telephone, shopping, finances)
  ③ Environmental support (housing, home maintenance)
  ④ Psychosocial support (socialization, companionship, recreation)
  ⑤ Advocates or facilitates patient's participation in appropriate medical care
  ⑥ Financial agent, power of attorney, or conservator of finance
  ⑦ Health care agent, conservator of person, or medical power of attorney
  Ⓤ UK-Unknown

SENSORY STATUS

27. **(M0390) Vision** with corrective lenses if the patient usually wears them:

  ⓪ Normal vision: sees adequately in most situations; can see medication labels, newsprint.
  ① Partially impaired: cannot see medication labels or newsprint, but <u>can</u> see obstacles in path, and the surrounding layout; can count fingers at arm's length.
  ② Severely impaired: cannot locate objects without hearing or touching them <u>or</u> patient non-responsive.

28. **(M0400) Hearing and Ability to Understand Spoken Language** in patient's own language (with hearing aids if the patient usually uses them):

  ⓪ No observable impairment. Able to hear and understand complex or detailed instructions and extended or abstract conversation.
  ① With minimal difficulty, able to hear and understand most multi-step instructions and ordinary conversation. May need occasional repetition, extra time, or louder voice.
  ② Has moderate difficulty hearing and understanding simple, one-step instructions and brief conversation; needs frequent prompting or assistance.
  ③ Has severe difficulty hearing and understanding simple greetings and short comments. Requires multiple repetitions, restatements, demonstrations, additional time.
  ④ <u>Unable</u> to hear and understand familiar words or common expressions consistently, <u>or</u> patient nonresponsive.

29. **(M0410) Speech and Oral (Verbal) Expression of Language** (in patient's own language):

  ⓪ Expresses complex ideas, feelings, and needs clearly, completely, and easily in all situations with no observable impairment.
  ① Minimal difficulty in expressing ideas and needs (may take extra time; makes occasional errors in word choice, grammar or speech intelligibility; needs minimal prompting or assistance).
  ② Expresses simple ideas or needs with moderate difficulty (needs prompting or assistance, errors in word choice, organization or speech intelligibility). Speaks in phrases or short sentences.
  ③ Has severe difficulty expressing basic ideas or needs and requires maximal assistance or guessing by listener. Speech limited to single words or short phrases.
  ④ <u>Unable</u> to express basic needs even with maximal prompting or assistance but is not comatose or unresponsive (e.g., speech is nonsensical or unintelligible).
  ⑤ Patient nonresponsive or unable to speak.

30. **(M0420) Frequency of Pain** interfering with patient's activity or movement:

  ⓪ Patient has no pain or pain does not interfere with activity or movement
  ① Less often than daily
  ② Daily, but not constantly
  ③ All of the time

31. **(M0430) Intractable Pain:** Is the patient experiencing pain that is <u>not easily relieved</u>, occurs at least daily, and affects the patient's sleep, appetite, physical or emotional energy, concentration, personal relationships, emotions, or ability or desire to perform physical activity?

  ⓪ No
  ① Yes

32. **(M0440)** Does this patient have a **Skin Lesion** or an **Open Wound?** This excludes "OSTOMIES."

ⓞ No
↓ [If No, go to *M0490* (Question 45)]
① Yes

33. **(M0445)** Does this patient have a **Pressure Ulcer?**

ⓞ No
↓ [If No, go to *M0468* (Question 37)]
① Yes

34. **(M0450) Current Number of Pressure Ulcers at Each Stage:** (one response for each stage.)

Pressure Ulcer Stages   **Number of Pressure Ulcers**

a) Stage 1: Nonblanchable erythema of intact skin; the heralding of skin ulceration. In darker-pigmented skin, warmth, edema, hardness, or discolored skin may be indicators.　　ⓞ ① ② ③ ④ **or more**

b) Stage 2: Partial thickness skin loss involving epidermis and/or dermis. The ulcer is superficial and presents clinically as an abrasion, blister, or shallow crater.　　ⓞ ① ② ③ ④ **or more**

c) Stage 3: Full-thickness skin loss involving damage or necrosis of subcutaneous tissue which may extend down to, but not through, underlying fascia. The ulcer presents clinically as a deep crater with or without undermining of adjacent tissue.　　ⓞ ① ② ③ ④ **or more**

d) Stage 4: Full-thickness skin loss with extensive destruction, tissue necrosis, or damage to muscle, bone, or supporting structures (e.g., tendon, joint capsule, etc.)　　ⓞ ① ② ③ ④ **or more**

e) In addition to the above, is there at least one pressure ulcer that cannot be observed due to the presence of eschar or a nonremovable dressing, including casts?　　ⓞ No　① Yes

35. **(M0460) Stage of Most Problematic (Observable) Pressure Ulcer:**

① Stage 1
② Stage 2
③ Stage 3
④ Stage 4
Ⓝ NA-No observable pressure ulcer

36. **(M0464) Status of Most Problematic (Observable) Pressure Ulcer:**

① Fully granulating
② Early/partial granulation
③ Not healing
Ⓝ NA-No observable pressure ulcer

37. **(M0468)** Does this patient have a **Stasis Ulcer?**

ⓞ No
↓ [If No, go to *M0482* (Question 41)]
① Yes

38. **(M0470) Current Number of Observable Stasis Ulcer(s):**

ⓞ Zero
① One
② Two
③ Three
④ Four or more

39. **(M0474)** Does this patient have at least one **Stasis Ulcer that Cannot be Observed** due to the presence of a nonremovable dressing?

ⓞ No
① Yes

40. **(M0476) Status of Most Problematic (Observable) Stasis Ulcer:**

① Fully granulating
② Early/partial granulation
③ Not healing
Ⓝ NA-No observable stasis ulcer

41. **(M0482)** Does this patient have a **Surgical Wound?**

ⓞ No
↓ [If No, go to *M0490* (Question 45)]
① Yes

42. **(M0484) Current Number of (Observable) Surgical Wounds:** (If a wound is partially closed but has <u>more</u> than one opening, consider each opening as a separate wound.)

- ⓪ Zero
- ① One
- ② Two
- ③ Three
- ④ Four or more

43. **(M0486)** Does this patient have at least one **Surgical Wound that Cannot be Observed** due to the presence of a nonremovable dressing?

- ⓪ No
- ① Yes

44. **(M0488) Status of Most Problematic (Observable) Surgical Wound:**

- ① Fully granulating
- ② Early/partial granulation
- ③ Not healing
- Ⓝ NA-No observable surgical wound

RESPIRATORY STATUS

45. **(M0490)** When is the patient dyspneic or noticeably **Short of Breath?**

- ⓪ Never, patient is not short of breath
- ① When walking more than 20 feet, climbing stairs
- ② With moderate exertion (e.g., while dressing, using commode or bedpan, walking distances less than 20 feet)
- ③ With minimal exertion (e.g., while eating, talking, or performing other ADLs) or with agitation
- ④ At rest (during day or night)

46. **(M0500) Respiratory Treatments** utilized at home: **(Mark all that apply.)**

- ① Oxygen (intermittent or continuous)
- ② Ventilator (continually or at night)
- ③ Continuous positive airway pressure
- ④ None of the above

ELIMINATION STATUS

47. **(M0510)** Has this patient been treated for a **Urinary Tract Infection** in the past 14 days?

- ⓪ No
- ① Yes
- Ⓝ NA-Patient on prophylactic treatment
- Ⓤ UK-Unknown

48. **(M0520) Urinary Incontinence or Urinary Catheter Presence:**

- ⓪ No incontinence or catheter (includes anuria or ostomy for urinary drainage)
  ↓ **[If No, go to *M0540* (Question 50)]**
- ① Patient is incontinent
- ② Patient requires a urinary catheter (i.e., external, indwelling, intermittent, suprapubic)
  ↓ **[Go to *M0540* (Question 50)]**

49. **(M0530) When** does **Urinary Incontinence** occur?

- ⓪ Timed-voiding defers incontinence
- ① During the night only
- ② During the day and night

50. **(M0540) Bowel Incontinence Frequency:**

- ⓪ Very rarely or never has bowel incontinence
- ① Less than once weekly
- ② One to three times weekly
- ③ Four to six times weekly
- ④ On a daily basis
- ⑤ More often than once daily
- Ⓝ NA-Patient has ostomy for bowel elimination
- Ⓤ UK-Unknown

51. **(M0550) Ostomy for Bowel Elimination:** Does this patient have an ostomy for bowel elimination that (within the last 14 days): a) was related to an inpatient facility stay, <u>or</u> b) necessitated a change in medical or treatment regimen?

- ⓪ Patient does <u>not</u> have an ostomy for bowel elimination.
- ① Patient's ostomy was <u>not</u> related to an inpatient stay and did <u>not</u> necessitate change in medical or treatment regimen.
- ② The ostomy <u>was</u> related to an inpatient stay or <u>did</u> necessitate change in medical or treatment regimen.

52. **(M0560) Cognitive Functioning:** (Patient's current level of alertness, orientation, comprehension, concentration, and immediate memory for simple commands.)

⓪ Alert/oriented, able to focus and shift attention, comprehends and recalls task directions independently.
① Requires prompting (cueing, repetition, reminders) only under stressful or unfamiliar conditions.
② Requires assistance and some direction in specific situations (e.g., on all tasks involving shifting of attention), or consistently requires low stimulus environment due to distractibility.
③ Requires considerable assistance in routine situations. Is not alert and oriented or is unable to shift attention and recall directions more than half the time.
④ Totally dependent due to disturbances such as constant disorientation, coma, persistent vegetative state, or delirium.

53. **(M0570) When Confused (Reported or Observed):**

⓪ Never
① In new or complex situations only
② On awakening or at night only
③ During the day and evening, but not constantly
④ Constantly
Ⓝ NA-Patient nonresponsive

54. **(M0580) When Anxious (Reported or Observed):**

⓪ None of the time
① Less often than daily
② Daily, but not constantly
③ All of the time
Ⓝ NA-Patient nonresponsive

55. **(M0590) Depressive Feelings Reported or Observed in Patient: (Mark all that apply.)**

① Depressed mood (e.g., feeling sad, tearful)
② Sense of failure or self reproach
③ Hopelessness
④ Recurrent thoughts of death
⑤ Thoughts of suicide
⑥ None of the above feelings observed or reported

56. **(M0600) Patient Behaviors (Reported or Observed): (Mark all that apply.)**

① Indecisiveness, lack of concentration
② Diminished interest in most activities
③ Sleep disturbances
④ Recent change in appetite or weight
⑤ Agitation
⑥ A suicide attempt
⑦ None of the above behaviors observed or reported

57. **(M0610) Behaviors Demonstrated <u>at Least Once a Week</u> (Reported or Observed): (Mark all that apply.)**

① Memory deficit: failure to recognize familiar persons/places, inability to recall events of past 24 hours, significant memory loss so that supervision is required
② Impaired decision-making: failure to perform usual ADLs or IADLs, inability to appropriately stop activities, jeopardizes safety through actions
③ Verbal disruption: yelling, threatening, excessive profanity, sexual references, etc.
④ Physical aggression: aggressive or combative to self and others (e.g., hits self, throws objects, punches, dangerous maneuvers with wheelchair or other objects)
⑤ Disruptive, infantile, or socially inappropriate behavior (**excludes** verbal actions)
⑥ Delusional, hallucinatory, or paranoid behavior
⑦ None of the above behaviors demonstrated

58. **(M0620) Frequency of Behavior Problems (Reported or Observed)** (e.g., wandering episodes, self abuse, verbal disruption, physical aggression, etc.):

⓪ Never
① Less than once a month
② Once a month
③ Several times each month
④ Several times a week
⑤ At least daily

59. **(M0630)** Is this patient receiving **Psychiatric Nursing Services** at home provided by a qualified psychiatric nurse?

⓪ No
① Yes

For M0640-M0800, complete the "Current" column for all patients. For these same items, complete the "Prior" column only at start of care and at resumption of care; mark the level that corresponds to the patient's condition 14 days prior to start of care date (M0030) or resumption of care date (M0032). In all cases, record what the patient is able to do.

60. **(M0640) Grooming:** Ability to tend to personal hygiene needs (i.e., washing face and hands, hair care, shaving or make up, teeth or denture care, fingernail care).

Prior Current

- ⓪ ⓪ Able to groom self unaided, with or without the use of assistive devices or adapted methods.
- ① ① Grooming utensils must be placed within reach before able to complete grooming activities.
- ② ② Someone must assist the patient to groom self.
- ③ ③ Patient depends entirely upon someone else for grooming needs.
- Ⓤ UK-Unknown

61. **(M0650) Ability to Dress Upper Body** (with or without dressing aids) including undergarments, pullovers, front-opening shirts and blouses, managing zippers, buttons, and snaps:

Prior Current

- ⓪ ⓪ Able to get clothes out of closets and drawers, put them on and remove them from the upper body without assistance.
- ① ① Able to dress upper body without assistance if clothing is laid out or handed to the patient.
- ② ② Someone must help the patient put on upper body clothing.
- ③ ③ Patient depends entirely upon another person to dress the upper body.
- Ⓤ UK-Unknown

62. **(M0660) Ability to Dress Lower Body** (with or without dressing aids) including undergarments, slacks, socks or nylons, shoes:

Prior Current

- ⓪ ⓪ Able to obtain, put on, and remove clothing and shoes without assistance.
- ① ① Able to dress lower body without assistance if clothing and shoes are laid out or handed to the patient.
- ② ② Someone must help the patient put on undergarments, slacks, socks or nylons, and shoes.
- ③ ③ Patient depends entirely upon another person to dress lower body.
- Ⓤ UK-Unknown

63. **(M0670) Bathing:** Ability to wash entire body. **Excludes grooming (washing face and hands only).**

Prior Current

- ⓪ ⓪ Able to bathe self in shower or tub independently.
- ① ① With the use of devices, is able to bathe self in shower or tub independently.
- ② ② Able to bathe in shower or tub with the assistance of another person:
    - (a) for intermittent supervision or encouragement or reminders, OR
    - (b) to get in and out of the shower or tub, OR
    - (c) for washing difficult to reach areas.
- ③ ③ Participates in bathing self in shower or tub, but requires presence of another person throughout the bath for assistance or supervision.
- ④ ④ Unable to use the shower or tub and is bathed in bed or bedside chair.
- ⑤ ⑤ Unable to effectively participate in bathing and is totally bathed by another person.
- Ⓤ UK-Unknown

64. **(M0680) Toileting:** Ability to get to and from the toilet or bedside commode.

Prior Current

- ⓪ ⓪ Able to get to and from the toilet independently with or without a device.
- ① ① When reminded, assisted, or supervised by another person, able to get to and from the toilet.
- ② ② Unable to get to and from the toilet but is able to use a bedside commode (with or without assistance).
- ③ ③ Unable to get to and from the toilet or bedside commode but is able to use a bedpan/urinal independently.
- ④ ④ Is totally dependent in toileting.
- Ⓤ UK-Unknown

65. **(M0690) Transferring:** Ability to move from bed to chair, on and off toilet or commode, into and out of tub or shower, and ability to turn and position self in bed if patient is bedfast.

Prior Current

- ⓪ ⓪ Able to independently transfer.
- ① ① Transfers with minimal human assistance or with use of an assistive device.
- ② ② Unable to transfer self but is able to bear weight and pivot during the transfer process.
- ③ ③ Unable to transfer self and is unable to bear weight or pivot when transferred by another person.
- ④ ④ Bedfast, unable to transfer but is able to turn and position self in bed.
- ⑤ ⑤ Bedfast, unable to transfer and is unable to turn and position self.
- Ⓤ UK-Unknown

66. **(M0700) Ambulation/Locomotion:** Ability to SAFELY walk, once in a standing position, or use a wheelchair, once in a seated position, on a variety of surfaces.

Prior Current

⓪ ⓪ Able to independently walk on even and uneven surfaces and climb stairs with or without railings (i.e., needs no human assistance or assistive device).
① ① Requires use of a device (e.g., cane, walker) to walk alone or requires human supervision or assistance to negotiate stairs or steps or uneven surfaces.
② ② Able to walk only with the supervision or assistance of another person at all times.
③ ③ Chairfast, unable to ambulate but is able to wheel self independently.
④ ④ Chairfast, unable to ambulate and is unable to wheel self.
⑤ ⑤ Bedfast, unable to ambulate or be up in a chair.
Ⓤ UK-Unknown

67. **(M0710) Feeding or Eating:** Ability to feed self meals and snacks. **Note: This refers only to the process of eating, chewing, and swallowing, not preparing the food to be eaten.**

Prior Current

⓪ ⓪ Able to independently feed self.
① ① Able to feed self independently but requires:
   (a) meal set-up; OR
   (b) intermittent assistance or supervision from another person; OR
   (c) a liquid, pureed or ground meat diet.
② ② Unable to feed self and must be assisted or supervised throughout the meal/snack.
③ ③ Able to take in nutrients orally and receives supplemental nutrients through a nasogastric tube or gastrostomy.
④ ④ Unable to take in nutrients orally and is fed nutrients through a nasogastric tube or gastrostomy.
⑤ ⑤ Unable to take in nutrients orally or by tube feeding.
Ⓤ UK-Unknown

68. **(M0720) Planning and Preparing Light Meals** (e.g., cereal, sandwich) or reheat delivered meals:

Prior Current

⓪ ⓪ (a) Able to independently plan and prepare all light meals for self or reheat delivered meals; OR
   (b) Is physically, cognitively, and mentally able to prepare light meals on a regular basis but has not routinely performed light meal preparation in the past (i.e., prior to this home care admission).
① ① Unable to prepare light meals on a regular basis due to physical, cognitive, or mental limitations.
② ② Unable to prepare any light meals or reheat any delivered meals.
Ⓤ UK-Unknown

69. **(M0730) Transportation:** Physical and mental ability to safely use a car, taxi, or public transportation (bus, train, subway).

Prior Current

⓪ ⓪ Able to independently drive a regular or adapted car; OR uses a regular or handicap-accessible public bus.
① ① Able to ride in a car only when driven by another person; OR able to use a bus or handicap van only when assisted or accompanied by another person.
② ② Unable to ride in a car, taxi, bus, or van, and requires transportation by ambulance.
Ⓤ UK-Unknown

70. **(M0740) Laundry:** Ability to do own laundry -- to carry laundry to and from washing machine, to use washer and dryer, to wash small items by hand.

Prior Current

⓪ ⓪ (a) Able to independently take care of all laundry tasks; OR
   (b) Physically, cognitively, and mentally able to do laundry and access facilities, but has not routinely performed laundry tasks in the past (i.e., prior to this home care admission).
① ① Able to do only light laundry, such as minor hand wash or light washer loads. Due to physical, cognitive, or mental limitations, needs assistance with heavy laundry such as carrying large loads of laundry.
② ② Unable to do any laundry due to physical limitation or needs continual supervision and assistance due to cognitive or mental limitation.
Ⓤ UK-Unknown

71. **(M0750) Housekeeping:** Ability to safely and effectively perform light housekeeping and heavier cleaning tasks.

Prior Current

⓪ ⓪ (a) Able to independently perform all housekeeping tasks; OR
   (b) Physically, cognitively, and mentally able to perform all housekeeping tasks but has not routinely participated in housekeeping tasks in the past (i.e., prior to this home care admission).
① ① Able to perform only light housekeeping (e.g., dusting, wiping kitchen counters) tasks independently.
② ② Able to perform housekeeping tasks with intermittent assistance or supervision from another person.
③ ③ Unable to consistently perform any housekeeping tasks unless assisted by another person throughout the process.
④ ④ Unable to effectively participate in any housekeeping tasks.
Ⓤ UK-Unknown

72. **(M0760) Shopping:** Ability to plan for, select, and purchase items in a store and to carry them home or arrange delivery.

Prior Current

⓪　⓪　(a) Able to plan for shopping needs and independently perform shopping tasks, including carrying packages; OR
　　　　(b) Physically, cognitively, and mentally able to take care of shopping, but has not done shopping in the past (i.e., prior to this home care admission).
①　①　Able to go shopping, but needs some assistance:
　　　　(a) By self is able to do only light shopping and carry small packages, but needs someone to do occasional major shopping; OR
　　　　(b) Unable to go shopping alone, but can go with someone to assist.
②　②　Unable to go shopping, but is able to identify items needed, place orders, and arrange home delivery.
③　③　Needs someone to do all shopping and errands.
Ⓤ　Ⓤ　UK-Unknown

73. **(M0770) Ability to Use Telephone:** Ability to answer the phone, dial numbers, and <u>effectively</u> use the telephone to communicate.

Prior Current

⓪　⓪　Able to dial numbers and answer calls appropriately and as desired.
①　①　Able to use a specially adapted telephone (i.e., large numbers on the dial, teletype phone for the deaf) and call essential numbers.
②　②　Able to answer the telephone and carry on a normal conversation but has difficulty with placing calls.
③　③　Able to answer the telephone only some of the time or is able to carry on only a limited conversation.
④　④　Unable to answer the telephone at all but can listen if assisted with equipment.
⑤　⑤　Totally unable to use the telephone.
Ⓝ　Ⓝ　NA-Patient does not have a telephone.
Ⓤ　Ⓤ　UK-Unknown

MEDICATIONS

74. **(M0780) Management of Oral Medications:** <u>Patient's ability</u> to prepare and take <u>all</u> prescribed oral medications reliably and safely, including administration of the correct dosage at the appropriate times/intervals. **Excludes injectable and IV medications. (NOTE: This refers to ability, not compliance or willingness.)**

Prior Current

⓪　⓪　Able to independently take the correct oral medication(s) and proper dosage(s) at the correct times.
①　①　Able to take medication(s) at the correct times if:
　　　　(a) individual dosages are prepared in advance by another person; OR
　　　　(b) given daily reminders; OR
　　　　(c) someone develops a drug diary or chart.
②　②　Unable to take medication unless administered by someone else.
Ⓝ　Ⓝ　NA-No oral medications prescribed.
Ⓤ　Ⓤ　UK-Unknown

75. **(M0790) Management of Inhalant/Mist Medications:** <u>Patient's ability</u> to prepare and take <u>all</u> prescribed inhalant/mist medications (nebulizers, metered dose devices) reliably and safely, including administration of the correct dosage at the appropriate times/intervals. **Excludes all other forms of medication (oral tablets, injectable and IV medications).**

Prior Current

⓪　⓪　Able to independently take the correct medication and proper dosage at the correct times.
①　①　Able to take medication at the correct times if:
　　　　(a) individual dosages are prepared in advance by another person, OR
　　　　(b) given daily reminders.
②　②　Unable to take medication unless administered by someone else.
Ⓝ　Ⓝ　NA-No inhalant/mist medications prescribed.
Ⓤ　Ⓤ　UK-Unknown

76. **(M0800) Management of Injectable Medications:** <u>Patient's ability</u> to prepare and take <u>all</u> prescribed injectable medications reliably and safely, including administration of correct dosage at the appropriate times/intervals. **Excludes IV medications.**

Prior Current

⓪　⓪　Able to independently take the correct medication and proper dosage at the correct times.
①　①　Able to take injectable medication at correct times if:
　　　　(a) individual syringes are prepared in advance by another person, OR
　　　　(b) given daily reminders.
②　②　Unable to take injectable medications unless administered by someone else.
Ⓝ　Ⓝ　NA-No injectable medications prescribed.
Ⓤ　Ⓤ　UK-Unknown

Patient's Name _____

Place Bar Code Here

FEED THIS DIRECTION

SCAN THIS SIDE UP

(M0030) Start of Care Date

Month	Day		Year			
○ Jan						
○ Feb						
○ Mar	⓪	⓪	⓪	⓪	⓪	⓪
○ Apr	①	①	①	①	①	①
○ May	②	②	②	②	②	②
○ Jun	③	③	③	③	③	③
○ Jul	④	④	④	④	④	④
○ Aug	⑤	⑤	⑤	⑤	⑤	⑤
○ Sep	⑥	⑥	⑥	⑥	⑥	⑥
○ Oct	⑦	⑦	⑦	⑦	⑦	⑦
○ Nov	⑧	⑧	⑧	⑧	⑧	⑧
○ Dec	⑨	⑨	⑨	⑨	⑨	⑨

(M0090) Date Assessment Completed

Month	Day		Year			
○ Jan						
○ Feb						
○ Mar	⓪	⓪	⓪	⓪	⓪	⓪
○ Apr	①	①	①	①	①	①
○ May	②	②	②	②	②	②
○ Jun	③	③	③	③	③	③
○ Jul	④	④	④	④	④	④
○ Aug	⑤	⑤	⑤	⑤	⑤	⑤
○ Sep	⑥	⑥	⑥	⑥	⑥	⑥
○ Oct	⑦	⑦	⑦	⑦	⑦	⑦
○ Nov	⑧	⑧	⑧	⑧	⑧	⑧
○ Dec	⑨	⑨	⑨	⑨	⑨	⑨

(M0032) Resumption of Care Date
○ Not Applicable

Month	Day		Year			
○ Jan						
○ Feb						
○ Mar	⓪	⓪	⓪	⓪	⓪	⓪
○ Apr	①	①	①	①	①	①
○ May	②	②	②	②	②	②
○ Jun	③	③	③	③	③	③
○ Jul	④	④	④	④	④	④
○ Aug	⑤	⑤	⑤	⑤	⑤	⑤
○ Sep	⑥	⑥	⑥	⑥	⑥	⑥
○ Oct	⑦	⑦	⑦	⑦	⑦	⑦
○ Nov	⑧	⑧	⑧	⑧	⑧	⑧
○ Dec	⑨	⑨	⑨	⑨	⑨	⑨

Caregiver ID Number

⓪	⓪	⓪	⓪	⓪	⓪	⓪	⓪	⓪	⓪
①	①	①	①	①	①	①	①	①	①
②	②	②	②	②	②	②	②	②	②
③	③	③	③	③	③	③	③	③	③
④	④	④	④	④	④	④	④	④	④
⑤	⑤	⑤	⑤	⑤	⑤	⑤	⑤	⑤	⑤
⑥	⑥	⑥	⑥	⑥	⑥	⑥	⑥	⑥	⑥
⑦	⑦	⑦	⑦	⑦	⑦	⑦	⑦	⑦	⑦
⑧	⑧	⑧	⑧	⑧	⑧	⑧	⑧	⑧	⑧
⑨	⑨	⑨	⑨	⑨	⑨	⑨	⑨	⑨	⑨

(M0064) Patient's SSN

⓪	⓪	⓪	⓪	⓪	⓪	⓪	⓪	⓪	⓪
①	①	①	①	①	①	①	①	①	①
②	②	②	②	②	②	②	②	②	②
③	③	③	③	③	③	③	③	③	③
④	④	④	④	④	④	④	④	④	④
⑤	⑤	⑤	⑤	⑤	⑤	⑤	⑤	⑤	⑤
⑥	⑥	⑥	⑥	⑥	⑥	⑥	⑥	⑥	⑥
⑦	⑦	⑦	⑦	⑦	⑦	⑦	⑦	⑦	⑦
⑧	⑧	⑧	⑧	⑧	⑧	⑧	⑧	⑧	⑧
⑨	⑨	⑨	⑨	⑨	⑨	⑨	⑨	⑨	⑨

EQUIPMENT MANAGEMENT

77. **(M0810) Patient Management of Equipment (includes ONLY oxygen, IV/infusion therapy, enteral/parenteral nutrition equipment or supplies):** Patient's ability to set up, monitor and change equipment reliably and safely, add appropriate fluids or medication, clean/store/dispose of equipment or supplies using proper technique. **(NOTE: This refers to ability, not compliance or willingness.)**

⓪ Patient manages all tasks related to equipment completely independently.
① If someone else sets up equipment (i.e., fills portable oxygen tank, provides patient with prepared solutions), patient is able
② to manage all other aspects of equipment.
③ Patient requires considerable assistance from another person to manage equipment, but independently completes portions
④ of the task.
⑤ Patient is only able to monitor equipment (e.g., liter flow, fluid in bag) and must call someone else to manage the equipment.
⑥ Patient is completely dependent on someone else to manage all equipment.
Ⓝ NA-No equipment of this type used in care
↓ [If NA, skip M0820 (skip question 78)]

78. **(M0820) Caregiver Management of Equipment (includes ONLY oxygen, IV/infusion equipment, enteral/parenteral nutrition, ventilator therapy equipment or supplies):** Caregiver's ability to set up, monitor, and change equipment reliably and safely, add appropriate fluids or medication, clean/store/dispose of equipment or supplies using proper technique. **(NOTE: This refers to ability, not compliance or willingness.)**

⓪ Caregiver manages all tasks related to equipment completely independently.
① If someone else sets up equipment, caregiver is able to manage all other aspects.
② Caregiver requires considerable assistance from another person to manage equipment, but independently completes
③ significant portions of task.
④ Caregiver is only able to complete small portions of task (e.g., administer nebulizer treatment, clean/store/dispose of
⑤ equipment or supplies).
⑥ Caregiver is completely dependent on someone else to manage all equipment.
Ⓝ NA-No caregiver
Ⓤ UK-Unknown

0065

B.2   Multicultural Nursing Assessment

There must be an awareness of one's own ethnocultural heritage, both as a person and as a nurse. In addition, an awareness and sensitivity must be developed to the health beliefs and practices of a client's heritage. This awareness and sensitivity can be developed through careful assessment of a client's heritage and cultural beliefs. The factors that must be explored during a multicultural nursing assessment are as follows:

Cultural

- What customs and values of the client may influence health behaviors and the provision of care?
- Could the client's communication process or language affect the provision of care? How?
- What health care beliefs and practices of the client may influence acceptance of and response to illness?
- Could nutritional variables and preferences or restrictions affect the provision of care?

Sociological

- Could the client's economic status affect the provision of care?
- Could educational status affect the provision of care?
- How does the client's social network affect the provision of care?

- What family structural variables may influence the provision of care?
- Are community support systems available, and do they help to fight against institutional racism?

Psychological

- Could self-concept and identity factors affect the provision of care?
- What are the client's defense mechanisms, and are they adaptive or maladaptive?
- Could religious or cultural considerations affect the provision of care?

Biological and Physiological

- Does the nurse need to take racial or anatomical characteristics or factors into account when providing care?
- Do growth and development patterns influence physical assessment findings?
- What variations in physical features and body systems are present?
- Are there any culturally specific diseases to note?
- Are there any diseases to which the client has increased (decreased) resistance?

From Potter PA, Perry AG: *Basic nursing: a critical thinking approach,* ed 4, St. Louis, 1999, Mosby.

Appendix C

Hepatitis Information

C.1   Summary Description of Hepatitis A-E and G

Type	Definition	Risk	Symptoms	Precautions	Prevention of Spreading
A	Liver disease caused by picornavirus, commonly called "infectious hepatitis"	Live in house with infected person Inject drugs Travel internationally to areas with high prevalence of hepatitis A Eat infected shellfish Consume contaminated food and water	Skin, eye yellowing Loss of appetite Nausea Vomiting Fever Fatigue Diarrhea Stomach/joint pain Unable to work for extended periods	Stricter handwashing by foodhandler Improved sanitary conditions Improved personal hygiene	Immune gamma globulin injections Hepatitis A vaccine
B	A major cause of acute and chronic liver disease that can lead to cirrhosis and hepatocellular cancer; "serum hepatitis"	Exposure to human blood Live with someone who is a carrier Inject drugs Have a sex partner infected with "B" Have sex with more than one partner A child born in Asia, Africa, Amazon, South America, Pacific Islands, or the Middle East	Skin, eye yellowing Loss of appetite Nausea Vomiting Diarrhea Stomach/joint pain No symptoms (carrier) Itching Skin eruptions	Vaccinate: • Babies at birth • Adolescents and others who have sex or inject drugs • Persons whose job places them at risk	Hepatitis B vaccine
C	Virus causing chronic liver disease, found in blood caused by non-A and non-B hepatitis virus. May develop cirrhosis and liver failure	Drug injection Exposure to human blood Hemodialysis patients Receipt of blood transfusion Multiple sex partners Live with person with "C"	Same as hepatitis "B"	Do not take blood, organs, tissue, or sperm from "C" person Do not share toothbrushes, razors, or other items possibly contaminated withblood (including needles) Cover open sores or other skin breaks	Practice safe sex Have only one sex partner Routine screening of blood/other donors

Type	Definition	Risk	Symptoms	Precautions	Prevention of Spreading
D	An incomplete virus requiring hepatitis B to be present to cause infection. This results in a more severe acute liver disease, leading to chronic liver disease with cirrhosis	Injection drug users Hemophilia clients Developmentally disabled persons who are hospitalized	Same as hepatitis "B"	Avoid sexual contact with injection drug users Do not use needle used by others Proper sterilization technique in institutions	Individual screening for hepatitis B Blood screening for "B" and "D" Early vaccination for hepatitis B
E	Enterically transmitted non-A and non-B hepatitis virus. Usually acute and does not usually cause chronic disease	Ingestion of fecally contaminated water Pregnant women International travelers Persons in Asia and Indian countries	Same as hepatitis "B"	Avoid contaminated waters	None at this time
G	Non A-E hepatitis virus described as a flavivirus. Present in 1%-2% of blood donors in USA. Causes acute liver disease	Any IV therapy Injected drugs End-stage renal disease Pregnancy Hemophilia	Same as B Liver inflammation Liver failure	Avoid multiple transfusions Avoid IV drug use Check new babies for perinatal transmission Avoid all unnecessary IVs Monitor persons for hemodialysis	Individual screening for HGV See precautions

Data from multiple sources provided by the Centers for Disease Control and Prevention, Atlanta, 1995; *Science News* 149(15):238, 1996; National Institutes of Health: HCV International Symposium, June 1999.

C.2 Recommended Prophylaxis of Hepatitis A

1. *Close personal contact.* Immune globulin (IG) is recommended for all household and sexual contacts of persons with hepatitis A.
2. *Day-care centers.* Day-care facilities with children in diapers can be important settings for hepatitis A virus (HAV) transmission. IG should be administered to all staff and attendees of daycare centers or homes if (1) one or more hepatitis A cases are recognized among children or employees, or (2) cases are recognized in two or more households of center attendees. When an outbreak (hepatitis cases in three or more families) occurs, IG should also be considered for members of households whose diapered children attend. In centers not enrolling children in diapers, IG need be given only to classroom contacts of an index case.
3. *Schools.* Contact at elementary and secondary schools is usually not an important means of transmitting hepatitis A. Routine administration of IG is not indicated for pupils and teachers in contact with a patient. However, when epidemiological study clearly shows the existence of a school- or classroom-centered outbreak, IG may be given to those who have close personal contact with patients.
4. *Institutions for custodial care.* Living conditions in some institutions, such as prisons and facilities for the developmentally disabled, favor transmission of hepatitis A. When outbreaks occur, giving IG to residents and staff who have close contact with patients with hepatitis A may reduce spread of disease. Depending on the epidemiologic circumstances, prophylaxis can be limited or can involve the entire institution.
5. *Hospitals.* Routine IG administration is not indicated. Rather, sound hygienic practices should be emphasized. Staff education should point out the risk of exposure to hepatitis A and emphasize precautions regarding direct contact with potentially infective materials. Outbreaks of hepatitis A among hospital staff occur occasionally, usually in association with an unsuspected index patient who is fecally incontinent. Large outbreaks have occurred among staff and family contacts of infected infants in neonatal intensive care units. In outbreaks, prophylaxis of persons exposed to feces of infected patients may be indicated.
6. *Offices and factories.* Routine IG administration is not indicated under the usual office or factory conditions for

persons exposed to a fellow worker with hepatitis A. Experience shows that casual contact in the work setting does not result in virus transmission.

7. *Common-source exposure.* IG might be effective in preventing food-borne or waterborne hepatitis A if exposure is recognized in time. However, IG is not recommended for persons exposed to a common source of hepatitis infection after cases have begun to occur in those exposed, because the 2-week period during which IG is effective will have been exceeded.

   If a food handler is diagnosed as having hepatitis A, common-source transmission is possible but uncommon.

IG should be administered to other food handlers but is usually not recommended for patrons. However, IG administration to patrons may be considered if (1) the infected person is directly involved in handling, without gloves, foods that will not be cooked before they are eaten; (2) the hygienic practices of the food handler are deficient; and (3) patrons can be identified and treated within 2 weeks of exposure. Situations in which repeated exposures may have occurred, such as in institutional cafeterias, may warrant stronger consideration of IG use.

For postexposure IG prophylaxis, a single intramuscular dose of 0.02 ml/kg is recommended.

C.3   Recommended Postexposure Prophylaxis for Percutaneous or Permucosal Exposure to Hepatitis B Virus

Vaccination and Antibody Response Status of Exposed Person	HBsAG Positive Source	HBsAg Negative Source	Source Not Tested or Status Unknown
Unvaccinated	HBIG $\times$ 1; initiate hepatitis B vaccine series	Initiate hepatitis B vaccine series	Initiate hepatitis B vaccine series
Previously vaccinated			
Known responder*	No treatment	No treatment	No treatment
Known non-responder	HBIG $\times$ 2 or HBIG $\times$ 1 and initiate revaccination	No treatment	If known high-risk source, treat as if source were HBsAg positive
Antibody response unknown	Test exposed person for anti-HBs 1. If adequate,* no treatment 2. If inadequate,* HBIG $\times$ 1 and vaccine booster	No treatment	Test exposed person for anti-HBs 1. If adequate,* no treatment 2. If inadequate,* initiate revaccination

*Responder is defined as a person with adequate levels of serum antibody to hepatitis B surface antigen (e.g., anti-HBs $\geq$10 mIU/mL); inadequate response to vaccination defined as serum anti-HBs <10 mIU/mL.
HBsAG, Hepatits B surface antigen; *HBIG,* hepatitis B immune globulin; dose 0.06 mL/kg intramuscularly; *anti-HBs,* antibody to hepatitis B surface.

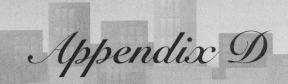
Immunization Information

D.1 Immunizations for Infants: A Guide for Parents

Age	Vaccine (Age Range in Which Vaccine Should Be Given)				
Birth	Hep-B (0-2 months)				
1-2 months	Hep-B (1-4 months)				
2 months	DTaP	Hib	IPV*	PCV7	
4 months	DTaP	Hib	IPV*	PCV7	
6 months	DTaP	Hib†	IPV (6-18 months)	PCV7	Hep-B (6-18 months)
12 months	MMR (12-15 months)	Hib (12-15 months)	Chickenpox (12-18 months)	PCV7 (12-15 months)	
15 months	DTaP (12-18 months)‡				

*As of January 1, 2000, inactivated polio vaccine (IPV), not oral polio vaccine, is recommended for routine vaccination.
†Depending on the brand of Hib vaccine used for the 1st and 2nd doses, a dose at 6 months of age may not be needed.
‡DTaP may be given as early as 12 months of age if 6 months have elapsed since the previous dose and if the child might not return by 18 months of age.

Check with your clinic to make sure your baby is getting immunized on time. Also make sure you ask your clinic to give you a record card with all the dates of your baby's shots and be sure to bring it to every visit.

Hep-B: protects against hepatitis B, a serious liver disease.
DTaP: protects against diphtheria, tetanus (lockjaw), and pertussis (whooping cough).
Hib: protects against *Haemophilus influenzae* type b.

IPV: inactivated (injected) polio vaccine protects against polio.
PCV7: pneumococcal conjugate vaccine protects against serious pneumococcal infections.
MMR: protects against measles, mumps, and rubella (German measles).
Chickenpox: varicella zoster vaccine protects against chickenpox.

Courtesy Immunization Action Coalition, St. Paul, Minnesota. Item #P4010 (rev 10/00).

D.2   When Do Children and Teens Need Vaccinations?

Age	Hep-B (Hepatitis B)	DTaP (Diphtheria, Tetanus, Pertussis)	Hib (*Haemophilus influenzae* Type b)	IPV (Polio)	PCV7 (Pneumococcal conjugate)	MMR (Measles, Mumps, Rubella)	Varicella (Chickenpox)
Birth	X 0-2 months*						
1 month	X 1-4 months*						
2 months		X	X	X†	X		
4 months		X	X	X†	X		
6 months	X 6-18 months*	X	X‡	X 6-18 months*,†	X		
12 months	All children 0 through 18 years of age need 3 doses of hepatitis B vaccine if they haven't already received them.§		X 12-15 months*		X 12-15 months* Children 16-59 months of age who have not been vaccinated may need 1 or 2 doses of PCV7. Talk to your health care provider.	X 12-15 months*	X 12-18 months* Children 12 months of age through 12 years of age (who have not had chickenpox or have not been previously vaccinated) need 1 dose.
15 months		X 12-18 months*,‖					
4-6 years		X		X†		X MMR #2 is given at 4-6 years of age. If dose #2 was not given at 4-6 years of age, it should be given at the next visit.	
11-12 years	X	X Td is given at age 11-12 if at least 5 years have passed since the last dose of DTaP/DTP.					
13-18 years	X						Children 13 years of age and older (who have not had chickenpox or have not been previously vaccinated) need 2 doses given 4-8 weeks apart.

Were you or your child born in a country where hepatitis B is a common disease? If so, your child should be vaccinated against hepatitis B right away, no matter what his or her age. Don't wait until your child reaches a certain age. Your child is at risk for this disease and needs protection now. Talk to your doctor.

*This is the age range in which the vaccine should be given.
†As of January 1, 2000, inactivated polio vaccine (IPV), not oral polio vaccine, is recommended for routine vaccination.
‡Depending on the brand of Hib vaccine used for doses #1 and #2, a dose at 6 months of age may not be needed.
§Some adolescents aged 11 through 15 years may be given two doses of hepatitis B vaccine. Check with your health care provider.
‖DTaP can be given at 12 months of age if 6 months have elapsed since the previous dose and if the child might not return by 18 months of age.

Talk to your health care provider about whether your child needs other vaccines: hepatitis A, influenza, Lyme disease, or pneumococcal polysaccharide vaccine. Certain children are at risk for these diseases and need to be immunized against them.

Courtesy Immunization Action Coalition, St. Paul, MN, www.immunize.org.

D.3   Summary of Rules for Childhood Immunizations*

Vaccine	Ages Usually Given and Other Guidelines	If Child Falls Behind (Minimum Intervals)	Contraindications (Mild Illness Is Not a Contraindication)
DTaP (diphtheria, tetanus, acellular pertussis) Give IM	• DTaP (not DTP) is recommended for all doses in the series. • Give at 2 months, 4 months, 6 months, 15-18 months, 4-6 years of age. • May give #1 as early as 6 weeks of age. • May give #4 as early as 12 months of age if 6 months have elapsed since #3 and the child is unlikely to return at age 15-18 months. • If started with DTP, complete the series with DTaP. • Do not give DTaP to children ≥7 years of age (give Td). • May give with all other vaccines but as a separate injection. • It is preferable but not mandatory to use the same DTaP product for all doses.	• #2 and #3 may be given 4 weeks after previous dose. • #4 may be given 6 months after #3. • If #4 is given before 4th birthday, wait at least 6 months for #5 (4-6 years of age). • If #4 is given after 4th birthday, #5 is not needed. • DO NOT restart series, no matter how long since previous dose.	• Anaphylactic reaction to a prior dose or to any vaccine component. • Moderate or severe acute illness. Do not postpone for mild illness. • Previous encephalopathy within 7 days after DTP/DTaP. *Precautions for DTP/DTaP:* The following are precautions, not contraindications. Generally when these conditions are present, the vaccine shouldn't be given. But in situations when the benefit outweighs the risk (e.g., community pertussis outbreak), vaccination should be considered. • T >105° F (40.5° C) within 48 hours after previous dose. • Continuous crying lasting ≥3 hours within 48 hours after previous dose. • Previous convulsion within 3 days after immunization. • Pale or limp episode or collapse within 48 hours after previous dose. • Unstable progressive neurologic problem (defer until stable).
DT Give IM	• Give to children <7 years of age if child had a serious reaction to "P" in DTaP/DTP or if parents refuse the pertussis component. • May give with all other vaccines but as a separate injection.		
Td Give IM	• Use for persons ≥7 years of age. • A booster dose is recommended for children 11-12 years of age if 5 years have elapsed since last dose. Then boost every 10 years. • May give with all other vaccines but as a separate injection.	• For those never vaccinated or with an unknown vaccination history: dose #1 is given now, dose #2 is given 4 weeks later, dose #3 is given 6 months after #2, then give booster dose every 10 years.	• Anaphylactic reaction to a prior dose or to any vaccine component. • Moderate or severe acute illness. Do not postpone for minor illness. • If the series is incomplete, continue from where you left off. DO NOT restart the series.

*The newer combination vaccines are not listed on this table but may be used whenever administration of any component is indicated and none is contraindicated. Read package inserts. For detailed information, see the ACIP statements published in the *MMWR*. Obtain from www.cdc.gov/nip/publications/ACIP-list.htm or from the Immunization Action Coalition's (IAC) website at www.immunize.org/acip. For recommendations of American Academy of Pediatrics (AAP), consult AAP's *2000 Red Book* and the journal *Pediatrics* or www.aap.org.
Modified from ACIP, AAP, and AAFP by the Immunization Action Coalition, March 2000.
Courtesy Immunization Action Coalition, St. Paul, Minn, www.immunize.org.

Continued

Vaccine	Ages Usually Given and Other Guidelines	If Child Falls Behind (Minimum Intervals)	Contraindications (Mild Illness Is Not a Contraindication)
MMR (Measles, mumps, rubella) Give SC	• Give #1 at 12-15 months of age. Give #2 at 4-6 years of age. • Make sure that all children (and teens) over 4-6 years of age have received both doses of MMR. • If a dose was given before 12 months of age it doesn't count as the first dose, so give #1 at 12-15 months of age with a minimum interval of 4 weeks between these doses. • If MMR and Var (and/or yellow fever vaccine) are not given on the same day, space them ≥28 days apart. • May give with all other vaccines but as a separate injection.	• 2 doses of MMR are recommended for all children ≤18 years of age. • Dose should be given whenever it is noted that a child is behind. Exception: If MMR and Var (and/or yellow fever vaccine) are not given on the same day, space them ≥28 days apart. • There should be a minimum interval of 28 days between MMR #1 and MMR #2. • Dose #2 can be given at any time if at least 28 days have elapsed since dose #1 and both doses are administered after 1 year of age. • DO NOT restart the series, no matter how long since previous dose.	• Anaphylactic reaction to a prior dose or to any vaccine component. • Pregnancy or possible pregnancy within next 3 months (use contraception). • Moderate or severe acute illness. Do not postpone for minor illness. • If blood, plasma, or immune globulin were given in past 11 months, see ACIP recommendations or 2000 Red Book (p. 390) regarding time to wait before vaccinating. • HIV is NOT a contraindication unless severely immunocompromised. • Immunocompromised persons (e.g., because of cancer, leukemia, lymphoma). NOTE: For patients on high-dose immunosuppressive therapy, consult ACIP recommendations regarding delay time. NOTE: MMR is not contraindicated if a PPD test was recently applied. If PPD and MMR were not given on same day, delay PPD for 4-6 weeks after MMR.
Var (Varicella [Chickenpox]) Give SC	• Routinely give at 12-18 months of age. • Vaccinate all children ≥12 months of age including all adolescents who have not had chickenpox. • May use as postexposure prophylaxis if given within 3-5 days. • If Var and MMR (and/or yellow fever vaccine) are not given on the same day, space them ≥28 days apart. • May give with all other vaccines but as a separate injection.	• Do not give to children <12 months of age. • Susceptible children <13 years of age receive 1 dose. • Susceptible persons ≥13 years of age receive 2 doses 4-8 weeks apart. • DO NOT restart series, no matter how long since previous dose.	• Anaphylactic reaction to a prior dose or to any vaccine component. • Moderate or severe acute illness. Do not postpone for minor illness. • Pregnancy or possibility of pregnancy within 1 month. • If blood, plasma, or immune globulin (IG or VZIG) were given in past 5 months, see ACIP recommendations or AAP's 2000 Red Book (p. 390) regarding time to wait before vaccinating. • Persons immunocompromised due to high doses of systemic steroids, cancer, leukemia, lymphoma, or immunodeficiency. NOTE: For patients with humoral immunodeficiency, HIV infection, or leukemia, or for patients on high doses of systemic steroids, consult ACIP recommendations. • For use in children taking salicylates, consult ACIP recommendations.

Courtesy Immunization Action Coalition, St. Paul, Minn, www.immunize.org.

Vaccine	Ages Usually Given and Other Guidelines	If Child Falls Behind (Minimum Intervals)	Contraindications (Mild Illness Is Not a Contraindication)
IV (Polio) Give SC or IM	• Give at 2 months, 4 months, 6-18 months, and 4-6 years of age. • May give #1 as early as 6 weeks of age. • Not routinely recommended for those ≥18 years of age (except certain travelers). • May give with all other vaccines but as a separate injection.	• All doses should be separated by at least 4 weeks. • #4 is given at 4-6 years of age. • If #3 of an all-IPV or all-OPV series is given at ≥4 years of age, dose #4 is not needed. • Those who receive a combination of IPV and OPV doses must receive all 4 doses. • DO NOT restart series, no matter how long since previous dose.	• Anaphylactic reaction to a prior dose or to any vaccine component. • Moderate or severe acute illness. Do not postpone for minor illness.
Hib Give IM	• HibTITER (HbOC) and ActHib or OmniHib (PRP-T): give at 2 months, 4 months, 6 months, 12-15 months. • PedvaxHIB (PRP-OMP): give at 2 months, 4 months, 12-15 months. • Dose #1 of Hib vaccine may be given as early as 6 weeks of age but no earlier. • May give with all other vaccines but as a separate injection. • Hib vaccines are interchangeable. • Any Hib vaccine may be used for the booster dose. • Hib is not routinely given to children ≥5 years of age.	*Rules for all Hib vaccines:* • The last dose (booster dose) is given no earlier than 12 months of age and a minimum of 2 months after the previous dose. • For children ≥15 months and <5 years of age who have never received Hib vaccine, give only 1 dose. • DO NOT restart series, no matter how long since previous dose. *Rules for HbOC (HibTITER) and PRP-T (ActHib, OmniHib) only:* • #2 and #3 may be given 4 weeks after previous dose. • If #1 was given at 7-11 months, only 3 doses are needed; #2 is given 4-8 weeks after #1, then boost at 12-15 months. • If #1 was given at 12-14 months, give a booster dose in 2 months. • Rules for PRP-OMP (Pedvax-HiB) only: • #2 may be given 4 weeks after dose #1. • If #1 was given at 12-14 months, boost 8 weeks later.	• Anaphylactic reaction to a prior dose or to any vaccine component. • Moderate or severe acute illness. Do not postpone for minor illness.

Continued

Vaccine	Ages Usually Given and Other Guidelines	If Child Falls Behind (Minimum Intervals)	Contraindications (Mild Illness Is Not a Contraindication)
Hep-B (hepatitis B) Give IM	• Vaccinate all infants at 0-2 months, 1-4 months, 6-18 months of age. • Vaccinate all children 0 through 18 years of age. • For older children/teens, spacing options include: 0, 1, 6 months; 0, 2, 4 months; or 0, 1, 4 months. • Children born (or whose parents were born) in countries of high HBV endemicity or who have other risk factors should be vaccinated ASAP. *If mother is HBsAg positive:* give HBIG and hep B #1 within 12 hours of birth, #2 at 1-2 months, and #3 at 6 months of age. *If mother's HBsAg status is unknown:* give hep B #1 within 12 hours of birth, #2 at 1-2 months, and #3 at 6 months of age. If mother is later found to be HbsAg positive, her infant should receive HBIG within 7 days of birth. • May give with all other vaccines but as a separate injection.	• DO NOT restart series, no matter how long since previous dose. • 3-dose series can be started at any age. • Minimum spacing for children and teens: 4 weeks between #1 & #2, and 8 weeks between #2 & #3. Overall there must be ≥16 weeks between #1 & #3. • Dose #3 should not be given earlier than 6 months of age. *Dosing of hepatitis B vaccines:* • Vaccine brands are interchangeable for 3-dose schedule. For Engerix-B, use 10 mcg for 0 through 19 years of age. For Recombivax HB, use 5 mcg for 0 through 19 years of age. • Alternative dosing schedule for adolescents aged 11 through 15 years: • For Recombivax HB only, use 10 mcg (adult dose) in two doses spaced 4-6 months apart. May only be given to adolescents 11 through 15 years of age.	• Anaphylactic reaction to a prior dose or to any vaccine component. • Moderate or severe acute illness. Do not postpone for minor illness.
Hep-A (hepatitis A) Give IM	• Vaccinate children ≥2 years old who live in areas with consistently elevated rates of hepatitis A, as well as children who have specific risk factors. (See ACIP statement and column 2 of this table for details.) • Children who travel outside of the U.S. (except Western Europe, New Zealand, Australia, Canada, or Japan). • Give dose #2 a minimum of 6 months after dose #1. • Dose #1 may not be given earlier than 2 years of age. • May give with all other vaccines but as a separate injection.	• DO NOT restart series, no matter how long since previous dose. • The minimum interval between dose #1 and #2 is 6 months. • Hepatitis A vaccine brands are interchangeable. • Consult your local or state public health authority for information regarding your city, county, or state hepatitis A rates. States with consistently elevated rates (average ≥10 cases per 100,000 population from 1987-1997) include the following: AL, AZ, AK, CA, CO, ID, MO, MT, NV, NM, OK, OR, SD, TX, UT, WA, and WY.	• Anaphylactic reaction to a prior dose or to any vaccine component. • Moderate or severe acute illness. Do not postpone for minor illness.

Courtesy Immunization Action Coalition, St. Paul, Minn, www.immunize.org.

Vaccine	Ages Usually Given and Other Guidelines	If Child Falls Behind (Minimum Intervals)	Contraindications (Mild Illness Is Not a Contraindication)
PCV7 (pneumococcal conjugate) Give IM	• Give at 2 months, 4 months, 6 months and 12-15 months of age. • For children 24-59 months of age, give 2 doses to high-risk children, and consider 1 dose for moderate-risk children. (See table footnote for list of high- and moderate-risk children.) • If both PCV7 and PPV23 are indicated, PPV23 is given ≥8 weeks after PCV7. • May give 1 dose to unvaccinated healthy children 24-59 months. • PCV7 not routinely given to children ≥5 years of age. • May give with all other vaccines but as separate injection.	• Minimum interval for infants ≤12 months of age is 4 weeks, for >12 months of age is 8 weeks. • For infants 7-11 months of age: If unvaccinated, give dose #1 now, give dose #2 4-8 weeks later, and boost at 12-15 months. If infant has had 1 or 2 previous doses, give next dose now, and boost at 12-15 months. • For infants 12-23 months: If not previously vaccinated or only one previous dose before 12 months, give 2 doses ≥8 weeks apart. If infant previously had 2 doses, give booster dose ≥8 weeks after previous dose. • DO NOT restart series, no matter how long since previous dose.	• Anaphylactic reaction to a prior dose or to any vaccine component. • Moderate or severe acute illness. Do not postpone for minor illness.
PPV23 (Pneumococcal conjugate) Give IM	There are children ≥2 years of age for whom pneumococcal polysaccharide vaccine (PPV23) is recommended. Give IM or SC. Consult the ACIP statement *Prevention of Pneumococcal Disease* (4/4/97) for details.		
Influenza	There are children ≥6 months of age for whom influenza vaccine is recommended. Give IM. Consult the current year's ACIP statement *Prevention and Control of Influenza* for details.		
Lyme	There are teenagers (≥15 years of age) for whom Lyme disease vaccine is recommended. Give IM. Consult the ACIP statement *Recommendations for the Use of Lyme Disease Vaccine* (6/4/99) for details.		
Meningococcal	Meningococcal disease risk and vaccine availability should be discussed with college students. Give SC. Consult the ACIP statement *Meningococcal Disease and College Students* (6/30/00) for details.		

High-risk children: Those with sickle cell disease; anatomic or functional asplenia; chronic cardiac, pulmonary, or renal disease; diabetes mellitus; CSF leak; HIV infection; or immunosuppression.
Moderate-risk children: Children ages 24-35 months; children ages 24-59 months who attend group daycare centers or are of Alaska Native, American Indian, or African-American descent.

D.4 Summary of Recommendations for Adult Immunizations

Vaccine Name and Route	For Whom It Is Recommended	Schedule for Routine and "Catch Up" Administration	Contraindications (Mild Illness Is Not a Contraindication)
Influenza Give IM	• Adults who are 50 years of age or older. • People 6 months-50 years of age with medical problems such as heart disease, lung disease, diabetes, renal dysfunction, hemoglobinopathies, immunosuppression, and/or people living in chronic care facilities. • People (≥6 months of age) working or living with at-risk people. • All health care workers and those who provide key community services. • Healthy pregnant women who will be in their 2nd or 3rd trimesters during influenza season. • Pregnant women who have underlying medical conditions should be vaccinated before influenza season, regardless of the stage of pregnancy. • Travelers to areas where influenza activity exists or when traveling among people from areas of the world where there is current influenza activity. • Anyone who wishes to reduce the likelihood of becoming ill with influenza.	• Given every year. • October through November is the *optimal* time to receive an annual flu shot to maximize protection. • Influenza vaccine may be given at any time during the influenza season (typically December through March) or at other times when the risk of influenza exists. • May give with all other vaccines but as a separate injection.	• Previous anaphylactic reaction to this vaccine, to any of its components, or to eggs. • Moderate or severe acute illness. NOTE: Pregnancy and breastfeeding are not contraindications to the use of this vaccine.
PPV23 (pneumococcal polysaccharide) Give IM or SC	• Adults who are 65 years of age or older. • People 2-64 years of age who have chronic illness or other risk factors, including chronic cardiac or pulmonary diseases, chronic liver disease, alcoholism, diabetes mellitus, CSF leaks, as well as people living in special environments or social settings (including Alaska Natives and certain American Indian populations). Those at highest risk of fatal pneumococcal infection are people with anatomic or functional asplenia, or sickle cell disease; immunocompromised persons including those with HIV infection, leukemia, lymphoma, Hodgkin's disease, multiple myeloma, generalized malignancy, chronic renal failure, or nephrotic syndrome; persons receiving immunosuppressive chemotherapy (including corticosteroids); and those who received an organ or bone marrow transplant. Pregnant women with high-risk conditions should be vaccinated if not done previously.	• Routinely given as a one-time dose; administer if previous vaccination history is unknown. • One-time revaccination is recommended 5 years later for people at highest risk of fatal pneumococcal infection or rapid antibody loss (e.g., renal disease) and for people ≥65 years of age if the 1st dose was given prior to age 65 and ≥5 years have elapsed since previous dose. • May give with all other vaccines but as a separate injection.	• Previous anaphylactic reaction to this vaccine or to any of its components. • Moderate or severe acute illness. NOTE: Pregnancy and breastfeeding are not contraindications to the use of this vaccine.

For specific ACIP immunization recommendations refer to the statements which are published in the *MMWR*. To obtain a complete set of ACIP statements, call (800) 232-2522, or to access individual statements, visit CDC's website: www.cdc.gov/nip/publications/ACIP-list.htm or visit IAC's website: www.immunize.org/acip.

This table is revised yearly due to the changing nature of U.S. immunization recommendations. Visit the Immunization Action Coalition's website at www.immunize.org/adultrules to make sure you have the most current version.

Modified from the Advisory Committee on Immunization Practices (ACIP) by the Immunization Action Coalition with reviews by ad hoc team, April 2001.

Courtesy Immunization Action Coalition, St. Paul, Minn; website: www.immunize.org.

Vaccine Name and Route	For Whom It Is Recommended	Schedule for Routine and "Catch Up" Administration	Contraindications (Mild Illness Is Not a Contraindication)
Hep-B (hepatitis B) Give IM Brands may be used interchangeably.	• All adolescents. • High risk adults including household contacts and sex partners of HBsAg-positive persons; users of illicit injectable drugs; heterosexuals with more than one sex partner in 6 months; men who have sex with men; people with recently diagnosed STDs; patients receiving hemodialysis and patients with renal disease that may result in dialysis; recipients of certain blood products; health care workers and public safety workers who are exposed to blood; clients and staff of institutions for the developmentally disabled; inmates of long-term correctional facilities, and certain international travelers. NOTE: Prior serologic testing may be recommended depending on the specific level of risk and/or likelihood of previous exposure. NOTE: In 1997, the NIH Consensus Development Conference, a panel of national experts, recommended that hepatitis B vaccination be given to all anti-HCV positive persons. EDITOR'S NOTE: Provide serologic screening for immigrants from endemic areas. When HBsAg-positive persons are identified, offer appropriate disease management. In addition, screen their sex partners and household members and, if found susceptible, vaccinate.	• Three doses are needed on a 0, 1, 6-month schedule. • Alternative timing options for vaccination include: • 0, 2, 4 months • 0, 1, 4 months • There must be 4 weeks between doses #1 and #2, and 8 weeks between doses #2 and #3. Overall there must be at least 16 weeks between doses #1 and #3. • *Schedule for those who have fallen behind:* If the series is delayed between doses, DO NOT start the series over. Continue from where you left off. • May give with all other vaccines but as a separate injection.	• Previous anaphylactic reaction to this vaccine or to any of its components. • Moderate or severe acute illness. NOTE: Pregnancy and breastfeeding are not contraindications to the use of this vaccine.
Hep-A (hepatitis A) Give IM Brands may be used interchangeably.	• People who travel outside of the U.S. (except for Western Europe, New Zealand, Australia, Canada, and Japan). • People with chronic liver disease including people with hepatitis C; people with hepatitis B who have chronic liver disease; illicit drug users; men who have sex with men; people with clotting-factor disorders; people who work with hepatitis A virus in experimental lab settings (not routine medical laboratories); and food handlers when health authorities or private employers determine vaccination to be cost-effective. NOTE: Prevaccination testing is likely to be cost effective for persons >40 years of age as well as for younger persons in certain groups with a high prevalence of hepatitis A virus infection.	• Two doses are needed. • The minimum interval between dose #1 and #2 is 6 months. • If dose #2 is delayed, do not repeat dose #1. Just give dose #2. • May give with all other vaccines but as a separate injection.	• Previous anaphylactic reaction to this vaccine or to any of its components. • Moderate or severe acute illness. • Safety during pregnancy has not been determined, so benefits must be weighed against potential risk. NOTE: Breastfeeding is not a contraindication to the use of this vaccine.

Continued

Vaccine Name and Route	For Whom It Is Recommended	Schedule for Routine and "Catch Up" Administration	Contraindications (Mild Illness Is Not a Contraindication)
Td (tetanus, diphtheria) Give IM	• All adolescents and adults. • After the primary series has been completed, a booster dose is recommended every 10 years. Make sure your patients have received a primary series of 3 doses. • A booster dose as early as 5 years later may be needed for the purpose of wound management, so consult ACIP recommendations.	• Give booster dose every 10 years after the primary series has been completed. • For those who are un-vaccinated or behind, complete the primary series (spaced at 0, 1-2 months, 6-12 months intervals). Don't restart the series, no matter how long since the previous dose. • May give with all other vaccines but as a separate injection.	• Previous anaphylactic or neurologic reaction to this vaccine or to any of its components. • Moderate or severe acute illness. NOTE: Pregnancy and breastfeeding are not contraindications to the use of this vaccine.
MMR (measles, mumps, rubella) Give SC	• Adults born in 1957 or later who are ≥18 years of age (including those born outside the U.S.) should receive at least one dose of MMR if there is no serologic proof of immunity or documentation of a dose given on or after 1st birthday. • Adults in high-risk groups, such as health care workers, students entering colleges and other post high school educational institutions, and international travelers, should receive a total of two doses. • Adults born before 1957 are usually considered immune but proof of immunity may be desirable for health care workers. • All women of childbearing age (i.e., adolescent girls and premenopausal adult women) who do not have acceptable evidence of rubella immunity or vaccination. • Special attention should be given to immunizing women born outside the United States in 1957 or later.	• One or two doses are needed. • If dose #2 is recommended, give it no sooner than 4 weeks after dose #1. • May be given with all other vaccines but as a separate injection. • If varicella vaccine and MMR are both needed and are not administered on the same day, space them at least 4 weeks apart. • If a pregnant woman is found to be rubella-susceptible, administer MMR postpartum.	• Previous anaphylactic reaction to this vaccine, or to any of its components. Pregnancy or possibility of pregnancy within 3 months (use contraception). NOTE: Breastfeeding is not a contraindication to the use of this vaccine. • HIV positivity is NOT a contraindication to MMR except for those who are severely immunocompromised. • Persons immunocompromised due to cancer, leukemia, lymphoma, immunosuppressive drug therapy, including high-dose steroids or radiation therapy. • If blood products or immune globulin have been administered during the past 11 months, consult the ACIP recommendations regarding time to wait before vaccinating. • Moderate or severe acute illness. NOTE: MMR is not contraindicated if a PPD test was recently applied. If PPD and MMR not given on same day, delay PPD for 4-6 weeks after MMR.

Vaccine Name and Route	For Whom It Is Recommended	Schedule for Routine and "Catch Up" Administration	Contraindications (Mild Illness Is Not a Contraindication)
Var (varicella [chickenpox]) Give SC	• All susceptible adults and adolescents should be vaccinated. It is especially important to ensure vaccination of the following groups: susceptible persons who have close contact with persons at high risk for serious complications (e.g., health care workers and family contacts of immunocompromised persons) and susceptible persons who are at high risk of exposure (e.g., teachers of young children, day care employees, residents and staff in institutional settings such as colleges and correctional institutions, military personnel, adolescents and adults living with children, non-pregnant women of childbearing age, and international travelers who do not have evidence of immunity). NOTE: People with reliable histories of chickenpox (such as self or parental report of disease) can be assumed to be immune. For adults who have no reliable history, serologic testing may be cost effective since most adults with a negative or uncertain history of varicella are immune.	• Two doses are needed. • Dose #2 is given 4-8 weeks after dose #1. • May be given with all other vaccines but as a separate injection. • If varicella vaccine and MMR are both needed and are not administered on the same day, space them at least 4 weeks apart. • If the second dose is delayed, do not repeat dose #1. Just give dose #2.	• Previous anaphylactic reaction to this vaccine or to any of its components. Pregnancy, or possibility of pregnancy within 1 month. • Immunocompromised persons due to malignancies and primary or acquired cellular immunodeficiency including HIV/AIDS. (See MMWR 1999, Vol. 28, No. RR-6.) NOTE: For those on high dose immunosuppressive therapy, consult ACIP recommendations regarding delay time. • If blood products or immune globulin have been administered during the past 5 months, consult the ACIP recommendations regarding time to wait before vaccinating. • Moderate or severe acute illness. NOTE: Breastfeeding is not a contraindication to the use of this vaccine. NOTE: Manufacturer recommends that salicylates be avoided for 6 weeks after receiving varicella vaccine because of a theoretical risk of Reye's syndrome.
IPV (polio) Give IM or SC	• Not routinely recommended for persons 18 years of age and older. NOTE: Adults living in the U.S. who never received or completed a primary series of polio vaccine need not be vaccinated unless they intend to travel to areas where exposure to wild-type virus is likely. Previously vaccinated adults can receive one booster dose if traveling to polio endemic areas.	• Refer to ACIP recommendations regarding unique situations, schedules, and dosing information. • May be given with all other vaccines as a separate injection.	• Refer to ACIP recommendations.

Continued

Vaccine Name and Route	For Whom It Is Recommended	Schedule for Routine and "Catch Up" Administration	Contraindications (Mild Illness Is Not a Contraindication)
Lyme disease Give IM	• Consider for persons 15-70 years of age who reside, work, or recreate in areas of high or moderate risk and who engage in activities that result in frequent or prolonged exposure to tick-infested habitat. • Persons with a history of previous uncomplicated Lyme disease who are at continued high risk for Lyme disease. (See description in the first bullet.) • See ACIP statement for a definition of high and moderate risk.	• Three doses are needed. Give at intervals of 0, 1, and 12 months. Schedule dose #1 (given in year 1) and dose #3 (given in year 2) to be given several weeks before tick season. See ACIP statement for details. • If given with other vaccines, give as a separate injection.	• Previous anaphylactic reaction to this vaccine or to any of its components. Pregnancy. • Moderate or severe acute illness. • Persons with treatment-resistant Lyme arthritis. • There are not enough data to recommend Lyme disease vaccine to persons with these conditions: immunodeficiency, diseases associated with joint swelling (including rheumatoid arthritis) or diffuse muscular pain, chronic health conditions due to Lyme disease.
Meningococcal disease	Meningococcal disease risk and vaccine availability should be discussed with college students. Consult the ACIP statement *Meningococcal Disease and College Students* (6/30/00) for details.		

Courtesy Immunization Action Coalition, St. Paul, Minn; website: www.immunize.org.

D.5   Recommended Immunizations for Specific At-Risk Populations

Vaccine	Indication	Notes
Hepatitis A	• Foreign travel to countries with intermediate to high endemic rates of disease • Children/adolescents residing in specific states or communities with high disease rates, as determined by the state public health officials • Persons with chronic liver disease • Homosexual and bisexual men/adolescents • Users of injection and noninjection illegal drugs • Persons with specific clotting factor disorders	• Not approved for children <2 years old

Influenza	Yearly administration in the fall for:
	• Targeted children/adolescents
	  1. Asthma or chronic pulmonary disease
	  2. Hemodynamically significant heart disease
	  3. Immunosuppressive disorders
	  4. HIV
	  5. Sickle cell anemia/other hemoglobinopathies
	  6. Diseases requiring long-term aspirin therapy (Kawasaki disease/rheumatoid arthritis)
	  7. Chronic renal dysfunction
	  8. Chronic metabolic disease (diabetes)
	• Children/adolescents who are members of households with high risk adults
	• Children/adolescents with underlying condition that may compromise resistance to influenza
	• Groups of persons whose close contact facilities transmission and spread of infection that may result in disruption of routine activities
	• Any health person who wishes to reduce the risk of infection with influenza
		• Indicated for children >6 months old
		• Children from 6 months to 12 years receive the split virus only
		• Children <9 years who have not had a previous vaccination require 2 doses administered one month apart

Meningococcal	• Children 2 years and older who are in high risk groups including asplenia and terminal complement or properdin deficiencies • College students, especially those living in dormitories or group housing	• Antibody persists about 5 years in adults/adolescents (3-5 years in children). • Reimmunization after that time is not usually recommended
Pneumococcal 23-valent	• Persons 2 years or older in high risk groups including sickle cell disease, asplenia, chronic renal failure or nephrotic syndrome, immunosuppression, HIV infection. CSF leaks, chronic cardiovascular disease, chronic pulmonary disease (not asthma), chronic liver disease or diabetes. • Persons 2 years or older living in specific environments where the risk of invasive disease or complications is high (e.g., Alaskan Native and certain Native American populations)	• Reimmunization may be recommended after 5 years (≥10 years old) or 3-5 years (<10 years) • Pneumococcal 7 valent vaccine is used for routine immunizations for infants and can be used for at risk children up to 9 years of age.

Appendix E

Guidelines for Practice

E.1 Infection-Control Guidelines for Home Care

The practice of universal precautions means that all blood and body fluids are treated as potentially infectious. Universal precautions procedures are implemented to prevent exposure and infection of caregivers. It is an important practice because many infections are subclinical.

- Use extreme care when handling needles, scalpels, and razors to prevent injuries. Do not recap, bend, break, or remove the needle from a syringe before disposal. Discard needles and syringes in puncture-resistant containers made of plastic or metal and dispose of them in a local landfill.

- Barrier precautions—such as gloves, masks, eye covering, and gowns—should be worn when contact with blood and body fluids is expected. Gloves must be worn when in contact with body fluids, mucous membranes, nonintact skin, and when drawing blood. Masks and eye coverings are recommended when droplets or splashes of blood or other body fluids are expected. Wear gowns, aprons, or smocks to protect regular clothing from splashes of blood or body fluids.

- Handwashing is the single most important practice in preventing infections. Handwashing should be done before and after providing client care and before and after preparing food, eating, feeding, or using the bathroom.

- Soiled dressings and perineal pads should be placed inside polyethylene garbage bags using two bags, one inside the other as a liner.

- HIV is easily decontaminated by common disinfectants such as Lysol and is rapidly killed by household bleach. Surfaces can be disinfected with a solution of 1 part bleach to 10 parts water. A new solution must be prepared daily to retain its disinfectant properties. Bathrooms and kitchens can be safely shared with persons infected with HIV, but towels, razors, and toothbrushes should not be shared. Household cleaning can be done in a regular manner unless there are spills of blood or body fluids. If a spill occurs, wear gloves and decontaminate the area by flooding the spill with a disinfectant, then use paper towels to remove visible debris, and reapply disinfectant.

- Kitchen counters, dishes, and laundry should be cleaned in warm water and detergent after use. Bathrooms may be cleaned with a household disinfectant.

E.2   Accident Prevention in Children

Age	Development	Major Accidents	Anticipatory Guidance
Neonate to 1 month	Is unable to protect self; when on abdomen can lift and turn head; dependent, requires protection; little control over body and movements.	Motor vehicles	• Use approved car seat. • Do not hold infant in lap. • Never leave infant in car unattended.
		Strangulation	• Spacing between crib bars should be no more than 2³⁄₈ inches apart. • Avoid tying anything, including pacifiers, around neck. • Fasten mobiles securely.
		Suffocation and injuries	• Crib mattress should fit firmly to sides. • Do not use pillows; use bumper pads. • Support infant's head when lifting, holding, or bathing.
		Burns, including sunburn	• Avoid bathing near hot water faucets. • Test water temperature before bath. • Set home water temperature less than 120°-130° F. • Avoid handling hot liquids, and do not smoke while handling infant. • Keep out of direct sunlight and use sunscreen. • Use flame-resistant clothing and furniture. • Have smoke detectors and fire extinguishers in the home. • Develop a fire plan for the home.
2-3 months	Begins gross motor movements of wiggling, squirming, thrashing, rolling.	Falls	• Never leave infant unattended (at any age) for any reason. • Keep one hand on infant while giving care. • Keep crib sides up. • Use infant seat on floor or playpen.
4-5 months	Mouths objects; brings hands to mouth.	Aspiration and choking	• Do not prop bottles (at any age). • Burp well before putting infant in crib. • Toys should be too large for infant to swallow, nonbreakable, and free of sharp edges, strings, and detachable parts. • Keep diaper pins closed during changing. • Keep small objects (e.g., buttons, coins) out of reach. • Use only one-piece pacifiers with a large shield.
		Suffocation	• Keep all plastic bags out of reach. • Keep stuffed animals out of crib.
		Lead poisoning	• Check toys and other objects for lead-free paint.
6-7 months	Sits without support; has a firm grasp; rolls and creeps.	Falls and falling objects	• Use safety strap in stroller or high chair. • Use sturdy high chair or feeding table. • Keep doors to stairs and outside locked; use safety gates. • Avoid use of hanging tablecloths. • Remove knickknacks and breakables.
		Ingestion	• Keep small objects, medicine, and plants out of reach. • Keep ipecac on hand and understand use. • Have poison control hotline number posted. • Lock up medicine, cleaning agents, insecticides, etc. • Keep trash cans out of reach or use locking lids.
		Injuries and electric shock	• Cover wall outlets. • Place furniture so cords are inaccessible. • Check furniture for sharp corners and add pads or remove furniture. • Inspect toys for breakage. • Keep sharp objects out of reach.

Continued

Age	Development	Major Accidents	Anticipatory Guidance
8-12 months	Pulls to stand; crawls, grabs; beginning to walk; enjoys exploring.	Burns	• Crawl around on floor and investigate what child could reach or get into. • Keep all hot food and drinks away from table edge; turn pot handles inward on stove. • Keep matches and lighters out of reach. • Keep kitchen closed up or gated. • Never leave child unattended near fireplace or stove. • Place guards around open hearths, registers, stoves, and fans. • Do not iron when child is crawling nearby.
		Choking	• Do not give child small hard foods such as peanuts, raw vegetables, popcorn. • Inspect toys for broken parts. • Keep floors, counters, tables free of small objects.
		Motor vehicle accidents	• Continue use of car seat. • Keep doors locked.
		Poisoning	• See previous discussion.
1-2 years	Walks up and down stairs; stoops and recovers; climbs; likes to take things apart.	Falls and injuries	• Supervise children in most activities, especially up and down stairs, outdoors, and at playgrounds. • Lock all windows; when opening, do so from top only. • Remove any objects or furniture in front of window that child could use as a ladder. • Permit climbing within child's capabilities. • Remove bumper pads or toys in crib that child could use to climb on. • Check toys, especially riding ones, for damage. • Keep small, pointed, or sharp objects out of reach. • Keep out of way of swings.
		Burns	• Teach child meaning of "hot." • Avoid use of baggy clothing.
		Drowning	• Continue to supervise bath/toilet use. • Supervise all water sport activity (e.g., wading pools, swimming, boating); use floats and/or life jackets. • Teach child to respect water and seek swimming lessons.
		Automobile-related accidents	• Continue to use appropriate car seat. • Keep doors and windows locked. • Do not permit child to hang out of windows. • Hold onto child when crossing street or in parking lots. • Do not permit child to ride toys near street.
		Poisoning and ingestion	• Have ipecac in any household the child frequents (e.g., baby sitter, grandparents). • Use childproof caps on medications. • Do not regard medicine as candy. • Do not give one child another child's prescription.
2-4 years	More adventuresome and curious; explores body orifices; more independent, with limited cognition; imitates.	Falls and injuries	• Teach child to be cautious around strange animals. • Supervise play at playground. • Keep out of reach small objects and foods (peanuts, beans) that can be inserted into orifices; check buttons on clothes and toys. • Discontinue use of crib when height of crib rail is 3/4 of toddler's height. • Keep stairs well lighted and free of clutter. • Give toys a safety check. • Discourage running in house and limit outdoor running to safe places. • Teach child to respect street and cars. • Teach child to stay away from and out of old appliances.

Age	Development	Major Accidents	Anticipatory Guidance
2-4 years—cont'd	Play increases to include rougher games and bike riding.	Drowning	• Continue to teach water safety. • Supervise all water activities. • Continue with swimming lessons.
		Automobile-related accidents	• See previous discussion.
		Burns	• Teach child what to do if fire breaks out; hold household drills. • Teach child to roll and smother fire if clothes catch on fire.
		Drowning	• Continue swimming lessons. • Use floats or life-jacket if child cannot swim. • Swim only where supervision is available (parent or lifeguard).
		Automobile-related accidents	• Teach pedestrian safety, providing example for child. • Do not permit playing in street. • Use adult seatbelt if child weighs >40 pounds. • If >55 inches tall, use shoulder restraints. • If <55 inches tall, only lap belt is used.
		Falls, injuries	• Make periodic checks on playground or play area used frequently. • Check on child when out playing. • Instruct child in safe use of toys; keep in good condition. • Keep away from driveways and streets. • If possible, provide fenced-in play area. • Set a good example by using seat belt, looking before crossing street, etc.
	Cognition improving and can identify good and bad.	Burns	• Teach child about danger of matches, lighters, stove. • Recheck radiators, space heaters, fireplaces, and protective guards.
		Poisoning and ingestions	• Do not become lax about keeping medication, etc., locked up. • Teach child to respect harmful objects and use a symbol to indicate "danger or harmful" to child. • Routinely check house, basement, and garage for harmful substances within reach.
4-6 years	Continues to be curious, daring, and imitative; frequently plays out of sight.		• Involve child in safety discussions. • Continue previously described activities when using household tools and equipment.

School age	Increased motor coordination and cognitive ability; increased peer and group activity and involvement in sports; assumes more responsibility for self and well-being.	Motor vehicle and bicycle accidents	• Involve child in safety discussion and planning.
			• Assign safety responsibilities, such as checking bike.
			• Teach child not to ride with strangers.
			• Teach child how to contact police and fire department and physician.
			• Be certain child knows address and phone number.
			• Discuss bicycle and pedestrian safety.
			• Discuss bicycle riding rules:
			  Always wear an approved bike helmet.
			  Do not hitch ride on moving vehicles.
			  Do not ride on dark street.
			  Use headlight or reflector light at night; wear bright clothes.
			  Do not dart from behind parked cars.
			  Do not carry passengers on bicycle.
			  Keep bike in good repair.
			• Do not use street as a playground.
			• Use seat belts.

Continued

Age	Development	Major Accidents	Anticipatory Guidance
School age—cont'd		Injuries	• Teach child to participate in sports safely using appropriate gear. • Permit only supervised sport activities. • Teach child proper use of household gadgets and equipment; supervise as necessary.
		Drowning	Teach the following swimming rules: • Swim only where a lifeguard is present. • Use buddy system. • Know water depth before diving. • Wear life jacket while boating or skiing or if nonswimmer. • No horseplay or calling for help jokingly.
		Falls	• See bicycle rules. • Discuss climbing trees: • Avoid slippery shoes. • Avoid weak or dead branches. • Keep a secure handhold.
		Burns	• Continue household drills. • Camp with supervision. • Teach proper campfire and barbecue care. • Use safe camping gear, including flame-retardant clothes.
Adolescence	Seeking identity and establishment of independence; subject to strong peer pressure; rejects unsought advice; has a need for physical activity; spends most of free time away from home.	Drowning	• Most important to have cooperation of adolescent when discussing and implementing safety measures. • See previous sections. • Never too late to learn to swim. • Enroll in lifesaving classes.
		Firearms accidents	• Avoid having loaded guns in household. • Learn safety handling if involved in sport hunting. • Keep guns in locked closet and ammunition in separate locked area. • Never assume gun is not loaded. • Never point gun at another.
		Automobile-related accidents	• Take driver education. • Use seat belts for self and passengers. • Practice pedestrian safety. • Do not drive under influence of drugs or alcohol. • Do not hitchhike or pick up hitchhikers.
		Alcohol, drugs, and tobacco	• Discuss effects of substance use and abuse. • Assist teen to identify other ways to achieve self-esteem, independence, and peer acceptance.

E.3   Guide for Evaluation of Group Effectiveness

The following questions focus evaluation on group task accomplishment, member satisfaction, conflict management, and group purpose. Answer each question for the group, then write a descriptive summary of group effectiveness.

1. Describe the group's task goal. List the steps proposed or acted on by members relative to the goal. How well do members achieve these steps?
2. Describe leadership behavior for the group. How well do members carry out other group roles?
3. Describe comfort level for group members. Do members support each other? Is the level of tension conducive to productive behavior?
4. Is disagreement expressed clearly and openly? How do members manage and resolve conflict?
5. By what bonds are members attracted to each other and to the group?
6. Are there implicit goals for the group, and do these goals interfere with the group's work toward the explicit goal?

Screening Tools

F.1 Infant Reflexes

Reflex	How to Elicit	Response of Infant	Clinical Implications
Acoustic blink	Produce a sharp loud noise (a clap of the hands) about 30 cm from the head.	By second or third day of life infant blinks both eyes. Disappearance of reflex is variable.	Absence may indicate decreased hearing.
Ankle clonus	Flex the leg at the hip and knee, sharply dorsiflex the foot, and maintain pressure.	Rhythmic flexions and extensions of the foot at the ankle.	Abnormal if more than 10 beats during the first 3 months or more than 3 beats after 3 months. Sustained clonus indicates upper motor neuron disease.
Babinski	Stroke lateral aspect of the plantar surface of foot from heel to toes. Use a blunt object.	Hyperextension or fanning of toes occurs. As myelinization is completed, the normal response becomes flexion (downward curling) of all toes; the positive (pathological) sign is hyperextension (dorsiflexion) of the great toe with or without fanning of the remaining toes.	After 2 years of age, a positive sign is the most significant clinical symptom of the presence of an upper motor neuron (pyramidal tract) lesion.
Blinking	Shine a light suddenly at the infant's open eyes.	Eyelids close in response to light. Disappears after first year.	Absence may indicate poor light perception or blindness.
Landau	Suspend infant carefully in prone position by supporting infant's abdomen with examiner's hand.	By 3 months of age the expected response consists of extension of head, trunk, and hips. Head is slightly above horizontal plane. Disappears by 2 years of age.	Result is abnormal if newborn collapses into a limp concave position.
Moro	With infant in supine position gently support head and lift it a few centimeters off the surface. As soon as neck relaxes, suddenly release the head and let it drop back to the surface. *or* Produce sudden loud noise, or jar the table or crib suddenly.	Normal response is present at birth and is one in which the arms extend outward, the hands open, and then are brought together in midline. The legs flex slightly. Usually disappears by 3 to 4 months. Infant may cry.	Asymmetry indicates possible paralysis. Absence suggests severe neurological problem. Persistence beyond 4 months may indicate neurological disease. If reflex lasts longer than 6 months, result is definitely abnormal.
Neck righting	With infant in supine position turn head to one side.	Infant's trunk rotates in direction in which head is turned. Appears at 4 to 6 months. Disappears at 24 months.	Absent or decreased reflex may indicate spasticity.
Palmar grasp	With infant's head positioned in midline, place examiner's index fingers from ulnar side into infant's palm and press against palm.	Normal response is flexion of all fingers around examiner's fingers. Present at birth and disappears by 4 months when infant is ready to reach.	Note symmetry and strength. Persistence of grasp beyond 4 months suggests cerebral dysfunction.

Continued

Reflex	How to Elicit	Response of Infant	Clinical Implications
Parachute	Infant is held in a prone position and is quickly lowered toward the surface of the examining table or floor.	Normal response is extension of arms, hands, and fingers, as if to break a fall. Appears by 9 months and persists.	Asymmetry or absence of response is abnormal.
Perez	Infant is held in a suspended prone position in one of the examiner's hands. The thumb of the other hand is moved firmly from sacrum along entire spine.	Normal response is extension of head and spine, flexion of knees on the chest, a cry, and emptying of the bladder. Present at birth and disappears by 3 months.	Absence indicates severe neurological disease.
Placing	Infant is held erect and the dorsum of one foot touches the undersurface of the examining table top.	Infant flexes hip and knee and places stimulated foot on top of the table. Present at birth and disappears at 6 weeks or variable.	Absent in paralysis or in infants born by breech delivery.
Plantar grasp	Examiner's finger is placed firmly across base of infant's toes.	Toes curl downward. Present at birth and disappears by 10 to 12 months.	Absent in defects of lower spinal column. Infant cannot walk until this reflex disappears.
Rooting	Infant is held in supine position with position with head in midline and hands against chest. Examiner strokes perioral skin at corner of mouth or cheek.	Infant opens mouth and turns head toward stimulated side. Present at birth and disappears by 3 to 4 months (awake); by 7 months (asleep).	Absence indicates severe central nervous system disease or depressed infant.
Rotation test	Infant is held upright facing examiner and rotated in one direction and then the other.	Infant's head turns in the direction in which the body is being turned. If head is restrained the eyes will turn in the direction in which the infant is turned.	If head and eyes do not move, it indicates a vestibular problem.
Spontaneous crawling (Bauer's response)	Infant is lying prone and examiner presses soles of feet.	Infant makes crawling movements. Present at birth.	Crawling is absent in weak or CNS depressed infants.
Stepping	Infant is held upright and soles of feet are put in touch with solid surface.	Infant "walks" along surface. Present at birth and disappears at 6 weeks.	Absence indicates depressed infant, breech delivery, or paralysis.
Sucking	With infant in supine position place nipple or finger 3 to 4 cm into mouth.	Vigorous sucking of finger or nipple. Present at birth and disappears by 3 to 4 months (awake) and 7 months (asleep). Tongue action should push finger up and back. Note rate of suck, amount of suction, and patterns or groupings of sucks.	Absence in term infants indicates central nervous system depression. Weak reflex may lead to feeding problems.
Tonic neck	With infant in supine position, passively rotate head to one side.	Arm and leg on side to which head is turned extend, and opposite arm and leg flex (fencer's position). Present sometimes at birth but usually by 2 to 3 months. Disappears by 6 months.	Obligatory response is always abnormal. Persistence beyond 6 months is abnormal and indicates central motor lesions (e.g., cerebral palsy).
Trunk incurvation (Galant's)	Infant is held prone in examiner's hand. With the other hand the examiner moves a finger down the paravertebral portion of the spine, first on one side, then on the other.	Infant's trunk should curve to the side being stimulated. Present at birth and disappears by 2 months.	Presence of spinal cord lesions interrupts this reflex.
Vertical suspension positioning	Infant is held upright, head is maintained in midline.	Legs are flexed at the hips and knees. Present at birth and disappears after 4 months.	Scissoring or fixed extension indicates spasticity.

F.2   Vision and Hearing Screening Procedures

Method	Age	Procedure	Normal Response
Vision			
Following	Infancy	Shine light or hold bright object directly in front of infant's line of vision; move slowly from side to side.	Follow light or bright object up to 180 degrees.
Turn to light response	Infancy	Hold back of head to bright light source.	Eyes turn toward source of light.
Optokinetic drum	Infancy	Twirl drum with stripes slowly in front of infant's eyes.	Nystagmus occurs.
Herschberg reflex (corneal light reflex)	Infancy through adolescence	Shine penlight into child's eyes; note where light reflex falls. For older children: have child focus and stare at point 14 inches and then 20 inches away before shining light into eyes.	Light reflex falls in same position in eye.
Cover test	Toddler through adolescence	Have child focus on specified spot first 14 inches, then 20 inches away. While child is focusing, one eye is completely covered for 5 to 10 seconds. Cover is then removed and eye observed for movement. Procedure repeated for other eye.	No wandering or sharp jerky movement of eyes noted, indicating ability to focus.
Snellen E	Preschool	Child is instructed to point finger in direction that the E or table legs are pointing from a distance of 20 feet. Test each eye separately, then together. Test as far down on chart as child can go.	Visual acuity of 20/30-20/40.
Snellen alphabet	School age through adolescence	Child stands 20 feet from chart and reads letters. Each eye is tested separately and then together. Testing usually started at 20/30 or 20/40 line and child allowed to test as far down chart as possible. Passing score consists of reading majority of letters (or Es) on each line.	Visual acuity of 20/20.
Hearing			
Startle reflex	Newborn	Loud noise or bang made near infant's ears.	Jumps at noise, blinks, cries or widens eyes.
Tracks sound	3-6 months	Make noise, call name, or sing.	Eyes shift toward sound; responds to mother's voice; coos to verbalization.
Recognizes sound	6-8 months	As preceding, from out of line of vision.	Turns head toward sound; responds to name, babbles to verbalization.
Localization of sound	8-12 months	Call name, or use tuning fork or say words.	Localizes source of sound; turns head (and body at times) toward sound, repeats words.
Pure tone screening—play	Toddler to preschool	Demonstrate to child by putting headphones on and making believe you hear sound. As you say "I hear it," put a block in box or ring on holder. Put headphones on child and give block or ring to use. Sound a 50 dB tone at 1000 Hz and guide child's hand with block to box. When child can do this alone, begin screening. Set at 25 dB at 1000 Hz. If child responds, go to 200, 4000, and 6000 Hz. Praise child and place new block in hand. Switch to other ear and test.	Should respond at 25 dB at any frequency.

Continued

Method	Age	Procedure	Normal Response
Hearing—cont'd			
Pure tone audiometry	School age through adolescence	Explain procedure to child. Place headphones on ears. Test one ear at a time in sequence as preceding (i.e., 25 dB at 1000, 2000, 4000 and 6000 Hz). Have child raise hand to indicate sound is heard.	Should respond at 25 dB at any frequency.
Tuning Fork Test	Some preschoolers; school age through adolescence		
Weber test		Strike tuning fork to make it vibrate and place the stem in midline of scalp. Ask child if sound is same in both ears or louder in either ear.	Sound heard equally well in both ears.
Rinne test		Strike tuning fork until it vibrates, place stem on child's mastoid until he no longer hears it. Then place vibrating fingers of fork 1 to 2 inches in front of concha. Ask child if he can still hear sound.	Sound from fingers of fork vibrating in air should be heard when child can no longer hear sound with stem against mastoid (i.e., air conduction is greater than bone conduction).

F.3   Screening for Common Orthopedic Problems

Deformity	Description	Screening
Congenital hip dislocation (CHD)	Complete or partial displacement of femoral head out of the acetabulum	*Barlow's maneuver* (for dislocation of femoral head): flex hip to 90 degrees; grasp symphysis in front and sacrum in back with one hand; with other hand, apply lateral pressure to medial thigh with thumb and longitudinal pressure to knee with palm; abduct flexed hip. A positive sign is sensation of abnormal movement. Reverse hands for examining other hip. (Figure F-1). *Ortolani's maneuver* (for reduction of femur): abduct hip to 80 degrees, lifting proximal femur anteriorly with fingers placed on lateral thigh. A positive sign is sensation of a jerk or snap with reduction into socket. (Figure F-2). *Limited full abduction of hips:* with child flat on back, abduct hips one at a time, then together. See Figure F-3 for degrees of hip abduction.

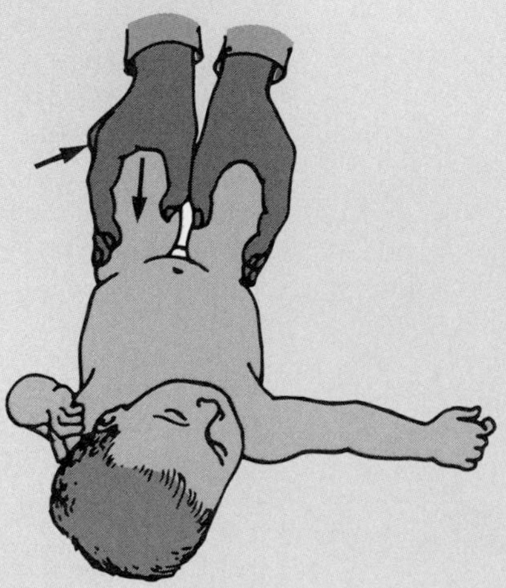

Figure F-1

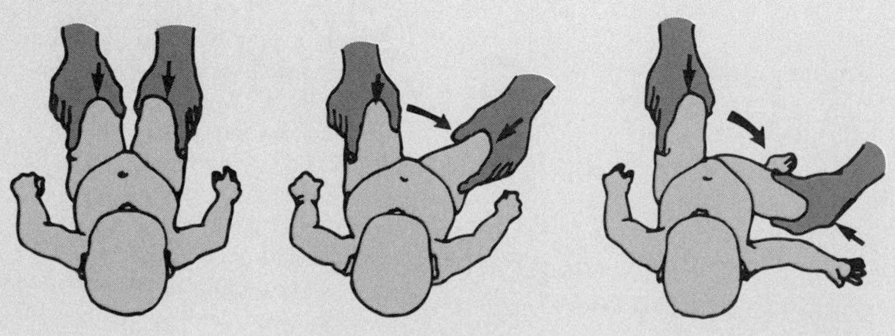

Figure F-2

Deformity	Description	Screening
Congenital hip dislocation (CHD)—cont'd		*Apparent shortening of femur:* 1. *Allis sign:* with child lying on back, pelvis flat, knees flexed and feet planted firmly, observe knees. If the knee projects further anteriorly, femur is longer; if one knee is higher, the tibia is longer. 2. With child on back, both legs are extended out with pressure on knees. Heels are matched and observed for equal or unequal length. 3. *Trendelenburg sign:* with child standing on one leg, observe pelvis. When child stands on abnormal leg, the pelvis drops on normal side. (Figure F-4).
Metatarsus adductus (varus)	Adduction or turning in of forefoot with high longitudinal arch and wide space between first and second toes. Commonly associated with tibial torsion.	Test foot for flexibility and elicit tonic foot reflexes. Rigidity is indicated by eversion or inversion when foot does not move beyond neutral position or does not respond to toe grasping or by dorsiflexing. Signs of metatarsus adductus are illustrated in Figure F-5.
Pes planus (flat feet)	When child is weight bearing, longitudinal arch of foot appears flat on floor *Pseudo flat feet:* very common until ages 2 to 3; created by plantar fat pad. Feet are flexible, exhibit hypermobility of joint, and have a low arch *Rigid flat feet:* Uncommon; created by tightness of heel cord or tarsal coalition (a cartilaginous fibrous or bony connection between bones)	1. Observe feet in weighted and unweighted position 2. Stand child on toes. Arch disappears with weight bearing in flexible flat foot and reappears when on toes (Figure F-6). 3. Elicit dorsal and plantar flexion to rule out tight heel cord. 4. Elicit eversion and inversion flexion to rule out tarsal coalition. Same as for preceding No. 1 (pseudo flat feet)

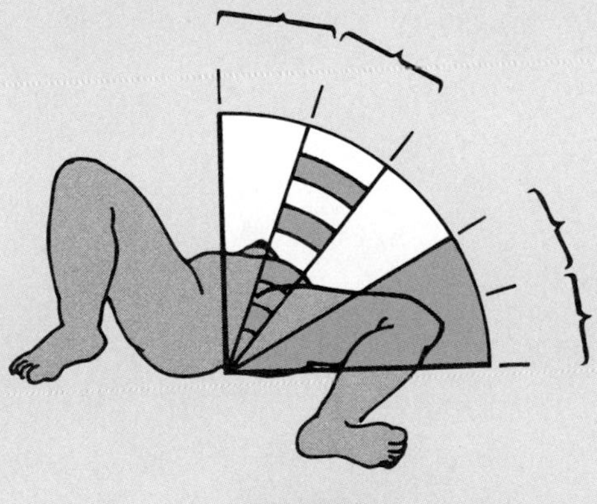

Figure F-3

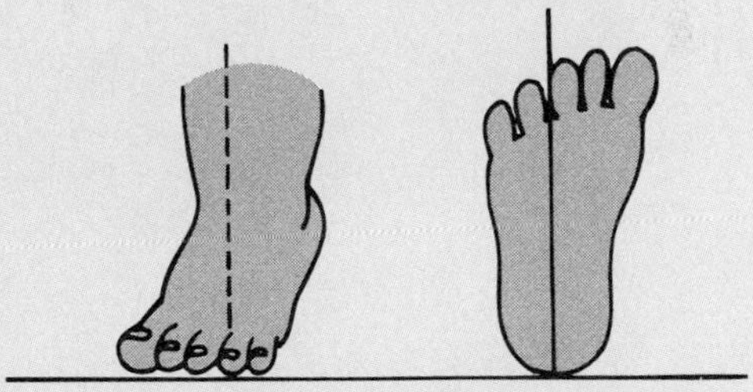

Figure F-5

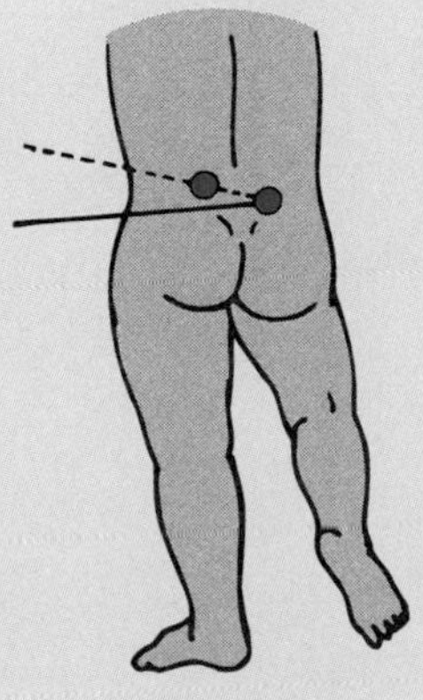

Figure F-4

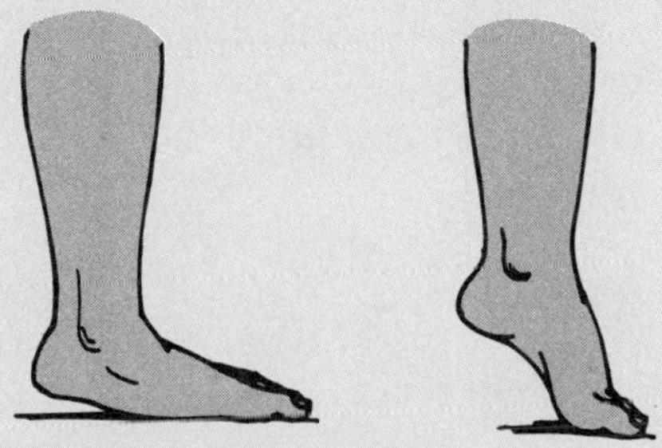

Figure F-6

Continued

Deformity	Description	Screening
Genu valgum (knock-knees)	A deviant axis of thighs and calves of more than 10 to 15 degrees; (normal from ages 2-6)	1. Observe axis of thighs and calves with child standing. Normally axes are parallel with 10 to 15 degrees deviance (Figure F-7). 2. Observe space between the knees from front to back. Normal spacing is 1½ inches. 3. Observe space between ankles from front and back. Normal spacing between medial malleoli at heel is 2 inches.
Genu varum (bowlegs)	Deviant axis of thighs and calves; is (1) Physiological: normal until ages 2 to 3; occurs with internal tibial torsion and genu valgum (2) Pathological	Same as for genu valgum.
Internal tibial torsion	Twisting or torsion of tibia usually accompanied by metatarsus adductus	1. Examine legs for range of motion, flexibility of ankle and elicit tonic foot reflexes. 2. Holding knee firmly with foot in neutral position, observe medial and lateral malleoli. The normal angle between them is approximately 15 to 20 degrees (Figure F-8). 3. Have child sit on examining table and draw a circle over patellar and external malleoli. With patella facing forward only anterior edge of malleolar circle should be seen (Figure F-9).
Scoliosis	S-shaped lateral curvature of spine with rotation of vertical bodies.	Screening is implemented as follows: 1. Ask the child to bend forward in a 50% flexing position with shoulders drooping forward, arms and head dangling. Observe the spine from above the head and inspect for any lateral curvature or prominent projection of the rib cage on one side (Figure F-10). 2. While the child is standing erect with weight equal on both feet, observe for: • Difference in levels of shoulders, scapula, and hips • Differences in the size of the spaces between the arms and the trunk • Prominence of either scapula or hip • A curve in the vertebral spinous process alignment. 3. Ask the child to walk and make observations discussed in No. 2 and observe for the presence of a waddle, limp, or tilt.

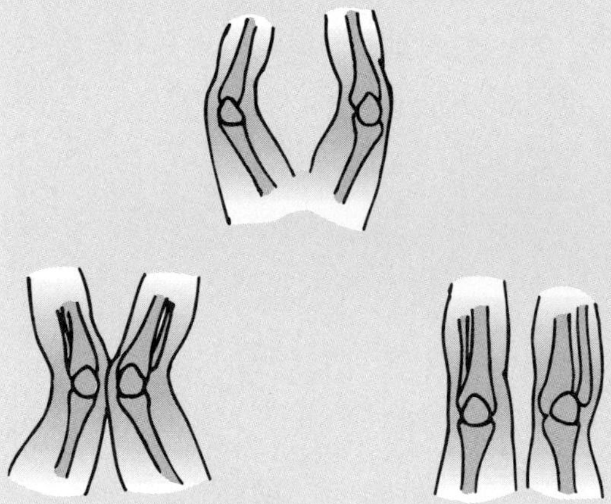

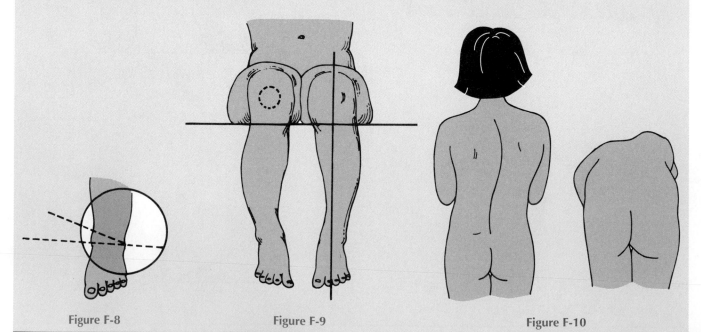

Figure F-7

Figure F-8

Figure F-9

Figure F-10

F.4   Development Characteristics: Summary for Children

Age	Physical and Motor Development	Intellectual Development	Socialization and Vocalization	Emotional Development
1 month	Physiologically more stable than in newborn period. Waves hands as clenched fists. Objects placed in hands are dropped immediately. Momentary visual fixation on objects and human face. Tonic neck reflex position frequent and Moro reflex brisk. Able to turn head when prone, but unable to support head. Responds to sounds of bell, rattle, etc. Makes crawling motions when prone. Sucking and rooting reflex present. Coordinates sucking, swallowing, and breathing.	Reflexive. No attempt to interact with environment. External stimuli do not have meaning.	Cries, mews, and makes throaty noises. Responds in terms of internal need states. Interested in the human face.	Response limited generally to tension states. Panic reactions, with arching of back and extension and flexion of extremities. Derives satisfaction from the feeding situation when held and pleasure from rocking, cuddling, and tactile stimulation. Maximum need for sucking pleasures. Quiets when picked up.
2 months	Moro reflex still brisk. Posture still toward tonic neck reflex position. Has visual response to patterns. Eye coordination to light and objects. Follows objects vertically and horizontally. Responds to objects placed on face. Listens actively to sounds. Able to lift head momentarily from prone position. Turns from side to back. Able to swallow pureed foods.	Recognition of familiar face. Indicates inspection of the environment. Begins to show anticipation before feeding.	Begins to vocalize; coos. Beginning of social smile. Actively follows movement of familiar person or object with eyes. Crying becomes differentiated. Vocalizes to mother's voice. Visually searches to locate sounds of mother's voice.	Maximum need for sucking pleasures. Indicates more active satisfaction when fed, held, rocked.
3 months	Frequency of tonic neck reflex position and vigor of Moro response rapidly diminishing. Uses arms and legs simultaneously but not separately. Able to raise head from prone position; may get chest off bed.	Shows active interest in environment. Can recognize familiar faces and objects such as bottle; however, objects do not have permanence. Recognition is indicative of recording of memory traces.	More ready and responsive smile. Facial and generalized body response to faces. Preferential response to adult voices. Has longer periods of wakefulness without crying.	Maximum need for sucking pleasure. Wishes to avoid unpleasant situations. Not yet able to act independently to evoke response in others.

From Waechter EH, Blake FG: *Nursing care of children*, ed 9, Philadelphia, 1976, JB Lippincott.

Continued

Age	Physical and Motor Development	Intellectual Development	Socialization and Vocalization	Emotional Development
3 months—cont'd	Holds head in fairly good control. Begins differentiation of motor responses. Hands are beginning to open, and objects placed in hands are retained for brief inspection; able to carry objects to mouth. Indicates preference for prone or supine position. Stepping reflex disappears. Landau reflex appears. Eyes converge as objects approach face. Has necessary muscular control to accept cereal and fruit.	Begins playing with parts of body. Follows objects visually. Begins to be able to coordinate stimuli from various sense organs. Shows awareness of a strange situation.	Begins to use prelanguage vocalizations, babbling and cooing. Laughs aloud and shows pleasure in vocalization. Shows anticipatory preparation to being lifted. Turns head to follow familiar person. Ceases crying when mother enters the room.	
4 months	Ability to carry objects to mouth. Inspects and plays with hands. Grasps objects with both hands. Turns head to sound of bell or bottle. Reaches for offered objects. Eyes focus on small objects. Begins to demonstrate eye-hand coordination. Ability to pick up objects. Rooting reflex disappears; tonic neck reflex disappearing. Sits with minimum support with stable head and back. Turns from back to side. Breathing and mouth activity coordination in relation to vocal cords. Holds head up when pulled to sitting position. Begins to drool.	Recognizes bottle on sight. Becomes bored when left alone for long periods of time. Actively interested in environment. Indicates beginnings of intentionality and interest in affecting the environment. Indicates beginning anticipation of consequences of action.	Vocalizes frequently and vocalizations change according to mood. Begins to respond to "no, no." Enjoys being propped in a sitting position. Turns head to familiar noise. Chuckles socially. Demands attention by fussing; enjoys attention.	Interest in mother heightens. Is affable and lovable. Shows signs of increasing trust and security.
5 months	Ability to recover near objects. Reaches persistently. Grasps with whole hand. Ability to lift objects. Begins to use thumb and finger in "pincer" movement. Able to sustain visual inspection.	Able to discriminate strangers from family. Turns head after fallen object. Shows active interest in novelty. Attempts to regain interesting action in environment.	Enjoys play with people and objects. Smiles at mirror image. More exuberantly playful but also more touchy and discriminating.	Other members of the family become important as the baby's emotional world expands. Begins to be able to postpone gratification. Awaits anticipated routines with happy expectation.

From Waechter EH, Blake FG: *Nursing care of children,* ed 9, Philadelphia, 1976, JB Lippincott.

Age	Physical and Motor Development	Intellectual Development	Socialization and Vocalization	Emotional Development
5 months—cont'd	Able to sit for longer periods of time when well supported. Begins to show signs of tooth eruption. Ability to sleep through night without feeding. Moro reflex and tonic neck reflex finally disappear.	Ability to coordinate visual impressions of an object. Begins differentiation of self from environment.		Begins to explore mother's body.
6 months	Ability to pick up small objects directly and deftly. Ability to lift cup by handle. Grasps, holds, and manipulates objects. Ability to pull self to sitting position. Begins to "hitch" in locomotion. Momentary sitting and hand support. When lying in prone position, supports weight with hands. Weight gain begins to decline. Ability to turn completely over.	Increasing awareness of self. Responds with attentiveness to novel stimuli. Begins to be able to recognize mother when she is dressed differently. Objects begin to acquire permanence; searches for lost object for brief period.	Very interested in sound production. Playful response to mirror. Laughs aloud when stimulated. Great interest in babbling, which is self-reinforcing. Begins to recognize strangers.	Begins to have sense of "self." Increased growth of ego
7 months	Ability to transfer objects from one hand to another. Holds object in one hand. Gums or mouths solid foods; exploratory behavior with food. Ability to bang objects together. Palmar grasp disappears. Bears weight when held in standing position. Sits alone for brief periods. Rolls over adeptly.	Ability to secure objects by pulling on string. Repeats activities that are enjoyed. Discovers and plays with own feet. Drops and picks up objects in exploration. Searches for lost objects outside perceptual field. Has consciousness of desires. Growing differentiation of self from environment. Rudimentary sense of depth and space.	Vocalizes four different syllables. Produces vowel sounds and chained syllables. Makes "talking sounds" in response to the talking of others. Crows and squeals.	Begins to show signs of fretfulness when mother leaves or in presence of strangers. Shows beginning fear of strangers. Orally aggressive in biting and mouthing.
8 months	Ability to ring bell purposefully. Ability to feed self with finger foods. Begins to experience tooth eruption. Sits well alone. Ability to release objects at will.	Uncovers hidden toy. Increased interest in feeding self. Differentiation of means from end in intentionality. Has lively curiosity about the world.	Listens selectively to familiar words. Says "da da" or equivalent. Babbles to produce consonant sounds. Vocalizes to toys. Stretches out arms to be picked up.	Plays for sheer pleasure of the activity. Anxiety when confronted by strangers indicates recognition and need of mother; attachment behavior begins to be obvious and strong.

Continued

Age	Physical and Motor Development	Intellectual Development	Socialization and Vocalization	Emotional Development
9 months	Rises to sitting position. Creeps and/or crawls; maybe backward at first. Tries out newly developing motor capacities. Ability to hold own bottle. Drinks from cup or glass with assistance. Begins to show regular patterns in bladder and bowel elimination. Good ability to use thumb and finger in pincer grasp. Pulls self to feet with help.	Ability to put objects in container. Examines object held in hand; explores objects by sucking, chewing, and biting.	Responds to simple verbal requests. Plays interactive games, such as peek-a-boo and patty cake.	Mother is increasingly important for her own sake; reacts violently to threat of her loss. Begins to show fears of going to bed and being left alone. Increasing interest in pleasing mother. Active search in play for solutions to separation anxiety.
10 months	Ability to unwrap objects. Pulls to standing position. Uses index finger to poke and finger and thumb to hold objects. Finger feeds self; controls lips around cup. Plantar reflex disappears. Neck-righting reflex disappears. Sits without support; recovers balance easily. Pulls self upright with use of furniture.	Begins to imitate. Looks at and follows pictures in book.	Extends toy to another person without releasing. Responds to own name. Inhibits behavior to "no, no" or own name. Begins to test reactions to parental responses during feeding and at bedtime. Imitates facial expressions and sounds.	Has powerful urge toward independence in locomotion, feeding; beginning to help in dressing. Experiences joy when achieving a goal and mastering fear.
11 months	Ability to hold crayon adaptively. Ability to push toys. Ability to put several objects in container; releases objects at will. Stands with assistance; may be beginning attempts to walk with assistance. Begins to be able to hold spoon. "Cruises" around furniture.	Works to get toy out of reach. Growing interest in novelty. Heightened curiosity and drive to explore environment.	Repeats performance laughed at by others. Imitates definite speech sounds. Uses jargon. Communicates by pointing to objects wanted.	Reacts to restrictions with frustration, but has ability to master new situations with mother's help (weaning).

From Waechter EH, Blake FG: *Nursing care of children,* ed 9, Philadelphia, 1976, JB Lippincott.

Age	Physical and Motor Development	Intellectual Development	Socialization and Vocalization	Emotional Development
12 months	Turns pages in book; can make marks on paper. Babinski sign disappears. Begins standing alone and toddling. "Cruises" around furniture. Lumbar curve develops. Hand dominance becomes evident. Ability to use spoon in feeding.	Dogged determination to remove barriers to action. Further separation of means from ends. Experiments to reach goals not attained previously. Concepts of space, time, and causality begin to have more objectivity.	Jabbers expressively. Has words that are specific to parents. Few, simple words. Experimentation with "pseudo-words" of great interest and pleasure.	Ability to show emotions of fear, anger, affection, jealousy, anxiety. Is in love with the world.
15-18 months	Uses spoon and cup with little spilling; builds 2-cube tower; can undress; has refined pincer grasp.	Stoops and recovers; walks well; pushes furniture to climb; walks up stairs one at a time with assistance.	Rolls ball back and forth with one other person; imitates household chores; indicates desires without crying; drinks from a cup.	Vocabulary of 10 to 20 words; understands simple questions; forms 2-word phrases; beginning to name pictures.
2 years	Builds a 6-cube tower; turns pages of a book one at a time; begins to dress self; washes and dries hands.	Runs; walks up and down stairs alone; walks backwards; jumps in place; throws ball overhand.	Removes clothes; awareness of ownership; helps out; eats with family but cannot sit through entire meal.	Points to body parts; has 300-400 word vocabulary; uses "my" pronouns and prepositions; forms 3- to 4-word phrases.
3 years	Opens and closes doors using knob by self; uses fingers to hold pencil; builds 8- to 10-block tower; zips zippers; does simple buttoning.	Walks up and down stairs alternating feet; rides tricycle; broad jumps; dresses with assistance.	May have imaginary playmates; can put on simple garment; washes and dries hands; likes to have a choice.	Uses plurals; forms 3- to 4-word sentences, using correct grammatical structures.
4 years	Draws a 3-part man; buttons easily; can cut out pictures.	Catches ball with hands; broad jumps; climbs up and down stairs, alternating feet; balances on one foot momentarily.	Separates easily from mother; can button clothing; plays interactive and associative games, demonstrating some control; able to share.	Comprehends and uses opposites; has increased vocabulary and about 90% comprehensibility; speaks in full sentences, using prepositions, pronouns, adverbs, and adjectives.
5 years	Copies a square accurately; draws a 5-part man; begins to tie shoelaces.	Runs with speed and agility; dresses without supervision; skips crudely.	Developing attachment outside of family; engages in cooperative play; strives for independence.	Vocabulary expanding to 3-syllable words; composition increasing to spoken paragraphs.

F.5   Developmental Behaviors: Summary for School-Age Children

Age (years)	Physical Competency	Intellectual Competency	Emotional-Social Competency	Play	Safety
6-12 (General)	Gains an average of 2.5-3.2 kg/year (5½-7 lb/yr). Overall height gains of 5.5 cm (2 in) per year; growth occurs in spurts and is mainly in trunk and extremities. Loses deciduous teeth; most of permanent teeth erupt. Progressively more coordinated in both gross and fine motor skills. Caloric needs increase with growth spurts.	Masters concrete operations. Moves from egocentrism; learns he is not always right. Learns grammar and expression of emotions and thoughts. Vocabulary increases to 3000 words or more; handles complex sentences.	Central crisis: industry vs. inferiority; wants to do and make things. Progressive sex education needed. Wants to be like friends; competition important. Fears body mutilation, alterations in body image; earlier phobias may recur, nightmares; fears death. Nervous habits common.	Plays in groups, mostly of same sex; "gang" activities predominate. Books for all ages. Bicycles a must. Sports equipment. Cards, board, and table games. Most of play is active games requiring little or no equipment.	Enforce continued use of safety belts during car travel. Bicycle safety must be taught and enforced. Teach safety related to hobbies, handicrafts, mechanical equipment.
6-7	Depth perception developed. Vision reaches adult level of 20/20. Gross motor skill exceeds fine motor coordination. Balance and rhythm are good—runs, skips, jumps, climbs, gallops. Throws and catches ball. Dresses self with little or no help.	Vocabulary of 2500 words. Learning to read and print; beginning concrete concepts of numbers, general classification of items. Knows concepts of right and left; morning, afternoon, and evening; coinage. Intuitive thought process. Verbally aggressive, bossy, opinionated, argumentative. Likes simple games with basic rules.	Boisterous, outgoing, and know-it-all, whiny; parents should sidestep power struggles, offer choices. Becomes quiet and reflective during seventh year; very sensitive. Can use telephone. Likes to make things: starts many, finishes few. Give some responsibility for household duties.	Still enjoys dolls, cars, and trucks. Plays well alone but enjoys small groups of both sexes; begins to prefer same-sex peers during seventh year. Ready to learn how to ride a bicycle. Prefers imaginary, dramatic play with real costumes. Begins collecting for quantity, not quality. Enjoys active games such as hide-and-seek, tag, jump rope, roller skating, kickball. Ready for lessons in dancing, gymnastics, music. Restrict TV time to 1-2 hours/day.	Teach and reinforce traffic safety. Still needs adult supervision of play. Teach to avoid strangers, never take anything from strangers. Teach cold prevention and reinforce continued practice of other health habits. Restrict bicycle use to home ground; no traffic areas; teach bicycle safety. Teach and set examples regarding harmful use of drugs, alcohol, smoking.

Age	Physical	Cognitive/Language	Social/Emotional	Activities	Safety
8-10	Myopia may appear. Secondary sex characteristics begin in girls. Hand-eye coordination and fine motor skills well established. Movements are graceful, coordinated. Cares for own physical needs completely. Constantly on move; plays and works hard; enforce balance in rest and activity. Vision and hearing fully developed.	Learning correct grammar and to express feelings in words. Likes books can read by oneself; will read funny papers, scan newspaper. Enjoys making detailed drawings. Mastering classification, seriation, spatial and temporal, numerical concepts. Uses language as a tool; likes riddles, jokes, chants, word games. Rules guiding force in life now. Very interested in how things work, what and how weather, seasons, etc., are made.	Strong preference for same-sex peers; antagonizes opposite sex peers. Self-assured and pragmatic at home; questions parental values and ideas. Has a strong sense of humor. Enjoys clubs, group projects, outings, large groups, camp. Modesty about own body increases over time; sex conscious. Works diligently to perfect skills he does best. Happy, cooperative, relaxed and casual in relationships. Increasingly courteous and well-mannered with adults. Gang stage at a peak; secret codes and rituals prevail. Responds better to suggestion than dictatorial approach.	Likes hiking, sports. Enjoys cooking, woodworking, crafts. Enjoys cards and table games. Likes radio and records. Begins qualitative collecting now. Continue restriction on TV time.	Stress safety with firearms. Keep them out of reach and allow use only with adult supervision. Know who the child's friends are; parents should still have some control over friend selection. Teach water safety; swimming should be supervised by an adult.
11-12	Vital signs approximate adult norms. Growth spurt for girls; inequalities between sexes increasingly noticeable; boys attain greater physical strength. Eruption of permanent teeth complete except for third molars. Secondary sex characteristics begin in boys. Menstruation may begin.	Able to think about social problems and prejudices; sees others' points of view. Enjoys reading mysteries, love stories. Begins playing with abstract ideas. Interested in whys of health measures and understands human reproduction. Very moralistic; religious commitment often made during this time.	Intense team loyalty; boys begin teasing girls and girls flirt with boys for attention; best-friend period. Wants unreasonable independence. Rebellious about routines; wide mood swings; needs some times daily for privacy. Very critical of own work. Hero worship prevails. "Facts of life" chats with friends prevail; masturbation increases. Appears under constant tension.	Enjoys projects and working with hands. Likes to do errands and jobs to earn money. Very involved in sports, dancing, talking on phone. Enjoys all aspects of acting and drama.	Continue monitoring friends; stress bicycle safety on streets and in traffic.

F.6   Tanner Stages of Puberty

Both sexes	Pubic hair
Stage 1	Prepubescent: no pubic hair
Stage 2	Sparse growth along labia or at base of penis; long, slightly pigmented, downy
Stage 3	Darker, coarser, curly hair spreading sparsely over junction of the pubes
Stage 4	Dark, coarse, adult-like in texture but smaller area of distribution
Stage 5	Adult-like in quantity and distribution; spread to medial surface of thighs
Stage 6	Spread up linea alba

Boys	Genitalia Development
Stage 1	Prepubescent: no change from childhood
Stage 2	Scrotum and testes enlarge; scrotal skin reddened and thicker in texture
Stage 3	Penis elongates; further enlargement of scrotum and testes
Stage 4	Penis enlarges with increased size of glans; scrotal skin continues to darken
Stage 5	Genitalia adult-like in size, shape, and pigmentation

Girls	Breast Development
Stage 1	Prepubescent: elevation of papilla only
Stage 2	Development of breast bud; diameter of areola increases; papilla and breast form small mound
Stage 3	Enlargement of breast and areola with no separation of contours
Stage 4	Areola and papilla form secondary mound above the level of the breast
Stage 5	Mature stage: Projection of papilla only, due to recession of the areola to the general contour of the breast

F.7   Sources of Screening and Assessment Tools

Denver Articulation Screening Examination (DASE) by AF Drumwright

Source: LADOCA Project and Publishing Foundation
East 51st Avenue and Lincoln Street
Denver, CO 80216

Denver Developmental Screening Test (Denver II) by WK Frankenberg, JB Dodds, A Fandal, E Kazuk, and M Cohrs

Source: LADOCA Project and Publishing Foundation
East 51st Avenue and Lincoln Street
Denver, CO 80216

Developmental Profile II by GD Alpern, TJ Boll, and MS Shearer

Source: Western Psychological Services
12031 Wilshire Blvd
Los Angeles, CA 90025

Early Language Milestone Scale

Source: Modern Educational Corp.
PO Box 721
Tulsa, OK 74101

Neonatal Behavioral Assessment Scale by TB Brazelton

Source: Spastics International Medical Publications
London, U.K.
Lippincott Publications
Philadelphia, PA 19106

Temperament Scales

Source: William Carey, MD
Division of General Pediatrics
Childrens Hospital of Philadelphia
Philadelphia, PA 19104

Appendix G

Individual Assessment Tools

G.1 Family Systems Stressor-Strength Inventory (FS³I)

Karen B. Mischke, RN, OGNP/WHCNP, PhD, CFLE

Hillsboro Women's Clinic
620 SE Oak Street
Hillsboro, OR 97123

Shirley M.H. Hanson, RN, PMHNP, PhD, FAAN, CFLE, LMFT*

Professor, School of Nursing
Department of Family Nursing
Oregon Health Sciences University
Portland, OR 97201
Telephone: (503) 494-3869
Fax: (503) 494-3878
E-Mail: hanson@ohsu.edu

INSTRUCTIONS FOR ADMINISTRATION

The Family Systems Stressor-Strength Inventory (FS³I) is an assessment/measurement instrument intended for use with families. It focuses on identifying stressful situations occurring in families and the strengths families use to maintain healthy family functioning. Each family member is asked to complete the instrument on an individual form prior to an interview with the clinician. Questions can be read to members unable to read.

Following completion of the instrument the clinician evaluates the family on each of the stressful situations (general and specific) and the available strengths they possess. This evaluation is recorded on the family member form.

The clinician records the individual family member's score and the clinician perception score on the Quantitative Summary. A different color code is used for each family member. The clinician also completes the Qualitative Summary synthesizing the information gleaned from all participants. Clinicians can use the Family Care Plan to prioritize diagnoses, set goals, develop prevention/intervention activities, and evaluate outcomes.

---

*Respondent to inquires.

From Mischke-Berkey K, Hanson SMH: *Pocket guide to family assessment and intervention,* St Louis, 1991, Mosby.

FAMILY SYSTEMS STRESSOR-STRENGTH INVENTORY (FS³I)

Family Name _____   Date _____

Family Member(s) Completing Assessment _____

Ethnic Background(s) _____

Religious Background(s) _____

Referral Source _____

Interviewer _____

Family members	Relationship in family	Age	Marital status	Education (highest degree)	Occupation
1.					
2.					
3.					
4.					
5.					
6.					

Families current reasons for seeking assistance?

_____

_____

_____

Part I: Family Systems Stressors (General)

DIRECTIONS: Each of the 25 situations/stressors listed here deals with some aspect of normal family life. They have the potential for creating stress within families or between families and the world in which they live. We are interested in your overall impression of how these situations affect your family life. Please circle a number (0 through 5) that best describes the amount of stress or tension they create for you.

Stressors:	Not applicable	Little stress		Medium stress		High stress	Clinician perception Score
1. Family member(s) feel unappreciated	0	1	2	3	4	5	____
2. Guilt for not accomplishing more	0	1	2	3	4	5	____
3. Insufficient "me" time	0	1	2	3	4	5	____
4. Self-image/self-esteem/feelings of unattractiveness	0	1	2	3	4	5	____
5. Perfectionism	0	1	2	3	4	5	____
6. Dieting	0	1	2	3	4	5	____
7. Health/Illness	0	1	2	3	4	5	____
8. Communication with children	0	1	2	3	4	5	____
9. Housekeeping standards	0	1	2	3	4	5	____
10. Insufficient couple time	0	1	2	3	4	5	____
11. Insufficient family playtime	0	1	2	3	4	5	____
12. Children's behavior/discipline/sibling fighting	0	1	2	3	4	5	____
13. Television	0	1	2	3	4	5	____
14. Over-scheduled family calendar	0	1	2	3	4	5	____
15. Lack of shared responsibility in the family	0	1	2	3	4	5	____
16. Moving	0	1	2	3	4	5	____
17. Spousal relationship (communication, friendship, sex)	0	1	2	3	4	5	____
18. Holidays	0	1	2	3	4	5	____
19. In-laws	0	1	2	3	4	5	____
20. Teen behaviors (communication, music, friends, school)	0	1	2	3	4	5	____
21. New baby	0	1	2	3	4	5	____
22. Economics/finances/budgets	0	1	2	3	4	5	____
23. Unhappiness with work situation	0	1	2	3	4	5	____
24. Overvolunteerism	0	1	2	3	4	5	____
25. Neighbors	0	1	2	3	4	5	____

Additional stressors: _____

Family remarks: _____

Clinician: Clarification of stressful situations/concerns with family members.
Prioritize in order of importance to family members: _____

Part II: Family Systems Stressors (Specific)

DIRECTIONS: The following 12 questions are designed to provide information about your specific stress producing situation, problem, or area of concern influencing your family's health. Please circle a number (1 through 5) that best describes the influence this situation has on your family's life and how well you perceive your family's overall functioning.

The specific stress producing situation/problem or area of concern at this time is _____

Stressors:	Family perception score			Clinician perception
	Little	Medium	High	Score

1. To what extent is your family bothered by this problem or stressful situation? 1   2   3   4   5   ____
   (e.g., effects on family interactions, communication among members, emotional, and social relationships)
   Family remarks: _____

   Clinician remarks: _____

2. How much of an effect does this stressful situation have on your family's usual pattern of living? 1   2   3   4   5   ____
   (e.g., effects on life-style patterns and family developmental tasks)
   Family remarks: _____

   Clinician remarks: _____

3. How much has this situation affected your family's ability to work together as a family unit? 1   2   3   4   5   ____
   (e.g., alteration in family roles, completion of family tasks, following through with responsibilities)
   Family remarks: _____

   Clinician remarks: _____

Has your family ever experienced a similar concern in the past?
   1. YES   If YES, complete question 4.
   2. NO   If NO, complete question 5.

4. How successful was your family in dealing with this situation/problem/concern in the past? 1   2   3   4   5   ____
   (e.g., workable coping strategies developed, adaptive measures useful, situation improved)
   Family remarks: _____

   Clinician remarks: _____

5. How strongly do you feel this current situation/problem/concern will affect your family's future? 1   2   3   4   5   ____
   (e.g., anticipated consequences)
   Family remarks: _____

   Clinician remarks: _____

6. To what extent are family members able to help themselves in this present situation/ problem/concern? 1   2   3   4   5   ____
   (e.g., self-assistive efforts, family expectations, spiritual influence, and family resources)
   Family remarks: _____

   Clinician remarks: _____

Stressors:	Family perception score					Clinician perception
	Little		Medium		High	Score
7. To what extent do you expect others to help your family with this situation/problem/concern? . . . . 1 (e.g., What roles would helpers play? How available are extra-family resources?)		2	3	4	5	_____
Family remarks: _____						
Clinician remarks: _____						

Stressors:	Family perception score					Clinician perception
	Poor		Satisfactory		Excellent	Score
8. How would you rate the way your family functions overall? . . . . 1 (e.g., how your family members relate to each other and to larger family and community)		2	3	4	5	_____
Family remarks: _____						
Clinician remarks: _____						
9. How would you rate the overall physical health status of each family member by name? (Include yourself as a family member; record additional names on back.)						
a. _____ 1		2	3	4	5	_____
b. _____ 1		2	3	4	5	_____
c. _____ 1		2	3	4	5	_____
d. _____ 1		2	3	4	5	_____
e. _____ 1		2	3	4	5	_____
10. How would you rate the overall physical health status of your family as a whole? 1		2	3	4	5	_____
Family remarks: _____						
Clinician perceptions: _____						
11. How would you rate the overall mental health status of each family member by name? (Include yourself as a family member; record additional names on back.)						
a. _____ 1		2	3	4	5	_____
b. _____ 1		2	3	4	5	_____
c. _____ 1		2	3	4	5	_____
d. _____ 1		2	3	4	5	_____
e. _____ 1		2	3	4	5	_____
12. How would you rate the overall mental health status of your family as a whole? 1		2	3	4	5	_____
Family remarks: _____						
Clinician perceptions: _____						

Part III: Family Systems Strengths

Directions: Each of the 16 traits/attributes listed below deals with some aspect of family life and its overall functioning. Each one contributes to the health and well-being of family members as individuals and to the family as a whole. Please circle a number (0 through 5) that best describes the extent that the trait applies to your family.

My family:	Not applicable	Seldom		Usually		Always	Clinician perception Score
1. Communicates and listens to one another 0		1	2	3	4	5	____
Family remarks: _____							
Clinician remarks: _____							
2. Affirms and supports one another 0		1	2	3	4	5	____
Family remarks: _____							
Clinician remarks: _____							
3. Teaches respect for others 0		1	2	3	4	5	____
Family remarks: _____							
Clinician remarks: _____							
4. Develops a sense of trust in members 0		1	2	3	4	5	____
Family remarks: _____							
Clinician remarks: _____							
5. Displays a sense of play and humor 0		1	2	3	4	5	____
Family remarks: _____							
Clinician remarks: _____							
6. Exhibits a sense of shared responsibility 0		1	2	3	4	5	____
Family remarks: _____							
Clinician remarks: _____							
7. Teaches a sense of right and wrong 0		1	2	3	4	5	____
Family remarks: _____							
Clinician remarks: _____							
8. Has a strong sense of family in which rituals and traditions abound 0		1	2	3	4	5	____
Family remarks: _____							
Clinician remarks: _____							
9. Has a balance of interaction among members 0		1	2	3	4	5	____
Family remarks: _____							
Clinician remarks: _____							
10. Has a shared religious core 0		1	2	3	4	5	____
Family remarks: _____							
Clinician remarks: _____							

My family:	Family perception score						Clinician perception
	Not applicable	Seldom		Usually		Always	Score
11. Respects the privacy of one another 0		1	2	3	4	5	____
Family remarks: _____							
Clinician remarks: _____							
12. Values service to others 0		1	2	3	4	5	____
Family remarks: _____							
Clinician remarks: _____							
13. Fosters family table time and conversation 0		1	2	3	4	5	____
Family remarks: _____							
Clinician remarks: _____							
14. Shares leisure time 0		1	2	3	4	5	____
Family remarks: _____							
Clinician remarks: _____							
15. Admits to and seeks help with problems 0		1	2	3	4	5	____
Family remarks: _____							
Clinician remarks: _____							
16a. How would you rate the overall strengths that exist in your family? 0		1	2	3	4	5	____
Family remarks: _____							
Clinician remarks: _____							

16b. Additional Family Strengths: _____

_____

_____

16c. Clinician: Clarification of family strengths with individual members: _____

_____

_____

_____

_____

SCORING SUMMARY

The Family Systems Stressor-Strength Inventory (FS^{3}I) Scoring Summary is divided into two sections: Section 1, Family Perception Scores and Section 2, Clinician Perception Scores. These two sections are further divided into three parts: Part I, Family Systems Stressors: General; Part II, Family Systems Stressors: Specific; and Part III, Family Systems Strengths. Each part contains a Quantitative Summary and a Qualitative Summary.

Quantifiable family and clinician perception scores are both graphed on the Quantitative Summary. Each family member has a designated color code. Family and clinician remarks are both recorded on the Qualitative Summary. Quantitative summary scores, when graphed, suggest a level for initiation of prevention/intervention modes: primary, secondary and tertiary. Qualitative summary information, when synthesized, contributes to the development and channeling of the Family Care Plan.

Section 1: Family Perception Scores

Part I   Family Systems Stressors (General)

Add scores from questions 1 to 25 and calculate an overall numerical score for Family System Stressors (General). Ratings are from 1 (most positive) to 5 (most negative). The Not Applicable (0) responses are omitted from the calculations. Total scores range from 25 to 125.

Family Systems Stressor Score: General

$$\frac{(\quad)}{25} \times 1 = \underline{\hspace{2cm}}$$

Graph score on Quantitative Summary, Family Systems Stressors: General, Family Member Perception. Color code to differentiate family members.

Record additional stressors and family remarks in Part I, Qualitative Summary: Family and Clinician Remarks.

Part II   Family Systems Stressors: Specific

Add scores from questions 1-8, 10, and 12 and calculate a numerical score for Family Systems Stressors: Specific. Ratings are from 1 (most positive) to 5 (most negative). Questions 4, 6, 7, 8, 10, and 12 are reverse scored.* Total scores range from 10-50.

Family Systems Stressor Score: Specific

$$\frac{(\quad)}{10} \times 1 = \underline{\hspace{2cm}}$$

Graph score on Quantitative Summary: Family Systems Stressor: Specific. (Family Member Perceptions). Color code to differentiate family members.

Summarize data from questions 9 and 11 (reverse scored) and record family remarks in Part II, Qualitative Summary: Family and Clinician Remarks

Part III   Family Systems Strengths

Add scores from questions 1 to 16 and calculate a numerical score for Family Systems Strengths. Ratings are from 1 (seldom) to 5 (always). The Not Applicable (0) responses are omitted from the calculations. Total scores range from 16 to 80.

Family Systems Strength Score

$$\frac{(\quad)}{16} \times 1 = \underline{\hspace{2cm}}$$

Graph score on Quantitative Summary: Family Systems Strengths (Family Member Perception).

Record additional family strengths and family remarks in Part III, Qualitative Summary: Family and Clinician Remarks.

---

*Reverse Scoring:
   Question answered as (1) is scored 5 points
   Question answered as (2) is scored 4 points
   Question answered as (3) is scored 3 points
   Question answered as (4) is scored 2 points
   Question answered as (5) is scored 1 point

Section 2: Clinician Perception Scores

Part I   Family Systems Stressors (General)

Add scores from questions 1 to 25 and calculate an overall numerical score for Family System Stressors (General). Ratings are from 1 (most positive) to 5 (most negative). The Not Applicable (0) responses are omitted from the calculations. Total scores range from 25 to 125.

Family Systems Stressor Score: General

$$\frac{(\quad)}{25} \times 1 = \underline{\hspace{2cm}}$$

Graph score on Quantitative Summary, Family Systems Stressors: General (Clinician Perception).

Record Clinicians' clarification of general stressors in Part I, Qualitative Summary: Family and Clinician Remarks

Part II   **Family Systems Stressors: Specific**

Add scores from questions 1-8, 10 and 12 and calculate a numerical score for Family Systems Stressors: Specific. Ratings are from 1 (most positive) to 5 (most negative). Questions 4, 6, 7, 8, 10, and 12 are reverse scored.* Total scores range from 10-50.

Family Systems Stressor Score: Specific

$$\frac{(\quad)}{10} \times 1 = \underline{\hspace{2cm}}$$

Graph score on Quantitative Summary: Family Systems Stressor: Specific. (Clinician Perception).

Summarize data from questions 9 and 11 (reverse order) and record clinician remarks in Part II, Qualitative Summary: Family and Clinician Remarks

Part III   **Family Systems Strengths**

Add scores from questions 1 to 16 and calculate a numerical score for Family Systems Strengths. Ratings are from 1 (seldom) to 5 (always). The Not Applicable (0) responses are omitted from the calculations. Total scores range from 16 to 80.

Family Systems Strength Score

$$\frac{(\quad)}{16} \times 1 = \underline{\hspace{2cm}}$$

Graph score on Quantitative Summary: Family Systems Strengths (Clinician Perception).

Record clinicians' clarification of family strengths in Part III, Qualitative Summary: Family and Clinician Remarks.

---

*Reverse Scoring:
    Question answered as (1) is scored 5 points
    Question answered as (2) is scored 4 points
    Question answered as (3) is scored 3 points
    Question answered as (4) is scored 2 points
    Question answered as (5) is scored 1 point

Scores for Wellness and Stability	Family Systems Stressors: General	
	Family Member Perception Score	Clinician Perception Score
5.0		
4.8		
4.6		
4.4		
4.2		
4.0		
3.8		
3.6		
3.4		
3.2		
3.0		
2.8		
2.6		
2.4		
2.2		
2.0		
1.8		
1.6		
1.4		
1.2		
1.0		

Scores for Wellness and Stability	Family Systems Stressors: Specific	
	Family Member Perception Score	Clinician Perception Score
5.0		
4.8		
4.6		
4.4		
4.2		
4.0		
3.8		
3.6		
3.4		
3.2		
3.0		
2.8		
2.6		
2.4		
2.2		
2.0		
1.8		
1.6		
1.4		
1.2		
1.0		

Sum of strengths available for prevention/ intervention mode	Family Systems Strengths	
	Family Member Perception Score	Clinician Perception Score
5.0		
4.8		
4.6		
4.4		
4.2		
4.0		
3.8		
3.6		
3.4		
3.2		
3.0		
2.8		
2.6		
2.4		
2.2		
2.0		
1.8		
1.6		
1.4		
1.2		
1.0		

Qualitative Summary Family and Clinician Remarks

Part I: Family Systems Stressors: General

Summarize general stressors and remarks of family and clinician. Prioritize stressors according to importance to family members.

_____

_____

_____

Part II: Family Systems Stressors: Specific

A. Summarize specific stressor and remarks of family and clinician.

_____

_____

_____

B. Summarize differences (if discrepancies exist) between how family members and clinician view effects of stressful situation on family.

_____

_____

_____

C. Summarize overall family functioning.

_____

_____

_____

D. Summarize overall significant physical health status for family members.

_____

_____

_____

E. Summarize overall significant mental health status for family members.

_____

_____

_____

Part III: Family Systems Strengths

Summarize family systems strengths and family and clinician remarks that facilitate family health and stability.

_____

_____

_____

Family Care Plan*

| Diagnosis general and specific family system stressors | Family systems strengths supporting family care plan | Goals family and clinician | Prevention/intervention mode | | Outcomes evaluation and replanning |
			Primary, secondary or tertiary	Prevention/intervention activities	

*Prioritize the three most significant diagnoses.

G.2 Friedman Family Assessment Model (Short Form)

FRIEDMAN FAMILY ASSESSMENT MODEL (SHORT FORM)

Before using the following guidelines in completing family assessments, two words of caution. First, not all areas included below will be germane for each of the families visited. The guidelines are comprehensive and allow depth when probing is necessary. The student should not feel that every sub-area needs to be covered when the broad area of inquiry poses no problems to the family or concern to the health worker. Second, by virtue of the interdependence of the family system, one will find unavoidable redundancy. For the sake of efficiency, the assessor should try not to repeat data, but to refer the reader back to sections where this information has already been described.

Identifying Data

1. Family Name
2. Address and Phone
3. Family Composition (see table)
4. Type of Family Form
5. Cultural (Ethnic) Background
6. Religious Identification
7. Social Class Status
8. Family's Recreational or Leisure-Time Activities

Developmental Stage and History of Family

9. Family's Present Developmental Stage
10. Extent of Developmental Tasks Fulfillment
11. Nuclear Family History
12. History of Family of Origin of Both Parents

Environmental Data

13. Characteristics of Home
14. Characteristics of Neighborhood and Larger Community
15. Family's Geographic Mobility
16. Family's Associations and Transactions with Community
17. Family's Social Support Network (ecomap)

Family Structure

18. Communication Patterns
    Extent of Functional and Dysfunctional Communication (types of recurring patterns)
    Extent of Emotional (Affective) Messages and How Expressed
    Characteristics of Communication within Family Subsystems
    Extent of Congruent and Incongruent Messages
    Types of Dysfunctional Communication Processes Seen in Family
    Areas of Open and Closed Communication
    Familial and External Variables Affecting Communication

19. Power Structure
    Power Outcomes
    Decision-making Process
    Power Bases
    Variables Affecting Family Power
    Overall Family System and Subsystem Power
20. Role Structure
    Formal Role Structure
    Informal Role Structure
    Analysis of Role Models (optional)
    Variables Affecting Role Structure
21. Family Values
    Compare the family to American or family's reference group values and/or identify important family values and their importance (priority) in family.
    Congruence Between the Family's Values and the Family's Reference Group or Wider Community
    Congruence Between the Family's Values and Family Member's Values
    Variables Influencing Family Values
    Values Consciously or Unconsciously Held
    Presence of Value Conflicts in Family
    Effect of the Above Values and Value Conflicts on Health Status of Family

Family Functions

22. Affective Function
    Family's Need-Response Patterns
    Mutual Nurturance, Closeness, and Identification
    Separateness and Connectedness
23. Socialization Function
    Family Child-Rearing Practices
    Adaptability of Child-Rearing Practices for Family Form and Family's Situation
    Who Is (Are) Socializing Agent(s) for Child(ren)?
    Value of Children in Family
    Cultural Beliefs That Influence Family's Child-Rearing Patterns
    Social Class Influence on Child-Rearing Patterns
    Estimation About Whether Family Is at Risk for Child-Rearing Problems and, if so, Indication of High-Risk Factors
    Adequacy of Home Environment for Child(ren)'s Needs to Play
24. Health Care Function
    Family's Health Beliefs, Values, and Behavior
    Family's Definitions of Health-Illness and Their Level of Knowledge
    Family's Perceived Health Status and Illness Susceptibility
    Family's Dietary Practices

Adequacy of family diet (recommended 24-hour food history record)

Function of mealtimes and attitudes toward food and mealtimes

Shopping (and its planning) practices

Person(s) responsible for planning, shopping, and preparation of meals

Sleep and Rest Habits

Physical Activity and Recreation Practices (not covered earlier)

Family's Drug Habits

Family's Role in Self-care Practices

Medically Based Preventive Measures (physicals, eye and hearing tests, and immunizations)

Dental Health Practices

Family Health History (both general and specific diseases—environmentally and genetically related)

Health Care Services Received
Feelings and Perceptions Regarding Health Services
Emergency Health Services
Source of Payments for Health and Other Services
Logistics of Receiving Care

Family Stress and Coping

25. Short- and Long-term Familial Stressors and Strengths
26. Extent of Family's Ability to Respond, Based on Objective Appraisal of Stress-producing Situations
27. Coping Strategies Utilized (present/past)
    Differences in family members' ways of coping
    Family's inner coping strategies
    Family's external coping strategies
28. Dysfunctional Adaptive Strategies Utilized (present/past; extent of usage)

Family Composition Form

Name (Last, First)	Gender	Relationship	Date and Place of Birth	Occupation	Education
1. (Father)					
2. (Mother)					
3. (Oldest child)					
4.					
5.					
6.					
7.					
8.					

From Friedman MM: *Family Nursing Research, Theory, and Practice,* Stamford, Conn, 1998, Appleton & Lange.

G.3   Case Example of Family Assessment

The Jeddi family is a real family in a real situation. They came to the attention of the nurse when the family was referred to the county home health agency for a baseline family assessment with their impending adoption of a 4-year-old boy from Russia. This upper middle class Caucasian family consists of Ben (age 51), Mare (age 43), and the son they will adopt, Alex (age 4). See Figure G-1 for the Jeddi family genogram and Figure G-2 for the Jeddi family ecomap.

Ben and Mare have been married for 8 years. Ben has a PhD in chemical engineering and does consulting work. His business is located in the caretaker apartment located in the basement of their home. Mare has a PhD, is a pediatric nurse, and teaches at a private university. They are adopting a 4-year-old boy from Russia. Mare has a diagnosis of infer-

tility after 2 years of trying to have a biological child and extensive testing. The infertility issue was a significant loss for both Ben and Mare. The couple considered in vitro fertilization. Mare decided against this approach because she felt the risks of failure of pregnancy and miscarriage were too great. Ben felt that this was Mare's decision to make since it more directly involved her physical and mental health. He supported Mare's decision to not pursue in vitro fertilization.

Mare initiated the discussions about adoption. The decision to adopt a child was reached in May of this year after a year a half of discussion and investigation. Initially, Ben was not equally committed to the concept of adoption and had a longer grieving process over their inability to have a child together than Mare. The issue of biological heritage and the

Date _____

Family name ___Jeddi family___

Completed by _____

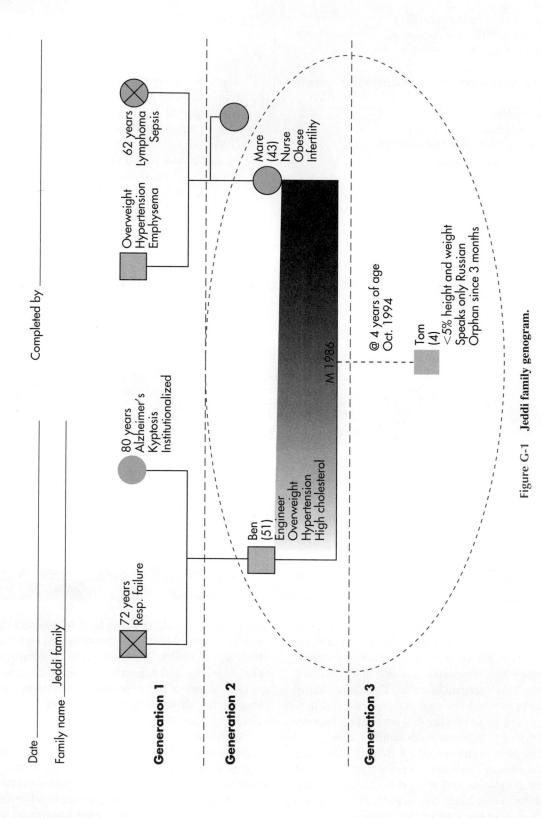

Generation 1

72 years
Resp. failure

80 years
Alzheimer's
Kyptosis
Institutionalized

Overweight
Hypertension
Emphysema

62 years
Lymphoma
Sepsis

Generation 2

Ben
(51)
Engineer
Overweight
Hypertension
High cholesterol

M 1986

Mare
(43)
Nurse
Obese
Infertility

Generation 3

@ 4 years of age
Oct. 1994

Tom
(4)
<5% height and weight
Speaks only Russian
Orphan since 3 months

Figure G-1   **Jeddi family genogram.**

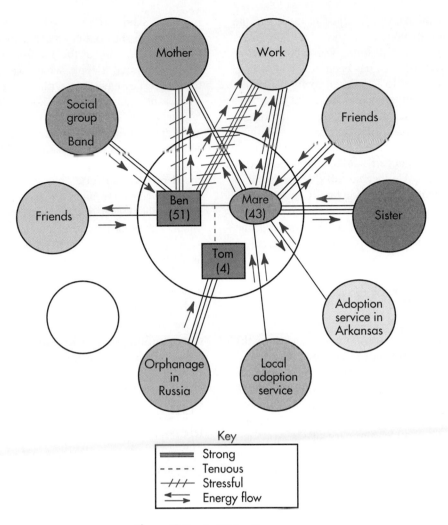

Figure G-2   Jeddi family ecomap.

loss of blood lineage were more significant to Ben. The significant issue for Mare was the loss of being a parent and raising a child.

The couple investigated several adoption agencies and attended potential adoptive parent classes a year and a half ago. At that time, Ben was not ready to make a commitment to adoption. The topic of adoption repeatedly was discussed by the couple over the course of the next year. This past January, the couple again seriously considered adoption. Mare investigated several adoption agencies again because she was not satisfied with the one they selected the last time. A local adoption agency was found to be supportive and informative for them. The couple attended an information meeting. After much intense emotional discussion, the couple pursued more information about adoption with the support personnel from the agency. At the end of May, Ben and Mare decided they wanted to adopt a child and completed the application process.

Both Ben and Mare feel this was an emotional time for them. After they made their decision to adopt, the next steps were to decide from which country they wanted to adopt a child, the child's age, and which child. They decided that given their lifestyles and personalities that they wanted to

adopt an older child between 3 and 5 years of age and not an infant. Ben wanted to adopt a son. Mare was not selective of the gender. Ben felt that the issue of race was important to him. He felt that he might have difficulty bonding with a child of dark skin. Because of Ben's immediate family origins from Finland, they decided to adopt a child from eastern Europe. Russia was selected because of its historical ties with Finland.

Mare reviewed video tapes of 40 children and selected the top male children for them to select from. Mare is a pediatric nurse and was determined to be the one to make the decisions about health. After viewing the films numerous times and reviewing a medical examination, Alex was the young child of choice. Ben and Mare made a formal petition to adopt Alex.

The process has taken 6 months. They are currently waiting for the final paperwork to arrive from the Russian government, which is expected in the next few days. They are in the midst of preparing their home for the arrival of Alex. They will both travel to Russia in 2 weeks to pick him up, complete the formal adoption process in Russia, and travel home together as a new family.

They are nervous and excited about the adoption. They

are concerned about how Alex will adjust to them and the move to America. They are concerned about how adopting a 4-year-old will change their lifestyle. The preparation of their home for the arrival of Alex has been time consuming. The arrangements for travel to Russia are being finalized. Ben took 2 years of Russian language classes 20 years ago, and both are currently taking individual language tutoring in Russian. Ben and Mare are currently working full time. Mare plans to continue working full time after they adopt Alex, but she does have reduced workload for the next 4 months. They plan to have Alex attend full-day preschool.

The initial assessment of the Jeddi family involved the use of two assessment approaches, with their respective instruments and guidelines, as well as a genogram and an ecomap. A summary of the findings from this assessment follows.

FAMILY SYSTEMS STRESSOR STRENGTH INVENTORY

The FS³I focused on the Jeddi family stressors and strengths to create a plan of action. Ben and Mare were interviewed together in their home by the nurse. Each person completed the FS³I, which provided individual and composite scores. Figure G-1 presents a completed genogram. Figure G-2 shows the Jeddi family ecomap. Figure G-3 and G-4 provide the scoring for the quantitative summary of stressors and strengths. A qualitative summary (Figure G-5) presents a brief picture of the family stresses and strengths and served as the guide for the family care plan (Figure G-6).

The general stressors of the family were the impending adoption of Alex, issues of family nutrition and dieting, and lowered self-image for both Ben and Mare. Mare was found to have a higher general stress level than Ben. She states that in addition to the above stressors, she is concerned about stress relative to housekeeping issues, an ongoing physical problem with her knee, and guilt for not accomplishing more than she presently is able. Ben noted that issues related to his mother, who has Alzheimer disease and lives in an assisted-living center, cause him additional stress. The nurse rated their general and specific stressors higher than both Ben and Mare rated themselves.

The specific stressor identified by Ben that is causing him the most stress is the impending adoption of Alex. He is concerned about time management with work and a new family member. The additional stress of his mother's care is requiring a lot of his time. She is well taken care of in an assisted-living center, but he is concerned about her advancing dementia. At present he is actively involved in renting out his mother's home. The specific stressor identified by Mare was how she is going to manage food preparations and mealtimes after they adopt Alex. She stated that cooking and meal preparation are currently a big problem for her. Mare stated that Ben does not help with food preparation or clean up now. They both eat on different schedules. She is concerned about family dinners and feels this is an important time for them with Alex. Food preparation is not a new issue

for them. She stated that she feels pressured and "like a failure" because she does not manage this aspect of their family life well now, without the addition of Alex. In the past the family has hired a cook, which was a "excellent solution" for them. They have been without a cook for 2 years now after their previous cook moved out of state.

The strengths of this family are many. They scored their individual strengths inventory almost identical, which demonstrates a similar perception of their family unit. Both Ben and Mare viewed their family and each other as experienced problem solvers. They have good open communication between them and feel that the adoption of Alex has brought them even closer together. They recognized that much of their current stress is related to the unknown about Alex. They feel that once they meet Alex, they will be able to work together to solve their problems.

The nurse concluded that this family has the strengths they need to adapt to their new family life cycle of a family with a preschooler. In looking at the ecomap, the family is found to be well supported by resources. They are responsive to information provided to them and ideas suggested by others for them to consider in their problem solving.

FRIEDMAN'S FAMILY ASSESSMENT FORM
Identifying Data

Ben and Mare Jeddi
Portland Maine
Type of family: Nuclear
Ethnic background: Ben comes from a Finnish background. Mare has no particular ethnic identity
Religious: No affiliation
Social Class: Upper middle class
Leisure activities: Travel, gardening, music
Occupations: Ben is a consulting chemical engineer. Mare is a pediatric nurse and university faculty member

Developmental Stage and History of Family

The family's present developmental stage cannot be defined in the conventional family life cycle. Ben and Mare have been married for 8 years, so they do not fit the categories for beginning families or families with children. However, they are in transition and with the adoption of a 4-year-old boy, the family will fit into the classical family life cycle stage of family with preschooler.

Ben comes from a nuclear family of origin; however, his parents were divorced after 30 years of marriage. Mare comes from a nuclear family of origin.

Environmental Data

The family live in an upper middle class urban neighborhood that is ethnically diverse. They are within close distance of schools, hospitals, fire department, and shopping

Text continues on p. 621.

Family Systems Stressor—Strength Inventory (FS³I)
Quantitative Summary
Family Systems Stressors: General and Specific
Family and Clinician Perception Scores

Directions: Graph the scores from each family member inventory by placing an **"X"** at the appropriate location. (Use first name initial for each different entry and different color code for each family member.)

Scores for Wellness and Stability	Family Systems Stressors: General		Scores for Wellness and Stability	Family Systems Stressors: Specific	
	Family Member Perception Score	Clinician Perception Score		Family Member Perception Score	Clinician Perception Score
5.0			5.0		
4.8			4.8		
4.6			4.6		
4.4			4.4		
4.2			4.2		
4.0			4.0		
3.8			3.8		
3.6			3.6		
3.4			3.4		MO
3.2			3.2	B X	B X
3.0			3.0		
2.8			2.8	MO	
2.6			2.6		
2.4		MO	2.4		
2.2	MO		2.2		
2.0			2.0		
1.8		B X	1.8		
1.6	B X		1.6		
1.4			1.4		
1.2			1.2		
1.0			1.0		

- **PRIMARY**   Prevention/Intervention Mode: Flexible Line   1.0 - 2.3
- **SECONDARY**   Prevention/Intervention Mode: Normal Line   2.4 - 3.6
- **TERTIARY**   Prevention/Intervention Mode: Resistance Lines   3.7 - 5.0

- Breakdown of numerical scores for stressor penetration are suggested values

Figure G-3   FS³I quantitative summary: stressors.

Family Systems Stressor—Strength Inventory (FS³I)
Quantitative Summary
Family Systems Strengths
Family and Clinician Perception Scores

Directions: Graph the scores from the inventory by placing an **"X"** at the appropriate location and connect with a line. (Use first name initial for each different entry and different color code for each family member.)

Sum of strengths available for prevention/ intervention mode	Family Systems Strengths	
	Family Member Perception Score	Clinician Perception Score
5.0		
4.8		
4.6		
4.4		
4.2		
4.0		
3.8		
3.6	M O B X	M O B X
3.4		
3.2		
3.0		
2.8		
2.6		
2.4		
2.2		
2.0		
1.8		
1.6		
1.4		
1.2		
1.0		

- **PRIMARY**   Prevention/Intervention Mode: Flexible Line   1.0 - 2.1
- **SECONDARY**   Prevention/Intervention Mode: Normal Line   2.2 - 3.6
- **TERTIARY**   Prevention/Intervention Mode: Resistance Lines   3.7 - 5.0

- Breakdown of numerical scores for stressor penetration are suggested values

Figure G-4   FS³I quantitative summary: strengths.

Family Systems Stressor—Strength Inventory (FS³I)
Qualitative Summary
Family and Clinician Remarks

Part I: Family Systems Stressors: General

Summarize general stressors and remarks of family and clinician. Prioritize stressors according to importance to family members.

Ben: General stressors are: Lower self image, dieting, and adopting new child.

Mare: General stressors are: Guilt for not doing more; adopting new child;

lower self image; dieting; housekeeping; lack of shared responsibility; knee problem

Part II: Family Systems Stressors: Specific

A. Summarize specific stressor and remarks of family and clinician.

Both Ben & Mare feel the adoption of new child is the most important stressor specifically,

Ben is concerned about time management and Mare about time management relative to

cooking healthy meals for the family. Nurse sees these stressors higher than Ben & Mare.

B. Summarize differences (if discrepancies exist) between how family members and clinician view effects of stressful situation on family.

Both Ben & Mare see this stressor similarly, but Mare also sees several other related

family stressors particularly lack of shared responsibilities.

C. Summarize overall family functioning.

Family overall is functioning well with this stressor, but as adoption gets closer the stress

level will continue to rise; both are perfectionists and first time parents; they communicate

well and are now open to help from the outside

D. Summarize overall significant physical health status for family members.

Ben — OK, but stressed

Mare — Stressed and concerned about knee problem which increases her emotional lability

Alex – Healthy, small for age both height and weight; mild developmental delay

E. Summarize overall significant mental health status for family members.

The family members are stressed but not in a crisis mode. They openly talk about concerns

and help each other emotionally.

Part III: Family Systems Strengths

Summarize family systems strengths and family and clinician remarks that facilitate family health and stability.

The major strengths are the open honest communication between Ben & Mare and their

experience with solving problems together and independently. They recently have opened

their closed family boundary to help from extended family, friends and professionals.

Figure G-5   **Qualitative summary.**

Family Systems and Stressor—Strength Inventory (FS³I)
Family Care Plan*

Diagnosis General and Specific Family System Stressors	Prognosis Goals Family and Clinician	Family Systems Strengths Supporting Family Care Plan	Prevention/Intervention Mode		Outcomes Evaluation and Replanning
			Primary, Secondary or Tertiary	Prevention/Intervention Activities	
1. Family life cycle transition: stress related to adoption of 4 yr old boy from Russia	1. Excellent prognosis with anticipatory guidance, information and history of problem solving	Family communication Family commitment to adoption	Primary	1.a. Offer educational material on families with preschool child 1.b. Introduce family to adoption support groups and networks	1.a. Discuss normal family stressors 1.b. Attend support group
2. Family nutrition management: Streseed related to adoption, ongoing eating patterns and family health problems	2. Good prognosis as had faced this problem before- Investigate prior problems family had with last cook. Poor self images will take time to affect	Family communication Family known problem solvers	Secondary	2.a. Provide sources to contact where family can hire a cook 2.b. Investigate why they did not follow through with their last cook 2.c. Education on nutrition for 4 yr old	2.a+b. Contact and hire a cook 2.c. Design healthy family meal plan for 1 month

*Prioritize the three most significant diagnoses

Figure G-6   Family care plan.

areas. The neighborhood is clean and relatively safe; there have been a few burglaries in the neighborhood. Both attend the neighborhood community meetings. The family is centrally located, only 8 blocks from freeways around town, 2 miles from downtown, and 5 blocks from a bus route. Ben works in the home, where the basement caretaker apartment has been converted into his office and labs. Mare works at the university, which is 4 miles away. She often rides her bike to work.

Their home is a 75-year-old brick home that has four levels. It is situated on the edge of a hollow. The home is well kept but is old. Both Ben and Mare enjoy their home and spend a lot of time there. They are gradually remodeling. The house is safe, but with the adoption of a 4-year-old boy, several safety factors need to be addressed. There is no medicine cabinet in the bathroom, and medicines are easily within reach of a 4-year-old. The cleaning solutions are kept under the sinks in the kitchen and the bathroom. The patio above the garage does have a railing, but a 4-year-old may be tempted to walk on it. A fire plan needs to be made for the family because all the bedrooms are on the top floor, which is three levels above the ground.

Family Structure

Communication is a strength of this family. There is an open relationship and communication pattern between Ben and Mare. Both are very verbal and expressive about their feelings, opinions and needs. Because of this openness, they state that there is often conflict and arguing between them. However, they feel that they are good at conflict resolution. At times however, the argument does get out of control and takes a personal attack format. When they realize this, usually Mare suggests that they take up the conversation at later time when they can both approach the topic more calmly. They are not worried about arguing in front of their son. They feel that their open honest communication will be helpful in raising their son.

The decision making of the family is by consensus for important issues that affect the lives of both members. Otherwise, the decision making style is accommodation. The power and decision making is more situational in that whoever has more experience with certain issues influences those decisions. For example, Mare is a nurse and has the referent power in health-related issues. Ben is a chemical engineer. He has referent power for concerns about fixing things in the house or with the cars. Both state that a strength of their family is that they are both known problem solvers.

The role structure is typical relative to gender. Mare does the cooking, laundry, house cleaning, shopping, and kinship roles. Ben does the lawn mowing, carries out the garbage, and services the cars. Mare feels that she has more roles and expected behaviors than Ben does. They both work full time, with Mare working outside the home. Both state they are concerned about role overload and time management issues with the adoption of their 4 year old. Mare knows that she

will be the primary caregiver, but she is not sure how much or in what way Ben will assist with these new role requirements. Ben is concerned about how much time the new child will demand and his ability to juggle all his work responsibilities and family responsibilities.

The family values are clear and shared by both Ben and Mare. The family values: education; open, honest communication; family; health; diversity; caring and compassion for others.

Family Functions

AFFECTIVE FUNCTION. Ben and Mare have a close caring relationship and demonstrate a reciprocal emotional relationship. They are a close cohesive family. They are excited about expanding their family with the adoption of Alex. They state that each of them is the major support person for the other. The family has closed boundaries, but does look to extended family members for needed support. They express concern about their son's adjustment to them as parents because he has lived in an orphanage in Russia since the age of 3 months. They have investigated as much as possible about how other children adapt to their new situations. They plan to go to Russia to pick up their son, which will give them access to information about rules and rituals he is familiar with in the orphanage, and they plan to institute them in their home.

SOCIALIZATION FUNCTION. Ben and Mare talk about the importance of parenting their son. They have openly discussed the type of discipline to be used, which will be time out. They plan to be involved in the child rearing practices of their son. Their son will be in full-day preschool. They plan to be active in the education process of their son.

HEALTH CARE FUNCTION. The family has a primary care physician for Ben and Mare, but they have not selected a pediatrician for their son. Ben sees the physician regularly for management of hypertension and high cholesterol. Mare rarely sees the doctor. They have a medical report for their son. He appears to be in good health, except that he is below the 5th percentile for height and weight. He is current on immunizations except hepatitis. They both have dental cleanings and exams every 6 months. They value health, yet both are overweight. Mare is obese. A major concern for Mare is regular meal preparation for their son. At present, Ben and Mare do not eat dinner together on a regular basis. In the past they have hired a cook to ensure that healthful meals were available, especially with Mare working full time.

Family Coping

The short-term stressors for this family are the imminent adoption of their 4-year-old son from Russia in 3 weeks. They are concerned about his adaptation to his new environment, his ability to learn English, and how their lives will change with this adoption. Long-term stressors are not an issue at this time.

The family has many successful coping strategies. They have a pattern of problem solving issues to the best of their ability. They are seeking out information and garnering support from people and resources acceptable to them. They are a well-adjusted family unit. The family is open to education and information.

SUMMARY OF ASSESSMENTS

In summary, both assessment approaches provided important information for the nurse and family to create a plan of action. There was some overlap of information, but the whole picture of the family was enhanced by merging data from both assessment tools.

G.4   Families With Physically Compromised Members: Assessment Tools

Assessment Tool	Purpose	Reference
The Caregiver Reaction Assessment (CRA)	Assess the reaction of family members caring for elderly persons with physical impairments.	Given CS, Given B, Stommel M, Collins C, King S, Franklin S: The Caregiver Reaction Assessment (CRA) for caregivers to persons with chronic physical and mental impairments, *Res Nurs Health* 15(4):271-283, 1992.
Coping Health Inventory for Parents (CHIP)	Assess parents' appraisal of their coping responses to management of family life when a child is seriously or chronically ill.	McCubbin HI, Thompson AI, McCubbin MA: *Family assessment: Resiliency, coping, and adaptation,* Madison, 1996, University of Wisconsin Publishers.
Demands-of-Illness Scale	Can be used with individuals or families to assess impact of disease on entire family's health, coping, and functioning.	Haberman MR, Woods NF, Packard NJ: Demands of chronic illness: Reliability and validity assessment of a Demands-of-Illness inventory, *Holistic Nurs Pract* 5(1):25-35, 1990.
Family Hardiness Index (FHI)	Measures the characteristic of hardiness as a stress-resistance and adaptation resource in families. Available in English and Spanish.	McCubbin HI, Thompson AI, McCubbin MA: *Family assessment: Resiliency, coping, and adaptation,* Madison, 1996, University of Wisconsin Publishers.
Family Needs Assessment Tool	Assesses needs of families of chronically ill children.	Rawlins PS, Rawlins RD, Horner M: Development of the Family Needs Assessment Tool, *West J Nurs Res* 12(2):201-214, 1990.
Family Pressures Scale–Ethnic (FPRES–E)	Assesses pressure related to life experiences of families of color; provides index of severity of these pressures on the family system.	McCubbin HI, Thompson AI, McCubbin MA: *Family assessment: Resiliency, coping, and adaptation,* Madison, 1996, University of Wisconsin Publishers.
Impact-on-Family Scale	Measures stressors related to childhood illness.	Stein R, Riessman C: The development of an Impact-on-Family scale: Preliminary findings, *Med Care* 18(2):324-330, 1980.
Parent/Caretaker Involvement Scale (P/CIS)	Assesses dyadic family interactions.	Comfort M, Farran DC: Parent-child interaction assessment in family-centered intervention, *Infants Young Children* 6(4):33-45, 1994.
Parents of Children with Disabilities Inventory (PCDI)	Measures perceived disability-related stress, to be used with mothers of children with physical disabilities.	Noojin AB, Wallander JL: Development and evaluation of a measure of concerns related to raising a child with a physical disability, *J Pediatr Psychol* 21(4):483-498, 1996.

G.5 Comprehensive Occupational and Environmental Health History

WORK HISTORY

1. List your current and past longest held jobs, including the military:

Company	Dates Employed	Job Title	Known Exposures

2. Do you work full-time?   NO ___ YES ___ How many hours per week? ___
3. Do you work part-time?   NO ___ YES ___ How many hours per week? ___
4. Please describe any health problems or injuries that you have experienced in connection with your present or past jobs:

5. Have you ever had to change jobs due to health problems or injuries?   YES ___ NO ___
   If yes, describe:

   Did any of your co-workers experience similar problems?

6. In what type of business do you currently work?

7. Describe your work (what you actually do).

8. Have you had any current or past exposure (through breathing or touching) to any of the following?

___ Acids	___ Chlorinated	___ Fiberglass	___ Noise (loud)	___ Styrene
___ Alcohols	naphthalenes	___ Halothane	___ PBBs	___ Talc
___ Alkalis	___ Chloroform	___ Heat (severe)	___ PCBs	___ TDI or MDI
___ Ammonia	___ Chloroprene	___ Isocyanates	___ Perchloroethylene	___ Toluene
___ Arsenic	___ Chromates	___ Ketones	___ Pesticides	___ Trichloroethylene
___ Asbestos	___ Coal dust	___ Lead	___ Phenol	___ Trinitrotoluene
___ Benzene	___ Cold (severe)	___ Manganese	___ Phosgene	___ Vibration
___ Beryllium	___ Dichlorobenzene	___ Mercury	___ Radiation	___ Vinyl chloride
___ Cadmium	___ Ethylene	___ Methylene	___ Rock dust	___ Welding fumes
___ Carbon	dibromide	chloride	___ Silica powder	___ X-rays
tetrachloride	___ Ethylene	___ Nickel	___ Solvents	
	dichloride			

9. Did you receive any safety training about these agents?   YES ___ NO ___
   Explain.

10. Are you involved in any work processes such as grinding, welding, soldering, or polishing that create dust, mists, or fumes?   YES ___ NO ___
    If yes, describe.

11. Did you use any of the following personal protective equipment when exposed?
__ Boots __ Coveralls __ Earplugs/earmuffs __ Glasses/goggles __ Gloves __ Respirator __ Safety shoes __ Shield __ Sleeves __ Welding mask

12. Is your work environment generally clean? YES __ NO __
If no, describe.

13. What ventilation systems are used in your workplace?

14. Do they seem to work? Are you aware of any chemical odors in your environment
If so, explain.

15. Where do you eat, smoke, and take your breaks when you are on the job?

16. Do you use a uniform or have clothing that you wear only to work? YES __ NO __
17. How is your work clothing laundered (at home, by employer, etc.)?

18. How often do you wash your hands at work and how do you wash them (running water, special soaps, etc.)?

19. Do you shower before leaving the work site? YES __ NO __
20. Do you have any physical symptoms associated with work? YES __ NO __
If yes, describe.

21. Are other workers similarly affected? YES __ NO __

HOME EXPOSURES

1. Which of the following do you have in your home?
__ Air conditioner __ Air purifier __ Central heating (gas or oil?) __ Fireplace __ Electric stove __ Wood stove

2. In approximately what year was your home built? _____

3. Have there been any recent renovations? YES __ NO __
If yes, describe.

4. Have you recently installed new carpet, bought new furniture, or refinished existing furniture? YES __ NO __
If yes, explain.

5. Do you use pesticides around your home or garden? YES __ NO __
If yes, describe.

6. What household cleaners do you use? (List most common and any new products you use.)

7. List all hobbies done at your home.

8. Are any of the agents listed earlier for work exposures encountered in hobbies or recreational activities? YES ___ NO ___

9. Is any special protective equipment or ventilation used during hobbies?   YES ___ NO ___
   Explain.

10. What are the occupations of other household members?

11. Do other household members have contact with any form of chemicals at work or during leisure activities?
    YES ___ NO ___
    If yes, explain.

12. Is anyone else in your home environment having symptoms similar to yours?   YES ___ NO ___
    If yes, explain.

COMMUNITY EXPOSURES

1. Are any of the following located in your community?
   ___ Industrial plant   ___ Landfill   ___ Major source of air polution   ___ Toxic spill   ___ Waste site   ___ Other
2. What is your source of drinking water? ___ Private well   ___ Public water source   ___ Other
3. Are neighbors experiencing any health problems similar to yours? YES ___ NO ___
   If yes, explain.

KEY OCCUPATIONAL AND ENVIRONMENTAL HEALTH QUESTIONS TO BE ASKED WITH ALL HISTORIES

1. What are your current and past longest-held jobs?

2. Have you been exposed to any radiation or chemical liquids, dusts, mists, or fumes?   YES ___ NO ___
3. Is there any relationship between current symptoms and activities at work or at home?   YES ___ NO ___

Modified from Pope AM, Snyder MA, Mood LH (editors): *Nursing, health, and environment: strengthening the relationship to improve the public's health,* Washington, DC, 1995, National Academy Press.

Answers to Clinical Applications

Chapter 1

C and G are population-focused, looking at the needs of their subpopulation and planning programs to meet their needs. A, B, D, and F are likely to be practicing community health nursing if their focus is health protection, health promotion, and disease prevention of the individuals and/or families in their subpopulations. B and D are more likely to be practicing community-based nursing, caring for clients who are ill.

Chapter 2

A. It is easier to use a population-focused approach to solving these problems. If a nurse can show through a community needs assessment that these are problems for a large number of people in the community and are putting the community at risk for increased health problems, more costly health care, and less social and economic growth, then it might be possible to convince policy makers to establish programs directed at these problems. With limited health care dollars, the emphasis is on the greatest good for the greatest number.

B. A historical approach will build understanding of the public policy elements limiting care of various populations. This involves exploring what attempts have been made in the past to innovate or reform services for these populations; determining what has limited these attempts; and identifying examples of programs or policies that have been successful.

Chapter 3

The correct answer is D. The nurse's responsibility is to educate clients about appropriate health care resources in their community and to allow families to choose care based on their own unique needs and preferences.

Chapter 4

The correct answer is A. The nurse should first find out from the client what he heard the doctor say. This is important because what the client heard would have a significant effect on his perception of health and what decisions he makes about treatment modalities.

Chapter 5

A. The nurse would include a Denver II in her assessment of Billy to determine the neurologic effects of the lead on his growth and development. An assessment of the population to find the total child population under 6 years of age who may benefit from screening and a community assessment to find the number of older homes in the community that may have lead-based paint would also be included.

B. Prevention strategies would include the following:

- Assisting the parents in enrolling Billy in Head Start to stimulate his development because of his altered growth and development state.
- Initiating a blood level screening program for children under 6 years of age in the community to determine other children who may need to be referred for treatment.
- Starting a community-wide lead poisoning prevention program that includes educational materials about where lead is found in home environments and how to test for it.
- Targeting parent group leaders, local newspapers, and the school system to distribute educational materials.

Chapter 6

A plan of action to influence the health department about its decision to close the prenatal clinic would include the following:

A. Reviewing the state register in the law library to see if regulations for the block grants had been finalized

B. Checking state health statistics, including vital statistics providing the current infant and maternity mortality rates in the state, and comparing these to national statistics

C. Reviewing the literature for research that would show the relationships between prenatal care, normal deliveries, and complications of pregnancy and delivery

D. After discussion, holding a group meeting with the state nurses association to create answers. Having the groups contact their local senators and representatives to ask for a meeting to discuss the issue is the next step

E. Contacting the legal aid society to find a lawyer interested in consulting with them in preparing written and oral testimony

F. Presenting the testimony to the state health department during the process of preparing the regulations for the block grants.

Chapter 7

A. Agencies are reimbursed for visits either by private insurance or Medicare or by clients through self-pay.

B. The payment for the visit is determined by using a cost basis or a charge basis. Cost basis reflects the actual cost to the agency to deliver the service. Charge basis reflects the cost plus additional monies charged for the visit, which may include indigent care visits or profit to be paid to stockholders if the agency is a for-profit agency.

C. Nursing care costs, while they may be known, are usually not used alone to determine the costs of a visit. The visit cost includes money for lights, water, supplies, secretarial and administrative salaries and benefits, as well as nurse salaries and benefits.

D. Rationing exists in all of health care. Home health visits are rationed by the criteria set by the federal government for Medicare clients, such as a limited number of visits per year; and by private insurance, which also limits the number of visits per year. The individual client who must pay out of pocket sets his or her own limits and self-rations the amount he or she may be willing to pay for home health visits.

Chapter 8

The correct answer is D. There are mixed opinions about prostate cancer screening. The revised American Cancer Society recommendations say that prostate cancer screening should be offered only after men are informed of their risk and benefits (von Eschenbach, 1997). Age recommendations for screening are 45 years and older in African-American men and 50 years and older in Caucasian men. Prostate cancer screening should be offered to men who have 10 years or more of life expectancy left.

Chapter 9

The correct answer is B. While all of the answers relate to the students' overall goal, this answer is directly related to their plan for collecting data for purposes of research. The plan for collection of the data would first need to be approved by the Institutional Review Board of the university.

Chapter 10

A. The nurse educator follows the educational process in developing a program for a community-based population.

B. The nurse would have needed to identify a reinforcer that he/she could control.

C. The nurse might pass out an evaluation tool to measure the success of the educational process.

D. The evaluation plan would be limited and would not enable the nurse to make significant changes in the program over time or determine the overall success in meeting program goals.

Chapter 11

The correct answer is B. A high level of community motivation is critical for any community-focused intervention and will help to ensure active community involvement in the planning process and commitment to the intervention itself.

Chapter 12

The correct sequence is C, B, A, D. The first piece of information (C) is essential to understanding the level, amount, and nature of services the client is eligible to receive. The client must be informed, her needs assessed, and her options discussed (B). Family care options must be understood to formulate resource possibilities for the client (A). Arrangement for a facility site visit may or may not be essential but may be preferred (D).

Chapter 13

The correct answer is A. Sharing her feelings with a trained professional who is familiar with the devastating circumstances in which Paula is involved will be most helpful. Although calling home might be comforting, family members with no experience in disaster work would not be able to fully appreciate the stress that Paula is experiencing.

Chapter 14

Eva would include all the steps in planning her project. She contacted the pastor of the church who was planning to open the soup kitchen to discuss the issue (formulation and assessment). She found him very receptive to the idea of developing a solution to the health care needs of the homeless. In her assessment, Eva found that no other health services were available to the homeless in the community. She looked at national data to estimate needs and size of the population. She talked with the community health nursing faculty to discuss potential solutions to the problem. She talked to members of the homeless population to get their perceptions of their needs.

On completing her assessment, Eva conceptualized the solutions. Several solutions were possible: work with the health department, attempt to provide better care through the local medical center, or open a clinic on site at the soup kitchen where most of the people gathered so that transportation would not be a problem.

After considering the solutions, Eva detailed the plan looking at the resources needed for opening a clinic at the soup kitchen. She considered supplies, equipment, facilities, and acceptability to the clients. She also considered the time involved, the activities required to implement a program, and funding sources.

In evaluating the possibilities, Eva considered the cost, the client and community benefits, and acceptability to clients, self, faculty, and the church. Although it would have been easier for her to choose to work with the health department or the medical center, she knew that the solution most acceptable to the clients would be to have a clinic located at the soup kitchen. The clinic would be more accessible, transportation would not be needed, and health services through the clinic could possibly prevent more costly hospital and emergency care (value).

Eva presented her plan to the faculty and the church. She convinced them that it would not be a costly endeavor. She had found nurses in the community who volunteered to help, she had contacted a carpenter who would donate his time to build an examining room in the back of the soup kitchen, and she had met with community physicians who had promised to provide equipment. The client assessment indicated that a first-aid and health assessment clinic was what was needed most. With approval from all (implementation), Eva began the clinic in 1981, seeing 25 to 35 clients a week, 1 hour per day for 5 days per week.

Eva evaluated the relevance of the program via the needs assessment process. She tracked the progress of the program by keeping records of her activities. She kept track of the resources in relation to the number of persons served (efficiency) and used these data to convince the church and the college of nursing to fund the ongoing clinic operation after she graduated. A summative evaluation of the clinic was completed by the faculty at the end of 4 years. The program's impact was outstanding. The clinic had grown. The client demand was high; most of the health problems could be handled at the clinic, which eliminated the cost burden to the community for more expensive health care; and it was highly acceptable to the clients (effectiveness). This clinic began as a service to 25 people for 1 hour per day. Today this clinic is open all day, 5 days per week, has more than 900 clients per year, and provides for more than 5000 client visits per year. The success of this clinic shows the effect that one community health nursing student can have on a community.

Chapter 15

Both of these questions would be important in determining outcome elements. After answering these questions with the committee, Margaret decides she would like to perform a self-evaluation or, preferably, have a peer review by fellow students to determine the quality of care she has given through the semester. She uses a client satisfaction survey to determine how the clients feel about the services she has delivered. She applies an audit instrument to review and evaluate several records of clients she has cared for. She interprets the data, makes adjustments in her care, and shares findings with her faculty advisor. Margaret feels good about the process and outcomes of her clients' care. She has

functioned under the agency policies and knows that she has contributed to the overall quality of care as defined by the agency.

Chapter 16

Several contributing factors should be considered, including each of the following. When the remaining student and parents "carried on" without confronting the students who seemingly disregarded their responsibility, it appears that:
- The group was unwilling to confront conflict when three members failed to carry out their expected parts.
- Member responsibilities may have been incompletely described when the agreement to work together was specified. The three students who failed to continue may not have known that they were expected to attend all sessions.
- Some students showed a lack of commitment to the project's purpose.

Chapter 17

A. No. The idealized version never existed. There have always been stressors that presented challenges for families. While not as prominent in the past, there have always been differing family structures within U.S. society.
B. According to a report from the National Commission on Children, people are both discouraged and encouraged about the status of America's families. The contradictions in this report indicate a disparity between people's perceptions of their own families (healthy) and the perception of families outside their own (unhealthy or dysfunctional).
C. There are liberal people in our society who believe the definition of family should include two-parent, single-parent, remarried, gay, adoptive, foster, and many other alternative family forms. That is, families are what people define them to be and the government with its health and economic sanctions should be supportive of all family groups. However, there are conservative people who believe that the definition of families should remain limited to the blood, legal, and adoptive guidelines.
D. How we ourselves define family will influence how we live, how we provide nursing care to families, and what health and welfare programs we are willing to support in the society.

Chapter 18

A. The home visit would allow for a more extensive assessment of the family within the four models of health: clinical, role-performance, adaptive, and eudaimonistic. The community health nurse phoned the home to make an appointment for a home visit. Amy's mother answered the phone and indicated that Amy was at school during the day. The nurse introduced herself and explained that the counselor at the high school had talked with Amy about the possibility of having a community health nurse from the health department help her to learn more about her pregnancy, labor and delivery, and caring for a new infant. Amy's mother sounded both relieved and enthusiastic about having the nurse visit. Although Amy was in school during the day, she could arrange to be at home so the nurse could meet her at the end of the agency working day. An appointment was made for later in the week to meet with Amy and her mother. At this point, the initiation and previsit phases of the home visit process were completed by the nurse.

B. At the first home visit, it became apparent that Amy and her mother were interested in continuing community health nursing service. During her visit with Amy and her mother, the nurse added to her assessment by exploring with them what they saw as problems and concerns. This is consistent with an approach focused on empowerment. Amy and her mother identified a number of questions and concerns. How could Amy finish her education and care for a child? What would labor and delivery be like? How could Amy and her boyfriend avoid unplanned pregnancies in the future? How could the family members be supportive and yet have their own needs met?

C. A second visit was scheduled to include Amy's boyfriend and stepfather. During the second visit, additional areas related to clinical health of the family, in terms of acute or chronic conditions, were assessed using a family genogram. Because it was apparent that there was a potential conflict between individual and family development needs that had implications for the adaptive processes of the family, time was spent identifying both family needs and individual needs and how best to meet these needs.

D. A contract was negotiated to continue visiting with Amy, but the visits would occur at school during a study period. The focus would be on prenatal teaching on the nurse's part, with Amy agreeing to attend group meetings for pregnant students offered at the school. Visits also were arranged with Amy's mother to discuss her concerns. These approaches reflected acknowledgment of the family's abilities to be actively and competently involved in resolving problems they had identified. Over time, the contract was modified and expanded to include well-child supervision during the year following the birth of a healthy baby boy.

Chapter 19

A. *Lab test:* CBC with differential, CD4+ T-cell count/percentage and CD4+/CD8+ ratio, HIV RNA viral load test, multichannel chemistry panel, urinalysis, TB test, and chest x-ray.

History and physical assessment: assess general appearance including weight changes and muscle wasting; eye examination; skin assessment and breakdown, including swollen, tender lymph nodes, mouth lesions, painful swollen gums, skin rashes, and lesions; neurologic and genitourinary examination; and nutrition screen.

B. Hyperthermia, social isolation, risk for infection, fluid volume deficit, ineffective coping, body image disturbance, altered nutrition, altered health maintenance, and altered family processes.

C. Ensure adequate hydration and nutrition, control fever and replace lost fluids, facilitate the restoration of usual bowel patterns, and prevent skin breakdown.

D. There is no cure at this time; however, goals should focus on the quality of life. Antiviral therapy suppresses the replication of HIV infection in the body. Retrovir is an antiviral agent most frequently used to treat AIDS. Monitor and treat opportunistic infections such as *Pneumocystis carinii* pneumonia as they occur. Develop an achievable plan that integrates psychosocial and health care goals. Link John to the needed services and continue to monitor/track the services for achievements.

E. Begin with the dietitian, social worker, and the clinical nurse specialist in HIV management at the local public health department. Community-based and national AIDS organizations that should be consulted and for assistance include Aids for AIDS, AIDS Service Center, HIV/AIDS legal organizations, homeless health care associations, and Project New Hope.

F. Outcome criteria include:
- Preservation and efficient use of energy
- Enhanced self-esteem
- Increased sense of personal control
- Maintenance of supportive family structure
- Decrease of anxiety to manageable levels.

Chapter 20

A. Check Ms. Green for proteinuria (because of her pitting edema and complaints of a mild headache). Contact the health department and arrange for her to be seen soon by the NP to determine what medication she needs, what dietary restrictions and additions she needs, what intervals of work/rest will help her, and whether she needs any meals brought to her or she needs to get some meals from a local shelter.

B. Ms. Green is likely approaching preeclampsia. She may be on the brink of an emergence of her psychotic illness. Her nutrition may be inadequate, with too much salt and fat. Her psychotropic medicine needs to be regulated and taken regularly. What help can she get to be able to afford the medicine? How can she get vitamins? Investigate whether she can really take care of this infant. Is the father a source of financial and emotional support?

Chapter 21

A. Assess his readiness for change, assess his educational needs regarding health effects of smoking, and provide any needed information, and evaluate the risks to family members from sidestream smoke.

B. Explain about support groups such as AA for Mr. Jones and Alanon for Anne and how this could be helpful.

C. Anne cannot make her grandfather stop drinking. She can provide him with information and refer him to professionals to help him. She does need to know where he drinks, what his behavior is like when he's drinking, health risks related to drinking, and the effects of his drinking on her children.

Chapter 22

A. The nurse needs to listen carefully to the pain and anguish the daughter felt about hitting her mother. She can convey a nonjudgmental attitude and help the daughter and mother explore ways in which both of their needs could be more effectively met. She can provide information and resources to allow the daughter some respite from constant caretaking and a way to continue her own activities.

B. The nurse should:
- Assess the situation
- Discuss options with the family
- Teach alternatives
- Make appropriate referrals and coordinate services.

C. Mrs. Jones will need to monitor the situation carefully for any further signs of abuse. Any further instance of violence must be discussed with the daughter and immediately reported. In a subsequent visit, the nurse evaluated the effectiveness of her teaching and learned that Mary and her mother were working more cooperatively on Mrs. Smith's care.

Chapter 23

A. The first step is to determine if a DOT program is needed. Historical and current TB surveillance data should be consulted to see if the number of TB cases has been increasing or not falling as would be expected and if noncompliance with treatment has been a contributing factor.

B. Justification for such a program would include a brief description of the difficulties in TB treatment, the resultant problems with noncompliance, the implications for development of resistance, and the potential for continued infection of the public.

C. Personally interview clients to determine potential incentives. The success of the incentive program appears to be linked with identifying an incentive that has a strong personal value to the client. Of course, the incentive must also be acceptable to all parties involved. For example, alcohol and tobacco would probably not be considered appropriate incentives.

D. Identifying contacts for treatment or prophylaxis is an important part of preventing the continued spread of TB infection. Clients may be reluctant (for personal reasons) to reveal contacts or they may simply not realize who all their contacts are. Observing client daily activity provides an opportunity to investigate all possibilities for transmitting disease.

Chapter 24

A. The nurse asks Yvonne about past injection-drug–using and sexual partners. The nurse evaluates Yvonne's comfort in sharing the information with Phil as she explores what she

thinks Phil's response might be. The nurse offers to role-play the situation of Yvonne telling Phil about the possibility of his infection, risks, and the importance of testing for the HIV antibody. Rather than contacting other previous sexual and drug-using partners herself, Yvonne requests that health department staff contact them about being tested for possible infection. She gives the nurse the names and addresses of two additional drug-using partners.

B. The most immediate concerns for Yvonne are the need to seek ongoing care to monitor the HIV infection and to decide whether to continue the pregnancy. The nurse asks Yvonne whether she has a primary health care provider. The information given to Yvonne includes a list of providers and counseling about the importance of establishing an ongoing relationship with a primary health care provider for follow-up of the HIV infection. She tells Yvonne that important information about her health may be identified that will help to determine her ability to carry and deliver the baby if she chooses to continue the pregnancy. Other important information includes the implications of the test results, such as how they may affect the infant's and mother's health.

The nurse explains that transmission to the fetus is possible during the pregnancy and she may have a greater chance of progressing from asymptomatic infection to symptomatic HIV disease but that medications would be given to try to prevent this from happening. The nurse explores possibilities with Yvonne about the decision regarding her ability to physically, emotionally, and financially cope with rearing a child that may be ill. Family members and other potential resources are assessed. The need for Yvonne to tell health care providers or blood handlers about the HIV infection is reviewed. The nurse schedules a second appointment for follow-up counseling 1 week after the initial test results are given. She also gives Yvonne the telephone number of the local AIDS support group and arranges to make a home visit to her in 2 days.

At the follow-up home and clinic visits, specific information is given regarding infection control in the home and safer sexual relations. The nurse ensures that Yvonne is taking steps toward getting prenatal care and medical care for the HIV infection. The nurse reviews information about how to maintain health and avoid stressors, and she contracts with Yvonne to initiate home visits to provide reinforcement of adequate prenatal nutrition and teaching and to assess Yvonne's physical health as the pregnancy progresses.

Chapter 25

The correct answer is C. The team was organized to develop the case definition, plan the interview questions and sampling, and organize the specimen collection. Interviews were used to determine characteristics of the illness and to attempt to identify the source by dietary recall and living arrangements. The dietary recall was focused on the food consumed during the three meals before illness onset. While the interviews were being conducted, an environmental investigation concentrated on food preparation, service, and storage, along with housekeeping procedures. The administrative staff of the retirement community kept a daily log documenting all interventions implemented to determine what effect the measures undertaken to stop the spread of illness may have actually had on controlling the spread of illness.

It was initially thought that the infectious agent was a "Norwalk-like" virus, classified under the heading of human caliciviruses (HCV). Specimen testing, however, confirmed the presence of a virus strain similar to the Mexican virus, also an HCV, but classified in a different genogroup than the Norwalk virus. Clinically, symptoms are indistinguishable. The outbreak was revealed to have been caused by a virus strain closely related to the Mexican virus. Fecal-oral spread through food contamination, close person-to-person contact, and possible respiratory spread were hypothesized for this highly contagious virus.

There is a great deal to be learned about the transmission from persons who are asymptomatic. A majority of the residents of the facility became ill even after the institutional precautions were implemented, such as closing the dining room and limiting contacts between residents, encouraging disinfection of common areas of the retirement community, and placing emphasis on personal hygiene and glove use by staff. Ill staff were told to stay home until at least 2 days after their symptoms subsided. Handwashing by the staff was emphasized using antibacterial soap and drying with paper towels. The use of disposable items was encouraged when possible. Due to the recent increase in gastrointestinal illness in older populations in the state and the fragile state of health of many of the residents, as a result of this investigation, recommendations for control measures during gastroenteritis outbreaks in institutions became incorporated into a checklist for long-term care facilities to increase the level of awareness of the importance of strict adherence to hygienic practices in institutional settings.

Chapter 26

Regardless of the earliest beginnings, the following elements are needed to shape the path:
- Discussions
- Questions
- Eliciting statements of healthy and unhealthy events in the lives of the members
- Surveying the physical, social, emotional, and spiritual environmental conditions of the faith community.

Formation of a broadly representative wellness committee will help to plan the formal and informal assessment methods and careful documentation of activities and communication.

Building on strengths of the congregation, gathering information on leaders and valued activities in the congregation, and becoming informed regarding lines of authority and communication help to provide a foundation for the service. The best answer is D, planning a congregational survey. This increases interest and involvement of the mem-

bers. Results assist in bringing a possible goal into focus. If the majority of the congregation is over age 55, it would be helpful to assess areas such as needs for retirement planning, current health status and adequacy of health financing options, involvement in caregiving for parents as well as adult children, needs for involvement in meaningful volunteer activities, and ability to holistically engage in activities appropriate for the life stage. Assessment would also include the impact of the over-55 age-group on the remainder of the congregation and the surrounding community. Information regarding resources within the church and geopolitical community is helpful.

Organizing and implementing a health fair to address identified needs often is beneficial in the following ways:
- Creating awareness of health needs
- Providing information to act on identified health concerns
- Increasing visibility of the value of health and faith connection
- Promoting interest for additional congregational members to become involved in the parish nurse/health ministry program.

The greater involvement by the members, the greater the ownership of the program by the total faith community. Evaluation of the activity will yield information regarding which areas or activities should be continued or reinforced, which need to change focus, and which should be omitted.

In addition to the group and population activities, the parish nurse meets regularly with the pastoral staff and coordinates with other committee chairs. Together, they identify individuals requiring further assessment or support; become aware of issues that need to be clarified, supported, or addressed; and determine individuals, groups, or issues that have not yet become a part of the parish nurse or congregational wellness program. Home visits, phone calls, and visits to hospitals or community agencies are also part of the parish nurse's weekly activities. Agendas might include advocacy and interpretation with a health care provider, monitoring dementia progress, supporting a new mother embarking on a "new" career at home, leading a support group, therapeutic touch, prayer, and visualization.

Chapter 27

A. The following strategies help to develop trust:
- Respecting the family's customs and space, as well as sensitivity to the timing of questions.
- Being flexible and keeping promises is even more important in the home.
- Giving the family a time range when making an appointment to allow for delays at other homes and for traffic.
- Providing the client and family information about the referral, the purpose of the visit, what services are available, and how to contact the agency.

- Dealing first with the issue that is uppermost on the client's mind, not what is first on the nurse's agenda. This strategy will decrease client anxiety and improve the ability to understand and focus on what the nurse needs to tell them.

B. The assessment in the home environment should include:
- Taking a detailed history
- Doing a physical assessment
- Walking through the important parts of the house (bedroom, bathroom, kitchen, and hallways) to obtain baseline data for forming the plan of care
- Listening to clients to get the most important clues to health status and effective teaching strategies
- Beginning to complete necessary forms to ensure the information is obtained. Some clients will not be able to complete all the forms and provide the required information on the first visit because of pain or fatigue. Focus on the essentials and complete the rest of the forms on a second visit.

C. Client contact must include the following:
- Setting short- and long-term goals with clients
- Having a plan for every visit to progress toward the goals
- Informing clients and families that home health services are time limited and that they need to learn to provide their own care
- Setting limits, modeling expected behaviors, and writing in the behaviors of the client
- Developing principles to facilitate and encourage self-care
- Planning for modifying care to allow as much independence as possible
- Writing plans to teach the client rather than do for the client.

D. Learning style is assessed by understanding adult learning principles and asking the client about the characteristics that indicate the preferred learning style.

Chapter 28

A. A school health program involves all three: health services, health education, and environmental health. School health services help to screen and identify children who have unmet health problems or need monitoring of chronic illnesses, either of which can affect the child's ability to learn. Health education is important and should begin in kindergarten so that children can understand the meaning of and begin practicing health habits early. Heath education throughout the school experience can affect how children learn and can lead to healthy productive adults. Attention to the physical environment of the school— climate, safety, esthetics—all affect the child's ability to pay attention and to want to learn. Reducing stress in the environment for teachers and students and creating a climate of acceptance for all may reduce violent acts and can improve attitudes toward learning.

B. The answer is 3. Creating a surveillance system will assist the nurse in defining the problem at the population level. The surveillance system will provide a system for tracking rates at each school and for the school system as a whole. Tracking students seen by the nurse, reviewing absence records, collecting data from teachers, and assessing students at risk through a personal life-style inventory are all a part of the surveillance system.

Chapter 29

The correct answer is D. This is an example of how the epidemiologic triad can be used to assess clients and plan nursing care. It illustrates the usefulness of approaching occupational health problems with an epidemiologic perspective.

Reference

von Eschenbach AC, et al: American Cancer Society guidelines for the early detection of prostate cancer: update 1997, *CA Cancer J Clin* 47:261, 1997.

Index

H

Menopause, 325
  defined, 316
Men's health; *See* Male population.
Mental health
  aging and, 340
  National Health Objectives 2010 and, 37, 536
Mental illness
  homelessness and, 354
  in women, 331
  National Health Objectives 2010 and, 536
Men/women death ratio, 316, 334, 335t
Mercury exposure, 77t, 83t
Message as education principle, 170b
Metatarsus adductus screening, 589
Methadone, 378
Metronidazole, 424t
Metropolitan Life Insurance Company, 16, 22, 23
Mexican-American population, 10
Microeconomic theory, 106, 107
Midwifery, 38-39, 40
Migrant farm worker, defined, 350, 355
Migrant workers, 355-356
Military Medical Care System, 91b
Mitigation
  defined, 217
  in disaster management, 219
Mi-Yuk Gook, 69f
MMR; *See* Measles-mumps-rubella.
Mock disaster, 221-222
Molecular technology in epidemiology, 133
Monitoring
  environmental, 76-77, 77b, 77t
  in case management, 204f, 205b
Moral
  defined, 50
  in ethics, 51, 56
Morbidity
  epidemiologic measurement of, 137-140, 138t
  in windshield survey, 192t
  new, defined, 488
Morbidity and Mortality Weekly Report, 400
Morning glory seeds, 371
Moro reflex, 585
Morphine abuse, 368
Mortality
  early, public health and, 6
  epidemiologic measurement of, 137-140, 138t
  from cancer, 77, 77b
  from cigarette smoking, 368, 369f
  from earthquake, 223
  from heart and vascular disease, 333t
  leading causes of
    from ages 11-24 years, 490f, 540
    from ages 25-64 years, 542
    from ages 65 and older, 544
    from birth to 10 years, 489, 490f, 539

Mortality—cont'd
  leading causes of—cont'd
    in male population, 332-337, 333t, 334f, 335t, 336t
    top ten, 132, 134f
Mortality rates, 34, 137-139, 138t
Motor function assessment of child, 591-595
Motor vehicle accident, 317
  alcohol use and, 337
  as cause of childhood death, 319, 319t
Multiadult household, 277b
Multiculturism, 50, 62
Mumps, 401b
  immunization against
    adulthood, 576
    childhood, 325t, 326t, 404, 568, 569
Mycobacterium tuberculosis, 412, 419t
Myocardial infarction
  in men's health, 333t
  in women's health, 328

N

National Academy of Certified Case Managers, 214t
National Board for Certification in Continuity of Care, 214t
National Case Management Task Force, 203
National Center for Nursing Research, 27, 127
National Disaster Medical System, 223
National Health Objectives; *See Healthy People 2010.*
National Health Quality Improvement Act of 1986, 243
National Health Service Corps, 33, 40
National Institute for Occupational Safety and Health, 512, 526, 527b
National Institute of Nursing Research
  defined, 88
  establishment of, 91, 127
    through legislative process, 99
  within Department of Health and Human Services, 40
National Institutes of Health, 39f, 40, 90, 327
National League for Nursing, 16, 26, 28, 245
National Notifiable Diseases Surveillance System, 400
National Organization for Public Health Nursing, 21, 22
National Women's Health Network, 327
Native American population, 68
Natural disaster, 217, 218, 218b
Natural history of disease in epidemiology, 130, 135
Natural immunity, 398, 399
NCNR; *See* National Center for Nursing Research.
NDMS; *See* National Disaster Medical System.
Neck righting reflex, 585
Needs assessment
  defined, 231
  in program management, 233
  in school nursing, 506, 507b
Negative predictive value, defined, 130
Negentropy, 281

Nutrition
cultural factors in, 68t, 69, 69b, 69f
in children, 322-324, 323f, 323t
in well child care, 318t
school-age, 489
in women's health, 327
National Health Objectives 2010 and, 536
teen pregnancy and, 355
Nutting, M, 22
NWHN; *See* National Women's Health Network.

O

OASDI; *See* Old Age Survivors and Disability Insurance.
OASIS; *See* Outcomes and Assessment Information Set.
Obesity
childhood, 489
in women, 330
National Health Objectives 2010 and, 37, 536
Objectives
defined, 184
educational, 173, 173t
in community-oriented practice, 195, 195t
in program management evaluation, 236-237
Observation, participant, 184, 190
Obstructive sleep apnea, 537
Occupational health hazard, 512, 524
Occupational health history, 522, 523f, 623-625
defined, 512
Occupational health nursing, 511-529
acquired immunodeficiency syndrome and, 422
application of epidemiologic model in, 516f, 516-520,
517b, 518t
definition and scope of, 512
disaster planning and management in, 527-528
early roots of, 21
Healthy People 2010 and, 526, 536
history and evolution of, 512-513
laws affecting, 102
legislation related to, 526-527, 527b
organizational and public efforts to promote worker
health and safety in, 520-522, 521b
professional roles and professionalism in, 513
worker assessment in, 522-524, 523f
workers as a population aggregate in, 513-516, 515f,
516b
workplace assessment in, 524-526, 525f
Occupational injury, 334, 335t
Occupational Safety and Health Administration, 526, 527b
defined, 88, 512
history of, 513
legal factors and, 102
on occupational exposure to bloodborne pathogens, 428
Occupational therapist, 474
Odocoileus virginianus, 409

Official health agency
defined, 16
establishment of, 22
in home health care, 466-467
Ofloxacin, 424t
Oklahoma City bombing, 224
Old Age Survivors and Disability Insurance, 95
Older Americans Act, 95
Omaha Visiting Nurses Association Problem Classification
System, 252
Omnibus Reconciliation Act, 478
Onchocerca volvulus, 411t
Open space in windshield survey, 192t
Opioids abuse, 368
Opium abuse, 368
Opportunistic infection of acquired immunodeficiency
syndrome, 419t
Optokinetic drum test, 587
Oral health, 536-537
Organic mercury exposure, 77t, 83t
Organic solvents, 77t
Organization in school nursing, 507
Orthopedics
impairment in elderly, 341t
screening for problems with, 588-590
Ortolani's maneuver, 588
OSA; *See* Obstructive sleep apnea.
OSHA; *See* Occupational Safety and Health
Administration.
Osteoporosis
defined, 316
in female population, 330-331
National Health Objectives 2010 and, 532
OT; *See* Occupational therapist.
Outcome
defined, 231, 242
in advocacy process, 209t
in case management process, 204t
in quality management, 249, 251-252
Outcome criteria, defined, 202
Outcomes and Assessment Information Set, 551-563
defined, 464
in home health nursing, 483
Outrage factors, 74, 83, 83t
Outreach in sexually transmitted disease prevention, 431
Outreach worker
defined, 439
public health nurse as, 446
Ovarian cancer, 328-329
Overeating, 330
Over-the-counter drugs
abuse of, 366
caffeine content in, 370t
Ozone
defined, 74
depletion of, 74
exposure to, 77b, 83t